McGraw-Hill Specialty Board Review

RADIOLOGY

Notice

McGraw-Hill Specialty Board Review

RADIOLOGY

Editor

Cheri L. Canon, MD

Professor of Radiology
Senior Vice Chair for Operations
Director, Division of Diagnostic Radiology
Chief, Gastrointestinal Radiology
University of Alabama at Birmingham
Birmingham, Alabama

McGraw Hill Medical

New York Chicago San Francisco Lisbon London Madrid
Mexico City Milan New Delhi San Juan Seoul
Singapore Sydney Toronto

McGraw-Hill Specialty Board Review
RADIOLOGY

1 2 3 4 5 6 7 8 9 0 QWD/QWD 14 13 12 11 10 9

ISBN 978-0-07-160164-1
MHID 0-07-160164-3

This book was set in Times by Aptara®, Inc.
The editors were Michael Weitz and Christie Naglieri.
The production supervisor was Catherine Saggese.
The illustration manager was Armen Ovsepyan.
Project management was provided by Sonia Taneja, Aptara®, Inc.
The cover designer was Aimee Davis.
Quebecor World was printer and binder.

This book is printed on acid-free paper.

Library of Congress Cataloging-in-Publication Data
Radiology / [edited] by Cheri L. Canon.
p. ; cm. – (McGraw-Hill specialty board review)
Includes bibliographical references and index.
ISBN-13: 978-0-07-160164-1 (hardcover : alk. paper)
ISBN-10: 0-07-160164-3 (hardcover : alk. paper)
1. Radiography, Medical–Examinations, questions, etc. 2. Radiologists–Licenses–United States–Examinations–Study guides. I. Canon, Cheri L. II. Series: McGraw-Hill specialty board review.
[DNLM: 1. Radiology–Examination Questions. 2. Technology, Radiologic–Examination Questions. WN 18.2 R1275 2009]
RC78.15.R275 2009
616.07'57076–dc22

2009003877

This book is dedicated to Malcolm, Olivia, and Evan, for their love and endless patience,

and

To Heather, who is my balance between work and family,

and

To Bob Koehler for his wisdom, enthusiasm, and above all else, his friendship.

CONTENTS

Section III
CARDIAC

Section IV
GASTROINTESTINAL TRACT

CONTRIBUTORS

Ahmed Kamel Abdel Aal, MD, MSc
Clinical Instructor
Department of Radiology
Chief of Vascular and Interventional Radiology
University of Alabama at Birmingham, VA Medical Center
Birmingham, Alabama

Rochelle F. Andreotti, MD
Associate Professor of Clinical Radiology
Assistant Professor of Obstetrics and Gynecology
Department of Radiology and Radiological Sciences
Vanderbilt University Medical Center
Nashville, Tennessee

Asim K. Bag, MD
Fellow
Department of Radiology
University of Alabama at Birmingham
Birmingham, Alabama

Sanjiv K. Bajaj, MD
Resident Physician
Mallinckrodt Institute of Radiology
St. Louis, Missouri

Jon A. Baldwin, DO, MBS
Assistant Professor of Radiology
Division of Nuclear Medicine
Program Director, Nuclear Medicine Residency Program
University of Alabama at Birmingham
Birmingham, Alabama

Lincoln L. Berland, MD, FACR
Professor of Radiology
Vice-Chairman for Quality Assurance and Patient Safety
Chief, Body CT and 3D Laboratory
University of Alabama at Birmingham
Birmingham, Alabama

Pradeep G. Bhambhvani, MD
Assistant Professor of Radiology
Division of Nuclear Medicine
University of Alabama at Birmingham
Birmingham, Alabama

Roderick F. Biosca Jr., MD
Resident
Department of Radiology
University of Alabama at Birmingham
Birmingham, Alabama

Michael A. Bruno, MS, MD
Associate Professor of Radiology & Medicine
Penn State University College of Medicine
Director of Quality Management Services
The Milton S. Hershey Medical Center
Hershey, Pennsylvania

Bao T. Bui, MD
Resident
Department of Radiology
University of Alabama at Birmingham
Birmingham, Alabama

Cheri L. Canon, MD
Professor of Radiology
Senior Vice Chair for Operations
Director, Division of Diagnostic Radiology
Chief, GI Radiology
University of Alabama at Birmingham
Birmingham, Alabama

Gregory S. Elliott, MD
X-Ray Associates of Louisville
Louisville, Kentucky

Andrew S. Ferrell, MD
Resident
Department of Radiology
University of Alabama at Birmingham
Birmingham, Alabama

Anne F. Fitzpatrick, MD
Fellow
Vascular and Interventional
Department of Radiology
University of Alabama at Birmingham Hospital
Birmingham, Alabama

Arthur C. Fleischer, MD
Professor of Radiology and Radiological Sciences
Professor, Department of Obstetrics and Gynecology
Vanderbilt University Medical Center
Nashville, Tennessee

Sibyll Goetze, MD
Assistant Professor of Radiology
Division of Nuclear Medicine
University of Alabama at Birmingham
Birmingham, Alabama

Allen B. Groves, MD
Fellow
Abdominal Imaging
Department of Radiology
University of Alabama at Birmingham
Birmingham, Alabama

Christopher J. Guion, MD
Clinical Professor of Radiology and Pediatrics
University of Alabama at Birmingham
Children's Health System of Alabama
Birmingham, Alabama

Heather L. Haddad, MD
Assistant Professor of Radiology
University of Alabama at Birmingham
Birmingham, Alabama

Kay M. Hamrick, MD
Associate Professor of Radiology
University of Alabama at Birmingham
Birmingham, Alabama

Camden L. Hebson, MD
Chief Resident
Department of Pediatrics
Emory University
Atlanta, Georgia

Cheryl R. Herman, MD
Assistant Professor of Radiology
Mallinckrodt Institute of Radiology at Washington University
St. Louis, Missouri

David E. Hogg, MD
Assistant Professor of Radiology
Medical Director Outpatient Radiology
University of Alabama at Birmingham
Birmingham, Alabama

Eric J. Howell, MD
Clinical Assistant Professor of Radiology and Pediatrics
University of Alabama at Birmingham
Children's Health System of Alabama
Birmingham, Alabama

Kenneth Hoyt, PhD
Assistant Professor of Radiology
University of Alabama at Birmingham
Birmingham, Alabama

Baljendra S. Kapoor, MD
Assistant Professor of Radiology
University of Alabama at Birmingham
Birmingham, Alabama

Philip J. Kenney, MD
Professor and Chair of Radiology
University of Arkansas for Medical Science
Little Rock, Arkansas

Robert E. Koehler, MD
Professor Emeritus of Radiology
University of Alabama School of Medicine
Birmingham, Alabama

Victoria E. Kraft
Undergraduate
University of Chicago
Chicago, Illinois

Matthew C. Larrison, MD
Assistant Professor of Radiology
Program Director, Musculoskeletal Fellowship
University of Alabama at Birmingham
Birmingham, Alabama

Reagan R. Leverett, MD
Instructor
Women's Imaging Fellow
Department of Radiology
Vanderbilt University Medical Center
Nashville, Tennessee

Mark D. Little, MD
Clinical Instructor of Radiology
University of Alabama at Birmingham
Birmingham, Alabama

Mark E. Lockhart, MD, MPH
Associate Professor of Radiology
Chief, Genitourinary Radiology
Program Director, Abdominal Imaging Fellowship
University of Alabama at Birmingham
Birmingham, Alabama

Robert Lopez-Ben, MD
Associate Professor of Radiology
University of Alabama at Birmingham
Birmingham, Alabama

Katherine P. Lursen, MD
Resident
Department of Radiology
University of Alabama at Birmingham
Birmingham, Alabama

Ian Malcolm, MD
Assistant Professor of Radiology
University of Alabama at Birmingham
Birmingham, Alabama

Richard S. Martin, MD
Clinical Assistant Professor of Radiology and Pediatrics
University of Alabama at Birmingham
Children's Health System of Alabama
Birmingham, Alabama

Michelle M. McNamara, MD
Assistant Professor of Radiology
University of Alabama at Birmingham
Birmingham, Alabama

Desiree E. Morgan, MD
Professor of Radiology
Vice Chair for Clinical Research
Chief, Body MRI
Medical Director, MRI
University of Alabama at Birmingham
Birmingham, Alabama

Robert S. Morrison III, MD, MS
Resident
Department of Radiology and Radiology Sciences
Vanderbilt University Medical Center
Nashville, Tenessee

Martha M. Munden, MD
Associate Professor of Radiology and Pediatrics
University of Alabama at Birmingham
Children's Health System of Alabama
Birmingham, Alabama

Emily R. Norman, MD
Resident
Department of Radiology
University of Alabama at Birmingham Hospital
Birmingham, Alabama

Robert P. Nuttall, MD, PhD
Clinical Assistant Professor of Radiology and Pediatrics
University of Alabama at Birmingham
Children's Health System of Alabama
Birmingham, Alabama

Rachel F. Oser, MD
Associate Professor of Radiology
Program Director, Vascular and Interventional Radiology Fellowship
University of Alabama at Birmingham
Birmingham, Alabama

Bhavik N. Patel, MD
Resident
Department of Radiology
University of Alabama at Birmingham
Birmingham, Alabama

Karthikram Raghuram, DNB, MD
Assistant Professor
Section of Neuroradiology and Interventional Neuroradiology
West Virginia University

Brenton D. Reading, MD
Resident
Department of Radiology
University of Alabama at Birmingham
Birmingham, Alabama

Michelle L. Robbin, MD, FACR
Professor of Radiology
Chief of Ultrasound
University of Alabama at Birmingham
Birmingham, Alabama

Jeremy T. Royal, MD
Resident
Department of Radiology
University of Alabama at Birmingham
Birmingham, Alabama

Stuart A. Royal, MS, MD, FACR
Clinical Professor and Chief of Radiology and Pediatrics
University of Alabama at Birmingham
Radiologist-in-Chief, Pediatrics
Children's Health System of Alabama
Birmingham, Alabama

Shyamsunder B. Sabat, MD
Fellow
Neuroradiology
Department of Radiology
University of Alabama at Birmingham
Birmingham, Alabama

Souheil Saddekni, MD, FSIR, FAHA
Professor of Radiology
Chief of Vascular and Interventional Radiology
Co-Medical Director, Heart and Vascular Center
University of Alabama at Birmingham
Birmingham, Alabama

Libby L. Shadinger, MD
Instructor
Diagnostic Radiology
Vanderbilt University Medical Center
Nashville, Tennessee

Ritu Shah, MD
Assistant Professor of Radiology
University of Alabama at Birmingham
Birmingham, Alabama

Satinder P. Singh, MD, FCCP
Associate Professor of Radiology
Chief Cardiopulmonary Radiology
Director, Cardiothoracic CT
University of Alabama at Birmingham
Birmingham, Alabama

Joshua P. Smith, MD
Resident
Department of Radiology
University of Alabama at Birmingham
Birmingham, Alabama

Clinton R. Smith, MD
Fellow
Vascular and Interventional Radiology
Department of Radiology
University of Alabama at Birmingham
Birmingham, Alabama

James S. Spann, MD
Resident
Department of Radiology
University of Alabama at Birmingham
Birmingham, Alabama

Joseph C. Sullivan III, MD
Assistant Professor of Neuroradiology
Residency Program Director
University of Alabama at Birmingham
Birmingham, Alabama

Mark Sultenfuss, MD
Resident
Department of Radiology
University of Alabama at Birmingham
Birmingham, Alabama

Kok C. Tan, MD, FRCR (UK)
Fellow
Interventional Radiology and Nuclear Medicine
Department of Radiology
University of Alabama at Birmingham
Birmingham, Alabama

Franklin N. Tessler, MD, CM
Professor of Radiology
Vice Chair for Radiology Informatics
Chief of Body Imaging
University of Alabama at Birmingham
Birmingham, Alabama

John C. Texada, MD
Fellow
Cardiothoracic
Department of Radiology
University of Alabama at Birmingham
Birmingham, Alabama

Heidi R. Umphrey, MD, MS
Assistant Professor of Radiology
University of Alabama at Birmingham
Birmingham, Alabama

Edgar S. Underwood, MD
Assistant Professor of Radiology
University of Alabama at Birmingham
Birmingham, Alabama

Yoginder N. Vaid, MBBS, DMRD, MD
Clinical Professor of Pediatrics and Diagnostic Radiology
University of Alabama at Birmingham
Children's Health System of Alabama
Birmingham, Alabama

Surjith Vattoth, MD, DMRD, DNB, FRCR
Fellow
Vascular and Interventional Radiology
Department of Radiology
University of Alabama at Birmingham
Birmingham, Alabama

Jonathan W. Walter, MD
Resident
Department of Radiology
University of Alabama at Birmingham
Birmingham, Alabama

Therese M. Weber, MD
Professor of Radiology
University of Alabama at Birmingham
Birmingham, Alabama

Jeffery R. White, MD
Resident
Department of Radiology
University of Alabama at Birmingham
Birmingham, Alabama

Daniel W. Young, MD, FACR
Clinical Professor of Radiology and Pediatrics
University of Alabama at Birmingham
Children's Health System of Alabama
Birmingham, Alabama

PREFACE

In recent years, there has been a paradigm shift in learning, specifically the manner in which information is gathered and ingested. This is particularly notable in subject matter that covers great breadth or is rapidly evolving, such as medicine, and more specifically, diagnostic imaging. Students and residents (and for that matter, practicing radiologists) quickly turn to the Internet to "Google™" unknown factoids, rapidly gathering information, in many cases without source validation. This has created silo learning where tidbits of information are immediately collected, answering the one specific question of concern. However, there is little depth or longevity afforded with this learning process, which in many cases does not drill down to the anatomic or pathophysiologic fundamental principles. As a result, there is a lack of complete understanding, or even worse, misunderstanding, and the information is often retained only long enough to address the question at hand.

This book is an attempt to address the silo learning afforded by the Internet. It is organized according to 10 subspecialties and includes overviews of imaging-based physics for ultrasound, MRI, and nuclear medicine. Content centers on the fundamentals of anatomy and pathophysiology with concise relevant imaging correlation. This, however, is not a text emphasizing image interpretation, as there are countless other references that do this quite well. At the end of each chapter, the reader is challenged with a set of questions written in single best answer, multiple-choice format. Detailed discussions of the answers enhance and enforce the reader's learning experience.

The goal of this text is to provide a firm foundation for learning and reference during residency training, and through lifelong learning. Its intent is to link together common concepts while presenting often complex material in a simple, straight-forward manner, hopefully balanced with enough depth so that fundamental concepts are reinforced so as to avoid piecemeal or silo learning.

ACKNOWLEDGMENTS

I am indebted to the contributing authors for their knowledge, insight, and perseverance. Their expertise has proven invaluable.

I would also like to thank Beth Parker, my assistant, for endless hours of editing and overall coordination of this project. Additionally, thanks goes to Rachel Metcalf, Toni Braddy, Brittany Harris, and Pat Moore for their support and to Tony Zagar for his illustrations. He has drawn clear, understandable figures despite my ambiguous and often conflicting instructions.

Finally, a note of appreciation goes to my fellow members of the Abdominal Imaging Section at the University of Alabama at Birmingham, Department of Radiology. Without your support and encouragement, this book would have never happened. It is a real pleasure to work with you each and everyday.

Section 1
CENTRAL NERVOUS SYSTEM

1 TECHNICAL ASPECTS OF CNS IMAGING

Joseph C. Sullivan III

Imaging used to evaluate the brain, head and neck, and spine primarily incorporates volume acquisition imaging, mainly CT and MRI. Conventional radiography remains useful in central nervous system (CNS) evaluation primarily in the realm of prescreening for indwelling metal foreign bodies and implants in patients undergoing MRI and initial imaging in an emergency setting.

CT

CT uses an x-ray transmission algorithm to mathematically reconstruct a cross-sectional image of the body from relative amounts of x-ray transmission. As the gantry of the CT scans spins around the patient, a narrow beam of x-rays is emitted to an associated row of rotating detectors on the opposite side of the gantry. Relative transmission is calculated and a cross-sectional image is created via computer algorithm. The use of multirow detectors with CT has nearly eliminated conventional (nonhelical) CT, as the speed at which helically acquired CT is now obtained allows for increased areas of coverage without breath-hold or with shorter breath-hold times. High-detail three-dimensional imaging can be obtained via postprocessing. Additionally, the larger number of detectors and overlap of the spiral acquisition nearly eliminates misregistration and volume-averaging artifacts.

The display of data with CT is a computer-based pixel assignment relative to water densities, Hounsfield unit (HU). This scale, named for Sir Godfrey Hounsfield assigns increasing HU to higher density materials with water being O. Therefore, fat and air have negative HU and bone is highly positive. Brain parenchyma and even CSF, which is slightly more dense than water, have HU somewhere between that of water and bone.

The basis of the display of this data is relative to the value given to each pixel and the display algorithm that is chosen. The midlevel, or area of interest based on tissue density, is the selected window level. A window width encompassing this level increases or decreases the surrounding variation of shades of gray displayed. Therefore, to evaluate a specific portion of the anatomy, the window is narrowed to a particular width to include the desired surrounding tissues. Therefore, multiple different window-width and window-level settings are used to evaluate for parenchyma (approximately 35–40 HU), blood (approximately 60–70 HU in a normal patient), bone (2000 HU or greater). Dedicated narrow windows are necessary to evaluate for stroke, specifically looking for edema within the parenchyma (25–40 HU); "subdural window" employs more of a soft-tissue window.

Image data can be reviewed in multiple ways and differing planes, allowing for increased information without subjecting the patient to additional radiation. It should be considered, however, that the imaging technique should be tailored for the specific clinical indication. Higher kVp provides improved resolution for more dense material such as bone, versus increased mA to give better resolution of soft tissue.

Ever-increasing multidetector helical acquisition and appetite for improved anatomical resolution must be balanced with risks of increased radiation dosage, particularly in those who are more susceptible to the adverse effects of radiation, that is, infants and children.

CT images are obtained with x-rays and are therefore subject to beam hardening and streak artifacts. As a beam of photons passes through a particular section of anatomy, it is attenuated so that the higher kVp photons are transmitted and registered by the detector on the contralateral side. This results in a misinterpretation by the detector that there was higher transmission than actually occurred, in turn calculated by the computer as an area of low density, thus lower HU. Streak artifact occurs when there are edges of sharp density delineation between adjacent objects. As the computer sees the large variation in x-ray attenuation, it misinterprets these regions and produces a "star" or a multistreak artifact as the gantry rotates around this interface. Motion artifact occurs when structures change position within the field of view as acquisition of the object changes position relative to the gantry. As the gantry encircles the patient, this causes a misregistration of the object in the field. This may be secondary to normal physiological motion in the case of heartbeat, respiration, vessel pulsation, or bowel gas peristalsis. Although CT scanners have improved in their speed of acquisition to the point this can be nulled or even gated, patient motion remains a continuing problem.

MRI

MRI is a completely different form of volume acquisition. There are different tissue characteristics based on its protons, resulting in differing T1 and T2 relaxation times. The T1 relaxation time is the time it takes for a tissue to become magnetized, while T2 indicates the time for loss of this magnetization. These differing relaxation times are localized within the field of the magnet depending on small variations in the radiofrequency applied and received by tailored antennas known as coils. Tissue within a field of localization may not remain within that field or may pass into that field under normal physiological conditions. Specifically, blood flow may demonstrate a flow void as blood flows through a blood vessel into and out of a magnetized field. Also, in variation with CT, which is acquired in a cross-sectional anatomic demographic plane and reconstructed via postprocessing, MRI can be acquired in multiple planes as the data is acquired volumetrically and presented in planes based on frequency encoding, corresponding to the *x*-axis, and phase coding, *y*-axis. Respectively, slice location is determined by slight variations and the gradient intensity along the *z*-axis.

MR is obtained in multiple varied sequence acquisitions, the primary of which is a spin echo pulse sequence. Standard T1- and T2-weighted images are created using a short time of repetition and time of echo versus longer times, respectively. Proton density sequences use a combination of long repetition time and short echo time, allowing for accentuation of hydrogen density differences between tissues. Variations of spin echo, called multiple spin echo, allow for the reduction of image acquisition time, typically referred to as fast-spin or turbo-spin echo. The trade-off is degradation of signal intensity and increased fat intensity on T2-weighted imaging. Fat-suppression techniques are often used to counter this effect and/or to allow for detection of underlying fluid latent pathology. Inversion recovery pulse sequences emphasize differences between T1 relaxation times as a delayed time of inversion is added to the time of repetition and time of echo; tissues with short T1 relaxation times such as fat are suppressed and tissues with an unexpected high water content (pathology) are accentuated. Fat-suppression techniques attempt to similarly depress the short T1 signal of fat; however, these are highly sensitive to magnetic field inhomogeneity, and do not work well with low field magnet strength. Fat suppression is performed using a saturation pulse at a resonant frequency of fat applied to each imaging plane. Although this is limited by its sensitivity for field inhomogeneity, this is better for use with postcontrast technique than those of inversion recovery as the latter suppresses all tissues with short T1 including those that may enhance after the administration of gadolinium. Echo planar imaging incorporates fast MR techniques for multislice studies with single radiofrequency excitation. It decreases motion artifact and continues to show improvement in high-resolution techniques such as blood perfusion and functional MR. Gradient recall echo imaging pulse sequences employ multiple short flip angles of less than 90 degrees to decrease the time taken to recover a signal. This, however, creates sensitivity to imperfections in the magnetic field from short T2 relaxation times, also known as T2 star.

Safety of the patient is the foremost concern. Ferromagnetic and magnetic susceptibility of implants, personal items carried by the patient, and support devices inadvertently taken into the field of the magnet must all be considered with each patient. Furthermore, although some implants may not have ferromagnetic components, the components of those implants should be carefully evaluated as wires or loops in a magnetic field can generate electric current. Such radiofrequency current can cause burns or false activation or failure of the implant. The strength of the magnet must also be considered as variations in magnetic field strength can have variable effects on all such devices. Some implants, although considered compatible with MR, may demonstrate artifacts associated with disruption of the magnetic field. This implies the object has some ferromagnetic quality. The safety considerations and compatibility of implants far exceeds the content of this text and should be considered on an individual case-by-case basis.

Motion artifacts in MR are also more prevalent than CT secondary to the longer acquisition time. Multiple techniques such as shorter acquisition time and computer reregistration are used for motion correction.

MYELOGRAPHY

Myelography is a useful tool in those who cannot be imaged adequately or safely with MRI. Although it is not nearly as prevalent as it once was, indications for and usefulness of myelography remain. A lumbar puncture is performed and once a spinal needle is advanced into the thecal sac, at a level that is deemed safe, the stylet is retracted. Upon the spontaneous return of cerebrospinal fluid, contrast media is carefully injected under direct visualization. Spot fluoroscopic imaging obtained at the time of contrast placement can reveal significant pathologic information by assessing contrast flow. Keeping in mind that all sections of the spinal thecal sac can usually be evaluated from a single puncture, it should be remembered that the density and amount of contrast material greatly varies based upon the clinical question at hand. Careful attention to the location of the contrast in the thecal sac, as this can have clinical side effects based on misplacement and/or its extension into the skull base, and the puncture site, as symptoms of skull-based headaches from cerebrospinal fluid leaks can be detrimental to the patient, must be demonstrated.

Myelographic imaging remains limited in that it only can delineate those things within the thecal sac or that impress upon the thecal sac but not pathology within the cord itself. However, in the patient in whom an MRI is contraindicated, localization of cord swelling or impression upon the cord or other neuroelements may be key to the surgical planning. Further usefulness of myelography is seen with postsurgical patients who have hardware that may not be tolerated in a magnetic field or may create artifacts to the point that evaluation of the adjacent neural elements may be precluded. Provided that the postmyelographic CT does not have substantial artifacts to limit its use, it must be remembered that the acquisition of fluoroscopic spot film at the time of actual myelography can give almost as much information as the postmyelographic CT.

SUGGESTED READING

Arena L, Morehouse H, Safir J. MR imaging artifacts that simulate disease: how to recognize them and eliminate them. *Radiographics*. 1995;15:1373-1394.

Association of University Radiologist. Abstracts from contrast media research symposium. *Acad Radiol*. 2005;12:S2-S85.

Frush D et al. Computed tomography and radiation: understanding the issues. *J Am Coll Radiol*. 2004;1:113-119.

Kanel E, Borgstede J, Barkovich A. American College of Radiology white paper on MR safety. *Am J Roentgenol*. 2002;178: 1335-1347.

McNitt-Gray M. Radiation dose in CT. *Radiographics*. 2002;22: 1541-1553.

Nguyen G et al. Adequacy of plain radiography in the diagnosis of cervical spine injuries. *Emerg Radiol*. 2005;11(3):158-161.

Pomper M et al. New techniques in magnetic resonance imaging of brain tumors. *Neuroimaging Clin N Am*. 2001;11(3):501-525.

Thompson M et al. Increased contrast, high spatial-resolution, diffusion-weightd, spin-echo, echo-planar imaging. *Radiology*. 1999;210:253-259.

White M. Cervical spine-magnetic resonance imaging techniques and anatomy. *Magn Reson Imag Clin N Am*. 2000;8:453-469.

QUESTIONS AND ANSWERS

1. What is the result when decreasing CT slice thickness with all other factors constant?
   A. Decreased radiation to the patient
   B. Decreased noise
   C. Decreased resolution
   D. Decreased tube heating
   E. Decreased motion sensitivity

   ANSWER: C. Resolution is decreased in the use of thinner slices if all other factors remain the same (unless kVp and/or mA are increased). A smoothing algorithm may be used to make the images more pleasing which may further limit sensitivity to subtly pathology. Radiation to the patient will increase unless kVp and/or mA is decreased. Tube heating therefore is also increased. The longer scan acquisition time increases risk for motion artifact.

2. Which one of the following artifacts is correctly paired with its modality?
   A. Beam attenuation–MRI
   B. Ring down–CT
   C. Streak–MRI
   D. Aliasing–MRI
   E. Partial-volume averaging–radiograph

   ANSWER: D. Aliasing is also known as wrap-around artifact. Ring down occurs with ultrasound. Beam attenuation can occur with any radiation-dependent imaging. Streak artifact occurs on CT at interfaces or secondary to motion at these interfaces.

3. What is an imaging benefit of CT versus conventional radiography?
   A. Decrease in artifacts
   B. Improved resolution
   C. Decreased noise
   D. Decreased contrast threshold
   E. All of the above

   ANSWER: D. CT is able to detect lower-contrast differences between tissues than conventional radiography. Radiography has fewer artifacts, better line pair resolution, and less noise than CT.

4. What is the basic measure of tissue variation in MRI?
   A. K-space
   B. Matrix
   C. NEX
   D. Proton density
   E. Proton rotation

ANSWER: D. The variability of T1 and T2 is primarily dependent on the differing density of protons in tissue. K-space is the image space from which an image is calculated from related to the area that is being imaged. The matrix is the rows and column that determine the resolution. NEX is the square root of the number of acquisitions and is related to signal noise. The spin of the protons allows the proton to give off signal as they align and precess in the field.

5. On MRI, what primarily affects the Larmor frequency?
   A. Strength of the magnetic field
   B. Orientation of the magnetic field
   C. Location within isocenter of the magnetic field
   D. Shimming of the magnetic field
   E. Bore size of the magnet

   ANSWER: A. Strength and isotope are the primary contributors to the Larmor frequency. Although location within a magnetic field cause a decrease in strength, this should occur while remaining within the isocenter.

6. Why are hydrogen (protons) molecules the ideal isotope for MRI?
   A. High spin density
   B. High tissue density
   C. High NMR sensitivity
   D. High abundance
   E. All of the above

   ANSWER: E. Spin and tissue density are the same thing. Protons have a high NMR sensitivity and are highly abundant in tissue as water.

7. What is the Hounsfield unit a measure of?
   A. Proton density
   B. Tissue density
   C. Spin density
   D. Hemoglobin density
   E. Bone density

   ANSWER: B. Density of tissue is measured in Hounsfield units (HU). Water is 0 HU. Those tissues less dense than water are given negative numbers, and those tissues more dense than water are positive, respectively.

8. How does increasing image noise impact an imaging study?
   A. Increased artifacts
   B. Increased blur
   C. Increased image distortion
   D. Decreased low-contrast resolution
   E. Increased radiation to the patient

   ANSWER: D. Increasing noise makes it more difficult to resolve images at lower contrast.

9. What modality has the best native resolution?
   A. MRI
   B. CT
   C. Conventional radiography
   D. Ultrasound

   ANSWER: C. Although modern CT scanners have improved their resolution capabilities substantially, the line pair resolution for conventional radiography continues to have the best inherent resolution.

10. Image resolution is a direct measure of what?
    A. Low-contrast objects
    B. High-contrast objects
    C. Anatomical detail
    D. Noisy images

    ANSWER: C. Resolution measures blurring associated with clarity of anatomical detail.

11. Of the following, what factor has the most significant effect on the majority of artifacts?
    A. Matrix size
    B. Gradient strength
    C. Magnetic field orientation
    D. Magnet strength
    E. NEX

    ANSWER: D. As magnet strength increases, the susceptibility and their respective artifacts also increase. Only motion artifacts may decrease with higher magnet strengths if additional parameters are constant.

2 BRAIN AND SPINE ANATOMY

Surjith Vattoth and Joseph C. Sullivan III

BRAIN ANATOMY

SCALP

The scalp consists of five layers: skin, connective tissue, aponeurosis, loose connective tissue, and pericranium. On T1-weighted images, scalp is hyperintense because of the fatty components.

The skin is attached to the third layer by fibrous septa, so that all three layers move together.

The second layer consisting of fibroadipose tissue lodges the blood vessels of scalp derived mainly from the external carotid artery and cutaneous sensory nerve supply derived from the second and third cervical nerves (the first cervical has no cutaneous branch) and from the trigeminal nerves, with the vessels attached to the fibrous septa. Wounds of the scalp bleed profusely because the vessels, being attached to fibrous septa, cannot retract and constrict. Posteriorly, the skin up to the vertex is supplied by the greater occipital and third occipital nerves (posterior primary rami of C2 and C3), while the skin behind the ear is supplied by the lesser occipital nerve (anterior primary rami of C2). The third layer consists mainly of galea aponeurotica, frontalis muscle anteriorly, and occipitalis muscle posteriorly. The fourth layer is loose areolar connective tissue between the upper three layers that move together and the periosteum of the skull vault. The periosteum or pericranium on the outer surface of the calvarium is continuous with that of the inner surface at the sutural connections between the bones of the skull.

CALVARIUM

The cranium consists of calvarial vault, base of skull, and facial skeleton. The calvarial vault is composed of frontal bone, paired parietal bones, squamous occipital bone, and paired squamous temporal bones. The coronal suture separates the frontal bone from the two parietal bones; the metopic suture seen in neonates separates the frontal bones in the midline which fuses later in life. The sagittal suture separates the two parietal bones, and the lambdoid suture separates the occipital bone from the two parietal bones.

On T1-weighted images, the calvarium is seen as hyperintense, fatty marrow, lined on inside and outside by low signal inner and outer tables of skull, respectively. The evaluation of the calvarial signals on the T1-weighted image is important to assess for marrow infiltrative disorders.

The base of skull and facial skeleton will be dealt with Chapter 13.

MENINGES

The dura (pachymeninges), arachnoid, and pia mater (combinedly called the leptomeninges) form the three meningeal layers covering the brain.

The dura mater has two layers, a superficial layer, which forms the periosteum of the inner skull and a deep layer, which forms the dura mater proper. The dura separates into two layers at dural reflections, two main dural reflections being falx cerebri and tentorium cerebelli.

The potential extradural or epidural space lies between the skull and dura and is seen as a biconvex space when collections or hematoma develops in this space. Epidural collections do not cross sutures, but may cross the midline. Epidural hematomas usually develop because of arterial bleeding from injury to the skull. The subdural space is a potential space between the dura and the arachnoid and the subdural collections have a concavo–convex appearance. Subdural collections cross sutures, but do not cross the midline. Subdural hematomas occur because of bleeding from the torn bridging veins in the subdural space.

Arachnoid lies inner to the dura and like the dura does not invaginate into the sulci. The subarachnoid space contains CSF and lies between the arachnoid and pia mater. The arachnoid villi are CSF reabsorbing endothelial-lined granulations of arachnoid and subarachnoid space extending into the dural sinuses.

Pia, which is the innermost meningeal layer, unlike the other two layers, invaginates into the sulci. It follows the penetrating cortical arteries into the brain to form the perivascular spaces also known as Virchow-Robin spaces. The subpial space is a potential space between the pia mater and the glia limitans of cortex.

PRACTICAL APPROACH TO IDENTIFICATION OF SULCI AND GYRI

First, at the top axial images, identify the anteroposteriorly oriented superior frontal sulcus joining the transversely oriented precentral sulcus. The premotor cortex of the frontal lobe lies anterior to this precentral sulcus. The central sulcus or Rolandic fissure, which separates the frontal and parietal lobes, is the next transversely oriented sulcus lying immediately posterior to precentral sulcus. The motor cortex of the frontal lobe lies between the central sulcus and precentral sulcus. The inverted omega or horizontal epsilon shaped posteriorly directed knob on the central sulcus/gyrus designates the motor cortex controlling hand function. The motor cortex for facial muscles lies lateral to the hand knob and the leg area lies medially in a parasagittal location. The sensory cortex lies posterior to the central sulcus in the parietal lobe. It is noteworthy that the precentral motor gyrus is thicker than the postcentral sensory gyrus with a mean cortical thickness ratio of 1.54. Also, in axial images, the posterior aspects (pars marginalis) of the right and left cingulate sulci form a horizontal bracket called pars bracket. In 97% of cases, the medial end of the central sulcus lies just anterior to this pars bracket and so it helps in central sulcus identification. However in 3% of cases, the postcentral sulcus may lie immediately anterior to this horizontal bracket, negating the value of this pars bracket sign.

The sylvian fissure in axial images helps to differentiate the frontal lobe anteriorly from temporal lobe posteriorly. On coronal images, the posterior ramus of sylvian fissure (lateral sulcus) separates the anterior part of parietal lobe superiorly from the temporal lobe inferiorly. Behind the point, where the posterior ramus of sylvian fissure ends (by turning superiorly into parietal lobe), there is no anatomic demarcation between the parietal and temporal lobes. A horizontal imaginary line is drawn posteriorly along the horizontal course of the posterior ramus of sylvian fissure to join another imaginary vertical line drawn between the end of the parietooccipital sulcus on the superomedial margin of the cerebral hemisphere and a notch on its inferolateral margin. This imaginary horizontal line separates the posterior aspect of the parietal lobe superiorly from the temporal lobe inferiorly. The imaginary vertical line separates the occipital lobe posteriorly from the parietal and temporal lobes anteriorly on the lateral parasagittal images. In medial sagittal images, the parietooccipital sulcus demarcates the occipital lobe posteriorly from the parietal lobe anteriorly. The occipital and temporal lobes on the inferomedial surface run into one another with no anatomic structures separating them.

On coronal images, the superior temporal gyrus lies between the sylvian fissure and superior temporal sulcus. The transverse temporal gyrus of Heschl, which is the primary auditory cortex, projects medially from the superior temporal gyrus. The Heschl gyrus can be easily identified in coronal images at the coronal level showing the tent formed by the convergence of fornices and presence of eighth cranial nerves and in axial images at the level of massa intermedia connecting the two thalami. The sensory speech area or Wernicke area is located in the superior temporal gyrus.

On coronal images, the middle temporal gyrus lies between the superior and middle temporal sulci. The inferior temporal gyrus lies between the middle and inferior temporal sulci. Further inferomedially, the fusiform gyrus, which continues posteriorly to join the occipital lobe, lies between the inferior temporal sulcus and collateral sulcus.

The mesial temporal structures of the limbic system lie medial to the collateral sulcus on coronal images with the parahippocampal gyrus inferiorly and hippocampus superiorly. If we follow the hippocampus anteriorly on serial coronal sections, we will reach the hippocampal head at the level of temporal horn of lateral ventricle. The amygdalla lies anterosuperomedial to the hippocampal head. As we follow the hippocampus posteriorly, we can see the head and body of hippocampus followed by its tail. The hippocampal white matter (alveus), which outlines the hippocampal gray matter, continues as fimbria and crus of the fornix on both sides alongside the lateral ventricles. The crura of fornices can in turn be traced anteriorly merging into the column of fornix.

On lateral sagittal images, the frontal lobe anterior to the precentral sulcus is divided by a series of sulci into superior, middle, and inferior frontal gyri. The posterior part of the inferior frontal gyrus is separated from the temporal lobe by the sylvian fissure that has an anterior horizontal and anterior ascending rami. This divides this portion of inferior frontal gyrus into an "M" shaped area, the anterior vertical line of M representing the pars orbitalis, the middle V of M representing the pars triangularis, and posterior vertical line of M representing the pars opercularis. The motor speech area or Broca's area is located in the opercula and triangular sections of the inferior frontal gyrus.

The lateral sagittal images are also helpful in demarcating the two component gyri of the inferior parietal lobule, namely the supramarginal gyrus and angular gyrus. The posterosuperior end of the posterior ramus of sylvian fissure is surrounded by a horseshoe-shaped gyrus, the supramarginal gyrus. Similarly, the posterior end of the superior temporal sulcus is surrounded by the horseshoe-shaped angular gyrus. The sulcus forming the superior border of these gyri is the intraparietal sulcus and the remainder of the parietal lobe superiorly is the superior parietal lobule.

The medial sagittal images help to demarcate the parietal lobe from the occipital lobe. The parietooccipital sulcus is bounded anteriorly by the precuneus (a parietal lobe gyrus) and posteriorly by the cuneus (an occipital lobe gyrus). Inferior to cuneus in the occipital lobe is the calcarine sulcus and the striate cortex in and around the calcarine sulcus serves as the primary visual cortex. The lingual gyrus of the occipital lobe lies inferior to calcarine sulcus. If we trace further anteriorly, the lingual gyrus becomes continuous with the mesial temporal parahippocampal gyrus. On the inferior surface of the occipital lobe, lateral to the lingual gyrus, lies the fusiform gyrus, which connects the temporal lobe with the occipital lobe. Thus as noted previously, the temporal and occipital lobes on the inferior surface run into one another with no anatomic structures separating them.

The anterior aspect of the medial sagittal images demonstrates the corpus callosum and is well demarcated superiorly by the callosal sulcus, which is continuous posteroinferiorly with the hippocampal sulcus. The cingulate gyrus lies parallel to and above the callosal sulcus and is demarcated superiorly by the cingulate sulcus. Near the region of splenium of corpus callosum, the cingulate sulcus gives the paracentral branch and marginal branch and then continues as the subparietal sulcus outlining the isthmus of cingulate gyrus (which becomes continuous with parahippocampal gyrus).

In the medial sagittal images, the paracentral lobule is divided by the medial end of the central sulcus into a larger anterior part belonging to the frontal lobe and a smaller posterior part that belongs to the parietal lobe. Anterior to the paracentral lobule lies the superior frontal gyrus and posterior to it lies the precuneus of parietal lobe.

BRAINSTEM

MIDBRAIN

Two large bundles of fibers called crura lie on either side of midline anteriorly divided by the interpeduncular or crural CSF cistern anteriorly and diverge to enter the corresponding cerebral hemispheres superiorly (cerebral peduncles). The third (oculomotor) cranial nerves emerge from the medial aspect of the crus on the same side and exit the midbrain via the interpeduncular cistern on their way to the cavernous sinus and superior orbital fissure to supply the four extraocular muscles, medial rectus, inferior rectus, superior rectus, and inferior oblique. The cerebral aqueduct of Sylvius divides the midbrain into tegmentum anteriorly and tectum or roof posteriorly.

The mesencephalic tegmentum contains the white matter tracts-medial longitudinal fasciculus (oculomotor/vestibular), medial (somatosensory) and lateral (auditory) leminisci, spinothalamic (somatosensory), and central tegmental motor tract including the reticular formation. The gray matter includes the substantia nigra, red nucleus, periaqueductal gray matter, and third/fourth cranial nerve nuclei. On thin section T2-weighted MRI, the pars compacta of substantia nigra can be seen as a hyperintense band between the hypointense band of pars reticularis of substantia nigra anterolaterally and hypointense nodular red nucleus posteromedially in paramidline location. The pars compacta atrophies in parkinsonian disorders. The third nerve nucleus lies at the superior colliculus level in a paramedian location anterior to cerebral aqueduct and posterior to the red nucleus. The parasympathetic nuclei of the third nerve, Edinger-Westphal nuclei, lie in the periaqueductal gray matter posterior to the third nerve nucleus. The fourth nerve nucleus lies at the inferior colliculus level in a paramedian location anterior to cerebral aqueduct and posterior to medial longitudinal fasciculus.

The tectal plate or quadrigeminal plate is composed of the paired superior colliculi for extraocular muscle coordination and inferior colliculi for hearing relay. Each colliculus is related laterally to a ridge called the brachium. The superior brachium connects the superior colliculus to the lateral geniculate body and the inferior brachium connects the inferior colliculus to the medial geniculate body on either side. The cistern posterior to the midbrain is called the quadrigeminal plate cistern as it is closely related the quadrigeminal plate. It is important to note that the persistent cavum veli interpositi (CVI) communicates with quadrigeminal cistern. The perimesencephalic or ambient cistern extends from the posterior margin of the interpeduncular cistern to the lateral edge of the midbrain colliculi, around the lateral surface of the upper portion of the brainstem. The ambient cistern mainly contain P2 segment of the posterior cerebral artery, superior cerebellar artery, anterior choroidal artery, basal vein of Rosenthal, and fourth cranial nerve.

Just below the colliculi lies the uppermost part of a membrane called the superior medullary velum, which stretches between the two superior cerebellar peduncles, forming the roof of the fourth ventricle. The fourth (trochlear) cranial nerve, which is the only cranial nerve that exits the brainstem dorsally, courses posteriorly around the cerebral aqueduct and decussates in the superior medullary velum, crosses over in the quadrigeminal cistern, and winds round the opposite side of the midbrain in the ambient cistern to reach its ventral aspect on the way to enter the contralateral cavernous sinus and orbit to supply the superior oblique muscle. During their course, both the third and fourth cranial nerves pass between the posterior cerebral artery and superior cerebellar artery and may be compressed by aneurysms. The superior cerebellar peduncles (brachium conjunctivum) decussate in the midbrain posterior to red nuclei, flank the upper fourth ventricle, and connect the midbrain to cerebellum.

PONS

The ventral surface of the pons is grooved by the sulcus basilaris along which the basilar artery passes. The fifth (trigeminal) cranial nerve emerges from the anterolateral surface of pons and passes through prepontine cistern to be connected to the Gasserian Ganglion in Meckel cave. The bulky middle cerebellar peduncles (brachium pontis) connect the pons with the cerebellum on each side. The sixth (abducens) cranial nerve emerges from the junction of pons and medulla anteromedially, just off the midline above the medullary pyramids, and passes through the prepontine cistern, penetrates dura of basisphenoid to enter the Dorello canal, arches over petrous apex below petrosphenoidal ligament into posterosuperior cavernous sinus, and then enters superior orbital fissure and orbit to innervate the lateral rectus muscle. The seventh (facial) and eighth (vestibulocochlear) cranial nerves emerge from the pontomedullary junction, laterally above the medullary olives, and enter the cerebellopontine angle cistern on their way to the internal auditory canal. The pons is separated from the cerebellum posteriorly by the fourth ventricle, which is continuous superiorly with the cerebral aqueduct.

The ventral pons, which forms the bellylike anterior projection on sagittal images, contain the longitudinal corticospinal, corticobulbar and corticopontine white matter tracts, and the multiple transverse pontine fibers, which make up the bulk.

The dorsal pontine tegmentum is composed of white matter tracts-medial longitudinal fasciculus (oculomotor/vestibular), medial (somatosensory) and lateral (auditory) leminisci, trapezoid body (auditory), spinothalamic tract (somatosensory), and central tegmental motor tract including the reticular formation. The gray matter includes the bulk of the motor, main sensory, and mesencephalic nuclei of fifth nerve located in the upper lateral dorsal pontine tegmentum in a location far anterolateral to fourth ventricle. The sixth nerve nucleus is located in lower dorsal pontine tegmentum near midline just anterior to fourth ventricle. The axons of facial nerve loop around the sixth nerve nucleus creating a bulge in the floor (anterior aspect) of the fourth ventricle, called the facial colliculus. The seventh nerve motor, superior salivatory, and tractus solitarius nuclei lie in the lower lateral dorsal pontine tegmentum in a location far anterolateral to fourth ventricle. The medial, lateral, inferior, and superior vestibular nuclei of eighth cranial nerve lie along the lateral aspect of the floor of the fourth ventricle at the pontomedullary junction. The dorsal and ventral cochlear nuclei of the eighth nerve lie dorsally and ventrally on the lateral aspect of the inferior cerebellar peduncle (restiform body) at the pontomedullary junction.

MEDULLA OBLONGATA

The ventral medulla is composed of the medullary pyramids and olives. The pyramids are two paramedian longitudinal projections anteriorly, composed of the corticospinal (pyramidal) tracts, and separated in the midline by ventral median fissure. Posterolateral to the pyramids, separated by the preolivary sulcus from which the rootlets of the twelfth (hypoglossal) cranial nerve exit on each side, lie the medullary olives that consist of inferior olivary nucleus (largest and forms the bulge on the surface of medulla), dorsal and medial accessory olivary nuclei, and superior olivary nucleus. The postolivary sulcus from which the rootlets of the ninth (glossopharyngeal), tenth (vagus), and eleventh (spinal accessory) cranial nerves exit the medulla lies posterolateral to olive.

The inferior cerebellar peduncle (restiform body) arises from the superior aspect of the dorsal medulla and connects the medulla with the cerebellum. As already stated, the cochlear nuclei lies on the lateral aspect of the inferior cerebellar peduncle at the pontomedullary junction. In the lower aspect of the dorsal medulla lies the paired gracile tubercles formed by the nucleus gracilis, separated in the midline by dorsal median sulcus. Immediately lateral to these lie the cuneate tubercles on each side, formed by the nucleus cuneatus and bounded anterolaterally by the postolivary sulcus. These are connected to the fasciculus gracilis and fasciculus cuneatus, respectively, and white matter tracts that enter the medulla from the posterior funiculus of the spinal cord. The lower part of the medulla, immediately lateral to fasciculus cuneatus, is another longitudinal elevation called the tuberculum cinereum formed by the spinal nucleus of the fifth (trigeminal) nerve. The spinal tract of the trigeminal nerve covers this and they actually extend into the upper cervical canal. The dorsal medullary tegmentum also contains the white matter tracts-medial longitudinal fasciculus (oculomotor/vestibular), medial (somatosensory) and lateral (auditory) leminisci, spinothalamic tract, spinocerebellar tract (somatosensory), and central tegmental motor tract including the reticular formation. The ninth and tenth cranial nerve nuclei, namely nucleus ambiguous and solitary tract nucleus, lie in upper and middorsal medullary tegmentum laterally. They have sensory fibers that terminate in spinal nucleus of trigeminal nerve. The ninth nerve also has the inferior salivatory nucleus and the tenth nerve has the dorsal vagal nucleus in addition. The eleventh nerve has bulbar nuclei in lower nucleus ambiguous in upper and midmedulla. The twelfth nerve nuclei in the middorsal medullary tegmentum paramedially produces the hypoglossal eminence, which is a bulge in the floor of fourth ventricle. The medulla is separated from the cerebellum posteriorly by the inferior portion of the fourth ventricle (obex), the outlet foramina of which is continuous with the cisterna magna through the Foramen of Magendie posteriorly in the midline, and with the cerebellopontine angles through the paired foramina of Luschka laterally. The obex communicates with the central canal of the spinal cord.

CEREBELLUM

Cerebellum consists of the median vermis and two lateral cerebellar hemispheres. The deepest fissures in the cerebellum are the primary fissure superiorly, horizontal fissure in the middle, and posterolateral fissure inferiorly. The cerebellar cortex lies superficial to white matter as in the cerebrum. Also, there are deep cerebellar nuclei embedded within the white matter, namely dentate nucleus, emboliform nucleus, globose nucleus, and fastigial nucleus. The white matter of the two sides is connected by a thin lamina of fibers that are closely related to the fourth ventricle. The upper part of this lamina forms the superior medullary velum and its inferior part forms the inferior medullary velum. Both these take part in forming the roof (posterior boundary) of the fourth ventricle. The cerebellar peduncles connecting the cerebellum with midbrain, pons, and medulla are already described in those sections.

DIENCEPHALON

The diencephalon consists of thalamus, hypothalamus, subthalamus, and epithalamus. The thalami lie on either side of the third ventricle. Massa intermedia or interthalamic adhesion connects the two thalami.

The hypothalamus lies around inferior aspect of the third ventricle and consists of the preoptic region adjoining the lamina terminalis, supraoptic region above the optic chiasm, infundibulotuberal region consisting of the pituitary infundibulum, tuber cinereum and the region above it, and mamillary or posterior region consisting of the mamillary bodies and the region above it. Of these, the preoptic region is actually a derivative of the telencephalon.

The subthalamus or ventral thalamus lies behind and lateral to the hypothalamus. Inferiorly it is continuous with the upper ends of substantia nigra and red nucleus of the midbrain and laterally it is related to the lowest part of the internal capsule.

The epithalamus consists of the pineal gland and habenular nuclei. The pineal gland lies anteroinferior to the splenium of corpus callosum and vein of Galen/-Internal cerebral vein and posterosuperior to the tectal plate/quadrigeminal cistern. Pineal masses elevate the vein of Galen/Internal cerebral veins and depress the tectal plate. The suprapineal recess of the third ventricle extends posteriorly immediately above the pineal gland. The quadrigeminal plate cistern lies posterior to the pineal gland and its anterior extension called the velum interpositum lies above the pineal gland/internal cerebral vein and extends anteriorly below the corpus callosum/fornix. The tentorial apex arches above and behind the pineal gland and the course of fourth cranial nerves lies in close relationship. The attachment of the pineal body to the posterior wall of the third ventricle is through a stalk that has two laminae, superior and inferior. The superior lamina is traversed by fibers of the habenular commissure and the inferior lamina by fibers of the posterior commissure.

BASAL GANGLIA

The caudate nucleus is a C-shaped mass of gray matter with a head abutting the lateral wall of the frontal horn of lateral ventricle and lies anteromedial to the lentiform nucleus separated by the anterior limb of internal capsule, a body that abuts the body of lateral ventricle, and a tail that continues anteroinferiorly with the lentiform nucleus.

The lentiform nucleus lies lateral to the internal capsule, the anterior limb of which separates it from the caudate nucleus, and the posterior limb from the thalamus. It consists of the globus pallidus medially and the putamen laterally. Laterally, the lentiform nucleus is separated from the claustrum by the external capsule.

Note that the so-called corpus striatum consists of caudate nucleus and putamen and has the main arterial supply from the medial and lateral striate branches of the middle cerebral artery (MCA). Also, their anteriormost parts including the head of caudate nucleus receive supply from the Heubner recurrent artery, a branch of anterior cerebral artery (ACA). Their posterior parts including tail of caudate nucleus also receive blood supply through anterior choroidal artery. The main blood supply of globus pallidus is from anterior choroidal artery. The medialmost part of globus pallidus receives branches from the posterior communicating artery (PCOM).

The claustrum is a thin lamina of gray matter lateral to the external capsule. Laterally, it is separated from the insula by the extreme capsule.

INTERNAL CAPSULE

The condensed projection fibers white matter structure, internal capsule, has an anterior limb, a genu that connects it to the posterior limb, a retrolentiform part, and a sublentiform part. The upper parts of the anterior limb, genu, and posterior limb are supplied by the lateral lenticulostriate branches of the middle cerebral artery. The lower parts have a different supply—the anterior limb by Huebner recurrent artery branch of anterior cerebral artery, genu by direct internal carotid artery branches/posterior communicating artery branches, and posterior limb by anterior choroidal artery branches. The retrolentiform and sublentiform parts of the internal capsule are also supplied by the anterior choroidal artery.

The internal capsule is continuous inferiorly with the white matter fibers of crus cerebri of the midbrain and superiorly with that of the corona radiata of the cerebral hemispheres. The corona radiata is continuous superiorly with the centrum semiovale.

CORPUS CALLOSUM

The corpus callosum is a large mass of commissural nerve fibers that connects the two cerebral hemispheres. It has a central body, anterior end bend on itself called the genu, and an enlarged posterior end called splenium. A thin lamina of nerve fibers called rostrum connects the genu to the upper end of lamina terminalis. The undersurface of corpus callosum gives attachment to septum pellucidum and this callososeptal interface is an area to be specifically looked for the dot–dash appearing T2 hyperintense demyelinating plaques in conditions like multiple sclerosis. The corpus callosum forms from anterior to posterior except for the rostrum, which is formed last. In partial callosal agenesis, splenium and rostrum are always missing.

The fibers of the genu run forward into frontal lobes forming the forceps minor and fibers of splenium run backward into occipital lobes forming the forceps major. The forceps major bulges into the upper aspect of occipital horn of lateral ventricles on each side, forming the bulb of the posterior horn. The fibers of the body and some from splenium run laterally and intersect the white matter fibers of corona radiata. As they pass laterally, some fibers of the body and splenium form a flattened band called the tapetum, which is closely related to the occipital and temporal horns of lateral ventricles.

VENTRICLES OF THE BRAIN

LATERAL VENTRICLES

The paired lateral ventricles have a frontal horn, body, atrium or trigone, temporal horn, and occipital horn. The body of lateral ventricle has a roof formed by body of corpus callosum, medial wall formed by septum pellucidum, and body of fornix and floor formed by thalamus medially and caudate nucleus laterally with thalamostriate vein and stria terminalis in between.

The atrium or trigone of the lateral ventricle connects the temporal horn inferiorly, the occipital horn posteriorly, and the body of the lateral ventricle anteriorly.

The frontal horn is bounded anteriorly by genu and rostrum of corpus callosum, roof is formed by anterior aspect of body of corpus callosum, floor is formed mainly by head of caudate nucleus and partially by rostrum of corpus callosum and medial wall by septum pellucidum.

The occipital horn has a roof and lateral wall formed by tapetum (fibers from splenium of corpus callosum) and a medial wall formed by an upper elevation called bulb of posterior horn (fibers of forceps major), and a lower elevation called calcar avis (white matter pushed in by formation of calcarine sulcus of occipital lobe).

The temporal horn has a roof or lateral wall formed by the tail of caudate nucleus laterally and stria terminalis medially (which extends from the floor of the body of lateral ventricle); the most anterosuperomedial part of roof is formed by amygdalla. The floor or medial wall is formed mainly by the hippocampus along with the alveus and fimbria medially and collateral eminence laterally (produced by inward bulging of collateral white matter lying deep to collateral sulcus).

THIRD VENTRICLE

The third ventricle is the cavity of the diencephalons situated in between the two thalami. It communicates with the two lateral ventricles through the interventricular foramina of Monroe anterosuperiorly just behind the columns of fornix. Posteroinferiorly, it is continuous with the cerebral aqueduct of Sylvius within the midbrain, which connects it to the fourth ventricle. The lateral walls are formed by the thalamus superiorly and hypothalamus inferiorly. The anterior wall is formed mainly by the lamina terminalis; and upper parts by the anterior commissure/columns of fornix. The posterior wall is formed by pineal gland and posterior commissure. The floor is formed from anterior to posterior by the optic chiasm, the hypothalamus including pituitary infundibulum, tuber cinereum and mamillary bodies, the posterior perforated substance, and the midbrain tegmentum. The roof is formed by ependyma stretching across the two thalami, tela chоridea and choroid plexuses. The interthalamic adhesion or massa intermedia pass through the cavity of the third ventricle. The cavity has many recesses including the optic recess that lies just above the optic chiasm, the infundibular recess that extends into the pituitary infundibulum, the pineal recess that lies between superior and inferior laminae of pineal stalk, and the suprapineal recess that lies above the pineal gland.

FOURTH VENTRICLE

The important features of fourth ventricle are already described in the section on brainstem.

TELA CHOROIDEA AND CHOROID PLEXUSES

The tela choroidea is a double-layered fold of pia mater that lies in the roof of the third ventricle. The posterior end of tela choroidea lies in the gap between (transverse fissure) the splenium of corpus callosum and the posterior part of roof of third ventricle. When traced further posteriorly, the two layers of pia mater separate with the upper layer curving upward over the posterior aspect of the splenium and the lower layer turning downward over the pineal body and tectum. The anterior end of the tela choroidea of third ventricle lies near the interventricular foramina of Monroe and passes through the gap (choroid fissure) between the fornix superiorly and thalamus inferiorly into the body of lateral ventricle on either side. The highly vascular choroid plexuses secrete CSF and are lined by a membrane formed by the fusion of ventricular ependyma with the pia mater of tela choroidea. The choroid plexus of the lateral ventricle extends into the temporal horn. It is noteworthy that the tela choroidea and the choroid plexus do not extend into the frontal horn. The fourth ventricle also possesses its own tela choroidea and choroids plexus, which also extends into the foramina of Magendie and Luschka.

PERSISTENT MIDLINE CSF CAVITIES

During intrauterine life, there are three potential midline cavities related to the cerebral ventricles that regress between the seventh month of intrauterine life and the second year of postnatal life. In adults, if they persist, cavum septum pellucidum (CSP), cavum vergae (CV), and cavum veli interpositi (CVI) occur from anterior to posterior. CSP lies within the two leaflets of septum pellucidum; CV extends further posteriorly and these usually do not communicate with the ventricles or cisterns. CVI is an anterior continuation of quadrigeminal plate cistern.

SELLA AND PITUITARY

The sella is a depression in the basisphenoid bone and contains the pituitary gland and inferior part of its stalk. Its anterior bony wall is called tuberculum sellae and is continuous anterosuperiorly with the anterior clinoid process. Its posterior bony wall is called dorsum sellae and is continuous posterosuperiorly with the posterior clinoid process. The sphenoid sinus lies directly below the sellar floor. The floor has thin bone called lamina dura.

The sella is bounded superiorly by a dural reflection called the diaphragma sellae. Suprasellar cistern above the diaphragma sellae is CSF filled and contains optic nerves/chiasm and upper part of infundibular stalk. The optic chiasm lies in the bony groove that leads to optic canal on each side, called sulcus chiasmaticus, anterior to tuberculum sellae. The hypothalamus and anterior third ventricular recesses lie just above the infundibular stalk. The suprasellar cistern is surrounded by the circle of Willis. The cavernous sinus lies lateral to the sella on either side and contains the cavernous internal carotid artery and sixth cranial nerve within it. The third, fourth, and ophthalmic and maxillary divisions of the fifth cranial nerve lie in the lateral wall of cavernous sinus.

The pituitary gland lies within the sella and has the anterior adenohypophysis and posterior neurohypophysis. The adenohypophysis, which comprises 75% of the pituitary volume appears isointense to gray matter on T1- and T2-weighted images and is composed of three parts—pars tuberalis (part of the infundibular stalk and median eminence of hypothalamus), pars intermedia, which is very small in humans, and pars distalis. which forms most of the intrasellar adenohypophysis. The posterior neurohypophysis appear-hyperintense on T1-weighted images and hypointense on T2-weighted images.

The height of the pituitary gland varies with age and sex. It measures up to 6 mm in children, 8 mm in males and postmenopausal females, 10 mm with upward bulge in young menstruating females, and 12 mm in pregnant or lactating females. The pituitary stalk measures up to 2 mm in maximum thickness near insertion on pituitary inferiorly and 3 to 3.5 mm near median eminence of hypothalamus superiorly. A rough guide to pituitary stalk thickness is that it should not be thicker than the adjacent basilar artery diameter.

SPINE ANATOMY

GENERAL CHARACTERISTICS

There are 33 spinal vertebrae: 7 cervical, 12 thoracic, 5 lumbar, 5 fused sacral, and 4 to 5 coccygeal. A typical vertebra has a body and posterior elements, namely two pedicles, two transverse processes, two laminae (one on each side), and a spinous process from anterior to posterior. Also the posterior elements have, on each side, articular processes consisting of a superior and inferior articular facet and pars interarticularis. The ligaments include the anterior longitudinal ligament, posterior longitudinal ligament, interspinous and supraspinous ligaments, ligamentum flavum, and the craniocervical ligaments namely alar ligament, transverse/cruciate ligaments, and membrane tectoria. The intervertebral disc is composed of inner nucleus pulposus and outer annulus fibrosus and adheres to the fenestrated hyaline cartilage of vertebral endplates. They are avascular except in children and the peripheral annular fibers in adults. The spine may also be divided into three columns for stability assessment—the anterior column consisting of anterior longitudinal ligament and anterior half of vertebral body, disc, and annulus; the middle column consisting of the posterior half of vertebral body, disc, and annulus and posterior longitudinal ligament; and the posterior column consisting of the posterior elements, ligamentum flavum, and inter-/supraspinous interconnecting ligaments.

MR SIGNAL INTENSITIES

In young children, the vertebral body has red marrow, which is isointense to paraspinous muscle on T1-weighted images. The marrow show marked enhancement postgadolinium in those younger than 2 years of age and gradually disappears by around 7 years of age. From 7 years to adolescence, the replacement of hematopoetic red marrow by fatty yellow marrow causes progressive change to hyperintensity on T1-weighted images and relative hypointensity on conventional spin echo T2-weighted images with mixed inhomogeneous signal in between. The intervertebral discs of infants are hyperintense on T2-weighted images except for small central hypointensity of notochord remnants. From the second decade onward, a hypointense band of compact fibrous tissue develops in the centre. In adults, the outer annulus is hypointense on both T1- and T2-weighted images and the inner nucleus pulposus appear hyperintense on T2-weighted images with a low-signal intranuclear cleft. As the disc degenerates, the nucleus pulposus loses its high signal.

VERTEBRAL BODIES

Lumbar: Large, more or less square-shaped vertebral bodies.

Thoracic: Vertebral bodies are slightly wedge-shaped from front to back and gradually increase in size from upper to lower thoracic spine.

Cervical: The typical cervical vertebrae are from C3 to C7 and their bodies gradually increase in size from C3 to C7. They have bilateral posterosuperolateral projections called uncinate processes that form the uncovertebral synovial joints of Luschka with the posterolateral margin of disc/vertebra above. The C2 or axis vertebra has an odontoid process that extends superiorly from its body and articulates anterosuperiorly with the anterior arch of atlas. The C1 or atlas vertebra has no body or spinous process. It has anterior and posterior arches, two lateral masses, and transverse processes. It is a bony ring with oblong or round inferior articular facets that articulate with superior facets of C2 and ellipsoid superior articular facets that articulate with the occipital condyles to form the atlantooccipital joints. The anatomy of the craniocervical junction is described in Chapter 13.

INTERVERTEBRAL DISCS

Lumbar: A normal lumbar disc is slightly concave posteriorly, but appears flat or slightly rounded at L5–S1.

Thoracic: The height of the thoracic discs is less than that of cervical or lumbar discs, but the annulus fibrosus is thicker.

Cervical: The discs are slightly thicker anteriorly than posteriorly.

PEDICLES, LAMINAE, AND SPINOUS PROCESSES

Thoracolumbar spine: The pedicles are thick bony pillars that are directed posterolaterally to join the broad and thick laminae in the thoracolumbar spine. In the lumbar spine, the interpedicular distance widens as we go down the spine, which is reversed in conditions like achondroplasia. The long spinous processes extend posteroinferiorly from the midline where the two laminae fuse.

Cervical spine: The laminae are thin in the cervical spine. The spinous processes are often bifid. C7 has the longest spinous process.

TRANSVERSE PROCESSES

Lumbar spine: Transverse processes project laterally on each side.

Thoracic spine: Transverse processes project superolaterally on each side from the articular pillars between the superior and inferior articular facets. The tip of each transverse process from T1 to T10 has an oval costal facet to form the costotransverse joint with the rib tubercle. Also from T2 to T9, the vertebral demifacets above and below the disc articulate with the rib head to form the costovertebral joint.

Cervical spine: The transverse processes project anteroinferolaterally from the vertebral bodies. The thin bony bar called costotransverse bar connects the anterior and posterior parts of the transverse process creating the transverse foramen for vertebral artery and vein.

ARTICULAR PILLARS AND FACET JOINTS

The articular pillars consist of the pars interarticularis, which is a bony plate that extends posteriorly from the pedicle and the superior and inferior articular facets that it gives rise to. The synovial facet joints are formed by the anteriorly positioned superior articular process of the lower vertebra and the posteriorly positioned inferior articular facet of the lower vertebra. A tough fibrous capsule covers the posterolateral aspect of the joint which is deficient ventrally, where the ligamentum flavum covers the joint.

LIGAMENTS

Anterior longitudinal ligament extends from basiocciput to S1, seen as a hypointense band in direct contact with the anterior surface of vertebral bodies and discs.

Posterior longitudinal ligament is a thinner band that extends from C1 to S1 vertebra and does not adhere to vertebral bodies. Epidural fat and veins are interposed between the posterior longitudinal ligament and vertebral bodies. The posterior longitudinal ligament widens laterally at the intervertebral discs attaching firmly to the annulus fibrosus reinforcing the mid-/ paramedian zones of the disc.

Ligamentum flavum arises from the anterior aspect of the lower margin of the lamina of the upper vertebra and attaches to the posterior surface of the lamina below. On axial MRI, it is seen as a hypointense structure that covers the facet joint anteriorly and sometimes filled with fat posteriorly. It thickens and buckles with degeneration and can become fat infiltrated or calcified.

NEURAL FORAMEN AND LATERAL RECESS

The neural foramen lies between the pedicles of the upper and lower vertebrae with the anterior margin formed by the vertebral body superiorly and the disc and posterior longitudinal ligament inferiorly. The posterior boundary is formed by the articular facet and ligamentum flavum. The lumbar nerve root exits the fat-filled foramen through the widest superior part of the foramen and on sagittal T1-weighted MRI looks like a bird's head and beak with the bird's eye formed by the dorsal root ganglion directly below the superior pedicle. The lateral recess is the region of the lumbar canal that is bordered laterally by the pedicle, posteriorly by the superior articular facet and ligamentum flavum, and anteriorly by the vertebral body, endplate margin, and disk margin. Measurements of the bone margins of the lateral recess suggest narrowing with possible root compression when the anteroposterior dimension is below 4 mm. It is important to remember that at the lumbar level, central disc protrusion produces compression of the descending lower nerve root and lateral recess/neural foramen compression impinges the exiting upper nerve root. For example, at L5–S1 level, central protrusion compresses S1 nerve root and lateral recess/neural foramen compression impinges on the L5 nerve root.

In the cervical spine, the nerve roots lie in the inferior aspect of the neural foramen just above the inferior pedicle and the dorsal root ganglia lies outside the neural foramen. This is because the nerve roots exit above the pedicles at the cervical level. At the cervical level, central disc protrusion produces compression of a still lower nerve root than that intervertebral level and neural foramen compression impinges the exiting lower nerve root. For example, at C5-6 level, central protrusion compresses C7 nerve root and neural foramen compression impinges on the C6 nerve root. The C5 nerve root is not compressed by a medial or lateral C5-6 compression.

As already stated, the nerve roots exit above the pedicles at the cervical level and so are seen in the lower aspects of the neural foramina. There are only seven cervical vertebrae, but there are eight cervical nerve roots. The C7 nerve root exits above the C7 pedicle and C8 nerve root exits below the C7 pedicle. From this level downward, the entire thoracic and lumbar nerves exit below the corresponding pedicle and so are seen in the upper aspect of the neural foramina. That is, T1 nerve root exits below T1 pedicle and L1 nerve root exits below L1 pedicle and lies within the upper part of neural foramen. (Remember that the neural foramen is bounded superiorly and inferiorly by the pedicles of the upper and lower vertebrae.)

SPINAL CORD AND CAUDA EQUINA

The spinal cord lies within the thecal sac and is anchored to dura by denticulate ligaments. It has a cervical enlargement for brachial plexus at C3-T2 and a lumbar enlargement at T9-12. The cord ends at the diamond-shaped conus medullaris between T12 and L2-3 (L1-2 being most common). A deep cleft called ventral median fissure is seen in anterior midline, a shallow dorsal median sulcus in posterior midline, paired dorsolateral sulci where dorsal nerve roots enter the cord, paired ventrolateral sulci from where the ventral nerve roots emerge from the cord, and the paired dorsal intermediate sulci separating the gracile and cuneate fasciculi.

Unlike the brain, the H-shaped gray matter of the spinal cord is centrally placed with the white matter superficial to it. The gray matter consists of the shorter thicker ventral horn containing multipolar motor neurons and longer narrower dorsal horn receiving sensory axons from dorsal root ganglia throughout the cord and small lateral horns from the T1 to conus medullaris. The white matter is divided into three columns (funiculi) on each side. The ventral funiculi lie between the ventral median fissure medially and the ventrolateral sulci and the lateral funiculi lie between ventrolateral and dorsolateral sulci. Both these funiculi have descending motor and ascending sensory tracts. The dorsal funiculi between the lateral funiculi and dorsal median sulcus contain fibers for position and discriminative touch.

After the spinal cord ends, the lower spinal nerve roots exit the conus medullaris and pass inferiorly within the thecal sac forming the cauda equina. On axial sections, the nerve roots lie with the lower sacral roots dorsally and the lumbar roots more anterolaterally.

SUGGESTED READING

Bartynski WS, Lin L. Lumbar root compression in the lateral recess: MR imaging, conventional myelography, and CT myelography comparison with surgical confirmation. *AJNR Am J Neuroradiol.* 2003;24(3):348-360.

Chen CY, Chen FH, Lee CC, et al. Sonographic characteristics of the cavum velum interpositum. *AJNR Am J Neuroradiol.* 1998; 19:1631-1635.

Dowd CF, Halbach VV, Barnwell SL, et al. Particulate embolization of the anterior choroidal artery in the treatment of cerebral arteriovenous malformations. *AJNR Am J Neuroradiol.* 1991; 12:1055-1061.

Grenier N, Greselle JF, Vital JM, et al. Normal and disrupted lumbar longitudinal ligaments: correlative MR and anatomic study. *Radiology.* 1989;171(1):197-205.

Held P, Nitz W, Seitz J, et al. Comparison of 2D and 3D MRI of the optic and oculomotor nerve anatomy. *Clin Imaging.* 2000; 24:337-343.

Naidich TP, Brightbill TC. Systems for localizing fronto-parietal gyri and sulci on axial CT and MRI. *Int J Neuroradiol.* 1996; 2:313-338.

Tanaka N, Fujimoto Y, An HS, et al. The anatomic relation among the nerve roots, intervertebral foramina, and intervertebral discs of the cervical spine. *Spine.* 2000;25(3):286-291.

Tohgi H, Satoshi T, Abe T, et al. Symptomatic characteristics of parkinsonism and the width of substantia nigra pars compacta on MRI according to ischemic changes in the putamen and cerebral white matter: implications for the diagnosis of vascular parkinsonism. *Eur Neurol.* 2001;46:1-10.

Yousry I, Camelio S, Wiesmann M, et al. Detailed MR anatomy of the cisternal segment of the abducens nerve: Dorello's canal, neurovascular relationships and landmarks. *J Neurosurg.* 1999;91:276-283.

Yousry TA, Schmid UD, Alkadhi H, et al. Localization of the motor hand area to a knob on the precentral gyrus: a new landmark. *Brain.* 1997;120:141-157.

QUESTIONS AND ANSWERS

1. What is the most medially located cranial nerve in the cavernous sinus?
   A. II
   B. III
   C. IV
   D. VI

   ANSWER: D. Sixth (abducens) nerve lies within the cavernous sinus whereas the third, fourth, and sixth and V2 nerves lie in its lateral wall. The ICA lies further medial to the sixth nerve. The second nerve is not closely related to cavernous sinus.

2. What is the blood supply of the anterior hippocampus?
   A. ACA
   B. MCA
   C. PCA
   D. Anterior choroidal

   ANSWER: D. Anterior choroidal arteries supply anterior hippocampus, lower part of posterior limb/subretrolentiform portions of the internal capsule, globus pallidus, and tail of caudate nucleus. The posterior hippocampus is supplied by PCA branches. The corpus striatum (caudate and putamen) and upper parts of anterior limb, genu, and posterior limb of internal capsule are supplied by lenticulostriate branches of MCA.

3. Which of the following best describes the appearance of the pituitary gland on MR imaging?
   A. Typically appears flat or with a mild concave anterosuperior surface
   B. Enhances less than adenoma
   C. Demonstrate early and prominent enhancement
   D. Typically dark on T2-weighted images

   ANSWER: C. After injection, enhancement is promptly noted on T1-weighted images in the anterior pituitary gland, the infundibulum, and the cavernous sinuses. The posterior pituitary is already high intensity on T1-weighted images. Pituitary microadenomas are generally hypointense compared with the normal gland on T1-weighted images and display variable intensity on T2-weighted images. Postcontrast, microadenomas generally appear initially hypointense to the normal gland; in delayed scanning (>20 minutes), the tumor may appear hyperintense. The pituitary gland can have variable appearance depending on sex and age. On noncontrast MR, the anterior pituitary is isointense to brain on T1- and T2-weighted images. The posterior pituitary is high intensity on T1-weighted images and of lower intensity on T2-weighted images.

4. Which one of the following is the motor strip?
   A. Calcarine gyrus
   B. Precentral gyrus
   C. Inferior frontal gyrus
   D. Postcentral gyrus

ANSWER: B. Postcentral gyrus of parietal lobe is sensory cortex, inferior frontal gyrus is Broca motor speech area, and calcarine cortex is primary visual cortex.

5. In a child, where does the conus end?
   A. T12
   B. L2
   C. L3
   D. L4

   ANSWER: B. The normal level of the conus medullaris in a child is L2. If the conus is below the L2/L3 disc interspace, it should be considered abnormal. In an adult, the cord ends above the L1/L2 disc level.

6. What symptoms would a patient have with far lateral disc herniation at L4-5?
   A. L4 radiculopathy
   B. L5 radiculopathy
   C. S1 radiculopathy
   D. No radiculopathy

   ANSWER: A. Above T1, spinal nerves course ABOVE pedicles for which they are named. (e.g., there is a C8 nerve root, but only a C7 vertebral body). Below T1, spinal nerves course below the pedicles for which they are named. Paracentral disk herniation in the lumbar region characteristically strikes the root exiting below the interspace. This is because the disk space is inferior to the exiting root at that level. Thus, an L4-5 disk herniation most often compresses the L5 root. Very lateral herniated disks may compress the upper root; that is, an L3-4 lateral herniation can compress the L3 root; or, in the case of this question, a far lateral L4-5 herniation can compress the L4 root. Larger disks can compress many roots in the thecal sac. Furthermore, disk fragments may migrate superiorly and compress the root exiting at the appropriate interspace. For example, an L3-4 free fragment can compress the L3 root or a combination of the L3 and L4 roots.

7. Which artery supplies the lower aspect of posterior limb of the internal capsule?
   A. Anterior choroidal
   B. Medial lenticulostriate
   C. Lateral lenticulostriate
   D. ACA

   ANSWER: A. Anterior choroidal artery originates from ICA. Cisternal segment: Passes through crural cistern, supplies hippocampus, optic tract, lower aspect of posterior limb, retro/sublentiform parts of internal capsule, globus pallidus, branches to midbrain, and lateral geniculate nucleus. Plexal segment: Supplies choroid plexus of anterior portion of temporal horn of lateral ventricles.

   Lateral lenticulostriate arteries of the MCA supplying basal ganglia structures: Part of head and body of caudate, putamen, lateral aspect of globus pallidus, upper *dorsal and ventrorostral* posterior limb, genu, and anterior limb of the internal capsule.

   Medial lenticulostriate (Heubner) arteries of the ACA: Supplies the caudate head, lower part of anterior limb of internal capsule, and septum pellucidum.

8. Of the following, what is the most echogenic structure in the fetal brain?
   A. Cerebellar vermis
   B. Corpus callosum
   C. Thalamus
   D. Caudate

   ANSWER: A. Cerebellar vermis. Vermis is the most echogenic structure on neonatal head sonogram of the ones listed above, but the glomus of the choroid plexus is the most echogenic structure. Not so echogenic structures are caudate and thalamus. Corpus callosum is a thin echogenic line.

9. What is the cavum veli interpositi?
   A. Anterior continuation of quadrigeminal plate cistern
   B. Posterior continuation of third ventricle
   C. Posterior continuation of cavum vergae
   D. Lies inferior to pineal gland

   ANSWER: A. The persistent fetal CSF cavities namely cavum septum pellucidum (CSP), cavum vergae (CV), and cavum veli interpositi (CVI) occur from anterior to posterior. CSP lies within the two leaflets of septum pellucidum; CV extends further posteriorly and these usually do not communicate with the ventricles or cisterns. CVI is an anterior continuation of quadrigeminal plate cistern and lies above the pineal gland/internal cerebral vein and extends anteriorly below the corpus callosum/fornix.

10. Which of the following regarding the fourth (trochlear) nerve is *true?*
    A. Exits the brainstem dorsally
    B. Passes between the posterior cerebral artery and superior cerebellar artery
    C. Each superior oblique muscle is innervated by contralateral trochlear nucleus.
    D. All of the above

ANSWER: D. The fourth (trochlear) cranial nerve, which is the only cranial nerve that exits the brainstem dorsally, courses posteriorly around the cerebral aqueduct and decussates in the superior medullary velum, crosses over in the quadrigeminal cistern, and winds round the opposite side of the midbrain in the ambient cistern to reach its ventral aspect on the way to enter the contralateral cavernous sinus and orbit to supply the superior oblique muscle. During their course, both the third and fourth cranial nerves pass between the posterior cerebral artery and superior cerebellar artery.

3 DEVELOPMENTAL DISORDERS

Surjith Vattoth and Joseph C. Sullivan III

EMBRYOLOGY

Stage 1 (dorsal induction): formation and closure of the neural tube. This occurs during 3 to 5 weeks of gestation, when the neural plate develops on the dorsal surface of the human embryo (approximately 18 days after fertilization). This invaginates forming the neural folds that later oppose in midline forming the neural tube. The tube closure begins in the medulla proceeding rostrally and caudally. Neurulation occurs in two phases in vertebrate embryos: primary and secondary neurulation. Primary neurulation, the formation of the neural plate and subsequent morphogenetic movements that transform it into a neural tube, forms the brain and trunk level of the spinal cord. Secondary neurulation, the formation of an epithelial cord and its subsequent cavitation to form a neural tube, forms the tail spinal cord. Failure of dorsal induction leads to conditions like anencephaly, iniencephaly, cephalocele, Chiari malformations, and spinal dysraphisms.

Stage 2 (ventral induction): formation of the brain segments and face. This occurs during 5 to 10 weeks of gestation, when three primary vesicles namely prosencephalon, mesencephalon, and rhombencephalon form the forebrain, midbrain, and hindbrain, respectively. The prosencephalon divides into telencephalon (future cerebrum) and diencephalon (future thalamic and hypothalamic regions). The rhombencephalon divides into metencephalon (future pons and cerebellum) and myelencephalon (future medulla). Failure of ventral induction leads to conditions like holoprosencephalies, septooptic dysplasia, Dandy-Walker spectrum, arrhinencephaly, cerebellar dysplasias, Joubert syndrome, rhombencephalosynapsis, tectocerebellar dysplasia, and facial anomalies.

Stage 3 (cortical development): neuronal and glial *proliferation* in the germinal matrix located in the subependymal embryologic layers during 2 to 4 months; neuronal *migration* of developing neurons along the radial glial units to the brain periphery during 3 to 5 months and *organization* of migrated neuronal bundles into the six-layered cortex from 5 months onward. Reduced *proliferation* leads to microcephaly and increased nonneoplastic proliferation leads to conditions such as tuberous sclerosis, balloon cell dysplasia (type II Taylor dysplasia), and hemimegalencephaly, whereas increased neoplastic proliferation leads to a dysembryoplastic neuroepithelial tumor (DNET), ganglioglioma, and gangliocytoma. Abnormal neuronal *migration* causes lissencephalies and heterotopias. Abnormal cortical *organization* leads to conditions such as polymicrogyria (PMG), schizencephaly, and nonballoon cell dysplasia (type I Taylor dysplasia).

In this chapter, we will discuss congenital brain malformations in four sections, namely disorders caused by failure of dorsal induction, ventral induction, cortical development, and miscellaneous/neurocutaneous syndromes.

FAILURE OF DORSAL INDUCTION—NEURAL TUBE CLOSURE DEFECTS AND CHIARI MALFORMATIONS

ANENCEPHALY

Anencephaly results from failure of neural tube closure at the cranial end of the developing embryo. The cerebrum and cerebellum are reduced or absent, but the hindbrain is present. Absence of the brain and calvarium may be partial or complete. Anencephaly leads to fetal loss, stillbirth, or neonatal death and is usually not associated with other malformations. Ultrasound diagnosis can be made as early as 20 weeks gestational age and is associated with polyhydramnios and high alphafetoprotein.

INIENCEPHALY

Iniencephaly is a rare neural defect involving the occiput and inion (external occipital protuberance) with rachischisis of the cervical and thoracic spine and retroflexion of the head. The main features of iniencephaly include a variable deficit of the occipital bones that results in an enlarged foramen magnum, partial or total absence of the cervical and thoracic vertebrae with an irregular fusion of those vertebrae that are present, and this is accompanied by incomplete closure of the vertebral arches and bodies, hyperextension of the malformed cervico-thoracic spine with significant shortening of the spinal column because of marked lordosis and an upward-turned face (star gazing fetus on ultrasound), and the mandibular skin being directly continuous with that of the chest owing to the short neck.

CEPHALOCELES

A herniation of cranial contents through a defect in the skull is termed a cephalocele. When the hernia consists of brain and meninges, it is called a meningoencephalocele; the absence of brain tissue characterizes a meningocele. Cephaloceles can be classified according to their location as occipital (between lambda and foramen magnum), parietal (between bregma and lambda), sincipital (at junction of frontal and ethmoidal bones), and basal (at junction of sphenoid and ethmoid bones). Sincipital cephaloceles can be further classified as nasofrontal, nasoethmoidal, and nasoorbital. Basal cephaloceles are subdivided into transethmoidal, sphenoethmoidal, sphenoorbital, sphenomaxillary, and transsphenoidal. An atretic cephalocele or meningocele manque, regarded as forme fruste of meningoencephalocele, is a skin-covered subcutaneous lesion that consists of meningeal, ectopic glial, or other CNS tissues such as anomalous blood vessels and has high incidence in conditions such as Walker-Warburg syndrome.

CHIARI MALFORMATIONS

The German pathologist Hans Chiari described the Chiari malformations I, II, and III in the 1890s based on autopsy studies. The so-called Chiari IV malformation is a form of severe cerebellar hypoplasia and occurs during a later developmental stage. Some authors reserve the term Chiari IV malformation for severe cerebellar hypoplasia associated with Chiari II.

Chiari I is characterized by herniation of the cerebellar tonsils through the foramen magnum into the cervical spinal canal. Herniation of at least one cerebellar tonsil that is 5 mm or more below the foramen magnum or of both tonsils that are 3 to 5 mm below the foramen magnum, accompanied by certain other features like small, crowded posterior fossa with effaced posterior fossa CSF cisterns, syringohydromyelia, pointed or peg-like appearance of the tonsils, and elongated but normally positioned fourth ventricle can point to this condition. As cerebellar tonsils ascend with age, the normal upper limit of tonsillar descent varies as follows: up to 6 mm in those aged 0 to 10 years, 5 mm in 10 to 30 years, 4 mm in 30 to 80 years, and 3 mm in 80 to 90 years. Syringohydromyelia seen in 25% (15%–75% depending on the series quoted) is most commonly observed between the C4–6 levels, even though any cord segment may be involved. Most common associated skeletal anomalies are platybasia, basilar invagination (25%–50%), and posteriorly angled odontoid process (26%) with brainstem compression and scoliosis (42%). Other skeletal anomalies include short clivus, short supraocciput, atlantooccipital assimilation, Klippel-Feil syndrome, incomplete C1 ring ossification, increased cervical lordosis, and thoracic kyphosis.

Chiari II malformation, also known as Arnold Chiari malformation, is a complex anomaly with skull, dural, brain, spinal, and spinal cord manifestations, almost always associated with myelomeningocele usually lumbar. The imaging findings in this condition are numerous and can be classified into four categories as skull and dural changes, brain changes, ventricular changes, and other associated changes. The skull and dural changes include lacunar skull or lückenschädel (areas of focal calvarial thinning and scooped out appearance that are most prominent near the vertex or torcular herophili, disappearing after 6 months of age), concave posterior aspects of a short clivus and petrous ridges, small posterior fossa and a large, round, gaping foramen magnum, low-lying transverse sinuses and torcular herophili, fenestrated falx with interdigitated cerebral gyri of two sides, hypoplastic tentorium attaching to the occipital bone far caudally just above the foramen magnum, and a heart-shaped tentorial incisura. The brain changes include inferiorly displaced cerebellar vermis through the foramen magnum, medullary spur and kinking inferiorly lying dorsal to the spinal cord, towering cerebellum projecting above the widened tentorial incisura, wrapping of the cerebellum around the brainstem anteriorly and laterally, beaking and inferior displacement of the tectal plate with variable degrees of fusion of the colliculi, and a prominent massa intermedia (interthalamic adhesion). The ventricular changes include a fourth ventricle that is elongated craniocaudally and narrowed in other dimensions, frequently enlarged third ventricle, obliterated posterior fossa cisterns, colpocephaly (enlarged occipital horns and atria of lateral ventricles because of maldeveloped occipital lobes), and anteroinferiorly pointed frontal horns. Hydrocephalus occurs in more than 90%. It is important to understand that the fourth ventricle is normally a thin vertical slit in Chiari

II malformation. A normal appearing or enlarged fourth ventricle in these patients suggests a shunt malfunction or an isolated fourth ventricle that needs CSF diversion. Most frequent associated anomalies include myelomeningocele (88%–100%), corpus callosal dysgenesis (80%–90%), syringohydromyelia (50%–90%), aqueductal stenosis (70%), contracted, narrow gyri or stenogyria (50%), and absent septum pellucidum (40%). Other rarer associated anomalies include heterotopias, diastematomyelia, low-lying tethered cord, and incomplete C1 arch.

Chiari III malformations have high cervical/low occipital encephaloceles that contain cerebellum or occipital lobes and other Chiari II features to a variable extent. They can be considered as Chiari II plus encephalocele.

SPINAL DYSRAPHISMS

Spinal dysraphism occurs in the first 8.5 weeks of fetal life. The neural tube develops from ectodermal cells, while mesoderm forms the bony elements, meninges, and muscle. The skin is separated from the neural tube by the mesoderm. Incomplete separation of ectoderm from the neural tube results in cord tethering, diastematomyelia, or a dermal sinus. Premature separation of the cutaneous ectoderm from the neural tube results in incorporation of mesenchymal elements between the neural tube and skin, which may result in the development of lipomas. If the neural tube fails to fuse in the midline posterior spinal abnormalities such as myelomeningoceles occur. Spina bifida can be divided into two categories, namely spina bifida cystica or aperta and spina bifida occulta.

The subtypes of spina bifida cystica are myelomeningocele, meningocele, rachischisis, lipomyelomeningocele, lipomeningocele, and terminal myelocystocele. *Myelomeningocele* is a condition in which the spinal cord and nerve roots herniate through the bony and musculocutaneous defect into a sac comprising the meninges. The spinal cord often ends in this sac in which it is splayed open, exposing the central canal. It is associated with conditions such as hydrocephalus and Chiari II malformation, intestinal, cardiac, and esophageal malformations, renal and urogenital anomalies. A *meningocele* is simply herniation of the meninges through the bony defect. The spinal cord and nerve roots do not herniate into this closed dorsal dural sac. It does not have associated neurologic malformations such as hydrocephalus or Chiari II. Rachischisis is the most severe form of spina bifida aperta and involves a widely patent dorsal opening of the spine with or without residual cord tissue. *Rachischisis* is usually associated with anencephaly. Lipomyelomeningocele or *lipomeningocele* has a lipomatous mass that herniates through the bony defect and attaches to the spinal cord, tethering the cord and often the associated nerve roots. The *lipomyelomeningocele* can envelop both dorsal and ventral nerve roots, only the dorsal nerve roots, or simply the filum terminale and conus medullaris. These lesions do not have associated hydrocephalus but have a more guarded prognosis than simple meningoceles with higher retethering rates following surgery. In *terminal myelocystocele*, the spinal cord has a large terminal cystic dilatation resulting from hydromyelia. The posterior wall of the spinal cord often is attached to the skin, giving rise to a large terminal skin-covered sac. The vast majority of the lesions are dorsal, the most common ventral variant being an anterior sacral meningocele. Posterior meningoceles, lipomyelomeningoceles, and myelocystocele are closed defects and may occur with a skin-covered back mass.

Spina bifida occulta does not have the meninges herniating through the bony defect and is covered by skin. They do not have associated hydrocephalus or Chiari II malformations. Frequently, a skin lesion such as a hairy patch, dermal sinus tract, dimple, hemangioma, or lipoma points to the underlying spina bifida and neurologic abnormality present in the thoracic, lumbar, or sacral region. Presence of these cutaneous stigmata above the gluteal fold signifies the presence of an occult spinal lesion. Dimples below the gluteal fold signify a benign, nonneurologic finding such as a pilonidal sinus.

A *dorsal dermal sinus* is a long, thin, epithelium-lined sinus that extends from the skin surface for a variable distance. This sinus may become symptomatic because of an infection if it has a connection within the thecal sac or compression of neural tissue if associated with a dermoid/epidermoid. An *intradural lipoma* has no anatomic connection with the subcutaneous fat and lies wholly within the dural space. This is similar to a lipomyelomeningocele except that the neural tube closes after the mesenchyme has entered.

A *split notochord* results from abnormal splitting of the notochord, which is usually associated with a persistent tract between the gut and the dorsal skin. The intervening tract may become obliterated at any point to create an enteric cyst, diverticulum, fistula, sinus, *neurenteric cyst*, or enteric duplication cyst.

Diastematomyelia refers to a complete or partial clefting of the spinal cord in a sagittal plane into two symmetric or asymmetric hemicords. The cord usually reunites more distally. Each of the hemicords has its own central canal and dorsal and ventral nerve roots. They are divided into two types: In type A (50%–60%), the hemicords are contained within a single dural and arachnoid lining without a dividing spur. In type B, each hemicord has its own dural and arachnoid sac with a spur or septum separating the two. The septum may be bony, cartilaginous, or fibrous. The most common site for this anomaly is the thoracolumbar region. Associated cutaneous stigmata at the site of the anomaly, cord tethering, and syringohydromyelia are common and therefore must be looked for in diastematomyelia. Whenever the conus lies below the L2-3 interspace in an infant, cord tethering should be considered. The term *tethered cord* implies that the cord may be attached to vertebral column or subcutaneous tissues by a thickened filum terminale, fibrous band, dermal sinus tract, diastematomyelia, or a lipoma (lipomyelomeningocele).

FAILURE OF VENTRAL INDUCTION—HOLOPROSENCEPHALIES AND POSTERIOR FOSSA MALFORMATIONS OTHER THAN CHIARI

HOLOPROSENCEPHALY

Holoprosencephaly (HPE) is a failure of ventral induction of the brain in which the developing forebrain (prosencephalon) fails to divide into two separate hemispheres and ventricles. They are classified into alobar, semilobar, and lobar subtypes. Midline facial malformations occur in most cases, which are correlated with the degree of HPE and vary from alobar to lobar as cyclopia (single, midline, fused eye beneath a proboscis), ethmocephaly (ocular hypotelorism with a proboscis), cebocephaly (ocular hypotelorism with a single nostril), ocular hypotelorism and midline clefting, or milder facial dysmorphic features. Also, there is a middle interhemispheric variant of HPE, which is associated with solitary median maxillary incisor tooth, prominent vomerine ridge in midpalate, and overgrowth of nasal process of maxilla producing nasal pyriform aperture stenosis.

Alobar HPE is the most severe form in which there is a single ventricle and no separation of the cerebral hemispheres. The interhemispheric fissure, falx cerebri, corpus callosum, septum pellucidum, and fornix are absent. The thalami and basal ganglia are fused.

Semilobar HPE has fused left and right frontal and parietal lobes and the interhemispheric fissure is only present posteriorly. A rudimentary falx may be present, and a primitive occipital horn may develop.

Lobar HPE is the mildest form, in which most of the right and left cerebral hemispheres and lateral ventricles are separated but the most rostral aspect of the telencephalon, the frontal lobes, are fused, especially anteroinferiorly. Sometimes, lobar HPE is limited to an absence of the septum pellucidum.

Septooptic dysplasia or De Morsier syndrome is the mildest form of lobar HPE in which there is no septum pellucidum and the optic nerves are very atrophic. Schizencephaly may be present in 50% of these cases. Corpus callosum agenesis may also be seen with this entity. They typically present with symptoms of hypothalamic–pituitary dysfunction.

Middle interhemispheric fusion variant (syntelencephaly) of HPE is a condition in which there is fusion of the posterior frontal and parietal lobes/sylvian fissures across the midline and absence of the body of the corpus callosum but presence of the genu and splenium of the corpus callosum. There is incomplete thalamic separation in one-third cases, but the hypothalamus and basal ganglia are usually separated.

ARRHINENCEPHALY

Arrhinencephaly is a condition where there is absence of the olfactory bulbs and tracts. Coronal MRI shows the olfactory sulci, but no olfactory bulbs or tracts. Most cases of HPE are associated with absent olfactory bulbs and tracts. Olfactory aplasia also occurs in Kallmann syndrome, which includes anosmia, hypogonadism, and mental retardation.

DANDY-WALKER SPECTRUM

The Dandy-Walker spectrum classically consists of Dandy-Walker malformation (DWM), Dandy-Walker variant, megacisterna magna. Dandy-Walker malformation is characterized by an enlarged posterior fossa, a high tentorial insertion (lambdoid–torcular inversion) with upward displacement of the transverse sinuses. The floor (anterior part) of the fourth ventricle is present, but the ventricle opens dorsally into a large posterior fossa cyst. There is generalized obstructive hydrocephalus in approximately 80% and colpocephaly (dilated occipital horns of lateral ventricles) if there is associated corpus callosal agenesis, which is seen in 20% to 25% cases. The hydrocephalus is not present at birth and frequently does not become evident until after the neonatal period. There is variable cerebellar vermian/hemispheric aplasia or hypoplasia with the cerebellar remnant everted anterosuperiorly above the cyst. In more severe case, the cerebellar hemispheres can appear winged outward and displaced anterolaterally against the petrous temporal bone. The brainstem may be hypoplastic or compressed. There can be other associated CNS anomalies in up to 70% cases including callosal agenesis, heterotopia, PMG, schizencephaly, and cephaloceles. In the absence of other associated anomalies, these children can have normal intelligence and lead normal lives if the hydrocephalus is controlled. Also the integrity of normal cerebellar vermian fissures and lobes is important in predicting outcome.

In Dandy-Walker variant, the posterior fossa is characteristically normal in size. There is mild inferior vermian hypoplasia with open communication of the posteroinferior fourth ventricle and cisterna magna through an enlarged vallecula (vallecula is the normal space in between the two cerebellar hemispheres beneath the vermis), producing a keyhole deformity. Some authors prefer to avoid using the term Dandy-Walker variant and describe it as a part of Dandy-Walker spectrum.

Megacisterna magna has a large posterior fossa with normal vermis and fourth ventricle. The cistern is crossed by falx cerebelli and tiny veins. Enlarged cisterna magna communicates freely with fourth ventricle and basal subarachnoid spaces.

Fourth ventriculocele variant of Dandy-Walker malformation is a condition in which the large cyst erodes occipital bone with the encysted fourth ventricle herniating into the occipital encephalocele.

Persistent Blake pouch cyst is a condition in which the inferior aspect of the fourth ventricle herniates through the foramen of Magendie into the vallecula and retrovermian cistern. The persistent Blake pouch cyst also freely communicates with fourth ventricle, but inferiorly under the vermis. The differentiating feature is that the vermis is normal in appearance even though rotated. Also, the basal cisterns are compressed posteriorly or effaced.

Posterior fossa arachnoid cysts are considered a separate entity. The cerebellar vermis is normal in this condition. It can produce scalloping of adjacent calvarium as does the megacisterna magna and also cause mass effect on the adjacent structures when large. It has closed fourth ventricle, not communicating freely with the cyst. The major imaging differentiation on MRI or contrast-enhanced CT scan is that the arachnoid cyst is not traversed by falx cerebelli or tiny veins, whereas the megacisterna magna can be traversed by these structures. True retrocerebellar arachnoid cysts displace the fourth ventricle and cerebellum anteriorly and show significant mass effect. Following instillation of intrathecal contrast in the lumbar subarachnoid space, the megacisterna magna will be readily opacified, whereas the arachnoid cyst will not opacify immediately (even though delayed opacification can occur by diffusion across the cyst membrane).

JOUBERT SYNDROME

In 1969, a French neurologist, Marie Joubert, reported a series of five cases of children with mental retardation, episodes of abnormally deep and rapid breathing, abnormal eye movements, and ataxia, which were associated with agenesis of the cerebellar vermis. The primary imaging features of Joubert syndrome are absence of the vermis, thickening and reorientation of the superior cerebellar peduncles, and fourth ventricle deformity. The molar tooth sign in axial images, which is considered pathagnomonic of this condition, is caused by a lack of normal decussation of superior cerebellar peduncular fiber tracts. A lack of decussation leads to enlargement of the peduncles. Also, the peduncles follow a more horizontal course as they extend perpendicularly to the brainstem between the midbrain and the cerebellum. The absence of crossing fibers is responsible for the decreased anteroposterior diameter of the midbrain and also causes the interpeduncular cistern to be deeper than that in the normal brain. The absence of a normal vermis creates a midline cleft (buttocks sign) between the two normal-appearing cerebellar hemispheres. The fourth ventricle shows a "batwing" appearance at the level of upper pons and a triangular shape at the level of midbrain.

RHOMBENCEPHALOSYNAPSIS

Rhombencephalosynapsis was first described by Obersteiner in 1914 and the first case diagnosed by MRI was reported in 1991. It is characterized by the absence or hypogenesis of the vermis and the midline fusion of the cerebellar hemispheres into a single mass. Unlike other vermian maldevelopment syndromes (such as Dandy-Walker complex, Joubert syndrome, or tectocerebellar dysraphia), there is no disconnection of the cerebellar hemispheres, rather they continue seamlessly through the midline. The most distinctive feature is agenesis or poor differentiation of the vermis, the rostral portion being the most severely affected, while the caudal vermis is better formed, usually with a well-developed flocculonodulus. Cerebellar hemispheres appear midline fused, with no intervening cyst; folia and fissures are transversely oriented (single-lobed cerebellum). Diagnosis is best made by axial images demonstrating the fused hemispheres, while coronal images show horizontal folial orientation. Superior and middle cerebellar peduncles may be fused as well as the dentate nuclei and the inferior colliculi, leading to a characteristic diamond-shaped fourth ventricle (narrowed and posteriorly pointing); however, this finding is not so constant. Olivary nuclei may be hypoplastic or absent. Hydrocephalus is the most frequently found supratentorial anomaly and may be associated with aqueductal stenosis. Other supratentorial findings include fused thalami, fornices and cerebral peduncles, absence of the septum pellucidum, dysgenesis of the limbic system, cortical malformations, and multiple suture synostoses.

Partial rhombencephalosynapsis is a still rarer entity with only two cases reported that involved the inferior (posterior) cerebellum and one that involved the superior (anterior) cerebellum.

TECTOCEREBELLAR DYSRAPHIA

The extremely rare tectocerebellar dysraphia consists of vermian hypoplasia or aplasia, occipital cephalocele, and dorsal traction of the tectal plate of midbrain, such that the hypoplastic cerebellar hemispheres are rotated around the brain stem to lie ventrolaterally to it.

MALFORMATIONS OF CORTICAL DEVELOPMENT

The malformations of cortical development can be further subdivided into three sections, namely malformations caused by neuronal and glial *proliferation,* neuronal *migration*, and *organization.*

MALFORMATIONS CAUSED BY ABNORMAL NEURONAL AND GLIAL *PROLIFERATION*

Reduced *proliferation* leads to microcephaly. The craniofacial ratio is reduced, the normal being 5:1 in premature infants, 4:1 in term infants, 3:1 at 2 years, 2.5:1 at 3 years, 2:1 at 12 years, and 1.5:1 in an adult. Primary or genetic microcephaly may have a small but grossly normal brain with gyral simplification or may be associated with cerebellar hypoplasia, pachygyria, lissencephaly, HPE, or hypomyelination. Secondary (nongenetic) microcephaly results from noxious agents that affect the fetal or infant brain growth like hypoxic ischemic encephalopathy, TORCH infection (Table 100-1), fetal alcohol syndrome, and nonaccidental head injury.

Increased nonneoplastic *proliferation* leads to conditions like tuberous sclerosis, balloon cell focal cortical dysplasia (type II Taylor dysplasia), and hemimegalencephaly. Pathologically, all these three have balloon cell proliferation. Balloon cells are giant progenitor cells that have characteristics of both neurons and astrocytes. Balloon cell anomalies typically have high signal intensity on long TR images. MR imaging features of balloon cell focal cortical dysplasia of Taylor include cortical thickening, homogeneous high signal intensity in the subcortical white matter, and abnormal signal intensity that extends to the ventricle and usually has a frontal lobe location. Hemimegalencephaly is a disorder with lobar or hemispheric enlargement associated with ipsilateral ventriculomegaly, white matter signal intensity changes, heterotopia, and cortical thickening. In cases with dissimilar size of two halves of the brain, it is important to see whether the smaller side or larger side has ventriculomegaly. If the smaller side has ventriculomegaly, it is hemiatrophy of that side whereas if the larger side has ventriculomegaly, then the size discrepancy is because of hemimegalencephaly of that side. Transmantle dysplasia is defined as any disorder with gray matter extending from the ventricular surface to the cortex.

Increased neoplastic *proliferation* leads to dysembryoplastic neuroepithelial tumor, ganglioglioma, and gangliocytoma. Dysembryoplastic neuroepithelial tumor (DNET) has abnormal proliferation of all three cell lines: neuronal, oligodendroglial, and astrocytic. It is a slow-growing benign neoplasm that is occasionally cystic and superficially located mainly in temporal lobe and often involves amygdalla and hippocampus. These are well-demarcated, wedge-shaped, multicystic, bubbly intracortical masses that scallop the inner table of skull and point toward the ventricle. Calcification can be seen in one-fourth cases and faint focal punctuate or ringlike enhancement in one-fifth. These almost always present with partial complex seizure disorders and with no focal neurologic deficit. Histologically, the lesion shows glioneuronal elements, a nodular component, or an association with cortical dysplasia. Gangliogliomas are partially cystic, cortical-based tumors that have a higher incidence of calcification and enhancement (approximately half the cases) than ganglioglioma. Temporal lobe is the most common location, followed by parietal and frontal lobes. They can occur as a circumscribed cyst with mural nodule, a solid tumor that often thickens and expands the gyri or rarely as an infiltrating poorly defined mass.

MALFORMATIONS CAUSED BY ABNORMAL *MIGRATION*

Abnormal neuronal *migration* causes lissencephalies and heterotopias. Arrest of migration leads to classical type 1 lissencephaly (agyria–pachygyria complex). It is usually associated with chromosome 17-LIS 1 gene mutation or X-linked DCX mutations in boys. Mothers with boys with X-linked lissencephaly who have the X-linked DCX mutation may develop the band heterotopia (double cortex) syndrome. Lissencephaly (smooth brain) or agyria pachygyria complex are terms used to denote brain with absent or reduced sulcation. Complete lissencephaly having a figure of eight or hourglass brain configuration because of smooth brain and shallow sylvian fissure is synonymous with agyria, whereas incomplete lissencephaly is synonymous with agyria–pachygyria. They are characterized by arrested neuronal migration, pachygyric (thick), four-layered cortex (instead of normal six layer), and smooth brain surface. There can be a cell-sparse white matter layer within the thick abnormal cortex which will be seen as hyperintense line outlined on both sides by lower signal intensity cortex in long TR images and this should not be mistaken for double cortex of band heterotopia. Lissencephaly is found in association with facial anomalies in Miller-Dieker syndrome or as an isolated finding in X-linked lissencephaly. Miller-Dieker syndrome can also have characteristic small midline septal calcification. The brain anomalies because of LIS1 mutation are more severe over the parietooccipital region whereas that owing to X-linked DCX mutation is more severe over the subfrontal and temporal regions. Band heterotopia seen in mothers of boys with X-linked lissencephaly shows symmetric subcortical gray matter ribbons embedded in white matter that parallels the cortex. In this case, the white matter, which separates the cortices, will have normal hypointensity in long TR images. Lissencephaly can also occur secondary to intrauterine cytomegalovirus infection in which case it is associated with periventricular and subcortical white matter calcifications. CMV-related lissencephaly usually does not have a thick cortex and the cortex is often polymicrogyric.

Overmigration results in cobblestone lissencephalies (type 2 lissencephaly). They are usually associated with congenital muscular dystrophy (CMD) subtypes 2, 3, and 4. These hypotonic infants have an abnormal Z-shaped brainstem on sagittal MRI images, which serve as an important diagnostic clue. CMDs comprise a heterogeneous group of autosomal recessive disorders of infancy. The CMDs are classified into four distinctive groups depending on MR imaging, namely CMD1 (merosin positive or negative), CMD2 (Fukuyama CMD), CMD3 (Muscle-eye-brain disease), and CMD4 (Walker-Warburg syndrome). Merosin-positive CMD1 cases have been described to show normal MRI or mild, nonspecific, periventricular white matter changes, cerebellar hypoplasia, or focal PMG. Merosin-negative CMD1 is known to cause bilateral white matter changes. In Fukuyama CMD (CMD2), diffuse central cerebral hypomyelination, cerebellar PMG with or without cysts, frontal PMG, variable degrees of pontine and cerebellar vermian hypoplasia, and occipital cobblestone cortex have been described. In this condition, PMG is seen primarily in frontal lobes and cobblestone lissencephaly is more prominent in occipital regions. Muscle-eye-brain disease (CMD3) is characterised by pachygyria with cobblestone cortex, midline defect, and hypoplastic pons and white matter changes in patients with muscle-eye-brain disease (CMD3). Patients with Walker-Warburg syndrome (CMD4) have diffuse cerebral cobblestone cortex, hydrocephalus, posterior cephaloceles, severe congenital eye malformations, absence of cerebral and cerebellar myelin, cerebellar PMG with or without cysts, pontine and cerebellar vermian hypoplasia, and variable callosal hypogenesis.

Other lissencephlay variants include X-linked lissencephaly with callosal agenesis and abnormal genitalia (XLAG) because of ARX gene mutation showing posterior agyria and anterior pachygyria. Females with this condition have callosal agenesis. Another lissencephalic variant is that secondary to reelin gene mutation in chromosome 7q22 and is called the Norman Roberts type of lissencephaly. No cell-sparse zone is seen in the thickened cortex. The brainstem and cerebellum are extremely small and hippocampus is incompletely rotated.

Gray matter heterotopia is another major group of migrational anomaly. They can be subependymal, subcortical, and band heterotopias and follow gray matter signal intensity in all MRI sequences. Subependymal nodular heterotopia is the most common subtype and produces a wavy outline of lateral ventricles. Differential diagnosis of the wavy outline of lateral ventricles includes the subependymal tubers of tuberous sclerosis (which have different signal intensity compared to gray matter), posthypoxic white matter loss producing wavy ventricular outline in periventricular leukomalacia, and the extremely rare subependymal metastasis. Subcortical heterotopia may have a thinned and dysplastic overlying cortex if the heterotopia is large. Band heterotopia has already been described along with lissencephaly.

MALFORMATIONS CAUSED BY ABNORMAL *CORTICAL ORGANIZATION*

Abnormal cortical *organization* leads to conditions like PMG, schizencephaly, and nonballoon cell dysplasia (type I Taylor dysplasia). PMG is a malformation of cortical development characterized by excessive small and prominent convolutions separated by shallow sulci, giving the cortical surface and cortical–white matter junction an irregular appearance. T2-weighted images of patients with PMG reveal two different cortical patterns; one in infants younger than 1 year showing a small, fine, and undulating appearance with normal cortical thickness (3–4 mm), and another pattern in children older than 18 months showing a thick and bumpy cortical appearance (5–8 mm). Pattern 1 seems to evolve into pattern 2 as the brain undergoes myelination. PMG can be associated with clefts and abnormal veins. The cleft (pial–ependymal seam) of schizencephaly is lined by polymicrogyric cortex. Intrauterine cytomegalovirus infection can cause lissencephaly, periventricular and subcortical calcifications, and PMG. Bilateral perisylvian PMG can be seen in Foix-Chavany-Marie syndrome (congenital bilateral perisylvian syndrome) and Zellweger syndrome.

Schizencephaly or split brain is divided into two types, namely closed-lip schizencephaly in which the cleft walls are in apposition and the more common open-lip schizencephaly in which the cleft walls are separated. The clefts can be located anywhere, but they commonly occur in the perisylvian regions and can be unilateral or bilateral, symmetric or asymmetric. Closed-lip schizencephaly can be identified by looking for the small nipple projecting from ventricle. The clefts are lined by heterotopic/pachy/polymicrogyric gray matter and extend from the pial surface to the ependyma of the lateral ventricle (pial–ependymal seam). The arachnoid membrane covering the cleft can be ruptured easily and hydrocephalus is seen especially in open-lip schizencephaly with ruptured membrane. Large primitive veins may be seen overlying the cleft. The septum pellucidum is absent in 80% to 90% of patients, and schizencephaly may coexist with septooptic dysplasia. In contrast to schizencephaly, the cleft of porencephaly caused by trauma or vascular insult is lined by gliotic white matter in MRI images and not dysplastic gray matter.

Non balloon cell cortical dysplasia (type I Taylor) is seen as a focal thickened area of cortex without underlying white matter changes (as compared to balloon cell type II dysplasia). A focal prominent convexity subarachnoid space overlying the focal area of thickened cortex can sometimes serve as an important diagnostic clue in MRI.

At this point, it would be interesting to review the differences between PMG, cobblestone cortex, and pachygyria in thin section high-resolution MR images. PMG is seen as irregularity of both the outer cortical surface as well as the inner cortical-white matter junction. Cobblestone cortex has a smooth outer cortical surface and an irregular inner cortical-white matter junction. In pachygyria (thick cortex), both the outer and inner margins are smooth, and in some cases, a layer of white matter can be detected in the cell-sparse zone within it.

MISCELLANEOUS/NEUROCUTANEOUS SYNDROMES

AGENESIS OF CORPUS CALLOSUM

The corpus callosum develops from the lamina reuniens in the telencephalon; it begins to appear between the anterior and hippocampal commissures at about 10.5 weeks and the adult form is achieved by 17 weeks gestational age. It begins in the genu and the body, progressing posteriorly, but myelinates from posterior to anterior. The anteriormost rostrum is also formed last. Therefore in partial callosal agenesis, the splenium and rostrum are usually absent. In contrast, in the middle interhemispheric variant of HPE, only the body of the corpus callosum is absent.

When the corpus callosum is absent, the third ventricle is often high riding, extending superiorly in between the lateral ventricles. On coronal imaging, a "viking helmet" or "bull's horn," "moose head," or "candelabra" appearance is seen. Probst bundles are longitudinal bundles of white matter seen medial to the lateral ventricles and represent nondecussated callosal fibers. Instead of crossing in the midline, these fibers deviate at the interhemispheric fissure to run along the medial borders of the lateral ventricles from the frontal paraolfactory cortex to the occipital region. Probst bundles are best seen on coronal or axial T1-weighted MRI and appear more slightly T1 hyperintense and T2 hypointense than other white matter. The occipital horns of the lateral ventricles are dilated (colpocephaly) and the frontal horns appear parallel on axial imaging. When the corpus callosum is absent, the cingulate sulcus is absent, and the medial cerebral sulci and gyri radiate toward the midline in a radial configuration. The hippocampal formations are frequently hypoplastic in patients with agenesis of corpus callosum, with resulting mild dilatation of the temporal horns.

The midline cysts associated with callosal agenesis may be a dilated third ventricle or a true arachnoid cyst. At autopsy, the lining of the cyst may contain ependymal or arachnoid cells. On MRI, the cyst may have a high protein content; in these cases, the signal intensity on T1-weighted images is greater than that of CSF. Barkovich et al. have classified these cysts into various subtypes. Type 1 cysts appear to be an extension or diverticulation of the third or lateral ventricles, whereas Type 2 cysts are loculated and do not communicate with the ventricular system. Type 1a cysts are associated with presumed communicating hydrocephalus but no other cerebral malformations. Type 1b cysts are associated with hydrocephalus secondary to diencephalic malformations prohibiting egress of CSF from the third ventricle into the aqueduct of Sylvius. Type 1c are associated with small head size and apparent cerebral hemispheric dysplasia or hypoplasia. Type 2a (multiloculated cysts) are associated with no abnormalities other than callosal agenesis/hypogenesis. Type 2b cysts are associated with deficiencies of the falx cerebri, subependymal heterotopia, and PMG and are almost all in patients diagnosed with Aicardi syndrome. Type 2c cysts are associated with subcortical heterotopia. Type 2d cysts consist of interhemispheric arachnoid cysts. Other than those with Type 2b cysts, gender predominance was overwhelmingly male. In complex types of multilocular interhemispheric cysts associated with callosal agenesis, a CT cystogram or ventriculogram may be obtained after iohexol is introduced into the cyst to establish which of the CSF collections communicate with each other or with the ventricular system.

Agenesis of corpus callosum may be associated with a multitude of other conditions including hydrocephalus, cephaloceles, lissencephaly, schizencephaly, gray matter heterotopias, pachygyria, PMG, Dandy-Walker syndrome, Aicardi syndrome, fetal alcohol syndrome, azygous anterior cerebral artery, trisomy 18, and lipomas. Intracranial lipomas result from lipomatous differentiation of the persistent meninx primitiva, the mesenchymal derivative of the embryonic neural crest, which envelops the developing embryo. Interhemispheric lipomas constitute 40% to 50% of intracranial lipomas and are frequently associated with a dysgenetic corpus callosum. Callosal lipomas are of two types: an anterior bulky tubulonodular variety, which is associated with forebrain and rostral callosal anomalies and a more posterior ribbonlike curvilinear lipoma, which is seen with a normal or nearly normal corpus callosum. CT scan shows findings of callosal agenesis with a fatty-density mass that is variably calcified, and on MR, the lipoma follows fat intensity. Prominent vessels often course directly through the more bulky anterior callosal lipomas and the lipomas show variable calcification.

NEUROFIBROMATOSIS TYPE 1 (VON RECKLINGHAUSEN DISEASE)

NF1 is an autosomal dominant phakomatosis with the gene locus on chromosome 17q11.2. NF1 constitutes approximately 90% neurofibromatosis cases. Neurofibromin, the NF gene product, is a tumor suppressor and its inactivation allows cell proliferation and tumor development. The neuroradiological manifestations of NF1 include osseous changes like sphenoid wing dysplasia (producing bare orbit sign in radiographs and causing pulsating exophthalmos because of herniation of temporal lobe with subarachnoid space into orbit), absence of the orbital floor, enlarged orbits, enlargement of cranial foramina, enlargement of orbital margins, sclerosis in the vicinity of the optic foramen because of optic nerve sheath meningioma, dural calcification especially at the vertex, and calvarial defects adjacent to the lambdoid suture. Macrocephaly can occur because of hydrocephalus or increased white matter volume.

Brain abnormalities include foci of abnormal signal intensity, hyperintense on T2-weighted images in the brainstem, cerebellar white matter, globus pallidus, and splenium of corpus callosum. These lesions are isointense on T1-weighted images and usually have no mass effect or edema. These are regions of myelin vacuolization and areas of separation of the layers of myelin as they spiral around the axon. The oligodendrocyte myelin glycoprotein gene is imbedded within the NF1 gene and neurofibromin is required for Schwann cell myelination. The vacuolization may develop in regions where the myelin is inherently dysplastic and the return of normal T2 signal on subsequent examinations later in life may represent myelin repair or remyelination. They become visible between ages 2 and 10 years, then regress by the second decade and are never seen after 20 years of age. If the T2 lesions show enhancement, glioma development should be suspected. Rarely, hyperintensities have been reported in the globus pallidus on T1-weighted images. Optic gliomas are seen in 15% of NF1 cases, and gliomas of other parts of the brain may be seen. Hydrocephalus in NF1 may be because of benign aqueduct stenosis or a glioma of tectum/tegmentum of the mesencephalon. Other intracranial findings include arachnoid cysts, arachnoid pouches, frontobasal meningocele, craniofacial plexiform neurofibromas, vascular intimal proliferation leading to occlusions, moyamoya (puff of smoke) pattern, aneurysms, and AVM.

Spine imaging findings include sharply angled kyphoscoliosis centered at the thoracolumbar junction with the kyphosis more pronounced than the scoliosis, enlargement of the intervertebral foramina and scalloping of the vertebral bodies, lateral thoracic meningocele, cord astrocytoma, and neurofibromas of spinal or peripheral nerves. The target sign showing hyperintensity on T2, with dark collagen centrally is highly suggestive of a peripheral or plexiform neurofibroma on MRI.

NEUROFIBROMATOSIS TYPE 2

The NF2 gene, which functions as a tumor suppressor gene is located in chromosome 22q12 and the gene product is merlin protein. NF2 is also known as MISME denoting multiple inherited schwannomas, meningiomas, and ependymomas. Bilateral eight nerve schwannomas is a definitive diagnostic criterion of NF2. Other definitive criteria include a first-degree relative with NF2 and either a unilateral CN VIII mass or two of the following: neurofibroma, meningioma, glioma, schwannoma, or juvenile posterior subcapsular lenticular opacity. Extensive calcifications of choroid plexus, cortical surfaces, and ventricular lining may be rarely seen.

TUBEROUS SCLEROSIS

Tuberous sclerosis complex has two distinct gene loci, TSC1 at chromosome 9q34.3 that encodes hamartin and TSC2 at chromosome 16p13.3 that encodes tuberin. The CNS manifestations include tubers or hamartomas, which are caused by abnormal neuronal and glial proliferation containing balloon cells. Subependymal nodules are seen in 98% of which about half calcify, the calcifications increase with age. About two-thirds of these lie along the striothalamic groove of lateral ventricles near the caudate nucleus, behind foramen of Monro. Subependymal giant cell astrocytomas occur in 15% cases, the majority of which enhance and are seen at the foramen of Monro region and can cause obstructive hydrocephalus. Cortical or subcortical tubers are seen as pyramidal-shaped gyral expansion. Approximately one-fifth of them have a central depression likened to an eye of potato. White matter hyperintensities on T2 are seen along the radial lines of neuronal migration as bands, wedge-shaped lesions, or cystoid brain degeneration. The tubers have high signal intensity compared to the nonmyelinated white matter on T1-weighted images and low on T2-weighted images in the neonate and young child. In older children and adults, the lesions are iso- to hypointense on T1 and hyperintense on T2-weighted images compared to both gray and white matter. There can be enhancement in 12% of cortical and subependymal tubers. Mild nonspecific ventriculomegaly even in the absence of subependymal giant cell astrocytomas can occur in 25% patients. Retinal phakomas occur in 50%. Other intracranial manifestations include aneurysms and vascular stenoses, bone islands in skull, and periosteal new bone formation.

STURGE-WEBER SYNDROME

Encephalotrigeminal angiomatosis or Sturge-Weber syndrome occurs because of a failure of normal fetal cortical venous development and the imaging features reflect chronic venous ischemia. Trigeminal nerve V1 and V2 distribution cutaneous nevus flammeus is seen in the vast majority of patients. Lack of superficial cortical veins leads to formation of enhancing pial angioma in the subarachnoid space and prominent enhancing medullary or subependymal veins and enlarged choroid plexus of that side. Orbital enhancement can be seen including choroidal angioma, periorbital soft tissues and bone. Later, the pial angiomas get burnt out with reduced enhancement and increasing cortical/subcortical atrophy and calcifications. The gyriform, curvilinear tram track cortical calcifications (not in the pial angioma) are most common in parietal and occipital lobes and are unusual before 2 years of age. It is unilateral in 80% and bilateral in 20%.

VON HIPPEL-LINDAU SYNDROME

Von hippel-lindau syndrome (VHL) gene is located at chromosome 3p25–26 and the CNS manifestations include hemangioblastomas, retinal angiomas, and endolymphatic sac tumors. Hemangioblastomas typically are multiple with half seen in spinal cord, more than one-third in cerebellum, one-tenth in brain stem, and 1% supratentorial in location along optic pathways or cerebral hemispheres. Two-thirds of hemangioblastomas are seen as cysts with an enhancing nodule abutting the pial surface. In one-third cases, they present as solid enhancing tumors. Retinal angiomas cause retinal detachment and vitreous hemorrhages and the VHL patients often present first with visual symptoms. Seven percent of VHL patients will develop endolymphatic sac tumor and if they are bilateral, VHL is present. Endolymphatic sac tumor is seen in CT scans as an aggressive soft-tissue mass that erodes the posterior wall of temporal bone. All of them have central speculated calcifications within the tumor matrix and most of them have a thin rim of calcification along the posterior margin. T1-weighted images shows foci of high signal suggestive of blood along the tumor margin when less than 3 cm in size and within the tumor matrix when larger in size.

HEREDITARY HEMORRHAGIC TELENGECTASIA (HHT OR OSLER-WEBER-RENDU SYNDROME)

The most common intracranial vascular malformation in hereditary hemorrhagic telengectasia (HHT) is AVM. Capillary telenegectasia can occur in scalp, nasopharynx, orbit, and brain. Multiple developmental venous anomalies (venous angiomas) can also occur in the brain. Brain abscess can occur in these patients with pulmonary AVM because of the right-to-left shunt.

LHERMITTE-DUCLOS DISEASE AND COWDEN SYNDROME

Lhermitte-Duclos disease or dysplastic cerebellar gangliocytoma is an uncommon cerebellar dysplasia with cellular disorganization, hypertrophied granular cell neurons, and axonal hypermyelination in the molecular layer of cerebellum. A nonenhancing mass in the posterior fossa with unilateral hemispheric expansion, hypointense on T1-weighted images, and hyperintense on T2-weighted images, with parallel linear striations on the surface of the lesion producing a tiger striped or corduroy appearance, should be considered specific for Lhermitte-Duclos disease in a middle-aged adult. They have no edema, little mass effect, variable calcification, and hydrocephalus and very rare enhancement. More than half of the patients with Lhermitte-Duclos disease have Cowden syndrome, which is a syndrome with multiple hamartomas/neoplasia in breast and thyroid, gastrointestinal polyps, mucocutaneous lesions, genitourinary malignancies, cataracts, macrocephaly, extremely high risk of meningiomas, and Lhermitte-Duclos disease.

NEUROCUTANEOUS MELANOSIS

Neurocutaneous melanosis is characterised by giant or multiple cutaneous melanocytic nevi and benign and malignant melanotic lesions of CNS. The melanocytes within the pia mater are responsible for the development of leptomeningeal melanosis. The dura is generally spared.

Diffuse intracranial leptomeningeal, intraspinal leptomeningeal, ventricular ependymal, and choroid plexus involvement also may occur. The cerebral parenchyma may be primarily or secondarily involved. Primary involvement may be caused by melanin-containing macrophages and melanocytes. Parenchymal melanosis usually occurs in the amygdalla, pons, basal ganglia, thalami, dentate nuclei, cerebellar hemispheres, and the basal frontal lobes. Secondary involvement of the cerebral parenchyma occurs from spread via the Virchow-Robin spaces; the deep cerebral parenchyma is usually spared. Malignant melanoma is most common in temporal lobes. Leptomeningeal melanosis show normal or diffuse leptomeningeal enhancement malignant melanoma of leptomeninges show diffuse leptomeningeal enhancement. Parenchymal melanosis shows no enhancement, whereas malignant melanoma shows avid often heterogeneous enhancement. They appear hyperintense on T1-weighted images and iso- to hyperdense on CT. Spinal involvement may be seen in as many as 20% of cases. Diffuse leptomeningeal thickening, arachnoiditis, and secondary syringomyelia may be seen.

SUGGESTED READING

Barkovich AJ, Simon EM, Walsh CA. Callosal agenesis with cyst. A better understanding and new classification. *Neurology.* 2001;56:220-227.

Bronen RA, Spencer DD, Fulbright RK. Cerebrospinal fluid cleft with cortical dimple: MR imaging marker for focal cortical dysgenesis. *Radiology.* 2000;214:657-663.

David DJ, Proudman TW. Cephaloceles: Classification, pathology, and management. *World J Surg.* 1989;13:349-357.

Ibrahim Abdulla JK, Vattoth S, Al Tawari AA, et al. Brain MRI features of merosin-negative congenital muscular dystrophy. *Australas Radiol.* 2007;51(Suppl 4):B221-B223.

Küker W, Mayrhofer H, Mader I, et al. Malformations of the midline commissures: MRI findings in different forms of callosal dysgenesis. *Eur Radiol.* 2003;13(3):598-604.

Kuzniecky RI. Magnetic resonance imaging in developmental disorders of the cerebral cortex. *Epilepsia.* 1994;35(6):S44-S56.

McGraw P. The molar tooth sign. *Radiology.* 2003;229:671-672.

McLone DG, Dias MS. The Chiari II malformation: cause and impact. *Childs Nerv Syst.* 2003;19(7-8):540-550.

Takanashi J, Barkovich AJ. The changing MR imaging appearance of polymicrogyria: a consequence of myelination. *AJNR Am J Neuroradiol.* 2003;24:788-793.

Vattoth S, Pandey T, Al Tawari AA, et al. Partial rhombencephalosynapsis of the superior cerebellum associated with GM1gangliosidosis. *J Neuroradiol.* 2007;20:182-185.

QUESTIONS AND ANSWERS

1. What is associated with NF2?
   A. Café au lait spots
   B. Optic gliomas
   C. Meningiomas
   D. None

   ANSWER: C. The diagnostic criteria for NF2 are bilateral eighth cranial nerve masses on CT or MRI or a parent, sibling, or child with NF2 and either a unilateral eight cranial nerve mass or any two of the following: neurofibroma, meningioma, glioma, schwannoma, or juvenile posterior subcapsular lenticular opacity. The mnemonic is "MISME"—multiple inherited schwannomas, meningiomas, and ependymomas.

2. Latex allergy is associated with what disease?
   A. Myelomeningocele
   B. Dandy-Walker malformation
   C. Rhombencephalosynapsis
   D. Neurocutaneous melanosis

   ANSWER: A. It is thought to happen secondary to the repeated surgeries that children with myelomeningocele undergo, with subsequent sensitization to the latex in the gloves.

3. What lines the cleft in schizencephaly?
   A. CSF
   B. Gray matter
   C. White matter
   D. Hamartomatous tissue

   ANSWER: B. The clefts are lined by heterotopic/pachy/polymicrogyric gray matter and extend from the pial surface to the ependyma of the lateral ventricle (pial ependymal seam). Large primitive veins may be seen overlying the cleft. In contrast to schizencephaly, the cleft of porencephaly caused by trauma or vascular insult is lined by gliotic white matter in MRI images and not dysplastic gray matter.

4. Which of the following is *not* a feature of tuberous sclerosis?
   A. Subependymal giant cell astrocytoma
   B. Angiomyolipoma
   C. Sphenoid wing dysplasia
   D. Cardiac rhabdomyomas

   ANSWER: C. Sphenoid wing dysplasia is a feature of NF1, not tuberous sclerosis.

5. MRI shows lobar atrophy, pial enhancement, and enlargement of the choroid plexus. What is the most likely diagnosis?
   A. Sturge-Weber
   B. Tuberous sclerosis
   C. NF2
   D. Osler-Weber-Rendu

   ANSWER: A. In Sturge-Weber syndrome, lack of superficial cortical veins leads to formation of enhancing pial angioma in the subarachnoid space and prominent enhancing medullary or subependymal veins and enlarged choroid plexus of that side. Orbital enhancement can be seen including choroidal angioma, periorbital soft tissues, and bone. Later, the pial angiomas get burnt out with reduced enhancement and increasing cortical/subcortical atrophy and calcifications. The gyriform, curvilinear tram track cortical calcifications (not in the pial angioma) are most common in parietal and occipital lobes and are unusual before 2 years of age. It is unilateral in 80% and bilateral in 20%.

6. Which of the following is most likely associated with a midline facial defect?
   A. Septooptic dysplasia
   B. Holoprosencephaly
   C. Dandy-Walker syndrome
   D. Tuberous sclerosis

   ANSWER: B. Midline defects of the face occur in greater than 80% of cases of holoprosencephaly. Midline facial malformations are correlated with the degree of holoprosencephaly and varies from alobar to lobar as cyclopia (single, midline, fused eye beneath a proboscis), ethmocephaly (ocular hypotelorism with a proboscis), cebocephaly (ocular hypotelorism with a single nostril), ocular hypotelorism and midline clefting, or milder facial dysmorphic features. Also, there is a middle interhemispheric variant of holoprosencephaly, which is associated with solitary median maxillary incisor tooth, prominent vomerine ridge in midpalate, and overgrowth of nasal process of maxilla producing nasal pyriform aperture stenosis.

7. In neurofibromatosis, what is the cause of pulsatile exophthalmos?
   A. Sphenoid wing dysplasia
   B. Enlargement of the optic canal
   C. Carotid cavernous fistula
   D. Buphthalmos

   ANSWER: A. Sphenoid wing hypoplasia is an osseous manifestation of NF1, which leads to temporal lobe herniation into the orbit. The temporal lobe with subarachnoid space herniation into orbit leads to pulsatile exophthalmos.

8. What is a fetus with small cisterna magna most likely to have?
   A. Meningomyelocele
   B. Dandy-walker syndrome
   C. Chiari I
   D. Chiari II

   ANSWER: D. Chiari II has abnormal neurulation that leads to a small posterior fossa, including obliteration of the cisterna magna (cerebellomedullary cistern). Chiari I does not cause a small posterior fossa. Myelomeningoceles do not have an association with small cisterna magna, other than being associated with Chiari II. Dandy-Walker syndrome is associated with an enlarged posterior fossa.

9. Which of the following is *not* associated with renal cysts?
   A. Tuberous sclerosis
   B. Chronic renal dialysis
   C. Von Hippel-Lindau
   D. NF1

   ANSWER: D. Renal cystic disease is associated with Von Hippel-Lindau disease and tuberous sclerosis. Patients on hemodialysis also develop renal cysts. Most renal cysts are simple cysts, seen in more than 50% of the population older than 50 years.

10. A child on MRI examination has abnormal high signal in the cerebellum and basal ganglia on T2-weighted images and an enlarged optic chiasm. What is the most likely diagnosis?
    A. NF2
    B. Tuberous sclerosis
    C. NF1
    D. Septooptic dysplasia

    ANSWER: C. NF1 typically has nonneoplastic hamartomas (80%–90%) that are foci of abnormal signal intensity hyperintense on T2 seen in cerebellar white matter, globus pallidus, and splenium of corpus callosum. These lesions are isointense on T1-weighted images and usually have no mass effect or edema. These are regions of myelin vacuolization, areas of separation of the layers of myelin as they spiral around the axon. The oligodendrocyte myelin glycoprotein gene is imbedded within the NF1 gene and neurofibromin is required for Schwann cell myelination. The vacuolization may develop in regions where the myelin is inherently dysplastic and the return of normal T2 signal on subsequent examinations later in life may represent myelin repair or remyelination. They become visible between ages 2 and 10 years, then regress by the second decade and are never seen after 20 years of age. If the T2 lesions show enhancement, glioma development should be suspected. Rarely, hyperintensities have been reported in the globus pallidus on T1-weighted images. Optic nerve gliomas occur in 15% NF1 patients.

4 CEREBROVASCULAR ANATOMY

Asim K. Bag and Joseph C. Sullivan III

ARTERIES OF ANTERIOR CIRCULATION

INTERNAL CAROTID ARTERY

Neuroradiologists, neurosurgeons, and neurologists now use anatomically correct Bouthillier classification to describe the course of the internal carotid artery. This classification system defines the internal carotid artery (ICA) course using a numerical scale from one to seven in the direction of blood flow. Each segment number identifies the segments of the ICA from its origin to the terminus according to anatomical compartments through which the artery travels, making it very useful clinical communication among clinicians.

Cervical Segment (C1)

The cervical segment of the ICA begins at the level of the common carotid artery bifurcation and ends at the entrance of the carotid canal into the petrous bone, anterior to the jugular foramen. The artery ascends perpendicularly upward encased in the carotid sheath with internal jugular vein and vagus nerve.

Branches

No branches from this segment.

Clinical Significance

Atherosclerotic Disease: The origin of the ICA is a very common location for atherosclerotic disease, the major culprit for the ischemic stroke. Carotid artery atherosclerotic disease is treated currently either by carotid endarterectomy or carotid artery stenting.

Management guideline for carotid stenosis (percent stenosis = 1 − minimal diameter/poststenotic diameter × 100%):

- Low-grade carotid stenosis (stenosis <50% in symptomatic patients and <60% in asymptomatic patients) → medical therapy rather than revascularization.
- Moderate-to severe-carotid stenosis:
  In symptomatic patients with >50% stenosis → carotid endarterectomy plus optimal medical therapy, if the patient has high perioperative risk, stenting is an alternative.
  In asymptomatic patients with >60% stenosis → carotid endarterectomy plus medical management as long as perioperative risk is low.
- Asymptomatic patients with carotid artery stenosis: stenting is not indicated.
- *Dissection*: May be spontaneous (particularly in women and also if the patient has inherent weakness in arterial wall such as in Marfan or Ehlers-Danlos syndromes) or traumatic. This may be asymptomatic. Typical presentation is partial Horner syndrome with ptosis and miosis, followed by symptoms of transient cerebral/retinal ischemia or stroke, most often in the MCA territory.
- The carotid artery may have a very medial course at the level of nasopharynx, where it may approximate the pharyngeal wall. Any instrumentation or biopsy may injure this segment. Also, phrayngeal infection may cause pseudoaneurysm of the ICA at this level.

Petrous Segment (C2)

The segment of the ICA within the carotid canal, called the petrous segment, ends at the posterior edge of the foramen lacerum, inferomedial to the Meckel cave. The petrous ICA runs within the periosteum of the carotid canal and is surrounded by areolar tissue, a venous plexus, and postganglionic sympathetic nerves.

Branches

Caroticotympanic and Mandibulo Vidian arteries.

Clinical Significance

Pathologies in this segment are very rare. Aneurysms may occur here, which can be surprisingly large. Dissections can continue into this segment. Size of the canal can be an indicator of developmental versus more acute pathologies.

LACERUM SEGMENT (C3)

The lacerum segment begins where the carotid canal ends, which is at a vertical line at the posterolateral margin of the exocranial foramen lacerum up to the superior margin of the petrolingual ligament. As in previous compartments, the lacerum segment is surrounded by areolar tissue, a venous plexus, and postganglionic sympathetic nerves.

Branches

Anterior meningeal.

Clinical Significance

This is a very important neurosurgical landmark for exposing Meckel cave through transfacial approach.

CAVERNOUS SEGMENT (C4)

The cavernous segment begins at the superior margin of the petrolingual ligament and ends at the proximal dural ring, formed by the junction of the medial and inferior periosteum of the anterior clinoid process. This segment of the ICA is surrounded by areolar tissue, fat, a venous plexus, and postganglionic sympathetic nerves.

Branches

Meningohypophyseal trunk posteriorly and inferolateral trunk anterolaterally.

Clinical Significance

There is a dangerous communication between the branches from the cavernous segment of ICA and ECA. These arteries may not be visible angiographically, however, utmost care should be taken during ECA branch embolization.

Aneurysms of cavernous carotid account for about 5% of total aneurysm. They are strongly associated with aging and hypertension. Most cavernous aneurysms identified during angiogram are incidental; asymptomatic small lesions usually do not warrant any treatment. When cavernous aneurysms rupture, which is an uncommon event, symptoms related to carotid–cavernous fistula, massive epistaxis, and subdural and much less likely subarachnoid hemorrhage.

More commonly, the cavernous carotid is affected by other sellar and parasellar pathologies that are discussed in a later chapter of this section.

CLINOID SEGMENT (C5)

The clinoid segment begins at the proximal dural ring and ends at the distal dural ring, where the ICA becomes intradural. The clinoid segment is short, coursing obliquely between the anterior clinoid, processing laterally and the carotid sulcus of the basisphenoid medially. This segment is not intracavernous.

Clinical Significance

At the end of this segment, the ICA becomes intradural, and also, this segment is closely related to the optic nerve. Ruptured aneurysms may present with subarachnoid hemorrhage (SAH). If the aneurysm is large and compresses the optic nerve, the patient may present with blindness. Because of the anatomic location, aneurysm of this segment is often surgically challenging.

OPHTHALMIC SEGMENT (C6)

The ophthalmic segment begins at the distal dural ring and ends just proximal to the origin of the posterior communicating artery (PComA). There are two major arterial branches from this segment: the ophthalmic and superior hypophyseal arteries.

Clinical Significance

This is a common site for aneurysm formation.

COMMUNICATING SEGMENT (C7)

The communicating segment begins just proximal to the origin of the PComA and ends at the ICA bifurcation.

Branches

In addition to the PcomA, this segment gives rise to anterior choroidal artery and occasional perforator branches. Anterior choroidal artery arises more distally and more laterally than the PComA. The anterior choroidal artery supplied critical brain structures of diencephalon and mesencephalon. It supplies the uncus, piriform cortex, tail of the caudate nucleus, hippocampus, amygdala, thalamus, lateral geniculate body, optic tract, cerebral peduncles, the subthalamic nucleus, genu, and posterior limb of internal capsule.

Clinical Significance

This is also a very common site for intracranial aneurysm formation. As this segment is closely related with the third cranial nerve, aneurysm may present with third nerve palsy.

The ICA terminates by dividing into anterior (smaller branch) and middle cerebral arteries.

VARIATION OF THE INTERNAL CAROTID ARTERY

- *Fetal origin of PCA:* PCA is supplied only from the ICA through the PComA with absent P1 segment.
- *Persistent trigeminal artery:* This is classified according to the location (medial or lateral) and presence or (Salzman type 2) absence (Salzman type 1) of PComA. Persistent trigeminal artery can increase the risk of intracranial aneurysm formation. The medial variant is

also very important surgically because it may have a transhypophyseal or intrasellar course.

- *Persistent hypoglossal artery:* This is the second most common anomaly. The persistent hypoglossal artery branches from the ICA as a large extracranial branch and passes through the hypoglossal canal. The basilar artery arises from this artery.
- *Persistent stapedial artery:* The stapedial artery is transiently present in normal fetal development, connecting the branches of the future external carotid artery (ECA) to the ICA. Postembryonic persistence of the stapedial artery is rare and presents as a pulsatile middle ear mass or may be found incidentally during middle ear surgery. This is diagnosed by absent foramen spinosum and soft-tissue prominence in the proximal aspect of the tympanic segment of the facial nerve.
- *Proatlantal intersegmental artery:* They are very rare.
- *Aberrant carotid artery:* Normally, tiny caroticotympanic branch of the internal carotid, a remnant of the embryologic hyoid artery, perforates the carotid plate to enter into the tympanic cavity. The inferior tympanic branch of the ascending pharyngeal artery enters the tympanic cavity through the inferior tympanic canaliculus. The aberrant carotid artery actually represents an enlarged inferior tympanic artery anastomosing with an enlarged caroticotympanic artery when the cervical segment of the ICA is undeveloped/underdeveloped. Consequently, the "aberrant carotid artery" enters the tympanic cavity, courses through the tympanic cavity, and then enters the horizontal carotid canal. This usually presents with pulsatile tinnitus.

ANTERIOR CEREBRAL ARTERY

The anterior cerebral artery (ACA) is the smaller terminal branch of the ICA. After its origin, it traverses anteromedially toward the interhemispheric fissure just above the optic chiasm. In most cases, the ACA joins its contralateral counter part at the level of interhemispheric fissure through the anterior communicating artery (AComA). The course of the ACA is divided into five segments: A1 is from the origin to the origin of AcomA; the A2 segment extends to the junction of the rostrum and genu of corpus callosum, the A3 extends around the genu of corpus callosum until the artery turns sharply posteriorly, and the A4 and A5 segments pass over the corpus callosum separated by the coronal fissure.

Normal Variant/Anomalies of ACA of Clinical Significance

Clinical Significance

Bihemispheric ACA: If the A2 segment is hypoplastic, the other A2 divides and supplies both the hemispheres, which may be difficult to differentiate by angiography from true azygos ACA.

Azygos anterior cerebral artery: If the embryonic median artery of corpus callosum persists, an azygos ACA is formed. This is an unpaired median trunk of the ACA, which supplies both the hemispheres. This variant is sometimes associated with the holoprosencephaly.

Unpaired A2 segments can increase the risk of distal ACA aneurysms particularly at the bifurcation of ACA into pericallosal and callosomarginal arteries.

Infraoptic ACA: When the ACA arises early from the intradural course of the ACA, near the origin of the ophthalmic artery, it courses below the optic chiasm and traverses medially and upward to join the normally positioned AComA. This variant has high prevalence of intracerebral aneurysm formation, particularly in the ACA–AComA complex.

Asymmetry of A1: Asymmetry (larger than the opposite side) of the A1 segment has an important impact on likelihood of aneurysm formation in the AComA. The end on hemodynamic impact of pulsatile flow through the larger A1 segment directed against the anterior wall of the A1–AComA junction is thought to explain high incidence of aneurysm formation in this location. This also explains why 70% of the AComA aneurysms are directed anteriorly. Up to 80% of the AComA aneurysms have significant A1 asymmetry.

Branches

Proximal ACA branches

- Anterior perforating branches: There are two sets of anterior perforating branches, inferiorly directed and superiorly directed, which arise from the A1, A2 segments, and sometimes also from the AComA. The inferiorly directed branches supply the optic chiasm and optic nerve. Superiorly directed medial lenticulostriate branches are 2 to 15 in number and supply anterior hypothalamus, septum pellucidum, columns of fornix and anterior commissure, genu of corpus callosum, and anterior aspect of striatum.
- Recurrent artery of Heubner: A prominent laterally directed lenticulostriate vessel (largest and longest of the perforating vessels) arising most commonly from the proximal A2 segment (may also arise from A1 and AComA). It is usually better demonstrated in the contralateral carotid injection. It supplies anterior aspect of the striatum, anterior limb of internal capsule, and the paraterminal gyrus. This is an important source of preservation of blood supply to the basal ganglia during occlusion of MCA. Occlusion of recurrent artery of Heubner causes hemiparesis that is most prominent in the face and superior extremity.

- Cortical branches: Usually do not arise from the pre-communicating segment. The first one or two orbital branches (aka orbitofrontal branches) arise from the proximal A2 segment and supply the orbital surface of the frontal lobe. There are also a group of branches arise from the mid A2; the largest one is frontopolar artery.

  Distal ACA branches: At the genu of the corpus callosum, the ACA bifurcates into two main vessels, pericallosal artery and callosomarginal artery. Pericallosal artery is rather continuation of the ACA trunk and courses posteriorly for a variable distance above the corpus callosum. The callosomarginal artery is the smaller branch that passes over the cingulate gyrus at the cingulate sulcus. The distal groups of branches, parietal branches, supply the precuneus and adjacent cortex.

Clinical Significance

The pericallosal artery can be compressed posteriorly (A5) in subfalcine herniation, angiographically appears as steplike deformity in the AP projection. The anterior part (A4) is usually displaced to the opposite side rather than being compressed in subfalcine herniation, because the artery is located well below the free margin of falx. Following trauma, there may be distal pericallosal artery pseudoaneurysm formation at the constraints of the free margin of the falx. In severe hydrocephalus, the pericallosal artery is displaced superiorly and takes a smooth curve, best demonstrated in lateral projection.

MIDDLE CEREBRAL ARTERY

The middle cerebral artery supplies most of the eloquent cortex including the somatosensory and motor cortex. The artery is divided into four segments: M1, from ICA bifurcation until the MCA turns superiorly into the insula (the genu); M2 segment extends from the genu to the circular sulcus; M3 extends from circular sulcus to the opercular turn of the branches; and the M4 segments are the branches visible in the lateral convexity of the hemisphere.

The MCA can divide into up to four branching patterns: a single trunk with no main division, a bifurcation, a trifurcation, and a quadrifurcation. The most common branching pattern is bifurcation with a superior and inferior division.

Most (70%) of the MCA aneurysms occur at its bifurcation. Aneurysm of the MCA trunk represents 10% of the aneurysms of this artery.

Branches

Lenticulostriate: There can be roughly 1 to 21 lenticulostriate branches, average being 10. Approximately 80% of the branches arise from the posterosuperior aspect of the MCA trunk, the remaining arise from the branches of the MCA. They supply the anterior commissure, internal capsule, dorsal aspect of head of caudate nucleus, putamen, lateral globus pallidus, and substantia inominata.

Cortical: The cortical branches supply most of the lateral convexity of cerebral hemisphere, the insular and opercular cortex, the lateral part of the orbital surface of the frontal lobe, and lateral and inferior part of the temporal lobe anteriorly. The borderline region between the distributions of the cerebral arteries is known as watershed zone. These regions are at risk for infarction in the case of severe hypotension, and also, these are the regions for lodging blood-borne diseases (i.e., infection [including mycotic anurysm] and tumor cell for metastasis).

Frontal lobe branches

- *Orbitiofrontal artery*: This branches anteriorly, superiorly, and laterally to vascularize the inferior frontal gyrus. Orbitofrontal branch supplies Brocas area, frontal eye field, and the premotor strip; patients with stroke involving these arteries in the dominant lobe will present with expressive aphasia.
- *Prefrontal arteries*: These arteries fan over the insula and supply the inferior and middle frontal gyrus. Near the suprior frontal gyrus, their anastomose with branches of pericallosal arteries.
- *Pre-Rolandic artery*: The artery courses over the media surface of the operculum and supplies the posterior parts of the middle and inferior frontal gyri as well as the lower parts of the precentral gyrus.
- *Rolandic arteries*: The artery supplies posterior precentral gyrus and the inferior portion of the postcentral gyrus coursing inside the central sulcus.

Parietal lobe branches

- *Anterior parietal*
- *Posterior parietal*
- *Angular*: The angular artery is a significant terminal branch of the anterior or middle trunk of the MCA. It emerges from the Sylvian fissure and passes over the anterior transverse temporal gyrus and usually divides into two branches supplying angular and supramarginal gyrus.
- *Temporaloccipital*: This is the longest cortical artery. It courses posteriorly after exiting from the Sylvian fissure parallel to the superior temporal sulcus and supplies the superior and inferior occipital gyri.

Temporal lobe branches

- *Temporopolar*
- *Anterior temporal*
- *Middle temporal*
- *Posterior temporal*

ARTERIES OF POSTERIOR CIRCULATION

VERTEBRAL ARTERIES

Of the two vertebral arteries, the left is the dominant artery in roughly 60% of cases. Both the vertebral arteries are equal in size in 25% of cases. The vertebral arteries are described in four segments. The first segment is from its origin at subclavian artery to its entry into the foramen transversarium usually at C6 vertebral body. The second segment is the course in the foramen transversarium from C6 to atlas. The third segment is a horizontal curvy course in superior surface of posterior arch of atlas. The fourth segment is the intracranial course after this pierces the atlantooccipital membrane and enters into the cranial cavity until the basilar confluence.

Clinical Significance

Vertebral artery injury: Vertebral artery injury occurs most commonly in the foraminal segment.

- Intimal tear: This is the most subtle form of injury. A free flap may be demonstrated within the lumen, or may not be seen in imaging.
- Dissection: When tear of the intima leads to dissection of the blood into the arterial wall.
    - Occlusion: If the blood accumulates between the intima and the media, which is more common, it will compress the arterial lumen.
    - Pseudoaneurysms: If the blood dissects between the media and adventitia, it will cause swelling of the arterial wall or pseudoaneurysm formation.
    - Transection: This is the most severe type, usually fatal.

Atherosclerotic disease: Atherosclerotic disease is common where the artery pierces the dura.

Dissecting aneurysms of the vertebrobasilar system: This is a special group of aneurysm, which involves the vertebral artery, particularly the V1 and V3 segments of the vertebral artery due to defect in the internal elastic lamina and development of a false lumen between internal elastic lamina and media of the arterial wall. The common angiographic findings are focal dilation of the lumen, luminal stenosis or occlusion, string of pearl-like (both occlusion and dilation), and double lumen.

Subclavian steal syndrome: Occurs in cases of proximal subclavian artery stenosis with retrograde flow in the vertebral artery toward the distal subclavian artery causing transient vertebrobasilar symptoms. Color Doppler ultrasound and phase-contrast MRA are useful to diagnose this condition.

Rotational vertebral artery syndrome: Consisting of attacks of vertigo, nystagmus, and tinnitus elicited by head-rotation-induced compression of the dominant vertebral artery.

Branches

Usually, classified as medial and lateral. Medial branches arise from the distal half of the vertebral artery and supply the anterior medulla and pyramid. The most prominent inferiorly directed medial branch is the anterior spinal artery. The lateral branches are posterior inferior cerebellar artery (PICA) and circumferential branches to the inferior cerebellar peduncle, lateral medulla, and olivary structures.

Clinical Significance

The PICA is the largest branch of the vertebral artery. Stroke involving the PICA territory has a classic spectrum of presentation which is also known as lateral medullary syndrome or Wallenberg syndrome, which includes contralateral deficits in pain and temperature sensation from body (involvement of lateral spinothalamic tract), ipsilateral loss of touch, pain, and temperature sensation from face (involvement of spinal trigeminal nucleus), dysphagia, hoarseness, diminished gag (involvement of nucleus ambiguus), vertigo, diplopia, nystagmus, vomiting (vestibular system involvement), ipsilateral Horner syndrome (descending sympathetic fiber involvement), and ipsilateral cerebellar sign (involvement of the inferior cerebellar peduncle).

BASILAR ARTERY

The basilar artery is formed by fusion of two vertebral arteries at the pontomedullary junction. It is about 32 mm in length and approximately 4 mm in diameter. The narrowest part of the artery is at the level of the origin of superior cerebellar artery, the embryologic junction between the anterior and posterior circulation.

Branches

Brainstem perforators: There may be up to 17 perforator branches from the basilar artery supplying the brainstem. There are two groups of arteries: short median branches, which enter in the pons in the midline in the median sulcus and penetrate up to the floor of the fourth ventricle; the other group encircles the brainstem and enters into the pons more laterally. These branches are very important as they supply the corticospinal and corticobulbar tracts, pontine nuclei, and motor nuclei of midbrain and pons.

Anterior inferior cerebellar artery: It usually arises from the proximal or middle third of the basilar artery. The artery of the internal auditory meatus arises from this artery. For chemoembolization of the posterior fossa tumor, the microcatheter should always be placed above the level of AICA as some of the chemotherapeutic drugs are toxic to the cochlea and can cause permanent hearing loss. About 8% (error) cases of trigeminal neuralgia due vascular compression of the trigeminal nerve roots is caused by this artery.

Superior cerebellar artery: It supplies the lower midbrain, upper pons, upper vermis, and superior aspect of the cerebellar hemisphere. SCA is the most common artery (50%) to cause trigeminal nerve root compression.

Posterior cerebral arteries (see below)

Clinical Significance

Atherosclerotic disease: Unlike the MCA strokes, which are more commonly embolic in nature, the acute vertebrobasilar strokes are usually thrombotic.

Basilar tip aneurysms: Approximately 10% to 18% of intracranial aneurysms occur in the posterior circulation, of which more than half occur at the basilar tip. These aneurysms are very difficult to approach surgically, particularly if they are directed anteriorly and if there is high basilar bifurcation of the basilar artery in relation to the posterior clinoid process.

POSTERIOR CEREBRAL ARTERIES

In fetal life, the posterior cerebral artery arises from ICA. But most commonly, by birth the main supply to the PCA artery is from the basilar artery.

SEGMENTATION

Like other cerebral arteries, the PCA is also described in three segments: P1 being the segment from the origin of PCA up to the junction of PComA; the P2 segment is from the PComA junction to the posterior aspect of midbrain, and the P3 segment being the lateral aspect of the quadrigeminal cistern around the pulvinar.

Clinical Significance

In the setting of asymmetric mass effect or severe temporal lobe herniation, the midbrain may become compressed against tentorium compressing the PCA or its branches, which normally travel between these two. If the branches are compressed between these two structures, there will be a midline brainstem hemorrhage, also known as Duret hemorrhage.

Branches

Branches to the thalamus and brainstem

- Thalamoperforator arteries: There are two groups of thalamoperforator arteries (anterior, 7 to 10 in number and posterior up to 8 in number). The anterior group supplies thalamic nuclei, posterior aspect of the optic chiasm, proximal part of the optic radiation, posterior hypothalamus, and part of the cerebral peduncle. The posterior group supplies thalamus, subthalamic nuclei, midbrain structures including substantia nigra, red nucleus, oculomotor and trochlear nuclei, the posterior portion of the internal capsule, and the cisternal segment of the oculomotor nerve. When a dominant thalamoperforator artery supplies the thalami bilaterally, it is sometimes referred to as artery of Percheron.
- Thalamogeniculate arteries: These may be up to 12 in number. They supply lateral thalamus, posterior limb of internal capsule, and part of the optic tract. Stroke involving these arteries give rise to classic lateral thalamic Dejerine-Roussy syndrome.
- Peduncular perforator arteries: These supply the peduncles.

Branches to the ventricles

- Medial posterior choroidal artery: This may be multiple in up to 40% of cases. Most commonly, it arises from the P2 segment. On lateral projection, it appears classically as "3" shaped. It supplies the choroids plexus of the third ventricle and may also supply the massa intermedia, stria medullaris, and fornix.
- Lateral choroidal arteries: These may be up to nine in number. They arise from P2 segment. They supply the glomus of the choroids plexus of the atrium and the body of the choroids plexus of the lateral ventricle.

Cortical branches

Proximal PCA (P2 segment):

- Anterior temporal artery: This is the first cortical branch and anastomoses with the anterior temporal branch of the MCA.
- Posterior temporal artery: This is the second cortical branch and arises from the middle of the P2 segment.
- Distal PCA (P3 & P4 segment): Distally PCA terminates into two trunks, which ultimately give rise to two sets arteries, medial and lateral:
- Medial arteries
  - Parieto-occipital: It supplies the cuneus, precuneus, and lateral occipital gyrus, and may occasionally extend to medial aspects of precentral gyrus and superior parietal lobule.
  - Calcarine: This supplies the primary visual cortex and may also supply to the lingual gyrus and cuneus. Unilateral occlusion causes homonymous hemianopsia with varying degree of macular sparing. Bilateral occlusion causes Anton syndrome, sudden bilateral cortical blindness with preserved pupillary reaction and denial of visual loss.
  - Splenial: It may arise either from the branches of the PCA or the PCA trunk itself. Sometimes, it is considered as the posterior pericallosal artery.

- Lateral arteries:
  - Anterior inferior temporal arteries.
  - Middle inferior temporal arteries.
  - Posterior inferior temporal arteries.

ARTERIES OF THE CIRCLE OF WILLIS

Circle of Willis is an intercommunicating arcade of collateral arteries (consisting of ICAs, A1 segments, AComA, PComA, P1 segments, and the basilar artery) at the base of the skull before reaching the brain. This arterial arcade balances flow in different regions of the brain. If one portion is hypoplastic, the blood flow is augmented by the collaterals. Complete circle of Willis is present at about one-fourth of the cases. Common variations include hypoplastic PComA, hypoplastic or absent A1, fetal origin of PCA, and infundibular origin of the PComA.

VENOUS SYSTEM OF THE BRAIN

SUPRATENTORIAL

Extradural

Diploic Veins

These are endothelial-lined vascular spaces within the diploic spaces. They do not have valves.

Dural Sinuses

Superior sagittal sinus (SSS): It is the largest dural sinus. It extends anteriorly from the crista galli to the torcular Herophili, the confluence of SSS, straight sinus, and occipital sinus. The sinus is covered by a fold of falx cerebri. The sinus gradually enlarges in size as it traverses posteriorly and receives numerous tributaries from the superficial veins draining the convexities. There are multiple prominent arachnoid granulations in the posterior aspect of the SSS, which may appear as filling defects in angiography (CTA and MRA) particularly, in old age.

The *inferior sagittal sinus* is much smaller structure than the SSS and runs posteriorly through the free edge of falx and meets the vein of Galen to form the straight sinus. It receives tributaries from the falx, cingulum, and medial hemisphere.

The union of the inferior sagittal sinus and the great vein of Galen form the *straight sinus*. It runs posteroinferiorly down to the torcular Herophili and receives multiple tributaries from the infratentorial veins.

Torcular Herophili is the confluence of SSS, straight sinus, and occipital sinus. It usually drains into two transverse sinuses. These may be equal in size or more often asymmetric, in which case the right transverse sinus is usually larger.

The transverse sinuses run anterolaterally from their origin at the torcula and meet the superior petrosal sinus and continue as sigmoid sinus.

Sigmoid sinus is the anteroinferior continuation of the transverse sinus down to the jugular bulb from where it continues as internal jugular vein.

Petrosal sinuses (superior and inferior) are two venous channels, which communicate with the cavernous sinus superiorly down to the ipsilateral sigmoid sinus and jugular bulb, respectively.

The *occipital sinus* is formed at the posterior margin of the foramen magnum by the confluence of the tributaries of the marginal plexus of vein.

Sphenoparietal sinus drains the superficial Sylvian vein into the cavernous sinus along the lesser wing of sphenoid.

Cavernous sinus is located on either side of the sphenoid body extending anteriorly from the superior orbital fissure to the petrous apex posteriorly. This sinus communicates extensively with extracranial and intracranial venous structures and sinuses. The ICA with sympathetic plexus is on the medial wall, the abducens nerve at the center of the sinus lateral to the ICA and medial to the oculomotor and trochlear nerves, as well as the ophthalmic and maxillary divisions of the trigeminal nerve in the lateral wall.

- Communications of the cavernous sinus:
  - *Anteriorly:* Receives the superior ophthalmic vein through the superior orbital fissure. Laterally, receives sphenoparietal sinus.
  - *Posteriorly:* Communicates with the transverse sinus by means of the superior petrosal sinus; with the internal jugular vein through the inferior petrosal sinus.
  - *Medially:* Communicates with each other by means of the anterior and posterior intercavernous sinuses. Also communicates with the pterygoid venous plexus through the foramen Vesalii, foramen ovale and foramen lacerum, and with the angular vein via the ophthalmic vein.
- *Cavernous sinus* syndrome: Cavernous sinus syndrome is symptom complex due to pathologies of the cavernous sinus (carotido–cavernous fistula, carotid artery aneurysm, infection, trauma, tumors, and inflammatory diseases involving the sinus). The symptoms include ophthalmoplegia, chemosis, proptosis, trigeminal sensory loss, and Horner syndrome.

Intradural

Deep

Medullary veins: Numerous angiographically undetectable small deep veins originatings 1 to 2 cm deep to the cortex, coursing medially through the subcortical white matter, and draining into the subependymal veins that course along the ventricular wall. These veins are prominent in susceptibility weighted imaging and the in the raw images of the perfusion weighted imaging in cases of tumefactive demyelination and also in some low-grade gliomas.

After receiving blood from the medullary veins, the subependymal veins aggregate to form the larger tributaries. The medial group consists of anterior septal vein that drains the deep frontal lobe and runs along the septum pellucidum; lateral group, veins that drain the caudate nucleus, are named as anterior/longitudinal caudate veins which drain into the thalamostriate vein. The anterior septal vein joins the thalamostriate veins at the foramen of Monro, the "venous angle," to form the internal cerebral vein. Internal cerebral veins are midline paired structures that run posteriorly in the roof of the third ventricle and meet below the tip of the splenium to form the great cerebral vein (of Galen).

The paired basal veins of Rosenthal are each formed in the region of anterior perforated substance by the union of the anterior cerebral veins, deep middle cerebral vein, and striate veins. After its formation, each basal vein passes posteriorly around the cerebral peduncle and terminates into the great cerebral vein (vein of Galen).

The great cerebral vein is a median venous trunk, about 2 cm long and is formed by the union of two internal cerebral veins. After its formation, the trunk abruptly turns upward around the splenium of the corpus callosum and then courses posterior and ends at the anterior end of the straight sinus near the tentorial apex.

Superficial

These include superior cerebral veins, superficial middle cerebral veins, and inferior cerebral veins. As these veins are so variable in number and configuration, most are unnamed.

Superior cerebral veins: About 8 to 10 in number, they collect the blood from superolateral and medial surfaces of the hemispheres and drain into the SSS. The veins course obliquely upward and forward to meet the SSS and drain against the flow of the blood flow in the SSS. This particular orientation helps prevent collapse of the mouth of the cerebral veins during raised intracranial pressure.

Superficial middle cerebral vein: This is a prominent but inconstant vein (or group of veins) that drains blood from the lateral surface of the hemisphere, runs along the posterior ramus and stem of the lateral sulcus, and empties into the cavernous sinus. The superior (vein of Trolard) and/or inferior (vein of Labbe) anastomotic veins connect the superficial middle cerebral veins with the SSS and transverse sinus, respectively.

Inferior cerebral veins: These veins drain the inferior surface and ventral part of the lateral surface of hemisphere. Those from the orbital surface join the sphenoparietal and cavernous sinuses and those from the tentorial surface terminate into the cavernous, superior petrosal, and transverse sinuses.

INFRATENTORIAL

The major infratentorial veins are described as superior (Galenic veins) that drain blood from the median cerebellum and brainstem usually into the vein of Galen; anterior (petrosal), which drain blood from cerebellum, pons, and medulla into the superior petrosal sinus; and the posterior (tentorial) drain blood from the cerebellar hemispheres and drain into the tentorial sinuses.

Venous sinus thrombosis: Venous sinus thrombosis is a relatively rare condition that occurs usually because of a hypercoagulable state but also may be because of slow flow, extrinsic compression or invasion of the sinus, dehydration and pregnancy/postpartum state. It presents with a myriad of clinical symptoms and imaging manifestations (delta sign in noncontrast CT and reverse/empty delta sign in CECT).

SUGGESTED READING

Fassett Daniel R, Dailey Andrew T, Vaccaro Alexander R. Vertebral artery injuries associated with cervical spine injuries: a review of the literature. *J Spinal Disord Tech.* 2008;21:252-258.

Hobson RW II, Mackey WC, Ascher E. Management of atherosclerotic carotid artery disease: clinical practice guidelines of the Society for Vascular Surgery. *J Vasc Surg.* 2008;48:480-486.

Redekop GJ, Extracranial carotid and vertebral artery dissection: *a review. Can J Neurol Sci.* 2008;35:146-152.

QUESTIONS AND ANSWERS

1. Which of the following is *true* regarding fibromuscular dysplasia of the carotids?
   A. Typically has string sign appearance in internal carotid artery
   B. Rarely associated with intracranial aneurysms
   C. More commonly involves external carotid artery than internal carotid artery
   D. Usually bilateral
   E. More common in men

   ANSWER: D. Sixty-five percent of cases are bilateral.

2. What is the predominant arterial supply for hippocampus?
   A. Anterior cerebral
   B. Middle cerebral
   C. Posterior cerebral
   D. Anterior choroidal
   E. Recurrent artery of Heubner

   ANSWER: C. Hippocampal artery branch of the PCA supplies the hippocampal gyrus.

3. Which artery supplies the posterior limb of the internal capsule?
   A. Anterior choroidal
   B. Recurrent artery of Heubner (Medial lenticulostriate)
   C. Lateral lenticulostriate
   D. Anterior cerebral

   ANSWER: C. The medial lenticulostriate artery supplies anterior limb of internal capsule.

4. A common carotid injection demonstrates occlusion of the ICA immediately above the bifurcation with subsequent filling of the ipsilateral intracranial internal carotid artery. What collateral supply does this most likely represent?
   A. Collaterals via the AComA
   B. Collaterals via the PComA
   C. Collaterals via the ophthalmic artery
   D. An intact circle of Willis
   E. Collaterals via the ipsilateral superficial temporal artery

   ANSWER: C. This is one of the common locations of collaterals from external carotid to internal carotid artery.

5. Which one of the following vessels is affected in the Wallenberg (lateral medullary) syndrome?
   A. Contralateral SCA
   B. Contralateral AICA
   C. Ipsilateral SCA
   D. Contralateral PICA
   E. Ipsilateral PICA

   ANSWER: E. Ipsilateral PICA typically causes Wallenberg syndrome.

6. You identify an enlarged tentorial branch of the meningohypophyseal trunk. What is the most likely etiology?
   A. Dural AVM
   B. Vestibular schwannoma
   C. Posterior fossa glioma
   D. Jugular paraganglioma
   E. Cerebellar hemangioblastoma

   ANSWER: A. It is unlikely to have blood supply from meningeal branches in other pathologies.

7. Patient presents with neck pain and Horner syndrome on the left after skiing and a fall, what is the most likely diagnosis?
   A. Vertebral dissection
   B. Internal carotid dissection
   C. Internal carotid occlusion
   D. Cerebral vascular accident
   E. Vertebral occlusion

   ANSWER: B. Sympathetic nerves supplying the ocular muscles course close to the ICA at the neck. Dissection may paralyze these sympathetic nerves.

8. What is the etiology of subclavian steal syndrome?
   A. Subclavian stenosis proximal to the origin of the vertebral artery
   B. Subclavian stenosis distal to the origin of the vertebral artery
   C. Stenosis of the ipsilateral vertebral artery
   D. Stenosis of the contralateral vertebral artery

   ANSWER: A. Subclavian stenosis proximal to the origin of the vertebral artery "steals" the blood from cranial circulation into the arm during exercise.

9. Which of the following is an example of carotid-basilar communication?
   A. Ophthalmic artery
   B. Posterior meningeal artery
   C. Recurrent artery of Hubner
   D. Otic artery
   E. Temporal artery

   ANSWER: D. Other arteries do not have any carotid-basilar communication.

10. A 37-year-old man was painting his roof when he acutely developed left tongue deviation, left facial numbness, ataxia, and right body weakness. What is the most likely diagnosis?
    A. Carotid artery dissection
    B. Vertebral artery dissection
    C. Middle cerebral artery infarct
    D. Wallenberg syndrome
    E. Anterior cerebral artery infarct

    ANSWER: B. Prolonged extension of the neck may cause the vertebral artery dissection, which produces these symptoms.

5 STROKE AND CEREBROVASCULAR DISEASES OF THE BRAIN

Ahmed Kamel Abdel Aal and
Joseph C. Sullivan III

STROKE

INTRODUCTION

Stroke is a general nonspecific term that indicates rapid loss of the brain functions because of disturbance in blood vessels. The major causes of stroke in children include congenital heart disease with emboli, dissection, hemorrhage from vascular malformation, idiopathic progressive arteriopathy of childhood, coagulopathy, and drug abuse. In middle-age and old adults, the causes of stroke include arterial thromboembolism, nontraumatic intracranial hemorrhage, intracranial veno-occlusive disorders, hemorrhage from vascular malformation, neoplasms, and coagulopathy.

The risk factors for stroke include hypertension, coronary heart disease, heart failure, atrial fibrillation, diabetes mellitus, high blood lipid levels, cigarette smoking, alcohol consumption, transient ischemic attack (TIA), and asymptomatic carotid atherosclerotic disease.

CEREBRAL ISCHEMIA AND INFARCTION

Ischemia and infarction remain the second most common cause of death worldwide. Cerebral ischemia and infarction have a variety of causes including thrombosis, embolism (from cardiac or noncardiac source), dissection, vasculitis, or generalized hypoperfusion.

The ischemic area consists of a central core of severe ischemia that will progress to infarction and has a cerebral blood flow (CBF) that is less than 12 to 18 mL/100 gm/min. This is surrounded by a peripheral less ischemic region "penumbra," containing cells that are still viable, but at risk of infarction if not salvaged, and with a CBF less than 20 to 23 mL/100 gm/min.

The most vulnerable parts of the brain to ischemia are the CA1 layer of the hippocampus, the third, fifth, and sixth layers of cortex, and the basal ganglia. Ischemia leads to energy depletion and failure of sodium/potassium pump leading to accumulation of intracellular sodium. High concentration of sodium draws water inside the cells by osmosis leading to cell swelling and cytotoxic edema. If the process continues, the cell membrane integrity is lost and the cells rupture leading to disruption and breakdown of the blood–brain barrier and the development of vasogenic edema.

Lacunar infarcts are small deep cerebral infarcts located predominantly in the basal ganglia and thalamus. They result from occlusion of small penetrating arteries in the deep gray matter because of various etiologies. They are strongly related to hypertension, and most of these lacunar infarcts are clinically silent.

Watershed or border-zone infarcts are caused by generalized hypoperfusion and/or hypoxic states resulting in insufficient blood flow and/or oxygenation to meet the metabolic demands of the brain. Causes include severe prolonged hypotension, resuscitation after cardiac arrest, and carbon monoxide inhalation. The process may be so severe involving the whole cerebral hemispheres. In less severe cases, the margins of major arterial territories will be involved. Watershed infarcts can also occur in the deep white mater watershed areas within the centrum semiovale leading to small infarcts in a linear orientation producing "string of pearls" appearance.

In the acute stage (6 hours–3 days), Noncontrast CT mainly serves to exclude hemorrhage as the cause of stroke, which will definitely alter the management of these patients. However, it may help in the diagnosis of infarction since it may show hyperdensity within an artery representing acute thrombus. "Dot sign" may also be seen and represents hyperdense dot in the sylvian fissure caused by thrombus in an MCA branch. Loss of gray–white matter distinction, with obscuration of the deep gray matter nuclei and loss of the cortical ribbon may also be noted. Hypodensity in a specific vascular territory, gyral swelling, and sulcal effacement are less commonly seen.

In the subacute stage (4 days–4 weeks), a wedge-shaped hypodense area is usually seen along the distribution of a vascular territory or in a watershed area depending on the etiology. Gyral swelling will start to decrease at 10 days. Hemorrhagic transformation of the infracted area can be seen in up to 25% of cases, especially large infarcts, and is primarily because of reperfusion of infracted areas with disrupted blood–brain barrier. The prognosis in this case is worse than bland infarct.

In the chronic stage (greater than 4 weeks), the infarct becomes more hypodense and there is prominence of the cortical sulci and dilatation of the adjacent portions of the ventricles.

In the acute stage, contrast-enhanced CT will demonstrate enhancement of the cortical vessels because of

TABLE 5-1 CBV, CBF, and MTT Values for Ischemia and Infarction

	CBF	CBV	MTT
Ischemia	Decreased (<20–23 mL/100 gm/min)	Normal	Increased
Infarction	Decreased (12–18 mL/100 gm/min)	Decreased (<2.0–2.5 mL/100 g)	Increased (>6 sec or >1.45% increase over contralateral normal side)

slow antegrade flow or retrograde flow from collaterals. Cortical gyral enhancement begins at 2 days, peaks at 2 weeks, and starts to disappear at 2 months. CT perfusion is done as part of the workup of these patients in some institutions. The cerebral blood volume (CBV), CBF, and mean transit time (MTT) values help determine infracted areas of the brain as well as the ischemic yet salvageable areas (Table 5-1).

CT angiography (CTA) will show stenosis or occlusion of the different arteries supplying the brain and the presence of collateral flow.

On MRI, diffusion imaging is the most sensitive sequence in detecting hyperacute infarction (<6 hours). Diffusion imaging mainly measures diffusion of water molecules in the extracellular space. In the hyperacute stage, cytotoxic edema leads to reduction in volume of extracellular space and restriction of motion of the water molecules in that space. The area of restricted diffusion is seen as hyperintense on DWI and hypointense on ADC maps. After 7 to 10 days, the cells start to rupture and vasogenic edema develops leading to increase in the volume of the extracellular space and the diffusion abnormalities will revert to normal. This is known as the "pseudonormal" stage and can last up to 4 weeks. The infracted area will be hyperintense on DWI because of "T2 shine-through" but will isointense on ADC maps that represent a more accurate measurement of diffusion. Thereafter and in the chronic stage, diffusion is increased because of continued increase in extracellular water, tissue cavitation, and gliosis. The area of restricted diffusion represents irreversible nonsalvagable ischemic area and correlates with the area of final infarct. However, some reports document reversibility of diffusion abnormality, but is not considered the general trend.

The combination of diffusion and perfusion imaging provide more information than either technique alone. In cases of arterial occlusion, areas of decreased diffusion and perfusion represent nonviable tissue or the core of the infarct. The more peripheral areas characterized by normal diffusion and decreased perfusion represent areas of "ischemic penumbra," which will progress to infarction unless early reperfusion occurs. In the infracted area, there is decreased rCBV, rCBF, and increased rMTT. In areas of "ischemic penumbra," the rCBV will be normal or increased. In the subacute stage, the rCBV will increase because of reperfusion hyperemia.

On conventional MRI sequences, acute infarction will demonstrate gyral swelling. The infracted area may appear normal in the hyperacute stage, but will be hypointense on T1-weighted images and hyperintense on T2-weighted image and FLAIR images in the acute stage. The presence of signal intensity within the arteries on these sequences indicates occlusion. In the subacute stage, blood products may be seen within the infarct if hemorrhagic transformation occurred, producing variable signal depending on the age of hemorrhage. In the chronic stage, encephalomalacia will ensue, producing CSF-like signal, which will be low on T1, high on T2, and low on FLAIR images. Encephalomalacia will be surrounded by gliosis that demonstrates high T2 and FLAIR signal. GRE images will show hypointense margin around the infarct because of hemosiderin in adjacent gliosis. Wallerian degeneration will lead to abnormal low T1 and high T2 signal along the course of the corticospinal tracts.

Postcontrast T1 images will show different enhancement patterns depending on the stage of the infarct. Intravascular enhancement may occur in the acute stage because of slow flow. In the subacute stage, meningeal and cortical enhancement will be seen and enhancement will start to disappear at 2 month.

MRA is helpful in demonstrating occlusion of large arteries. Conventional (catheter) angiogram is usually reserved for case that will benefit from interventional treatment. Abrupt arterial cut-off or arterial tapering may be seen. There may be slow antegrade flow or retrograde flow from collaterals. Intra-arterial infusion of recombinant tissue plasminogen activator (r-TPA) is used to thrombolyse the clot if the patient presents within 6-hours window. Alternatively, it can be infused intravenously, with a window of 3 hours only. The use of r-TPA significantly improves the outcome and prognosis. The main factors that affect the outcome include administration within the therapeutic window, nonhemorrhagic infarct, and infarct size that is less than one-third of the MCA territory. Devices that retrieve clots are also used but are associated with a high complication rate if clot fragmentation occurred.

NONTRAUMATIC INTRACRANIAL HEMORRHAGE

This accounts for approximately 10% of stroke cases. The causes of nontraumatic intracranial hemorrhage according to different age groups are listed (Table 5-2).

TABLE 5-2 Causes of Nontraumatic Intracranial Hemorrhage by Age Group

AGE GROUP	CAUSES
Premature infants	Germinal matrix hemorrhage
Term infants	Trauma during delivery
	Hypoxic ischemic injury
Young adults	Aneurysm
	Vascular malformation
	Hemorrhagic infarct
	Hypertensive intracerebral hemorrhage
	Hemorrhagic neoplasm
	Drug abuse (e.g., cocaine)
	Vasculitis
Elderly adults	Hypertensive intracerebral hemorrhage
	Amyloid angiopathy
	Hemorrhagic infarct
	Coagulopathy
	Hemorrhagic neoplasm

HYPERTENSIVE INTRACEREBRAL HEMORRHAGE

Hypertensive intracerebral hemorrhage is the most common cause of nontraumatic intracerebral hemorrhage in adults accounting for 70% to 90% of cases. The most common location is in the basal ganglia and is because of rupture of lenticulostriate artery aneurysm (Charcot–Bouchard aneurysm). Other less common locations include the thalamus, pons, cerebellum, and white matter.

HEMORRHAGIC INFARCTION

It is usually owing to hemorrhagic transformation of bland infarct as a result of reperfusion. However, arterial infarcts can be primarily hemorrhagic and will usually have an embolic etiology. Venous infarcts are more commonly hemorrhagic and caused by veno-occlusive disease such as dural venous sinus, cortical venous, and deep venous thrombosis.

AMYLOID ANGIOPATHY

It results from extracellular deposition of amyloid in the media and adventitia of small- and medium-sized arteries. Pathologically, there are microaneurysms and fibrinoid degeneration. There is loss of elasticity and increased fragility secondary to replacement of internal elastic lamina by amyloid deposits leading to intracerebral hemorrhage. Amyloid angiopathy accounts for approximately 10% to 20% of nontraumatic intracerebral hemorrhages and is considered the second most common cause in elderly adults. Lobar hemorrhages at different ages may be seen most commonly in the frontal and parietal lobes. Multifocal tiny subcortical hypointensities may also be seen on T2-weighted and GRE images representing chronic microbleeds.

VENO-OCCLUSIVE DISORDERS

These include dural venous sinus, cortical venous, and deep venous thrombosis. A variety of predisposing factors may lead to veno-occlusive disease and are listed (Table 5-3).

DURAL SINUS THROMBOSIS

Thrombosis may involve the dural venous sinus and extend into cortical vein tributaries. The most commonly involved in the superior sagittal sinus, and females are more commonly affected than males.

On noncontrast CT, the thrombosed sinus appears hyperdense, and if the thrombus extends into a cortical vein, a hyperdense linear cordlike structure may be seen. Because of obliteration of the venous drainage of the brain parenchyma, a venous infarct may be seen in 50% of cases, and has a high tendency to be initially hemorrhagic or shows hemorrhagic transformation on follow-up scans. On contrast-enhanced CT, enhancement of the dura surrounding the nonenhancing thrombus will produce the "empty delta" sign which is seen in 25% of cases. With the advent of multidetector CT scanners, CT venography may be performed and will show complete occlusion or intraluminal filling defect within the sinus.

On MRI, the normal flow void within the sinus is replaced by intraluminal thrombus. The signal intensity of the thrombus will depend on its age. It is difficult to detect the thrombus in the acute phase, since deoxyhemoglobin will be isointense on T1-weighted images and hypointense on T2 images and therefore indistinguishable from normal flow voids in most cases. In the subacute stage, the thrombus will appear hyperintense on both T1 and T2 images. The cortical veins may also be involved and will display similar signal intensity to thrombosed venous sinus. Venous infarct may occur producing gyral swelling and T2 and FLAIR hyperintensity in the

TABLE 5-3 Predisposing Factors for Intracranial Venous Thrombosis

Trauma
Neoplasms
Infection: sinusitis, mastoiditis
Pregnancy and oral contraceptives
Dehydration
Metabolic: thyrotoxicosis, cirrhosis
Coagulopathy: factor V Leiden, protein S deficiency
Vasculitis: Behcet

involved brain parenchyma. In case of hemorrhagic infarction or hemorrhagic transformation, the signal intensity will be complex and will depend on the age of hemorrhage. Diffusion imaging may show the infarct earlier than conventional sequences, and unlike arterial infarcts, the signal abnormality is reversible in most cases. Postcontrast images will show peripheral enhancement around the acute thrombus. GRE images will demonstrate blooming in the thrombosed sinus and within a hemorrhagic infarct. In chronic sinus thrombosis, heeling by organizing fibrous tissue will produce isointense to hypointense signal in the sinus that will enhance on postcontrast images.

MRV is very helpful in establishing a diagnosis in most cases. 2D or 3D time of flight (TOF) may be used and will show absence of flow in the thrombosed sinus. If there is partial recanalization, the sinus will have a shaggy or frayed appearance. Enlarged collateral venous channels may also be seen. TOF MRV is limited in the subacute stage by the T1 hyperintensity of the thrombus, which falsely appears as patent sinus with normal flow. Therefore, TOF MRV images should always be evaluated alongside the source images and conventional sequences, or alternatively, phase-contrast MRV may be performed, which does not have this limitation.

The 3D contrast-enhanced MRV (CE-MRV) is a more flow-insensitive technique relying on vascular enhancement, after contrast administration, for vessel detection. This technique has shown to provide much better depiction of normal venous structures, better outline of the thrombus, and is much faster relative to TOF MRV. However, its utilization in the diagnosis of chronic thrombosis has been questioned because of possible intense enhancement of the chronic thrombus that will produce an erroneous appearance of a patent sinus.

Catheter angiography may show occlusion of the involved sinus, with slow flow in the adjacent patent cortical veins. Collateral venous channels may also be seen. Partial recanalization in the subacute or chronic stage may produce irregular shaggy outline of the dural venous sinus. Percutaneous catheter directed thrombolysis or mechanical fragmentation can be performed.

Cortical Venous Thrombosis

Thrombosis of a cortical vein may be isolated or result from extension of thrombus from dural sinus. On NECT, the cortical vein will appear as hyperdense linear cord-like structure. Associated hypodensity in the brain parenchyma suggests venous infarct.

CECT and CT venography will show a filling defect within the thrombosed vein and will depict collateral venous channels. However, they have a limited value in chronic cases, since a chronic thrombus will also enhance simulating a patent vein. The appearance of a thrombosed cortical vein on MRI depends on age and is similar to that of a thrombosed sinus described above. Venous infarction may be seen. Catheter angiography appears to be more sensitive than MRI in the detection of cortical venous thrombosis, and the ability to perform percutaneous treatment is another advantage. This can be achieved by transcatheter administration of thrombolytics and/or mechanically fragmentation of the clot.

Deep Venous Thrombosis

This involves thrombosis of the internal cerebral veins, and the thrombus may extend into the vein of Galen, basal veins of Rosenthal, and then into the draining dural venous sinuses. Deep vein thrombosis is more commonly bilateral. If the internal cerebral veins are thrombosed, venous infarcts will involve the thalami and basal ganglia, producing abnormalities on CT and MRI. The imaging features of deep venous thrombosis on CT and MRI are similar to those described above for the dural sinus thrombosis.

CEREBROVASCULAR DISEASES OF THE BRAIN

ATHEROSCLEROTIC DISEASE

Atherosclerotic disease of is a major cause of disability and is ranked third among the most common causes of death in industrialized countries. It accounts for 90% of cerebral thromboembolic infarcts. Atherosclerosis affects arteries of all size including the aorta and cerebral microvasculature. A variety of predisposing factors are known including hypertension, diabetes, smoking, high lipid profile, obesity, and old age.

The pathogenesis of atherosclerosis involves injury to the vascular endothelium and LDL deposition in the arterial intima. After a series of changes in the arterial wall, an atherosclerotic plaque is finally formed, which is a complex fibrotic lesion formed of a variety of cells including monocytes, macrophages and smooth muscle cells, as well as connective tissue and lipid deposits. Neovascularization occurs at the center of the plaque. Luminal narrowing occurs because of rupture of neovacularization leading to intraplaque/subintimal hemorrhage. Fracture and ulceration of the fibrous cap and intima at the surface of the plaque invites platelet aggregation and activates the coagulation cascade leading to the formation of thrombus on the surface of the plaque. The thrombus may shower emboli distally, that lodge in smaller arteries leading to infarction. Alternatively, the whole plaque may rupture leading to distal embolization.

The most common location for atherosclerosis is the CCA bifurcation and the proximal ICA. Intracranially, atherosclerotic disease is most commonly seen in the carotid siphons and vetebrobasilar arteries. The clinical presentation is variable and patients may be asymptomatic or present with carotid bruit, TIAs, or stroke.

Sonography is the most important noninvasive technique for visualization of extracranial cerebrovascular atherosclerotic disease. The use of real time gray scale and color Doppler ultrasound (US) provides more information than each technique alone. With gray scale US, the presence of calcification in the plaque can be determined. A hypoechoic plaque will have less calcium and more lipid than content than a hyperechoic plaque and is considered a potential risk factor for embolic stroke. Using peak systolic velocity (PSV) measurement in the CCA and ICA, and obtaining an ICA:CCA PSV ratio, the degree of stenosis can be determined.

Just like any other technique, ultrasound has falsies and disadvantages and is operator-dependant. Estimation of the degree of stenosis based on velocities may sometimes be inaccurate, especially in the presence of tandem severe stenoses, severe stenosis leading to decreased rather than increased PSV, contralateral CCA occlusion, ipsilateral external carotid artery (ECA) occlusion, or cardiac valve disease.

On noncontrast CT, calcification in the involved vessels may be seen. The plaque may display hypodense foci caused by their lipid content. Contrast-enhanced CT will opacify the residual artery lumen and may obscure visualization of calcified plaques on standard brain windows. With the advent of multidetector CT scanners, CTA has become an important tool for visualization of plaques and in determining the degree of stenosis and is a useful alternative for conventional angiography in patients who are at high risk of developing stroke during the procedure or those who refuse to do it. CTA can also characterize the constituents of the plaque by assigning different colors for different densities within the plaque. Plaques with high lipid contents are generally associated with more ischemic symptoms than calcified plaques and are therefore considered potential markers for ischemic stroke.

On MRI, the absence of flow voids in any pulse sequence indicates occlusion of the arterial lumen. T1 appears to be the most helpful sequence in visualizing vessel wall thickening and luminal narrowing caused by plaque formation. Complication of atherosclerotic vascular disease such as large or lacunar ischemic infarcts can also be seen.

Several MR angiographic techniques are used by different institutions. The 2D TOF MRA technique is usually used for imaging the extracranial neck arteries and the degree of stenosis may be determined. However, this technique tends to overestimate the degree of stenosis because of turbulence and eddy currents occurring at the stenotic lesion leading to loss of signal. In case of severe stenosis, there is usually severe loss of signal leading to "flow gap." Furthermore, blood flowing in a direction parallel to, and in the plane of acquisition, will be subject to saturation and loss of signal, which is known as "in-plane saturation." Therefore, this technique cannot be used to image the intracranial cerebral arteries. This technique is also very sensitive to motion artifact that can be caused by arterial pulsation or swallowing.

The 3D TOF MRA technique is usually used for imaging the intracranial circulation. In this technique, thin slices are achievable and the technique is relatively fast. However, similar to 2D TOF MRA, it tends to overestimate the degree of stenosis for two main reasons. One is the presence of turbulence and eddy currents at the stenotic lesion that causes loss of signal. Second is the slow flow, leading to saturation of the fresh blood protons and loss of signal. Severe stenosis will therefore produce significant loss of signal and "flow gap." The technique also has the disadvantage of poor background suppression of fat and hemorrhage and high sensitivity to motion artifact.

The 3D contrast-enhanced MRA (CE-MRA) is a more flow-insensitive technique relying on vascular enhancement after contrast administration for vessel detection. The center of the K-space is filled first to provide more contrast to the image. Images should be acquired during the arterial phase to avoid venous contamination and therefore timing of image acquisition is important. Several methods such as test bolus or smart prep are therefore used. The tightness of the bolus is also important and is achieved by injection of about 40 mL of gadolinium (at a rate of 2 mL/sec) followed by a bolus of saline. A fast scanner is required since the set of images should be acquired within 10 to 15 seconds. This technique has several advantages. It is a much faster imaging technique, and therefore, several sets of images may be acquired, and the optimum images without venous contamination are selected. It is not affected by "in-plane saturation" as in 2D TOF. It is not affected by saturation because of slow flow as in 3D TOF. Therefore, it is less affected by flow artifacts, and the degree of stenosis is therefore more accurately depicted than TOF techniques. It is performed in the coronal plane with a large field of view that enables visualization of the arterial origins from the aorta as well as the intracranial circulation.

Conventional angiography is the gold standard imaging technique and allows visualization of degree of stenosis and surface of the plaque. Irregularity of the surface of the plaque is usually associated with increased risk of stroke at all degrees of stenosis. North America symptomatic carotid endarterectomy trial (NASCET) criteria are used by most institutions to determine the degree of stenosis. The maximum luminal diameter stenosis is compared to the diameter of a normal distal segment of the ICA beyond the bulb. The greatest value for diameter stenosis of the two standard views is used. According to NASCET, symptomatic patients with luminal diameter stenosis of >70% will benefit from carotid endarterectomy. The asymptomatic carotid atherosclerosis study (ACAS) showed surgical benefit in asymptomatic patients with luminal diameter narrowing of 60% or more. Angiography has the advantage of assessing collateral circulation and identifying tandem lesions. Interventional procedures, such as angioplasty and stent placement, can also be performed.

NONATHEROSCLEROTIC ARTERIAL DISEASES

There are several congenital and acquired diseases that cause cerebrovascular arterial disease and narrowing (Table 5-4). Vasculopathy is a general term.

Hypoplasia or Aplasia

The A1 and P1 segments of the anterior and posterior cerebral arteries respectively are most commonly seen. The A2 segment is fed by the contralateral anterior cerebral artery via a patent Acom. The P2 segment is fed through a prominent Pcom, which is known as "fetal origin" of the posterior cerebral artery.

TABLE 5-4 Nonatherosclerotic Causes of Cerebrovascular Arterial Disease

Congenital	Hypoplasia or aplasia
	Neurofibromatosis
	Tuberous sclerosis
	Idiopathic progressive arteriopathy of childhood (Moyamoya)
Traumatic	Dissection
Vasospasm	Subarachnoid hemorrhage
	Catheter manipulation
	Migraine
Neoplastic	Compression by tumor
	Radiation vasculitis
Hematologic	Sickle cell disease
Infectious vasculitis	Tuberculosis
	Syphilis
	Fungal: aspergillosis
	Viral: Herpes simplex and HIV
Noninfectious vasculitis	Sarcoid
	Collagen vascular disease: SLE, rheumatoid, and scleroderma
	Primary arteritis of CNS
	Polyarteritis nodosa
	Giant cell (temporal) arteritis
	Wegener granulomatosis
	Takayasu arteritis
	Behcet disease
	Drug-induced
	Radiation
Compressive	Skull base fracture involving carotid canal
	Cervical spine fracture or subluxation involving the transverse foramina
	Osteophyte from cervical spine degeneration
	Neoplasm
Idiopathic	Fibromuscular dysplasia

Neurofibromatosis

Although uncommonly affects the cerebrovascular circulation, it is considered the most common neurocutaneous syndrome that produce vascular abnormality. In this case, basal arterial stenosis is seen with a Moyamoyalike pattern of collateral blood flow. There are four pathologic types: pure intimal, advanced intimal, intimal aneurysmal, and nodular. Many of the lesions have features of more than one of the pure types. It is proposed that the pathogenesis of all of the types of arterial lesions is proliferation of Schwann cells within arteries with secondary fibrosis.

Tuberous Sclerosis

It rarely affects the cerebrovascular circulation. There is ectasia and aneurysms of the intracranial circulation seen in these cases.

Idiopathic Progressive Arteriopathy of Childhood (Moyamoya)

There is progressive narrowing of the distal supraclinoid ICA and proximal anterior and middle cerebral arteries. The posterior circulation is less commonly involved with stenosis seen in the distal basilar and proximal posterior cerebral arteries. Multiple punctuate hypodensities are seen in the basal ganglia that enhance following the administration of contrast and represent enlarged lenticulostriate and thalamoperforate arteries providing collateral flow. CTA shows the stenotic lesions and collateral flow.

On MRI, the basal ganglia collateral circulation will be seen as flow voids on all pulse sequences. Flow void basal cisternal wormlike filling defects are best seen on T2-weighted images. The sulci will appear bright on FLAIR images because of slow flow within engorged pial collaterals. MRI may also show infarcts. Postcontrast images will demonstrate enhancement of the basal ganglia and leptomeningeal collateral vessels. MRA will show similar findings to CTA. On conventional angiography, the lateral views will demonstrate the lenticulostriate and thalamoperforate collateral vessels appearing as a "puff of smoke" (Moyamoya).

Sickle Cell Disease

It is caused by abnormality in hemoglobin (Hb) synthesis leading to the formation of Hb S, which produces sickling of the RBCs and capillary occlusion leading to ischemia and infarction. Sickle cell disease is the most common cause of infarction in African American children, and the incidence of stroke is significantly decreased by blood transfusion.

Vasculopathy occurs in approximately 50% of cases and involves the distal ICA and proximal ACA and MCA, similar to Moyamoya disease. The adherence of the abnormal sickled RBCs to the endothelium initiates endothelial injury, which is then followed by fragmentation of the internal elastic lamina and degeneration of the media.

The imaging findings are related to two factors: vasculopathy resulting in stenosis, and capillary occlusion leading to ischemia and infarction. On CT, infarctions may be cortical caused by vascular occlusion. Watershed ACA–MCA infarcts may also occur because of vascular stenosis. Multiple punctuate hypodensities are seen in the basal ganglia because of lenticulostriate arteries collateralization and will enhance on postcontrast images. On MRI, cortical and deep white matter watershed infarcts are seen and diffusion imaging better delineates acute infarcts. Basal ganglia collateral circulation will be seen as flow voids on all pulse sequences. The sulci will appear bright on FLAIR images because of slow flow within engorged pial collaterals. MRI may also show infarcts. Postcontrast images will demonstrate enhancement of the basal ganglia and leptomeningeal collaterals. CTA, MRA, and conventional angiography will demonstrate stenosis of the supraclinoid ICA and proximal ACA and MCA, with a Moyamoyalike pattern on lateral views.

Primary Arteritis of Central Nervous System

Idiopathic primary vasculitis that is only confined to the intracranial cerebrovascular circulation and characterized by ischemic lesions and small petechial hemorrhages. Pathologically, the presence of mononuclear inflammation with necrosis of the blood vessel wall is characteristic. The disease may involve any vessel (arteries and veins), of any size and can occur in childhood through adulthood. The affected vessels may show alternating stenosis and dilatation, and the degree of vessel narrowing may range from mild stenosis to complete occlusion resulting in infarction. Involvement of the venules may lead to parenchymal hemorrhage.

Areas of infarction are usually seen in the deep gray matter and subcortical white matter on CT and MRI. Patchy areas of enhancement may also be seen, while GRE images may show hypointense areas from petechial hemorrhage. On angiography, alternating areas of stenosis and dilatation are usually demonstrated in the affected vessels; however, long segment stenosis or complete occlusion may also be seen.

Vasculitis

Vasculitis can be classified as infectious and noninfectious (Table 5-4). It can also be classified according to the size of the involved arteries into large, medium, and small vessel vasculitis (Table 5-5).

TABLE 5-5 Classification of Vasculitis Based on the Size of the Affected Vessel

Large vessel vasculitis (ICA, BA, A1,M1 and P1)	Viral: Herpes simplex type 1, HZV, and HIV
	Tuberculosis
	Syphilis
	Bacterial meningitis
	Sarcoid
	Primary arteritis of CNS
	Scleroderma
	Takayasu arteritis
	Giant cell (temporal) arteritis
	Idiopathic progressive arteriopathy of childhood (Moyamoya)
Medium vessel vasculitis (distal to MCA bifurcation/trifurcation, distal to Acom and Pcom)	SLE Polyarteritis nodosa Kawasaki disease Behcet's disease
Small vessel vasculitis	SLE
	Rheumatoid
	Henoch-Schoenlein purpura
	Wegener granulomatosis
	Churg-Strauss syndrome

The imaging features of vasculitis include direct and indirect signs. Direct signs include vessel wall thickening and enhancement which is best seen on high resolution thin section contrast-enhanced T1 fat-suppressed images. Evaluation of large vessel vasculitis may be done using this technique, while medium and small vessel vasculitis is usually beyond the resolution of this technique. With thin sections, the walls of the arteries are normally invisible and any thickening in the wall should be considered abnormal. Enhancement is usually restricted to the walls of acutely inflamed arteries; however, it may extend into the adjacent leptomeninges.

Indirect signs include perfusion deficits, multiple infarcts of different ages, intracerebral or subarachnoid hemorrhage, and vascular stenosis atypical for atherosclerosis. Nonspecific patchy areas of enhancement may also be seen. MRI is the imaging modality of choice in these cases and may be supplemented by MR perfusion sequence to detect perfusion deficits. MRA of the neck and brain arteries will demonstrate arterial irregularities or alternating stenosis and dilatations of the affected arteries. Arterial occlusion can also be seen.

Conventional angiography is the technique of choice for medium vessel vasculitis which is usually beyond the resolution of MRA. Irregularity, stenosis, dilatation, and occlusion can be seen in the involved second- and third-order branches. Microaneurysms may be seen in polyarteritis nodosa.

TABLE 5-6 Types of Fibromuscular Dysplasia

TYPE	INCIDENCE	ANGIOGRAPHIC FEATURE
Intimal fibroplasia	1%	Ringlike stenosis Smooth tubular stenosis
Medial fibroplasia: Three subtypes		
a. Medial dysplasia	65%	Alternating webs and aneurysms resulting in classic "string of beads"
b. Perimedial fibroplasia	20%	Alternating webs and aneurysms resulting in "string of beads," but the beads (aneurysms) are not larger than the diameter of the original vessel
c. Medial hyperplasia	10%	Tubular smooth stenosis
Adventitial fibroplasia	<1%	Tubular smooth stenosis

FIBROMUSCULAR DYSPLASIA

Fibromuscular dysplasia (FMD) is a nonatherosclerotic, noninflammatory arterial disease of unknown etiology. It is a collection of fibrotic disorders that can involve the intima media or adventitia of medium-sized arteries. In the cerebrovascular circulation, the disease more commonly affects the extracranial cervical ICA in 75% of cases. The external carotid artery and the cervical vertebral artery are less commonly involved. Bilateral ICA affection is seen in approximately 65% of cases. The disease is more common in young females. The disease is associated with intracranial aneurysms in 30% of cases and with spontaneous carotid artery dissection in as many as 10% to 20% of cases. Therefore, patients may present with Horner syndrome, TIAs, ischemic stroke, or subarachnoid hemorrhage.

There are five types of FMD (Table 5-6). Medial dysplasia is by far the most common type, and it should be noted that the incidence of the various types of FMD outlined in the table is from large renal studies and may not reflect the incidence of different FMD types in carotid disease.

SUGGESTED READING

Eastwood JD, Engelter ST, MacFall JF, et al. Quantitative assessment of the time course of infarct signal intensity on diffusion-weighted images. *AJNR Am J Neuroradiol*. 2003;24: 680-687.

Gonzalez RG. Imaging-guided acute ischemic stroke therapy: from "Time is Brain" to "Physiology Is Brain". *AJNR Am J Neuroradiol*. 2006;27:728-735.

Kadkhodayan Y, Alreshaid A, Moran CJ, et al. Primary angiitis of the central nervous system at conventional angiography. *Radiology*. 2004;233:878-882.

Kuker W. Cerebral vasculitis: imaging signs revisited. *Neuroradiology*. 2007;49:471-479.

Lansberg MG, Thijs VN, O'Brien MW, et al. Evolution of apparent diffusion coefficient, diffusion-weighted, and T2-weighted signal intensity of acute stroke. *AJNR Am J Neuroradiol*. 2001;22:637-644.

Leach JL, Wolujewicz M, Strub WM. Partially recanalized chronic dural sinus thrombosis: findings on MR imaging, time-of-flight MR venography, and contrast-enhanced MR Venography. *AJNR Am J Neuroradiol*. 2007;28:782-789.

Salyer WR. The vascular lesions of neurofibromatosis. *Angiology*. 1974;25(8):510-519.

Schaefer PW, Ozsunar Y, He J, et al. Assessing tissue viability with MR diffusion and perfusion imaging. *AJNR Am J Neuroradiol*. 2003;24:436-443.

Slovut DP, Olin JW. Fibromuscular dysplasia. *N Engl J Med*. 2004;350:1862-1871.

Sunshine JL, Bambakidis N, Tarr RW, et al. Benefits of perfusion MR imaging relative to diffusion MR imaging in the diagnosis and treatment of hyperacute stroke. *AJNR Am J Neuroradiol*. 2001;22:915-921.

QUESTIONS AND ANSWERS

1. In acute infarction, all the following are *true* except:
   A. Noncontrast CT mainly serves to exclude hemorrhage as the cause of stroke.
   B. Hyperdensity within an artery on noncontrast CT represents acute thrombus.
   C. Loss of gray–white matter distinction, with obscuration of the deep gray matter nuclei are seen on noncontract CT.
   D. Hypodensity in a specific vascular territory is by far the most common finding.

   ANSWER: D. Hypodensity in a specific vascular territory is less commonly seen.

2. Which of the following is the most correct about enhancement patterns in acute infarction on contrast-enhanced CT?
   A. Enhancement of the cortical vessels may be secondary to slow antegrade flow.
   B. Cortical gyral enhancement usually begins at 2 weeks.
   C. Enhancement of the cortical vessels may be because of retrograde flow from collaterals.
   D. Cortical gyral enhancement starts to disappear at 2 months.

   ANSWER: B. Cortical gyral enhancement usually begins at approximately 1 week and peaks at 10 days to 2 weeks. This usually subsides by 4 months. As the blood brain barrier breaks down, the tissues and residual supply vessels become leaky. This results in a mix of enhancement and sometimes overlapping laminar necrosis. Laminar necrosis may have some precontrast hyperdensity from calcification. Enhancement of the vessels in stroke is seen better on MRI (T1 shortening) than CT. On CT, the hyperdense appearance may be from clot and not enhancement.

3. On CT perfusion, which of the following is *true*?
   A. The CBV and MTT are decreased and CBF is increased in the infarct.
   B. The CBV, CBF, and MTT are decreased in the ischemic area.
   C. The CBV and CBF are decreased and MTT is increased in infarct area.
   D. CBV and MTT are decreased and CBF is normal or increased in ischemic area.

   ANSWER: C. The CBV and CBF are decreased and MTT is increased in infarct area. The CBF is decreased, MTT is increased, and the CBV is normal or slightly increased in the ischemic area.

4. On diffusion MRI, which of the following is *false*?
   A. Diffusion imaging is the most sensitive sequence in detecting hyperacute infarction.
   B. Cytotoxic edema leads to restriction of motion of the water molecules mainly in the extracellular space.
   C. After 7 to 10 days, pseudonormalization occurs.
   D. The area of restricted diffusion is seen as hypointense on DWI and hyperintense on ADC maps.

   ANSWER: C. The area of restricted diffusion is seen as hyperintense on DWI and hypointense on ADC maps.

5. Concerning nontraumatic intracranial hemorrhage, which of the following is *true*?
   A. Intracerebral hemorrhage in adults accounts for 25% of cases.
   B. The most common location is in the basal ganglia.
   C. Amyloid angiopathy accounts for approximately 60% of nontraumatic intracerebral hemorrhages.
   D. Lobar hemorrhages in the same age may be seen most commonly in the occipital and temporal lobes.

   ANSWER: B. Intracerebral hemorrhage in adults accounts for 70% to 90% of cases. The most common location is in the basal ganglia. Amyloid angiopathy accounts for approximately 10% to 20% of nontraumatic intracerebral hemorrhages. Lobar hemorrhages are seen in different ages and most commonly in the frontal and parietal lobes.

6. In dural venous sinus thrombosis, which of the following is *false*?
   A. Most commonly involved is the superior sagittal sinus.
   B. Females are more commonly affected than males.
   C. "Empty delta" sign is seen in almost all cases.
   D. Venous infarct may be seen in 50% of cases.

   ANSWER: A. "Empty delta" sign is seen in 25% of cases.

7. In dural venous sinus thrombosis, which of the following is *true*?
   A. The thrombus can be easily seen in the acute phase.
   B. In the subacute stage, the thrombus will appear hypointense on both T1 and T2 images.
   C. In the chronic stage, the thrombus will not enhance on postcontrast images.
   D. TOF MRV is limited in the acute stage by the T1 hypointensity of the thrombus.
   E. CE-MRV is limited in evaluation of chronic thrombus.

   ANSWER: E. It is difficult to detect the thrombus in the acute phase, since deoxyhemoglobin will be isointense on T1 and hypointense on T2 images and therefore indistinguishable from normal flow voids in most cases. In the subacute stage, the thrombus will appear hyperintense on both T1- and T2-weighted images. In chronic sinus thrombosis, heeling by organizing fibrous tissue will produce enhancement on postcontrast images. TOF MRV is limited in the subacute stage by the T1 hyperintensity of the thrombus, which falsely appears as patent sinus with normal flow. The utilization of CE-MRV in the diagnosis of chronic thrombosis has been questioned because of possible intense enhancement of the chronic thrombus that will produce an erroneous appearance of a patent sinus.

8. Regarding atherosclerotic vascular disease, which of the following is *true*?
   A. It accounts for 50% of cerebral thromboembolic infarcts.
   B. The most common location for atherosclerosis is the distal ICA.
   C. CTA can be used to characterize the constituents of the plaque by assigning different colors for different densities within the plaque.

   ANSWER: C. It accounts for 90% of cerebral thromboembolic infarcts. The most common location for atherosclerosis is the CCA bifurcation and the proximal ICA. Intracranially, atherosclerotic disease is most commonly seen in the carotid siphons and vetebrobasilar arteries.

9. Regarding idiopathic progressive arteriopathy of childhood, which of the following is *false*?
   A. There is progressive narrowing of the distal supraclinoid internal carotid artery and proximal anterior and middle cerebral arteries.
   B. Basal ganglia collateral circulation will be seen as flow voids.
   C. The lateral views of conventional angiography will demonstrate the lenticulostriate and thalamoperforate collateral vessels appearing as a "puff of smoke".
   D. FLAIR images will be normal.

   ANSWER: D. Basal ganglia collateral circulation will be seen as flow voids on FLAIR. The sulci will appear bright on FLAIR images because of slow flow within engorged pial collaterals.

10. Regarding fibromuscular dysplasia, which of the following is *false*?
    A. FMD is a nonatherosclerotic, noninflammatory arterial disease of unknown etiology.
    B. In the cerebrovascular circulation, the disease more commonly affects the extracranial cervical ICA in 75% of cases.
    C. Bilateral ICA affection is seen in approximately 35% of cases.
    D. The disease is associated with intracranial aneurysms in 30% of cases.
    E. The disease is associated with spontaneous carotid artery dissection in as many as 10% to 20% of cases.

    ANSWER: C. Bilateral ICA affection is seen in approximately 65% of cases.

6 INTRACRANIAL ANEURYSMS AND VASCULAR MALFORMATIONS

Ahmed Kamel Abdel Aal and Joseph C. Sullivan III

INTRACRANIAL ANEURYSMS

Aneurysms are usually asymptomatic until they rupture, and they account for approximately 80% to 90% of nontraumatic subarachnoid hemorrhage, resulting in unfavorable outcome in most cases with mortality and morbidity as high as 50%. There are three general types of aneurysms: saccular (berry), fusiform, and blisterlike aneurysms. Pseudoaneurysms are a pathologically different entity.

SACCULAR ANEURYSM

Saccular aneurysms are rounded berrylike outpouchings, the wall of which is formed only of intima and adventitia. The intima protrudes through a defect in the media and internal elastic lamina. Approximately 95% arise from the circle of Willis (COW), most commonly at the arterial bifurcation or trifurcation, since these areas are subject to high biomechanical shear stress. Approximately 90% arise in the anterior circulation at the ICA, PCOM junction, at the ACOM, or at the ICA bifurcation/trifurcation. Other less common sites include basilar apex aneurysms and PICA, which constitute around 5% to 10% of cases.

Aneurysms are rare in children; peak age is between 40 and 60 years. Multiple aneurysms are seen in approximately 20% of cases. Although there is no evidence for congenital origin of these aneurysms and the proposed etiology is biomechanical arterial wall stress, there is increased incidence among patients with positive family history. Predisposing factors include adult polycystic kidney disease, coarctation of the aorta, fibromuscular dysplasia, Marfan syndrome, Ehler-Danlos syndrome, and connective tissue disorders such as systemic lupus erythematosus.

The most common clinical presentation is SAH secondary to aneurysm rupture. Cranial neuropathy may also be seen and will preferentially involve the occulomotor nerve in case of ICA–PCOM junction aneurysm. The outer fibers of the nerve are affected first, leading to pupillary dilatation. Patients may also present with stroke related to infarction caused by either emboli showering from the aneurysm sac or by SAH-induced vasospasm. Another cause of stroke in these patients is rupture of the aneurysm into the brain parenchyma leading to intracerebral hemorrhage.

The size of the aneurysm ranges from few millimeters to several centimeters. Giant aneurysms are defined as those larger than 2.5 cm in diameter. The risk of rupture depends primarily on the size of the aneurysm. Generally, the risk of rupture is minimal for aneurysms less than 7 mm and is very high for those greater than 2.5 cm. Other factors that predispose to aneurysm rupture include the configuration of the aneurysm, its location, and presence of hypertension. A multilobed aneurysm, the presence of a "tit" or "daughter aneurysm" at its apex, and a sac-to-neck ratio of greater than 1.6 also increase risk of rupture.

On noncontrast CT, ruptured aneurysm may produce regional SAH that helps predict aneurysm location. Predominance of SAH in the suprasellar cistern suggests ruptured ICA–PCOM junction aneurysm, while interhemispheric SAH and sylvian fissure SAH suggest ruptured ACOM and MCA aneurysms, respectively. Other complications include parenchymal hemorrhage, infarction, and hydrocephalus. CTA is the modality of choice for evaluating suspected aneurysms and is positive in roughly 95% of patients with ruptured aneurysms.

The appearance of aneurysms on MRI is more complex and depends on the flow within and the patency of the aneurysm sac. An aneurysm sac with high flow will appear signal void on T1- and T2-weighted images. The partial or complete obliteration of the aneurysm sac will produce a signal abnormality dependent on the age of the clot. Sometimes a laminated appearance is seen corresponding to different ages of layered thrombus. Diffusion imaging may demonstrate infarctions related to SAH-induced vasospasm. Gandolinium-enhanced MR may demonstrate hyperintensity in a patent aneurysm with significantly slow flow. Pulsation artifacts in the phase-encoding direction are helpful in localizing small aneurysms. 3D TOF MRA is valuable in showing patent aneurysms. MRA using spoiled gradient technique appears to be more sensitive than 3D TOF MRA for peripheral, smaller aneurysms, although not routinely performed by many institutions. With the improvements in multidetector CTA, digital subtraction angiography (DSA) is performed only when endovascular treatment using detachable coils is considered. Following coil placement, 3D TOF MRA without and with contrast using short TE and subtraction technique may help show residual lumen on follow-up studies.

FUSIFORM ANEURYSM

Fusiform aneurysm is usually caused by atherosclerosis in older patients. However, other etiologies include collagen vascular disease, HIV, Marfan syndrome, Ehler-Danlos syndrome, and neurofibromatosis (NF) type 1, mostly in young patients. Clinically, patients present with symptoms and signs related to mass effect of the dilated artery. They may also present with stroke from emboli showering from clots formed within the aneurysm.

CTA and MRA reveal a long segment of fusiform arterial dilatation usually involving a nonbranching segment. The basilar artery is more commonly involved. On MRI, the aneurysm will appear as flow void on T1, T2, and FLAIR images, unless a clot is formed giving a laminated appearance. Diffusion imaging helps depict infarction related to embolic complications.

BLISTERLIKE ANEURYSM

These are small broad-based aneurysms arising from the arterial wall, primarily composed of fibrous tissue. The most common location is the supraclinoid ICA. These aneurysms usually occur in middle-aged patients and tend to rupture at an earlier age and smaller size than saccular aneurysms. CTA shows asymmetric broad-based bulge of the supraclinoid ICA.

PSEUDOANEURYSM

The walls of these aneurysms are formed of organized clot and fibrin without any layers of the normal arterial wall. These are formed by rupture of an artery leading to the formation of a focal perivascular hematoma. The hematoma then cavitates and communicates with the arterial lumen through a narrow neck. The most important etiologies for pseudoaneurysm are infections (mycotic aneurysms), trauma, neoplasm, and drug abuse. They commonly occur at the distal MCA or, less commonly, the distal ACA branches. Pseudoaneurysms can occur at any age of life.

On noncontrast CT, perivascular high-density hematoma can be seen. On CTA, a focal collection of contrast within the hematoma is noted and communicates with the lumen of the adjacent parent artery. The appearance of the perivascular hematoma on MRI is variable and depends on its age. Flow void within the hematoma corresponds to the focal collection of contrast identified on CTA. The hematoma will appear hypointense on GRE images. Diffusion imaging may demonstrate infarction related to emboli showering from clots formed in the pseudoaneurysm. On 3D TOF MRA, the hematoma will appear hyperintense because of T1 shortening and will therefore obscure the pseudoaneurysm. Therefore, CE-MRA or phase-contrast MRA is better in this context.

VASCULAR MALFORMATIONS

Cerebrovascular malformations are a heterogeneous group of congenital anomalies affecting the blood vessels of the brain. The traditional classification of vascular malformations was historically based on their dominant pathologic features, either precapillary or postcapillary vascular malformations. Precapillary vascular malformations include arteriovenous malformations (AVM). Postcapillary vascular malformations include developmental venous anomaly, cavernous malformation, and capillary telangiectasia. With advances in endovascular therapy and the need to identify arteriovenous shunting before intervention, vascular malformations were reclassified. Vascular malformations with arteriovenous shunting include arteriovenous malformation, dural arteriovenous fistula, and vein on Galen malformation. Vascular malformations without arteriovenous shunting include developmental venous anomaly, cavernous malformation, capillary telangiectasia, and sinus pericranii.

ARTERIOVENOUS MALFORMATION

AVM are congenital lesions, although they are rarely diagnosed early in life. There is no familial association or associated specific gene mutation. AVM is most likely caused by dysregulated angiogenesis. Pathologically, this lesion is characterized by large feeding arteries supplying a nidus of thin dysplastic vessels devoid of any capillary bed. The draining veins are enlarged, often with a venous varix or stenosis related to high-velocity blood flow. There is absent normal brain within the nidus. The adjacent brain may show perinidal capillary network as well as hemorrhagic residue.

Approximately 85% AVM occur in the cerebral hemispheres, while 15% occur in the posterior fossa. Multiple lesions are extremely rare and likely seen in hereditary hemorrhagic telangiectasia. AVM is the most common symptomatic vascular malformation, usually presenting between 20 and 40 years of age. Intracranial hemorrhage is the most common presentation occurring in approximately 50% of patients, including intraparenchymal, intraventricular, or subarachnoid hemorrhage. Patients may also present with seizures or other neurologic symptoms.

Spetzler graded these lesions using points for size, location in eloquent brain, and pattern of venous drainage (Table 6-1). Grades 1 to 3 are considered low morbidity for surgical intervention, while grade 6 is considered inoperable. The risk of hemorrhage is increased if there is associated intranidal aneurysm, venous varix, stenosis of the draining vein, central venous drainage, and periventricular location.

Noncontrast CT may show intracranial hemorrhage. The AVM may appear as serpentine isodense or hyperdense lesion without mass effect or surrounding edema. Calcification may also be present, and the lesion will enhance avidly on contrast-enhanced CT. On MRI, the appearance is complex and depends on the flow rate and the presence and age of hemorrhage. Classically, AVM appears as serpentine flow voids, a "bag of worms," without mass effect or edema. Adjacent hyperintense gliosis can extend around the lesion, identified on T2 and FLAIR images. GRE images will demonstrate blooming hypointense blood products. Contrast-enhanced images may demonstrate hyperintensity in an AVM with a significantly slow flow. MRA and MRV generally do not provide additional information.

TABLE 6-1 Spetzler Classification of AVM

Size	Small <3 cm = 1
	Medium 3–6 cm = 2
	Large >6 cm = 3
Location	Noneloquent area = 0
	Eloquent area = 1
Venous drainage	Superficial = 0
	Deep = 1

Cerebral angiogram is valuable in delineating the feeding arteries, draining veins, as well as the angioarchitecture of the AVM. It appears as a tightly packed mass of vessels. Arterial feeders could be pial, dural, or both. The presence of intranidal aneurysm, venous varix, or stenosis in the draining vein should be sought in these studies, since these are associated with high risk of hemorrhage. Treatment includes percutaneous embolization, radiosurgery or microvascular surgery, or a combination of the above.

DURAL ARTERIOVENOUS FISTULA

Dural arteriovenous fistula (DAVF) account for only 15% of intracranial vascular malformations and consist of a network of tiny vessels in the wall of a dural venous sinus. Consensus is that these are acquired lesions, likely caused by venous sinus thrombosis, supported by the fact that most cases have a history of prior local trauma or hypercoagulability state. Regardless of the cause, neoangiogenesis occurring in granulation tissue create a network of proliferating capillaries and microfistulae that drain into the dural venous sinus, a cortical vein, or both.

The most common location for DAVF is the transverse (sigmoid) sinus followed by the cavernous sinus (carotid–cavernous fistula). Middle-aged patients are usually affected and the clinical presentation depends upon the location. Transverse sinus lesion presents with pulsatile tinnitus, while carotid–cavernous fistula presents with pulsatile exophthalmus, papilledema, and loss of vision. In severe cases, venous hypertension may ensue leading to thrombosis and ischemia. Intracranial hemorrhage may occur in aggressive lesions. Cognard classified DAVF according to the pattern of venous drainage, which correlates with the risk of hemorrhage (Table 6-2). Barrow classified carotid–cavernous fistulas according to their arterial supply (Table 6-3).

Noncontrast CT is usually normal and contrast CT may show tortuous dural arterial feeders and enlarged dural venous sinus. In carotid–cavernous fistula, the superior and sometimes the inferior ophthalmic veins are enlarged. CTA is valuable in detecting small lesions and demonstrating with greater conspicuity the arterial feeders. Aggressive DAVF can create enlarged cortical veins.

TABLE 6-2 Cognard Classification of Dural Arteriouvenous Fistula

TYPE	PATTERN OF VENOUS DRAINAGE	RISK OF HEMORRHAGE (%)
Type I	Drains into the sinus with antegrade flow	
Type II A	Drains into the sinus with retrograde flow into the sinus but not cortical veins	
Type II B	Drains into the sinus with retrograde flow into the sinus and cortical veins	10
Type III	Drains into cortical vein without venous ectasia	40
Type IV	Drains into cortical vein with venous ectasia	65
Type V	Spinal perimedulary veins	

On MRI, thrombosed dural venous sinus will appear hyperintense on T1- and T2-weighted images and will enhance on post contrast images. Tiny flow voids at the wall of the sinus represent DAVF and hyperintensity in the adjacent brain parenchyma on FLAIR images is related to venous hypertension or infarction. The appearance of associated parenchymal hemorrhage depends on its age. MRV shows the occluded sinus and 3D PC MRA, especially when low velocity encoding is implemented and depicts the arterial feeders and the direction of flow in the draining sinuses or veins.

On angiography, multiple arterial feeders are usually identified, supplying "cracklike vessels on a dural venous sinus wall" and draining into the sinus or cortical vein. The most common arterial feeders are the meningeal branches of the ECA. Other arterial feeders may arise from the dural and tentorial branches of the ICA, especially the tentorial branch of the meningohypophyseal trunk (artery of Bernasconi Casinary), and from the vertebral artery. The draining venous sinus is either thrombosed or appears deformed because of recanalization. If the DAVF drains into a cortical vein, the high flow may lead to venous stenosis and hemorrhage. The DAVF may drain into a cortical venous collecting pouch that is separable from the normal venous drainage of the adjacent brain and in such a case it can be amenable to percutaneous transvenous embolization.

TABLE 6-3 Barrow Classification of Carotid–Cavernous Fistula

TYPE	ARTERIAL FEEDERS
Type A	No DAVF Direct flow from cavernous segment of ICA Usually secondary to trauma and skull base fracture
Type B	DAVF supplied by ICA branches
Type C	DAVF supplied by ECA branches
Type D	DAVF supplied by ICA and ECA branches

VEIN OF GALEN MALFORMATION

Vein of Galen malformation (VOGM) is an arteriovenous fistula draining into an aneurysmally dilated median prosencephalic vein of Markowski and is therefore a misnomer. Median prosencephalic vein is part of the fetal venous system that normally drains the choroid plexus and is the precursor of vein of Galen. At about the 10th week of gestation, the cranial aspect of the vein regresses, while the caudal portion persists and joins the internal cerebral veins to become the vein of Galen. Arteriovenous fistula occurs around the 10th to 12th week gestational age and leads to dilatation of the median prosencephalic vein, producing what is known as vein of Galen malformation. The arterial feeders are most commonly the posterior choroidal arteries, followed by the anterior cerebral arteries. In 50% of cases, the dilated median prosencephalic vein drains into a persistent embryonic falcine sinus, and as such, the straight sinus will be absent or severely hypoplastic. High flow within the draining venous sinuses may lead to stenosis or thrombosis.

VOGM is located in the quadrigeminal cistern or velum interpositum cistern. It usually presents in infants and is twice more common in males than females. The high-flow arteriovenous shunt causes cranial bruit and subsequently will lead to high output congestive heart failure. Ischemia or infarction can be seen secondary to arterial steal or because of chronic venous hypertension related to dural venous sinus stenosis. Hydrocephalus may also occur and is also related to impaired drainage caused by dural venous sinus stenosis.

On noncontrast CT, the enlarged venous pouch in the quadrigeminal cistern will appear hyperdense and calcification may be seen. On contrast-enhanced CT and CTA, the feeding arteries appear enlarged; the dilated median prosencephalic vein will appear as a venous pouch that significantly enhances. On MRI, the arterial feeders and dilated median prosencephalic vein will appear signal void. Complex signal is sometimes seen in median prosencephalic vein related to turbulence. Hydrocephalus may be seen and diffusion images are helpful in demonstrating areas of infarction. MRA is also helpful in demonstrating the arterial feeders.

Conventional angiograms are very important in differentiating VOGM from vein of Galen dilatation. In VOGM, there is persistence of the fetal circulation, and the thalamostriate veins will drain into the thalamic and subtemporal veins, which eventually drain in the superior petrosal sinus, producing "epsilon vein" on the venous phase of lateral angiograms. The arteriovenous fistula will drain into median prosencephalic vein that is not connected to the deep venous system. The median prosencephalic vein will drain into transverse sinus or the falcine sinus. In vein of Galen dilatation, there is an AVM located in the cerebellum, brainstem, or in the deep supratentorial territories that drains into one of the tributaries of the vein of Galen. The vein of Galen is fully developed and drains not only the lesion but also the adjacent brain parenchyma. The dilatation of the vein of the vein of Galen is variable and depends on the outflow obstruction caused by stenosis or thrombosis that usually occurs at the junction of the vein with the straight sinus.

DEVELOPMENTAL VENOUS ANOMALY

Developmental venous anomaly (DVA) is congenital venous vascular malformation resulting from arrest of medullary vein development. It can be viewed as an extreme anatomic venous variant rather than a true vascular malformation. It is the most common of all vascular malformations, representing approximately 60% to 70% of cases. Pathologically, it is formed from multiple medullary veins that are radially oriented forming "caput medusae," which drain into a larger "collector" vein. The "collector" vein may drain superficially into a dural sinus or cortical vein or may drain deeply into a subependymal vein. The intervening and surrounding brain is normal, and these venous malformations are physiologically important since they provide normal venous drainage. DVA may be complicated by spontaneous thrombosis of the draining vein or sinus leading to parenchymal hemorrhage or infarction of the region of the brain that it drains.

DVA is typically solitary; multiple lesions are extremely uncommon. DVA can occur at any age. Approximately 65% of cases occur in the supratentorial compartment with the frontal lobe being the most common location. Patients are most commonly asymptomatic, and these lesions will be seen incidentally on imaging studies performed for unrelated indications. Occasionally, the patients may present with seizure, headache, or other neurologic deficit, particularly if DVA is associated with other vascular malformation. DVA may be complicated by spontaneous thrombosis of the draining vein or sinus leading to parenchymal hemorrhage or infarction of the region of the brain drained by the anomaly.

Noncontrast CT is usually normal, but may show calcification if DVA is associated with other vascular malformations. On contrast-enhanced CT, the collector vein may be seen as a linear enhancing structure. CTA may show the "caput medusae" near the angle of a ventricle as well as the drainage pathway of the "collector" vein.

The appearance of DVA on MRI is variable depending on the flow rate and will appear classically as linear signal void structure on T1 and T2 in its characteristic location. A thrombosed draining vein or dural venous sinus will appear hyperintense on T1, T2, and FLAIR images, and the resultant parenchymal hemorrhage will show variable signal depending on the age of the clot. Diffusion images are important in showing early venous infarction also related to draining pathway thrombosis. On postcontrast T1 images, the "collector" vein enhances, since the blood flow is slow enough to produce T1 shortening. In large developmental venous anomaly, the "caput medusae" pattern may be delineated. MRV may be diagnostic, while the venous phase of MRA may show high-flow DVA. On conventional angiography, the arterial phase is usually normal, while the venous phase shows the anomaly and demonstrates its drainage pathway. It is important to emphasize that approximately 10% are angiographically "occult," with studies completely normal.

CAVERNOUS MALFORMATION

Also known as cavernoma, cavernous malformation is a benign vascular hamartoma. Pathologically, it is formed of large closely packed thin walled vascular channels, lined by endothelium and lacking muscular and elastic layers. There is no normal brain within the lesion. The surrounding brain parenchyma shows a mixture of gliosis and chronic hemorrhagic residue.

Single lesion is seen in approximately 85% of cases; multiple lesions are rare and are thought to be a familial form. The most common associated vascular malformation is developmental venous anomaly, although it may also be associated with café au lait spots and cherry angiomas. The most common location is the subcortical white matter in the supratentorial compartment occurring in approximately 80% of cases. However, it can occur anywhere in the CNS including the spine, nerve roots and dural venous sinuses (especially the cavernous sinus). Patients usually present between 20 and 40 years of age. The most common presentation is seizure occurring in approximately 50% of cases, although patients may present with variable neurologic deficits. The size is variable ranging from 0.5 cm to greater than 6 cm.

On noncontrast CT, calcification may be identified in one-half of the cases, and contrast CT may reveal faint enhancement. CTA is usually negative. MRI is the modality of choice for diagnosis, which is classically described as "popcornlike" lesion. The lesion consists of a central area of multiloculated blood-containing spaces, with mixed hyper- and hypointensity on T1- and T2-weighted images and a peripheral zone of hypointense hemosiderin rim on T2-weighted and FLAIR images. There is no mass effect or surrounding edema. Cavernous malformation may be complicated by hemorrhage. In this instance, signal will depend on the age of hemorrhage. Similar to contrast CT, gadolinium-enhanced T1-

weighted images will demonstrate faint enhancement. GRE shows hypointense blooming lesion and is valuable in demonstrating small lesions that are not well seen on other sequences. MRA and MRV demonstrate no abnormality, unless there are other vascular malformations.

Cavernous malformation is the most common angiographically "occult" lesion and the study is usually normal. Rarely, a faint contrast blush may be seen in the venous phase.

CAPPILARY TELANGIECTASIA

Cappilary telangiectasia is the second most common vascular malformation following developmental venous anomaly. Pathologically, capillary telangiectasia represent cluster of ectatic capillaries, which is normal intervening brain parenchyma. The walls of the dilated capillaries are histologically identical to normal capillaries, lacking smooth muscles and elastic fibers. There is no gliosis, calcification, or residual hemorrhagic blood products in pure capillary telangiectasia.

Cappilary telangiectasia usually coexist with other vascular malformations, are usually clinically silent and are discovered incidentally with imaging for other indications. Symptomatic lesions are usually associated with other vascular malformation. They can be seen at any age and can be associated with hereditary hemorrhagic telangiectasia. The most common location is in the infratentorial compartment, particularly the brainstem. The spinal cord may also be involved.

CT is usually normal. On CTA, "brushlike" enhancement may be seen. MRI is the modality of choice, and the lesion may be seen as hyperintense on T2 and FLAIR images in about one-half of cases. GRE images are helpful in lesion diagnosis, which appears hypointense, but also serves to identify other smaller lesions that are otherwise occult. Postcontrast T1 images will show faint "brushlike" enhancement.

Similar to cavernous malformations, these lesions are angiographically "occult" in most cases and the study is usually normal. Rarely, a faint contrast blush may be seen in the venous phase.

SINUS PERICRANII

Sinus pericranii represents a communication between a dural venous sinus and the extracranial venous system, either directly (through a transcalvarial vein) or indirectly (through an intervening intracranial cortical vein and transcalvarial vein). Venous varix is usually seen on both sides of the calvarium.

The lesions are secondary to congenital failure of closure of the cranial sutures over venous sinuses or abnormal bone ossification. Those that are acquired may be caused by trauma, skull fracture, and emissary vein tear, or can be spontaneous. Associated abnormalities include systemic vascular malformations and blue rubber-bleb nevus syndrome.

Patients can present at any age, usually with nontender expansile scalp mass that increases in size in the prone position and on Valsalva maneuver and regresses in the upright position. The overlying skin is usually hairless and blue-tinged. There is a potential lifetime risk of hemorrhage and air embolism.

The superior sagittal sinus is most commonly involved, and therefore, sinus pericranii is usually seen in midline or paramedian location. On noncontrast CT, it appears as a soft-tissue mass representing venous varix, adjacent to a well-defined bone defect. Contrast CT and CT venography will demonstrate the enhancing varix and the transcalvarial vein passing through the bone defect. On MRI, the signal in the varix will depend on the flow rate, and classically, signal void is seen in high-flow lesions. The lesions will enhance on postcontrast T1-weighted images. Angiographically, sinus pericranii is identified on the venous phase.

SUGGESTED READING

Alvarez H, Monaco RG, Rodesch G, et al. Vein of Galen aneurysmal malformations. *Neuroimag Clin North Am*. 2007;17:189-206.

Brown RD, Jr., Flemming KD, Meyer FB, et al. Natural history, evaluation, and management of intracranial vascular malformations. *Mayo Clin Proc*. 2005;80(2):269-281.

Buxton N, Vloeberghs M. Sinus pericranii. Report of a case and review of literature. *Pediatr Neurosurg*. 1999;30:96-99.

Byrne JV. Cerebrovascular malformations. *Eur Radiol*. 2005;15:448-452.

Choi JH, Mohr JP. Brain arteriovenous malformations in adults. *Lancet Neurol*. 2005;4:299-308.

Clatterbuck RE, Hsu FPK, Spetzler RF, et al. Supratentorial arteriovenous malformations. *Neurosurgery*. 2005;57(1):164-167.

Kwon BJ, Han MH, Kang HS, et al. MR imaging findings of intracranial dural arteriovenous fistulas: relations with venous drainage patterns. *AJNR AM J Neuroradiol*. 2005;26:2500-2507.

Vattoth S, Purkayastha S, Jayadevan ER, et al. Bilateral cerebral venous angioma associated with varices: a case report and review of the literature. *AJNR AM J Neuroradiol*. 2005;26:2320-2322.

QUESTIONS AND ANSWERS

1. What is the most common clinical presentation of aneurysm?
   A. Subarachnoid hemorrhage
   B. Cranial neuropathy involving the occulomotor nerve

C. Infarction
D. Intracerebral hemorrhage

ANSWER: A. The most common clinical presentation is SAH that occurs with aneurysm rupture. Ruptured aneurysms account for approximately 80% to 90% of nontraumatic SAH. Cranial neuropathy may also be seen and will preferentially involve the occulomotor nerve in case of ICA–PCOM junction aneurysm.

2. What arterial layer(s) compose(s) the wall of saccular aneurysms?
   A. Media
   B. Media and adventitia
   C. Media, intima and adventitia
   D. Intima and adventitia

   ANSWER: D. The wall of saccular aneurysms is formed only of intima and adventitia. The intima protrudes through a defect in the media and internal elastic lamina.

3. A patient presents with suprasellar cistern haemorrhage on CT. What is the most likely aneurysm location?
   A. ACA aneurysm
   B. MCA bifurcation aneurysm
   C. ICA–PCOM aneurysm
   D. ACOM aneurysm

   ANSWER: C. Predominance of SAH in the suprasellar cistern suggests ruptured ICA–PCOM junction aneurysm, while interhemispheric SAH and sylvian fissure SAH suggest ruptured ACOM and MCA aneurysms, respectively.

4. Which of the following is *not* related to the risk of rupture of saccular aneurysms?
   A. Size of the aneurysm
   B. Configuration of the aneurysm
   C. Location of the aneurysm
   D. Age of the patient

   ANSWER: D. There is no relation between the risk of aneurysm rupture and the age of the patient.

5. What is the most common cause of fusiform aneurysm?
   A. Marfan syndrome
   B. Atherosclerosis
   C. Collagen vascular disease
   D. Ehler-Danlos syndrome

   ANSWER: B. Fusiform aneurysms are usually caused by atherosclerosis in the elderly. However, other etiologies include collagen vascular disease, HIV, Marfan syndrome, Ehler-Danlos syndrome, and neurofibromatosis (NF) type 1, and these mostly affect young patients.

6. What is the most common location of arteriovenous malformations?
   A. Midbrain
   B. Medulla
   C. Cerebral hemispheres
   D. Cerebellar hemispheres

   ANSWER: C. Approximately 85% AVMs occur in the cerebral hemispheres, while 15% occur in the posterior fossa.

7. According to Cognard classification, what is the type of dural arteriovenous fistula if it drains into an ectatic cortical vein?
   A. Type I
   B. Type IIB
   C. Type III
   D. Type IV

   ANSWER: D. Type IV has 65% risk of hemorrhage.

8. According to Barrow classification, what is the type of a carotid cavernous fistula if it is supplied by the ICA?
   A. Type A or B
   B. Type A, B, or C
   C. Type A, B, or D
   D. Type D

   ANSWER: C. Types A, B, and D have ICA involvement (Table 6-3).

9. What percentage of vascular malformations do developmental venous anomalies constitute?
   A. 10%–20%
   B. 30%–40%
   C. 60%–70%
   D. 80%–90%

   ANSWER: C. DVA is the most common of all vascular malformations, representing approximately 60% to 70% of cases.

10. What is the most common malformation associated with cavernous malformation?
    A. DVA
    B. Café au lait spots
    C. Cherry angiomas
    D. Capillary telangiectasia

    ANSWER: A. The most common associated vascular malformation is DVA, although it may also be associated with café au lait spots and cherry angiomas.

7 HEAD TRAUMA

Ahmed Kamel Abdel Aal and Joseph C. Sullivan III

INTRODUCTION

Trauma is the most common cause of death in children and young adults, with head injury being the major cause in 50% of cases. Motor vehicle collision is the most common cause of trauma; however, falls in anticoagulated elderly patients and nonaccidental injury in infants and children are other contributors.

PRIMARY MANIFESTATIONS OF HEAD TRAUMA

These include extra-axial manifestations such as epidural hemorrhage, subdural hemorrhage, and subarachnoid hemorrhage, and intra-axial manifestations such as diffuse axonal injury (DAI), cerebral cortical contusion, subcortical injuries, and intraventricular hemorrhage.

EXTRA-AXIAL MANIFESTATIONS

These are because of hemorrhage occurring outside the brain parenchyma.

Epidural hemorrhage is caused by forceful impact. It creates a hematoma that collects between the calvarium and dura (epidural space). Approximately 90% of cases are caused by arterial injury, usually the middle meningeal artery, while the remainders are caused by transgression of one of the sinuses by the fracture, resulting in venous bleed. The epidural hematoma occurs at the impact site (coup). Approximately 95% of cases are unilateral and supratentorial, of which two-thirds will be located at the temporoparietal region because of injury of the middle meningeal artery. Approximately 50% of cases will be associated with other injuries such as cerebral contusions or skull fractures.

About half of the patients will present after asymptomatic "lucid" interval following initial loss of consciousness. On nonenhanced CT, acute epidural hematoma will appear as biconvex or lentiform hyperdense extra-axial collection. If there is active hemorrhage at the time of scanning, mixed hyper/hypodense areas will be seen caused by low-density unclotted blood. Epidural hematoma does not cross the sutures (unless large with diastatic fracture), but will cross the dural reflections including the falx and the tentorium. Vertex epidural hematoma can occur, however it is rare and caused by injury of the superior sagittal sinus. In that case, the fracture is seen crossing the sinus. Subacute and chronic epidural hematoma will be isodense and hypodense on nonenhanced CT and both will demonstrate marginal enhancement following contrast administration. With MR imaging, the appearance of blood products depends on its temporal stage (Table 7-1).

Subdural hemorrhage occurs between the dura and arachnoid meningeal layers and usually results from trauma tearing the bridging cortical veins that cross the subdural space to drain into a dural venous sinus. Other less common causes include vascular malformations, extension of intracerebral hemorrhage into the subdural space, aneurysm rupture, and coagulopathy. The hemorrhage then spreads diffusely over the convexity of the cerebral hemispheres. Approximately 85% of cases are unilateral, and 95% are supratentorial. Nearly two-thirds of cases will be associated with other injuries, more commonly subarachnoid hemorrhage. Similar to epidural hematoma, patients may present after asymptomatic "lucid" interval following initial loss of consciousness.

On noncontrast CT, subdural hematoma appears as a crescent-shaped, extra-axial collection overlying the cerebral convexity. Subdural hematoma may cross the sutures, but will not cross the dural reflections such as the falx and the tentorium (Table 7-2). In the acute stage, the collection appears hyperdense, however, mixed hyper/hypodensity may be seen in cases of active bleeding (producing the "swirl" sign) and in cases of anemia and coagulopathy. In the subacute stage, the collection becomes isodense to the brain parenchyma, making it difficult to identify. Medial displacement of the gray–white matter junction may help in their identification unless the lesions are bilateral and symmetrical. Other signs

TABLE 7-1 CT and MRI Appearance of the Various Stages of Intracranial Hemorrhage

TIME	BLOOD PRODUCT	NECT	CECT	T1	T2	GRE
Hyperacute: 4–6 h	Intracellular oxy-Hgb	Hyperdense		Isointense	Hyperintense	Hypointense
Acute: 6 h-3 d	Intracellular deoxy-Hgb	Hyperdense		Isointense	Hypointense	Hypointense
Early subacute: 4–7 d	Intracellular met-Hgb	Isodense		Hyperintense	Hypointense	Hypointense
Late subacute: 1–4 wk	Extracellular met-Hgb	Isodense	Rim	Hyperintense	Hyperintense	Hypointense
Chronic: >4wk	Hemosiderin	Hypodense	Rim	Hypointense	Hypointense	Hypointense

TABLE 7-2 Epidural Versus Subdural Hemorrhage

EPIDURAL HEMORRHAGE	SUBDURAL HEMORRHAGE
Does not cross sutures	May cross sutures
May cross dural reflections (falx and tentorium)	Does not cross dural reflections
Biconvex or lentiform-shaped	Crescent-shaped
95% Unilateral	85% Unilateral
95% Supratentorial (two-thirds temporoparietal)	95% Supratentorial
90% Arterial bleed (middle meningeal artery) 10% Venous bleed (lacerated venous sinus)	More commonly caused by tear of bridging veins in the subdural space

that might help in the diagnosis include medial displacement of the effaced sulci (appearing as tiny hypodensities) and medial displacement of the cortical vein together with rim enhancement (seen on contrast-enhanced CT). In the chronic stage, the collection appears hypodense to the brain parenchyma and will demonstrate rim enhancement following contrast administration because of encapsulation by neomembrane formed of granulation tissue. However, they have a high tendency to rebleed from fragile neovascularity formed in the membrane, producing variable complex density. Eventually, the membrane will stabilize and the collection will undergo resorption.

On MRI, subdural hemorrhage will generally follow the usual signal changes seen in any intracranial hemorrhage (Table 7-1). FLAIR images are particularly useful and appear to be the most sensitive sequence capable of detecting small subdural hemorrhage. The appearance of hemorrhage on diffusion images is complex and nonspecific and involves many factors including the relative amounts of different blood products; therefore, producing a heterogeneous nonspecific signal in most cases. However, diffusion images are valuable in differentiating subdural hemorrhage from other subdural collections, such as sterile subdural effusion that is most commonly associated with meningitis and shows increased diffusion (hypointense on diffusion-weighted imaging (DWI) and hyperintense on apparent diffusion coefficient (ADC) as well as subdural empyema, which shows restricted diffusion (hyperintense on DWI and hypointense on ADC).

Subarachnoid hemorrhage (SAH) is usually seen in severe head trauma and typically associated with worse prognosis. Bleeding occurs between the pia and arachnoid membranes and results from tearing of veins in the subarachnoid space. Traumatic SAH is more common than nontraumatic causes. It may be associated with other injuries such as subdural hemorrhage and brain contusions.

Traumatic SAH may be complicated by vasospasm leading to ischemia and possibly infarction. It usually occurs within 3 to 15 days after subarachnoid hemorrhage. Another complication is hydrocephalus because of obstruction of the basal foramina or arachnoid granulations.

On nonenhanced CT, there is high-density blood in the sulci and basal cisterns. This is usually seen adjacent to other traumatic brain lesions such as brain contusions or subdural hemorrhage. Bleeding in the interpeduncular cistern may be the only sign in subtle cases. "Pseudodelta" sign may be seen on nonenhanced CT because of presence of high-density SAH surrounding the hypodense superior sagittal sinus.

On MRI, FLAIR images appear to be the most valuable, and it is very sensitive to detecting subtle SAH that appears hyperintense. On T1-weighted and T2-weighted images, SAH appears isointense to brain parenchyma. Diffusion images are very important to detect early complications related to vasospasm including ischemia and infarction. Angiography may also be helpful to demonstrate SAH-induced vasospasm and offers additional therapeutic advantage through intra-arterial calcium channel blockers (nicardipine) administration.

The differential diagnosis of traumatic SAH includes meningitis, meningeal metastasis (carcinomatosis), gadolinium administration in patients with or without renal failure, oxygen therapy, diffuse cerebral edema (pseudo-SAH), and various causes of nontraumatic SAH (Table 7-3).

TABLE 7-3 Differential Diagnosis of Subarchnoid Hemorrhage on MRI

Nontraumatic SAH	Causative lesion is usually detected, most commonly aneurysm or vascular malformation
	Other causes include perimesencephalic venous hemorrhage, ruptured dissecting aneurysm, hemorrhagic transformation of bland infarct, and hypertensive intracranial hemorrhage
	History may suggest coagulopathy
Meningitis	WBCs in the subarachnoid space
	High FLAIR signal
	Meningeal enhancement
	CSF analysis shows infectious pattern
Meningeal metastasis (carcinomatosis)	Malignant cells in the subarachnoid spac High FLAIR signal
	Irregular meningeal enhancement
	CSF cytology shows malignant cells
Oxygen therapy	Administration of 100% O_2
	High FLAIR signal
Gadolinium administration	In patient with lesions causing blood–brain barrier disruption
	In patient with or without renal insufficiency
	High FLAIR signal
Diffuse cerebral edema	Diffusely hypodense brain
	Relatively hyperdense meninges

INTRA-AXIAL MANIFESTATIONS

These are caused by hemorrhage occurring within brain parenchyma.

Cerebral cortical contusion is injury of the cortical gray matter of the brain caused by impaction of gyri against osseous ridges or dural reflections. The temporal and frontal lobes are therefore more commonly involved. Focal cortical injury may also result from depressed fractures. Cerebral contusions are multiple and bilateral in approximately 90% of cases and can occur in regions of direct trauma (coup) and indirect trauma (countercoup). It is important to realize that the lesion usually starts as a focal area of brain edema showing multiple areas of punctate or linear hemorrhages. Within the next 24 to 48 hours, the size of hemorrhagic component may substantially increase in size and may involve the superficial subcortical white matter, accounting for increased mass effect and clinical deterioration. Therefore, the possible progression of these lesions justifies close follow-up imaging of these patients.

On nonenhanced CT, there are usually patchy cortical hypodense areas of brain edema with small punctate and linear hyperdense foci of petechial hemorrhages. SAH in the adjacent sulci is common. In the next 24 to 48 hours, the petechial hemorrhages may progress to parenchymal hematoma, and new lesions at different locations may also be seen. In the chronic stage, hypodense encephalomalacia is seen with parenchymal volume loss and ex vacuo dilatation of adjacent CSF spaces.

On MRI, T1-weighted images will show heterogeneous hypointense and hyperintense signal in the acute stage, while in the chronic stage hypointense gliosis and parenchymal volume loss will be seen. On T2-weighted and FLAIR images, hyperintense areas of edema and hypointense foci of hemorrhage can be seen. FLAIR images can also show adjacent SAH. On GRE images, just like any other hemorrhage, blood products appear hypointense and will bloom. On diffusion images, there is restricted diffusion (hyperintense on DWI and hypointense on ADC) because of cytotoxic edema and is seen to extend beyond the boundaries of the lesion seen on conventional imaging.

DAI results from high-velocity deceleration injury from high-velocity head impact leading to tear of the neuronal axons and blood vessels. The most common location is at the frontotemporal gray–white matter junction constituting approximately 75% of cases. It can also occur in the body and splenium of the corpus callosum, upper brainstem, and basal ganglia. These patients usually present by loss of consciousness at the time of injury that might progress to a persistent vegetative state.

Nonenhanced CT is usually normal; however, tiny foci of hypodensity (representing edema) or hyperdensity (representing hemorrhage) may be seen at the site of injury. On MRI, T1-weighted images are usually normal, while T2-weighted and FLAIR images will show tiny hyperintense foci in the characteristic locations. If hemorrhage is seen in these lesions, the blood products will produce signal abnormalities dependant on their age (Table 7-1). GRE is the most sensitive sequence in showing DAI, appearing as hypointense lesions even in subtle cases.

Subcortical injury refers to cerebral contusion occurring at the basal ganglia, thalami, and brainstem, secondary to disruption of the penetrating vessels in these areas by shearing forces. Similar to cerebral contusions, these lesions consist of focal areas of parenchymal edema containing linear and punctate foci of petechial hemorrhage. Radiologically, they are similar to cerebral contusions except for the location, but are clinically associated with worse prognosis.

Intraventricular hemorrhages primary hemorrhage within the ventricular system is most commonly because of disruption of the subependymal veins. Less commonly, it can occur because of choroid plexus hemorrhage or can be secondary to rupture of intraparenchymal hemorrhage into the ventricles.

On nonenhanced CT, intraventricular blood appears hyperdense producing CSF-blood level. Bleeding may be extensive, filling and expanding the ventricles. On MRI, the blood products appear hyperintense to the CSF on T1-weighted images, hypointense to CSF on T2-weighted images, hyperintense to the attenuated CSF on FLAIR images, and hypointense with blooming on GRE images.

Shaken baby syndrome refers to nonaccidental brain and skull injuries related to child abuse. There is usually discrepancy between the stated history by parents (minimal trauma) and the degree of brain injury on CT. It can occur at any age but is more common in the first 6 months of life and is more common in males. These children may present with apnea, loss of consciousness, or retinal hemorrhages. These are specific imaging findings suggesting diagnosis (Table 7-4).

TABLE 7-4 Cranial Imaging Findings in Child Abuse

Scalp injuries
Multiple, complex, depressed, diastatic, unexplained skull fracture at different ages of healing
Subdural, subarachnoid, and intraventricular hemorrhage in different stages and locations
Epidural hemorrhage is rare
Cerebral cortical contusions and shear injuries
Global or focal infarction
Other skeletal injuries of different ages and other injuries in the body

SECONDARY EFFECTS OF HEAD TRAUMA

These occur after the initial trauma and represent damage to the neurons caused by systemic physiologic responses to the initial trauma. Secondary effects include cerebral herniation, cerebral edema, cerebral infarction, arterial dissection, and carotid cavernous fistula. Secondary effects of trauma may be more serious and have a worse prognosis than primary effects.

In order to easily understand the concept of brain herniation, it is important to realize that after closure of the skull sutures the intracranial cavity becomes functionally divided by the dural reflections into three compartments: two supratentorial and one infratentorial compartments. Space-occupying lesions such as hemorrhage or neoplasms in one compartment may exert significant mass effect leading to displacement of the brain parenchyma, CSF spaces including ventricles, and blood vessels from one compartment to the other. There are six types of brain herniation.

Subfalcine herniation is the most common type of cerebral herniation and is caused by mass effect on the frontal lobe by a space-occupying lesion. The cingulate gyrus herniates beneath the falx. The ipsilateral ventricle is compressed because of the mass effect, while the contralateral ventricle is enlarged because of obstruction of the foramen of Monro. Severe herniation may occlude the anterior cerebral artery leading to infarction along its territory.

Unilateral descending transtentorial herniation is the second most common type and is caused by mass effect on the temporal lobe due to herniation of the medial temporal lobe through the tentorial incisura. In mild cases, the uncus and parahippocampal gyrus will be displaced medially, partially effacing the suprasellar cistern. The ipsilateral ambient and cerebellopontine angle cisterns will enlarge, as will the contralateral temporal horn because of entrapment. In more severe cases, the suprasellar cistern will be completely obliterated by the herniating brain and the brainstem will be displaced and compressed against the contralateral tentorial margin (Kernohans notch). The occulomotor (III) nerve may be compressed, which in mild cases will manifest with ipsilateral pupillary dilatation because of compression of the parasympathetic fibers, which are located peripherally within the nerve. In more severe cases, the ipsilateral eye globe will be deviated outward and downward because of compression of the motor fibers which are located in the center of the nerve. Severe herniation may occlude the posterior cerebral artery leading to occipital infarction. Duret hemorrhages may occur and these are delayed hemorrhages in the ventral and paramedian aspects of the upper brainstem, resulting in fatal outcome in most cases. The pathophysiology of duret hemorrhage remains under debate and can be either arterial or venous in origin. Arterial origin results from stretching and laceration of pontine perforating branches of the basilar artery, while venous origin results from venous obstruction and thrombosis resulting in venous infarction with subsequent hemorrhagic conversion

Bilateral descending transtentorial herniation is caused by mass effect on both temporal lobes resulting in bilateral herniation of the medial temporal lobes through the tentorial incisura. The thalami, midbrain, optic chiasm, and hypothalamus will be displaced inferiorly and the angle between the midbrain and pons will become more acute. In severe cases the basal arteries may occlude leading to basal infarcts.

Ascending transtentorial herniation is secondary to a space-occupying lesion in the posterior fossa resulting in herniation of the vermis and cerebellar hemispheres superiorly through the tentorial incisura. The quadrigeminal cistern will be effaced and the tectal plate of the midbrain will appear compressed and deformed. The aqueduct may be obstructed leading to hydrocephalus.

Tonsillar herniation is secondary to a space-occupying lesion in the posterior fossa resulting in herniation of the cerebellar tonsils through the foramen magnum into the spinal canal. Patients usually have concurrent ascending transtentorial herniation since both are caused by lesions in the same compartment. There is inferior displacement of the tonsils >5 mm below the foramen magnum, with "peglike" configuration. The tonsillar folia are vertically oriented instead of their normal horizontal orientation. The cisterna magna appears effaced and the fourth ventricle may become elongated and in severe cases may become obstructed leading to hydrocephalus.

Transalar herniation is a rare entity caused by herniation of brain parenchyma and MCA across the sphenoid wing. In ascending transalar herniation, mass effect on the temporal lobe leads to herniation of the anterior temporal lobe and MCA anterosuperiorly over the sphenoid wing, with upward displacement of the sylvian fissure. In descending transalar herniation, mass effect on the frontal lobe leads to posteroinferior displacement of the frontal lobe over the sphenoid wing and posterior displacement of the MCA.

Diffuse cerebral edema occurs in the setting of severe trauma and may lead to diffuse vasogenic and cytotoxic edema, resulting in increased intracranial pressure. The prognosis is usually poor with mortality up to 50%. Diffuse cerebral edema can occur at all ages and is usually associated with other traumatic injuries. Compression of the ventricles and effacement of the sulci are seen. On nonenhanced CT, the cerebral hemispheres appear hypodense compared to the cerebellum that appears relatively hyperdense. The surrounding meninges may also appear relatively hyperdense leading to pseudo-SAH appearance. On MRI, the cerebral hemispheres appear hypointense on T1-weighted images and hyperintense on T2-weighted and FLAIR images. MRA and MRV may demonstrate compression and thinning of the arteries or dural sinuses caused by increased intracranial pressure.

A variety of causes may lead to posttraumatic cerebral infarction. These include systemic hypoperfusion, arterial compression secondary to brain herniation, arterial injury (dissection or transection), SAH-induced vasospasm, diffuse cerebral edema causing marked increase in intracranial pressure, and venous compression or thrombosis by epidural hemorrhage. The location of the infarct will depend on the vessel involved, with the posterior cerebral artery being most commonly involved followed by the anterior and middle cerebral arteries in a descending order of frequency. Regardless of the cause, the imaging findings will be those of acute infarction. Nonenhanced CT does not show the infarct in the acute stage, but other signs of brain injury will be evident. CT perfusion may be helpful in cases where infarction is suspected based on clinical or imaging findings, but not evident on nonenhanced CT and will demonstrate decrease in CBF and CBV, with increase in MTT.

On MRI, diffusion images are the most sensitive in detecting early changes related to cerebral infarction. Hyperacute infarcts will show restricted diffusion (hyperintense on DWI and hypointense on ADC maps). On conventional images, infarcts show hypointense T1-weighted and hyperintense T2-weighted and FLAIR signal, and postcontrast images may demonstrate enhancement in the subacute chronic stage. MRA and MRV may be helpful in delineating the occluded vessel or dural venous sinus. MR perfusion has similar role to CT perfusion and demonstrates similar changes in CBF, CBV, and MTT.

Arterial dissection is defined as disruption of the arterial wall continuity by a hematoma in the subintimal or subadventitial planes, splitting the arterial wall and narrowing the true lumen. The traumatic event may be severe as in penetrating injuries or may be very trivial and not recognized by the patient, such as chiropractic maneuvers and violent sneezing and coughing.

Intracranial dissection is the most common location by far is in the vertebral arteries accounting for approximately 75% of cases. Complete disruption of the arterial wall may ensue leading to arterial rupture in the subarachnoid space with resultant subarachnoid hemorrhage. However, the most common complication seems to be infarction related to narrowing or occlusion of the true lumen. The patient may present with acute or delayed symptoms.

Nonenhanced CT is useful in demonstrating complications (infarction and SAH). CTA is crucial to the diagnosis and should be performed whenever dissection is suspected. Complete occlusion of the artery may be seen in severe cases. In milder cases, there may be fusiform dilatation of the arterial contour with narrowing of the true lumen by an intramural hematoma. Alternatively, an intimal flap may be seen as a filling defect separating the true and false lumens.

On MRI, the absence of flow voids in an artery may suggest the diagnosis. On T1-weighted images, the intramural hematoma appears hyperintense and will be more conspicuous if fat suppressed images were used. Diffusion images and FLAIR are helpful in showing acute infarcts and SAH, respectively. MRA and conventional angiograms may demonstrate arterial occlusion or narrowing. An intimal flap may also be seen as a thin filling defect.

Extracranial dissection can occur in the carotid or vertebral arteries. In the carotid arteries, the most common location is in the cervical segment of the internal carotid artery (ICA), above the bulb to the skull base. In the vertebral artery (VA), it usually occurs at the level of C1-C2. The most common complication of extracranial dissection is infarction related to arterial occlusion or severe stenosis. The patient presents with severe headache in most cases. Horner syndrome may occur and is related to injury of the sympathetic plexus around the ICA from the fusiform dilatation. Underlying vascular abnormalities such as fibromuscular dysplasia, Marfan syndrome, Ehler-Danlos syndrome, cystic medial degeneration, and syphilis may predispose patients to dissection. The imaging findings are similar to intracranial dissection but in extracranial characteristic locations.

Suggested Reading

Al-Nakshabandi NA. The swirl sign. *Radiology*. 2001;218(2):433.

Ashikaga R, Araki Y, Ishida O. MRI of head injury using FLAIR. *Neuroradiology*. 1997;39:239-242.

Beitsch P, Weigelt JA, Flynn E, et al. Physical examination and arteriography in patients with penetrating zone II neck wounds. *Arch Surg*. 1994;129:557-581.

Gean AD. Brain herniation. In: *Imaging of Head Trauma*. New York, NY: Raven Press; 1994:249-297.

Itoyama Y, Fujioka S, Ushio Y. Kernohan's notch in chronic subdural hematoma: findings on magnetic resonance imaging. *J Neurosurg*. 1995;82:645-646.

Numerow LM, Fong TC, Wallace CJ. Pseudo-delta sign on computed tomography: an indication of bilateral interhemispheric hemorrhage. *Can Assoc Radiol J*. 1994;45:23-27.

Orrison WW, Gentry LR, Stimac GK, et al. Blinded comparison of cranial CT and MR in closed head injury evaluation. *AJNR*. 1994;15:351-356.

Osborn AG. Intracranial hemorrhage. In: *Diagnostic Neuroradiology*. St Louis: Mosby; 1994:154-198.

Pfleger MJ, Hardee EP, Contant CF, Jr., et al. Sensitivity and specificity of fluid-blood levels for coagulopathy in acute intracerebral hematomas. *AJNR*. 1994;15:217-223.

Wilms G, Marchal E, Geusens C. Isodense subdural hematomas on CT: MRI findings. *Neuroradiology*. 1992;34:497-499.

QUESTIONS AND ANSWERS

1. What vessel is disrupted in temporoparietal epidural hematomas?
   A. Superficial temporal artery
   B. Cortical veins
   C. Middle meningeal artery
   D. Sphenoparietal venous sinus

   ANSWER: C. Approximately 90% of cases are because of arterial injury, usually the middle meningeal artery, while the remainders are caused by transgression of one of the sinuses by the fracture, resulting in venous bleed. The epidural hematoma occurs at the impact site (coup). Approximately 95% of cases are unilateral and supratentorial, of which two-thirds will be located at the temporoparietal region because of injury of the middle meningeal artery.

2. On T1-weighted and T2-weighted MRI, what are the signal characteristics of subacute hemorrhage?
   A. Hypointense on T1-weighted and hypointense on T2-weighted images
   B. Hyperintense on T1-weighted and hypointense on T2-weighted images
   C. Hyperintense on T1-weighted and hyperintense on T2-weighted images
   D. Hypointense on T1-weighted and hyperintense on T2-weighted images

   ANSWER: B. Subacute hematoma appears isodense on nonenhanced CT. It shows hyperintense signal on T1-weighted and hypointense signal on T2-weighted images because of intracellular methemoglobin. Progression occurs from periphery to center.

3. Which type of extra-axial hemorrhage *does not* cross the skull sutures?
   A. Epidural hemorrhage
   B. Subdural hemorrhage
   C. Subarachnoid hemorrhage

   ANSWER: A. Epidural hematoma does not cross the sutures (unless large with diastatic fracture), but will cross the dural reflections including the falx and the tentorium.

4. In cerebral contusion, what is the time frame for progression of the petechial hemorrhages to parenchymal hemorrhage?
   A. 2–4 months
   B. 1–2 months
   C. 1–2 weeks
   D. 1–2 days

   ANSWER: D. The size of hemorrhagic component may substantially increase in 24 to 48 hours, accounting for increased mass effect and clinical deterioration. Therefore, the possible progression of these lesions justifies close follow-up imaging of these patients.

5. What is the most common location for DAI?
   A. Corpus callosum
   B. Brain stem
   C. Frontotemporal gray–white matter junction
   D. Basal ganglia

   ANSWER: C. The most common location of DAI is at the frontotemporal gray–white matter junction constituting approximately 75% of cases. It can also occur in the body and splenium of the corpus callosum, upper brainstem, and basal ganglia.

6. What is the most common cause of intraventricular hemorrhage?
   A. Disruption of the subependymal veins
   B. Choroid plexus hemorrhage
   C. Rupture of intraparenchymal hemorrhage into the ventricle
   D. Extension from subarachnoid hemorrhage

   ANSWER: A. Primary intraventricular hemorrhage is most commonly caused by disruption of the subependymal veins. Less commonly, it can occur because of choroid plexus hemorrhage or can be secondary to rupture of intraparenchymal hemorrhage into the ventricles.

7. What is the location of the mass effect leading to subfalcine herniation?
   A. Temporal lobe
   B. Frontal lobe
   C. Cerebral hemispheres and vermis
   D. Cerebellar tonsils

   ANSWER: B. Subfalcine herniation is the most common type of herniation and caused by mass effect on the frontal lobe by a space-occupying lesion. Descending transtentorial herniation is the second most common type and caused by mass effect on the temporal lobe. Ascending transtentorial herniation is caused by a space-occupying lesion in the posterior fossa resulting in herniation of the vermis and cerebellar hemispheres superiorly through the tentorial incisura. Tonsillar herniation is caused by a space-occupying lesion in the posterior fossa resulting in herniation of the cerebellar tonsils through the foramen magnum into the spinal canal.

8. Which anatomic structure of the brain herniates in descending transtentorial herniation?
   A. Cerebellar tonsils
   B. Cerebellar hemispheres
   C. Cingulate gyrus
   D. Uncus and hippocampus

   ANSWER: D. In a transtentorial herniation the cingulate guyms descends secondary to it's anatomic location just cephalad and lateral to the tentorial let leaflet.

9. Which vessel is intracranial dissection more likely to involve?
   A. Vertebral artery
   B. Intracranial ICA
   C. MCA
   D. ACA

   ANSWER: A. The most common location by far is in the vertebral arteries accounting for approximately 75% of cases.

10. Extracranial dissection can present with Horner syndrome if it involves which vessel?
    A. Vertebral artery
    B. ICA
    C. Subclavian artery
    D. ECA

    ANSWER: B. Extracranial dissection may present with Horners syndrome and is related to injury of the sympathetic plexus around the ICA from the fusiform dilatation.

8 SPINE TRAUMA

Joseph C. Sullivan III

MECHANISM OF INJURY

Spine trauma is best described by location (cervical, thoracic, or lumbar) and mechanism. Cervical spine fracture mechanism includes flexion, extension, compression, and complex fractures (Table 8-1). Flexion fractures are further subdivided into anterior, flexion subluxation, and facet dislocation (unilateral or bilateral), wedge compression, flexion teardrop, and clay shovelers fractures. Extension type fractures include hangman (traumatic spondylolisthesis), extension teardrop, and hyperextension dislocation fractures. Compression fractures are further divided into burst fractures and Jefferson fractures. Complex fractures are often seen at the craniocervical junction as well as mixed fractures, various combinations of fractures, primarily involving the odontoid process, as well as alanto-occipital junction.

TABLE 8-1 Cervical Spine Fracture Types

Flexion fractures	Anterior
	Flexion subluxation
	Facet dislocation (unilateral, bilateral)
	Wedge compression
	Flexion teardrop
	Clay shoveler
Extension fractures	Hangman (traumatic spondylolisthesis)
	Extension teardrop
	Hyperextension dislocation
Compression fractures	Burst
	Jefferson

CERVICAL SPINE

With conventional radiography, all seven vertebral bodies should be well seen without motion, limitation of visualization from other anatomical parts, or foreign material obscuring sections of the cervical spine. Additional images, such as a swimmer view or CT may be required. Normal curvature of the spine is lordotic. This however can be reduced even in normal patients depending on positioning, muscular spasm, or in the setting of collar placement. Loss of normal lordosis may be the first indication of a fracture, ligamentous injury, or instability. Multiple papers have described the use of parallel lines to evaluate the cervical spine and its alignment (Fig. 8-1). These lines include the prevertebral space, anterior longitudinal and posterior longitudinal lines, a line along spinolaminar line, as well as a line that may intercede the tips of the spinous processes. An easy way to remember the prevertebral soft-tissue normal thickness is "6 mm at C2 and 2 cm at C6." The predental space should be less than 3 mm in the adult and less than 4 to 5 mm in the child. When evaluating the base of dens at its synchondrosis with the body of C2, a normal variant, os odontoideum may be visualized and should not be mistaken for a fracture line. Lateral masses of C1 and C2 should be symmetric and aligned. The disk spaces should be maintained barring degenerative change. Transverse processes are better evaluated

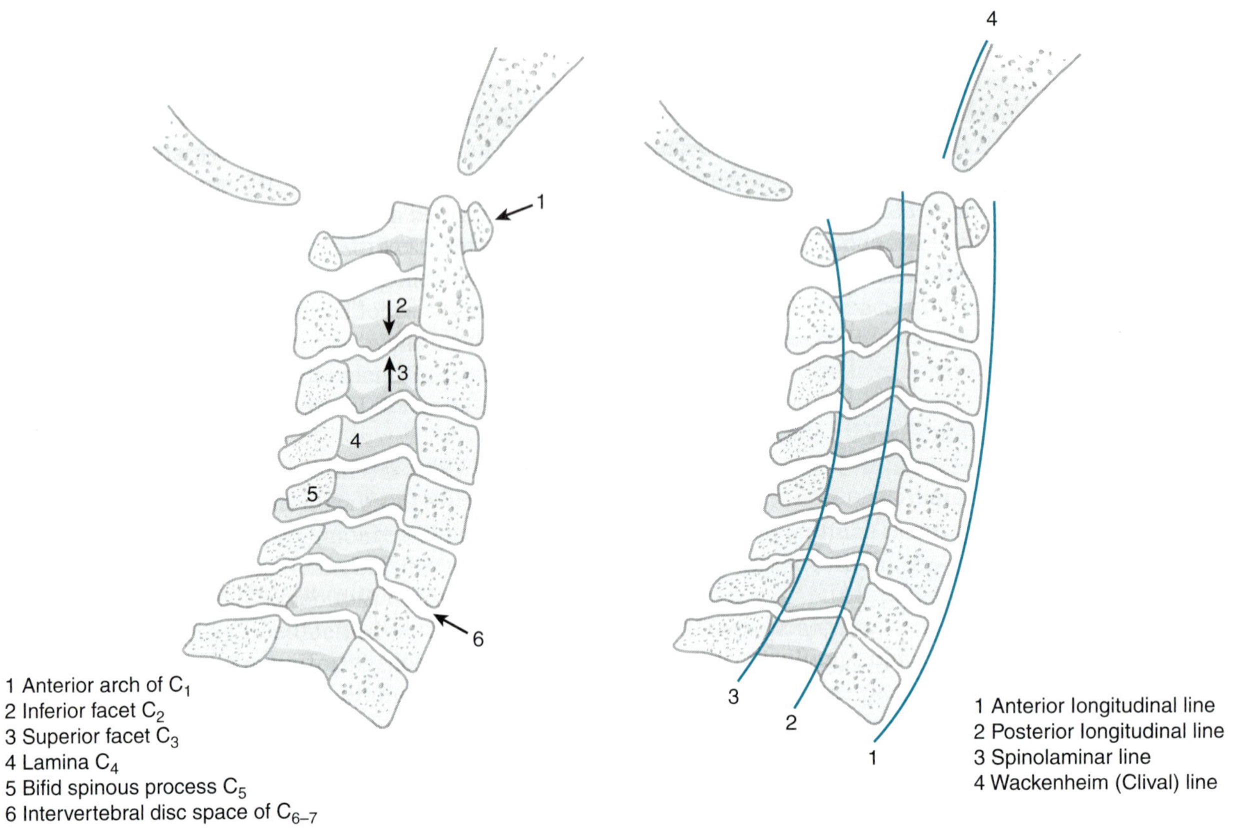

FIG. 8-1 Evaluation of lateral cervical spine alignment.

on axial and frontal projections, and cervical transverse processes should have a caudal angulation, while thoracic transverse processes angulate slightly cephalad.

Many emergency departments have abandoned conventional radiographs for CT in evaluation of spinal trauma, particularly of the cervical spine. Some, however, obtain an initial lateral view to search for significant fractures. In this scenario, further imaging with CT should be performed unless there is absolutely no clinical indication. If the question is of cord or ligamentous injury, MRI is the modality of choice.

In the setting of anterior subluxation, kyphotic angulation, relative widening of the interspinous space, and facet subluxation should be evaluated. As this can sometimes be difficult to assess in patients realigned by collar placement, voluntary extension films may be obtained for demonstration of stability.

Facet dislocations have a multitude of possible presentations: unilateral or bilateral, complete or perched, and with other associated fractures. When there is a facet dislocation, the associated disk and the posterior longitudinal ligament at the level of fracture might also be injured. The existence of bilateral facet dislocations would indicate disk and posterior longitudinal involvement with concern for an unstable fracture. Some widening of the posterior elements can occur with flexion compression injuries without an associated disk injury. However, these patients, secondary to compression, may be susceptible to traumatic ruptured disk and can present with spinal cord injury without radiologic abnormality (SCIWORA).

A flexion teardrop fracture usually occurs with major shear injury resulting in disrupted ligamentous stability and canal compromise. Conversely, if there is no ligamentous injury or tearing, there may be spinous fractures. Flexion type injuries of such are more likely to cause cord injury as the cephalad fragments sublux over the caudad portions of the vertebral bodies that move relatively posteriorly to impinge upon the canal. By definition, flexion teardrop type fractures are unstable. Clay shoveler fracture is a mild variant of flexion type injury occurring when the cervical spine is in a straightened or flexed position with movement of the body upward relative to a fixed shoulder girdle. This leads to interspinous ligamentous injury and fracture from the downward pull against the spinous processes. As such, it is similar to patients lifting their body while having their arms fixed upon a shovel in the clay, hence the name.

Hangman type fracture is otherwise known as traumatic spondylolisthesis. It is an extension type fracture with a minor flexion variant. As in the setting of a hanging, there is a forward flexing motion of the head depending on the positioning of the knot posteriorly. Today, this is most commonly seen with ejection associated with motor vehicle collisions and an impact of the posterior calvarium on the windshield or roof, creating a traumatic spondylolisthesis at C2 with separation of the posterior elements of the C2 ring. This in effect widens the cervical canal at this level and may actually result in a lower occurrence of cord injury in the event; this is an isolated injury. However, any oblique movement may cause a secondary shearing of the cervical cord. Historically, the hanging knot correctly placed behind one ear would create an oblique motion that would sever the cord in addition to fracturing the spine. However, if the knot was left more posteriorly, it would lead to fracture without cord injury with subsequent death by asphyxiation.

Extension teardrop injuries cause an avulsion of the anterior and inferior corner of the vertebral bodies secondary to hyperextension. This may have a lesser degree of cord injury as the patient extends, and there is some allowance of the posterior elements to collapse upon one another without causing a subluxation posteriorly. This can have a similar appearance as flexion teardrop without the misalignment that is commonly seen with the cephalad portion of the cervical spine moved anteriorly with flexion type injuries. This is not to say that hyperextension dislocation cannot occur, as this being an unstable fracture can also result in cord injury.

In a burst fracture, the vertebral body collapses with multiple fragments that can dislocate posteriorly and impinge the cord. It should be noted that the involvement of two of the three columns of the spine indicates an unstable injury. A compression type fracture involving only the anterior column of the vertebral body is considered stable. One variant of a cervical burst type fracture, Jefferson fracture, occurs in the ringed vertebra of C1. The lateral masses of C1 are laterally displaced, and there can be widening of the predental space, leading to atlanto-axial instability.

Odontoid fractures are classified into three subtypes, depending upon fracture location (Table 8-2). Type I is an avulsion fracture at the superior aspect of the dens; type II is a transverse fracture across the base of the dens; and type III is fractures through the base of C2. A developmental normal variant, os odontoideum, can mimic at type II dens fracture.

Atlanto-occipital dislocation is an unstable ligamentous injury that may not have associated fracture. It results in a stretching of the cord, which may or may not result in neurologic deficit depending upon the amount of dislocation and degree of cord stretching. Previously, this diagnosis was identified by conventional radiographs when the distance between the basion and the apex of the dens was greater than 12 mm. More recent studies define the distance as 8 to 10 mm with cross-sectional imaging. Magnification on conventional radiographs may explain the discrepancy. Traditionally, the powers ratio was used to describe atlanto-occipital dislocation: distance from the basion to the posterior ring of C1 divided by the distance from the anterior ring of C1 to the opisthion. If this is greater than 1, then dislocation should be suspected. However, trauma patients are often placed in a C-collar, which elevates and aligns the cranium relative to the cervical spine. This may result in a false-negative powers ratio. Cases such as this have been seen in the pediatric population without initial cord injury, suggesting this ratio may not be the best indicator of injury.

TABLE 8-2 Odontoid Fractures

Type I	Superior dens
Type II	Base of dens; mimicks os odontoideum
Type III	Base of C2

THORACIC SPINE

Determining stability is a key feature in imaging of spinal trauma. The spine can be considered in three anatomic columns. If two of the three columns are fractured, then the fracture is considered unstable. The three columns include the anterior and posterior aspects of the vertebral body and the posterior column formed from the posterior elements. The anterior longitudinal ligament stabilizes the anterior column, the posterior longitudinal ligament stabilizes the middle column, and the intraspinous and ligamentum flavum ligament stabilize the posterior column.

Because of the stability lent to the thoracic spine by the rib cage, there is a much higher-energy requirement for thoracic spine flexion, extension, and dislocation injuries. Axial loading injury is much more common in the thoracic spine, creating a wedge-type deformity. As a result, most thoracic spinal fractures are usually compression and/or burst fractures. However, Chance fractures secondary to shearing injuries and flexion distraction can also occur, although they require greater impact.

In the setting of compression fractures, flexion associated with axial loading involves only the anterior column resulting in a stable fracture. In the setting of a burst fracture, there is at least anterior and middle column involvement with possible posterior involvement as well, which can be stable or unstable. There can also be posterior longitudinal ligament disruption with associated impingement of the cord by fracture fragments.

In the setting of a Chance fracture, transverse forces result in spinal injury (bone and/or ligamental) that involves all three columns at either a single level or multiple levels. Keep in mind that fracture lines can extend from the vertebra body through the pedicles into the posterior elements, giving a so-called "open mouth" appearance at the pedicle.

Flexion distraction injuries tend to occur with a higher-energy injury, resulting in instability at all three columns with anterior wedge abnormality of the inferior vertebral body as well as middle and posterior column instability with possible rotational axis posterior to the anterior longitudinal ligament.

LUMBAR SPINE

The lumbar spine undergoes similar mechanisms of injury as the thoracic spine with a slightly more common occurrence of flexion–distraction injuries. However, compression type injuries remain substantially more common because of the stability provided by the chest, rib cage, and muscular abdominal girdle. Higher mass load is placed on the lumbar spine as it is the fulcrum between the upper and lower body and because of the higher weight of the more cephalad body.

Direct injury to the cord can result in injury to small blood vessels, tears of the pia, or axial disruption. Indirect injury includes reactive effects of venous congestion, perivascular edema, and subsequent decreased blood flow resulting in necrosis or hemorrhage. Not all injuries are immediately visible (SCIWORA). There tends to be improvement in the amount of neurologic deficit over time in the setting of purely edematous cord and/or those with mixed edematous and hemorrhagic changes, with less improvement in the setting of primarily hemorrhagic injury. When there is extradural impingement of the canal, it is important to remember that not all cord injuries occur at the level of the osseous abnormality. It is also important to note that injuries can occur as the spine returns to its normal alignment. This can occur in the setting of hematomas, disks herniations, or when bony fragments impinge on the cord at the time of reduction.

Spine trauma should initially be evaluated via conventional radiography even in today's setting of MDCT. Radiographic evaluation should quickly progress to cross sectional imaging if the mechanism of trauma is such or there are unexplained neurologic deficits. Concomitantly in the setting of head trauma, there is a strong possibility that there will be related cervical injury. CT imaging can quickly establish normal alignment of the vertebral bodies as well as maintenance of the normal vertebral heights, vertebral disk space heights, and appropriate perispinal soft tissues. MR imaging can further contribute with additional information of cord injury or edema indicating microinjuries, or the osseous elements or ligamentous instability, which can be obscured by collar placement. This is aided by the use of inversion recovering imaging. MRI can diagnose epidural hematoma or traumatic disk injuries, and gradient recall echo imaging increases sensitivity of diagnosis of hematomyelia and bone or disk fragments within the canal. T1-weighted imaging delineates anatomy and identifies cord swelling and hematomas, while fast and echo T2 techniques essentially provide an MR myelogram pattern for evaluation of cord and canal.

In the setting of spinal injuries, the perispinal soft tissues should be evaluated for adjacent ligamentous, muscular, and vascular abnormalities, with consideration of the energy and mechanism of injury. This can help identify an underlying malignant process complicating spinal fracture. In the setting of single level injury, the location of the fracture should be considered; for example, pedicle fracture is more likely a malignant process. A compression fracture will maintain the normal volume of the bone, whereas a pathologic fracture may present itself as an expanse of soft tissue at the level of compression.

Follow-up imaging is indicated if there are continued or new neurologic symptoms or if there are persistent symptoms of compression post/reduction. This is best performed with MRI as cord changes can be evaluated and/or posttraumatic progressive myelopathy can be diagnosed. The latter includes myelomalacia and syrinx formation. Subarachnoid cysts, scarring, and/or fibrosis can also be seen. These complications can be delayed in onset with progressive motor and sensory loss. Specifically, syrinx and/or syringomyelia onset can be as late as 10 to 15 years after the initial injury.

Imaging in spinal trauma continues to advance as reconstruction techniques improve and increased scanner speed decreases motion artifacts and increases patient throughout. MRI imaging also continues to improve with decreased acquisition times and improved signal to noise ratio with the smaller fields of view needed for the spine.

SUGGESTED READING

Chakeras DW et al. MR Imaging of acute spinal cord trauma. *AJNR Am J Neuroradiol*. 1987;8:5-10.

Cornelius R. Imaging of acute cervical spine trauma. *Semin Ultrasound CT MRI*. 2001;22:108-124.

Davis P et al. Spinal injuries in children: Role of MR. *AJNR AM J Neuroradiol*. 1993;14:607-617.

Gray L, Vandermark R, Hays M. Thoracic and lumbar spine trauma. *Semin Ultrasound CT MRI*. 2001;22:125-134.

Nguyen G et al. Adequacy of plain radiography in the diagnosis of cervical spine injuries. *Emerg Radiol*. 2004;11(3)158-161.

White M. Cervical spine—magnetic resonance imaging techniques and anatomy. *Magn Reson Imaging Clin N Am*. 2000;8:453-469.

QUESTIONS AND ANSWERS

1. Which of the following fractures is most likely to be stable?
   A. Jefferson
   B. Hangman
   C. Occipital condyle avulsion
   D. Unilateral facet dislocation
   E. Flexion teardrop

   ANSWER: D. Only a single column is likely to be involved in unilateral facet dislocation, and there is no definite ligamentous injury.

2. Which of the following fractures is most likely to cause neurologic deficit?
   A. Jefferson
   B. Hangman
   C. Occipital condyle avulsion
   D. Unilateral facet dislocation
   E. Flexion teardrop

   ANSWER: E. Flexion injuries are more likely to cause cord injury, and the remainder, although unstable, are less likely to impinge in the cord.

3. With MRI finding suggests increased likelihood of traumatic cord injury?
   A. Increased T1; increased T2
   B. Increased T1; isointense T2
   C. Isointense T1; increased T2
   D. Isointense T1; hypointense T2
   E. Hypointense T1; hypointense T2

   ANSWER: C. Isointense signal with T1-weighted images and increased T2 signal imply only edema and not hematomyelia, which usually show improvement as the edema abates.

4. Which of the following is *not* an indication of ligamentous injury?
   A. Asymmetry of the dens in the C1 ring
   B. Widening of the posterior elements
   C. Unilateral facet dislocation
   D. Occipital condyle avulsion
   E. Widening of the basion-odontoid interspace

   ANSWER: C. Bilateral facet dislocation implies ligamentous injury. Unilateral does not.

5. When dealing with compression fractures, which of the following is a good indicator of benignity?
   A. Nitrogen formation in the adjacent disc
   B. Paraspinal soft-tissue thickening
   C. Complete midline collapse
   D. Isointense signal on STIR imaging
   E. Mild enhancement soon after the believed compression causing event

   ANSWER: A. Gas in the absence of infection, juxtaposed to a fracture most likely indicates a degenerative collapse.

6. Which of the following is the best indication for MR imaging of the cord?
   A. High-speed MVC in an inebriated patient
   B. Patient with seat belt sign on their neck
   C. Patient with pain 2 days after the accident
   D. Patient with parasthesia and normal CT examination
   E. Patient with micturition at the scene of the accident

   ANSWER: D. Unexplained deficit, even with normal CT, may indicate cord injury. MRI may also be unimpressive in mild cord injuries.

7. Which of the following is most likely to demonstrate a vertebral artery injury?
   A. Patient with seat belt sign to the neck
   B. Patient with fracture involvement of the sixth foramen transversarium
   C. Patient with C3-4 grade II traumatic listhesis without other fracture
   D. Patient with hangman fracture
   E. Patient with atlantal occipital dislocation

   ANSWER: C. The vertebral artery is likely to be injured by the pulling cased by separation of the C3 and C4 transverse components.

8. Which vertebral level fracture implies the greatest force of injury?
   A. C1
   B. C2
   C. C4
   D. T4
   E. L4

   ANSWER: D. T4 is the most supported vertebral body listed. It is reinforced by the rib cage.

9 CENTRAL NERVOUS SYSTEM NEOPLASMS

Asim K. Bag and Joseph C. Sullivan III

INTRODUCTION

The incidence of primary neoplasm of brain in the United States is 14.4 per 100 000 persons. Women are affected slightly more than men. Pathologists classify brain tumors according to histopathologic behavior, but tumors can be heterogeneous and have different histologic elements. For purposes of this chapter, classification will be based on location and epidemiology.

In adult patients, the most common primary intra-axial supratentorial neoplasm tumor is glioblastoma multiforme, and metastasis is the most common tumor in the posterior fossa. In pediatric population, brain tumors are exceedingly common among all tumors. These are the second most common site of tumor after leukemias. Tumors in the first year of life may be congenital or de novo and usually of high grade. In the prepubescent child, the most common tumors are infratentorial, 75% involve the cerebellum and 25% arise from the brain stem.

ADULT BRAIN TUMORS

INTRAPARENCHYMAL

Superficial Cortical

- Ganglioglioma/gangliocytoma: More common in children.
- Pleomorphic xanthoastrocytoma: More common in children.
- Dysembryoplastic neuroepithelial tumor: More common in children.
- Dysplastic cerebellar gangliocytoma (Lhermitte-Duclos syndrome): Holohemispheric cerebellar hamartoma is composed of dysplastic ganglion cells. This is a very rare tumor associated with Cowden disease, and usually presents in adults with dysmetria. On T2-weighted sequences, it appears as hyperintense mass with thickened folia and heterogeneous hyperintense stripes.
- Desmoplastic infantile ganglioglioma: Only in infants.

Diffuse Cortical

Astrocytoma

Astrocytoma is the most common type of primary brain tumor in adults. The most consistent finding of this tumor both histologically and on imaging is heterogeneity. The natural history of this tumor is a continuous evolution from most benign tumor to most malignant tumor. It is very difficult to identify the transition period of this tumor with imaging and also sometimes histologically. The tumor grade depends upon the most malignant part of the tumor. If most of the tumor histology is grade II and one corner shows features of grade III tumor, the tumor is labeled and treated as grade III tumor.

Diffuse astrocytoma is a diffuse, benign slow-growing tumor of young adults occurring predominantly in the supratentorial cortex. It is composed of mature astrocytes but over time dedifferentiates into anaplastic astrocytoma and ultimately to glioblastoma. It accounts for 10% to 15% of all astrocytic tumors and most commonly occurs in the 30 to 40 years age range. There is a slight male predominance. It can occur in any part of the neural axis but most commonly occurs in frontal and temporal lobes, with the most common presentation of seizures.

Diffuse astrocytoma is a grade II tumor. The histological signature of grade II tumors is cellular atypia (variation in nuclear shape or size associated with hyperchromasia). Pathologically, they may be fibrillary (most common type), gemistocytic, and protoplasmic (rare).

Diffuse astrocytoma is usually a homogenous mass in the cerebral hemispheres, hypodense in CT, and hyperintense on T2-weighted images. There may be a focal area of heterogeneity. It usually has well-defined margins; however, there is microscopic infiltration of the peritumoral areas not identified by the MR. There may be infrequent intratumoral calcification, usually not evident in MR. Classically, it does not enhance; however, subtle enhancement may occur occasionally. There is no correlation between tumor enhancement and tumor grade. Diffusion restriction and increased rCBV indicate higher-grade tumors. These sequences should be included to guide prebiopsy primary brain tumors imaging to identify the most aggressive part of the tumor.

Anaplastic astrocytoma is a diffuse and malignant tumor. The average age at diagnosis is 45 to 51 years. It preferentially involves the cerebral hemisphere but can occur anywhere. Symptoms are similar to those of diffuse astrocytoma.

Anaplastic astrocytoma is a grade III tumor. The histological signature of grade III tumors is cellular atypia, anaplasia, and unequivocal mitotic activity. These tumors may evolve from grade II diffuse astrocytoma or de novo without any evidence of a less malignant precursor lesion. These tumors have an inherent tendency to dedifferentiate into glioblastoma.

CT is not useful in differentiating grade II from grade III tumor. There are a few MRI features that suggest a more malignant tumor. (Again it is difficult to differentiate anaplastic astrocytoma from glioblastoma.) This tumor is heterogeneous without the features of necrosis. Contrast enhancement is extremely variable in extent and pattern. As described earlier in the chapter, there is no correlation between tumor enhancement and tumor grade. There is a significant area of peritumoral T2 signal hyperintensity that is a mixture of edema, tumor infiltration, and rarely demyelination. On diffusion imaging, it may show diffusion restriction. On perfusion imaging, there may be focal area of increased rCBV compared to the contralateral normal-appearing white matter. MR spectroscopy may show a low NAA peak and high choline peak usually not associated with a lipid/lac peak. An intratumoral focus with low ADC value, high rCBV, and high choline peak is the best place for biopsy.

Glioblastoma multiforme is the most common primary brain tumor, with mean age of presentation between 45 and 75 years. This tumor most commonly occurs in cerebral hemispheres predominantly in the subcortical white matter with slight preference for the temporal and frontal lobe.

The clinical history is short (less than 3 months). The usual clinical features are headache, nausea/vomiting, seizures, and/or papilledema and may include other localizing signs depending upon the location of the tumor.

Glioblastoma multiforme is a grade IV tumor with all the histologic features of grade III tumors and microvascular proliferation, necrosis, and vascular thrombosis. Most commonly, it is a rapidly developing de novo tumor. Less commonly, it secondarily develops into low-grade tumors.

Glioblastoma multiforme is usually a cerebral hemisphere tumor but may involve brain stem, cerebellum, and rarely even spinal cord. It may cross the midline to involve the opposite lobe usually along myelinated structures such as the corpus callosum and fornices. This tumor may be very large and extremely heterogeneous on T2 associated with necrosis, focal area of hemorrhage, and hypercellularity. The hypercellular area appears as relatively hypointense in T2 than the rest of the well known tumor and shows diffusion restriction in DWI because of compromised extracellular space. The necrotic area is hypointense in T1, hyperintense in T2, and shows facilitated diffusion in DWI. There is extensive peritumoral T2 signal hyperintensity because of mixture of tumor infiltration and edema. There may be signal void in the T2 demonstrating hypervascular tumor. Neoangiogenesis, the hallmark of the glioblastoma, is reliably identified in perfusion imaging. This consistently shows high rCBV in the region of the neoangiogenesis (development of new tumor blood vessel). One important concept is that there is no strong correlation between neoangiogenesis and enhancement in T1. Contrast enhancement is due to the T1 shortening of the tissue by the leaked gadolinium in the tissue through the disrupted blood brain barrier. High rCBV in the area of neoangiogenesis is due to high blood vessel density. In fact, contrast leakage may paradoxically lower the rCBV value. Intratumoral hemorrhage is not uncommon and is best evaluated by susceptibility-weighted imaging. However, GRE and T2 are also sensitive to detect the hemorrhage.

Gliomatosis cerebri is a diffuse glioma with exceptionally extensive infiltration of a large region of the CNS, with at least three-lobe involvement, usually bilateral. The age range varies from neonatal period till ninth decade of life, the peak incidence being fifth to sixth decade. Any part of the brain may be involved by this tumor. The most common areas of involvement are cerebral hemispheres, mesencephalon, pons, thalamus basal ganglia, cerebellum, and medulla, in descending order of frequency. The spinal cord can also be involved by this tumor.

Presentation depends upon the site of involvement. It may be changes in the mental status, seizures, pyramidal symptoms, cranial nerve dysfunction, and signs of increased intracranial pressure.

The involved areas of brain are edematous, firm, and blurred distinction of grey–white matter interface. They most commonly express an astrocytic phenotype, but oligodendroglioma can also present with a gliomatosis growth pattern. Glioblastoma cerebri is a grade III tumor.

These are Poorly differentiated hypodense lesions with little mass effect and mild blurring of grey–white differentiation. MR imaging shows extensive white matter T2 hyperintensity, with minimal mass effect. Contrast enhancement is not a typical feature unless there is dedifferentiation. However, irregular small enhancement in parts of the tumor is not uncommon. Sometimes the diagnosis may be confused with diffuse demyelinating or dysmyelinating diseases. Presence of subtle mass effect, diffuse sulcal, or ventricular effacement should prompt thought of this diagnosis instead of demyelination.

Oligodendroglioma

Oligodendroglioma is a diffusely infiltrating, well-differentiated tumor of oligodendroglial lineage of adults, typically located in the cerebral hemispheres. It comprises 2.5% of all brain tumors and 5% to 6% of all gliomas. The majority of these tumors occur in adults, with peak age of presentation being 40 to 45 years. It preferentially occurs in the cortex and white matter of cerebral hemispheres. The frontal lobe is involved in 50% to 65% of cases, followed in decreasing order of frequencies by temporal, parietal, and occipital lobes. If the tumors of oligodendroglial lineage show focal or diffuse features of malignancy (cellular atypia, mitoses, vascular hypertrophy, pleomorphism necrosis, and so on), they are called anaplastic astrocytoma. They are approximately 20% to 35% of all the oligodendrogliomas. Very rarely, tumors may have mixed astrocytic and oligodendroglial lineage; such tumors are called oligoastrocytoma. Oligoastrocytomas do not have any specific clinical or radiological findings.

Concurrent deletion of the 1p and 19q chromosomal arms constitutes the genetic hallmark of oligodendroglioma, which may be found in up to 80% of cases. Most tumors show losses of one entire copy of 1p and

19q as a result of unbalanced translocation. Tumors with 1p/19q loss have distinct clinical, histologic, and radiological findings from those tumors without. The following characteristics are more commonly found in tumors with 1p/19q loss:

- Better response to chemotherapy.
- More indolent clinical behavior.
- Longer-lasting response to radiotherapy.
- Tumors with 1p/19q loss occur more commonly in frontal and parietal lobes compared to the temporal lobe and diencephalon.
- Usual oligodendroglial morphology instead of mixed oligoastrocytic component.
- More indistinct border in MRI and heterogeneous appearance on T1 and T2.
- Diffuse patchy enhancement instead of ring enhancement and necrosis.
- Median survival is improved.

Approximately two-thirds of patients will present with seizures. Other common presenting symptoms are headache, signs of increased intracranial pressure, focal neurological deficit, and cognitive or mental changes.

Oligodendroglioma is diffusely infiltrating tumors of moderate cellularity with oligodendroglial lineage. An important histological finding is presence of microcalcification. Classically, it is a grade II tumor.

Peripheral location, presence of characteristic calcification (linear or nodular or clumped), and occasional findings of modeling defect of the adjacent calvaria are suggestive of diagnosis. Calcification may be seen in 70% to 90%. It is heterogeneous in T2-weighted sequence. The intensity is less compared to the astrocytoma of similar grade because of high cellularity. The most specific MR feature is cortical infiltration and marked thickening, which usually is not seen in astrocytoma. Small cystic changes and intratumoral hemorrhage are common. Contrast enhancement is common but does not have any specific morphology. Oligodendroglioma may be confused with dysembryoplastic neuroepithelial tumors in young adults, but it is more hyperintense and homogenous in T2.

Primary CNS Lymphoma

By definition, primary CNS lymphoma arises in the CNS with no systemic disease. The incidence of primary CNS lymphoma has increased in the past few years. It can occur in immunologically intact and immunocompromised patients. Before HAART therapy, the tumor was highly prevalent in the end-stage HIV infection/AIDS. This tumor also occurs in posttransplant patients. This tumor can occur at any ages with a peak incidence in immunocompetent patient being sixth to seventh decade and a male predominance. In immunocompromised patients, it may occur much earlier in life. Immunodeficiency, either acquired or congenital, predisposes to primary CNS lymphoma. Epstein-Barr virus plays a significant role in the development of the tumor. Approximately 60% of the tumors are supratentorial and can involve cerebral cortex, deep gray matter, and periventricular region. Approximately 10% to 25% of the tumors are multiple (60%–85% in AIDS). Secondary meningeal spread occurs in roughly 25% of patients. Secondary lymphoma, however, predominantly involves the meninges. Around 50% to 80% of these lymphomas present with focal neurological signs. Neuropsychiatric symptoms are also common.

The classic imaging finding is intensely and homogenously solid-enhancing mass in the earlier mentioned locations. In AIDS patients, it may appear as multiple ring-enhancing lesions with peritumoral T2 signal hyperintensity, which is often difficult to distinguish from toxoplasmosis. The presence of subependymal spread is in favor of lymphoma rather than toxoplasmosis. CNS lymphoma usually follows the signal intensity of the cortex. However, it may be hypo- or hyperintense on T2-weighted images. Peritumoral T2 signal hyperintensity is much less intense than that of gliomas. There is usually no tumor infiltration beyond the tumor margin. It causes moderate severe diffusion restriction because of severely compromised extracellular space secondary to hypercellularity. One other common presentation is perivascular enhancement. Both extra-axial and parenchymal sarcoidosis mimic primary CNS lymphoma.

Metastatic Tumors

Metastatic tumors are the most common CNS neoplasms. Brain metastases occur in approximately 25% of patients who die of cancer, leptomeningeal metastases occur in 4% to 15% of patients, and dural metastases occur in 8% to 9% of patients. The most common source of brain metastasis is the lung followed by breast, melanoma, and cancer of unknown primary source. More than 80% of the tumors are located in the cerebral hemispheres at the gray–white matter interface secondary to abrupt change in the caliber of the arterioles in this location. Usually all metastatic foci have significant peritumoral vasogenic edema. There is also no infiltration of the tumor beyond the tumor margin.

On CT, they are usually hypodense ring-enhancing masses with significant peritumoral vasogenic edema. On MR, they present similar to that on CT. The edema associated with the tumor usually does not cross the corpus callosum. Cortical metastasis may not have any edema. One characteristic feature of melanoma metastasis is T1 hyperintensity in precontrast imaging because of paramagnetic melanin content. Metastases from melanoma, small cell lung carcinoma, thyroid cancer, choriocarcinoma, and renal cell cancer are prone to have intratumoral hemorrhage.

INFRATENTORIAL

Medulloblastoma

See "Pediatric Brain Tumors" section.

Pilocytic Astrocytomas

See "Pediatric Brain Tumors" section.

Hemangioblastoma

Hemangioblastoma is a relatively uncommon tumor. It may occur sporadically or may have familial association with von Hippel-Landau (Table 9-1). It usually occurs in adults, in the fifth to sixth decade of life. If it is associated with von Hippel-Landau, it may occur in much younger patients. Sporadic tumors are usually single and occur in the cerebellum. Tumors associated with von Hippel-Landau may be multiple and may involve cerebellum, brain stem, and/or spinal cord. They may present with cerebellar symptoms. They frequently cause hydrocephalus by obstructing cerebrospinal fluid (CSF) outflow.

TABLE 9-1 Familial Tumor Syndromes Involving the CNS

NF1	CNS tumors: Neurofibroma, malignant peripheral nerve sheath tumor, optic nerve glioma, astrocytoma
	Other tissue involvement: Iris hamartoma, osseous lesions, pheochromocytoma, leukemia, café au lait spots, axillary freckling
NF2	CNS tumors: Bilateral vestibular schwannoma, peripheral schwannoma, meningioma, meningiomatosis, spinal ependymoma, astrocytoma, glial hamartomas, cerebral calcification
	Other tissue involvement: Posterior subcapsular ventricular opacities, retinal hamartomas
von Hippel-Landau syndrome	CNS tumor: Hemangioblastoma (brain and retina)
	Other tissue involvement: Renal cell carcinoma, pheochromocytoma, visceral cysts
Tuberous sclerosis	CNS tumor: subependymal giant cell astrocytoma (SEGA), cortical tubers
	Other tissue involvement: Cardiac rhabdomyoma, adenomatous polyps of the duodenum and the small intestines, cysts of the lung and kidney, lymphangioleiomyomatosis, renal angiomyolipoma, cutaneous angiofibroma, subungual fibroma
Li-Fraumeni syndrome	CNS tumors: Astrocytoma, PNET
	Other tissue involvement: Breast cancer, bone and soft-tissue sarcoma, adrenocortical carcinoma, leukemias
Nevoid basal cell carcinoma syndrome (Gorlin)	CNS tumor: Medulloblastoma
	Other tissue involvement: Jaw cysts, ovarian fibroma, skeletal abnormalities, basal cell cancer of skin
Turcot syndrome	CNS tumors: Glioblastoma medulloblastoma
	Other tissue involvement: Adenomatous colon polyps, café au lait spots
Cowden disease	CNS tumors: Dysplastic cerebellar gangliocytoma, megalencephaly
	Other tissue involvement: Hamartomatous polyps of the colon, thyroid neoplasm, breast cancer, multiple trichilemmoma, fibroma
Rhabdoid tumor predisposition syndrome	CNS tumors: AT/RT
	Other tissue involvement: Bilateral renal rhabdoid tumors

Abbreviations: PNET, primitive neuroectodermal tumors.

Pilocytic astrocytomas are well-demarcated cystic lesions with a highly vascular nodule in the wall. They are composed of large vacuolated cells and vascular cells. They are grade I tumors.

Pilocytic astrocytomas are usually large, sharply marginated cystic masses of the cerebellar hemisphere with a pial-based mural nodule with very minimal to no peritumoral edema. There is usually no calcification. A cystic posterior fossa mass, brightly enhancing pial-based nodule, and a prominent vessel (flow void) within or adjacent to the tumor on MR, in combination, are consistent with hemangioblastoma. The mural nodule produces intense blush in angiography. The cyst fluid may appear hyperintense to normal CSF because of presence of hemorrhage and protein contents.

Dysplastic Cerebellar Gangliocytoma

This is a childhood tumor. See "Pediatric Brain Tumors" section.

INTRAVENTRICULAR

Lateral Ventricular

Ependymoma

This is more common among children (See "Pediatric Brain Tumors" section).

Subependymoma

Subependymomas are WHO grade I tumors and are usually asymptomatic. They are more common in males with peak age of presentation being the fourth through sixth decade. They are well-circumscribed, lobulated intraventricular masses. The most common locations are the foramen of Monro and the fourth ventricle. Subependymomas of the foramen of Monro or at the region of aqueduct may obstruct CSF flow and can present with hydrocephalus. They are hypodense in CT with or without calcification. They are hyperintense to gray matter in T2, with no enhancement.

Central Neurocytoma

Central neurocytomas are rare, benign intraventricular tumors attached to the septum pellucidum and/or the lateral ventricular wall often arising from the region of the foramen of Monro. They usually occur in early adulthood. On microscopy, they look like oligodendroglioma. Calcification is a common finding. Their enhancement is variable but common.

Xanthogranuloma
They are benign choroid plexus masses. They are usually bilateral and typically occur in adults.

Meningioma
See "Meningeal" section.

Metastasis
See "Intraparenchymal" section.

Anterior Third Ventricle

Subependymal Giant Cell Astrocytoma
This is usually a tumor of pediatric age group (Table 9-1).

Colloid Cyst
Colloid cysts are well-capsulated neuroepithelial cysts in the roof of the third ventricle found almost exclusively in the anterior part of the third ventricle right behind the foramen of Monroe. They occur in both sexes and are frequently asymptomatic. Sometimes they present with headache. They may obstruct the foramen of Monroe and can cause hydrocephalus. There are reported cases of sudden death after acute onset hydrocephalus.

On CT they are usually well-capsulated and round. They are typically hypodense, but if there is higher protein concentration, these may be hyperdense of variable degree. The capsule may enhance. On MR, they are hypointense in T1 unless they contain highly proteinaceous fluid, blood products, or cholesterol crystal when they become hyperintense. They are typically hyperintense on T2, unless they contain blood products or highly proteinaceous fluid. Endoscopic removal is the treatment of choice.

Metastases of the anterior third vehicle are benign, unilocular, smooth, round, epithelial-lined (derived from endoderm), mucin-containing cysts of the anterior third ventricle between the columns of fornix. They represent the most common type and location of neuroepithelial cysts. They may present with headache, sudden transient paralysis of lower extremity, incontinence, and personality changes. Hydrocephalus, which may be positional and intermittent, is also common. They are usually seen in young adult and middle-age patients. They are hyperdense in CT. The MR signal characteristics are variable depending upon the protein content and also frequent presence of different paramagnetic substances. The signal intensity may vary from markedly hypointense to markedly hyperintense in T2. They can also be of high or low signal intensity on T1. Rarely, there may also be rim enhancement. Solid enhancement should suggest other diagnoses.

SELLAR/PARASELLAR/SUPRASELLAR

Pituitary Adenoma

Pituitary adenomas are slow-growing tumors arising from the adenohypophysis. They are the most common tumor of the sella turcica. They are primarily tumors of adults. Only about 3% occur in children less than 18 years. They can be of variable size from less than a centimeter up to several centimeters. Tumors less then 10 mm in size are known as microadenoma. Most of the functional adenomas are prolactin secreting. Prolactinomas occur predominantly in women. ACTH-secreting adenomas constitute 15%. Approximately 25% tumors are nonfunctional.

Prolactinomas in women cause presenting clinical symptoms like menstrual irregularity and galactorrhea. Women tend to seek medical attention much earlier than men, thus explaining the comparatively smaller tumor size in women. The clinical symptoms in men can be subtle (decreased libido) precluding early tumor detection. Symptoms owing to mass effect on adjacent structures (visual field defect, ptosis) are more common in men. Growth hormone–secreting tumors present with gigantism in children; in adults, they present as acromegaly. ACTH-secreting tumors present with Cushing syndrome, predominantly in women. Nonfunctional adenomas are usually clinically silent until they become large enough to impinge the adjacent structures.

The best imaging modality is MRI as the soft-tissue resolution is greatly superior to CT, and there are no bone artifacts. Coronal plane is the best plane for evaluation of the pituitary/sella. Almost 80% of tumors present as focal T1 hypointensity and T2 hyperintensity with or without contour abnormality of the gland. Tumoral calcification is rare. The best sequence for evaluation of microadenoma is coronal postcontrast dynamic T1-weighted sequence. As the tumors uptake contrast at much slower rate than the normal pituitary tissue, tumors appear as focal hypointense defect. A laterally located tumor may displace the pituitary stalk; if the tumor is large enough it may invade the cavernous sinus and impinge on the internal carotid arteries and surrounding cranial nerves, which is of great importance in preoperative planning. There are many MR signs described for detection of the invasion of the cavernous signs. The definite signs of noninvasion are normal pituitary tissue between the tumor and cavernous sinus, less than 25% of the ICA encasement, and intact medial venous compartment. A large tumor may show demineralization of the adjacent bone. Intratumoral hemorrhage can occur in 20% to 30% of adenomas, mostly in macroadenomas. Most of the time the hemorrhage is subclinical but may also present as pituitary apoplexy. The incidence of hemorrhage is higher in patients treated with bromocriptine.

Craniopharyngioma

In adults, papillary craniopharyngiomas are more common. They are solid, without calcification. Unlike the adamantinomatous form, they are encapsulated with absent desmoplasia and are easily separable from the adjacent structures. This also explains less recurrence after surgery compared to the adamantinomatous form. They frequently involve the third ventricle.

Rathke Cleft Cyst

Rathke cleft cysts are usually incidental on autopsy findings. They are rarely symptomatic, except when they are large and compress the adjacent structures. They may appear with variable signal intensity in both T1- and T2-weighted sequence depending upon the protein concentration of the cyst. They may be T1 hyperintense and T2 hypointense compared to the cortex, if the protein concentration is very high. They are usually hypodense in CT but may be hyperdense as well. They usually do not enhance.

Meningioma

Approximately 10% of meningiomas occur in the parasellar region. See "Meningeal" section.

Chordoma

The clivus is the most common site of cranial chordomas. Chordomas originate from the embryologic remnant of the notochord or ectopic cordal foci. They usually present in the sixth decade. They are benign, locally aggressive masses causing extensive bony destruction. If large enough, they may cause compression of the visual pathways, cranial nerve palsies, and brain stem compression. If they grow laterally, they can present as a CP angle mass or inferiorly; they can present as pharyngeal mass. They are hypointense in T1 with replacement of the normal high T1 signal intensity of fat within the bone marrow. Characteristically, they are moderate to severely hyperintense in T2. They may be heterogeneous because of calcification and bone destruction.

Suprasellar Germinoma

This is a tumor of childhood. See "Pediatric Brain Tumors" section.

Hypothalamic Hamartoma

A disease of childhood. See "Pediatric Brain Tumors" section.

Dermoid Cysts

Dermoid cysts are ectodermal inclusion cysts, which usually occur at midline or near the midline. They may have epidermal derivative like hair and sweat glands. They usually occur in the third decade. Midline structures such as the vermis or fourth ventricle are the most common locations of this tumor followed by sellar/suprasellar region and frontobasal regions. The cysts usually contain lipoid material, and that is why they appear as hypodense mass in CT and very bright in noncontrast T1-weighted sequence. One important feature of dermoids is that they may rupture and spread in the CSF spaces. This can result in chemical meningitis with seizures, which can be fatal. Headaches and seizures are common presenting features. They usually do not enhance with contrast.

Dermoid cysts constitute approximately 8% of the primary intracranial tumors. The most common site is the intracanalicular portion of the vestibular division of the eighth nerve complex with or without extension into the CP angle. They are associated with NF2.

Pathologically, dermoids are well encapsulated and arise from the outer nerve sheath layer and grow eccentrically outward and this is the reason they most commonly present with hearing loss due to compression of the cochlear division by the growing tumors. They more commonly arise from the sensory nerves. Histologically, they may be of two types: Antoni A cell type with compact stroma and Antoni B type with loose matrix. They usually appear as heterogeneously T2 hyperintense mass with bright enhancement in the postcontrast images. The Antoni B type is usually hyperintense in T2-weighted sequence. High-resolution heavy T2-weighted sequences (CISS, FIESTA) allow excellent delineation of the tumor.

Hypothalamic and Chiasmatic Glioma

See "Pediatric Brain Tumors" section.

CEREBELLAR PONTINE ANGLE

Acoustic Neuroma

Meningioma

See "Meningeal" section.

Epidermoid Cysts

Epidermoid cysts may be congenital and acquired. Congenital tumors occur as an inclusion cyst. They probably arise from the ectopic epithelial inclusion at the time of neural tube closure. Acquired tumors arise after trauma. They are soft tumors that have an inherent tendency to insinuate along the CSF spaces rather than compress the surrounding structures. They usually contain squamous epithelium, keratin debris, and sometimes cholesterol crystal. Unlike dermoid, they lack dermal elements and are usually off midline rather than midline. They are more common than dermoid cysts. They usually occur in the fourth or fifth decade of life. Usual symptom is headache.

Epidermoid cysts follow the CSF density and intensity in CT and MR respectively. Rarely, there may be mural calcification. They usually do not enhance in the post contrast scan. The most consistent and characteristic finding is diffusion restriction in DWI. Unlike arachnoid cysts, they appear hyperintense in FLAIR.

Cranial Nerve Schwannomas

These are benign nerve sheath tumors that arise from myelin support cells. These displace but do not invade the nerve.

Metastasis

See "Meningeal" section.

MENINGEAL

Meningioma

Meningiomas arise from the meningothelial cells. They account for approximately 30% of the primary intracranial tumors. There is an association with NF2 (may be multiple) (Table 9-1). This is a tumor of adulthood, with peak age being the sixth and seventh decades. There is a slight female predominance. Spinal meningiomas show a marked female predominance. Radiation to the head is known to cause meningiomas. Sex hormones may also have some role. The most common location is over the cerebral convexities, often parasagittal (Table 9-2). Others common locations are olfactory groove, sphenoid ridges, sellar/parasellar region, optic nerve sheaths, petrous ridge, posterior fossa. The predilection to these common sites may be explained by the predominance of the arachnoid granulations in these locations.

Meningiomas are slow-growing tumors, usually present with headache, and may also be associated with seizures and nerve palsies. They are mostly WHO grade I tumors, but may also be grade II or III. There are numerous pathologic subtypes. The most common type is the meningothelial subtype.

On conventional radiograph, there may be bone erosion, localized bone thickening, enlarged vascular channels, and enlarged paranasal sinuses (in skull-base meningiomas).

On noncontrast CT, meningiomas are usually homogenously isodense or can be hyperdense (to brain parenchyma). They are well-circumscribed dural-based masses. There may be calcification in approximately 25% of cases. Hyperostosis is a common finding. Contrast-enhanced CT shows intense homogenous enhancement (as these tumors develop from dura which does not have blood–brain barrier).

On MR, the tumor is isointense to cortex in T1 and isointense to cortex in T2 in 50% and hyperintense to cortex in 50%. These tumors enhance brilliantly after contrast administration. The CSF cleft is commonly seen. There may be vasogenic edema in the adjacent cortex. There is no definite imaging finding to differentiate typical meningiomas from atypical meningiomas.

TABLE 9-2 Imaging Findings in Favor of Extra-Axial Tumors

A CSF cleft around the tumors
Vessel interposed between brain and tumor
Displaced/Compressed (with or without edema) gray matter between white matter and the mass
Enlarged CSF spaces, particularly at the margins of the tumor
In posterior fossa mass, compression and displacement of the brain stem opposite to the tumors
Peripheral broad dural based

Abbreviations: CSF, cerebrospinal fluid.

Hemangiopericytoma

These are soft tissue sarcomas that originate from the pericytes of blood vessels. They can apppear similar to a vascular aggressive meningioma on imaging.

Metastasis

The most common type of metastasis to the dura is from breast cancer. Other common primary sites are lungs, lymphoma, prostate, and less likely neuroblastoma. Very rarely, extensive dural involvement with or without multiple cranial nerve palsies, carcinomatous meningitis, may occur. They usually appear as enhancing lesions of the dura with or without thickening.

Lymphoma/Leukemia

Their involvement of the meninges is primarily from metastatic or cranial extension.

Sarcoidosis

Secondary intracranial involvement in sarcoidosis is not uncommon. Intracranial sarcoidosis may be of two types: granulomatous meningitis (more common) and parenchyma space-occupying lesions. The leptomeningeal involvement may involve the cranial nerves causing cranial nerve palsy. The facial nerve is the most common. Leptomeningeal lesion present as an irregular thickening/lobular dural mass, which is isointense in T1, hypointense in T2, and brightly enhancing in T1+c. Parenchymal lesions are rare.

PEDIATRIC BRAIN TUMORS

TUMORS IN THE FIRST YEAR OF LIFE

Teratoma

These are tumors containing all three germ cell lines.

Atypical Teratoid and Rhabdoid Tumor

Although these represent only 32% of CNS pediatric tumors, they are one of the more common solid CNS childhood malignancies, with roughly two-thirds occurring in the posterior fossa. See "Supratentorial" section.

Desmoplastic Infantile Ganglioglioma and Astrocytoma

The tumors listed here are large cystic tumors of infants that involve the superficial cerebral cortex and leptomeninges with a favorable prognosis. They are rare tumors of infancy and early childhood. They usually present within the first year of life. They always arise in the supratentorial region and usually involve more than one lobe, preferentially the frontal and parietal lobes.

These tumors of childhood usually present with increasing head circumference, tense and bulging fontanelles, and lethargy. They are huge tumors that are mostly cystic and almost always associated with a focal hyperenhancing superficial solid portion. The solid portion is primarily extracerebral and involves the leptomeninges and superficial cortex. This solid portion is hyperdense to cortex in CT and isointense to cortex in T1 and T2.

Choroid Plexus Cancer/Papilloma

Choroid plexus cancer/papilloma constitutes approximately 10% to 20% of all brain tumors in the first year of life.

EARLY ADULTHOOD TUMORS

Parenchymal Tumors

Infratentorial

Medulloblastoma

Medulloblastomas are malignant tumors of cerebellum presenting in early childhood and with an inherent tendency to metastasize via CSF pathways. They comprise 15% to 20% of intracranial tumors in children and 30% to 40% of infratentorial tumors in early childhood. The peak age at presentation is 7 years. There is a slight male predominance. Two-thirds of childhood medulloblastomas arise in the vermis and project into the fourth ventricle. Involvement of the cerebellar hemispheres increases with age. This tumor is associated with basal cell nevus syndrome.

Medulloblastomas usually present with cerebellar signs and signs of increased intracranial pressure. The duration of symptoms is usually short because of the aggressive nature of the tumor. In infants, there may be enlarged head circumference due to hydrocephalus. Spinal metastasis is present at the time of initial diagnosis in 30% of tumors.

Medulloblastomas are composed of densely packed, primitive, undifferentiated small round cells with cellular signature of high-grade tumors. Homer-Wright rosettes are seen in 40% of tumors. They are WHO grade IV tumors with multiple histologic variants.

On CT, medulloblastomas typically appear as well-circumscribed hyperdense masses involving only vermis, or vermis and cerebellum. More peripherally located tumors may have exophytic growth pattern and may extend to the CP angle. Calcifications may be seen in 20% and intratumoral cysts are found in about half of the cases. The mass appears heterogeneous in both T1 and T2. The solid portion is isointense to grey matter in T1 and hypo- to isointense in T2. CSF metastasis is common with the most common location as the basilar cisterns and in the ependyma of lateral ventricles. In the spinal cord, the most common location is the dorsal surface of the thoracolumbar spinal cord (intradural extramedullary or intramedullary). The caudal most part of the thecal sac is also a common location. Complete imaging of the spinal cord at diagnosis is always required for assessment of disease burden.

Cerebellar Astrocytoma

Cerebellar astrocytoma constitutes 5% to 6% of all gliomas. This is the most common glioma in children, occurring most commonly in the cerebellum. The most common supratentorial site in children is visual pathways/hypothalamus. This tumor most commonly develops in the first two decades of life. This tumor can arise from any part of neural axis containing glial tissue. Common locations are the optic nerves (optic nerve glioma), hypothalamus, thalamus, basal ganglia, hemispheres, cerebellum (cerebellar astrocytoma), brain stem (dorsal exophytic glioma). Intracranial visual pathway PAs are often associated with NF1 (Table 9-1).

Clinical features depend upon the location of the tumor. Cerebellar astrocytoma usually does not present with seizures as it infrequently involves the cerebral cortex. Posterior fossa tumors present with cerebellar symptoms, such as clumsiness, problems in balance and coordination. Tumors involving the optic pathways present with visual difficulty. Tumors of the sella usually present with endocrinologic abnormality or cranial nerve palsies.

Cerebellar astrocytoma is well circumscribed, partially cystic, often with a mural nodule of solid vascular tissue. The cause of cyst formation within the tumor is not known but may be proteinaceous. This is a WHO grade I tumor and does not show features of a high-grade tumor. There is low to moderate cellularity with loose-textured cells and microcysts.

The cystic part appears as hypodense (denser than CSF because it contains protein) on CT, hypointense in T1, and hyperintense in T2 (may be more hyperintense than CSF if it contains protein). Intratumoral calcification is not common. Mural nodule is slightly hyperintense in T2 and hypointense in T1 in comparison to normal brain tissue and enhances brightly and homogenously in the postcontrast images. The wall of the cyst may or may not enhance (as most of the time the wall is the compressed normal brain tissue or reactive glial tissue). The solid portion of the tumor is usually homogenous and isointense to normal brain on T2. It displaces and therefore compresses the fourth ventricle. Visual pathway gliomas may be completely solid without any cystic component. Brain stem pilocytic astrocytomas are usually dorsal, exophytic with variable enhancement instead of symmetric pontine enlargement as seen in diffuse fibrillary astrocytomas.

Ependymoma

Ependymomas constitute 8% to 12% of all primary pediatric CNS tumors. They may occur at any age, but the mean age at presentation is 6.4 years. There is a second peak in the fourth and fifth decades. They can occur at any ventricle and the spinal cord. The most common location is the fourth ventricle (both from the roof and floor of the fourth ventricle with frequent extension into the foramen of Luschka and Magendie) and the spinal cord followed by the lateral and third ventricles. Supratentorial ependymomas occur particularly in children and they are usually parenchymal.

Presentation depends upon the location, but fourth ventricle ependymomas usually present with hydrocephalus and signs of raised intracranial pressure.

Ependymomas arise from the ependymal cells. They are so-called plastic tumors that fill the fourth ventricle and emerge out of the fourth ventricle through the foramen of Luschka and Magendie. There are many histologic subtypes of the tumor. They are usually WHO grade II tumors. In 10% to 12% cases, there may be CSF spread. CSF spread is usually associated with higher-grade tumors (grade III or ependymoblastoma).

The typical CT appearance is iso- to hyperdense fourth ventricular mass with both solid and cystic component, calcification, heterogeneous enhancement, and extension through the foramen of Luschka and Magendie. On MR, the mass is extremely heterogeneous with solid portions, cystic portions, calcification, and hemorrhage. In preoperative evaluation, spinal MR should be included to exclude the possibility of CSF dissemination.

Brain Stem Tumor

Brain stem tumors represent 15% of all pediatric tumors and about one-third of all posterior fossa tumors. The peak age at presentation is between 3 and 10 years, although they can present at any age. Brain stem tumors are broadly classified as medullary, pontine, mesencephalic, and tumors associated with NF1 (Table 9-1). Although brain stem tumors may be of any histology, astrocytoma is the most common.

Medullary tumors may be of pilocytic astrocytoma variety, which typically involve dorsal medulla with exophytic growth, or it may be diffuse fibrillary astrocytoma involving pons rostrally and cervical cord caudally with or without enhancement.

Pons is the most common location of brain stem tumor. The usual histology is high-grade fibrillary glioma. It usually presents with multiple cranial nerve palsy and cerebellar signs. It is hypodense to cortex on CT and hypointense to cortex on T1 and hyperintense on T2 and FLAIR with expansion of the pons. There is a blurry margin of pons with subtle or no enhancement. The imaging appearance is so typical that biopsy is not required to start treatment. However, the presence of any atypical sign (marked enhancement before treatment or presence of hemoglobin degradation product) should always be carefully searched for alternate diagnosis.

Hemangioblastoma

Usually this tumor occurs in the older age group (Table 9-1). See "Infralentorial" section.

Supratentorial

Astrocytoma

The presentation, clinical feature, and imaging features are similar to that of adult astrocytoma. See "intraparenchymal" section.

Ganglioglioma/Cangliocytoma

Ganglioglioma/gangliocytoma represents 1.3% of all brain tumors. The age of presentation is wide ranging: from 2 to 70 years of age, with a mean age of presentation 8.5 to 25 years. They can occur in any part of the CNS but occur mostly at the supratentorial superficial cortex. The most common location is the temporal lobe (greater than 70%). Parietal and frontal lobes are the next most common location.

Tumors of the cerebrum present with refractory seizures. They are the most common tumors presenting with seizures.

Gangliogliomas/gangliocytomas are well-differentiated slowly growing tumors containing neoplastic mature ganglion cells and glial cells. They are usually solid/cystic lesions with minimal mass effect. They are usually WHO grade I tumors and may be rarely of higher grade.

Typically ganglioglioma/gangliocytoma is well circumscribed and solid or partially cystic often with focal calcification. There is no specific imaging sign. Usually it is hypodense in CT and heterogeneously T2 hyperintense tumors of varying sizes and varying contrast enhancement with little mass effect. On rare occasions, there may be remodeling of the adjacent bone, confirming the slow-growing nature of the tumor. Sometimes the tumor cannot be differentiated from the gangliocytoma both histologically and by MR. When this occurs, they are loosely called as ganglion cell tumors.

This lesion presents as a central solid mass with multiple surrounding large cysts. It usually presents in the first 24 months and involves more than one lobe of the cerebrum.

Desmoplastic Infantile Astrocytoma and Ganglioglioma
Dysembryoplastic Neuroepithelial Tumor

Dysembryoplastic neuroepithelial tumors are uncommon benign supratentorial intracortical tumors that occur preferentially in children and young adults, mainly at the temporal lobe.

Typically, these tumors present with drug-resistant partial seizures, with or without secondary generalization, and no neurological deficit.

Dysembryoplastic neuroepithelial tumors are grade I tumors containing glioneural elements; the histologic hallmark is the column of tumor cells perpendicular to the cortical surface. Focal cortical dysplasia is associated in 80% of cases.

Classically, these tumors selectively involve the cortex. There may be enhancement in approximately 20% of cases. They are hypodense on CT. There may be calcification in about one-third of patients. In some lesions, there may be focal remodeling changes in the adjacent calvarium. On MRI, there may be multiple small focal intratumoral cysts.

Pleomorphic Xanthoastrocytoma

Pleomorphic xanthoastrocytoma is a relatively rare tumor that accounts for approximately 1% of all astrocytic tumors. This is a tumor of children and young adults. Seventy-five percent of tumors present in persons less than 18 years. This is a superficial cortical tumor and involves the meninges. It is almost always supratentorial, and the most common location is temporal lobe.

As this tumor preferentially involves the cerebral cortex, the most common presentation is long-standing seizures.

Pleomorphic xanthoastrocytomas are frequently associated with cysts (in 50%) and a mural nodule. Pleomorphic refers to variable histologic appearances. Xanthoastrocytoma refers to presence of xanthomatous cells showing intracellular lipid accumulation. They are WHO grade II tumors.

Typical imaging appearance is well-circumscribed peripheral temporal lobe mass with cystic and solid component without any calcification. The solid portion is isodense to gray matter in CT and isointense to gray matter in T1 and T2. The solid portion enhances homogenously but may be heterogeneous if there are microcystic changes. There is usually no peritumoral T2 signal hyperintensity. The tumor frequently invades the leptomeninges. Like other superficial tumors, this tumor may also produce bony remodeling in the adjacent calvarium.

Gliomatosis Cerebri

Subependymal giant cell astrocytoma is a specific tumor that is characteristically associated with tuberous sclerosis. It occurs in 5% to 10% of tuberous sclerosis patients. The tumor may occur at any age but the median age at diagnosis is 5 to 10 years. It typically arises from the wall of the lateral ventricle near the foramen of Monro and frequently present with hydrocephalus by obstructing the foramen. The tumor is most likely originated from the subependymal hamartomas of tuberous sclerosis because they are identical histologically. It is hypo- to isodense in CT (hypo- to isointense in MR) with frequent calcification, and enhances homogenously with contrast.

Primitive Neuroectodermal Tumor

Primitive neuroectodermal tumors (PNET) are embryonal tumors of undifferentiated or poorly differential neuroepithelial cell origin with capacity for divergent differentiation. Ninety to 95 percent of tumor cells are undifferentiated or poorly differentiated. Histologically, they are similar to medulloblastoma, pinealoblastoma, and peripheral neuroblastoma.

Exact incidence is not known, as there is frequent overlap with above-mentioned pathologies. The tumor may occur between 4 weeks and 20 years of life but median age of presentation is 5.5 years. They usually occur in the deep cerebral white matter of cerebrum.

The clinical presentation depends upon the location of the tumor. Most are very large at presentation and contain poorly differentiated cells. PNET are WHO grade IV tumors. They can metastasize outside CNS.

They are an extremely heterogeneous tumor, usually located either in the cerebral hemisphere or in the lateral ventricles. They may be mixed having solid and cystic components, and solid tumors with central necrosis with frequent calcification. The solid portion of the tumor is hyperdense in CT (isointense to gray matter in T2 and FLAIR). There is frequent enhancement in postcontrast images.

Supratentorial Ependymoma

Supratentorial ependymomas constitute 20% to 40% of childhood ependymoma. They usually occur early in childhood with a slight male predominance.

Presentation depends upon the location of the tumor, but seizure is a common presenting symptom.

These tumors are histologically identical to the infratentorial counterpart. The imaging appearances are variable. They may be completely solid and/or containing cystic component and calcification. They are iso- to hyper dense on CT (usually follow the signal characteristics of grey matter in T1, T2, and FLAIR images). The heterogeneity and peritrigonal location raises the suspicion of this tumor. Oligodendroglioma is rare in children, and constitutes 1% of all pediatric brain tumors.

Atypical Teratoid/Rhabdoid Tumor

Atypical teratoid/rhabdoid tumors are highly malignant rare tumors of early childhood (Table 9-1). They rarely occur in patients older than 6 years of age, median age of presentation is 2 years. They may be both supra- and infratentorial, supratentorial being slightly more common. The usual supratentorial location is cerebral hemispheres. They can involve the cerebellum, CP angle, and brain stem infratentorially.

The clinical presentation depends upon the tumor location, size, and age at presentation. Usual presentations are lethargy, failure to thrive, and signs of increased intracranial pressure.

Atypical teratoid/rhabdoid tumors are grade IV tumors containing rhabdoid cells and any type of cells arising from the ecto-, endo-, and mesoderm. They are usually large at presentation. Typically, they are angry-looking solid tumors with heterogeneous enhancement and variable necrosis. The solid portion is usually hyperdense to normal gray matter in noncontrast CT owing to hypercellularity. Sometimes they are difficult to differentiate from primitive neuroectodermal tumors.

Ventricular Tumors

Choroid Plexus Papilloma/Carcinoma

Choroid plexus papillomas (CPP) are intraventricular papillary tumors. They represent 2% to 4% of brain tumors in children younger than 15 years of life. Approximately 80% of the lateral ventricle tumors present before 20 years of age. The fourth ventricle tumor can occur at any age. CPP occurs more commonly in males, but there is no sexual predilection in choroid plexus carcinoma (CPC). The tumor involves the lateral ventricles in approximately 50% (the trigone is the most common location), the fourth ventricle in 40%, and third ventricle in 5%.

Typically, the child presents with hydrocephalus because of obstruction of CSF flow and/or overproduction of CSF.

CPPs are cauliflower-like masses of the ventricle that may involve the ventricular wall. They do not involve the adjacent brain tissue unlike CPC. CPP is a WHO grade I tumor. If there is an atypical feature, it is considered to be grade II. CPC is grade III tumor.

On CT, the typical papilloma appears as a multilobulated intraventricular hypodense mass with occasional calcification but almost always with intense enhancement. Occasionally the papilloma grows through the ependyma and involves/infiltrates periventricular white matter. CPC usually invades and infiltrates adjacent white matter with extensive T2 signal hyperintensity. Usually CPC are heterogeneous with loss of lobulation in appearance and also they enhance heterogeneously. The central portion of the tumor is hypointense to the grey matter in T2. Intratumoral hemorrhage is common and can be identified on MR. Based on imaging appearances, most of the time it is impossible to correctly identify CPP versus CPC. However, CPP may have aggressive features, and the malignant looking mass may turn out to be an atypical CPP in histology.

Ependymoma

See “Infratentorial” section.

Colloid Cyst

See “Anterior Third Ventricle” section.

Pineal Region Tumors

Germinoma

There is geographic variance in incidence. Germinomas are more common in Far East Asia. They account for 2% to 3% of all primary CNS neoplasms and up to 15% of all pediatric tumors in Japan. The respective numbers for the west is 0.3% and 3% to 4%. Approximately 90% of CNS germ cell tumors occur in patients younger than 25 years with a peak age of incidence 10 to 14 years. There is an interesting sexual distribution of the tumor. The great majority of the pineal germinomas occur in boys, but the suprasellar tumors are common in girls. Of all the germinomas, teratomas occur in males in approximately 90% of cases. The majority of the germinomas arise around the third ventricle. The most common location is pineal region followed by suprasellar region.

The clinical presentation and duration of symptoms depend upon the histology and the location of the tumor. The pineal region tumor presents with progressive hydrocephalus owing to compression of the aqueduct. If the tumor involves the tectal plate, characteristic paralysis of upward gaze and convergence (dorsal Parinaud syndrome) occur. Suprasellar germinomas may compress the optic chiasm producing characteristic bitemporal hemianopsia. They also frequently present with hormonal disturbances (diabetes insipidus, pituitary failure) owing to interference with hypothalamic-pituitary functions. Precocious puberty is also a known manifestation because of secretion of hCG.

Germinomas are predominant in the suprasellar compartment. Nongerminatous germ cell tumors predominate in other locations. Multifocal germinomas usually involve the pineal and suprasellar region either simultaneously or sequentially. Characteristic CT finding is a midline pineal/suprasellar mass containing both fat and calcification with variable contrast enhancement. On MR, the lesion is heterogeneous in both T1- and T2-weighted images because of different contents. However, germinomas can present as homogenous soft-tissue density/intensity mass with variable contrast enhancement in the typical location and typical age group. A more malignant variant may be associated with vasogenic edema.

Pineal Parenchymal Tumors

Pineal parenchymal tumors are less common than germinomas. They may be of two types: pineocytomas and pinealoblastomas. Pineocytomas are rare in childhood, but pinealoblastomas usually present in the pediatric age group. Pineocytomas are well-circumscribed, noninvasive slow-growing tumors composed of differentiated cells and pinealoblastomas are highly malignant, invasive tumors composed of small round undifferentiated cells. Pineal parenchymal tumors commonly disseminate through the CSF. Imaging features are like that of primitive neuroectodermal tumors in the pineal region.

Sellar/Suprasellar Tumors

Craniopharyngioma

Craniopharyngioma is partially cystic epithelial tumor of the sellar region. These tumors account for 1.2% to 4.6%. The incidence is higher in Japan and Nigeria. Craniopharyngioma may be of two types: adamantinomatous and papillary. There is a bimodal age distribution of the adamantinomatous form with peaks in children 5 to 15 years and adults aged 45 to 60 years. Papillary craniopharyngioma occurs almost exclusively in adults with mean age of presentation 40 to 55 years. The most common location is suprasellar cistern with a minor intrasellar component.

Clinical features are nonspecific and depend on the involvement of the adjacent structures caused by mass effect. It may present with visual field defects (most common presentation) because of compression of the optic chiasm/nerve/tract and endocrine abnormality because of interference with hypothalamic-hypophyseal functions. Cognitive impairment and personality changes are also common.

Typically, they are lobulated cystic masses with solid component in adamantinomatous variety. On sectioning, there is a typical greenish-brown liquid like "machine oil." They often extend beyond anatomic confinement and produce dense desmoplasia causing superficial brain penetration and adhering to the adjacent vessels and nerves. They are very difficult to resect surgically. On the other hand, papillary variety is well-circumscribed solid, rarely cystic tumor with absence of calcification. They are WHO grade I tumors.

The imaging appearance depends upon the histologic type. Adamantinomatous form appears as a mixed solid and cystic mass with calcification in most. The CT density of the cyst may be hypo-, iso- or hyperdense to cortex. The calcification may be circumferential at the wall or dense calcification in the solid portion. There is variable enhancement in most. A cystic or solid/cystic enhancing mass with calcification at the suprasellar region with intrasellar extension is consistent with a craniopharyngioma. Large tumors may extend to middle/anterior/posterior cranial fossa.

Rathke Cleft Cyst

See "Sellar/Parasellar/Suprasellar" in "Adult Brain Tumors" section.

Pituitary Adenoma

See "Sellar/Parasellar/Suprasellar" in "Adult Brain Tumors" section.

Hypothalamic Hamartoma

Hypothalamic hamartomas are congenital lesions of the normal neuronal tissue involving the hypothalamus and pituitary stalk. There is a markedly male predominance. The most common presentation is isosexual precocious puberty. Usual presentation is less than 2 years. The other common clinical presentation is seizure, typically of gelastic type. They are well-defined masses from the hypothalamus extending down to suprasellar cistern following the density/signal intensity of normal gray matter without any enhancement.

Chiasmatic/Hypothalamic Astrocytomas and Optic Nerve Tumor

Astrocytomas at these locations constitute approximately 10% to 15% of the supratentorial tumors. Once the tumor grows beyond the margin of the primary location, it is difficult to identify the exact origin. Males and females are affected equally. Usual age of presentation is 2 to 4 years. One interesting behavior of the astrocytomas of the optic nerve and chiasm is that they can resolve spontaneously over time. This is true both with and without the setting of the NF1.

The usual clinical presentation is visual field defects, optic atrophy, and short stature. If the tumor is large, it can present with hydrocephalus and signs of increased intracranial pressure.

Up to 50% of the astrocytomas at this location are associated with NF1. The majority of the tumors at this location are pilocytic astrocytomas; the pathology and imaging findings are similar to the pilocytic astrocytomas of the cerebellum.

Bone artifacts in the CT scan prevent accurate evaluation of the tumor extent. MRI is very helpful for defining the extent of the tumor and also involvement of the optic pathways. The tumor primarily arising in the optic nerve causes fusiform enlargement of the optic nerve. Astrocytomas of this location are almost always hypodense to brain on CT and hypointense to gray matter in T1-weighted sequence and hyperintense to gray matter in T2-weighted sequence. In postcontrast images, the tumor enhances heterogeneously to a variable extent. The sagittal plane is optimal for evaluation of the optic nerve and coronal plane is very good for evaluation of the chiasm and brain involvement.

Langerhans Cell Histiocytosis

Langerhans cell histiocytosis (LCH) is a heterogeneous group of tumors and tumorlike masses composed of histiocytosis. LCH shows features of dendritic Langerhans cells, whereas most of various non-LCH show macrophage lineage. LCH is a disease of childhood and presents most commonly as a solitary lytic lesion of the skull bones. The mean age of presentation is 12 years. If there are multifocal lytic bony lesions associated with involvement of the hypothalamus, it is known as Hand-Schüller-Christian disease. Histiocytosis of the lymph node, skin, and viscera without brain involvement is otherwise known as Letterer-Siwe disease.

The most common intracranial location is at the involvement of the pituitary stalk. Diabetes insipidus is a known clinical feature and can occur from 5% to 50% of cases. Usually the first deposit is in the subarachnoid space, but gradually the pituitary stalk is involved. In the later stage of the disease, there is granulomatous involvement of the brain parenchyma too. The hypothalamic involvement may vary from slight thickening of the stalk to a frank mass. There is usually enhancement of the pituitary stalk/mass. One characteristic finding is absent T1 bright signal in the posterior pituitary.

Suprasellar Germ Cell Tumor

Unlike pineal region germ cell tumors, suprasellar germ cell tumors are more common in girls.

Suggested Reading

Barkovich AJ, ed. Intracranial, orbital, and neck masses of childhood. In: *Pediatric Neuroimaging*. 4th ed. Philadelphia, PA: Lippincott Williams & Wilson; 2005:506-659.

CBTRUS. *Statistical Report: Primary Brain Tumors in the United States, 1998-2002.* 2005.

Koeller KK, Henry JM. From the archives of the AFIP. Superficial gliomas: radiologic-pathologic correlation. *Radiographics.* 2001;21:1533-1556.

Koeller KK, Rushing EJ. From the archives of the AFIP. Oligodendroglioma and its variants: radiologic-pathologic correlation. *Radiographics.* 2005;25:1669-1688.

Koeller KK, Sandberg GD. From the archives of the AFIP. Cerebral intraventricular neoplasms: radiologic-pathologic correlation. *Radiographics.* 2002;22:1473-1505.

Louis DN, Ohgaki H, Wiestler OD, Cavenee WK, eds. *WHO Classification of Tumors of the Central Nervous System.* 4th ed. IARC; 2007. World Health Organization. WHO Press Geneva, Switzerland.

Provenzale JM, ed. Advanced imaging of brain tumors. *Neuroimaging Clin N Am.* 2002;12(4). p477-699

Rees JH, Smirniotopoulos JG, Jones RV, et al. Glioblastoma multiforme: radiologic-pathologic correlation. *Radiographics.* 1996;16:1413-1438.

Smith MA, Friedlin B, Gloeckler-Ries LA, et al. Trends in reported incidence of primary malignant brain tumors in children in the United States. *J Natl Cancer Inst.* 1998;90: 1269-1277.

Wen PY, Schiff D, eds. Brain tumors in adults. *Neurologic Clin N Am.* 2007;25(4): p867-1258.

QUESTIONS AND ANSWERS

1. What is the most likely location of a lesion that causes homonymous hemianopsia?
   A. Optic nerve
   B. Optic chiasm
   C. Lateral geniculate body
   D. Postchiasmic optic pathways

   ANSWER: D. Homonymous hemianopsia can occur as a result of lesions anywhere in the postchiasmatic visual pathways including optic tract, lateral geniculate body, optic radiation, and visual cortex. Lateral geniculate body is correct and is a better option because it includes all possible causes and is more appropriate. The nasal fibers, responsible for the temporal visual fields, decussate at the optic chiasm. Lesions in the optic chiasm cause bitemporal hemianopsia. Unilateral optic nerve lesions cause unilateral visual disturbances.

2. Where is intraventricular meningioma most commonly located?
   A. Frontal horn
   B. Fourth vent
   C. Atria of the lateral ventricle
   D. Third ventricle

   ANSWER: C. Intraventricular meningioma arises from the choroid plexus stromal cells. Choroid plexus is voluminous at the atria of the lateral ventricles, explaining this is to be the most common location.

3. CT scan demonstrates focal calcifications at the junction of the optic nerve and the globe in a patient with unilateral papilledema. Which of the following is the most likely diagnosis?
   A. Retinoblastoma
   B. Optic glioma
   C. Drusen
   D. Hemangioma with phleboliths

   ANSWER: C. Calcification classically occurs at this location in Drusen. Calcification retinoblastoma occurs within the tumor of the retina. Optic glioma usually does not calcify. Hemangioma usually does not involve the optic nerve.

4. Which of the following is the most likely cause of drop metastases?
   A. Epidermoid
   B. Medulloblastoma
   C. Dysgerminoma
   D. Oligodendroglioma
   E. Hemangioblastoma

   ANSWER: B. Medulloblastoma is the most common to drop metastasize. Rarely, oligodendroglioma can have drop mets. Other tumors do not produce drop metastasis.

5. Which of the following is the most likely diagnosis of a high-density mass on head CT?
   A. Lymphoma
   B. Astrocytoma
   C. Schwannoma
   D. Paraganglioma

   ANSWER: A. Because of densely packed cells, lymphomas appear hyperdense on CT.

6. Which of the following is *not* associated with renal cysts?
   A. Tuberous sclerosis
   B. Chronic renal dialysis
   C. von Hippel-Landau
   D. Neurofibromatosis I

   ANSWER: D. The other three conditions are known to be associated with renal cysts.

7. Imaging reveals cerebellar lesion with increased T2 signal involving the cerebral peduncles and optic nerves. Which of the following is the most likely diagnosis?
   A. Neurofibromatosis II
   B. Neurofibromatosis I
   C. Tuberous sclerosis
   D. von Hippel-Landau

   ANSWER: B. NF1 typically causes multiple astrocytomas. Cerebellum and optic nerve are common locations of astrocytomas in the setting of NF1.

8. Which of the following is the most likely cause of an enhancing suprasellar mass in a 1-year-old?
   A. Neuroblastoma metastasis
   B. Glioma
   C. Craniopharyngioma
   D. Pituitary adenoma
   E. Dysgerminoma

   ANSWER: C. Of all these, the incidence of craniopharyngioma is much higher than other pathologies.

9. A 34-year-old female presents with sudden-onset headache. MR shows fluid-fluid level in sella. Which of the following is the most likely diagnosis?
   A. Pituitary apoplexy
   B. Pituitary abscess
   C. Carotid aneurysm
   D. Lymphocytic hypophysitis

   ANSWER: A. Pituitary apoplexy classically presents acutely in women. On imaging it shows enlarged pituitary with or without intragland hemorrhage, which appear as fluid-fluid level on MR. The other three conditions usually do not present so acutely.

10. A 1-year-old boy develops ataxia and vomiting. MRI shows enhancing mass in the cerebellar vermis extending into the fourth ventricle. Which of the following is the most likely diagnosis?
    A. Medulloblastoma
    B. Glioma
    C. Ependymoma
    D. Brain stem glioma

    ANSWER: A. This is the classic age, location, and imaging appearance for the medulloblastoma.

10 INTRACRANIAL INFECTIONS

Ahmed Kamel Abdel Aal and Joseph C. Sullivan III

CONGENITAL/NEONATAL INFECTIONS

Although the causative organisms might be somewhat similar, the radiological presentation of intracranial CNS infections in neonates is significantly different than adults (Table 10-1).

INTRODUCTION

The gestational age of the fetus at the time of infection is the most important determining factor that will eventually dictate the degree and type of brain damage. If the fetus is infected during the first two trimesters, a resulting congenital brain malformation is likely to ensue. If the fetus is infected thereafter, the brain is likely to undergo an encephaloclastic response that will ultimately lead to brain destruction.

The TORCH infections refer to the most common organisms involved in congenital/neonatal infections and include toxoplasmosis, rubella, cytomegalovirus (CMV), and herpes simplex virus type 1 (Table 100-1). With the increased prevalence of human immunodeficiency virus (HIV) in the general population, congenital HIV infection has also become a common pathogen in CNS infections.

TABLE 10-1 Comparison of Neonatal Infections

	CMV	TOXOPLASMOSIS	RUBELLA	HSV TYPE 2	HIV
Incidence	Most common	Second-most common	—	—	—
Mode of transmission	Hematogenous, transplacental	Hematogenous, transplacental	Hematogenous, transplacental	During transvaginal delivery	Hematogenous, transplacental, during delivery, and during lactation
Increased frequency	—	Late in pregnancy	During early pregnancy	Maternal genital disease at delivery	High maternal viral load
Increased severity	—	Infection during early pregnancy	—	—	—
Calcification	Periventricular	Basal ganglia	Cortical and basal ganglia	Superficial and deep gray matter	Basal ganglia
Microcephaly	Present	Present	Present	Present	—
Enhancement				Cortical	Basal ganglia
Cerebellar hypoplasia	Present	—	—	—	—
Migrational anomalies	Present	—	—	—	—

CYTOMEGALOVIRUS

CMV has been implicated as the most common cause of congenital CNS infections, at least three times as frequent as toxoplasmosis, which is the second most common organism. The virus affects about 1% of newborns. The virus is transmitted in utero through hematogenous/transplacental route. In the neonatal period, the virus can be acquired from the mother during delivery or thereafter through breast milk. It is to be noted that about 40% of mothers who acquire the infection during pregnancy transmit the virus to their fetuses.

CMV has a predilection for the germinal matrix as well as the capillary endothelium, producing periventricular tissue necrosis, thrombosis, ischemia, and subsequently periventricular dystrophic calcification. When fetal infection occurs at an early age, migrational abnormalities are likely to occur including lissencephaly, heterotopias, and cortical dysplasia.

On nonenhanced CT, the most common finding is periventricular subependymal calcification occurring in 40% to 70% of cases. Microcephaly as well as ventricular dilatation secondary to white matter loss are also noted. Migration anomalies as previously described can be seen together with cerebellar hypoplasia. On MRI, tiny periventricular pseudocysts can be seen together with focal white matter areas of high T2 signal representing gliosis.

TOXOPLASMOSIS

Toxoplasmosis is the second most common CNS infection following CMV. It is caused by a parasite, *toxoplasma gondii*. Maternal infection occurs following direct or indirect contact with oocytes in cat feces or ingestion of undercooked meat containing tissue cysts.

The fetus acquires infection through hematogenous/transplacental spread. The disease is transmitted more frequently in the later stages of pregnancy, while the severity and prognosis of the disease are related to disease transmission in early pregnancy.

On nonenhanced CT, punctate calcification can be seen predominantly in the basal ganglia. As with CMV, microcephaly is a predominant feature. On MRI, hydrocephalus caused by aqueduct stenosis, porencephaly, and hydranencephaly can be seen.

RUBELLA

Fetal infection usually occurs if maternal infection occurs during pregnancy. Infection with rubella virus has significantly declined following the widespread use of rubella vaccine. The frequency and severity of the disease are greatest if infection occurs in the first trimester. Similar to CMV, it has a predilection for the germinal matrix and vascular endothelium resulting in tissue necrosis.

On nonenhanced CT, cortical and basal ganglia calcification can occur but appear less prominent than other TORCH infections. Microcephaly, ventriculomegaly, and brain atrophy can also be seen. On MRI, focal high T2 signal might be seen in the white matter related to vasculopathy and ischemic injury.

HERPES SIMPLEX VIRUS

There are two types of herpes simplex virus. Type 1 account for 10% of neonatal infection, while type 2 accounts for 90%. The virus is transmitted during delivery by contact of the fetus with vaginal or cervical maternal herpetic lesions, and therefore, the frequency of infection is higher if genital disease was present during delivery. Unlike adults, the virus does not have a predilection to the limbic system, but usually involves the endothelial cells resulting in thrombosis and hemorrhagic infarction with subsequent encephalomalacia and atrophy.

On nonenhanced CT, superficial and deep gray matter punctate calcification is noted. Patchy white matter hypodensities are also seen that demonstrate edema pattern (low T1 and high T2) on MRI. Following administration of contrast, there is patchy cortical enhancement on CT and MRI.

HUMAN IMMUNODEFICIENCY VIRUS

Infection is caused by HIV type 1 virus, encountered during pregnancy, at delivery, or through breast-feeding. Thirty percent of mothers infected with HIV transmit the infection to their newborns. The risk of transmission is proportional to maternal viral load. In infants and children, CNS manifestations are primarily caused by HIV encephalitis and less commonly caused by secondary infections or tumors.

On nonenhanced CT, there is brain atrophy predominantly in the frontal lobes. There is faint basal ganglia enhancement seen on CT and MRI preceding the appearance of basal ganglia calcification.

ACQUIRED INFECTIONS

EXTRA-AXIAL PRESENTATIONS

Extra-axial presentations are caused by a variety of organisms and include meningitis, subdural empyema, and epidural abscess.

MENINGITIS

Inflammation of the meningeal coverings of the brain is the most common CNS infection and is divided into three general categories: acute pyogenic meningitis (usually bacterial), lymphocytic meningitis (usually viral), and chronic meningitis that could be infectious (as in tuberculosis [TB] and fungal infections) or noninfectious (sarcoidosis) (Table 10-2).

Acute pyogenic meningitis is the most common organism causing acute pyogenic meningitis and varies according to the age of patient. In neonates, it is most commonly caused by Group B streptococcus and *Escherichia coli,* which in addition to meningitis, can also present with cerebritis, ventriculitis, vasculitis, and subdural empyema. In infants and children, the most causative organism is *Neisseria meningitidis* . In adults, *Streptococcus pneumoniae* is by far the most common organism involved.

The various organisms may reach the meninges through various routes. Hematogenous spread appears to be the most common route. Direct extension from adjacent foci of inflammation such as otitis media, mastoiditis, and sinusitis is the second most common. Other possible routes include penetrating head trauma, neurosurgery, extension of intra-axial infectious process such as cerebritis or brain abscess, or extension through a preexisting congenital communication with the CSF space (as in dermal sinus).

Complications include venous thrombosis caused by stasis and thrombophlebitis, arterial vasospasm that may result in infarctions, subdural sterile effusion that is more commonly seen in infants, epidural empyema, ventriculitis/ependymitis, choroid plexitis, obstructive (communicating or noncommunicating hydrocephalus), cerebritis, and abscess formation.

Acute lymphocytic meningitis is most commonly caused by enteroviruses such as echoviruses and coxsackie viruses. Viral meningitis occurs more frequently in adults and children and is uncommon in neonates.

Chronic infectious meningitis is most commonly caused by tuberculosis. Other frequent causative organisms include cryptococcosis (especially in immunocompromised patients) and coccidiodomycosis.

Chronic noninfectious meningitis is most commonly caused by sarcoidosis. Others include histiocytosis, Wegner granulomatosis, and rheumatoid meningitis.

On nonenhanced CT, there is hardly any abnormality. Effacement of the basal cisterns may be noted. On contrast-enhanced CT, dural or leptomeningeal enhancement may be noted along the brain convexities or

TABLE 10-2 Causative Organisms and Etiologies in Different Types of Meningitis

ACUTE PYOGENIC	ACUTE LYMPHOCYTIC	CHRONIC INFECTIOUS	CHRONIC NONINFECTIOUS
Neonates: Group B streptococcus *E. coli* Infants and children: *N. meningitidis* Adults: *S. pneumoniae*	Enteroviruses (echoviruses and coxsackie viruses)	Tuberculosis Fungal infections (cryptococcosis and coccidiodomycosis)	Sarcoidosis Histiocytosis Wegners granulomatosis Rheumatoid pachymeningitis

basal cisterns, although it is much less apparent in case of acute lymphocytic meningitis related to viral infection. MRI is more sensitive than CT in detecting meningitis as well as early complications. The exudate appears isointense on T1 and hyperintense on T2 and FLAIR images. There is thickening and enhancement of the meninges following administration of contrast. Diffusion images are useful in detecting infarcts related to vasospasm, and gradient images will show hypointense blood products in the setting of hemorrhagic infarcts related to venous thrombosis. Superior sagittal sinus thrombosis may be recognized as a central triangular nonenhancing thrombus surrounded by enhancing meninges and flowing blood producing the "delta sign" on contrast-enhanced CT. On MRI, this will appear as hyperintensity along the course of the superior sagittal sinus on noncontrast T1 images. MRA and MRV are also helpful and may be obtained if arterial and venous complications are evident or clinically suspected. Other complications such as hydrocephalus, abscess, and extra-axial collections/empyema are also evident. The imaging features of tuberculous and cryptococcal meningitis will be discussed separately later in this chapter.

Subdural empyema is more common than epidural abscess and usually caused by a penetrating wound or following surgery. Less commonly, it may result from extension of infection from nearby focus such as otitis media, mastoiditis, sinusitis, or meningitis. The most common causative organisms are *S. pneumoniae* and *Staphylococcus aureus*. It is to be noted that meningitis in infants may be complicated by sterile subdural effusions that might later become infected producing subdural empyema. Complications are seen in 10% of cases and include cortical venous and dural venous thrombosis that may result in infarction. Adjacent parenchymal abscess/cerebritis is also a potential complication. In general, complications are more commonly seen in subdural empyema than in epidural abscess.

Subdural empyemas follow the same rules as subdural hemorrhage and will cross the dural attachments at cranial sutures but will not cross the falx. On nonenhanced CT, crescentic extra-axial collection is noted that might be hyperdense compared to CSF. Sterile effusions will appear isodense to CSF if not secondarily infected. On contrast-enhanced CT, peripheral rim enhancement will be evident. On MRI, the extra-axial collection may appear hyperintense to CSF on T1 and FLAIR images and will show restricted diffusion. Similar to CT, postcontrast MR images will show strong peripheral enhancement and possible loculation caused by internal fibrous septae. MRA and MRV may show arterial and venous complications.

Epidural abscess, together with subdural empyema, account for 30% of intracranial infections. The routes of infections are similar to that of subdural empyema. In contrast to subdural empyema, it can cross the falx but cannot cross the dural attachment at cranial sutures, abiding by the same rules as epidural hematoma. Apart from being lentiform (lens) shaped, it usually follows the same signal intensity and pattern of enhancement as subdural empyema. On T2-weighted images, the collection may be seen displacing the hypointense dural line inward.

INTRA-AXIAL INFECTION

Intra-axial infections are caused by a variety of organisms and include cerebritis, abscess, and ventriculitis/ependymitis.

Cerebritis is the earliest stage of intra-axial purulent parenchymal infection and in most cases will progress to abscess formation if not treated early. Routes of infection include hematogenous spread, direct spread from nearby focus of infection, penetrating trauma, neurosurgery, right-to-left shunts such as congenital cardiac or pulmonary arteriovenous malformations, or extension through a preexisting congenital communication with the CSF space (as in dermal sinus).

Early cerebritis (during first week) presents as a low-density lesion at the gray/white matter junction on CT, that shows low T1 and high T2 signal on MRI. There is minimal or no enhancement on both CT and MRI. As such, the appearance is similar to low-grade gliomas, and distinction should be based on clinical presentation. In late cerebritis (1–2 weeks), there is usually patchy or ill-defined peripheral enhancement on CT and MRI scans.

Pyogenic abscess results from progression of cerebritis, which was not treated or was unsuccessfully treated. The routes of infection and location (at the gray/white matter junction) are therefore the same as cerebritis. The causative organism is usually polymicrobial including streptococci, staphylococci, and anaerobes. Risk factors include diabetes, immunosuppression, septicemia, and infective endocarditis.

In the early stages of abscess formation (greater than 2 weeks), a central necrotic core surrounded by a well-defined collagen capsule is noted. The capsule is surrounded by edema and gliosis. In the late stages (weeks to months), the cavity shrinks, the collagen capsule thickens, and the surrounding edema decreases.

Early abscess demonstrates hypodense epicenter on CT, with well-defined, thin, smooth-enhancing capsule, which appears thinner toward the ventricles. On MRI, the abscess shows a hypointense center compared to

TABLE 10-3 Early and Late Appearance of Cerebral Abscess on CT and MRI

	EARLY ABSCESS				LATE ABSCESS			
	CECT	T1	T2	T1+C	CECT	T1	T2	T1+C
Epicenter	Hypodense	Hypointense	Hyperintense	—	Smaller			
Capsule	Thin enhancing	Iso-/hyperintense	Hypointense	Thin enhancing	Thick and irregular, decreased T2 hypointensity, decreased enhancement			
Edema	Hypodense				Decrease			

brain parenchyma (yet hyperintense when compared to CSF) on T1-weighted images, with a thin peripheral rim of isointense to hyperintense signal compared to brain parenchyma representing the capsule (Table 10-3). On T2-weighted images, the center will definitely appear hyperintense to brain parenchyma, while the capsule will appear hypointense. The T2-weighted shortening of the capsule is explained by the presence of collagen and, the paramagnetic effect of free radicals resulting from macrophage activity. Postcontrast T1-weighted images demonstrate smooth, thin-enhancing capsule. Diffusion imaging shows restrained diffusion within the central area of necrosis, which helps differentiate it from other ring-enhancing lesions. MR spectroscopy will show high concentration of lactate, and PET FDG will demonstrate increased metabolism.

Late abscess will show decrease in size of the central cavity on both CT and MRI, with thickening and slight irregularity of the surrounding capsule. With resolution of the abscess, the surrounding edema will diminish as will the T2 hypointensity of the capsule. Enhancement of the capsule may persist for several months but will definitely decrease on serial scans.

Ventriculitis/ependymitis describes inflammation of the ependymal lining the ventricles. It usually results as a complication of shunt procedures, intraventricular surgery, or intrathecal chemotherapy; however, it can also occur as a complication of meningitis or abscess. The incidence is by far more common in young age especially neonates and infants. Causative organisms include a variety of bacterial, fungal, and parasitic infections. In shunt procedures, staphylococci and streptococci seem to be the most common organisms, while in neonates, *E. coli* is the commonest. In the immunocompromised patients, a variety of fungal and parasitic infections may be involved, the most common of which is CMV.

On contrast-enhanced CT, there is thickening and enhancement of the ventricular wall with faint hypodensity seen in the surrounding periventricular brain parenchyma. There may be intraventricular fluid/fluid level caused by layering of debris. On MRI, periventricular T1 hypointensity and T2/FLAIR hyperintensity is noted with thickening and enhancement of the ventricular wall. Choroid plexitis is rare and is seen as enlarged and markedly enhancing choroid plexus. Obstruction at the level of the basal foramina or aqueduct by debris may occur and lead to hydrocephalus. Obstruction of the foramina of Monro may lead to entrapment of either or both lateral ventricles. Septations or adhesions may be noted that eventually lead to loculated areas within the ventricles.

INFECTIONS WITH SPECIFIC PRESENTATIONS

TB has been increasing in the last decade as a result of immunocompromised states, intravenous drug abuse, resistant strains, and increased crowding in certain populations such as prisons, nursing homes, and similar facilities. It is to be noted that 20% of patients with HIV have TB, while 30% of patients with TB have HIV. CNS infection is mostly caused by mycobacterium tuberculosis and results from hematogenous spread of pulmonary TB or less likely from GI or GU tracts. In the pediatric population, the infection is typically primary, while in adults, it is mostly because of reactivation/reinfection. In CNS, TB presents with meningitis or tuberculoma that may progress to tuberculous abscess.

Tuberculous meningitis is the most common presentation, with the same imaging features as meningitis, but it has a predilection for basal cisterns and may be associated with dystrophic calcification. Rarely T2 hypointense nodules can be seen along the meninges representing granulomas. On FLAIR images, there is increased intensity in the basal cisterns and sulci because of proteinaceous exudate. Enhancement of the basal meninges is seen on postcontrast images with minimal nodularity.

Tuberculoma is a localized parenchymal infection, usually multiple, supratentorial at the gray–white matter junction. Tuberculomas may be noncaseating, caseating with nonnecrotic center, or caseating with a necrotic center (Table 10-4).

Vasculitis caused by basal meningitis and extension of infection into the perivascular space may lead to

TABLE 10-4 CT and MR Imaging Features of Tuberculoma

	CECT/T1+C	T1	T2
Noncaseating	Nodular enhancement	Hypointense to brain	Hyperintense to brain
Caseating with nonnecrotic center	Ring enhancement	Iso-/hypointense to brain	Isointense center with hypointense rim
Caseating with necrotic center	Ring enhancement	Hypointense center with isointense rim	Hyperintense center with hypointense rim

thrombosis and infarction. The lenticulostriate and thalamoperforate arteries are frequently involved producing punctate or linear basal ganglia enhancement on postcontrast MR images. Diffusion images are helpful in detecting infarctions related to vasculitis.

Herpes and other encephalitides: encephalitis is a diffuse brain inflammation characterized by increased water content of the brain parenchyma. It can be caused by various organisms although usually viral (Table 10-5). Viruses spread to the brain hematogenously or through cranial nerves (as in case of HSV). Most viral encephalitides will present radiologically with nonspecific imaging appearance with high T2-weighted signal in the gray and/or white matter and variable enhancement. As such, the diagnosis is usually based on the clinical presentation and laboratory findings.

The exception to this rule is HSV, which has a specific radiological appearance on brain imaging that helps distinguish it from other similar disease processes. In adults and children HSV type 1 (orofacial herpes) is involved, as compared to HSV type 2 (genital herpes) in neonates, which shows different radiological features than type 1 (see neonatal infections). Initial infection occurs in the oronasopharynx through infected secretions. The virus then travels in retrograde fashion along the lingual branch of the mandibular division of the trigeminal nerve to the trigeminal ganglion, where it remains dormant. Reinfection or reactivation (because of immunosuppression) will cause the virus to become active causing hemorrhagic necrotizing encephalitis. Mortality rate is as high as 70% if untreated. PCR of CSF samples is usually performed to establish the diagnosis. However, the PCR protocols and quality control vary tremendously from laboratory to laboratory. A negative CSF result cannot absolutely exclude HSV. Therefore, if MRI shows compatible temporal lobe findings and no alternative diagnosis is established, early and continued treatment with acyclovir should be strongly considered.

TABLE 10-5 Location of Brain Abnormalities in Encephalitides

CAUSATIVE ORGANISM	LOCATION OF ABNORMALITY
HSV-1	Limbic system (see below)
CMV	Periventricular white matter
VZV (Varicella)	Cortex
VZV (Herpes zoster)	Cortex, brainstem, and cranial nerves
Eastern equine virus	Basal ganglia and thalami
Coxsackie and polio viruses	Midbrain and anterior spinal cord
St Louis virus	Substantia nigra
West Nile virus	Substantia nigra, brainstem, cerebellum, and anterior spinal cord
Japanese virus	Cortex, thalami, brainstem, cerebellum, and spinal cord
Listeria	Brainstem and cerebellum
Rabies	Cortex, white matter, hippocampus, hypothalamus, and brainstem

HSV has a predilection to involve the limbic system (temporal lobes, subfrontal area, cingulate gyrus, and insula). Cerebral convexities, especially the occipital cortices, are less commonly involved. Bilateral involvement is common but usually asymmetric. Rarely, the virus might involve the brainstem.

On CT, there is usually hypodensity and mild mass effect in the medial temporal lobes, with patchy or gyriform enhancement after contrast administration. MRI is more sensitive and specific in diagnosing HSV, because of higher ability to outline involvement of different structures of the limbic system. On T1 images, there is edema with mild mass effect of the involved regions. High signal intensity on T1 indicates hemorrhage, which can also be demonstrated as hypointensity on GRE images. High T2 and FLAIR signal in typical areas is seen and involves the cortex and subcortical white matter. Postcontrast images will show patchy or gyriform enhancement, with meningeal involvement and enhancement. Diffusion images will show restricted diffusion in involved areas. Differential diagnosis of HSV encephalitis is broad (Table 10-6).

Lyme disease is caused by *Borriella burgdorferi*, a tick-borne spirochete. The intermediate hosts are deer and mice. Clinically, it presents with arthralgia, erythema chronicum migrans, adenopathy, and facial nerve symptoms with or without Bells palsy. Periventricular white matter hypodense lesions are seen on CT that might enhance after contrast administration. On MRI, these lesions are best seen on T2-weighted and FLAIR sequences. Gray matter lesions are rarely seen. Meningeal involvement is less common and can be detected as meningeal enhancement on postcontrast images. Facial nerve thickening and enhancement correlates with clinically symptomatic facial neuritis. Diagnosis is usually confirmed by ELISA or PCR. Differential diagnosis

TABLE 10-6 Differential Diagnosis of Herpes Encephalitis

Limbic encephalitis	Paraneoplastic syndrome Limbic system involved Bilateral and symmetric Insidious onset
Glioma	Low-grade gliomas: Unilateral Gliomatosis cerebri: Bilateral and asymmetric Insidious onset
Infarction	MCA distribution More acute onset
Status epilepticus	Active seizures Unilateral
Syphilis	Involve medial temporal lobes, meninges, and arteries

includes multiple sclerosis, vasculitis, lacunar infarcts, and age-related white matter changes.

Rocky Mountain spotted fever is also a tick-borne rickettsial disease caused by *Rickettsia rickettsii*. Similar to Lyme disease, it has a predilection to involve the white matter and cauda equina. The white matter lesions appear similar to those of Lyme disease on CT and MRI, with similar enhancement of the lower thoracic cord and cauda equine roots.

Neurocysticercosis is caused by the helminthic cestodes tinea solium and tinea saginata, and the intermediate hosts are pigs and cattle, respectively. Infection is transmitted to human beings by eating undercooked pork or beef. It is considered the most important cause of acquired seizures. The most common location is the convexity subarachnoid space, basal cisterns, brain parenchyma, and ventricles in a descending order of frequency. Amongst all, those located in the basal cisterns carry the worst prognosis since they incite vasculitis and leptomeningitis, resulting in communicating hydrocephalus.

There are four pathologic stages that correlate with the imaging findings (Table 10-7). In the vesicular stage, the larva is alive and seen as a small marginal nodule in a small cyst with clear fluid. There is little or no inflammation around the cyst. It can remain in that stage for years before it degenerates. In the colloidal vesicular stage, the larva dies and the cyst starts to degenerate exciting inflammation and edema in the surrounding tissue. The cyst shrinks and its contents become turbid and the capsule thickens. In the granular nodular stage, the shrinkage of the cyst and thickening of the capsule progresses, and the surrounding inflammation and edema start to subside and the scolices begin to calcify. In the nodular calcified stage, the cyst becomes small and completely calcified with resolution of the adjacent inflammation.

FUNGAL INFECTIONS

A variety of fungal infections can involve the CNS such as aspergillosis, candidiasis, histoplasmosis, and coccidiodomycosis. Although immunocompromised states are the major predisposing factors for fungal infection, they still can occur in immunocompetent patients. The only manifestation may be diffuse brain edema. The lesions are usually multiple and widely distributed throughout the brain parenchyma. They appear as discrete solid-enhancing or ring-enhancing lesions that are low on T1 and high on T2 and FLAIR images. Meningeal involvement is also typical. Fungal infections are often seen to cause vasculitis with subsequent thrombosis or infarction, which can be seen on diffusion images and MRA. Cryptococcosis is discussed separately with HIV infection.

CNS MANIFESTATIONS OF HIV INFECTION

Approximately 40% to 50% of patients with AIDS have neurologic symptoms throughout their life span. Approximately 5% to 10% of patients with AIDS present

TABLE 10-7 CT and MRI Appearance of Stages of Neurocysticercosis

	VESICULAR	COLLOIDAL VESICULAR	GRANULAR NODULAR	NODULAR CALCIFIED
NECT	Well-defined, thin-walled cyst	Hyperdense cyst	Cyst shrinks and wall thickens	Small calcified lesion
CECT	Minimal or no capsule enhancement	Thick, ring-enhancing capsule	Cyst shrinks and wall thickens	No enhancement
T1	Isointense to CSF, scolex may show eccentric hyperintensity	Slightly hyperintense to CSF and capsule thickens	Cyst shrinks and wall thickens	Calcified lesion of variable intensity
T2	Isointense to CSF	Hyperintense to CSF	Cyst shrinks and wall thickens	Calcified lesion of variable intensity
FLAIR	Isointense to CSF (oxygen therapy increase conspicuity)	Hyperintense to CSF	Cyst shrinks and wall thickens	Calcified lesion of variable intensity
T1+C	Minimal or no capsule enhancement	Thick, ring-enhancing capsule and enhancing eccentric scolex	Cyst shrinks and wall thickens and enhances	Calcified lesion +/− persistent enhancement
GRE	Hypointense calcified scolex			Hypointense calcified lesion
Edema	None	Present	Decrease	Resolve

initially with CNS disease. CNS disease in AIDS is primarily infectious or neoplastic. Infections are the most common pathologies in patients with AIDS, with HIV infection being the most common. The most common opportunistic infection in patients with AIDS is toxoplasmosis, and the most common fungal infection is cryptococcosis. Other common infections include JC papovavirus causing progressive multifocal leucoencephalopathy (PML) and CMV. Uncommon infections include a variety of other fungal organisms, TB, syphilis, HSV and varicella-zoster virus. Neoplastic lesions in AIDS include primary and secondary lymphoma which unlike their appearance in immunocompetent patients have imaging findings similar to some of the AIDS infections. Other less common neoplastic lesions include glioblastoma multiforme, plasmacytoma, and Kaposi's sarcoma. Radiologically, CNS manifestations of HIV infections have two distinct presentations, diffuse or patchy white matter abnormalities and/or focal or multifocal lesions.

Diffuse or patchy white matter abnormalities can be seen in HIV encephalitis, PML, and CMV infection. Less commonly these can be due to vasculitis caused by neurosyphilis or a variety of viral and fungal infections such as varicella-zoster virus, candidiasis, or aspergillosis (Table 10-8).

HIV encephalitis is caused by HIV type 1, which is the most common infectious agent in AIDS patients followed by toxoplasmosis and cryptococcosis. Approximately 50% of adult patients and 40% of pediatric patients with AIDS have HIV encephalitis. Usually, it affects AIDS patients with CD4 counts less than 200/mm^3; clinically, it presents with AIDS dementia complex, which is a triad of cognitive, motor, and behavioral dysfunction.

On CT, there is typically generalized cerebral and cerebellar atrophy with diffuse or patchy white matter hypodensities. On MRI, T1-weighted images usually show no abnormality, while T2 and FLAIR images will demonstrate the high signal diffuse or patchy white matter changes. These lesions do not enhance following contrast administration on either CT or MRI. Similar lesions in the basal ganglia, brainstem, and cerebellum may be seen later in the disease.

PML is caused by JC virus (named after the first patient diagnosed with PML), which belongs to the papovavirus group. PML occurs in 5% of AIDS patients, usually with CD4 counts less than 50/mm^3.

On CT, there is usually single or multiple areas of white matter hypodensity in the subcortical frontal or parieto-occipital lobes without mass effect. On T1 images, the lesions appear hypointense as opposed to the normal T1 images in HIV encephalitis. On T2 and FLAIR images, the lesions appear hyperintense, with predilection for the subcortical U-shaped fibers. Usually, the lesions do not enhance, although faint enhancement can be rarely seen. Multiple lesions may enlarge along the course of the disease and later become confluent. Even when the lesions are multiple and bilateral, they are asymmetric differentiating them from the white matter lesions in HIV encephalitis. Although the lesions are more common in the white matter, any myelinated areas can be affected, and the lesions can be seen less commonly in the basal ganglia, thalami, brainstem, and cerebellum, with the later presenting with a comma-shaped lesion, caused by sparing of the dentate nucleus.

CMV belongs to the herpes virus family. In addition to encephalitis and ependymitis, the virus can produce myelitis, vasculitis, cranial neuritis, peripheral neuritis, and chorioretinitis in AIDS patients.

On CT, there is usually generalized cerebral and cerebellar atrophy, with periventricular low-density lesions. On MRI, these lesions appear hyperintense on T2 and FLAIR images. There will be ependymal enhancement seen on CT and MRI following contrast administration. Table 10-9 lists the causes of ependymal enhancement in AIDS patients.

Neurosyphilis is a sexually transmitted disease caused by the spirochete treponema pallidum. There is

TABLE 10-8 White Matter Abnormalities in Patients with HIV

	HIV ENCEPHALITIS	PML	CMV	NEUROSYPHILIS
Location	Diffuse deep WM	Fronto-parieto-occipital subcortical WM (U-fibers)	Periventricular WM	No specific predilection
Distribution	Bilateral symmetric	Bilateral asymmetric	Bilateral symmetric	Bilateral
T1 Signal	Normal	Hypointense	Hypointense	Hypointense
Enhancement	No enhancement	May show faint enhancement	Ependymal and subependymal enhancement	Enhancement of parenchymal lesions (gummas)
Brain atrophy	Cerebral and cerebellar		Cerebral and cerebellar	
Other locations	Basal ganglia, brainstem, and cerebellum, later in the disease	Basal ganglia, thalami, brainstem, and cerebellum (sparing the dentate nucleus)	None	Gray matter, meninges, cranial nerves, and cord

TABLE 10-9 Etiology of Ependymal Enhancement in Patients with AIDS

Cytomegalovirus	Periventricular lesions and smooth ependymal enhancement
Lymphoma	Thick, irregular, and nodular ependymal enhancement and ring-enhancing lesions Tumoral enhancement.
Intraventricular spread of infection	TB or pyogenic
Glioblastoma multiforme	

an association between HIV and syphilis infections since both have the same predisposing factors and routes of infection. Although it is still unclear whether AIDS increases the risk of acquiring syphilis, it is usually seen at a younger age and is more aggressive in AIDS patients. The most common intracranial manifestations of syphilis are encephalitis and meningovasculitis. In the later, there is small- and medium-sized artery involvement.

On imaging, there may be white matter lesions that appear hypodense on CT and hyperintense on T2 and FLAIR images related to vasculitis. Discrete, enhancing lesions can also be detected in the brain parenchyma representing gummas. These lesions are peripherally located and may show adjacent meningeal thickening and enhancement. MRI is more sensitive in showing cranial neuritis particularly optic and vestibulocochlear neuritis. Diffusion images are useful in showing infarcts that more commonly occur along the distribution of the middle cerebral artery and are related to vasculitis.

FOCAL OR MULTIFOCAL LESIONS

Toxoplasmosis is caused by the protozoan parasite *toxoplasma gondii* that is acquired through ingestion of undercooked meat containing the cysts or exposure to cat feces. Approximately 70% of the general population has positive serology. The parasite later reactivates when the host immunity is decreased. It is the most common opportunistic infection in patients with AIDS.

On CT, there is single or multiple isodense or hypodense ring-enhancing lesions located in the basal ganglia or gray–white matter junction, particularly of the frontal lobe, with surrounding edema. The lesions are usually 1 to 3 cm in diameter (smaller than lymphoma) (Table 10-10) and may show intralesional hemorrhage especially after treatment. On MRI, the lesions appear hypointense on T1 and hyperintense on T2 and diffusion images. MR perfusion studies shows decreased cerebral blood volume (CBV) in toxoplasmosis which may help differentiate these lesions from lymphoma, since the later usually show increased CBV, although recent reports have shown decreased CBV in lymphoma as well. Thallium-201 SPECT shows increased tracer uptake in lymphoma but not in toxoplasmosis. Despite the efforts to differentiate these two entities using various imaging modalities, clinicians usually administer a course of antitoxoplasma therapy initially and reimage the patients to see the response.

Cryptococcosis is the most common fungal infection in patients with AIDS, although it may occur in immunocompetent patients, usually with underlying chronic illness such as diabetes, alcoholism, collagen

TABLE 10-10 Imaging Findings of Toxoplasmosis Versus Lymphoma in Immunocompromised Patients

	TOXOPLASMOSIS	LYMPHOMA
Size	Smaller 1–3 cm	Larger, greater than 3 cm
Number	Single or multiple. If multiple, more numerous	Mostly multiple and less numerous
Location	Basal ganglia, gray–white matter junction at the frontal lobe	Periventricular with subependymal extension
CT	Isodense or hypodense	Hyperdense in one-third of cases
T1	Hypointense	Isointense/hypointense
T2	Hyperintense	Isointense/hypointense (because of high nuclear:cytoplasmic ratio
FLAIR	Hyperintense	Isointense/hypointense
DWI	Hyperintense	Hyperintense
Enhancement	Less than 1 cm: 75% solid	Less than 1 cm: 75% solid
	More than 1 cm: 75% ring	More than 1 cm: 50% ring +/− ependymal enhancement
Hemorrhage	More common, usually after treatment	Less common, usually after steroid or radiotherapy
Thallium-201 SPECT	Decreased tracer uptake	Increased tracer uptake
PET	Hypometabolic	Hypermetabolic
MR perfusion	Decreased CBV	Increased or decreased CBV

vascular disease, or neoplasms. It ranks the third after HIV and toxoplasmosis as a cause of CNS infection in AIDS and is seen in approximately 10% of patients. It is caused by Cryptococcus neoformans, a fungus that enters the body through the respiratory tract. Following entry, the organism spreads hematogenously to the CNS. As a result of the host immune response, the organism becomes encapsulated with acidic polysaccharide capsule that produce mucoid deposits. The most common presentation is meningitis that usually affects the base of the brain. The infection can spread along the perivascular spaces that become dilated with mucoid material forming gelatinous pseudocysts. Further spread may cause parenchymal lesions, particularly in the basal ganglia, thalami, and midbrain, known as cryptococcomas.

On CT, hypodense lesion can be seen in the basal ganglia representing cryptococcomas. These lesions appear hypointense on T1-weighted and hyperintense on T2-weighted and FLAIR images and may show ring enhancement especially in immunocompetent patients. Leptomeningeal enhancement is the most common presentation. Dilated perivascular spaces that follow CSF intensity may also be seen, representing gelatinous pseudocysts, which do not enhance since they are extra-axial and do not compromise the blood–brain barrier.

Suggested Reading

Balakrisbnan J, Becker PS, Kumar A, et al. Acquired immunodeficiency syndrome: correlation of radiologic and pathologic findings in the brain. *Radiographics*. 1990;10:201-215.

Barkovich AJ, Lindan CE. Congenital cytomegalovirus infection of the brain: imaging analysis and embryologic considerations. *AJNR Am J Neuroradiol*. 1994;15:703-715.

Benator RM, Magill HL, Gerald B, et al. Herpes simplex encephalitis: CT findings in the neonate and young infant. *AJNR Am J Neuroradiol*. 1985;6:539-543.

Caldemeyer KS, Mathews VP, Edwards-Brown MK, et al. Central nervous system cryptococcosis: parenchymal calcification and large gelatinous pseudocysts. *AJNR Am J Neuroradiol*. 1997;18:107-109.

Chang KH, Han MH. MRI of CNS parasitic diseases. *J Magn Reson Imaging*. 1998;8(2):297-307.

Chiang FL, Miller BL, Chang L, et al. Fulminant cerebral lymphoma in AIDS. *AJNR Am J Neuroradiol*. 1996;17(1):157-160.

Chrysikopoulos HS, Press GA, Grafe MR, et al. Encephalitis caused by human immunodeficiency virus: CT and MR imaging manifestations with clinical and pathologic correlation. *Radiology*. 1990;175:185-191.

Dina T. Primary central nervous system lymphoma versus toxoplasmosis in AIDS. *Radiology*. 1991;179:823-828.

Enzmann DR, Chang Y, Augustyn G. MR findings in neonatal herpes encephalitis type II. *J Comput Assist Tomogr*. 1990; 14:453-457.

Ferreira NDF, Otta GM, Amaral LLFD, et al. Imaging aspects of pyogenic infections of the central nervous system. *Top Magn Reson Imaging*. 2005;16 (2).

QUESTIONS AND ANSWERS

1. What is the most common cause of congenital CNS infection?
   A. CMV
   B. Toxoplasmosis
   C. Rubella
   D. Herpes

   ANSWER: A. CMV is the most common cause of congenital CNS infection, and toxoplasmosis is the second.

2. In which of the following infections are cerebellar hypoplasia and migration anomalies most common?
   A. HSV
   B. Toxoplasmosis
   C. CMV
   D. Rubella

   ANSWER: C. CMV has a predilection for the germinal matrix as well as the capillary endothelium, producing periventricular tissue necrosis, thrombosis, ischemia, and subsequently periventricular dystrophic calcification. When fetal infection occurs at an early age, migrational abnormalities are likely to occur including lissencephaly, heterotopias, and cortical dysplasia.

3. In which neonatal infection is basal ganglia calcification most commonly seen?
   A. Rubella
   B. Toxoplasmosis
   C. HIV
   D. All of the above

   ANSWER: D. In neonatal toxoplasmosis and HIV, calcification is usually seen in the basal ganglia. In neonatal rubella infection, calcification is usually seen in the cortex and basal ganglia.

4. What is the most common causative organism of acute pyogenic meningitis in adults?
   A. *E. coli*
   B. *N. meningitides*
   C. *S. pneumonia*
   D. *S. aureus*

   ANSWER: C. *E. coli* is the most common agent in neonatal pyogenic meningitis, while *N. meningitides* is common in infants and children.

5. What are the MRI characteristics of a pyogenic abscess in its early stage?
   A. Thin and well-defined
   B. Irregular
   C. Hyperintense on T2-weighted images
   D. Hypointense on T1-weighted images

   ANSWER: A. Early abscess shows thin, well-defined enhancing capsule that appears iso/hyperintense on T1-weighted and hypointense on T2-weighted images. The T2-weighted hypointensity of the capsule is explained by the presence of collagen and the paramagnetic effect of free radicals resulting from macrophage activity.

6. What is the most common intracranial presentation of TB?
   A. Noncaseating tuberculoma
   B. Caseating tuberculoma with nonnecrotic center
   C. Caseating tuberculoma with necrotic center
   D. Tuberculous meningitis

   ANSWER: D. Tuberculous meningitis is the most common presentation, with the same imaging features as meningitis but it has a predilection for basal cisterns and may be associated with dystrophic calcification.

7. All of the following regions of the brain are involved in herpes virus infection, *except*
   A. Insula
   B. Cingulate gyrus
   C. Temporal lobes
   D. Cerebellum

   ANSWER: D. HSV has a predilection to involve the limbic system (temporal lobes, subfrontal area, cingulate gyrus, and insula). Cerebral convexities, especially the occipital cortices, are less commonly involved. Bilateral involvement is common but usually asymmetric. Rarely the virus might involve the brainstem.

8. What is the most commonly affected cranial nerve in Lyme disease?
   A. Optic nerve
   B. Occulomotor nerve
   C. Facial nerve
   D. Vestibulecochlear nerve

   ANSWER: C. Facial nerve is the most commonly involved cranial nerve. Facial nerve thickening and enhancement correlate with clinically symptomatic facial neuritis.

9. In which stage of neurocysticercosis is the larva alive?
   A. Vesicular stage
   B. Colloidal vesicular stage
   C. Granular nodular stage
   D. Nodular calcified stage

   ANSWER: A. In the vesicular stage, the larva is alive and seen as a small marginal nodule in a small cyst with clear fluid. In the colloidal vesicular stage, the larva dies and the cyst starts to degenerate.

10. What is the most common opportunistic infection in AIDS?
    A. Toxoplasmosis
    B. Cryptococcosis
    C. CMV
    D. TB

    ANSWER: A. The most common opportunistic infection in patients with AIDS is toxoplasmosis, and the most common fungal infection is cryptococcosis.

11 NEURODEGENERATIVE AND WHITE MATTER DISEASES

Ritu Shah and Joseph C. Sullivan III

WHITE MATTER DISEASES

White matter diseases are conventionally classified into "demyelinating" and "dysmyelinating" disorders. Demyelination refers to the destruction of normally formed myelin, whereas dysmyelination indicates a defect in the formation or maintenance of myelin. In the following text, we will focus primarily on disorders of myelination while briefly mentioning other processes that may also cause white matter lesions. White matter lesions can be further categorized as multifocal (Table 11-1) or diffuse (Table 11-2).

MULTIFOCAL WHITE MATTER LESIONS

Age-related white matter hyperintensities are subcortical, central, and periventricular, commonly identified on T2-weighted MR scans in an otherwise healthy elderly patient. Cognitive function is not related to the presence or absence of the white matter hyperintensities. Patients with hypertension, diabetes, hyperlipidemia, and heart disease have more white matter hyperintensities compared to patients without these risk factors.

Virchow-Robin spaces (perivascular spaces) are found in the basal ganglia and centrum semiovale in patients of all ages and are considered a normal anatomic variant. These become more frequent and larger with

TABLE 11-1 Differential Diagnosis of Multifocal White Matter Lesions

Common	Age-related white matter hyperintensities (also known as microangiopathic changes)
	Virchow-Robin spaces
	Multiple sclerosis
	Lacunar infarcts
	Reversible posterior leukoencephalopathy syndrome
Less common	Acute disseminated encephalomyelitis
	Cerebral arteritis caused by collagen vascular or granulomatous disease
	Migraine
	Traumatic shear injuries
	Osmotic demyelination syndrome
	PML

advancing age. Virchow-Robin spaces appear as round or linear smoothly marginated foci that follow CSF on all pulse sequences on MRI.

Lacunar infarcts result from occlusion of deep perforating arteries in the basal ganglia, thalami, and brainstem. These are usually less than 1 cm in diameter, hypointense on T1-weighted images, and hyperintense on T2 and FLAIR images. Acute lesions may enhance.

Multiple sclerosis (MS) is the most commonly acquired demyelinating disease. Its precise etiology remains unknown although it is believed to be due to autoimmune-mediated demyelination in genetically susceptible individuals. Onset of disease is usually between 20 and 40 years of age with a female-to-male ratio of 1.7–2:1. In children, there is no sex predominance.

On the basis of the natural history, multiple sclerosis is classified as relapsing-remitting (85%), secondary-progressive, primary-progressive (5%–10%), and progressive-relapsing types.

Presentation with a single episode of neurologic deficit such as optic neuritis, transverse myelitis, or brainstem syndrome is also common. Progression to multiple sclerosis occurs in approximately 57% of patients with isolated brainstem syndrome and in 42% of patients with spinal cord syndrome. Risk of developing MS following optic neuritis has been estimated to be 75% or more. Presence as well as number of asymptomatic lesions on MRI markedly increase the risk of progression. Seventy percent of patients have elevated CSF IgG levels and approximately 90% have elevated oligoclonal bands.

TABLE 11-2 Differential Diagnosis of Diffuse or Confluent White Matter Lesions

Common	AIDS encephalopathy
	Advanced, deep white matter ischemia
Uncommon	Radiation injury
	Chemotherapeutic toxicity
	Severe PRES
	Leukodystrophies (adrenoleukodystrophy, Krabbe, globoid cell, Alexander disease, Canavan disease, etc.)
	Gliomatosis cerebri
	Lymphoma

MRI Findings

- Ovoid and periventricular lesions oriented perpendicularly to the long axis of the brain and lateral ventricles are characteristic of MS. These lesions are present in 85% of patients and are believed to represent inflammatory changes along long axis of medullary vein (Dawson fingers).
- The callososeptal interface is involved in 50% to 90% of patients; it is optimally imaged on the sagittal FLAIR images. Callososeptal lesions have 93% sensitivity and 98% specificity in differentiating MS lesions from vascular diseases.
- Ten percent of MS plaques in adults are infratentorial, mostly located in the brainstem or surrounding the fourth ventricle. In children, posterior fossa involvement is more common.
- Enhancement can be solid or ringlike and represents active demyelination. An open-ring pattern of enhancement is considered characteristic for MS. Delayed imaging (15–60 minutes following injection) and triple dose of gadolinium (0.3 mmol/kg versus 0.1 KG/kg) increases detection of enhancing MS lesions.
- Acute lesions can demonstrate restricted diffusion.
- MR spectroscopy: ↓ NAA, ↑ Cho. Abnormalities also present in normal-appearing white matter.
- Magnetization transfer is decreased in MS plaques and in normal-appearing white matter. Magnetization transfer ratio is highest in homogenously enhancing lesions, lower in nonenhancing lesions, and lowest in central portion of ring-enhancing lesions.
- Uncommonly, multiple sclerosis may appear as a large mass, which can be mistaken for a neoplasm (tumefactive MS). However, this mass effect is usually relatively less than expected for the size of the lesion. Tumefactive MS lesions have leading edge of enhancement and an incomplete horseshoe-shaped ring. Veins are displaced by neoplasm but course through MS lesions. Perfusion is not increased. Single-voxel MR spectroscopy utilizing a PRESS protocol with a short echo time (30 milliseconds) has been reported to demonstrate elevation of glutamate/glutamine peaks, which can aid differentiation of tumefactive demyelinating lesions from tumors.
- Solitary spinal cord involvement is seen in 5% to 24% of patients; however simultaneous brain and spinal cord involvement is more common. Sixty percent of

spinal cord lesions are in the cervical region. Spinal cord lesions in MS tend to be peripherally located, do not respect white and gray matter boundaries, and the overwhelming majority are less than two vertebral body segments in length. Associated spinal cord swelling occurs in 6% to 14% of patients and atrophy in 2% to 40% of patients.

MRI criteria for diagnosis of MS suggested by Fazekas and colleagues include three or more lesions with presence of at least two of the following lesion characteristics:

1. Size greater than 5 mm
2. Periventricular
3. Infratentorial

Multiple Sclerosis Variants

Devic disease, or neuromyelitis optica, consists of both transverse myelitis and optic neuritis, which can occur simultaneously or be separated by days or weeks. It is controversial whether this represents an acute variant of multiple sclerosis or a separate demyelinating disease.

Balo concentric sclerosis represents lesion with alternating concentric regions of demyelination and normal brain.

Schilder disease is an acute, rapidly progressive form of MS with bilateral, relatively symmetric demyelination. It is seen in childhood and rarely after the age of 40 years and is characterized by large confluent areas of demyelination involving supra- and infratentorial parenchyma.

Marburg variant is a fulminant form affecting younger patients. It has a febrile prodrome and poor prognosis with death in months.

Persons younger than 40 years and with migraine can have high signal abnormalities predominantly in the centrum semiovale and subcortical white matter, which extend into the deeper white matter at the level of the basal ganglia.

Acute disseminated encephalomyelitis (ADEM) is a monophasic demyelinating disease, usually caused by infection, vaccination, or exanthematous diseases of childhood. Suspected etiology is based on an allergic or autoimmune cross-reaction with a viral protein. MRI findings in ADEM include multiple large T2-hyperintense lesions, which enhance in a nodular or ring pattern. However, enhancement is usually mild or spotty in nature. Bilateral but asymmetric involvement of peripheral gray-white matter junction is seen. Lesions do not usually involve callososeptal interface. No new lesions should appear on MR after 6 months from initial diagnosis of the disease.

Acute hemorrhagic leukoencephalitis (Hurst disease) is a fulminant form of ADEM with rapid progression from confusion to stupor and coma in less than a week. The hemorrhages although seen on autopsy may not be seen on MRI. There is massive brain swelling and high intensity on T2WI. Enhancement may not be prominent.

Progressive multifocal leukoencephalopathy (PML) is caused by JC virus infecting the oligodendrocyte. It is associated with immunosuppressed state (most commonly AIDS) but can also be seen in autoimmune diseases, cancer, immunosuppressive therapy, lymphoproliferative disorders, myeloproliferative disorders, sarcoid, transplantation, tuberculosis, and Whipple disease. The prognosis is poor with death within 6 months to 1 year after onset. However with highly active antiretroviral therapy (HAART), longer survival has been reported. MRI typically reveals T1-hypointense and T2-hyperintense nonenhancing lesions without mass effect with predilection for parietooccipital region and posterior fossa. Brainstem and cerebellar regions are involved in approximately one-third of patients. The disease eventually becomes multifocal and confluent. Sparing of cortical ribbon and deep gray matter is common. Uncommonly, mass effect and enhancement can be seen especially as a result of immune reactivation after HAART therapy.

Reversible posterior leukoencephalopathy or posterior reversible encephalopathy syndrome (PRES) is associated with hypertension, immunosuppressive and chemotherapeutic agents (including cyclosporine, ARA and ARA-C, tacrolimus and cisplatin), preeclampsia–eclampsia, renal disease, systemic lupus erythematosus, cryoglobulinemia, hemolytic-uremic syndrome, and severe hypercalcemia. Patients present with headaches, seizures, confusion, and visual disturbances. MRI reveals reversible bilateral asymmetric cortical and subcortical white matter edema in the parietal occipital region, which can extend into temporal and frontal lobes, pons, and cerebellum. Typically, these are not restricted on diffusion, although small areas with restricted diffusion can be seen in up to 17% of cases. These may reverse or continue onto infarction. Minimal gyriform enhancement and hemorrhage are less common.

Many other diseases, including collagen vascular diseases, sarcoidosis, Lyme disease, Behcet disease, and vasculitis, result in multifocal white matter lesions that can mimic MS.

DIFFUSE OR CONFLUENT WHITE MATTER LESIONS

In advanced stages, all multifocal white matter diseases can progress to a more diffuse, confluent pattern. However, there are other conditions that more frequently have a confluent pattern of white matter abnormality.

TABLE 11-3 CNS Abnormalities Produced by Drugs and Toxins

AGENT	PATHOLOGIC FINDINGS
Heroin inhalation	Symmetric signal abnormality in cerebellar and posterior cerebral white matter and posterior limb internal capsule
Cocaine	Increased T2/FLAIR hyperintensities, hemorrhagic and ischemic stroke
Amphetamines	Hemorrhage, vasculitis, infarcts, pseudoaneurysm information
Alcohol	Chronic vermian atrophy and generalized atrophy; Wernicke encephalopathy: mamillary body, medial thalamus, hypothalamus, and periaqueductal gray signal abnormality and enhancement; Marchiafava-Bignami syndrome: signal abnormality, swelling, and enhancement involving the genu and splenium of the corpus callosum; restricted diffusion may occur in the acute form
Methanol	Optic nerve atrophy, hemorrhagic putaminal and subcortical white matter necrosis, less commonly caudate in hypothalamus
Ethylene glycol	Thalamus and pons showing T2 hyperintensity
Toluene	Cerebrum, corpus callosum, and cerebellar vermis atrophy; diffuse white matter T2 hyperintensity
Carbon monoxide	Globus pallidus, white matter, and hippocampus

CNS insults from a wide variety of recreational drugs and toxins affect white matter. The imaging abnormalities encountered often include but are not limited to the white matter (Table 11-3).

Radiation-induced demyelination is seen as T2 white matter hyperintensity and atrophy, conforming to the radiation portal. Other radiation-induced findings include hemosiderin deposition, telangiectasia, and mineralizing microangiopathy seen as calcification affecting basal ganglia and subcortical white matter. Young age at the time of treatment is associated with worse prognosis.

Disseminated necrotizing leukoencephalopathy results in diffuse demyelination after cranial spinal radiation in combination with intrathecal methotrexate for leukemia in children and adults, bone and soft tissue sarcoma, and small cell carcinoma of lung. Progressive decline in mental status and seizures are seen. MRI findings include diffuse T2 hyperintensity throughout the white matter with predilection for periventricular region and centrum semiovale with sparing of U fibers. Enhancement is rarely reported.

Postanoxic encephalopathy is an allergic demyelination caused by exposure to a myelin antigen during anoxic injury. It occurs after a severe anoxic episode, followed by recovery in 24 to 48 hours and then precipitous decline within a 2-week period. MRI findings reveal diffuse T2 hyperintensity throughout the white matter, particularly involving corpus callosum, subcortical U fibers, and internal and external capsules. Restricted diffusion is seen. Similar findings can be produced by carbon monoxide exposure but with a propensity for bilateral symmetric globus pallidus lesions.

Osmotic demyelination syndrome occurs in alcoholic, malnourished patients, who have rapid correction of hyponatremia. It is also associated with chronic renal failure, liver failure, diabetes mellitus, rapid dialysis, and syndrome of inappropriate antidiuretic hormone secretion. In children, this syndrome has been associated with orthotopic liver transplantation, acute myelogenous leukemia, Hodgkin disease, Wilson disease, and craniopharyngioma. T1 hypointense and T2 hyperintense nonenhancing signal abnormalities are seen on MRI in pons with sparing of periphery and descending corticospinal tracts. Involvement of extrapontine structures, including basal ganglia; internal, external, and extreme capsules; amygdala and cerebellum, is also seen. No mass effect or enhancement is typically present. Features of some common dysmyelinating disease have been described in Table 11-4.

TABLE 11-4 Dysmyelinating Diseases

DISEASE	INHERITANCE/ENZYMATIC DEFICIENCY	DISTINGUISHING FEATURES
Metachromatic leukodystrophy	Autosomal recessive, arylsulfatase A deficiency	Symmetric diffuse white matter hyperintensity in cerebrum and cerebellum
Adrenoleukodystrophy	X-linked or autosomal recessive, acyl-coA synthetase deficiency	Parietooccipital white matter abnormalities progressing anteriorly, enhancement along leading edge; can have enhancement in major white matter tracts
Alexander disease	Unknown	Megalencephaly in infantile form; diffuse white matter abnormality; enhancement early in course of disease
Canavan disease	Autosomal recessive, *N*-acetylaspatoacylase deficiency	Megalencephaly, diffuse white matter signal abnormality, high levels of NAA on MR spectroscopy
Krabbe disease	Unknown, beta-galactocerebrosides deficiency	Diffuse cerebral and cerebellar white matter signal abnormality; symmetric thalamic hyperdensity can be seen; optic nerve enlargement reported
Pelizaeus-Merzbacher disease	X-linked, unknown	Diffuse white matter signal abnormality and atrophy; iron deposition in lentiform nuclei, substantia nigra, dentate nuclei and thalamus, tigroid pattern

NEURODEGENERATIVE DISORDERS

Alzheimer disease (dementia Alzheimer type or DAT) accounts for 60% to 90% of the dementing disorders. Vascular dementia (15%–30%) and alcohol are the second and third most common causes of dementia, respectively. Senile plaques and neurofibrillary tangles are the diagnostic pathologic features. Abnormal accumulation of tau protein is thought to play a key role. Five to ten percent of cases are familial, and early onset of familial Alzheimer disease is associated with mutations in amyloid precursor protein gene on chromosome 21, presenilin-1 gene on chromosome 1, and presenilin-2 gene on chromosome 14. Late onset of familial and sporadic forms of Alzheimer disease is associated with ApoE-ε4 allele on chromosome 19.

Parietal and temporal cortical atrophy with disproportionate hippocampal volume loss is identified on cross-sectional imaging. Temporal horn dilatation of more than 3 mm is seen in more than 65% of patients with Alzheimer type dementia. Width of the temporal horn is also found to be the most sensitive discriminator. Subiculum of the parahippocampal region is most severely affected. In absence of cardiovascular risk factors, white matter changes are less frequent in patients with Alzheimer-type as compared to normal age-matched controls. MR spectroscopy reveals decreased NAA and increased myoinositol levels and is useful to follow progression of disease by monitoring decrease in NAA. With MR perfusion, relative values of temporoparietal CBV (as a percentage of cerebellar rCBV) are reduced by 20% in patients with DAT compared to normal controls.

Multi-infarct dementia (vascular dementia) is the second most common cause of dementia. It is clinically characterized by a progressive, episodic, stepwise decline. MRI shows cortical infarcts, with white matter ischemia and lacunar infarctions, in patients with long-standing hypertension or other risk factors for atherosclerotic disease.

Multisystem atrophy, progressive supranuclear palsy, cortical-basal ganglionic degeneration, and dementia with Lewy bodies are together known as Parkinson-plus syndromes. They also share the findings of pars compacta atrophy with Parkinson disease. Globus pallidus internus and subthalamic nucleus are usually targeted for stereotactic stimulator implantation in Parkinson disease. Table 11-5 describes unique clinical and MRI features of Parkinson syndromes, and other uncommon dementias.

AIDS–dementia complex is characterized by atrophy and white matter hyperintensity without mass effect in an AIDS patient. MR spectroscopy shows decrease in NAA and elevated choline. HAART therapy can reverse cognitive decline; however, imaging response is often delayed and may even progress initially before stabilizing eventually. Basal ganglia and brainstem manifestations respond to the greatest degree.

Binswanger disease (subcortical arteriosclerotic encephalopathy) is a demyelinating disease affecting patients older than 55 years. It is associated with hypertension (98%) and lacunar infarction. Patients may present with acute stroke followed by declining mental status or a slow, insidious decline. MRI shows broad regions of T2-hyperintense abnormalities in white matter

TABLE 11-5 Distinctive Clinical and MRI Features of Other Idiopathic Dementias

DEMENTIA	DISTINCTIVE CLINICAL FEATURE	DISTINCTIVE MRI FEATURE
Frontotemporal dementia (FTD)	Early behavioral changes with intact visual and spatial skills	Frontal and temporal lobe atrophy
Pick disease	Same as FTD, but this term is reserved for pathological variant with cytoplasmic inclusion "Pick bodies"	Anterior temporal and frontal involvement with posterior temporal and parietal sparing; "knifelike gyri"
Parkinson disease	Bradykinesia, shuffling gait, rigidity and involuntary tremors, which precede onset of dementia by >1 y	Decrease in width of pars compacta of substantia nigra on T2WI
Multisystem atrophy (MSA)	Autonomic system dysfunction and parkinsonian symptoms; dementia is usually not a prominent component of MSA	Marked cerebellar atrophy; abnormal iron deposition (T2 hypointensity) in putamen and caudate nucleus; "hot-cross bun sign" in pons on T1 and T2
Progressive supranuclear palsy	Supranuclear ophthalmoplegia (impaired downward gaze) and pseudobulbar palsy after onset of parkinsonian symptoms	Midbrain atrophy (diameter on axial scans <17 mm), enlargement of the interpeduncular cistern, third ventricular dilatation, atrophy of superior colliculi, periaqueductal high intensity
Cortical-basal ganglionic degeneration	Postural instability, dystonia, akinesia, apraxia, myoclonus, bradykinesia, and limb rigidity	Asymmetrical atrophy involving posterosuperior frontal and parietal regions ("knife blade" atrophy)
Dementia with Lewy bodies	Dementia preceding or accompanying parkinsonism, visual hallucinations, cognitive fluctuation	Brainstem and substantia nigra atrophy is seen; greater degree of cortical atrophy than the Parkinson disease; SPECT scans show occipital hypoperfusion

or frontal–parietal–occipital regions in the centrum semiovale with sparing of subcortical U fibers.

Cerebral autosomal dominant arteriopathy with subcortical infarcts and leukoencephalopathy (CADASIL) is an inherited disease caused by mutations of Notch 3 gene on chromosome 19. The disease onsets in the fourth decade, with mean age of death being 59. Recurrent transient ischemic attacks, strokes, dementia, and depression characterize this neurodegenerative disorder. It mainly affects frontal, temporal lobes, and insula. T2-hyperintense and T1-hypointense white matter lesions are seen typically with involvement of subcortical U fibers in anteroinferior temporal lobes and inferior frontal lobes.

Creutzfeldt-Jakob disease (CJD) is a rare dementing disorder thought to be due to a prion. The sporadic form is mostly seen more commonly and presents with rapid cognitive decline and cerebellar dysfunction. A new variant Creutzfeldt-Jakob disease (nvCJD), a human disease thought to be due to the same infectious agent as for bovine spongiform encephalopathy, or mad cow disease, presents at young age with more frequent psychiatric and sensory abnormalities. Prognosis is poor with 1-year survival rate of only 10%. CSF 14-3-3 is 95% sensitive and 93% specific in diagnosis of sporadic CJD.

CT studies may be normal or show atrophy. FDG PET may show cerebral hypometabolism even before MRI abnormalities are seen. Bilaterally symmetrical increased T2 hyperintensity in putaminal and caudate nuclei and cortex is seen on MRI in sporadic CJD. Restricted diffusion in cortex and basal ganglia is usually the earliest abnormality. The pulvinar sign (bilaterally symmetrical hyperintensity of the pulvinar of the thalamus) and "hockey stick" sign (symmetrical pulvinar and dorsomedial thalamic nuclear FLAIR hyperintensity) are characteristic of nvCJD.

Other related prion diseases include kuru in brain-eating cannibals, scrapie in New Guinea sheep, and Gerstmann-Straussler-Scheinker disease, which manifests with severe cerebellar dysfunction.

Amyotrophic lateral sclerosis (ALS) is a degenerative upper motor neuron disease causing progressive loss of motor, facial, limb, and diaphragmatic musculature. MRI findings reveal signal abnormality in the corticospinal tract at the level of the internal capsules. Abnormalities may extend through the full length of the corticospinal tracts from motor cortex to posterior limb of internal capsule, cerebral peduncles, and brainstem. Atrophy of anterior horn cell region of the spinal cord can also be seen.

Cerebrotendinous xanthomatosis is an autosomal recessive disorder affecting the bile acid synthesis pathway as a result of deficiency of sterol 26-hydroxylase. Mental retardation, epilepsy, polyneuropathy, and spasticity result from neurologic involvement. Combination of cataract, symmetric deep gray matter lesions and a posterior column involvement in a young individual suggests diagnoses. Focal areas of T2 hyperintensity in the globus pallidus and supratentorial white matter structures (especially corticospinal tracts in the cerebral peduncles) are identified on MRI and dentate nucleus calcification on CT. Enlargement of Virchow-Robin spaces in the spine can be seen; posterior and lateral columns may be selectively affected.

DEGENERATIVE DEEP GRAY NUCLEI DISORDERS

Unlike the cortical neurodegenerative disorders described above, these disorders usually present with movement disorders and incoordination.

Huntington chorea is an autosomal dominant genetic disorder resulting from a defect in the short arm of chromosome 4. Severe memory impairment and involuntary choreoathetoid movements are seen. It results in selective atrophy of the caudate nuclei resulting in dilated frontal horns of lateral ventricles. Increased signal intensity on MR in putaminal and globus pallidus has been described in the juvenile form of Huntington disease and frontal atrophy is usually present.

Hallervorden-Spatz syndrome is an autosomal recessive disorder associated with involuntary movements, spasticity, and progressive dementia. On MRI, T2 hypointensity in globus pallidus, red nuclei, and substantia nigra results from iron accumulation. Although normal iron deposition in these structures can be seen with increasing age, its presence in a young adult with bradykinesia, muscle rigidity, and choreoathetoid moments of the body is suggestive of the disease. "Eye of the tiger sign" is described as an area of linear high signal in a dark globus pallidus on T2WI and is considered characteristic but can be also seen in other diseases as well.

Wilson disease (hepatolenticular degeneration) is an autosomal recessive disorder caused by abnormal ceruloplasmin metabolism. Classic Kayser-Fleischer rings due to copper deposition are identified in cornea on ophthalmologic examination. CT reveals caudate nuclei and brainstem atrophy and hypodensity in basal ganglia and thalami. Bilateral symmetric FLAIR hyperintensity in caudate nuclei and putamina, T1 hyperintensity in putamina, and caudate nucleus atrophy are typical MR findings. Signal abnormalities in the midbrain on T2WI have been described as "face of the giant panda" sign. Table 11-6 given the differential diagram of T1 hyperintense in basal ganglia.

TABLE 11-6 Hyperintense Basal Ganglia on T1-Weighted Imaging

Common	Hepatic encephalopathy
	Parenteral nutrition
	Calcium-phosphate metabolic disorders (hyperparathyroidism, hypoparathyroidism, pseudohypoparathyroidism, pseudopseudohypoparathyroidism)
	Hypoxic ischemic encephalopathy
	Neurofibromatosis type I
Uncommon	Japanese encephalitis
	Wilson disease
	Hallervorden-Spatz syndrome
	Carbon monoxide poisoning
	AIDS
	Fucosidosis

METABOLIC DISORDERS

Metabolic disorders affecting the brain comprise of a large number and variety of diseases, which include mucopolysaccharidoses, lipidoses, mitochondrial defects, aminoacidopathies, and lysosomal disorders.

MUCOPOLYSACCHARIDOSES

Mucopolysaccharidoses (MPS) clinically manifest as mental retardation, peculiar facies, and musculoskeletal deformities. MRI findings include diffuse atrophy, enlargement of Virchow-Robin spaces, white matter signal abnormality with cribriform appearance, and dural thickening. Arachnoid cysts due to deposition of glycosaminoglycans in the meninges can be seen. Macrocrania can be seen with Hunter syndrome (MPS II). Atlantoaxial subluxation and cord compression due to ligamentous hypertrophy can be seen in Morquio (MPS IV) and Maroteaux-Lamy (MPS VI) syndromes.

LIPIDOSES AND OTHER STORAGE DISORDERS

Cerebellar atrophy and ataxia are seen with Tay-Sachs disease and Niemann-Pick disease. Bilateral thalamic hyperdensity on CT is characteristic of Sandhoff disease and Tay-Sachs disease. Fabry disease is an X-linked recessive disorder caused by deficiency of α-galactosidase A. It is characterized by angiokeratoma, corneal and lenticular abnormalities, acroparesthesia, renal and cardiac dysfunction, and stroke. Imaging findings include multiple infarcts, vascular stenoses and thromboses, and lacunar infarcts. T1 hyperintensity in the pulvinar likely representing calcification has been described as pathognomonic of Fabry disease.

MITOCHONDRIAL DEFECTS

Leigh disease (necrotizing encephalomyelopathy) is caused by pyruvate carboxylase/dehydrogenase deficiency. Majority of patients present by age of 2 with psychomotor delay/regression and progressive brainstem and basal ganglia dysfunction. Elevated blood and CSF lactate levels aid diagnosis. Diagnosis is made by mitochondrial analysis of muscle biopsy or cultured skin fibroblasts. MRI features include increased T2/FLAIR hyperintensity in the putamen and periaqueductal gray matter. Substantia nigra and dorsomedial nuclei of thalami can also be involved. MR spectroscopy demonstrates increased choline and decreased NAA with presence of lactate.

MELAS (mitochondrial myopathy, encephalopathy, lactic acidosis, and strokelike episodes) is characterized by onset of strokelike episodes in childhood/early adulthood with mean age of onset at 15. Male-to-female ratio is 2:1. CSF lactate is elevated. MRI findings in the acute stage include gyriform cortical swelling, not limited to vascular territories. In the chronic stage, multiple lacunar infarcts and atrophy are seen. MR spectroscopy is useful in demonstrating elevated lactate doublet peak at 1.3 ppm in 60% cases.

Other less common mitochondrial disorders also include MERRF syndrome, Kearns-Sayre syndrome, Alpers disease, Leigh disease, Menkes kinky hair disease, Zellweger syndrome, and Refsum disease.

SUGGESTED READING

Anderson JC, Costantino MM, Stratford T. Basal ganglia: anatomy, pathology, and imaging characteristics. *Curr Probl Diagn Radiol*. 2004;33:28-41.

Gasperini C. Differential diagnosis in multiple sclerosis. *Neurol Sci*. 2001;22(suppl 2):S93-S97.

Grossman RI, Yousem DM. Neurodegenerative diseases and hydrocephalus. In: Grossman RI, Yousem DM, eds. *Neuroradiology: The Requisites*. 2nd ed. Philadelphia: Mosby; 2003: 369-410.

Hesselink JR. Differential diagnostic approach to MR imaging of white matter diseases. *Top Magn Reson Imaging*. 2006; 17: 243-263.

Wallace CJ, Sevick RJ. Multifocal white matter lesions. *Semin Ultrasound CT MR*. 1996;17:251-264.

QUESTIONS AND ANSWERS

1. What is a characteristic feature of multiple sclerosis plaques in the cord?
   A. Less than two vertebral segments in length
   B. Solitary

C. Central cord involvement
D. Cord swelling

ANSWER: A. Plaques in MS typically involve peripheral cord and are less than 2 vertebral segments in length.

2. Which MRI feature supports the diagnosis of tumefactive multiple sclerosis rather than tumor?
   A. Mass effect excessive for the size of the lesion
   B. Increased perfusion
   C. Elevation of glutamate/glutamine peak on single-voxel MRS using PRESS
   D. Absence of enhancement

   ANSWER: C. Tumefactive MS lesions have less mass effect relative to size of lesion, decreased perfusion, and have an open-ring pattern of enhancement, which aid differentiation from tumor. Absence of enhancement can be seen with low-grade tumors or demyelinating lesions and does not support one diagnosis over the other.

3. What causes progressive multifocal leukoencephalopathy in AIDS patients?
   A. Autoimmune reaction to HIV
   B. JC virus infection of oligodendrocyte
   C. Prion reactivation
   D. Toxicity due to HAART therapy

   ANSWER: B. PML is caused by JC virus infecting the oligodendrocyte.

4. A 59-year old diabetic woman presents with a 2-month history of rapid cognitive decline and ataxia. MRI shows restricted diffusion and T2 hyperintensity in bilateral caudate nuclei and putamina. What is the most likely diagnosis?
   A. Hypoxic-ischemic encephalopathy
   B. Viral encephalitis
   C. Creutzfeldt-Jakob disease
   D. Uremic encephalopathy

   ANSWER: C. While hypoxic-ischemic encephalopathy, hypoglycemia, and encephalitis can all result in bilateral basal ganglia showing T2 signal abnormalities, the history together with MRI findings makes CJD the most likely diagnosis.

5. Which dysmyelinating disorder is characterized by elevated levels of NAA on MR spectroscopy?
   A. Alexander disease
   B. Canavan disease
   C. Adrenoleukodystrophy
   D. Metachromatic leukodystrophy

   ANSWER: B. Canavan disease has elevated levels of NAA on MR Spectroscopy.

6. What is the most likely diagnosis in a patient with parkinsonian features and "hot cross bun" sign on MRI?
   A. Idiopathic parkinson disease
   B. Multisystem atrophy
   C. Progressive supranuclear palsy
   D. Corticobasal degeneration

   ANSWER: B. "Hot-cross bun" sign is considered characteristic of multisystem atrophy in a patient with parkinsonian symptoms.

12 SELLA AND PARASELLAR PATHOLOGY

Joseph C. Sullivan III

CAVERNOUS SINUS ANATOMY

The sella is essentially formed by the base of the sphenoid bone and its more medial wings, with a reflection of dura surrounding this, as it encompasses the inferior hypothalamic region of the brain and the medial cranial fossa. It is bordered inferiorly by the sphenoid sinuses and anteriorly by clinoid processes at the posterior aspect of the ethmoid bone. The orbital plate also lends structure to the anterior aspect of the sella and parasellar regions. Within the cavernous sinus, there is essentially a mixed plexus of venous sinusoidal components encircling the anatomical structures, which reside and traverse the cavernous sinus. The pituitary gland proper is a central point within this sinus. Its infundibulum traverses inferiorly from the hypothalamus bordered on its anterior aspect by the posterior optic chiasm. The internal carotid arteries essentially occupy four corners of the cavernous sinus when viewed in a coronal plane (Fig. 12-1). The inferior aspects of the cavernous portions of the internal carotid artery course anteriorly after coming cephalad past the foramen lacerum from the petrous segment extending into the vertical portion. ICA it then turns anteriorly in the horizontal cavernous aspect before coming to an anterior genu, which curves the internal carotid artery more posteriorly. This gives off branches, including the meningohypophyseal trunk as well as the inferior lateral trunk. They supply the meninges. More superiorly, the ophthalmic and superior hypophyseal arteries branch off as the internal carotid artery turns more vertically at the anterior genu and then more posteriorly as it penetrates the dura.

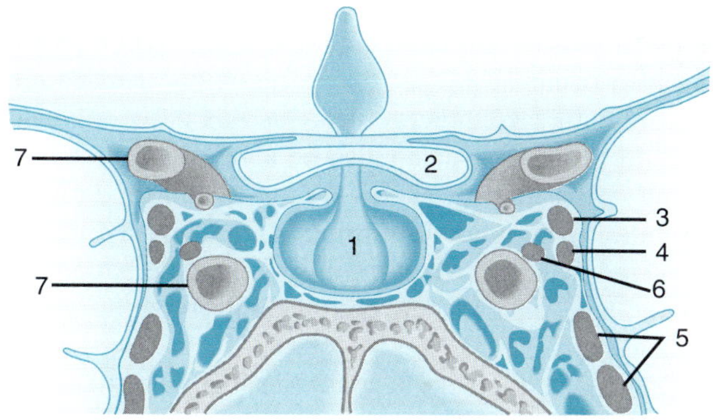

1 Pituitary gland
2 Optic chiasm
3 CN III
4 CN IV
5 CN V_1 & V_2
6 CN VI
7 ICA

FIG. 12-1 Anatomy of cavernous sinus, coronalplane.

In the coronal plane, the cranial nerves horizontally traverse through the cavernous sinus, with the sixth cranial nerve the most medial. Lesions in the central portion of the central cavernous sinus, may present with a sixth nerve palsy before impinging the more lateral cranial nerves. In a cephalad to caudad arrangement, the third, fourth, and first two components of the fifth cranial nerve course along the lateral aspect of the cavernous sinus. Another difference is that these lateral cranial nerves are encircled by a membranous layer of internal and external dural reflection. It should also be noted that the second component of the fifth cranial nerve may actually reside inferiorly in an extended reflection of the dura anterior to Meckel cave. Therefore, lesions occurring within the lateral intradural wall of the cavernous sinus, such as schwannoma, epidermoid, or less likely metastatic disease and to have a more smooth contour and shape with medial displacement of the intracavernous components and normally occur without internal carotid involvement, unless the lesion is aggressive. This is in contrast to lesions that occur in a more medial intracavernous sinus, such as meningioma or adenoma, which actually *encase* the carotid arteries.

PITUITARY GLAND

The pituitary gland itself is essentially divided into anterior and posterior lobes. The anterior lobe is further subdivided into the pars distalis, pars intermedia, and pars tuberalis more cephalad at the insertion at the infundibulum. The pars distalis is the more anterior portion with the pars intermedia being the more posterior portion of the anterior lobe abating the posterior lobe. The pars intermedia is felt to be the origin for Rathke cleft cysts, whereas pars distalis is the primary component of hormonal secretion and therefore the source of most functioning microadenomas. However, the pars tuberalis can also be a source for adenomas and may actually function after transsphenoidal hypophysectomy of the pars distalis and the pars intermedia. This may present as an adenoma, which appears to be above the diaphragma sella at the roof of the sella above the pituitary. The posterior pituitary gland or neurohypophysis is further subdivided into an infundibulum or stem, a more medium imminence, and a posterior (neural) lobe. The posterior lobe has a more direct arterial supply. The meningeal hypophyseal trunk and the inferior hypophyseal arteries arise directly from cavernous internal carotid artery. This may explain the near immediate enhancement of the posterior lobe while there is a delayed, more portal supply, enhancement of the anterior lobe. This further explains why the anterior lobe is more susceptible to ischemia and infarction, such as in the postpartum setting (Sheehan syndrome). Sheehan syndrome is a variation of pituitary apoplexy, which occurs with acute onset of infarction, necrosis, and hemorrhage into the pituitary gland. This is secondary to an adenoma in true pituitary apoplexy. Although the patient history may differ, clinical onset, however, is very similar with the acute onset of headache, visual changes, nausea, and possible ptosis. MRI is the modality of choice for diagnosis.

CONGENITAL AND DEVELOPMENTAL LESIONS

Congenital and developmental lesions consist of cyst and midline abnormalities including lipoma, teratoma, and dermoid/epidermoid. As previously mentioned, the Rathke cleft cyst develops most commonly from the pars intermedia. This is felt to be a remnant of a pouch with diverticulum from the stomodeum or primitive buccal cavity as it extends cephalad to meet the inferior migrating portion of neuroectoderm, which will form the posterior pituitary. It is this remnant connection with the oral cavity that is felt to be trapped and form a Rathke pouch cyst. However, debate remains whether this may be similar or the same lesion of a more ventral cyst of neuroectodermal origin. There can also be a continuous tract called the craniopharyngeal canal extending into the sphenoid sinus in a very small number of individuals. Similarly, there can be entrapped arachnoid-forming arachnoid cysts. Other developmental lesions such as midline lipomas or mixed mesodermal origin lesions can form as they do in other parts of the neuroaxis. Another congenital variant may be ectopic pituitary in which there is focal pituitary-enhancing tissue most commonly just at the posterior aspect of the optic chiasm at the upper infundibulum without identifiable connection into the sella. These patients may present with an overall delayed hormonal development.

NEOPLASM

Adenomas are divided into two subgroups: functioning and nonfunctioning. The functioning or hormonally active adenomas tend to present with smaller size because of their overt clinical signs secondary to abnormal hormonal effect. These can be difficult to visualize on MRI, even with the use of dynamic contrast evaluation. These adenomas have a slight delay in enhancement, resulting in a relative hypointense signal character on T1-weighted postcontrast MRI. However, again, their small size may preclude identification. Nonfunctioning adenomas tend to exert mass effect on local tissues, such as the optic chiasm, presenting with classic bitemporal hemianopsia or sixth nerve palsy with lateral rectus palsy because of this sixth cranial nerve's medial location within the sella. The macroadenoma may distort the local anatomy displacing the infundibulum to the contralateral direction as it still remains attached to the normal pituitary tissue. Even in the setting of macroadenoma, diagnosis can be difficult with CT. Secondary signs such as extension into the sphenoid sinus via erosion of the floor, bulging of the cavernous sinus at the lateral walls, or mass effect on the chiasm, infundibulum or hypothalamus may be the first imaging signs.

Glioma (astrocytoma) can arise along the optic pathways or the hypothalamus. The differentiation between a parasellar lesion with local extension versus hypothalamic origin of a tumor is critical. It should also be evaluated in the correct clinical setting because hamartomas of the tuber cinereum can have a similar appearance but a different clinical presentation consisting of gelastic seizures and possible precocious puberty. Although fairly different in appearance, a germinoma can have a similar appearance early on in young adults.

Cancer can invade (or metastasize) to the cavernous sinus. Metastasis to the anterior skull base is more commonly seen with breast and lung carcinoma but can also be seen with prostate cancer. While prostate metastases tends to be more osteoblastic and lung metastasis more lytic, breast carcinoma, although more commonly lytic, has variable presentations within the skull base. Other lesions within the clivus can be mistaken for metastasis, such as chloromas in patients with leukemia, chordomas, or even Wegener granulomatosis. Inflammation from the petrous apex, Gradenigo syndrome, can spread to the lateral petroclival junction. Chondroid lesions such as chondrosarcoma or chondroid chordomas can also occur at the petroclival junction, usually presenting with a sixth nerve palsy as this nerve traverses Dorello canal. There can also be spread of tumor from below in the inferior skull base sinuses in the younger patients. Juvenile angiofibroma is an aggressive vascular lesion usually presenting in young male patients. It can extend into the cavernous sinus via the pterygopalatine fossa.

Other paracavernous lesions or lesions that extend into the cavernous sinus, such as meningiomas, may be difficult to initially evaluate based on their location. These should be traceable to a central aspect from a localized clinoid process, reflection of dura across the diaphragma sellae, or extending from the clivus or planum sphenoidale. Lesions such as these tend to cause symptoms secondary to mass effect more than infiltration. Schwannomas rising along the cranial nerves may traverse through the cavernous sinus. If involved in the third, fourth, or first two sections of the fifth cranial nerves, they may have more of a rounded tubular appearance because of their location in the lateral cavernous dural sheath. In contrast, if these lesions are in the sixth cranial nerve, they may appear elongated and compressed, secondary to their resistance to expansion because of their more medial location within the sella. The cranial nerves should be evaluated for perineural spread from craniofacial lesions. Most frequently, this occurs with the more common squamous cell carcinoma, although adenoid cystic carcinoma has a greater propensity for perineural spread earlier in the course of the disease.

INFLAMMATION AND INFECTION

There are a multitude of inflammatory and infectious processes that can affect the pituitary gland. The sella and cavernous sinus can be affected by infectious processes within the intracranial vault of the meninges, such as basilar infectious processes from contiguous extent into the sella and cavernous sinus from the sinuses. The sella and cavernous sinus can also be affected by idiopathic inflammatory processes, such as the so-called Tolosa-Hunt syndrome. Such processes can present alone or in concert with involvement with surrounding structures such as thrombosis of the cavernous sinuses or its drainage pathways. These are of interest because their diagnostic dilemma is the entity of eosinophilic granuloma, which can present as a simple thickening of the infundibular stalk. This, as well as adenomas, can be confused with lymphocytic hypophysitis, which is an inflammatory process involving the pituitary gland or the infundibulum. This is most often seen in the classic postpartum setting; however, it can also occur in men. The enlarged pituitary gland and/or stalk may regress spontaneously or with steroid treatment. Other granulomatous processes such as giant cell granulomas and sarcoidosis can have a similar appearance as any other pituitary lesion and may also appear even similar to an adenoma of the pituitary gland. Diagnoses are often made in association with other extracranial findings. It should also be noted that although uncommon, in the correct clinical setting (immunosuppression or postoperative state), abscesses could exist in this location.

MISCELLANEOUS

In discussing the postoperative appearance within the sella and cavernous sinus and its juxtaposed sphenoid sinuses, fat saturation imaging is critical for the evaluation of the postsurgical fat patch, which is used during transsphenoidal hypophysectomy. It is also important to evaluate the optic pathways for tethering or scarring after reduction removal of large sella and suprasellar lesions.

Similar in appearance, although separate in etiology, the empty sella may occur with dehiscence of diaphragma sellae. This can be associated with increased intracranial pressure of an idiopathic nature or so-called pseudotumor cerebri. Careful attention to the optic nerve sheaths and optic heads, which can be other signs of increased intracranial pressure, should be paid when the sella appears pancaked inferiorly within the sella. Careful attention should also be paid to the native size of the sella itself so as not to mistake this appearance with previous disease.

SUGGESTED READING

Ahmadi J. Cavernous sinus invasion by pituitary adenomas. *Am J Neuroradiol.* 1985;6:893-898.

Chakeras DW et al. Magnetic resonance imaging of pituitary and parasellar abnormalities. *Radiol Clin North Am.* 1989;27(2): 265-282.

Drevelegas A. *Imaging of Brain Tumors with Histological Correlations.* New York: Springer; 2002.

El-Kalliny et al. Tumors of the lateral wall of the cavernous sinus. *J Neurosurg.* 1992;77(4):508-514.

Harrison MJ et al. Epithelial cystic lesions of the sella and parasellar region: a continuum of epithelial derivatives. *J Neurosurg.* 1994;80:1018-1025.

Hershey BL. Suprasellar masses: diagnosis and differential diagnosis. *Semin Ultrasound CT MRI.* 1993;14:215-231.

Kattath J, Silgala R, et al. Presentation and management of parasellar and suprasellar metastatic mass lesions. *J Neurol Neurosurg Psychiatry.* 1985;48:44-49.

Schwartzberg D. Imaging of pituitary gland tumors. *Semin Ultrasound CT MRI.* 1992;13:207-223.

QUESTIONS AND ANSWERS

1. Which of the following clinical signs would *not* indicate the possibility of a sella/cavernous lesion?
   A. Unilateral in turned eye
   B. Unilateral jaw pain
   C. Anisocoria
   D. Inability to close one eye
   E. Amenorrhea

   ANSWER: D. Bell palsy of the seventh cranial nerve. This is a common presentation of Bell palsy and should not be confused for the presentations seen with impingement of the cranial nerves: III supplies pupillary and upper eye lid opening, which may cause anisocoria; IV supplies the superior oblique muscle, which contributes to the ability to look down and medially; V is responsible for sensation to the face; VI supplies the lateral rectus, which is used for abduction of the globe. Amenorrhea could imply a lesion with pituitary involvement.

2. Which of the following is a lesion *least* likely seen in a parasellar distribution?
   A. Metastasis
   B. Schwannoma
   C. Adenoma
   D. Glioma
   E. Epidermoid

   ANSWER: E. Epidermoid is more typical in the cerebellar pontine angle or fourth ventricle. Cholesteatoma, a lesion similar to an epidermoid, can be seen in the petrous ridge. A schwannoma can involve the nerves traversing the cavernous sinus. Gliomas can involve the hypothalamic axis of the optic distributions.

3. Which of the following about craniopharyngiomas is *not* true?
   A. Tend to have a cystic and solid component.
   B. Childhood type (adamantinomatous) is more amenable to resection.
   C. Cyst contains a mixed proteinaceous material.
   D. Enlarging cyst may be symptomatic.
   E. Recurrences can occur with both types.

   ANSWER: B. The adamantanomatous type tends to be more adhesive to normal structures as opposed to the squamous-papillary type thought to be a cause for its said greater rate of recurrence. The squamous-papillary type, which occurs more commonly in adults, is said to be less lobulated with smaller, more watery cysts.

4. Which of the following is *not* true about aneurysms in the parasellar cavernous sinus distribution?
   A. Opthalmic complaints may be the only presenting sign.
   B. If they rupture distal to the ophthalmic segment, they will present with subarachnoid hemorrhage.
   C. Anisocoria can be caused by a posterior communicating aneurysm.
   D. If they rupture within the cavernous sinus, it will likely tamponade.
   E. Any of the cavernous cranial nerves can be affected by an ICA aneurysm.

   ANSWER: D. Rupture into the cavernous sinus most often results in a C-C fistula. This will result in arterialized flow within the opthalmic veins, presenting with ophthalmic symptoms. This is as opposed to the subarachnoid hemorrhage that occurs once the ICA penetrates the dura. Anisocoria can be caused by impingement of the pupillary control running along CN III by a PComm origin aneurysm.

5. Which of the following about schwannomas is *true*?
   A. It expands from the central nerve.
   B. Often seen in the cavernous sinus.
   C. Tubular shape indicates a lateral cavernous nerve involvement.
   D. Usually detected early.
   E. Primarily presents with vascular occlusion.

   ANSWER: C. The tubular nature is caused by restriction of the dural reflection in the lateral cavernous sinus. It originates from the support Schwann cells along the nerve. It is not that common within the cavernous sinus and when it does, Schwannomas can be silent for some time because of the dura reflection encasing the lateral cranial nerves within the cavernous sinus. They tend to present from neuronal compression.

6. What is the most sensitive imaging study for pituitary adenoma?
   A. Dynamic post-gadolinium T1 imaging
   B. Thin section T2-fast spin echo
   C. Delayed postcontrast T1-fat saturation imaging
   D. Evaluation of secondary signs (infundibular displacement)
   E. Coronal thin section inversion recovery imaging

   ANSWER: A. Dynamic postcontrast imaging uses the delay in enhancement to demonstrate the late enhancing adenoma. The anterior pituitary lobe is supplied primarily by a portal system. The adenoma will see a delayed contrast enhancement as well as a slightly slower wash out of contrast. This is useful for finding microadenomas as well as differentiating normal gland displaced by large macroadenomas.

7. Which of the following is *true* about pituitary hemorrhage?
   A. Only occurs after pregnancy
   B. More likely to occur in the posterior pituitary gland
   C. More likely to occur in an adenoma
   D. Usually presents with subarachnoid hemorrhage
   E. Usually presents with acute onset of sixth nerve palsy

   ANSWER: C. It occurs more often in adenomas as a result of a more tenuous blood supply with a classic presentation of acute onset of blindness and headache. Although it is more often described in pregnant women, it can occur in nonpregnant women or even men.

8. Which of the following is *true* about postoperative imaging of the sella/pituitary?
   A. If the chiasm is tethered, the patient will have visual defects.
   B. Delayed contrast enhanced T1-fat saturation imaging is the key.
   C. Dynamic gadolinium enhanced T1 imaging is the most beneficial for recurrence.
   D. Infundibulum will point toward the removed lesion.
   E. Sinuses do not need to be included for examination.

   ANSWER: B. As fat packing is usually used after transsphenoidal hypophysectomy, fat saturation should be used. The patient does not always have visual defect with tethering of the chiasm. Dynamic T1-postcontrast imaging may be difficult with the packing in the sella and sphenoid sinuses.

9. Which of the following is the most common cranial nerve affected by a pituitary macroadenoma?
   A. CN III
   B. CN IV
   C. CN V
   D. CN VI
   E. CN I

   ANSWER: D. Although the optic nerve (CN II) is commonly the nerve impinged by a macroadenoma at presentation, it should be remembered that CN VI is the most medial one in the cavernous sinus.

Commonly, a degree of lateral rectus palsy can be detected on examination at the time of presentation with visual symptoms. It is not covered by a reflection of dura unlike those cranial nerves in the lateral cavernous sinus.

10. What is the most common isolated cranial nerve palsy secondary pathology outside of the cavernous sinus to of those that traverse the cavernous sinus?
    A. CN I
    B. CN III
    C. CN IV
    D. CN V
    E. CN VI

    ANSWER: E. The sixth cranial nerve traverses the longest distance and is more tethered than other cranial nerves that traverse the cavernous sinus. It travels cephalad from a long course within the brainstem, exiting at the caudal pons and turns anterosuperiorly at Dorello canal at the petroclival junction. This means that it is susceptible to subtle mass effect on the brainstem as well as a multitude of skull base processes.

13 FACE AND NECK ANATOMY

Surjith Vattoth and Joseph C. Sullivan III

FACIAL SKELETON: THE BUTTRESS CONCEPT

The facial skeleton can be conceptualized as four transverse and four paired vertical buttresses, which is important from a surgeon's perspective. The buttresses represent areas of relative increased bone thickness that support the functional units of the face, including muscles, eyes, dental occlusion, and airway, in an optimal relation and define the form of the face by projecting the overlying soft-tissue envelope. As structural units that support the face, the buttresses must either directly or indirectly interface with the skull base or cranium as a stable reference. Any significant buttress displacement is treated surgically using reduction and rigid internal fixation. Transverse buttress reduction restores facial profile and width while vertical buttress reduction restores facial height. Buttress reduction establishes a functional support for the teeth and globes.

The upper transverse maxillary buttress runs from the squamous temporal bone, across the zygomatic arch and the inferior orbital rim, to the nasofrontal junction. The orbital floor is the posterior extension of this buttress. The lower transverse maxillary buttress runs along the maxilla above the alveolar ridge. The hard palate is the posterior extension of this buttress. The paired lateral vertical midface buttresses are the columns of bone from above the posterior maxillary molars across the zygomaticomaxillary suture and body of the zygoma, extending superiorly along the lateral orbital rim and across the zygomaticofrontal suture to the frontal bone. The posterior projections of these buttresses include the lateral orbital wall and the lateral wall of the maxillary sinus. The paired medial maxillary buttresses are the columns of bone from the anterior nasal spine, extending along the rim of the piriform aperture, up the frontal process of the maxilla, and across the nasofrontal junction to the frontal bone. The posterior projection of these buttresses includes the medial orbital wall and the anterior projection includes the lateral nasal wall. The paired posterior maxillary buttresses are the columns of bone at the pterygomaxillary junction where the pterygoid processes of the sphenoid join the posterior maxilla.

Naso-orbitoethmoid (NOE) fractures involve the central upper midface, disrupting the confluence of the medial maxillary buttress with the upper transverse maxillary buttress as well as their posterior extensions along the medial orbital wall and floor. The eyelids insert around the lacrimal fossa through the medial canthal tendon. Even if the frontal process of the maxilla, which is the superior portion of the medial maxillary buttress, is anatomically reduced, there can still be a residual rotation deformity that splays the posterior extension of this buttress resulting in telecanthus and globe malposition. It is important to note that in axial CT scan sections, the frontal process of maxilla lies immediately posterior to the lacrimal bones and it is a common mistake to describe these as nasal bones. Radiologic reports of NOE fractures should describe the degree of comminution of the medial vertical maxillary buttress, specifically in the region of the lacrimal fossa, where the medial canthus attaches. The distance between the two lacrimal fossae in the coronal plane is also important for the surgeon to assess the need for a medial canthoplasty. NOE fractures include damage to the ethmoid sinus and walls. If there is bilateral comminution and displacement in this region, the nasofrontal ducts that drain the frontal sinus are also likely disrupted. Although the frontal sinus may not be directly injured, if the nasofrontal ducts are disrupted, then frontal sinus surgery is needed to prevent a mucocele in the future. NOE fractures can include orbital damage. NOE fractures are distinguished from simple nasal fractures by posterior disruption of the medial canthal region, the ethmoids, and the medial orbital walls.

The two major buttresses of the zygomaticomaxillary complexes are the upper transverse maxillary (across the zygomaticomaxillary and zygomaticotemporal sutures) and the lateral vertical maxillary (across the zygomaticomaxillary and frontozygomatic sutures). The zygomaticomaxillary complexes relate to the temporal bone, maxilla, frontal bone, and skull base and are therefore a quadripod (not truly a tripod) structure. Fractures typically occur across these three buttress-related sutures, leading to the term tripod fracture. Tripod fractures consist of fracture of the zygomatic arch, the lateral orbital wall, and the inferior orbital floor. This term fails to recognize the posterior relationship of the zygoma with the sphenoid bone of the skull base and its extension inferiorly down the lateral wall of the maxillary sinus. A displaced zygomaticomaxillary complex (ZMC) fracture is a quadripod fracture. If the two buttresses of the zygoma are reduced and fixated, it is still possible to have a rotational deformity of the zygoma about the zygomaticosphenoid suture. Fractures of the zygomatic complex frequently result in sensory disturbances in the infraorbital nerve because fractures generally occur in the vicinity of the infraorbital foramen and canal.

Another accepted system of facial fracture description is the Le Fort classification. It is easy to identify the Le Fort fractures if we know the following anatomic concepts. Pterygoid process fracture is common to all Le Fort fractures, and it is rare for the pterygoid processes to be fractured in the absence of a Le Fort fracture. Each of the Le Fort fractures has a unique component. Le Fort I fracture is the only one that involves the anterolateral margin of the nasal fossa just above the maxillary alveolar process. This fracture of the anterolateral margin of the nasal fossa is easily seen on coronal or three-dimensional CT images of the face. If the pterygoid processes are broken and this portion of the maxilla is broken, a Le Fort I fracture most likely is present. If the anterolateral margin of the nasal fossa is intact, a Le Fort I fracture is excluded. Le Fort II fracture is the only one that involves the inferior orbital rim. The inferior orbital rim is also easily seen on coronal or three-dimensional CT images of the face. If the pterygoid processes are broken and the inferior orbital rim is broken, a Le Fort II fracture is probably present. If the inferior orbital rim is intact, a Le Fort II fracture is then excluded. Le Fort III fracture is the only one that involves the zygomatic arch. The zygomatic arch is easily seen on axial or three-dimensional CT images of the face. If the pterygoid processes are broken and the zygomatic arch is broken, probably a Le Fort III fracture is present. If the zygomatic arch is intact, a Le Fort III fracture is excluded.

NASAL CAVITY AND PARANASAL SINUSES

The nasal cavity has a roof formed by the cribriform plate of ethmoid; a floor formed by the palate; lateral walls formed by the turbinates/meatuses; and a midline septum formed by the perpendicular plate of ethmoid posterosuperiorly, vomer posteroinferiorly, and septal cartilage anteriorly. The meatuses of the lateral walls lie below the respective turbinates. The superior meatus receives drainage from the posterior ethmoidal air cells at the sphenoethmoidal recess. The vertical lamella of middle turbinate attaches superiorly to the cribriform plate of ethmoid and its basal lamella or ground lamella attaches posterolaterally to the lamina papyracea (lateral ethmoid sinus wall/ medial orbital wall) and forms the junction of anterior and posterior ethmoid sinuses. The surgical relevance is that the anterior ethmoid cells drain into the hiatus semilunaris of the middle meatus, while the posterior ethmoid cells drain into the superior meatus. The classical anatomy of dividing the ethmoid sinus into anterior, middle, and posterior group of cells is no longer surgically relevant. The hiatus semilunaris of the middle meatus also receives the drainage from the maxillary sinuses. The inferior meatus receives drainage from the nasolacrimal duct anteriorly.

Concha bullosa is a pneumatized middle turbinate and sometimes may be large enough to cause obstruction in the middle meatus or the infundibulum. The middle turbinate usually curves medially toward the nasal septum. However, in one-fourth of patients, the convexity is directed laterally resulting in a paradoxical middle turbinate.

The frontal sinuses are funnel-shaped cavities with a central septum dividing the frontal sinus into two parts but several septa may also be seen. The frontal recess is the drainage pathway of the frontal sinus bordered by the agger nasi cell anteriorly, lamina papyracea/agger nasi/ethmoid bulla laterally, and middle turbinate medially. It drains directly into the anterior aspect of middle meatus if the uncinate process inserts on lamina papyracea. Alternatively, the frontal recess drains into the ethmoid infundibulum and then to the middle meatus if the uncinate process inserts on middle turbinate or skull base. On coronal CT, the frontal recess is seen superior and medial to the agger nasi. Reconstructed sagittal images are the best to see the frontal recess.

The posterior limit of the frontal recess is defined by the location of the anterior ethmoidal artery. The anterior ethmoidal artery is a branch of the ophthalmic artery. From the orbit, it passes through a canal into the anterior ethmoid sinus just posterior to the frontal recess. It then crosses the sinus and enters the anterior cranial fossa before exiting and reentering the nasal cavity via the cribriform plate.

Frontal recess (Kuhn) cells are the cells that extend from the anterior ethmoid labyrinth into the frontal recess posterosuperior to the agger nasi.

1. Type I cell is a single frontal recess cell above the agger nasi but below the floor of the frontal sinus.
2. Type II cells are a tier of cells in the frontal recess above the agger nasi that might extend into the frontal sinus.
3. Type III cell is a single massive frontal recess cell that pneumatizes superiorly into the frontal sinus.
4. Type IV cell is a single isolated cell within the frontal sinus. Intersinus cell is derived from the frontal sinus, seen between the frontal sinuses, and can have mass effect on the frontal recess.

Agger nasi (meaning nasal mound in Latin) cells lie anterior and inferior to the frontal recess. They are constant extramural cells and represent the most anterior ethmoid cells. On coronal CT, they appear inferior to the frontal recess and lateral to the middle turbinate and form important surgical landmarks. When inflamed, the agger nasi cells may obstruct the frontal recess causing isolated opacification of frontal sinus without involving anterior ethmoid or maxillary sinuses. Opening these cells at endoscopic surgery usually gives access to the frontal recess.

Haller (infraorbital ethmoid) cells are ethmoid cells that extend along the floor of the orbit. They lie lateral to ethmoid (maxillary) infundibulum and when inflamed can obstruct the infundibulum producing isolated maxillary sinus disease sparing the ethmoid sinuses, the so-called infundibular pattern of sinus disease.

Onodi (sphenoethmoid) cells are posterior ethmoid cells that extend lateral and superior to the sphenoid sinus and abut the optic nerve with an endoscopically visible bulge of the optic canal.

Supraorbital cells arise from the anterior ethmoid air cells and extend between the medial orbital wall and ethmoid roof resulting in pneumatization of the orbital plate of frontal bone posterior to frontal recess and lateral to frontal sinus.

The ethmoid roof is formed by the fovea ethmoidalis of the frontal bone laterally and the lateral lamella of cribriform plate of the ethmoid bone medially. The medial aspect is 10 times thinner than the lateral aspect. Because of the delicate attachment of the middle turbinate to the cribriform plate anteriorly, surgery in this area should be performed carefully as detachment of the middle turbinate may damage the dura, resulting in cerebrospinal fluid leak. Keros has classified ethmoid roof into three types, according to the vertical height of the lateral lamella with the resultant depths of olfactory fossa. Keros type I: olfactory fossa is 1 to 3 mm deep, lateral lamella is nearly nonexistent; type II: olfactory fossa is 4 to 7 mm deep; and type III: olfactory fossa is 8 to 16 mm deep with the longest vertical height of lateral lamella of cribriform plate. Keros type III has the highest risk for iatrogenic injury to the lateral lamella of the cribriform plate at endoscopic surgery. Also the anterior ethmoidal artery is vulnerable to injury at the cribriform plate, which may cause catastrophic bleeding into the orbit.

The ostiomeatal unit is the complex anatomic region superolateral to the middle meatus where drainage of frontal, anterior, ethmoid, and maxillary sinuses occurs. It includes the superomedial maxillary sinus, maxillary sinus ostium, ethmoid (maxillary) infundibulum, hiatus semilunaris, ethmoid bulla, anterior ethmoid cells, and the frontal recess. The ethmoid infundibulum is bound laterally by the inferomedial wall of the orbit, superiorly by the hiatus semilunaris and ethmoid bulla, and medially by the uncinate process. As the maxillary sinus ostium opens into the floor of the ethmoid infundibulum, it is not possible to see the ostium endoscopically without removing the uncinate process. If an ostium is seen endoscopically, it is most likely to represent an accessory ostium. The hiatus semilunaris runs obliquely in a posteroinferior direction between the uncinate process and the ethmoid bulla and is best seen on parasagittal reconstructions. On CT, it is bound superiorly by the ethmoid bulla, laterally by the medial bony orbit, inferiorly by the uncinate process, and medially by the middle meatus. The gap between the tip of the uncinate process and the ethmoid bulla constitutes the hiatus semilunaris. In short, the maxillary sinus ostium opens into the inferior aspect (floor) of the ethmoid (maxillary) infundibulum, which runs superomedially to drain into the hiatus semilunaris, which in turn is continuous into the middle meatus of nasal cavity.

The uncinate process forms the upper medial maxillary sinus wall. It can be seen attached inferiorly to the inferior turbinate with the free edge representing the posterior free margin. Superiorly, the uncinate process may be attached to the lamina papyracea, the skull base, or the middle turbinate. As already stated, if the uncinate process is attached superiorly to the skull base or the middle turbinate, the frontal recess opens into the ethmoid infundibulum on its way to the middle meatus and infection in the infundibulum may affect the frontal sinus, resulting in the involvement of the frontal, ethmoid, and maxillary sinuses. Alternatively, if the uncinate process inserts into the lamina papyracea, the frontal recess drains directly into the anterior aspect of middle meatus, the ethmoid infundibulum being closed superiorly by a blind-ending pouch known as recessus terminals. Therefore, ethmoid infundibular inflammation does not result in concomitant frontal sinusitis. The free edge of the uncinate process may be deviated medially, which may narrow the middle meatus, or deviated laterally, which may obstruct the ethmoid infundibulum. Pneumatization maybe seen in a minority, but this uncinate process variant rarely compromises the infundibulum. A bent uncinate process may simulate a double middle turbinate on endoscopy. An atelectatic uncinate process is a condition in which the edge of the uncinate process approximates the orbital floor or the inferior aspect of the lamina papyracea and is usually associated with a hypoplastic ethmoid bulla or maxillary sinus. Uncinectomy may therefore result in injury to the orbital contents.

The ethmoid bulla is a dominant anterior ethmoid cell that protrudes inferomedially into the ethmoid infundibulum and upper middle meatus. The degree of pneumatization varies considerably ranging from failure of pneumatization (torus ethmoidalis) to a giant ethmoid bulla insinuating between the middle turbinate and uncinate process, displacing the uncinate process medially. The ethmoid bulla is bordered inferomedially by the hiatus semilunaris and ethmoid infundibulum, laterally by the lamina papyracea, and posterosuperomedially by the basal or ground lamella of middle turbinate, with the aerated gap called the sinus lateralis in between.

The sphenoid sinus is situated in the body of the sphenoid bone below the sella turcica. Its ostium is seen in the anterosuperomedial portion of the anterior sinus wall and communicates with the sphenoethmoidal recess and the posterior portion of the superior meatus. The carotid artery is related to its lateral walls, the optic nerve lies superolaterally, and the Vidian canal in its floor. The carotid artery may bulge into the sinus in approximately two-thirds of patients and rarely, the thin sinus wall separating the two may be absent. The intersphenoid septum is often deflected to one side and may be attached to the bony wall covering the carotid artery predisposing it to injury when the septum is avulsed during surgery. The maxillary (V2) nerve is closely related to the lateral aspect of the roof of the sphenoid sinus and hence, sphenoid sinusitis can produce trigeminal neuralgia. The posterior ethmoid sinus has a variable relationship with the sphenoid sinus and is intimately related to the optic nerve. The sphenoid sinus need not be directly posterior to the posterior ethmoid sinus, and the posterior ethmoid cell may extend laterally or superiorly beyond the anterior wall of the sphenoid sinus and may lead to the potential injury to the optic nerve at endoscopy. Also, there may be complete bony dehiscence of the optic canal exposing the nerve to injury.

ORBIT

The orbital roof, the floor of the anterior cranial fossa, and the frontal sinus are formed by the orbital plate of the frontal bone. The orbital surface of the zygomatic bone and greater wing of the sphenoid constitute the lateral orbital wall. The medial wall is made from anterior to posterior by the frontal process of the maxillary bone, the lacrimal bone, and the lamina papyracea of the ethmoid bone with a small contribution by the lesser wing of the sphenoid. The floor is formed by the orbital surfaces of the zygomatic bone and maxilla as well as minimally by the palatine bone medially. Medially, the superior orbital rim ends in the spine of the lacrimal bone lying posterior to the infraorbital margin, which ends in the spine of the maxillary bone. The fossa of the lacrimal sac is between these two spines. Note that the lacrimal gland lies in the lacrimal fossa, a recess of the frontal bone anterolaterally in the orbit.

The extraocular muscles are comprised of four rectus muscles, the levator palpebrae superioris and the inferior and superior oblique muscles. Other than the inferior oblique muscle, which originates at anteroinferior orbital rim, all other extraocular muscles arise from a common fibrous ring, the annulus of Zinn, which overlies the optic foramen and the medial end of the superior orbital fissure. All four rectus muscles insert into the globe behind the limbus or sclerocorneal junction. The superior oblique muscle passes medially along the roof of the orbit to the trochlear, a tendinous sling attached to the orbital roof posterior to the superomedial orbital rim. It then passes posterolaterally between the superior rectus and globe where it inserts into the sclera in the middle of the globe. The inferior oblique arises from the medial orbital floor lateral to the lacrimal sac, passing posterolaterally beneath the inferior rectus and between the lateral rectus and globe to insert into the sclera adjacent to the superior oblique. The levator palpebrae superioris is not always identified discretely from the superior rectus on conventional imaging and the two muscles are often referred to as the superior muscle complex. Extraocular muscle thickness based on CT data are inferior rectus 4.8 mm, medial rectus 4.2 mm, superior rectus 4.6 mm, and lateral rectus 3.3 mm. The muscular cone divides the orbit into an extraconal, a conal, and an intraconal compartment.

The optic foramen is formed by the lesser wing of sphenoid and is separated inferomedially from the superior orbital fissure by the optic strut, which may have high signal marrow, seen separating the optic nerve from the oculomotor and other cranial nerves (CN) on high-resolution T1-weighted MRI of the orbital apex. The superior orbital fissure is limited by the lesser wing of sphenoid superomedially and the greater wing of sphenoid inferolaterally and connects the orbit and the middle cranial fossa via the cavernous sinus. The superior orbital fissure contains ophthalmic division of trigeminal nerve; CN III, IV, and VI; superior ophthalmic vein; orbital branch of the middle meningeal artery; and sympathetic fibers. The oculomotor nerve (III) divides into superior and inferior divisions within the superior orbital fissure. The superior division supplies the superior rectus and levator palpebrae superioris, lying deep to their respective muscles. The inferior division has three branches supplying the medial and inferior rectus and the inferior oblique. The trochlear nerve (IV) lies above the oculomotor nerve in the orbital apex. It enters the orbit lateral to the annulus of Zinn above the frontal division of V1, runs medially between the superior muscle complex and the orbital periosteum, and then along the superior oblique muscle, which it supplies. The sensory ophthalmic division of the trigeminal nerve divides into three branches (frontal, lacrimal, and nasociliary) within the distal cavernous sinus before entering the orbit. The abducens nerve (VI) supplies the lateral rectus muscle.

The inferior orbital fissure lies between the floor and the greater wing of sphenoid. It communicates with the pterygopalatine fossa (PPF) and the masticator space (MS) and contains infraorbital nerve and zygomatic branch of the maxillary branch of the trigeminal nerve and emissary veins between inferior ophthalmic vein and pterygoid plexus. The infraorbital groove traverses the orbital floor, ending in the infraorbital canal and foramen.

The optic nerve sheath complex is formed by the optic nerve and the dural and leptomeningeal coverings. The intracanalicular portion of the optic nerve enters the orbit through the optic foramen with the ophthalmic artery lying inferiorly. The ciliary ganglion lies between the optic nerve and the lateral rectus muscle, usually lateral to the ophthalmic artery. The ophthalmic artery lies inferolateral to the intracanalicular optic nerve within the dural sheath. It leaves the dura inferiorly, crossing perpendicularly above the optic nerve from lateral to medial sides. In contrast, the ophthalmic vein crosses with lesser obliquity, enabling the distinction from the ophthalmic artery. The central retinal artery arises from the ophthalmic artery as it winds around the nerve and runs centrally within the optic nerve. The superior ophthalmic vein is larger and lies lateral to the superior oblique muscle anteriorly, passing backward over the optic nerve and beneath the superior muscle complex where it can be seen on coronal imaging. The inferior ophthalmic vein lies on the orbital floor between the lateral and inferior rectus muscles. It communicates through the inferior orbital fissure with the pterygoid venous plexus and the PPF.

PTERYGOPALATINE FOSSA

PPF is a fat-filled space between maxillary sinus anteriorly and pterygoid bone posteriorly. Its contents are pterygopalatine ganglion, maxillary nerve (V2) entering via foramen rotundum, and distal internal maxillary artery entering via pterygomaxillary fissure.

Pterygomaxillary fissure is the lateral opening of PPF into nasopharyngeal MS. Sphenopalatine (nasopalatine) foramen is its medial opening into superior meatus of nose, covered by mucosa. This is the region where nasopharyngeal angiofibromas arise. Inferior orbital fissure is its anterosuperior opening into orbit, which transmits infraorbital nerve (V2 branch) and artery. Foramen rotundum is the posterosuperolateral canal along which intracranial maxillary nerve (V2) passes into PPF. It can be easily identified if we search for the canal connecting the PPF to middle cranial fossa at the lateral wall of cavernous sinus. Vidian canal (running through the body of sphenoid bone) is a posteroinferomedial canal below foramen rotundum, connecting PPF to foramen lacerum. (Remember that the foramen lacerum is the anteroinferomedial cartilaginous floor of horizontal petrous previously defined ICA canal, between sphenoid and temporal bones).

Pterygopalatine canal is the inferior canal leading from PPF through greater palatine foramen to hard palate. Lesser palatine foramen, another communication of PPF to palate, is posterior to greater palatine foramen.

JUGULAR FORAMEN AND HYPOGLOSSAL CANAL

The double eagle appearance of the occipital condyles of both sides is an important landmark, which can be easily identified in coronal sections roughly at the level of the dens. The eagle's head and beak is formed by the jugular tubercle. The hypoglossal canal passes through the occipital condyle along the undersurface of the beak. The beak separates the inferomedial hypoglossal canal from the superolateral jugular foramen. The jugular foramen actually lies between the occipital and temporal bones and is anteriorly connected with the petrooccipital fissure. The carotid space (CS) extends directly up to jugular foramen.

The jugular foramen has two parts partially divided by the jugular spine, the smaller anteromedial pars nervosa and the larger posterolateral pars vascularis. The pars nervosa transmits the ninth (glossopharyngeal) cranial nerve, Jacobson nerve, and inferior petrosal sinus. The pars vascularis transmits the tenth (vagus) and eleventh (spinal accessory) cranial nerves, Arnold's nerve, jugular bulb, and posterior meningeal artery. The hypoglossal canal transmits the twelfth (hypoglossal) cranial nerve and can be seen in contrast-enhanced MRI as linear low signal–intensity structures surrounded by enhancing high signal basiocciput venous plexus. As soon as the nerve exits the hypoglossal canal, it immediately enters the nasopharyngeal CS to join CN IX, X, and XI, which come from the jugular foramen. Both the hypoglossal canal and jugular foramen empty into the cephalad–CS and therefore, the upper CS contains CN IX to XII and the internal jugular vein (IJV).

CRANIOCERVICAL JUNCTION

The articulations of the craniocervical junction include the middle atlantoaxial joint, which consists of two synovial compartments that surround the dens and allow rotation of C1 and C2 with respect to each other and the paired lateral atlantoaxial and atlanto-occipital articulations. These joints are bound and supported by several ligaments, including the anterior longitudinal ligament, the anterior atlantoaxial and atlanto-occipital ligaments, the cruciform ligaments, the alar ligaments, the apical ligament, and the tectorial membrane, which extend cranially as the cephalic extension of the posterior longitudinal ligament. The alar ligaments can be identified in coronal thin section T2/PD MRI as they extend from the lateral surface of tip of dens to anteromedial occipital condyles on each side. The transverse fibers of the cruciate ligament called the transverse atlantal ligament can be seen in T2 W axial images extending between the lateral masses of C1 passing behind the dens. On the open-mouth anteroposterior view of the craniocervical junction, the lateral masses of C1 should align exactly with the lateral margins of C2 when degenerative spurring is ignored. The posterior axial line is a line drawn along the posterior cortex of the body of the axis and extended cranially. The basion axial interval is the distance between the basion and this line and measured in the midsagittal plane. The basion axial interval is difficult to reproduce on CT images. The basion-dens interval is the distance from the most inferior portion of the basion to the closest point of the superior aspect of the dens in the midsagittal plane. In plain radiographs, 95% of adults have the basion-dens interval less than 12 mm and in 98%, the basion is situated no more than 12 mm anterior or 4 mm posterior to the posterior axial line. An abnormal distance between the dens or posterior axial line and the basion suggests failure or insufficiency of the alar ligaments, tectorial membrane, or both. In a recent CT scan series, 95% of the population was found to have a basion axial interval less than 8.5 mm with a maximum of 9.1 mm, compared with 12 mm on data from plain radiographs. The power ratio is obtained by dividing the distance between the tip of the basion to the spinolaminar line of the atlas by the distance from the tip of the opisthion to the midpoint of the posterior aspect of the anterior arch of C1. It is normal when the value is less than 1 and there is no significant difference compared with data obtained by plain radiographs. Power ratio is only sensitive in the evaluation of anterior atlanto-occipital dissociation. A posterior dissociation or vertical distraction injury could result in a normal value and consequently go undiagnosed. The atlantodental interval is measured by drawing a line from the posterior aspect of the anterior arch of C1 to the most anterior aspect of the dens at the midpoint of the thickness of the arch in craniocaudal dimension in the midsagittal plane. In plain radiographs, enlargement of the predental space, which should be less than 5 mm in children younger than 9 years of age and less than 3 mm in adults, points to injury of the transverse atlantal ligament. In CT scan, 95% of the population was found to have an atlantodental interval less than 2 mm, compared with 3 mm, the previously accepted plain radiograph measurement. The atlanto-occipital interval is calculated by drawing a line perpendicular to the articular surfaces of the occipital condyle and the lateral mass of C1, drawn at the center of the articulation by correlating the sagittal and coronal images. Measurements of the AOI are performed bilaterally and the values averaged. The atlanto-occipital interval in 95% of the population ranged between 0.5 and 1.4 mm.

The important lines and indices used for assessment of basilar invagination are Wackenheim line, Welcher basal angle, Klaus index, Chamberlain line, McGregor line, McRae line in lateral projection and atlanto-occipital joint angle in anteroposterior projection. The Wackenheim line is drawn along the posterior surface of clivus. The dens should lie anteroinferior to this line normally and any intersection of dens by this line is abnormal. The Welcher basal angle is the angle between the line drawn along the posterior surface of clivus and a line drawn anteriorly along the plane of sphenoid bone. Normal measurement is less than 140 degrees and signifies platybasia above that. Klaus index measures the perpendicular height from the tip of the dens to the twining's line. The twining's line is an anteroposterior line drawn from the tuberculum sellae to the internal occipital protuberance. If the Klaus posterior fossa height index is less than 30 mm, it suggests platybasia and basilar invagination. Chamberlain (palato-opisthion) line is drawn between hard palate and opisthion, the posterior margin of foramen magnum. Odontoid tip lying more than 5 mm above this line is abnormal. McGregor (palato-suboccipital) line is drawn from the hard palate to base of occipital bone. odontoid tip lying more than 7 mm above this line is abnormal. McRae line is drawn between the anterior and posterior margins of foramen magnum, that is, basion and opisthion. It is normally 35 mm in diameter and dens does not extend above it. In the frontal view, the angle formed at the junction of the lines traversing atlanto-occipital joints of both sides normally measures 125 to 130 degrees. It may reflect occipital condyle hypoplasia if the angle is less than 124 degrees.

TEMPORAL BONE

The external auditory canal which is a slightly S-shaped canal measuring approximately 2.5 cm in length has a fibrocartilaginous lateral third and bony medial two-thirds, without periosteum, formed mainly by the tympanic portion of temporal bone. The external auditory canal is lined by closely adherent skin, which contains hair follicles, ceruminous and sebaceous glands at the cartilaginous portion. Medially, the canal ends at the tympanic membrane, which separates the external ear from the middle ear cavity. The membrane slants inferomedially at an angle with the floor of the external auditory canal, stretching superiorly from the thin sharp-edged scutum down to the tympanic annulus. The scutum is one of the bony structures eroded or blunted early by a cholesteatoma. The tympanic membrane consists of an upper pars flaccida and a larger lower pars tensa. The pars tensa consists of an outer thin layer of squamous cells, an intermediate layer of fibrous tissue, and an inner layer of mucosal cells continuous with the middle ear cavity. The pars flaccida lacks the intermediate fibrous layer. The scutum, the tympanic membrane, and the tympanic annulus are best demonstrated on coronal images at the mid bony portion of the external auditory canal.

The middle ear cavity is divided into three compartments in the coronal plane. A line drawn from the lower edge of the scutum to the tympanic portion of the facial nerve divides the superior compartment, the epitympanum (attic), from the middle compartment, the mesotympanum (tympanic cavity proper). A line drawn parallel to the floor of the external auditory canal further divides the mesotympanum from the inferior compartment, the hypotympanum. On the axial images lines drawn parallel to the anterior and posterior walls of the external auditory canal are also used to divide the middle ear cavity into three compartments, from anterior to posterior, the protympanum, the mesotympanum, and the posterior tympanum.

The epitympanum contains the head of the malleus, the malleoincudal articulation, and the body and short process of the incus, which are best demonstrated on axial images at about the level of the vestibule. The roof of the epitympanum forms an important bony landmark, the tegmen tympani, which separates the middle ear cavity from the middle cranial fossa and is best evaluated on coronal images. The space situated between the scutum and pars flaccida laterally and the neck of the malleus medially is called the Prussak space or the lateral epitympanic recess. This is the site where the pars flaccida cholesteatoma arises and is best seen on the coronal plane. Posteriorly, the epitympanum opens into the mastoid antrum via the aditus ad antrum, which is well demonstrated on both the axial and coronal images. The Koerner septum separates the mastoid antrum medially from squamous portion of the mastoid air cells laterally. The medial wall of the epitympanum is the bone overlying the lateral semicircular canal and is an area to evaluate for fistula in cholesteatoma in the epitympanum. The tympanic portion of the facial nerve runs posterolaterally inferior to the lateral semicircular canal. In this area, the bony floor of the facial nerve canal is very thin and may not be visualized on coronal CT scan images. The tympanic segment of the facial nerve can also be identified on the axial images running from the anterior genu posterolaterally, just below the lateral semicircular canal, to the posterior genu. Coronal CT scan images at the lateral semicircular level shows three important landmarks from superior to inferior, namely, lateral semicircular canal, tympanic segment of facial nerve, and oval window. Below the oval window on coronal scan are the mesotympanic structures, namely cochlear promontory and the round window.

The mesotympanum contains the rest of the ossicular chain. On coronal images, the long process of incus is vertically oriented parallel to the malleus manubrium, continuing as the rounded lenticular process with the "hockey stick" appearance and with the facet to articulate with the head of the stapes. The stapes consists of the head and the neck (hub), the anterior and posterior crura, and a footplate. The stapes neck and crura are best demonstrated on axial images at the level of the oval window. The stapes footplate sits in the oval window niche. Both the malleoincudal and the incudostapedial articulations are synovial joints and may be afflicted with diseases involving other synovial joints of the body. At the posterior wall of the mesotympanum is a bony protuberance called the pyramidal eminence where the stapedius muscle exits to its tendinous attachment at the head or posterior crus of the stapes. Lateral to the pyramidal eminence is the facial recess which contains the descending (mastoid) segment of the facial nerve. Medial to the pyramidal eminence is the sinus tympani which may be a blind spot for the surgeon during transmastoid cholesteatoma surgery. The oval window is seen just anterior to the sinus tympani in axial images. Anteriorly just above the entrance into the eustachian tube is the bony canal for the tensor tympani muscle which inserts to the malleus. Both the stapedius and tensor tympani muscles serve to dampen the effect of high-intensity sound waves. The tensor tympani muscle is supplied by the mandibular branch of the trigeminal nerve (V3), while the stapedius muscle is supplied by the facial nerve. There is a bony prominence on the medial wall of the mesotympanum called the promontory which is caused by protrusion of the basal turn of the cochlea. Above the promontory is the oval window and posteroinferior to which is the round window niche; these relationships are well seen in coronal images through the cochlear promontory. The round window is seen at the posterolateral aspect of the basal turn of cochlea in axial images.

Anatomy of ossicular chain can be adequately evaluated in temporal bone CT scan by assessing three axial levels and a coronal level as follows. Axial section at epitympanum (attic) shows an ice cream cone appearance with the malleus head forming the anterior ice cream and the incus body/short process forming the posterior cone. Axial section at mesotympanum shows two parallel lines with the tensor tympani tendon leading to malleus neck forming the anterior line and the incus lenticular process, incudostapedial joint, and stapes head forming the posterior line. Axial section of the mesotympanum at the oval window level shows the anterior and posterior crura of stapes and its footplate fitting into the oval window. A coronal section of mesotympanum should show the ossicular "L" or hockey stick formed by the vertically oriented long process of incus and horizontally oriented lenticular process of incus.

The inner ear includes the membranous labyrinth within the bony labyrinth. The membranous labyrinth consists of the utricle, saccule, cochlear duct, and the membranous channels within the semicircular canals and the endolymphatic duct. The membranous labyrinth contains endolymph and is surrounded by perilymph, which together appear as low attenuation on CT and high-fluid signal on T2-weighted images. Perilymph connects to subarachnoid space via cochlear aqueduct, which is seen in the medial wall of temporal bone inferior to the internal auditory canal (IAC) in axial images. The bony labyrinth consists of the cochlea, the vestibule, the semicircular canals, and the cochlear and vestibular aqueducts. The cochlea consisting of two and half turns contains the organ of Corti and is the auditory end organ receiving sound waves transmitted by the ossicular chain. The base of the cochlea is at the lateral end of the IAC. The basal turn opens into the round window niche. Cochlear implants are inserted through a new opening made into the basal turn of cochlea just anterior to the round window niche. The opening to cochlea from the IAC is called the cochlear aperture. Modiolus is the central bony axis of cochlea, which lodges the spiral ganglion containing cell bodies of cochlear nerve. The osseous spiral lamina is a thin bony plate projecting to basilar membrane from modiolus and provides support and allows organized transmission of cochlear nerve fibers to each segment of the cochlea. The cochlea has three spiral chambers, namely, the perilymph containing ascending anterior spiral called scala vestibuli, the perilymph containing descending posterior spiral called scala tympani, and the endolymph containing scala media (cochlear duct) in between. The scala media is separated from the anterior scala vestibule by the vestibular (Reissner) membrane and from the posterior scala tympani by the basilar membrane on which sits the organ of Corti.

The vestibule is the largest component of the membranous labyrinth. It consists of the superior utricle and the inferior saccule. The semicircular ducts open into the utricle. There are three semicircular canals, namely, the superior (anterior), lateral (horizontal), and posterior semicircular canals. They are perpendicular to each other. The plane of the posterior semicircular canal is parallel to the petrous ridge while that of the superior semicircular canal is perpendicular to it, although both are in the vertical plane. All the semicircular canals join the vestibule with posterior limbs of the superior and posterior canals sharing a common crus. The vestibule is separated from the middle ear cavity by the oval window niche. The superior semicircular canal forms a bony ridge at the roof of the petrous bone called the arcuate eminence giving a landmark to the surgeon entering through the middle cranial fossa. The subarcuate canal is an osseous canal seen just below the superior semicircular canal passing through its arch and contains the subarcuate artery, which is a branch of labyrinthine artery, from basilar artery or anterior inferior cerebellar artery. It connects the subarachnoid space of IAC to the mastoid antrum and is a potential route of spread of infection. The subarcuate canal should not be mistaken for a congenital lesion in a child or fracture in an adult. As already stated, the cochlear aqueduct contains the perilymphatic duct and runs inferiorly to the IAC from the basal turn of the cochlea to the subarachnoid space superomedial to the jugular foramen. The vestibular aqueduct contains the endolymphatic duct and the intraosseous portion of the endolymphatic sac. It arises from the posteromedial aspect of the vestibule and runs first posterosuperiorly and then posteroinferiorly in an arc to open at the posterior aspect of the petrous temporal bone. The extraosseous portion of the endolymphatic sac lies outside the vestibular aqueduct between the layers of the posterior fossa dura.

The IAC contains the facial nerve, the cochlear nerve, the superior vestibular nerve, the inferior vestibular nerve, and the artery of the IAC. The medial opening of the IAC is called the porus acousticus. The IAC is divided at its most lateral end by the horizontal crista falciformis and the vertical crests (Bill's bar) into four compartments.

The facial nerve is in the anterosuperior compartment, the cochlear nerve is in the anteroinferior compartment, while the superior and inferior vestibular nerves are in the posterior superior and inferior compartments respectively. The facial nerve from the lateral end of the IAC enters the petrous bone as the labyrinthine portion running anterolaterally, superior to the cochlea, and toward the anterior genu (geniculate ganglion) where it makes an abrupt turn to then run posterolaterally along the medial attic wall beneath the lateral semicircular canal as the tympanic portion toward the posterior genu at the fossa incudis. It then turns inferiorly as the descending (mastoid) portion to exit at the stylomastoid foramen. Coronal images just posterior to the plane of the geniculate ganglion will show both the distal labyrinthine (medial) and proximal tympanic (lateral) portions in tangent giving the "cobra-eye" sign. The greater superficial petrosal nerve arises from the geniculate ganglion and supplies secretomotor fibers to the lacrimal gland and taste fibres from the palate. The chorda tympani nerve arises from the descending segment of the facial nerve running anterosuperiorly passing through the tympanic cavity to transmit taste fibres from the anterior two-thirds of the tongue to the lingual nerve as well as secretomotor fibres to the submandibular and sublingual glands. The singular canal is a tiny canal in the temporal bone seen parallel and posteroinferior to the IAC in axial CT scan and contains a branch of the inferior vestibular nerve that travels to posterior semicircular canal.

ORAL CAVITY

Oral cavity is the area of the suprahyoid neck below the sinonasal region and anterior to the oropharynx. It is separated from the oropharynx by soft palate, anterior tonsillar pillars, and circumvallate papillae. Note that the lingual and palatine tonsils are both contents of oropharynx, not oral cavity. The oral cavity consists of four distinct regions, namely, oral mucosal space, sublingual space, submandibular space, and root of tongue. There is no fascia covering the oral cavity regions, except the submandibular space, which is lined by superficial layer of deep cervical fascia. Also, no fascia separates the posterior submandibular and sublingual spaces from inferior parapharyngeal space (PPS).

The oral mucosal space extends from skin-vermilion junction of lips to junction of hard and soft palate above and to line of circumvallate papillae below. It includes the mucosal lip, upper and lower alveolar ridge mucosal surface, retromolar trigone, buccal mucosa, mucosal surface of floor of mouth, mucosal surface of hard palate, and mucosal surface of anterior two-thirds of the tongue (oral tongue). The posterior one-third of the tongue (base of tongue) contains the lingual tonsil and is a part of the oropharynx, not oral cavity. The retromolar trigone is a triangular mucosal area posterior to last mandibular molar tooth that covers the anterior surface of lower ascending ramus of mandible. Beneath the mucosa of the retromolar trigone lies the pterygomandibular raphe, which is a thick band of middle layer of deep cervical fascia extending between posterior border of mandibular mylohyoid ridge inferiorly and hamulus of medial pterygoid plate superiorly. The pterygomandibular raphe provides superior and inferior routes of early spread of squamous cell carcinoma involving the retromolar trigone. If carcinoma spreads directly into mandible from retromolar trigone, anterior perineural spread along inferior alveolar nerve in the mandibular inferior alveolar canal may occur. The mucosal surface of the floor of the mouth overlies the mylohyoid and hyoglossus muscles. Its posterior boundary is the base of anterior pillar of tonsil. It is divided into two sides by the frenulum of the tongue and has ostia of submandibular and sublingual salivary ducts.

Root of tongue is the undersurface of oral tongue at its junction with the anterior floor of mouth and mandible. It includes the lingual septum, inferior portion of genioglossus muscles, and geniohyoid muscles. It ends superiorly at the intrinsic tongue muscles, inferiorly at mylohyoid sling, and anteriorly at mandibular symphysis.

The sublingual space includes part of the oral tongue between mylohyoid muscle inferolaterally and geniohyoid muscle of root of tongue medially. The non–fascia-lined sublingual spaces of either side communicates anteriorly under the frenulum of tongue. Posteriorly, the sublingual space communicates with the submandibular space and inferior PPS at the posterior margin of mylohyoid muscle. Lesions of sublingual space may also extend to the anterior submandibular space in front of submandibular gland through the variably sized cleft at the junction of anterior one-third and posterior two-thirds of the mylohyoid muscle. The posterior aspect of the sublingual space is divided into medial and lateral compartments by the hyoglossus muscle attaching to the side of tongue. The lateral compartment lateral to hyoglossus and medial to mylohyoid contains hypoglossal nerve, lingual nerve, sublingual glands and ducts, deep portion of submandibular gland, and the submandibular (Wharton's) duct. The medial compartment of the posterior sublingual space medial to hyoglossus muscle and lateral to genioglossus muscle of root of tongue contains glossopharyngeal nerve, lingual artery and vein.

The submandibular space lies inferolateral to mylohyoid muscle sling, deep to platysma muscle, and superior to hyoid bone. It continues inferiorly into infrahyoid neck as anterior cervical space. Its contents include anterior belly of digastric muscle, superficial portion of submandibular gland, submandibular and submental lymph nodes, facial artery and vein, fat, and inferior loop of the hypoglossal nerve on its way to the tongue muscles. The tail of parotid gland may sometimes hang down into the posterior submandibular space.

PHARYNX

The pharynx is a musculomembranous tube extending from the skull base to the level of the cricoid cartilage. It is subdivided into the nasopharynx, oropharynx, and hypopharynx. The wall of the pharynx is composed of circular constrictor muscles—the superior, middle, and inferior constrictors—and inserts posteriorly in the midline on a median raphe, which is attached superiorly to the pharyngeal tubercle at the skull base. The other muscles of the pharynx include the salpingopharyngeus, stylopharyngeus, palatopharyngeus, tensor veli palatini, and levator veli palatini, all of which aid in movement of the pharynx during swallowing. The junctional zone between the hypopharynx and esophagus is demarcated by the cricopharyngeus muscle at C5-6 level, which is approximately 1 cm wide and attaches like a sling to the lamina of the cricoid cartilage and is the major element to the upper esophageal sphincter.

The boundaries of the nasopharynx are the basisphenoid and clivus superiorly, the retropharyngeal and prevertebral space (PVS) posteriorly, the nasal choanae anteriorly, the oropharynx inferiorly, the PPS laterally. Anteriorly, the soft palate separates the nasopharynx from the oropharynx with the posterior side of the soft palate belonging to the nasopharynx and its inferior side to the oropharynx. Posteriorly, there is no clear separation between the nasopharynx and oropharynx; on imaging studies, this separation can be made by drawing a horizontal line along the superior edge of the anterior arch of C1 or through the atlantoaxial articulation. The nasopharyngeal mucosa consists of epithelium delineating the pharyngeal mucosal space (PMS). The submucosal space also contains lymphoid tissue, accessory salivary glands, cellular notochord remnants, and tensor and levator veli palatini muscles. There are two main mucosal-lined recesses, namely, the eustachian tube orifice, just in front of the torus tubarius, and the lateral pharyngeal recess or fossa of Rosenmüller, located posterosuperior to the torus tubarius. Because of the configuration of the torus tubarius, the fossa of Rosenmüller appears posterior on axial images and superior on coronal images to the eustachian tube orifice.

The oropharynx contains the palatine (faucial) tonsils bound by anterior and posterior tonsillar pillars. The anterior tonsillar pillar is formed by mucosa over the palatoglossus muscle and the posterior tonsillar pillar is formed by mucosa over the palatopharyngeus muscle. The soft palate, posterior oropharyngeal wall, and the posterior third of the tongue (tongue base) posterior to the circumvallate papilla extending inferiorly to the vallecula, containing the lingual tonsils, are the other components. The epiglottic vallecula is the air space seen anterior to the free superior margin of epiglottis and pharyngoepiglottic folds divided in the midline by the glossoepiglottic fold and are considered a part of oropharynx.

The adenoids or pharyngeal tonsils, which are prominent in children, consist of lymphatic tissue located midline in the roof of the nasopharynx.

The fascia covering the outside of the posterior of the pharynx is the buccopharyngeal fascia (that is continuous with the fascia covering buccinator muscle). The interior fascia is the pharyngobasilar fascia. The pharyngobasilar fascia is a tough aponeurosis that surrounds the pharynx and attaches to the skull base, anteriorly to the medial plate of the pterygoid process and superiorly to the inferior part of the petrous apex. The foramen ovale is lateral to this fascia while the foramen lacerum is within the attachment of this fascia to the skull base. Posteriorly, the pharyngobasilar fascia attaches to the occipital pharyngeal tubercle and the prevertebral muscles. The eustachian tube and levator veli palatini muscle enter the nasopharynx through a posterolateral defect of the pharyngobasilar fascia, which is known as the sinus of Morgagni. The strong pharyngobasilar fascia limits tumor spread, but this protection is weak at the foramen lacerum where skull base and intracranial spread may occur despite the closure of this orifice by a fibrocartilage and at the sinus of Morgagni where posterolateral spread may occur.

Hypopharynx is the caudal continuation of the PMS between the oropharynx and esophagus and extends from the level of glossoepiglottic and pharyngoepiglottic folds superiorly to cricopharyngeus muscle at the inferior cricoid cartilage level inferiorly. The roof of the hypopharynx is formed by the glossoepiglottic fold in midline anteriorly and paired pharyngoepiglottic folds on each side laterally at the axial level of hyoid bone. These folds connect the free upper margin of epiglottis to the tongue and lateral pharyngeal walls respectively. Note that the epiglottic vallecula is the air space seen anterior to the free superior margin of epiglottis and pharyngoepiglottic folds divided in the midline by the glossoepiglottic fold.

The hypopharynx consists of three regions: paired pyriform sinuses, which are its anterolateral air containing outpouchings, posterior wall of hypopharynx, which is continuous inferiorly with the esophagus, and postcricoid region, which is the anterior wall of lower hypopharynx continuous inferiorly with the larynx. The anteromedial wall of pyriform sinus is formed by the aryepiglottic fold, which is actually a supraglottic laryngeal structure and has been referred to as marginal supraglottis. The pyriform sinus apex extends further inferiorly and is seen at the axial level of true vocal cords of the glottis.

LARYNX

The larynx has three subunits, namely, supraglottis, glottis, and subglottis. Embryologically, the supraglottic larynx develops from the primitive buccopharyngeal anlage and has rich lymphatics. The laryngeal ventricle separates it from the glottic and subglottic larynx, which forms from tracheobronchial buds and has few lymphatics.

The supraglottis consists of epiglottis, aryepiglottic folds, false vocal cords, and laryngeal ventricles. Epiglottis is a leaf-shaped cartilage with an upper suprahyoid free margin and a lower infrahyoid fixed portion. The aryepiglottic folds project superiorly from the upper tip of arytenoid cartilages to the inferolateral margin of epiglottis. As already stated, they form the superolateral margin of the supraglottis, separating it from pyriform sinuses of the hypopharynx on each side. The air-filled laryngeal ventricle separates the false vocal cord of supraglottis above from the true vocal cord of glottis below, which is well seen on coronal CT reconstructions. When a tumor crosses laryngeal ventricle to involve true and false vocal cords, it is called transglottic spread and has important treatment implications.

The glottis consists of true vocal cords, anterior commissure, and posterior commissure. During quiet respiration, the larynx is open and the anterior commissure is well demonstrated. The anterior commissure connecting the true vocal cords of two sides should not be more than 1 mm in thickness normally. In breath-hold CT scans, the vocal cords adduct and the laryngeal airway is closed. The subglottis extends from the undersurface of true vocal cords to inferior surface of cricoid cartilage.

The laryngeal cartilages include thyroid cartilage, cricoid cartilage, and paired arytenoid and corniculate cartilages. The thyroid cartilage shields the larynx. The cricoid cartilage has posterior lamina and anterior arches. It forms the inferior margin of the larynx and is the only complete laryngeal cartilage ring. The paired arytenoid cartilages are seen on the superior edge of posterior cricoid lamina. The vocal ligament attaches to the vocal process of arytenoid cartilage and marks the level of the true vocal cord. The thyroarytenoid muscle forms the bulk of the true vocal cord. Its medial fibers constitute the vocalis muscle. The corniculate cartilage lies on top of superior process of arytenoid cartilage within the aryepiglottic folds.

The paraglottic space of the glottis (true cord level) shows soft-tissue density on CT that is due to the thyroarytenoid muscle and the paraglottic space of supraglottis (under the mucosa of false cord) shows low-density fat. The preepiglottic space is a fat-filled space anterior to epiglottis and is contiguous with the paraglottic space. These spaces cannot be seen on endoscopy and imaging is required to detect occult masses.

SUPRAHYOID NECK SPACES

Suprahyoid neck spaces other than the already described sublingual and submandibular spaces are PMS, retropharyngeal space (RPS), PVS, PPS, CS, MS, parotid space, and buccal space.

There are two main fascial layers in the suprahyoid neck, namely, superficial cervical fascia that covers the subcutaneous tissues and the deep cervical fascia. The deep cervical fascia in turn has a superficial layer, a middle visceral or pharyngomucosal layer, and a deep prevertebral layer. In the suprahyoid neck, the middle visceral or pharyngomucosal layer of the deep cervical fascia encloses the pharynx. Thus the oropharynx and nasopharynx are collectively called the visceral or pharyngeal mucosal space. In the infrahyoid neck, the visceral fascia also encircles the hypopharynx, larynx, and thyroid gland and these structures are also components of visceral space.

The RPS is located directly behind the pharynx. It is a potential space bound anteriorly by the visceral fascia and posteriorly by the prevertebral fascia. The RPS is divided into anterior and posterior compartments by a very thin fascial layer called alar fascia, which may be identified in patients with edema of RPS following radiation therapy. The anterior compartment located between the visceral fascia and alar fascia is the true RPS. This space extends from the skull base to the location where the alar fascia fuses with the visceral fascia, which varies between C6 and T4. The posterior compartment between the alar fascia anteriorly and prevertebral fascia posteriorly is referred to as the danger space. This space extends from the skull base to the diaphragm and provides a direct pathway for head and neck infections to spread to posterior mediastinum. Fat and retropharyngeal lymph nodes (nodes of Rouviere), which may extend from skull base to C3 level, are the main contents of RPS. The retropharyngeal lymph nodes which are contained in the true RPS can be divided into a lateral group that overlie the prevertebral fascia at the level of transverse processes of upper cervical vertebrae and a median group that are smaller and not consistently present. The lateral nodes are more commonly involved by pathology especially from squamous cell carcinomas of nasopharynx, oropharynx, nasal cavity, and hypopharynx and present as rounded mass more than 1 cm diameter. There are no RPS lymph nodes in the infrahyoid neck. It is important to note that an RPS abscess does not elevate the prevertebral muscles, whereas PVS abscess does so.

The PVS is enclosed by prevertebral fascia. It lies directly posterior to RPS. The contents in suprahyoid neck are prevertebral muscles longus colli capitis, vertebral body, cervical intervertebral disc, spinal canal, vertebral artery, and phrenic nerve. Large rhabdomyosarcomas arising in PVS may cause diagnostic confusion with large neuroblastomas arising in CS. Erosion of adjacent anterior portion of vertebral body favors a PVS tumor and erosion along the lateral aspect of vertebra favors neuroblastoma.

The PPS lies anterior to styloid process and extends from skull base to approximately hyoid bone level. Its contents are fat, small branches of mandibular nerve, internal maxillary artery, ascending pharyngeal artery, pharyngeal venous plexus, and less commonly lymph nodes and ectopic minor salivary gland rests. Most common lesions in PPS result from extension of pathology from adjacent spaces like deep extension of tonsillar carcinoma or abscess from PMS or medial extension of odontogenic infection arising in MS. A primary PPS mass typically displaces the lateral wall of the PMS medially, the deep lobe of parotid gland laterally, and the contents of the CS posteriorly. It is important not to confuse a primary PPS mass with a mass arising from the deep lobe of parotid gland. A deep lobe of parotid mass may be surrounded medially by a thin rim of parotid tissue and may extend to superficial lobe of parotid. PPS masses are usually unifocal and parotid masses may be multifocal. Also, a primary PPS mass should not be confused with a primary MS lesion. Primary PPS masses arise medial to medial pterygoid muscle. Large masses may displace the medial pterygoid laterally, but usually do not invade it. A mass that appears to replace the medial pterygoid and involve the PPS is likely to be a MS mass that has extended into the PPS.

The CS is the poststyloid PPS that extends from the jugular foramen superiorly to the aortic arch inferiorly. It is bound anteriorly by the styloid process and PPS, laterally by the posterior belly of digastric muscle and parotid space, and medially by the lateral margin of RPS. Its contents are ICA, IJV, and CN IX and XII in the nasopharyngeal CS. Only the tenth (vagus) cranial nerve is seen from the oropharyngeal CS inferiorly. The vagus nerve is seen in the posterior notch between ICA and IJV. The sympathetic plexus runs outside the CS closely attached and medial to CS and lateral to RPS. The suprahyoid neck CS lesions typically displace the PPS fat anteriorly, styloid process anterolaterally, and the posterior belly of digastric (which separates it from the deep lobe of parotid gland) laterally. The carotid sheath is made up of components of all three layers of deep cervical fascia.

The MS contains the muscles of mastication, namely, medial and lateral pterygoids, masseter and temporalis, ramus of mandible, and the mandibular division of fifth cranial (trigeminal) nerve as it passes from the cranial cavity through foramen ovale into suprahyoid neck. The superficial layer of deep cervical fascia splits to enclose this space. The space extends inferiorly to the attachment of medial pterygoid and master muscles onto the mandible, superomedially abuts the skull base with the foramen ovale and foramen spinosum included in this space, and superolaterally extends high along parietal calvarium up to where the temporalis muscle inserts. The suprazygomatic MS or temporal fossa contains only the belly of temporalis muscle and the infrazygomatic MS or nasopharyngeal MS or infratemporal fossa is the MS proper.

The parotid space contains the parotid gland, retromandibular vein, external carotid artery, and intraparotid lymph nodes. The parotid gland is divided into superficial and deep lobes by the plane of the facial nerve, the location of which can be suggested on imaging, as it is situated just lateral to the retromandibular vein. The external carotid artery is the smaller, medial vessel of the two vessels seen within the parotid gland just behind the mandibular ramus and the retromandibular vein is the larger lateral vessel. The PPS is directly medial to parotid space, the CS posteromedial, and the MS anterior to it. A mass of the deep lobe of parotid gland displaces the PPS medially with widening of the stylomandibular gap. The upper parotid space is separated from the CS by the posterior belly of digastric muscle.

The buccal space is bound medially by the buccinator muscle, which attaches to the outer cortex of maxillary alveolar ridge, posteriorly by the MS, laterally by the parotid space, and anteriorly by the superficial muscles of facial expression and the investing fascia and inferiorly it blends imperceptibly with the submandibular space. The buccal space does not have complete fascial coverings that separate it from adjacent spaces and therefore easy spread of infections occurs. Its contents are minor salivary glands; parotid duct; lymph nodes; facial vein; facial, angular, and buccal arteries; and buccal branches of facial and mandibular nerves. The parotid (Stenson) duct emerges from the anterior parotid gland, runs along the surface of the masseter muscle, arches through the buccal space to pierce the buccinator muscle, and opens into oral cavity at the level of upper second molar tooth. The facial artery and vein that lie just anterior to the buccal segment of the parotid duct divide this space into anterior and posterior compartments. The fat of deep buccal space is a special form of adipose tissue syssarcosis, a remnant of succatory fat pad in infants, which appear on CT to have lower attenuation compared with fat of anterior buccal space and subcutaneous tissue of face.

INFRAHYOID NECK SPACES

Infrahyoid neck spaces are mainly extensions of the suprahyoid spaces, including the visceral space, CS, RPS, and perivertebral space. Other spaces are the posterior cervical space, which is a posterolateral fat containing neck space extending from mastoid tip to clavicle on both sides, and the anterior cervical space, which is the inferior continuation of the submandibular space lying lateral to the visceral space on both sides. The eleventh (spinal accessory) cranial nerve and dorsal scapular nerve lie in the floor of the posterior cervical space. Spinal accessory nodes are the main components of this space. The visceral space, which is the largest infrahyoid neck space, contains hypopharynx, larynx, trachea, esophagus, thyroid, and parathyroid glands.

NECK LYMPH NODE CLASSIFICATION

Level I nodes are submental and submandibular nodes. Level IA represents the submental nodes that lie between the medial margins of the anterior bellies of the digastric muscles. Level IB represents the submandibular nodes that lie posterior and lateral to the medial edge of the anterior belly of the digastric muscle, and anterior to a transverse line drawn on each axial image tangent to the posterior surface of the submandibular gland on each side of the neck.

Level II nodes are suprahyoid internal jugular nodes. It extends from the skull base, at the lower level of the bony margin of the jugular fossa, to the level of the lower body of the hyoid bone. Level II nodes lie anterior to a transverse line drawn on each axial image through the posterior edge of the sternocleidomastoid muscle and lie posterior to a transverse line drawn on each axial scan through the posterior edge of the submandibular gland. If a node situated within 2 cm of the skull base lies anterior, lateral, or posterior to the carotid sheath, it is classified as a level II node. If the node lies medial to the ICA, it is classified as a retropharyngeal node. Caudal to 2 cm below the skull base, level II nodes can lie anterior, lateral, medial, and posterior to the IJV. Level IIA nodes are upper internal jugular nodes that lie posterior to the IJV and are inseparable from the vein or that lie anterior, lateral, or medial to the vein. Level IIB nodes are upper spinal accessory nodes that lie posterior to the IJV and have a fat plane separating the nodes and the vein.

Level III or midjugular nodes lie between the level of the lower body of the hyoid bone and the level of the lower margin of the cricoid cartilage. These nodes lie anterior to a transverse line drawn on each axial image through the posterior edge of the sternocleidomastoid muscle. Level III nodes also lie lateral to the medial margin of either the common carotid artery or the ICA. On each side of the neck, the medial margin of these arteries separates level III (lateral) nodes from level VI (medial) nodes.

Level IV or low jugular nodes lie between the level of the lower margin of the cricoid cartilage arch and the level of the clavicle on each side as seen on each axial scan. These nodes lie anterior and medial to an oblique line drawn through the posterior edge of the sternocleidomastoid muscle and the posterolateral edge of the anterior scalene muscle on each axial image. The medial aspect of the common carotid artery is the landmark that separates level IV nodes (lateral to this artery) from level VI nodes (medial to this artery).

Level V nodes are posterior triangle nodes that extend from the skull base, at the posterior border of the attachment of the sternocleidomastoid muscle, to the level of the clavicle as seen on each axial scan. Level V nodes all lie anterior to a transverse line drawn on each axial scan through the anterior edge of the trapezius muscle. Between the levels of the skull base and the bottom of the cricoid arch, these nodes are situated posterior to a transverse line drawn on each axial scan through the posterior edge of the sternocleidomastoid muscle. Between the axial level of the bottom of the cricoid arch and the level of the clavicle, level V nodes lie posterior and lateral to an oblique line through the posterior edge of the sternocleidomastoid muscle and the posterolateral edge of the anterior scalene muscle. Level VA (upper level V) nodes lie between the skull base and the level of the lower margin of the cricoid cartilage arch, behind the posterior edge of the sternocleidomastoid muscle. Level VB (lower level V) nodes on each side lie between the level of the lower margin of the cricoid cartilage arch and the level of the clavicle as seen on each axial scan. They are behind an oblique line through the posterior edge of the sternocleidomastoid muscle and the posterolateral edge of the anterior scalene muscle.

Level VI and VII nodes are anterior neck nodes. Level VI or visceral nodes lie inferior to the lower body of the hyoid bone, superior to the top of the manubrium, and between the medial margins of the left and right common carotid arteries or the ICAs.

Level VII nodes lie caudal to the top of the manubrium in the superior mediastinum, between the medial margins of the left and right common carotid arteries. These superior mediastinal nodes extend caudally to the level of the innominate vein.

Supraclavicular nodes lie at or caudal to the level of clavicle, lateral to carotid artery, above and medial to the ribs. The nodes seen lateral to the ribs represent axillary nodes.

Suggested Reading

Ahuja AT, Yuen HY, Wong KT, et al. Computed tomography imaging of the temporal bone—normal anatomy. *Clin Radiol.* 2003;58:681-686.

Aviva RI, Casselman J. Orbital imaging. Part 1. Normal anatomy. *Clin Radiol.* 2005;60:279-287.

Coates, MH, Whyte AM, Earwaker JWS. Frontal recess air cells: spectrum of CT appearances. *Australas Radiol.* 2003;47(1):4-10.

Curtin HD, Williams R. Computed tomographic anatomy of the pterygopalatine fossa. *Radiographics.* 1985;5(3):429-440.

Hopper RA, Salemy S, Sze RW. Diagnosis of midface fractures with CT: what the surgeon needs to know. *Radiographics.* 2006;26(3):783-793.

Mukherji S, Castillo M. A simplified approach to the spaces of the suprahyoid neck. *Radiol Clin North Am.* 1998;36(5): 761-780.

Rhea JT, Novelline RA. How to simplify the CT diagnosis of Le Fort fractures. *AJR Am J Roentgenol.* 2005;184:1700-1705.

Rojas CA, Bertozzi JC, Martinez CR, et al. Reassessment of the craniocervical junction: normal values on CT. *AJNR Am J Neuroradiol.* 2007;28:1819-1823.

Som PM, Curtin HD, Mancuso AA. Imaging-based nodal classification for evaluation of neck metastatic adenopathy. *AJR Am J Roentgenol.* 2000;174:837-844.

Tan HM, Chong VFH. CT of the paranasal sinuses: normal anatomy, variants and pathology. *CME Radiol.* 2001;2(3): 120-125.

QUESTIONS AND ANSWERS

1. Which of the following is *true* regarding orbital anatomy?
   A. Trochlear nerve innervates the inferior oblique muscle
   B. Trochlea of superior oblique muscle is in the lateral wall
   C. Ophthalmic vein is superior to ophthalmic artery
   D. Annulus of Zinn separates the anterior and posterior compartments
   E. Superior orbital fissure contains the maxillary division of the trigeminal nerve

   ANSWER: C. Superior ophthalmic vein is superior to the ophthalmic artery. The trochlear nerve supplies the superior oblique muscle. The trochlea for the superior oblique muscle is in the medial wall. Other than the inferior oblique muscle, which originates at anteroinferior orbital rim, all other extraocular muscles arise from a common fibrous ring, the annulus of Zinn; the anterior and posterior compartments are not defined. The superior orbital fissure contains ophthalmic division of CN V; CN III, IV, and VI; superior ophthalmic vein; orbital branch of the middle meningeal artery; and sympathetic fibers. The maxillary division of CN V exits through foramen rotundum. CN III innervates all extraocular muscles except lateral rectus (supplied by CN VI) and superior oblique muscle (by CN IV).

2. A patient with head and neck carcinoma presents with a submental node. According to the Sloan-Kettering classification, which of the following is the nodal station?
   A. I
   B. II
   C. III
   D. V
   E. VI

   ANSWER: A. Sloan-Kettering classification groups are (I) submental and submandibular, (II) internal jugular nodes above hyoid including jugulodigastric (upper pharyngeal node adjacent to posterior belly of digastric muscle), (III) jugular between hyoid and cricoid cartilage, (IV) jugular below cricoid (most nodes will be in group II–IV), (V) posterior triangle (deep and posterior to the sternocleidomastoid and above the clavicle), (VI) anterior jugular visceral chain in front of the thyroid. See text for more details on imaging classification of cervical lymph nodes.

3. Which of the following statements is *false* regarding the position of the facial nerve in the IAC?
   A. Anterior to the vestibular nerve
   B. Above the crista falciformis
   C. Below the crista falciformis
   D. Superior to the cochlear nerve

   ANSWER: C. The IAC is separated into four quadrants by the transverse crista falciformis and vertically by Bill's bar. The facial nerve is in the anterosuperior compartment, the cochlear nerve is in the anteroinferior compartment, while the superior and inferior vestibular nerves are in the posterior superior and inferior compartments, respectively.

4. Regarding the facial nerve, all are *true* except:
   A. Superior to cochlear nerve
   B. Can enhance on MR
   C. Goes through stylomastoid foramen
   D. Separates superficial and deep portions of parotid
   E. Innervates posterior two-thirds of tongue

   ANSWER: E. Taste from the anterior two-thirds of the tongue is carried by the chorda tympani—a branch of the seventh cranial nerve that runs with fibers of the third division of CN V as the lingual nerve. Fibers run through the otic and geniculate ganglion to end at the cell bodies in the nucleus solitarius. The posterior one-third is supplied by CN IX. These fibers run through the petrosal ganglion to also reach the cell bodies of the nucleus solitarius. The facial nerve courses through the middle ear after entering the IAC. It exits through the stylomastoid foramen. It may normally show some enhancement at the geniculate ganglion and its horizontal and descending portions. Seventy-six percent enhance in one or more portions and this may be very asymmetric. Enhancement in the IAC is always abnormal. The normal enhancement is thought to be caused by a circumferential arteriovenous plexus, which is not present in the intralabyrinthine and extracranial portions. Bell palsy tends to enlarge and enhance the nerve.

5. What sinuses are involved in the ostiomeatal sinus occlusion pattern?
   A. Frontal
   B. Ethmoid and maxillary
   C. Maxillary and frontal
   D. Frontal, anterior ethmoids and maxillary sinuses

   ANSWER: D. Blockage of just the maxillary sinus ostium will result in obstruction of the maxillary sinuses, but obstruction of the hiatus semilunaris in the middle meatus will affect the frontal, maxillary, and anterior and middle ethmoids. The ostiomeatal unit is the complex anatomic region superolateral to the middle meatus where drainage of frontal, anterior ethmoid and maxillary sinuses occurs. It includes the superomedial maxillary sinus, maxillary sinus ostium, ethmoid (maxillary) infundibulum, hiatus semilunaris, ethmoid bulla, anterior ethmoid cells, and the frontal recess. Haller (infraorbital ethmoid) cells are lateral to ethmoid (maxillary) infundibulum, and when inflamed can obstruct the infundibulum producing isolated maxillary sinus disease sparing the ethmoid sinuses, the so-called infundibular pattern of sinus disease. When inflamed, the agger nasi cell may obstruct the frontal recess causing isolated opacification of frontal sinus without involving anterior ethmoid or maxillary sinuses. The posterior ethmoid sinuses and sphenoid sinus opens via the sphenoethmoidal recess into the superior meatus nose.

6. A lesion in which of the following areas will not cause in homonymous hemianopsia?
   A. Lateral geniculate body
   B. Anterior to the chiasm
   C. Posterior to the chiasm
   D. In the occipital lobe

   ANSWER: B. Homonymous hemianopsia is defined as a visual field defect involving one-half of the visual field in both eyes. Interruption of the optic tract as well as injury to the lateral geniculate nucleus results in homonymous hemianopsia. Injury to the optic nerve causes ipsilateral monocular blindness. Damage to the middle of the chiasm will cause bitemporal hemianopsia and damage to the lateral edge will cause ipsilateral nasal hemianopsia. Injury to the occipital lobe will also cause contralateral homonymous hemianopsia, but with macular sparing. Thus, an injury posterior to the chiasm will cause homonymous hemianopsia. Lesions anterior to the chiasm will cause either blindness of one eye if affecting the optic nerve or bitemporal or ipsilateral nasal hemianopsia if affecting the anterior chiasm.

7. What is the caudal extent of imaging in a patient with left vocal cord paralysis?
   A. Thyroid gland
   B. Thoracic inlet
   C. Aortopulmonary window
   D. Subclavian artery level

   ANSWER: C. Recurrent laryngeal nerves which are branches of X (vagus) cranial nerve loop under the aortic arch (ligamentum arteriosum) on the left and under the subclavian artery on the right. They supply all laryngeal muscles except for the cricothyroid, which is innervated by the external laryngeal branch of the superior laryngeal nerve (a vagal branch in the neck). Above the vocal folds the sensory innervation of the larynx is via the internal laryngeal branch of the superior laryngeal nerve. Below the vocal folds it is by way of branches of the recurrent laryngeal nerve.

8. Which of the following is *true* regarding hypopharynx?
   A. Vallecula is a part of hypopharynx.
   B. Aryepiglottic folds are hypopharyngeal structures.

C. Cricopharyngeus muscle forms the junctional zone of hypopharynx with esophagus.
D. Pyriform sinus apex is seen at the level of oropharynx.

ANSWER: C. The hypopharynx consists of three regions the names of which start with the letter "p"—the paired pyriform sinuses, which are its anterolateral air containing outpouchings, posterior wall of hypopharynx, which is continuous inferiorly with the esophagus, and postcricoid region, which is the anterior wall of lower hypopharynx continuous inferiorly with the larynx. Note that the epiglottic vallecula is the air space seen anterior to the free superior margin of epiglottis and pharyngoepiglottic folds divided in the midline by the glossoepiglottic fold and is considered a part of oropharynx. The anteromedial wall of pyriform sinus is formed by the aryepiglottic fold, which is actually a supraglottic laryngeal structure and has been referred to as marginal supraglottis. The pyriform sinus apex extends further inferiorly and is seen at the axial level of true vocal cords of the glottis. The junctional zone between the hypopharynx and esophagus is demarcated by the cricopharyngeus muscle at C5-6 level, which is approximately 1 cm wide and attaches like a sling to the lamina of the cricoid cartilage. It is the major element to the upper esophageal sphincter.

9. Which of the following is *true* regarding the epitympanum?
   A. Tegmen tympani form the floor of epitympanum.
   B. Prussak space is the medial epitympanic recess.
   C. Tympanic portion of facial nerve runs superior to lateral semicircular canal.
   D. Medial wall of epitympanum is formed by the bone overlying lateral semicircular canal.

ANSWER: D. The roof of the epitympanum forms an important bony landmark, the tegmen tympani, which separates the middle ear cavity from the middle cranial fossa and is best evaluated on coronal images. The space situated between the scutum and pars flaccida laterally and the neck of the malleus medially is called the Prussak space or the lateral epitympanic recess. This is the site where the pars flaccida cholesteatoma arises and is best seen on the coronal plane. Posteriorly, the epitympanum opens into the mastoid antrum via the aditus ad antrum, which is well demonstrated on both the axial and coronal images. The Koerner septum separates the mastoid antrum from squamous portion of the mastoid air cells. The medial wall of the epitympanum is the bone overlying the lateral semicircular canal and is an area to evaluate for fistula in cholesteatoma in the epitympanum. The tympanic portion of the facial nerve runs posterolaterally inferior to the lateral semicircular canal.

10. Which of the following is *true* regarding suprahyoid neck spaces?
   A. Anterior belly of digastric muscle separates the parotid space from CS.
   B. A mass of the deep lobe of parotid gland displaces the PPS medially with widening of the stylomandibular gap.
   C. A primary PPS mass typically displace the lateral wall of the pharyngomucosal or visceral space laterally.
   D. An RPS abscess elevates the prevertebral muscles.

ANSWER: B. A mass of the deep lobe of parotid gland displaces the PPS medially with widening of the stylomandibular gap. The upper parotid space is separated from the CS by the posterior belly of digastric muscle. The anterior belly of digastric muscle is seen in submandibular space. A primary PPS mass typically displace the lateral wall of the pharyngomucosal or visceral space medially, the deep lobe of parotid gland laterally, and the contents of the CS posteriorly. An RPS abscess does not elevate the prevertebral muscles, whereas a PVS abscess does so.

14 HEAD AND NECK PATHOLOGY

Asim K. Bag and Joseph C. Sullivan III

TEMPORAL BONE

PETROUS APEX

Asymmetric marrow: This is an asymmetric aeration of one petrous apex with nonpneumatized marrow on the opposite side, which appears as a pseudomass, particularly in T1-weighted images.

Cholesterol granuloma: This is due to inflammatory response caused by the cholesterol crystal deposition in a trapped apical air cell in the petrous apex probably from recurrent subclinical hemorrhage. This may present with sensorineural hearing loss and tinnitus. Most common imaging appearance is well-defined expansile lesion in the petrous apex with high signal in both T1- and T2-weighted images. Large lesions may extend to the clivus medially, carotid canal anteriorly, and internal auditory canal (IAC) posteriorly.

Cholesteatoma: Cholesteatoma in this location arises either from the embryonal epithelial cell rest or from extension from the middle ear cavity. They are smooth expansile masses. The most common presentation is sensory neural hearing loss. They usually follow the cerebrospinal fluid (CSF) signal, and there is prominent diffusion restriction in DWI.

Cephalocele: This is usually due to lateral prolapse of Meckel cave into the petrous apex caused by dehiscence of bone. This is usually an incidental finding; however, this may present with recurrent meningitis.

Apical petrositis: This is due to extension of the middle ear cavity/mastoid infection in the aerated petrous apex typically with meningeal involvement. This usually presents with deep pain and otorrhea. The classic clinical triad of Gradenigo syndrome (otalgia as a result of fifth nerve involvement, lateral rectus palsy as a result of sixth nerve involvement, and otomastoiditis) is rarely present.

Internal carotid arteries aneurysm: This is a very rare location for internal carotid arteries aneurysm. As this aneurysm usually does not produce any symptom, it may be surprisingly large at presentation with thrombus in the aneurysm sac.

INNER EAR

CONGENITAL

Labyrinthine aplasia: There is absence of the entire inner ear structure. There is amorphous bone in place of the cochlea, vestibule, and semicircular canal. Usually the IAC is small, but in severe cases the entire IAC may be absent. Facial nerve canal is prominent.

Cochlear aplasia/hypoplasia: The entire cochlea is absent. The vestibule and semicircular canals may be normal, hypoplastic, or with cystic changes.

Cystic common cavity of inner ear: There is fluid-filled cystic cavity in the region of the semicircular canal and cochlea that is due to incomplete development and presents with congenital sensory neural hearing loss.

Incomplete partition and dilatational defect: In this condition, there is only the basilar turn of cochlea and a dilated cavity in the region of the middle and apical turn. It may be associated with other inner ear abnormalities.

Isolated semicircular canal aplasia/hypoplasia: Aplasia/hypoplasia is a very rare congenital anomaly. The lateral semicircular canal is most commonly involved.

Endolymphatic hydrops: Endolymphatic hydrops is an abnormal dilation of the endolymphatic space because of failure of the endolymphatic sac to reabsorb the endolymph, resulting in dilation of the sac with or without communication between endolymph with perilymph. This can be congenital or acquired or idiopathic. Any congenital malformation can ultimately lead to the endolymphatic hydrops, the most common being the large vestibular aqueduct syndrome (dilated endolymphatic duct [greater than 1.5 mm in the mid bony aqueduct] and sac, presenting with hearing loss and vertigo). Any inflammation and infection of inner ear can also end up with hydrops. Ménière disease is the idiopathic form of the hydrops presenting with fluctuating SNHL with or without vertigo. This is most often unilateral, and there may be enhancement of the endolymphatic sac in the post contrast scan.

INFECTION AND INFLAMMATION

Labyrinthitis: Labyrinthitis is an inflammation of the membranous labyrinth, mostly caused by virus but can also be immune and drug mediated. There is enhancement of the cochlea and semicircular canals on the postcontrast T1-weighted scans. The enhancement on the postcontrast T1 images may not be well appreciated because of high precontrast T1 signal from the proteinaceous inflammatory exudates. Postcontrast FLAIR may be helpful in these cases.

Labyrinthitis ossificans: There is ossification of the membranous labyrinth as a healing response to inflammation or trauma. They usually occur in children in the age 2 to 18 months after an episode of acute meningitis. The most common presenting symptom is bilateral sensorineural hearing loss with or without vertigo.

Otosclerosis: Otosclerosis is a disorder of bony labyrinth and stapes. This is bilateral in 80% of cases and presents with slowly progressive disorder affecting predominantly females. It typically presents with hearing loss with or without tinnitus. The hearing loss is predominantly conductive with or without sensorineural component. The disease has two distinct presentations:

- *Fenestral:* Typical presentation of this condition is slowly progressive conductive hearing loss. Conductive hearing loss is due to impingement of the footplate with the oval window. The most common location is just anterior to oval window at the fissula ante fenestram. Pathologically, there is initial resorption of the bone followed by deposition of spongy vascular bone in the early stage. In the late stage of the disease, there is restoration of bone density due to sclerosis. In otoscopy, there is normal tympanic membrane and no sign of middle ear inflammation. There may also be a pink hue in the otoscopy reflecting the vascularity of the abnormal bone. On CT, there is subtle focal demineralization of otic capsule at the region of fissula ante fenestram (a small focus anteromedial to the oval window). With progression of disease, the demineralized bone enlarges and encroaches and causes narrowing of the oval window and ultimately the footplate of stapes is thickened and fixed to the oval window. Rarely, in late stage, the bone density gradually returns and then demineralization may not be identified in CT.

- *Retrofenestral:* This is a more severe condition with extensive demineralization of around the cochlea in addition to the involvement of the fissula ante fenestram. HRCT is required for the diagnosis. There are multiple radiolucent arcs in the otic capsule. There is almost always a sensorineural component in the hearing loss. The disease is bilateral symmetric in almost all cases. There is no definite MR feature of this condition.

Tumors

Endolymphatic sac tumor: This tumor is usually locally invasive and large at presentation. This may be solitary, but more frequently is associated with von Hippel-Lindau. This presents with sensorineural hearing loss with or without facial nerve dysfunction. The presentation may be acute as a result of intratumoral hemorrhage or chronic as a result of progressive local invasion. This is heterogeneous on T2-weighted images and enhances with contrast.

Schwannoma: This may be in the seventh or eighth nerve with usual appearance.

Squamous cell carcinoma (SCC)/adenoid cell carcinoma: They are rare primary tumors.

Rhabdomyosarcoma: It may involve the soft tissue.

Middle Ear/Mastoid

Otitis media (OM) is a common childhood disease. Acute OM with effusion is an infection of the middle ear with fluid in the middle ear cavity. The infection of the upper airway secondarily involves the middle ear, mastoids, and pneumatized petrous bone as they are interconnected to each other with the eustachian tube. In most cases, OM is treated with antibiotics with no need for imaging. The usual pathogens are *Streptococcus*, *Hemophilus*, *Moraxella*. Acute OM may go on to the chronic phase. By definition, if there is persistent fluid in the middle ear cavity for more than 3 months, it is considered as chronic. Chronic suppurative OM is otorrhea more than 6 weeks.

Complication of Acute OM

Coalescent mastoiditis: This is defined as erosion of mastoid septae with or without intramastoid abscess.

Facial nerve palsy: Mostly caused by inflammation of the tympanic segment.

Dural sinus thrombosis: Bony defect/dehiscence in mastoid exposes the infected material to sigmoid sinus and dura, which may result in thrombophlebitis or thrombosis of the sinus. This may progress and secondarily involve the other sinus. This may appear as "empty delta sign" on contrast-enhanced CT when involving the sagittal sinus.

Venous infarction: This infarction occurs secondary to sinus thrombosis causing venous hypertension and ultimately venous infarction.

Meningitis: Meningeal infection occurs either from bony defect/osteomyelitis or venous thrombophlebitis. They may be complicated with empyema, subdural abscess, or brain abscess.

Otitic hydrocephalus: This is secondary to sinus thrombosis probably caused by obstruction in the arachnoid granulation.

Labyrinthitis: The bacteria or endo-/exotoxin may spread either through the oval or round window. The membranous labyrinth may enhance after contrast on postcontrast T1.

Cholesteatoma: Cholesteatoma is a sac of exfoliated debris of growing skin in a wrong place. It may be either congenital or acquired. The congenital cholesteatoma (same is epidermoid in other places) of the temporal bone due to epithelial cells rests of embryonal origin. Acquired disease is by far more common than congenital disease and most commonly occurs in Prussak's space secondary to perforation of the pars flaccida of tympanic membrane either secondary to chronic OM or trauma. The growing cholesteatoma medially displaces the malleus head, laterally erodes the scutum, posteriorly extends into the incudal space and posterolateral attic, and from there to mastoid through aditus ed antrum.

Pars tensa cholesteatoma: This is less common and has a tendency to grow medially. The inner ear structures are involved early and more commonly in this variant. The hallmark of imaging manifestation is bone erosion along the line of the growth of the tumor. This frequently erodes the middle ear ossicles, approximately 75% in pars flaccida cholesteatoma and approximately 90% in pars tensa cholesteatoma. The long process of incus is the most common segment of the ossicular chain eroded by both the two types.

Labyrinthine fistula: This is another severe complication where the lateral semicircular canal is most commonly involved. The growing lesion also involves the facial nerve canal, most commonly the tympanic segment, in 1% of cases. There may be erosion of the tegmen tympani and sigmoid sinus plate increasing the chance of sinus thrombosis and intracranial complications as described before.

Tumors

Glomus tympanicum is a small paraganglioma of the middle ear cavity. It is very small at the time of presentation.

EXTERNAL EAR

Infection/Inflammation

Necrotizing External Otitis

Necrotizing external otitis is a locally aggressive infection of the external ear usually from the pseudomonas. The usual predisposing factors are older patients with diabetes and AIDS. Usually the infection starts insidiously at the osteocartilaginous junction as a focal ulcer. The tympanic membrane is resistant to infection. The infection spreads through the cartilaginous part into the soft tissue and ultimately involves all structures of the base of the skull. CT and MRI both are necessary for evaluation of the disease extension. CT is required for evaluation bony changes. MRI is needed for evaluation of the soft-tissue involvement.

Diffuse Petrous Diseases

Osteogenesis imperfecta is a disease of abnormal type I collagen formation. The typical presentation is fragile bone, blue sclera, and deafness. CT shows thickened bone around the otic capsule and narrow middle ear cavity with the footplate of stapes embedded in the dysplastic bone. The facial nerve canal may also be obstructed. The imaging appearance is similar to the retrofenestral otospongiosis but the demineralization is more extensive.

Osteopetrosis: Osteopetrosis is a rare hereditary defect of bone remodeling caused by abnormal osteoclastic activity resulting in thick, dense fragile bone. There is increased density of the temporal bone with absent mastoid air cells. The internal auditory canal is shortened. The middle ear ossicles may be thickened and enlarged.

Paget disease: Paget disease can be a uni- or multifocal disease caused by exaggerated bony remodeling. Temporal bone Paget disease presents with hearing loss, which may be conductive, sensorineural, or mixed. Facial nerve dysfunction may also occur as a result of compromised facial nerve canal. In temporal bone, the disease begins in the petrous apex. The otic capsule is the last structure to be involved. The stapedial footplate may be thickened.

Fibrous dysplasia: Fibrous dysplasia is a disease of unknown cause in which the normal bone is replaced by fibro-osseous tissue. This may be mono-/polyostotic. In fibrous dysplasia of temporal bone, there is increase in the size of the temporal bone causing compression of the bony foramina and ostia. It usually presents with progressive hearing loss. The facial nerve may be entrapped. The common CT finding is increased bone thickness and loss of trabecular pattern.

SKULL BASE

ANTERIOR SKULL BASE

Congenital

Cephaloceles: By definition, cephaloceles are congenital herniations of intracranial contents through cranial defects. There are various developmental concepts. They may arise because of incomplete separation of neural and surface ectoderm at the site of final closure of the anterior neuropore during the final phase of neurulation in the fourth week of gestation. Another theory is excess outgrowth of the surface ectoderm might act as an outward vector to the attached neuroectoderm and may drag out the neuroectodermal tissue. They can be classified according to the contents of the sac.

- *Meningocele:* If there is herniation of meninges and CSF.
- *Meningoencephalocele:* If there is herniation of CSF, meninges, and brain.
- *Glioceles:* If the glial-lined cysts contain CSF only.
- *Atretic cephalocele:* This is forme fruste of cephalocele consisting of dura, fibrous tissue, and dysplastic neural tissue.

The most common location is occipital region, followed by frontonasal, basal cephaloceles, in descending order of frequency. Cephaloceles may be associated with microphthalmos, anomalies of the corpus callosum, interhemispheric lipomas/arachnoid cyst, migrational anomalies, and so on. They usually present as externally visible frontonasal masses in newborns or infants with broadening of the nasal bridge and hypertelorism. They commonly enlarge with crying and with jugular compression (Furstenberg sign). They may also present with nasal obstruction, CSF leakage, or meningitis. Basal cephalocele may mimic an intranasal polyp or other nasal masses.

MR is the preferred method for evaluation. Continuity of herniated tissue and/or fluid with the brain is crucial to the diagnosis. On T1-weighted images, they are isointense to grey matter and also CSF signal. On T2-weighted images, they are hyperintense due to gliosis and CSF signal. They do not enhance with contrast.

Developmental cysts: Incomplete separation of the dura from the skin elements can result in pulling in the dermal contents with the involuting dural diverticulum and result in dermal sinus, congenital dermal inclusion cysts (epidermoid and dermoid), and tumor (teratoma). The peak age of presentation is 23 months. Roughly one half of these children of these children have a dimple or pit over the nasal bridge. Occasionally hairs/sebaceous discharge emanate from the pit. A palpable mass is found in 30% of children. Broad nasal bridge and hypertelorism are in 50% of children. They may be associated epidermoid and/or dermoid cysts and are usually extracranial. Rarely, they may present with infection.

MR is the preferred modality of evaluation. Epidermoid follows the signal intensity of CSF but appears as a lightbulb in DWI. Dermoid cyst is variably hyperintense in both T1 and T2; hence it does not show up in DWI. Subtle dermal sinus may be detected well by highly T2-weighted sequences (also known as MR cisternography). A bifid crista galli or enlarged foramen cecum, if present, can be a clue.

Nasal glioma: Developmentally, nasal glioma can be conceptualized as cephaloceles with lost intracranial connection. By definition, they do not contain any CSF-filled space that is connected with subarachnoid space/ventricles. Histologically, they are congenital masses of glial tissue that occur intra-/extranasally at or near nasal root. They resemble reactive gliosis instead of any glial proliferation.

They constitute approximately 4.5% of nasal masses. They occur sporadically with no familial tendency. There is no sexual predilection. Up to 15% may have associated cerebral heterotopias. Of all the lesions, 60% are extranasal, 14% to 30% are intranasal, and 10% to 14% are mixed (with both intra- and extranasal component). They usually present early in infancy as nonpulsatile skin-covered mass, which does not change size with Valsalva, and tends to grow along with the child. Intranasal heterotopias present as polypoid mass typically medial to middle turbinate and attached to the turbinates. They may cause blockage of NLD. They are commonly confused with inflammatory polyps.

MRI is the preferred method of evaluation. The nasal glioma is typically well circumscribed, rounded, or polypoid in shape; hypointense in T1-weighted images; and hyperintense in T2-weighted images. On postcontrast scan, they do not enhance but may have peripheral enhancement.

INFECTION/INFLAMMATION

Sinusitis: Complicated sinusitis can involve the anterior skull base.

Epidural abscess/empyema: Epidural empyema is the collection of pus between dura and skull and occurs secondary to sinusitis at this location. The falx and dural sinuses may be displaced. Hypointense peripheral rim is seen in T2, which reflects the inflamed edematous dura, which shows moderate enhancement in postcontrast scan.

TUMORS

SCC of sinuses: Invasive frontal and ethmoid sinus cancer, which can involve the anterior cranial fossa.

Meningioma: Olfactory groove, sphenoid wing, and optic pathway meningioma are common in this location.

Metastasis: Usual primary are sinonasal, breast, lung, prostate, and vascular mets.

Rhabdomyosarcoma: Head and neck are the most common location of this tumor. They usually involve nasal cavity, paranasal sinuses, orbit, and nasopharyngeal musculature. They are highly malignant masses with local invasion and distal lymph nodal metastasis. These are the most common extracranial masses invading the skull base in children. They are heterogeneous masses isodense to brain parenchyma. They enhance moderately with contrast.

Sinonasal undifferentiated cancer (SNUC): This is a highly malignant mass of nasal cavity and paranasal sinuses.

Lymphoma: The usual primary mass is in the nasopharynx. The sphenoid can secondarily be involved.

Esthesioneuroblastoma: These are the tumors of the primitive neuroectodermal tumor family.

Plasmacytoma: This is an extramedullary tumor.

CENTRAL SKULL BASE

CONGENITAL

Cephalocele in this location is very rare.

INFECTION/INFLAMMATION

Sinusitis: Sphenoid sinus infection and complications involve the central skull base.

Langerhans cell histiocytosis (LCH): LCH frequently involves calvarial bones; however, the skull base may also be involved. The lesions are typical "punched out" with sharp margin. CT is best to demonstrate the typical punched out lesion. On MRI, they are usually associated with T2 hyperintense soft tissue.

TUMORS

Squamous cell cancer of sinuses: Invasive squamous cell cancer can involve the central skull base.

Meningioma: Sphenoid wing is a common location.

Pituitary adenoma: Pituitary macroadenoma can be surprisingly large and can involve the sphenoid bone. Usually there is demineralization of the involved bone.

Chordoma: Clival chordoma frequently involves the central skull base.

Chondrosarcoma: When large in size, they frequently encroaches the central skull base from the petroclival junction.

Aneurysmal bone cyst: Aneurysmal bone cysts are occasionally seen in the sphenoid bone. They frequently hemorrhage and have characteristic multiple intratumoral hemorrhagic cysts and fluid-fluid levels which are easily identified on MRI.

Giant cell tumors: Giant cell tumors can involve the sphenoid bone.

POSTERIOR SKULL BASE

TUMORS

Nasopharyngeal cancer (NPC): Advanced-stage NPC involves the sphenoid bone with bony lysis.

Chordoma: Chordoma is a tumor of remnant notochord elements. The most common location is the sacrum. The clivus is the most common cranial location. They are locally aggressive masses of the posterior and central skull base with a tendency to involve anterior structures, like the nasopharynx. The peak age at presentation is 20 to 40 years with a male predominance. They are highly vascular tumors with frequent destruction of the bone and also with frequent tumoral calcification. They are hypointense on T1-weighted images and heterogeneously hyperintense on T2-weighted images with bright enhancement with contrast. Combined CT and MR evaluation is required in some cases where there is only subtle contrast enhancement.

Chondrosarcoma: Chondrosarcoma also predominantly arise at the posterior skull base at petroclival junction. They are similar to chordoma both on imaging and on histology. The typical location is off midline in the region of petroclival synchondrosis. They can occur at any age but the usual age of presentation is fifth to sixth decade. The clinical presentation is headache and the symptoms related to the secondary involvement of structures by the tumors (like multiple cranial nerve palsies). The CT finding is variable. Typically they are slightly hyperdense (to surrounding muscles) with variable enhancement. Chondroid matrix with typical chondroid calcification is the characteristic finding but may not be found always. They are usually very bright on T2-weighted images with moderate enhancement. If there is dense calcification, the tumor may appear as heterogeneous.

Plasmacytoma: Plasmacytoma is a rare tumor of this location.

Meningioma: CP angle meningioma and meningioma around the foramen magnum may involve the posterior skull base.

JUGULAR FORAMEN

CONGENITAL

High-riding jugular bulb: Jugular bulb is considered "high riding" when it extends to the middle ear, above the level of the floor of the IAC or tympanic annulus.

Dehiscent jugular bulb: There is absence of the bony margin separating the jugular bulb from the posteroinferior aspect of the jugular foramen causing forward displacement of the jugular bulb into the tympanic cavity. They usually present with pulsatile tinnitus.

INFECTION/INFLAMMATION

LCH may involve the jugular foramen with usual features.

TUMORS

Paraganglioma: Paragangliomas in this location have different names according to the nerve involved. Glomus tympanicum is small paraganglioma of the middle ear cavity arising from the nerve of Jacobson. Glomus jugulare is the paraganglioma of the jugular foramen and skull base arising from paraganglia of the adventitia of the jugular bulb. Glomus vagale (paraganglioma of the vagus nerve) are tumors arising from the vagus nerve and they are usually parapharyngeal masses.

Paragangliomas usually present between the fourth and fifth decades of life. They are more common in women. Rarely they are familial. The clinical presentation is myriad and depends upon the infiltration of the adjacent structure and also chemical activity of the tumor. The usual presentations are pulsatile tinnitus, conductive hearing loss, jugular foramen syndrome with or without involvement of the hypoglossal or facial nerve. Acoustic symptoms are more frequent than the lower cranial nerve palsies. The size of the tumor at the time of diagnosis varies from a few millimeters (glomus tympanicum) to several centimeters. The glomus tympanicum most commonly occurs at the promontory, but can be anywhere along the course of the Jacobson's nerve at the medial wall of the middle ear cavity. The extension of the tumor involving surrounding bone is evaluated better in CT but MR is much better for appreciation of contrast enhancement. The earliest imaging feature of glomus jugulare is erosion of the anterior bony wall of the jugular foramen. This tumor sometimes becomes very large and can grow along the course of the jugular vein and even obstructs the vein either partially or completely. They usually enhance intensely with contrast. Sometime it is difficult to differentiate a small tumor from the normal jugular bulb in CECT. On T2 images, there may be "salt and pepper" appearance because of the signal voids from the tumor vessels.

Metastasis: Metastasis at this location is usually from renal or thyroid.

Schwannoma/neurofibroma: Schwannoma at this location arises from the ninth and tenth cranial nerves and spinal accessory nerve. The tumor may be predominantly intracranial or may be predominantly at the jugular foramen. Intracranial tumors present with cerebellar symptoms but predominantly jugular foramen masses present with jugular foramen syndrome (aka Vernet syndrome), which includes paralysis of the ninth and tenth cranial nerves and spinal accessory nerve. They usually expand the foramen and can appear like CP angle schwannoma.

ORBIT

VASCULAR LESIONS

Orbital Cavernous Malformation

Orbital cavernous malformation is the most common vascular abnormality of the orbit in adults. It usually occurs in the second to fourth decade of life. There is a gradually enlarging mass (usually intraconal), presenting as gradual-onset painless proptosis. Histologically, they are enlarged vascular space lined by endothelium, with no feature of endothelial proliferation. They are sharply marginated, lobular homogenous soft-tissue mass of increasing density with variable enhancement. Phlebolith is not common. They are usually isointense to muscles and enhance variably.

Capillary Hemangioma

Capillary hemangioma is primarily diseases of the first year of life and slightly more common in girls. Microscopically, there is endothelial and capillary proliferation. They enlarge rapidly in the initial 6 to 18 months and usually after 1 year they start to regress. They are mostly extraconal mass of varying sizes with well-/ill-defined margin and variable enhancement.

Venolymphatic Malformation

The term lymphangioma is not technically correct, as there is no cellular proliferation. The best term to describe this condition is lymphatic malformation or venolymphatic malformation as this condition is often mixed with vessels with venous characteristics. They are relatively large, progressively enlarging, ill-defined extra-/intraconal masses of childhood or young adulthood. They are frequently associated with intracranial vascular abnormality, most common being developmental venous anomaly. They are not well encapsulated and may infiltrate surrounding structures. They are heterogeneous in density/intensity. The enhancement is also heterogeneous. On MR, fluid-fluid levels and hemorrhages of different ages could be identified. If the lesion is purely lymphatic, it does not enhance with contrast.

Orbital Varix

Primary orbital varix may involve a vein, a small segment of a vein, a tangle of venous structures with massive dilation that is due to weakness of the venous wall. There is painless intermittent proptosis, which enlarges with Valsalva. Orbital varix may be associated with intracranial AVM. Supine CT scan or MR may be normal. In suspicious cases, scan in prone position is required. Sometimes scanning during Valsalva is required for demonstration of varix. There may be phleboliths.

CAROTID–CAVERNOUS FISTULA

Carotid–cavernous fistula can present with pulsating exophthalmos, chemosis, venous engorgement, and restricted ocular motility. It may occur because of trauma or surgery or may occur spontaneously. On imaging, there is engorgement of the superior ophthalmic vein with or without engorgement of the extraocular muscles. Angiogram is often needed for exact localization of the fistula and planning of treatment.

INFLAMMATORY AND INFECTIOUS LESIONS

Thyroid Orbitopathy

Dysthyroid ophthalmopathy (of Grave disease) is the most common cause of both unilateral and bilateral proptosis. The average age at presentation is the fifth decade of life; women are commonly involved but involvement in men is more commonly severe. Thyroid orbitopathy is an autoimmune process with infiltration of the ocular muscles and retrobulbar compartment presenting with proptosis, limitation of the eye movement, and upper and lower lid retraction. This occurs in patients with hyperthyroidism but may also occur in the setting of hypothyroidism, euthyroidism, and also in Hashimoto thyroiditis.

In the acute stage, there is bilateral swelling of the retrobulbar contents and enlargement of the extra ocular muscles (best visualized in coronal planes) sparing the tendons. The enlarged muscles are hypodense in CT and shows increased signal intensity on T2-weighted images.

Idiopathic Orbital Inflammatory Disorder

Idiopathic orbital inflammatory disorder, aka orbital pseudotumor, is nongranulomatous inflammation of the eye/orbit, which can present acutely or may present as subacute and chronic disorder. This is the second most common ophthalmologic disorder after thyroid orbitopathy. This condition can be bilateral in up to one-third of cases. It usually presents acutely with orbital pain, restricted ocular movement, proptosis, visual abnormality, conjunctival/scleral congestion. Histologically, there is polymorphous infiltration of the inflammatory cells into the involved areas. Depending upon the location they are described as follows:

- *Anterior orbital inflammation*: There is involvement of the anterior orbit and the globe. The symptoms are usual with conjunctival hyperemia and lid swelling. MRI is better than CT to identify the scleral thickening. There may be accumulation of fluid in Tenon's capsule, which can be easily picked up by ultrasound. There is enhancement of the thickened sclera and also the optic nerve junction. In some cases there may be retinal detachment.
- *Diffuse orbital inflammation:* Diffuse orbital inflammation was classically described as orbital pseudotumor. There is diffuse infiltration of the retrobulbar fat with polymorphous inflammatory cells. This diffuse infiltration causes proptosis and surrounds the globe without any deformation. There is enhancement of the entire infiltrated areas. The presentation may be acute or subacute.
- *Orbital myositis:* Orbital myositis is an idiopathic inflammation of the extraocular muscles. This may be acute, subacute, or recurrent in presentation, usually present with painful extraocular movement, diplopia, and proptosis. The superior muscle complex and the medial rectus are the most common muscles to be involved. The involvement can be bilateral. The close differential diagnosis is dysthyroid involvement of the muscles. In thyroid myopathy, the onset is painless, slowly progressive, and usually with systemic stigmata of hyperthyroidism. In idiopathic myositis, the enlargement extends anteriorly to involve the tendons with ragged and ill-defined margin of the enlarged muscle. The fat plane between the muscle cone and periosteum is also lost because of inflammation/infiltration. There may inward bowing of the muscle belly immediately posterior to the globe.
- *Perineuritis and periscleritis:* This condition can mimic the clinical presentation of optic neuritis. Pressing the globe may exacerbate the pain. There is enlargement of the optic nerve sheath complex with irregular margin. There may be involvement of the retrobulbar fat adjacent to the nerve.
- *Lacrimal:* Isolated involvement of the lacrimal gland is also possible. It can mimic viral adenitis. There is pain in the superolateral compartment of the orbit. On imaging, there is enlargement of the gland and enhancement with contrast.
- *Apical orbital inflammation:* In this condition, there is typical orbital apex syndrome with painful ophthalmoplegia, mild proptosis, and pain.

Tolosa-Hunt syndrome, a granulomatous inflammation of the orbital apex extending posteriorly up to the cavernous sinus, is now considered in the spectrum of the idiopathic orbital inflammation syndrome. There is also involvement of the cavernous carotid with narrowing of the lumen and thrombosis of the ophthalmic vein. There are recurrent attacks of deep orbital pain with painful paralysis of the third, fourth, and sixth cranial nerves including the ophthalmic and maxillary divisions of the trigeminal nerve. It is usually bilateral but may be unilateral.

Orbital Cellulitis

Sinusitis is the most common cause of the orbital cellulitis. Infection from the sinuses involves the orbit through direct involvement through the disruption of the thin bony medial orbital wall or through the valveless intercommunicating veins. The orbital/periorbital infection can be classified into five stages:

- *Inflammatory edema:* There is swelling and hyperemia of the eyelid.
- *Preseptal cellulitis:* The infection is limited to the skin and subcutaneous tissue anterior to the orbital septum, usually the medial aspect the upper eyelid. There are no signs of orbital involvement.
- *Postseptal cellulitis:* This is infection of the orbit proper. There is diffuse edema of the orbital contents. Usual presentation is pain, restricted extra ocular movement, no/minimal proptosis but usually no visual deficit. There is stranding of the orbital fat in noncontrast CT. In fat-suppressed T2-weighted images, the edema is prominent and there is diffuse enhancement in the fat suppressed T1-weighted images with contrast

- *Subperiosteal abscess:* The edema is more generalized with more severe symptoms. In postcontrast images, there may be infiltration/abscess cavity between the involved sinus and the periorbital region.
- *Orbital abscess:* The abscess occurs within the orbit proper. The symptoms are more severe with visual loss. With progressive involvement there is ophthalmic vein and/or cavernous sinus thrombosis.
- *Cavernous sinus thrombosis:* This occurs either as a late complication of infection of the central face (areas of face that has venous drainage to cavernous sinus) or as extension of epidural infection. *Staphylococcus* is the most common organism. Angioinvasive fungi (such as Rhizopus) also cause this, particularly in the setting of diabetic ketoacidosis. The patients usually present with severe headache; dysfunction of the third, fourth, and fifth cranial nerves; and first and second division of trigeminal nerve associated with symptoms and signs related to primary site of infection. In noncontrast CT, there is loss of low density in the cavernous sinus. In contrast-enhanced images, there is enhancing cavernous sinus mass with filling defects. The lateral margin of the cavernous sinus may be convex. The enlarged ophthalmic vein is also seen. MRV can show absent flow in the ophthalmic vein and in the cavernous sinuses.

Sarcoidosis

This is a systemic disease with myriad manifestations. Ocular involvement occurs in approximately 25% of patients. Any part of the orbit or orbital contents (including optic nerve) can be involved. The most common orbital presentation is chronic dacryoadenitis, which may present with dry eye. The involved areas are usually isointense and enhance with contrast. Optic nerve involvement presents with progressive loss of vision with or without disc change. Imaging features include enhancement of the optic nerve including the intracranial segment.

Optic Neuritis

The most common cause is multiple sclerosis. Devic disease, clinicopathologically different from multiple sclerosis, involves the optic nerve and spinal cord specifically without/with periventricular brain involvement. This can also occur after viral infection. The intraorbital portion of the optic nerve is the most common location. The optic nerve is focally enlarged. There is focal T2 hyperintensity, best appreciated by coronal STIR sequence. In more than 90%, there is enhancement in T1+c.

TUMORS

Optic nerve sheath meningioma: Optic nerve sheath is a relatively uncommon site for meningioma. Meningioma circumferentially involves the orbital or canalicular optic nerve. In most of the cases, the optic nerve sheath is secondarily involved from the meningioma arising from the meninges in relation to the optic nerve course. They may be associated with NF2. The peak age of presentation is fourth to fifth decade with significant female preponderance (2–4:1). Usually, they present with exophthalmos and gradually progressive painless unilateral loss of vision. The classic triad of presentation is visual loss, optic atrophy, and optocilary shunt vessels from the occlusion of the central retinal vein. Histologically, they are similar to intracranial meningioma. There is enlargement of the optic nerve sheath with bright enhancement, which on axial scans appear as "tram track." Calcification also occurs within the tumor in one-third to one-half of the cases, which often helps to differentiate the condition from optic nerve glioma, perineuritis, sarcoidosis. "Perioptic cyst," dilation of the subarachnoid space between the distal edge of an optic nerve sheath meningioma and the eyeball, is a specific finding but is not commonly seen.

Retinoblastoma: Retinoblastoma is the most common intraocular tumor of the childhood. This can be isolated or familial (autosomal dominant) because of mutation of the Rb1 tumor suppressor gene. The familial tumors are usually bilateral. This tumor is highly malignant, arising from the nuclear layer of the retina. The earliest presentation is leukocoria. Later on, they develop vision loss, proptosis, or strabismus. The average age at presentation is 18 months. Bilateral and familial disease usually present earlier.

Calcification is the most dominant feature and is found in more than 90% of cases. There is homo- or heterogeneous enhancement on the postcontrast scans. On MR, they are moderately hypointense (to vitreous) mass with homo-/heterogeneous enhancement. If bilateral retinoblastoma is associated with midline intracranial neuroblastic tumor (usually pinealoblastoma), the condition is known as trilateral retinoblastoma.

Orbital melanoma: The most common location is choroid, but it can arise from ciliary body or iris. The peak age of incidence is 50 years, with a slight male preference. They usually present with painless vision disturbance. They are small soft-tissue density mass with moderate enhancement. They are very bright in noncontrast T1 and hypointense (to vitreous) in T2. There is diffuse enhancement in the postcontrast scan. The associated retinal/choroid detachment is also well evaluated by MR.

Lymphoma: The most common neoplasm of orbit is lymphoma. B-cell NHL is the most common type. Usually they are primary orbital lymphoma but there may be secondary involvement of the orbit, too. Usual age of presentation is the seventh decade. They usually present with gradually enlarging painless orbital mass. Most commonly they are intraconal well-defined masses with diffuse enhancement.

Optic nerve glioma: Optic nerve gliomas are relatively uncommon and usually occur in children and may be associated with NF1. When associated with NF1, they usually involve the anterior optic nerve; otherwise chiasmatic or retrochiasmatic involvement is more common. Enhancement and signal intensity are variable. They are described in detail in the brain tumor chapter.

Rhabdomyosarcoma: Rhabdomyosarcoma is the most common primary orbital malignancy in the childhood. The peak age at presentation is 2 to 5 years. Orbital rhabdomyosarcoma is almost always unilateral and involves the superior aspect of the orbit. There is usually a short history of progressive proptosis. They usually arise from the mesenchymal tissue, not from the extraocular striated muscles. Depending upon the stage of the disease, the mass can be homo-/heterogeneous, well/ill defined, without/with bone destruction. CT is better for demonstration of bone destruction; however, on fat-saturated T2, there is edema in the bone marrow. They are usually isodense to muscles and frequently show intratumoral hemorrhage. There is usually intense enhancement in the postcontrast scans.

Schwannoma/neurofibroma: Schwannoma is a well-defined benign peripheral nerve sheath tumor growing eccentrically from the nerve. It typically arises from a sensory nerve, most commonly from the V1 division. It is usually extraconal but if it arises from the nasociliary nerve or rarely from the ocular motor nerves, it can be intraconal. Unlike neurofibroma, there may be occasional hemorrhage within the schwannoma best identified in MR.

- Circumscribed neurofibromas also most commonly arise from the V1 division of the trigeminal nerve and usually involve the nerve circumferentially. On T2, they are homogenously hyperintense or there may be occasional "target sign" with hyperintense periphery and central hypointensity.
- Plexiform neurofibromas usually occur in association with NF1. They are ill-defined masses of the orbit and are usually associated with sphenoid wing dysplasia. They are usually hypointense (to muscles) on T1-weighted images and show hyperintense (to muscles) signal on T2-weighted images. They may enhance intensely with contrast.

Metastasis: The most common primary to metastasize in the orbit is the breast cancer. Others may be lung, colon, or prostate. In children, common tumors that metastasize to orbits are neuroblastoma, leukemia, and Ewing sarcoma. In children, the usual location is the orbital wall, and in adults they usually start at highly vascular choroid.

Developmental cysts: Dermoid cysts are most common congenital benign orbital masses. They usually occur in early childhood and present with proptosis and eyelid swelling. They usually result from trapped ectodermal elements within the sutures during orbital development. This explains their frequent location in relation to the sutures and frequent bony erosions. They usually show fat density/intensity in MR.

Epidermoid cysts are less common, well-defined tumors that follow the signal intensity of CSF.

SINONASAL CAVITIES

CONGENITAL

Choanal atresia is a rare congenital anomaly; may be uni-/bilateral. Bilateral choanal atresia is a medical emergency. The choana may be obstructed by fibrous tissue or rarely by a bony ridge.

INFECTION

Rhinosinusitis: This is acute inflammation of the sinonasal mucosa lasting less than 4 weeks of duration. They may occur in both young and adult people usually after upper respiratory tract viral infection. Usual presentations are nasal congestion, thick postnasal discharge, headache, olfactory disturbance. They are most common in ethmoid sinus followed by maxillary sinuses. On imaging, there is thickening of the paranasal sinus mucosa with or without obstruction of the drainage pathway. There may be air-fluid level with bubbly appearance. The inflamed mucosa usually enhances avidly with contrast.

If the inflammation continued beyond 12 consecutive weeks, it is defined as chronic sinusitis. The symptoms of the acute inflammation continue. On imaging, there is mucosal thickening or opacification of sinus without expansion of sinus. There is sclerotic and thickened sinus wall. The secretion may become hypo-, iso- to hyperdense (to the muscles) depending upon the protein content of the secretion. With chronic obstruction, the water in the secretion is reabsorbed, and there is Goblet cell metaplasia of the mucosa, which further secretes protein-rich secretion. On T2-weighted images, the signal intensity drops as the protein content of the secretion increases. If the protein concentration is greater than 35%, there is signal void on T2 images. Evaluation of the disease with only MRI may underestimate the extent of the disease.

Allergic fungal sinusitis: This is a severe form of the chronic sinusitis, probably resulting from type I hypersensitivity reaction. Multiple sinuses may be involved. There is expansion of the involved sinus. The disease may invade the orbits. They are usually hyperdense on CT and typically hypointense on T2 images. There is enhancement of the mucosa with contrast.

Invasive fungal sinusitis: This is rapid-progressing fungal infection in immunocompromised (including diabetic) patients with spread of the disease from the sinuses to the vessels caused by angioinvasive fungi (*Mucor*, *Aspergillus*, and *Rhizopus*). They most commonly occur in the setting of the uncontrolled diabetes. The most common presentation is acute-onset fever, epistaxis, sinus pain, headache, cough, and nasal mucosal ulceration. Orbital and intracranial extension is the most dreaded complication. In diabetic patients, there is black crusting of the nasal mucosa. There is complete or partial obstruction of the sinus. There is also infiltration of the fat and soft tissue around the sinuses. On contrast-enhanced images, there is enhancement of the mucosa and also the inflamed fat and soft tissue around the sinuses. There can be narrowing of the arterial and venous lumen because of vasculitis. CTA can demonstrate this finding very well. MRI is better for demonstration of disease beyond the sinuses.

Sinonasal polyposis: This is due to nonneoplastic proliferation of the nasal and paranasal mucosa. They may be associated with asthma, cystic fibrosis, aspirin sensitivity, and also allergic fungal sinusitis. They usually present with nasal stuffiness and nasal obstruction. They are usually diseases of adulthood. On CT scan, they appear as multiple polypoid soft tissue within nasal cavity and paranasal sinuses. If associated with allergic sinusitis, there may be bone erosion. On MR they are usually hyperintense on T2 images. If the obstruction is chronic, the signal intensity on T2-weighted images drops.

Mucocele: Mucocele is expansion of the sinus cavity caused by obstruction of the drainage pathway. The frontal sinus is most commonly affected, in approximately 60% of cases. On CT, there is expansion of the sinus with thinned sinus wall containing hypodense material. Early mucocele are hyperintense in T2 but lately, they are hyperintense on T2 images.

TUMORS

Juvenile angiofibroma: This benign but locally aggressive highly vascular tumor occurs almost exclusively in adolescent males. Common presenting symptoms are unilateral nasal obstruction and spontaneous epistaxis. The typical location is at or around the sphenopalatine foramen at the lateral nasopharyngeal wall. The classic imaging findings are widening of the pterygopalatine fossa, anterior displacement of the posterior wall of the maxillary sinus, erosion of the medial pterygoid plate. Thin-section CT scan in axial plane with coronal reformation is required for complete evaluation. On MR, the mass is heterogeneous on T2 images with numerous flow voids. They also enhance brightly. Conventional angiography is required for delineation of vascular anatomy (supplied from the internal maxillary, ascending pharyngeal and palatine arteries) and also for presurgery embolization of the tumor.

Inverted papilloma: Typically, they occur in males between 40 to 70 years. The typical location is lateral nasal wall near the middle turbinate and usually extends into the sinuses (more commonly into the maxillary than ethmoid). Very rarely, they may be purely intrasinus or arise from the nasal septum. Usual presenting symptoms are nasal obstruction and epistaxis. Microscopically, there is hyperplastic squamous epithelium. There is also squamous metaplasia in the surrounding mucosa, explaining frequent recurrence after resection and need for en block resection. Carcinoma may rarely develop from these papillomas. Imaging features are variable from small nasal polyp to an expansile mass. There is no specific CT or MR imaging sign.

Osteoma: This is a benign, expansile proliferation of mature bone. They are almost exclusively found in relation to the membranous bones of the skull and face, most commonly frontal sinuses followed by ethmoid sinus. They are usually incidental but may obstruct the ostium and need early decompression. Multiple osteomas are associated with Gardner syndrome. They arise either from the wall of the sinus or from the septum. They are usually hyperdense well-defined masses on CT and on MR they are hypo- to isointense.

SCC: This is the most common cancer of the nasal cavity and paranasal sinuses. The most common location is the maxillary antrum. Occupational exposure to nickel, chromium, and wood fibers increases the chance of cancer development. There may be metachronous or synchronous development. They usually occur in the sixth or seventh decade of life. When they are small, they may be misdiagnosed as chronic sinusitis, nasal polyposis. Cancer of the frontal and sphenoid sinuses is rare. They usually present with symptoms of chronic sinusitis. On CT, they are heterogeneous masses with irregular margin with variable enhancement. They are intermediate to hyperintense in T2-weighted images with mild to moderate enhancement.

Approximately 10% of the sinonasal cancers may be adenocarcinoma.

Esthesioneuroblastoma: This is a neural crest–derived highly malignant tumor. They have bimodal age distribution in the second and sixth decades of life. The common locations are superior nasal cavities, superior turbinates, and ethmoid. On CT, they are homogenous hyperenhancing masses with bone destruction/remodeling. They frequently invade the base of the skull and involve the anterior/middle cranial fossa. There are multiple cysts at the interface of normal brain and the tumor. There may be intratumoral calcification. On MR, the signal intensity varies but they enhances brightly.

SNUC: SNUC is a highly malignant tumor with undifferentiated cellular lineage. These are rare tumors occur usually after the fifth decade of life. Most of the SNUCs occur at the same location of the esthesioneuroblastoma and usually present with nasal obstruction, epistaxis, and pain with or without orbital symptoms. The radiologic features are similar to the SCC with destruction of the bones. They are highly cellular tumors; on diffusion-weighted imaging, they may appear hyperintense.

Lymphoma: Lymphoma in head and neck most commonly involves the lymph nodes, 10% being extranodal. Sinonasal lymphoma is most common in Asia. This can be either B-cell or T-cell lymphoma. On imaging, they are bulky soft-tissue masses that enhance to a moderate degree. They tend to remodel bone, but bone erosion is not unknown. Most often the disease involves the nasal fossa and the maxillary sinuses. They are of intermediate signal intensity on all MR sequences.

Plasmacytoma: They are rare extramedullary tumors, which predominantly occur in the head and neck. The most common location is the nasal cavity followed by paranasal sinuses. On CT they are a homogenous hyperenhancing mass of the nasal cavity and paranasal sinuses. They are highly vascular and may have flow voids on MR.

JAW PATHOLOGIES

Odontogenic cyst: Periapical cyst is the most common odontogenic cyst, which can occur at any time of life. The condition is usually associated with tooth infection. The infection extends to the pulp, and from there ultimately extends outside the apex and causes apical periodontitis, which ultimately becomes a periapical or a radicular cyst. They are well-defined lucent/hypodense periapical masses surrounded by thin cortical rim.

Dentigerous cyst: This is the second most common odontogenic cyst. They develop from the crown of an unerupted tooth. They are most commonly identified in the mandible at the third or fourth decade of life. Dentigerous cyst may also develop from the maxilla. The cyst usually develops between the epithelium or between the enamel and the epithelium. The typical imaging appearance is a lucent/lytic mass in relation to the crown of an unerupted tooth in the mandible surrounded by thin cortical rim.

Cherubism: This is an autosomal dominant disease presented with bilateral painless enlargement of jaw. This is a disease of early childhood. The mandible is involved first followed by the maxilla. On CT there are multiple expansile cystic masses at the mandibular junction.

Other pathologies bone (like ABC, simple cyst) can also involve the jawbones.

Ameloblastoma: They are locally aggressive benign epithelial odontogenic tumors. They are more common in the mandible, mostly at the molar region. The usual time of presentation is from the fourth to sixth decade. They usually present with painless jaw swelling. They are thought to arise from the ameloblast. They may also develop from the dentigerous cyst. They may be uni- or multilocular. The multilocular tumor often has bubbly appearance. There may be focal cortical invasion end involvement of the soft tissue. On MR, these are solid cystic lesions with a thick enhancing wall.

UPPER AERODIGESTIVE TRACT

PHARYNX

Tornwaldt cyst: They are midline, well-circumscribed developmental cysts of the posterior wall of the nasopharynx anterior to the longus colli muscles. They are usually asymptomatic. They may sometime present with pain and halitosis if there is infection. They are low-density lesions in the typical location with minimal thin rim enhancement.

Peritonsillar abscess: Acute tonsillitis is usually a self-limited process. The most common offending agent is *Streptococcus pneumoniae*. Suppurative uncontrolled infection of the tonsil may lead to abscess in the peritonsillar region. The peritonsillar abscess may spread to the parapharyngeal or lateral retropharyngeal space. Trismus may develop if the medial pterygoid muscle is involved. On CT, there is homogenous swelling of the tonsillar region. There may be stranding of parapharyngeal fat. If there is development of an abscess, it appears as ugly ring-enhancing lesion.

Retropharyngeal infections: Retropharyngeal space infections are rare but may be potentially life threatening. Infection of the retropharyngeal abscess used to be due to lymphatic spread of infections from sinonasal cavities, tonsil, oral cavity, and middle ear. Nowadays, the most common cause of infection in this region is due to penetrating trauma or extension from the cervical osteomyelitis. They are more common in immunocompromised patients. Retropharyngeal space infection may spread to the mediastinum via the danger space, which is located immediately posterior to the retropharyngeal space. Patients usually present with sore throat, fever, pain, odynophagia, chills, neck pain, and stiffness. Both CT and MR are excellent for the evaluation of the retropharyngeal space infection. Though MR has best soft-tissue resolution, CT is most commonly performed for evaluation of retropharyngeal infection. Retropharyngeal abscess is a low-density lesion with enhancing walls and expansion of the retropharyngeal space. Retropharyngeal adenitis appears as low-density lesion with subtle enhancement of the wall.

NPC: Squamous cell cancer is the most common tumor in this location, followed by the lymphoma and adenocarcinoma. The squamous cell variety is much more common in Asia than the Americas. This is more common in males. Unlike squamous cell cancers at other sites of the head and neck, the etiology of NPC is not usually related to tobacco and alcohol use, but is multifactorial with viral, genetic, and environmental factors. Epstein-Barr virus is strongly associated with NPC. Immunoglobulin A antibodies against the capsid antigen of EBV is widely used as a tumor marker with 80% to 90% sensitivity.

NPC occurs most commonly at the fossa of Rosenmuller. It can extend anteriorly into the nasal cavity, anterosuperiorly to the ethmoid sinus and orbits, superiorly into the sphenoid sinus and foramen lacerum, laterally into the parapharyngeal space and pterygoid muscles, and inferiorly into the oral cavity.

CT and MR are complementary to each other for evaluation and staging of NPC. CT is best for determination of cortical involvement. MR is best for determination of tumor spread. The tumors are hyperintense in T2 signal compared to the muscles. They usually enhance brightly with contrast. Imaging of cervical lymph node is essential as 90% of the cancers go to the lymph node at the time of the initial diagnosis. Retropharyngeal and level II lymph node are most commonly involved.

Oropharyngeal cancer: The most common cancer is the squamous cell cancer followed by lymphoma and minor salivary gland tumor. For a definite description of the tumor, they are described as cancer of anterior tonsillar pillar, posterior tonsillar pillar, tonsillar fossa, soft palate, and base of tongue.

Hypopharyngeal cancer: More than 95% of cancers are SCC. Risk factors include tobacco, alcohol, and previous radiation therapy. Plummer-Vinson syndrome is an independent risk factor for development of cancer at this location. Seventy-five percent of the SCC at this location has lymph node spread at the time of diagnosis. Up to 15% of the tumor has a second primary, which may be synchronous or metachronous.

ORAL CAVITY

Vascular Malformation

As there is no cellular proliferation, vascular lesions are not tumors per se. They are developmental anomalies. They may involve the capillary level, the veins, the arteries, and the lymphatic system.

Capillary malformation: These lesions were previously called port wine stain, capillary hemangioma, nevus flammeus. They may be associated with Sturge-Weber syndrome. There is hypertrophy of the involved part.

Venous malformation: They are sometimes called cavernous malformation. They do not involute with age. They may involve the bone too. They are the most common vascular lesions of the oral cavity. They may be enormous in size. They may involve multiple fascial planes and may be purely intramuscular. They are usually muscle density masses, which enhance variably with contrast. There may be phlebolith within these lesions. On MR, there may be vascular flow void from high flow arterial or venous lesions.

Arteriovenous malformation: Arteriovenous malformation or fistula is a high-flow common developmental anomaly of the head and neck area. Angiographically, there is an arterial part and an early draining vein.

Lymphatic malformation: Lymphatic malformation used to be called lymphangioma. As there is no cellular proliferation microscopically, so these lesions are better called lymphatic malformation or venolymphatic malformation, if there is a venous part associated within the lesion. They are usually poorly marginated lesions and may involve multiple fascial planes. They may contain subacute blood, which is easily picked up in MR.

Infection of the Oral Cavity

Infection of the oral cavity is a very common clinical condition and has numerous causes. The most common is secondary extension of the infection from the teeth. Other causes include bad oral hygiene, infection of the salivary gland, and involvement from osteomyelitis. CT is the preferred modality as it can depict small calculus and clearly delineate osteomyelitis. It typically appears as a low-density uni- or multilocular ring-enhancing lesions with stranding of the adjacent fatty tissue. On MR, the abscess has typical hypointense lesions on T1, which is hyperintense in T2 with rim enhancement of the abscess wall.

Ludwig Angina

Ludwig angina is extensive infection of the floor of the mouth by oral flora. The most common source of this infection is a mandibular molar. This usually presents as extensive transfascial cellulitis often with bilateral involvement from floor of mouth downward. This infection is spread by contiguous involvement rather than lymphatic spread. Any structure in the course of the infection can be involved. The salivary glands are usually spared.

Ranula

These are mucous retention cysts of the floor of the mouth and may be of two types:

Simple ranula is lined by true epithelium in the region of sublingual space above the mylohyoid muscle. Most probably, they arise from the obstruction of the minor salivary glands. Diving/plunging ranula is due to rupture of the simple ranula and is lined by granulation or fibrous tissue. The lesion typically grows posteriorly into the submandibular region. On imaging, they typically appear as cysts. The plunging component usually enters into the submandibular space medially and displaces the submandibular gland laterally. By comparison, the second branchial cleft cyst, which is sometimes confused with the plunging ranula without any sublingual component, arises from the posterior aspect of the gland and displaces the gland medially.

Oral Cavity Cancer

Oral cavity cancer is a potentially devastating condition, typically first identified as small painful nonhealing ulcers. It is commonly associated with tobacco and alcohol use. Oral cavity is a large space. Description of the locations of the oral cavity cancers are described separately: lips, buccal mucosa, floor of the mouth, retromolar trigone, oral tongue, hard palate, soft palate, alveolar ridge. The most common cancer is SCC, followed by minor salivary gland cancer, lymphoma, and sarcomas.

Complete radiologic evaluation of the head neck cancer, including PET/CT and MR, should be obtained before biopsy for baseline record of the tumor and lymph node status as biopsy may alter the original uptake pattern. MRI is clearly the imaging modality of choice as it can depict the extension of the tumor very well. Noncontrast T1-weighted scans are very helpful for detection of tumor extension. PET has emerged as a powerful adjunct for the detection of the tumor both for pretreatment staging and also for screening of head and neck metastasis.

Adenoid Cystic Carcinoma

Adenoid cystic carcinomas are cancers of the minor salivary glands. They are present in the entire upper aerodigestive tract but concentrated at the buccal, labial, palatal, and lingual region. They typically occur in middle age. On imaging, it is not possible to differentiate this lesion from SCC. This tumor is notorious for spreading along the nerves. On CT, perineural spread is demonstrated as enlargement of the cranial nerve foramina at the base of the skull, enlarged pterygomaxillary fissure. On MR, the involved nerve is thickened, they are hyperintense in T2, and enhance with contrast.

LARYNX AND TRACHEA

Laryngomalacia: In the nontraumatic setting, laryngomalacia is due to delayed development of laryngeal support system. The inherent supporting structures are weak. Usually the supraglottic larynx is involved.

Vocal cord paralysis: The vocal cord is supplied by the superior laryngeal nerve and recurrent laryngeal nerve. Vocal cord paralysis may be due to paralysis of either of the two nerves. Superior laryngeal nerve palsy causes the arytenoid to rotate toward the paralyzed site. The more common cause is paralysis of recurrent laryngeal nerve, which supplies all of the laryngeal muscles, except the cricothyroid. On cross-sectional imaging, there is enlargement of the ventricle as the thyroarytenoid muscle atrophies.

Laryngocele: The enlarged saccule of the laryngeal ventricle in the paraglottic region of the supraglottic larynx containing air or fluid, or both is known as laryngocele. It can be internal, external, or mixed. An internal laryngocele is within the larynx and presents as a mass in the supraglottic larynx. The mixed one has both internal and external component. The internal mass comes out through the thyrohyoid membrane. Most of these lesions are mixed type. The can be easily identified in CT, MR, and x-rays. The CT density/MR intensity changes with the protein contents. Although laryngocele is benign, it may be associated with malignancy. Careful examination of the ventricle should be done.

Epiglottitis: Epiglottitis is a disease of early childhood; the peak age of presentation is 2 to 4 years. The typical organism is *Haemophilus influenzae*. The classical presentation is sore throat and inability to swallow and the epiglottis appears as cherry red. The epiglottis is thickened in the lateral radiograph. This is a medical emergency and the child should be under strict surveillance.

Rheumatoid and other connective tissue disorders: The cricoarytenoid and cricothyroid joints are synovial joints and therefore may be involved in rheumatoid arthritis. In rheumatoid arthritis, there will be variable mixture of erosion and sclerosis in and around the joint associated with soft tissue. They usually present with hoarseness. In late stage, there may be joint fixation.

SCC: The most common cancer of the larynx is SCC. The most common offending agents are tobacco and alcohol. Laryngeal papilloma may also be turned into malignancy. For complete description, the laryngeal cancers are described as supraglottic, glottic, and subglottic.

- Supraglottic carcinomas usually involve the aryepiglottic fold, epiglottis, and periepiglottic areas. The usual clinical presentation is sore throat with or without hoarseness. The peak age of presentation is the sixth decade with a male predominance. These carcinomas are moderately enhancing infiltrating masses of these regions. In late stage of the disease, the carcinomas can involve the laryngeal cartilage. On MR, there is diffuse enhancement with contrast. One treatment option of this tumor may be supraglottic laryngectomy. However, the contraindications are bilateral arytenoid involvement, involvement of cartilages, invasion of the vocal cord involvement of the pyriform sinus, and involvement of the base of the tongue.
- Glottic cancer arises in the vocal cords. Most common presenting symptom is hoarseness. The demography is the same as that of supraglottic cancers. On imaging, there is thickening of the true vocal cords. They are hyperintense lesions of the vocal cord with homogenous enhancement. As they arise from the vocal cord, they present very early with hoarseness.
- Laryngeal cancer arising from inferior to the true vocal cord down to the cricoid cartilage is considered as subglottic cancer. As they don't produce any symptom in the early stage of the disease, they are usually large at presentation with lymph node involvement.

PAROTID SPACE

INFECTION/INFLAMMATION

Acute parotitis: Acute infection of the gland may be viral or bacterial. Bacterial infections are due to direct spread from the oral cavity. Obstruction to the flow of secretion is the single most common cause of acute parotitis. The infection of the parotid gland is more common than that of the submandibular gland because of larger orifice and small diameter of the Stensen's duct, and the disadvantageous position makes the distal duct and orifice prone to injury. Acute infection of the salivary gland is very painful. The entire gland swells and is very tender to touch. This usually occurs in dehydrated patients with bad oral hygiene. The common organisms are *Staphylococcus aureus, Streptococcus viridans, and H. influenzae*. Usually the patient presents acutely. A CT scan shows dilated ductular system with diffuse enhancement of the gland and duct walls. It is also very good to demonstrate small calculus. Sialography is contraindicated in this acute setting. Mumps is the most common virus that infects the parotid gland. The presentation may be acute or chronic.

Sialolithiasis: Eighty to ninety percent of sialolithiasis occurs in the submandibular gland as a result of the orientation (and vertical course) of the duct, thick mucoid secretion, alkaline pH, and narrower orifice. Parotid gland calculus is not uncommon. Smaller stone presents with intermittent pain during increased salivation. Larger stone presents with deep aching pain. The calculus can be identified in x-rays as they are made up of calcium phosphate. On CT, the dilated ductular system obstructed by the calculus could be easily identified.

Benign lymphoepithelial disease: In this condition, there are bilateral benign mixed solid and cystic lesions in the diffusely enlarged parotid glands in the setting of HIV. It is usually associated with lymphadenopathy, fatigue, night sweats, diarrhea, and weight loss. Associated opportunistic infections might not be present in this early stage. The lymph nodes in the parotid glands are known to contain salivary gland acini and ducts. Since lymphoid tissue is vulnerable to HIV infection, intranodal epithelial proliferation can occur, causing cyst formation. Parotid gland lymphoepithelial cysts are painless and slow growing. They can suggest the presence of HIV infection in a patient with cervical lymphadenopathy. These cysts usually involve the superficial parotid lobe bilaterally. Multiple cysts are more common than single cysts. Their size varies from 0.5 to 5 cm in diameter. There may be thin rim enhancement.

Sjögren syndrome: Sjögren syndrome is an autoimmune disorder of the exocrine glands in which there is lymphocyte-induced destruction of the glands resulting in decreased secretion and dryness. It may be primary when it manifests alone or it may be secondary if occurs along with other connective tissue disorders.

The mean age of diagnosis is the sixth decade of life. It occurs more frequently in women. It presents with recurrent acute episodes of tender glandular swelling and chronic glandular enlargement with superimposed acute attacks. There is dry mouth and dry eyes because of involvement of the exocrine glands. There is increased risk of development of non-Hodgkin lymphoma (usually MALT type) in the setting of Sjögren syndrome.

In the early stage of the disease, the gland appears normal in cross-sectional imaging. With time, the gland gradually enlarges in size and becomes increasingly dense. In later stage, there will be development of honeycomb appearance. This is a characteristic finding of Sjögren syndrome but not pathognomonic. Like cross-sectional imaging, the sialograms are usually normal in the early stage of the disease with normal-appearing central ducts. Later on there are multiple globular areas of contrast accumulation close to the dilated central ducts.

TUMORS

Pleomorphic adenoma: This is the most common salivary gland tumor of the major salivary glands and accounts for 70% to 80% of all the benign tumors. Of all, approximately 85% occur in parotid glands and approximately 10% in submandibular gland, approximately 5% in the minor salivary glands (this is the most common tumor in the minor salivary glands), and less than 1% in sublingual glands. Ninety percent of the parotid pleomorphic adenomas arise from the superficial parotid gland.

Typically they present as painless slow-growing tumors. They may be a few millimeters to several centimeters in size. The usual presentation is fifth decade onward with slight female predominance. Microscopically, they contain both glandular and ductular elements. They are well-marginated, high-density spherical tumors with variable enhancement. Smaller tumors tend to be homogeneous in appearance but larger tumors are heterogeneous in both pre- and postcontrast study. Usually the tumors enhance with time, so a delayed postcontrast scan is helpful. On MR they are hypointense in T1 and hyperintense on T2 images, with T2 hypointense periphery.

There is a high recurrence rate of this tumor after resection, so they are typically treated with partial parotidectomy. Part of the tumor may be dedifferentiated to carcinoma expleomorphic adenoma.

Warthins tumor: This is the second most common benign tumor of the parotid gland. This is also a slow-growing benign tumor, which occurs almost exclusively in the parotid gland. They are commonly cystic. Like pleomorphic adenoma, they occur after the sixth decade of life. They are the most common bilateral parotid tumors (occurs in 5%–14%). They are small oval tumors, usually at the posterior aspect of the superficial lobe of the parotid gland. They are homogeneous iso- to hypodense lesions, if not cystic. There is no dystrophic calcification. The solid tumor is hypointense on T1-weighted images and, hyperintensive on T2-weighted images. The cystic tumors may be heterogeneous and demonstrate uptake 99mTc pertechnetate. Oncocytoma is the only other parotid tumor which also uptakes 99mTc pertechnetate.

Mucoepidermoid carcinoma: This is the most common malignant tumor of the minor salivary glands. They present earlier than the benign tumors, usually from the fourth decade and slightly more common in women. Radiation can cause the tumor. The tumors may be of low grade, intermediate grade, and high grade. The imaging appearance varies with tumor grade. The low-grade tumors are homogenous and benign looking; however, the high-grade tumors are aggressive looking with soft-tissue involvement beyond the gland and spread along the nerves. Noncontrast T1 is the best modality because of inherent contrast of intraglandular fatty tissues.

Adenoid cystic carcinoma: Though this more commonly occurs in minor salivary glands, the most common location of the tumor in the major salivary glands is the parotid gland. They usually occur fourth decade onward. They are slow-growing malignant tumors with potential for extensive infiltration of the surrounding tissues. These tumors are notorious for perineural spread along the cranial nerves into the skull base and cranial cavity. Microscopically, there are multiple subtypes of the tumor. On imaging, the tumor may appear benign or malignant looking, depending upon the grade of the tumor. MRI is the best modality for detection of the perineural spread and also to define the extensive soft-tissue involvement. Usually the tumor enhances with contrast as is the involved soft tissue and perineural spread.

Lymphoma: Primary lymphoma of the salivary gland is a rare entity. They most commonly involve the parotid glands. The lymphomas are usually MALT type. However, secondary involvement of the parotid gland from systemic lymphoma may also occur. There is no specific imaging sign of the lymphomas. They may be solitary or multiple, usually homogenous masses. They usually enhance with contrast. There may be cystic degeneration. They may be benign-looking nodular masses or there may rarely be invasive infiltrating tumor of the entire gland. MRI is better modality for the evaluation of the tumor.

CAROTID SPACE

Carotid body paraganglioma (carotid body tumor): They are tumors arising from the neural crest cell and mesenchymal cell of the third branchial arch. They typically arise from the adventitial layer at the carotid bifurcation. They may be familial; bilateral and multiple tumors are common in familial diseases. They may be associated with pheochromocytoma and other head and neck paragangliomas. These tumors appear as slowly growing, asymptomatic palpable masses in the anterior triangle of the neck. In late stage, they may surround the external and internal carotid arteries characteristically without any significant compression. Large tumors may involve cranial nerve of the carotid sheath, pharyngeal compression and skull base, and intracranial invasion. Uncommonly, the tumor may present with pain, hoarseness, dysphagia, Horner syndrome, tongue paresis, and vertigo. Functional paragangliomas are rare. The peak age of presentation is 40 to 50 years.

On ultrasonography, the demonstration of a solid, well-defined, weakly echogenic mass located within the carotid bifurcation safely differentiates and excludes purely cystic masses. High-frequency high-resolution ultrasonography depicts accurately the location, shape of the disease process and anatomic relationship of the tumor with the vessels of the neck, and demonstrates multiplicity of nodules if any. Doppler analysis of the mass demonstrates low-resistance arterial blood flow within the mass.

CT demonstrates a hypodense solid mass that shows intense homogenous enhancement on intravenous contrast administration. The large tumor vessels may also be visualized.

There is intense tumor-blush in the region of carotid bifurcation. This tumor can be embolized preoperatively to decrease the bleeding from the surgery.

On MR, they are heterogeneous both in T1- and T2-weighted images that is due to flow voids from the prominent tumor vessels.

Schwannoma: Schwannoma in the carotid space is not uncommon. In the nasopharyngeal carotid space, they may arise from ninth to twelfth cranial nerves and from tenth cranial nerve from oropharynx downward. The imaging features are similar to its cranial counterpart.

VISCERAL SPACE

THYROID GLAND

Acute thyroiditis is rare and is usually due to suppurative infection, the most common organism being *Staphylococcus*. The most common associated lesion is pyriform sinus in children and young men. Necrosis within a thyroid malignancy is usually commonly associated in elderly people. The usual clinical presentation is thyroid pain with referred pain in the throat and ears. CT and ultrasound help to localize the tumor.

GOITER

Goiter is enlarged thyroid gland. The gland can be enlarged because of numerous causes. Goiter is classified as follows:

Diffuse nontoxic goiter: There is diffuse enlargement of the gland with no hyperfunctioning or nodularity.

Nontoxic multinodular goiter: Multinodular goiter is diffuse nodularity of the enlarged gland, which is hormonally inactive.

Toxic multinodular goiter: In this condition there is enlargement of the thyroid gland with nodularity associated with subclinical or mild thyrotoxicosis.

THYROID MALIGNANCY

Malignant thyroid tumors are classified as follicular epithelial cells, C-cell malignancy and lymphomas, metastasis, and sarcomas. Follicular epithelial cell carcinomas are again subdivided into papillary carcinoma, follicular carcinoma, and undifferentiated carcinomas. The most common tumor is papillary cancer, which constitutes approximately 80% to 90% of cancer.

LYMPH NODE DISEASE

There are numerous lymph nodes in the head and neck region. They are systemically classified into seven stages according to the international staging system.

Level I: IA, submental; IB, submandibular

Level II: Jugulodigastric, from the base of the skull to the level of the hyoid bone.
- A: Closely related to the carotid vessels
- B: Related posterior, away from the carotid vessel

Level III: Jugulodigastric lymph nodes from hyoid bone down to the lower border of cricoid cartilage.

Level IV: Jugulodigastric lymph nodes from the lower border of cricoid cartilage to the supraclavicular region.

Level V: Lymph nodes of the posterior triangle.
- A: Above the level of hyoid
- B: Below the level of hyoid

Level VI: Level VI lymph nodes are suprasternal lymph nodes between sternomastoid heads.

Level VII: These are superior mediastinal lymph nodes.

PEDIATRIC DISEASES

BRANCHIAL CLEFT ANOMALIES

First branchial cleft cyst: They are derived from the first branchial arch around the ear and can be of two types: periauricular and periparotid. They are well-circumscribed low-density masses with or without enhancement of the wall. They usually present in children as a painless swelling.

Second branchial cleft cyst: They are derived from the second branchial arch, and may be fistula, sinus, or cyst or any combination of the three. They are most commonly located anteromedial to the sternomastoid lateral to the carotid space. They usually present early in childhood. Unless they are treated early, they may get infected.

Third branchial arch cyst: They are thin-walled cystic lesions in the posterior triangle along the border of the sternomastoid.

Fourth branchial anomaly: They are epithelial-lined cysts lateral to the left lobe of thyroid usually attached to the thyroid cartilage. There may be associated sinus or fistula. They usually present in infants.

Thyroglossal duct cyst: They are developmental aberrations of the thyroglossal duct and can occur anywhere from the foramen cecum to the thyroid gland. Most of them are related to the hyoid bone. They are usually midline except in the infrahyoid neck, where they are usually paramedian. On CT, they are hypodense structures with or without enhancement of the wall. If they are infected, there is usually enhancement of the wall. They are usually asymptomatic swellings of early childhood. If infected, they may present with pain. The surgical treatment is a Sistrunk procedure.

Lymphangioma (cystic hygroma): They are transfascial multicystic soft masses of the posterior triangle. Usual age of presentation is less than 2 years. Large lesions may present with respiratory obstruction. They are ill-defined lesions with multiple fluid-fluid levels, usually with no significant enhancement.

SUGGESTED READING

Benson MT, Dalen K, Mancuso AA, et al. Congenital anomalies of the branchial apparatus: embryology and pathologic anatomy. *Radiographics.* 1992;12:943-960.

Caldemeyer KS, Mathews VP, Azzarelli B, et al. The jugular foramen: a review of anatomy, masses, and imaging characteristics. *Radiographics.* 1997;17:1123-1139.

Caldemeyer KS, Mathews VP, Righi PD, et al. Imaging features and clinical significance of perineural spread or extension of head and neck tumors. *Radiographics.* 1998;18:97-110.

Chung EM, Murphey MD, Specht CS, et al. From the archives of the AFIP: Pediatric orbit tumors and tumorlike lesions: osseous lesions of the orbit. *Radiographics.* 2008;28:1193-1214.

Laine FJ, Nadel L, Braun IF. CT and MR imaging of the central skull base. Part 2. Pathologic spectrum. *Radiographics.* 1990; 10:797-821.

Mafee MF, Valbassori GE, Becker M. *Valbassori's Imaging of the Head and Neck.* 2nd ed. New York and Stuttgart Germany: Georg Thieme Verlag; 2004.

Meyer JS, Harty MP, Mahboubi S, et al. Langerhans cell histiocytosis: presentation and evolution of radiologic findings with clinical correlation. *Radiographics.* 1995;15:1135-1146.

Rao AB, Koeller KK, Adair CF. From the archives of the AFIP: Paragangliomas of the head and neck: radiologic-pathologic correlation. *Radiographics.* 1999;19:1605-1632.

Sigal R, Zagdanski AM, Schwaab G, et al. CT and MR imaging of squamous cell carcinoma of the tongue and floor of the mouth. *Radiographics.* 1996;16:787-810.

Smirniotopoulos JG, Yue NC, Rushing EJ. Cerebellopontine angle masses: radiologic-pathologic correlation. *Radiographics.* 1993;13:1131-1147.

QUESTIONS AND ANSWERS

1. Which of the following is most likely to present with symptoms other than pulsatile tinnitus?
   A. Dehiscence of jugular foramen
   B. Glomus tumor
   C. Cholesteatoma
   D. Aberrant carotid artery
   E. Temporal bone tumor

   ANSWER: C. Vascular lesions produce pulsatile tinnitus. Cholesteatoma is not a vascular lesion.

2. You identify a new cystic mass in the carotid space in a 55-year-old patient who smokes. Which of the following is the most likely diagnosis?
   A. Abscess
   B. Branchial cyst
   C. Metastasis
   D. Paraganglioma

   ANSWER: C. New-onset cystic mass in the carotid space in an older patient who smokes is most likely due to a lymph node metastasis with cystic degeneration.

3. A patient with head and neck carcinoma presents with a submental node. According to the WHO lymph node classification, at which level is this node located?
   A. I
   B. II

C. III
D. IV
E. V

ANSWER: A. Submental lymph nodes are considered as level Ia.

4. Which of the following does *not* present with leukokoria?
A. Optic glioma
B. Retinoblastoma
C. Coat disease
D. PHPV
E. Congenital cataract

ANSWER: A. Optic gliomas do not usually involve the optic disc or retina unless very far advanced. This is retrobulbar pathology not seen in ophthalmoscopy. Other four conditions are known to produce leukokoria.

5. What is the most common cause of facial hemipalsy?
A. Ramsey Hunt
B. MS
C. Vertebrobasal dolichoectasia
D. Bell palsy
E. Facial nerve schwannoma

ANSWER: D. Bell palsy is the most common cause of facial nerve palsy. Others are rare conditions.

6. Which of the following is the cause of pulsatile exophthalmos in NF1?
A. Plexiform neurofibroma
B. Venous malformation
C. Sphenoid wing dysplasia
D. Optic nerve glioma

ANSWER: C. Sphenoid wing dysplasia allows for direct transmission of the intracranial carotid pulsation through the absent sphenoid wing. Plexiform neurofibroma, venous malformation, and optic nerve glioma cause exophthalmos but typically not pulsatile.

7. A young woman with a history of sore throat presents with four weeks of irritability and weight loss. A radioactive thyroid iodine uptake tests less than 1% uptake. Which of the following is the most likely diagnosis?
A. Grave disease
B. Acute suppurative thyroiditis
C. Subacute nonsuppurative thyroiditis
D. Hashimoto thyroiditis
E. Thyroid carcinoma

ANSWER: C. This is the classic presentation of early-stage subacute nonsuppurative thyroiditis when there is destruction of the gland that releases the T3 and T4, which decreases the TSH level causing low iodine uptake. In Graves disease, the feature of hyperthyroidism is more prominent. Acute suppurative thyroiditis presents with thyroid pain and swelling.

8. What is the *least* common presentation of juvenile nasopharyngeal angiofibroma?
A. Origination in the nasal cavity
B. Involves pterygopalatine fossa
C. Involves sphenoid sinus
D. Contains calcifications
E. Presents with epistaxis

ANSWER: D. Angiofibromas are highly vascular tumors, but they do not calcify. They typically arise in the pterygopalatine fossa but may involve the nasal cavity and sphenoid bone.

9. Which of the following is the *most* likely diagnosis in a 35 year-old man with bilateral painless parotid enlargement and cervical adenopathy?
A. Benign lymphoepithelial cysts
B. Warthin tumor
C. Mumps
D. Sjögren syndrome
E. Sialoadenitis

ANSWER: A. Warthin tumor is bilateral but rarely associated with adenopathy. Mumps is not common in adult patients. Sjögren syndrome is more common in women and not associated with adenopathy. Benign lymphoepithelial cysts are a common presentation in HIV.

10. Which of the following is the *least* likely presentation of Tolosa-Hunt syndrome?
A. Bilateral orbital apex involvement
B. Granulomatous inflammation in the cavernous sinus
C. Narrowing of cavernous carotid artery
D. Thrombosis of the ophthalmic vein

ANSWER: A. It is usually a unilateral granulomatous process that can cause these vascular complications.

15 SPINAL CORD PATHOLOGY

Joseph C. Sullivan III

DEVELOPMENTAL LESIONS

Developmental lesions of the cord include a whole host of processes associated with neural tube closure.

In an adult patient, a tethered cord or low-lying conus below the level of L2 is difficult to distinguish from a thickened filum (thickness greater than 2–3 mm). This may be associated with spinal dysraphism, such as spina bifida occulta, an intradural lipoma, or cutaneous presentation such as a sinus tract or hairy patch on the back. The mildest form can be referred to as lipomatous infiltration of the filum terminale.

Cysts that occur within the spinal canal and cord tend to present with mass effect on the cord. Of these, the most common is the arachnoid cyst. It has a smooth contoured displacement of the cord and demonstrates similar signal characteristics to CSF on all sequences. Clinical presentation tends to be secondary to mass effect with myelopathic symptoms. Other cysts commonly seen are Tarlov cysts. These are truly cystic dilatation of the perineural root pouches generally associated with sacral roots. These are caused by a so-called ball-valve effect at the junction of the osseous elements and the nerve root sheath with underlying cause thought to be secondary to CSF pulsation from respiration and/or arterial fluctuations. These tend to have direct connection with the thecal sac. Differentiation from meningocele, traumatic avulsion, arachnoid cyst, and dural ectasia should be considered.

Epidural cysts may be extramedullary or rarely can be intramedullary in location. The congenital type is the result of ectodermal inclusion of trapped ectoderm at time of neural tube closure. The acquired variant is secondary to intervention displacing ectodermal tissue into the spinal canal or possibly into the cord itself. This, along with epidermoids, may reflect complication of lumbar punctures, providing the teaching of leaving the stylet within the spinal needle until one has traversed the thecal sac. These lesions tend to be discreet and have variable signal intensity on MRI. If there is associated peripheral enhancement, it is likely a reactive response.

Cysts and syrinx formations within the cord develop by one of two processes. In the first type, a syrinx can arise centrally because of dilatation of the central canal. This can occur either above or below the craniocervical junction. The former results from an intracranial obstruction distal to the outflow of the fourth ventricle, and the latter is formed below the craniocervical junction secondary to changes in CSF flow from intramedullary or extramedullary effect. This can be seen with dilation of the central canal or cysts thought to be formed from Chiari I malformations, resulting in impingement of the craniocervical junction with effacement of the foramen magnum. It can also occur in the setting of with intra- or extramedullary lesions such as tumor, and arachnoid cyst, which may form in the association of trauma or canal stenosis, or inflammatory process such as arachnoiditis. This central canal dilatation may be focal or more diffuse. It tends to have a smooth dilatation without abrupt changes in morphology and follows CSF signal on all sequences. CSF flow artifacts may be seen on FLAIR imaging. These cysts/syrinxes tend to expand the overall cord's circumference, as there is displacement of the surrounding normal cord. The second type, which is not centrally located and can be more asymmetric, is thought to originate within the parenchyma of the cord itself. It is uncertain if the mass effect creates myelomalacia of the surrounding cord as in some cases edema and swelling of the cord may present prior to true syrinx formation. Eccentric syrinx formation may also be associated with myelomalacia from direct trauma or asymmetric expansion of the central canal and fissures within the ependymal margin allowing for CSF pulsation to form an eccentric cyst. These may also simply represent arachnoid cysts formed from other etiologies or changes in CSF dynamics from inflammatory processes or adhesions, which can occur in the setting of trauma or ischemia. It is a clinical conundrum as to whether the myelomalacia associated with cord injury is cystic or noncystic in nature. A noncystic myelomalacia implies cord parenchyma loss and, therefore, would not benefit from shunt placement. However, there would be a role for shunt placement if it is a true cyst with mass effect.

INFECTIOUS AND INFLAMMATORY DISORDERS

Inflammatory and infectious processes of the spinal cord traditionally present with symptoms of radiculitis, radiculopathy, or paresthesia and paresis. However, pain may be the only complaint. These inflammatory processes, including multiple sclerosis or connective tissue diseases including Sjögren syndrome, lupus, or rheumatoid arthritis, can lead to rapidly progressive neurologic dysfunction. In transverse myelitis, there may be dysfunction of a portion or the entirety of the spinal cord.

Sarcoidosis, vasculitis, or idiopathic processes can also present with radiculitis, as does disseminated encephalomyelitis, although it has a very different etiology.

B_{12} (cobalamin) deficiency can present as an acute combined degenerative myelitis, including paresthesia of the hands and feet and loss of protopathic and epicritic sensation, leading to ataxia, spasticity, and lower motor neuroweakness. However, it can also present with lesions in the optic tracts, cerebrum, and peripheral nerves. T2 hyperintensity is identified in the nucleus gracilis and cuneatus, primarily within the cervical and thoracic spine, and there may or may not be associated cord swelling. This tends to be a long segment lesion and can be confused with multiple other etiologies such as those seen with folic acid deficiency, tabes dorsalis (syphilis), certain chemotherapeutic agents such as vincristine, and carcinomatous radiculopathy. The causes of B_{12} insufficiency include autoimmune reaction toward the gastric parietal cells in the gastric fundus and proximal gastric body. These cells produce an intrinsic factor that is used to bind B_{12} and allow its subsequent absorption from the terminal ileum. This can also be a complication of extended gastrectomy or decreased intake, which can occur in strictly limited diets (vegan). In such settings, changes within the marrow appearance resulting in benign hyperplastic marrow secondary to pernicious anemia may be an indication of its etiology.

Systemic lupus erythematosus can present as a traditional transverse myelitis with paraparesis or quadriparesis, sensory loss, or back pain. This tends to occur over several segments within the cord without predilection for location. Involved segment tends to be slightly longer than in multiple sclerosis and it may enhance. Etiology is believed to be autoimmune-related, vacuolar degeneration, or ischemia.

Multiple sclerosis tends to occur over a shorter segment, usually two to three vertebral body lengths. It can produce myelopathic signs with only spinal signs and symptoms in up to one-fourth of the cases. Multiple sclerosis has a predilection for the cervical spine and although may commonly affect the lateral cord, it does not have a limitation with respect to the gray or white boundaries. There may be enhancement if there is ongoing demyelination. Over time this can lead to parenchymal loss. However, rarely there is mild edema depending on the acuity of the lesion. A large amount of spinal cord edema and swelling should raise suspicion of other etiologies.

Although unusual, sarcoidosis can present within the spinal cord, also with a predilection for the cervical region. Sarcoidosis can imitate multiple diseases: nodules on the surface of the cord (metastatic disease), a plaque on individual nerve roots (infectious or metastatic disease), or rarely as an intramedullary lesion, which may be diffuse or discreet. Sarcoid lesions have a mixed pattern of enhancement.

Tuberculosis usually affects the lower spine and thoracolumbar region; it can be an indolent process presenting late in its progression with epidural components or soft-tissue involvement with Pott disease. Pott disease leads to vertebral body destruction with sparing of the disk space, giving the impression of malignant processes. The disease may result in severe alignment deformities. Diagnosis, although usually one of exclusion, requires the difficult isolation and growth of the *tuberculum bacillus*.

Epidural abscess can indirectly compress the spinal cord or create an inflammatory response that secondarily affects the cord. Most commonly, epidural abscesses are caused by direct extension from vertebral or paraspinal infection, which are commonly due to the blood-borne spread of infectious source, such as cardiac or urinary tract infection or other cause of septicemia. Immunosuppression or intravenous drug abuse can also serve as an etiology. Rarely, epidural abscess can be associated with trauma to the spine belong with hematoma formation and subsequent superinfection or can be iatrogenic (spinal surgery or instrumentation). Although nuclear scintigraphy may be beneficial to evaluate for infection on inflammatory processes or osseous involvement, MRI remains the mainstay of imaging and diagnosis because of improved morphologic evaluation. This can also allow the surgeons to plan their operative approach and posttherapy reconstruction.

Diskitis and osteomyelitis are usually blood-borne infections, typically seeding at the endplate, which may result in focal back pain or radicular pain. This may impinge or create inflammatory response in the meningeal or neural elements. Most commonly, diskitis and osteomyelitis are caused by skin pathogens that have penetrated into the blood such as staphylococcus, streptococcus, or less likely *Escherichia coli*. Although gallium nuclear scintigraphy can be very sensitive for this inflammatory process, MRI remains a more conclusive diagnostic tool. If there is extension into the epidural space, ischemia at the neural elements from vascular inflammatory response should be entertained. Vertebral osteomyelitis is also well delineated with a three-phase bone scan. These processes are more frequent in the setting of immunodeficiency but they are not limited to the immunocompromised.

Subacute necrotizing myelopathy can present with clinical symptoms similar to transverse myelitis. It can occur with a multitude of infections: herpes zoster, mononucleosis, mumps, rubeola, toxoplasmosis, or TB. However, it can also be seen in vascular malformations, with dural AVM and venous hypertension.

VASCULAR DISORDERS

Cord ischemia or infarction may occur at any level. However, the blood supply at the junctions of upper thoracic spine and the thoracolumbar junction is more tenuous and so these are the areas most likely to be involved. These areas have the greatest demand for blood by the arms, neck, chest; and within the thoracolumbar junction, where the aorta supplies multiple solid and hollow organ systems and has a tenuous vascular supply (artery of Adamkiewicz) to the spinal cord anteriorly. Spinal cord ischemia and infarction tend to be anterior because of its singular supply. The posterior spinal cord has a dual artery supply, precluding it from ischemia except in the setting where multiple vessels may be involved, for example in vasculitis. Ischemia or infarction of the cord may present in a multitude of clinical scenarios, although lower extremity claudication may be the earliest and mildest presentation. Cord swelling in the upper thoracic or thoracolumbar junction may be the earliest imaging presentation. This cord compromise can be the result of a multitude of clinical etiologies (Table 15-1).

Arteriovenous malformations (AVM) of the spinal cord divided into three categories: spinal dural AVF spinal cord AVM either of a predominately intramedullary type or a mixed intra- or extramedullary, and extraspinal type; and spinal cord AVF.

Spinal dural AVF consists of a single nidus associated with the nerve root. This is the most frequent vascular malformation associated with the spine and is seen more commonly in the dorsal lower thoracic cord. Foix-Alajouanine is a specific myelopathy associated with spinal dural AVF. Arterial pressure creates a kink in the normal venous outflow, resulting in venous hypertension, which leads to edema and possibly ischemia from swelling. This eventually restricts arterial inflow within the cord. A large venous varix can be mistaken for a mass on imaging. However, the most common imaging appearance is a so called peppered or (multiple nodules) along the cord because of the dilated venous plexus. Treatment of a dural AVF, which arises at the same level as an anterior spinal artery, should be performed surgically because endovascular treatment is contraindicated. Treatment is usually aimed at the ligation occlusion of the arterial supply to the fistula, as removal of the venous plexus at surgery can actually be more detrimental to the cord.

TABLE 15-1 Etiologies of Cord Compromise

Atherosclerosis of the aorta
Thromboembolic source from the aorta
Dissecting aneurysm of the abdominal aorta
Vertebral artery dissection or occlusion
Vasculitis
Vascular malformations
Pregnancy
Diffuse hypertension
Caisson disease
Infection
Sickle cell disease
Diabetes

Spinal cord AVM is fed by a single or multiple branches of the anterior and posterior spinal arteries, with an intramedullary nidus of arterial flow extending into multiple spinous veins. This is considered a true AVM. Unlike spinal dural AVF, with its insidious onset, spinal cord arterial venous fistula tends to have a more acute onset usually as a presentation of intramedullary hemorrhage. A variant of the spinal cord AVM, the so-called juvenile type, tends to have extensive involvement of intramedullary, extramedullary, and possibly extraspinal components. These AVM tend to occur earlier in life and have a poor prognosis.

The third type of vascular malformation, spinal cord AVF (type 4 spinal AVM) is an intradural, extramedullary AVF without an intervening capillary network. This is located on the pial surface. It can involve the anterior and posterior spinal arteries or can have a single arteriovenous connection. It may present with progressive myelopathy and/or hemorrhage, as a result of increase in venous pressure. This hemorrhage can often present in a similar fashion as intracranial hemorrhage and is a source of nonaneurysmal intracranial subarachnoid hemorrhage.

Cavernous angiomas are also seen within the spinal cord and are of similar appearance as those seen within the cerebral and cerebellar parenchyma. Their presentation is variable depending on their location.

Soft tissues associated with the neural axis can be injured, creating neural symptoms without direct cord injury. Injuries such as a nerve root avulsion may be caused by seemingly mild spinal trauma. An avulsed nerve root can form an empty pseudomeningocele at the site of injury. These injuries can be diagnosed either with MR imaging or myelography. However, particularly later on, the posttraumatic myelomeningocele may no longer connect with the thecal sac. Other secondary injuries may be associated with prior events such as siderosis from hemorrhage associated with spinal AVM or other medullary or leptomeninges processes. Typical imaging appearance is described as a dark line outlining the neural structures as if they were "dipped in oil." Other injuries associated with the spinal cord may be secondary to injuries to its sleeve, the so-called tears in the dura, a risk for spinal cord herniation, and adhesion, leading to which can present as a tethered type of myelopathy.

NEOPLASMS

Neoplastic lesions of the cord are considered intramedullary, extramedullary–intradural, and extradural. Of those to be considered here are primarily the intramedullary and extramedullary–intradural. Intramedullary type is a small percent roughly 5% to 10% of CNS tumors, and 90% to 95% of these are glial in origin. Ependymomas are the most common (roughly two-thirds) of these glial lesions with astrocytomas predominating in the other one-third. Ependymomas present more likely within the cervical spine and conus as opposed to the astrocytomas, which occur more commonly in the thoracic spine. Ependymomas tend to be more central secondary to the lining of the central canal with ependymal cells as opposed to the astrocytoma, which is eccentric. Ependymomas tend to be more short segment averaging approximately four segments but tending to be less than six; astrocytomas tend to be seven segments or longer. Cysts associated with these lesions tend to be at the polar aspects with ependymomas. Astrocytomas tend to have intratumoral cysts. Ependymomas occur in adults with a slightly lower grade, while astrocytomas present in children with higher grade. Hemorrhage occurs with ependymomas and not with astrocytomas. Enhancement can be variable in both but is more focal and intense with ependymomas. Therefore, astrocytoma has eight letters prior to "oma" and tends to be longer segment. Ependymoma has fewer letters and tends to be of shorter (six or less) segments. The cysts associated with ependymomas tend to be on the "end" as opposed to astrocytomas, which occur more often in the central aspect. Furthermore, the use of the end can be applied to their age of onset. The appearance of being well-defined with ependymomas tends to go along with the lower grade as opposed to poor definition appearance with astrocytomas, which tends to be of the higher grade. Beyond these glial neoplasms, more common lesions are the hemangioblastoma with dilated tortuous vessels and vascular appearance, which can have cysts and associated syrinx formation. These lesions are associated with von Hippel-Lindau. Spinal paragangliomas are neural-independent, encapsulated lesions that are peripheral and located on the extramedullary surface. Spinal cord metastases are difficult to discern from primary neoplasm. Lymphoma tends to affect the epidural space and vertebral bodies as opposed to an intramedullary lesion. Primitive neural ectodermal tumors tend to be long segment and undifferentiated with a poor prognosis.

The extramedullary–intradural lesions create symptoms by cord displacement. These have a sharp border between the mass and CSF or intrathecal contrast in the setting of myelography. They also enlarge the ipsilateral subarachnoid space. Of these, approximately 90% are nerve sheath tumors (schwannomas and meningiomas). Paraganglion, dermoids, and epidermoid cysts encompass the remaining 10% of these lesions. Approximately three-quarters of the nerve sheath tumors are intradural, although some can present as a dumbbell shape with extradural extension. Meningiomas are the second most common intraspinal tumors with a slight female predilection. These are more commonly solitary but can be multiple in neurofibromatosis type 2 and are more commonly seen within the thoracic spine. Of those lesions that are extradural but can have an indirect effect on the cord, the differential includes disks, blood, bone, tumor, and sometimes puss. There are three more common primary neoplasms that may affect neural elements by compression: chordoma, lymphoma, and sarcoma. Chordoma is a layered but slow growing, locally aggressive tumor arising from notochordal elements, more commonly seen within the sacrum and clivus, but can be seen within the vertebral body secondary to inclusion at time of neural tube closure. Lymphoma can have multiple appearances within the vertebral body and tends to be secondary when it involves the spine. The "ivory vertebra" is one particular manifestation of Hodgkin disease. Metastatic disease to the vertebral elements may have a similar appearance and effect on the neural elements.

SUGGESTED READING

Baker L et al. Benign versus pathologic compression fractures of vertebral bodies. *Radiology*. 1990;174:485-502.

Barnwell S et al. Cryptic vascular malformations of the spinal cord: diagnosis by MRI and outcome of surgery. *J Neurosurg*. 1990;72:403-407.

Bourgouin P et al. A pattern approach to the differential diagnosis of intramedullary spinal cord lesions on MR imaging. *AJR Am J Roentgenol*. 1998;170:1645-1649.

Kim R. Necrotizing myelopathy. *AJNR Am J Neuroradiol*. 1992;12:1084-1086.

Masaryk T. Neoplastic disease of the spine. *Radiol Clin North Am*. 1991;29:829-846.

Okumar R et al. Fatty filum terminale: assessment with MR imaging. *J Comput Assist Tomogr*. 1990;14:571-573.

Tims S, Cure J, Kurant J. Subacute combined degeneration of the spinal cord: MR findings. *AJNR*. 1993;14:1224-1228.

Zimmerman R, Bilaniuk L. Imaging of tumors of the spine canal and cord. *Radiol Clin North Am*. 1988;26:965-1007.

QUESTIONS AND ANSWERS

1. MRI of the cord identifies a mass. What finding suggests the tumor is an astrocytoma rather than an ependymoma?
   A. Polar cyst
   B. Hemorrhage at the cap

C. Seven vertebral segments in length
D. Mixed enhancement
E. Adult patient

ANSWER: C. Astrocytomas tend to be longer than six vertebral segments. Their cysts tend to be within the lesion and rarely have hemorrhage at the margins. Astrocytomas occur more often in younger patients and both may have a mixed enhancement pattern.

2. Compression of the thecal sac on myelography could indicate all of the following diagnoses *except*
   A. Hematoma
   B. Abscess
   C. Disc herniation
   D. Astrocytoma
   E. Metastasis

   ANSWER: D. Astrocytomas are intramedullary and would expand the thecal sac. The remaining are part of the extradural differential that typically include disc, blood, bone, tumor, and sometimes pus.

3. Which of the following image findings is a contraindication to endovascular therapy of a spinal vascular malformation?
   A. Multiple arterial supplies to the nidus
   B. Anterior spinal artery supplied at the same level as an AV fistula
   C. Involvement of the posterior and anterior supply at the same level
   D. Only one dominant venous outflow noted
   E. Asymptomatic patient at time of AVM discovery on imaging

   ANSWER: B. Embolization of an artery that also supplies the anterior spinal artery could cause cord infarction if the only arterial supply is at the same level and is treated endovascularly.

4. Sarcoidosis has a predilection for which region of the spinal cord?
   A. Cervical
   B. Thoracic
   C. Lumbar
   D. Central cord
   E. Peripheral cord

   ANSWER: A. Sarcoidosis appears more commonly within the cervical region, but may be seen any where in the cord and can imitate most lesions.

5. Which of the following are the *least likely* to be the origin of an epidural abscess?
   A. Hematoma after trauma with subsequent degradation of products
   B. Instrumentation
   C. IV drug abuse
   D. UTI in an immune competent patient
   E. Psoas abscess

   ANSWER: A. Although a degrading hematoma is the perfect place for bacteria to grow, as long as it is sterile, it is less likely to result in infection. The remainder may seed the epidural space by direct or hematogenous spread.

6. Which of the following is more commonly associated with osteomyelitis than discitis?
   A. Tuberculosis
   B. Streptococcus
   C. Staphylococcus
   D. *E. coli*

   ANSWER: A. TB is more often seen to spread to the bone and epidural components contiguously. While the remaining choices spread to the disc as well, the disc is fairly resistant to involvement by TB.

7. What is the mildest form of developmental spinal abnormality?
   A. Caudal sac lipoma
   B. Spina bifida occulta
   C. Lipomatous infiltration of the filum terminale
   D. Meningocele
   E. Myelomeningocele

   ANSWER: C. Fatty filum is the mildest form of developmental spinal abnormality with minimal lipomatous replacement. The remaining options are considered more significant developmental abnormalities.

8. What is the most common cause of cord ischemia?
   A. AVM
   B. Infection
   C. Hypertension
   D. Vasculitis
   E. Thromboembolic

   ANSWER: E. Thromboembolic disease (usually from the aorta) can commonly occur in atherosclerosis and/or aneurysms, while the remainder can contribute to cord ischemia, but are not commonly the sole cause.

9. What is the most common spinal location for cord astrocytoma?
   A. Cervical
   B. Thoracic
   C. Lumbar
   D. Sacral

   ANSWER: A. Cervical. These tumors develop from astrocytes within the spinal cord. They occur at any age, but are more common during the early years of life. In children younger than 10 years of age, they account for 90% of all intramedullary tumors. In adolescents, they account for about 60% of all intramedullary tumors. Most astrocytomas are located in the spinal cord near the neck and upper chest.

10. What is the most common spinal location for cord ependymomas?
    A. Cervical
    B. Thoracic
    C. Lumbar
    D. Sacral

ANSWER: C. Ependymomas develop from ependymal cells. They are most often seen in adults aging 20 to 40 years. This is a relatively common and usually slow-growing spinal tumor, accounting for more than half of adult spinal cord tumors. Ependymoma can develop anywhere along the spinal cord, but up to 40% are found near the tailbone.

11. What is the most common location for chordomas?
    A. Clival
    B. Cervical spine
    C. Thoracic spine
    D. Lumbar spine
    E. Sacral spine

ANSWER: A. Chordomas arise from notochordal remnants of the axial skeleton and constitute less than 3% of primary malignant bone tumors. Approximately 50% arise in the sacrococcygeal region, the second commonest site is the base of the skull. They are most common in the fifth and sixth decades and have a male preponderance.

Section 2
PULMONARY

16 NORMAL ANATOMY AND VARIANTS

John C. Texada and Satinder P. Singh

LUNGS

DEVELOPMENT

The embryonic stage begins around day 26, when the lung bud forms at the ventral foregut. Over the next 2 to 3 days, it divides into left and right buds, and the tracheobronchial and esophageal guts separate via transverse ingrowths. By days 32 to 34, the lobar bronchi have appeared. In the pseudoglandular stage, the 5th to 16th weeks of development, additional bronchial tree ramifications develop. By week 16, almost all airways are present but are blind tubules. Cartilage appears in the seventh week and develops distally. In the canalicular stage, the 17th through 24th or 25th weeks of development, the peripheral bronchial tree forms canaliculi that will become the transitional airways. Capillaries grow into the mesenchyme and air spaces form. At around 28 weeks, type I and type II pneumocytes begin to differentiate and resulting blood–gas barrier is capable of gas exchange. In the saccular stage, from the 25th week through birth, acini develop. By the 28th week, several generations of respiratory bronchioles are present, and thereafter the saccules continue to proliferate and increase in vascularity. Alveolar development begins early in this stage. The alveolar period is from 36 weeks to term. Alveolar tissues have been found as early as 30 weeks, but by 36 weeks they are always present. The typical acinus at birth has three generations of respiratory bronchioles, one of transitional ducts, and three of saccules. Most alveoli have developed by 2 years of age, but some development continues until 8 years.

FUNCTIONAL ZONES

The conducting zone includes airways without alveoli and no gas exchange: the trachea (with 16–20 incomplete cartilage rings), bronchi (varying cartilage), and membranous bronchioles (no cartilage). There are about 25 generations of conducting airways from the trachea, the smallest about 0.8 mm indiameter. Ciliated cells are more numerous than secretory epithelial cells, increasingly so in the distal airways. Airways in the transitional zone participate in both conduction and respiration: the respiratory bronchioles and alveolar ducts. There are typically six to nine generations of airway and an average of 10 to 20 alveoli per duct. Up to 40% of alveoli may arise directly from the transitional airways. Upon reaching the alveolar ducts, only minimal connective tissue is left. The respiratory zone is composed of alveoli, whose function is to carry out gas exchange. Approximately 87% of lung volume is alveoli: 6% of which is tissue and the remainder is gas.

CELL TYPES AND ALVEOLAR CONNECTIONS

Alveolar pores are small (2–10 μm) alveolar wall discontinuities, more numerous in older tissue and at the apices and subpleural parenchyma; there are 5 to 20 pores per alveolus, probably covered by surfactant. Alveolar fenestrae are larger (20–100 μm), probably pathologic in nature and perhaps a forme-fruste emphysema. The canals of Lambert are proposed collateral pathways, epithelialized tubes connecting alveoli to distal bronchioles, 0 to 30 μm.

Goblet cells secrete mucus and become more numerous in inflammation. Basal cells at the basement membrane populate the epithelium. Brush cells are rare and may serve in secretion–absorption. Clara cells produce lipids and proteins, including surfactant proteins, and possibly are a progenitor for epithelial redevelopment. Neuroendocrine K cells produce neurosecretory granules and may function in mediation of hypoxia, fetal–neonatal transition, and/or epithelial growth and repair regulation. Dendritic and Langerhans cells process and present antigens.

Type I alveolar cells, membranous pneumocytes, are only 8% of all parenchymal lung cells, but cover 95% of the alveolar surface. Their function is primarily gas exchange, but they may participate in particle uptake. They are thought to be incapable of cell division. Type II alveolar cells, the granular pneumocytes, are the source of alveolar surfactant. They are capable of undergoing mitosis and are the source for replacement of type I cells. They also function in protein synthesis and maintenance, possible immune response, and fluid uptake.

PRIMARY LUNG UNITS

The primary lobule is composed of the parenchyma distal to the last respiratory bronchiole. There may be as many as 20 to 25 million primary lobules, too small to image. The secondary lobule is the smallest portion of the lung surrounded by a septum, typically 5 to 15 mm. The interlobular septa are best developed at the lung periphery, where they are continuous with the pleura. Normal secondary lobules are visible in high-resolution CT (HRCT), the smallest normal structures identifiable; only with interlobular septal thickening do the secondary lobules become radiographically visible. The acinar unit is the tissue distal to the terminal bronchiole: respiratory bronchioles, alveolar ducts and sacs, and alveoli, and their connective tissue. An acinus may be 6 to 10 mm, and a person may have thousands. Radiographically, a filled acinus may appear as a rosette or a sphere, but normal acini are not apparent even in HRCT.

TRACHEA

The normal trachea is 6 to 9 cm long. It is midline, sometimes with slight rightward deviation at the aortic arch, generally about halfway between the sternum and the spine but occasionally more anterior or posterior. The walls are smoothly corrugated by the tracheal cartilages and are parallel except possible left-sided aortic indentation just above the bifurcation. In cross section, the trachea is generally round or oval, though it may have other shapes. Its dimensions range from 13 to 25 mm and 13 to 27 mm (coronal and sagittal) in men and from 10 to 21 mm and 10 to 23 mm in women. The normal intrathoracic trachea does not change dimensions with changes in pleural pressure.

BRONCHI

The right main bronchus is slightly larger than the left at total lung capacity, 15 versus 13 mm, but it is shorter, 2.2 versus 5 cm. The subcarinal interbronchial angle measures about 60 degrees, with range about 40 to 70 degrees. The angle decreases slightly as the chest lengthens.

BRONCHOPULMONARY SEGMENTAL ANATOMY

Subsegmental and even segmental and lobar bronchial branching may vary, generally without clinical significance. The bronchopulmonary segments are relatively constant despite any airway variation.

The right lung has 10 segments. The right upper lobe bronchus arises 2 cm from the carina and divides into apical, anterior, and posterior segmental bronchi; this bronchus or one of its branches may arise directly from the lateral trachea in bronchus suis. The bronchus intermedius continues 3 to 4 cm and then bifurcates into middle and lower lobe bronchi. The right middle lobe bronchus divides into medial and lateral segmental bronchi; the right lower lobe bronchus into superior, medial basal, anterior basal, lateral basal, and posterior basal segmental bronchi.

The left lung has eight segments. The left upper lobe bronchus arises 5 cm from the carina and soon bifurcates or trifurcates into lingular and upper-division (or independent apicoposterior and anterior) bronchi. The lingular bronchus splits into superior and inferior bronchi and the left lower lobe bronchus into superior, anteromedial, lateral basal, and posterior basal bronchi.

PLEURA

The visceral pleura invests the lungs and parietal pleura invests the chest wall, diaphragm, and mediastinum. The two join at the pulmonary hila. Visceral pleural extensions form the fissures.

The visceral pleura has three layers: the superficial endopleura, the chief layer of collagen and elastic tissue, and the vascular or interstitial layer, containing connective tissue with lymphatic and blood vessels and continuous with the interlobular septal interstitium. The visceral pleura is perfused partly by bronchial artery branches; the costal and diaphragmatic portions may be bronchial or pulmonary. Bronchial veins drain the hilar regions; pulmonary veins drain the rest of the visceral pleura. Innervation is by branches of the vagus nerve and sympathetic nerves.

The parietal pleura is adjacent to the fascia of the chest wall. It has two parts, separated by a layer of fibroelastic tissue, with most of the blood vessels in the most external layer. Perfusion is via branches of chest wall arteries. The parietal pleura is innervated by intercostal nerves.

FISSURAL ANATOMY

Normal Fissures

The major fissures begin near the fifth thoracic vertebral body and course anteroinferiorly along the sixth rib. The left lower lobe usually extends slightly higher than the right. Both fissures face slightly laterally and are slightly undulating. The minor fissure separates the right upper and middle lobes; it is variably oriented but roughly horizontal at the level of the anterior fourth rib, commonly lower anteriorly and laterally. Incomplete normal fissures are common: partial right upper and middle lobe fusion is found in up to 88% of patients; right upper and lower lobe fusion, in 70%; and others range 40% to 50%.

Accessory Fissures

Any segment of lung may be partially or completely separated from adjacent lung. The azygous fissure is formed by downward migration of the azygous vein through the apical right upper lobe, visible in 0.5% of radiographs and in 1% of anatomic specimens. If a patient with an azygous fissure develops a right-sided pneumothorax, the apical pleural surfaces will not separate and sometimes fluid or pneumothorax can get loculated in azygous fissure creating bizarre radiographic appearance. Its presence may also be a potential impediment to thoracotomy and extrapleural approach to surgery for esophageal atresia and endoscopic thoracic sympathectomy done for hyperhiderosis. The inferior accessory fissure (right or left) separates the medial basal segment from the rest of the lower lobe, visible in 30% to 45% of autopsies and 8% of radiographs. The superior accessory fissure (right or left) separates the superior segment from the basal segments of the lower lobe. Less commonly the left upper lobe fissure is similar to the azygous fissure caused by the left superior intercostal vein; and the left minor fissure separates the lingula from the rest of the left upper lobe.

PULMONARY LIGAMENT

The pulmonary ligament is a double layer of pleura connecting the medial lower lobe to the mediastinum and diaphragm, formed by the mediastinal parietal pleura as it reflects over the hilar bronchovascular structures onto the surface of the lung as the visceral pleura. It is visible in 60% to 70% (left) and 40% to 60% (right) of CT, where it usually appears as a small peak on the mediastinal surface, extending as a thin line inferiorly, usually coursing obliquely posterior.

CHEST WALL

SOFT TISSUES

The pectoral muscles form the anterior axillary fold, which should curve smoothly from the axilla to the ribcage. Congenital absence of the pectoralis muscle is rare and may be associated with multiple abnormalities including Sprengel deformity (pathologically fixed scapular elevation). In this deformity, a cervical rib may articulate with the scapula (an omovertebral bone) but its presence is not required; 60% to 70% of patients with Sprengel deformity lack this bone.

The sternocleidomastoid muscles are sometimes visible paralleling the spine in the medial third of the apices, curving down and laterally to meet the clavicular companion shadow; this measures 2 to 3 mm, parallels the superior clavicle, and is formed by the skin and subcutaneous tissues overlying the bone. Isolated asymmetric absence of the companion shadow suggests supraclavicular mass.

The transversus thoracis courses from the inferior sternum to the second through fifth costal cartilages, visible in CT at the level of the heart as a thin line, internal to the anterior costal cartilage. Other muscles are clearly visible with CT: the pectoralis major and minor; the serratus anterior, immediately superficial to the lateral ribs; and the superficial, middle, and deep muscles of the back.

PRIMARY RESPIRATORY MUSCLES

In inspiration, the diaphragm is the main primary muscle; the others are the parasternal, scalene, and external intercostal muscles. The parasternal and external intercostal muscles are tonically active, preventing inward rib movement with diaphragm contraction. This ceases with anesthesia, REM sleep, or high spinal cord injury, allowing the ribcage to fall inward with diaphragm contraction. Accessory muscles are recruited when ventilatory demand increases: sternocleidomastoid, pectoralis, serratus anterior, trapezius, and latissimus dorsi.

Expiration is passive in normal people, with activity needed when ventilation exceeds 50% of maximum voluntary ventilation or with increased load. The rectus and transversus abdominis, internal and external obliques, internal intercostals, and triangularis sterni act when needed.

BONES

Twelve thoracic vertebrae are present, and twelve paired ribs are normally present. On lateral chest radiograph, lucency should increase as the spine progresses caudally; any increase should suggest intrathoracic disease ("spine sign"). Hypoplasia of the first rib may be found in 1.2% of patients, and supernumerary C7 ribs may be found in 1.5%, nearly all bilaterally. An intrathoracic rib is a rare asymptomatic congenital accessory rib arising from the anterior surface of a rib or a vertebral body, and usually extending downward and laterally to end near the diaphragm. Inferior rib indentation near the tubercles is normal and not the pathologic rib notching of coarctation and other processes. Rib cartilage calcification is common and not pathologic; the costal cartilages of men tend to calcify further at the margins, whereas costal cartilages of women tend to calcify centrally first.

The clavicle may have an inferomedial indentation called the rhomboid fossa, where costoclavicular (rhomboid) ligaments attach. The sternum should be visible in its entirety in the lateral projection; in the posteroanterior (PA) projection, only the superior and lateral walls of the manubrium are visible. The scapulae sometimes have well-defined lucencies surrounded by cortical bone: sites of incomplete bone formation, not to be reported as fracture or lytic lesion.

NONCARDIAC VASCULAR MEDIASTINUM

PULMONARY ARTERIES

DEVELOPMENT

The pulmonary artery develops from the sixth aortic arch. The proximal sixth arch on each side develops into the proximal right and left arteries; the right side loses its connection with the aortic arch, whereas the left side keeps the connection as the ductus arteriosis. Branches from each side grow toward the lung buds and form the pulmonary hila, then ramify with airway development. Most preacinar branches are present by 16 weeks gestation.

HISTOLOGY

The pulmonary arteries have thinner walls than systemic arteries of the same diameter, and the intima is very thin. The main, lobar, segmental, and subsegmental arteries are elastic but their elastin is more irregular and fragmented than in systemic elastic arteries. As vessel diameter decreases to 0.5 mm the elastic tissue is lost forming, the muscular arteries. Beginning at around 0.1 mm the smooth muscle starts to disappear forming, the arterioles. By 70 μm, the vessels have only a thin intima and a single elastic lamina; the arterioles continue to divide in the acinus. The capillaries are composed of endothelium with a basement membrane shared with the pulmonary epithelium.

GROSS ANATOMY

The pulmonary trunk extends cranially, posterior, and slightly leftward for 4 to 5 cm from the right ventricle. It divides within the pericardium into left and longer right pulmonary arteries. The main pulmonary artery diameter range is 22 to 26 mm. The left pulmonary artery continues in the same direction to the hilum; it arcs over the left main bronchus and into the vertical left interlobar artery posterolateral to the lower lobe bronchus. The left interlobar artery then typically divides into segmental branches. The right pulmonary artery courses horizontally posterior to the aorta and anterior to the right main bronchus, and divides into the truncus anterior and interlobar artery. The right pulmonary artery diameter range is 12 to 15 mm. The truncus anterior supplies the upper lobe, and the interlobar artery the middle and lower lobes; in 90% of people a part of the upper lobe posterior segment has its own arterial branch from the interlobar artery. The right interlobar artery runs between the superior vena cava (SVC) and the bronchus intermedius, then in the major fissure before dividing into middle- and lower-lobe segmental branches. The upper limit of interlobar artery diameter is 16 mm in men and 15 mm in women, decreased by 1 to 3 mm in expiration. Segmental branching is variable but one pulmonary artery always follows each bronchial division. Supernumerary arteries are common.

PULMONARY VEINS

DEVELOPMENT

Embryonic pulmonary venous blood flows initially to splanchnic plexus. The cranial sinoatrial heart outpouching develops into the common pulmonary vein, which extends to the developing lungs; it eventually becomes incorporated into the left atrial wall, generally leaving the separate pulmonary veins. The splanchnic–pulmonary connections eventually regress.

HISTOLOGY

Small pulmonary venules are identical to arterioles. Veins are clearly recognizable by a diameter of 60 to 100 μm. They have variable numbers of elastic laminae and small irregular smooth muscle and collagen bundles. There is no external elastic lamina. No valves are present, but there are focal constrictions created by rings of smooth muscle.

Gross Anatomy

The veins arise from alveolar and pleural capillaries, not associated with the airways. Their course is variable but they usually end up as two main superior and two main inferior veins. Numerous supernumerary veins are present. The right-sided veins course beneath the pulmonary artery posterior to the SVC. The right superior vein drains upper lobe segmental veins to the superoposterior left atrium. The middle lobe vein generally enters at the base of the superior pulmonary vein but may enter separately. The right inferior vein drains the lower lobe separately into the posterior inferior left atrium. The left-sided veins pass anterior to the descending aorta. The left superior vein arises from the left upper lobe segmental veins. The lingular vein then joins it and it enters the posterosuperior left atrium. The left inferior vein drains the left lower lobe. It may enter the left atrium separately or join the left superior vein within the pericardium.

VASCULAR PEDICLE

The pedicle extends from the thoracic inlet to the top of the heart. Its boundaries are the right brachiocephalic vein and SVC, and the left subclavian artery. Its width is normally 38 to 58 mm, measured from the SVC-right main bronchus intersection to the left subclavian artery origin. A widened pedicle may reflect vascular enlargement or processes such as hemorrhage.

PULMONARY HILA

The hila may be defined as the areas that connect the mediastinum to the lungs, composed of pulmonary arteries and veins, bronchi, nodes, and connective tissue. The proximal left pulmonary artery is almost always higher than the right interlobar artery and never lower. In lateral radiography, the hila are superposed. The carina projects at thoracic vertebral body level T4-T5. The right upper lobe bronchus can be seen end-on in about half of patients; the left upper lobe bronchus is visible more caudally in 75%. The former is not as well-circumscribed by tissue as the latter; if it is clearly visible that suggests surrounding soft-tissue prominence, usually lymphadenopathy.

BRONCHIAL ARTERIES

The bronchial arteries are variable in number, with patients typically having 2 to 4 bronchial arteries. Commonly one right bronchial artery arises from the right third intercostal artery and two on the left arise from the anterolateral aorta at the thoracic level T5/T6. They may originate elsewhere along the aorta or from the subclavian, innominate, internal mammary, or coronary arteries. They anastomose with other mediastinal arteries, then encircle the main bronchi. The true bronchial arteries radiate from these rings, course along the bronchi, and branch with the airways. Two or three arteries are generally present along each bronchus, connecting with adventitial and submucosal plexuses.

BRONCHIAL VEINS

The trachea and large bronchi drain via bronchial veins to the azygous and hemiazygous systems. Most intrapulmonary bronchial drainage is via anastomoses into the pulmonary venous system.

LEFT SUBCLAVIAN ARTERY

This is located in the supra-aortic middle mediastinum. It courses superiorly touching the left mediastinal pleura, visible in PA radiographs as a concave edge extending from the arch to the medial clavicle. Aberrant right subclavian artery (approximately 0.5% prevalence) may be visible as an edge ascending from the aortic arch obliquely to the right. The proximal part of this artery is often dilated, called the diverticulum of Kommerell.

LEFT SUPERIOR INTERCOSTAL VEIN

The first left intercostal space drains via the supreme intercostal vein; the second to fourth intercostal veins drain via the left superior intercostal vein. In most patients, this drains into the accessory hemiazygous vein and then into the left brachiocephalic vein. It may be visible as the aortic nipple as it passes interiorly adjacent to the arch or at its paraspinal and retroaortic portions.

LEFT SUPERIOR VENA CAVA

The normal right-sided SVC develops from the right anterior cardinal vein. If the left anterior cardinal vein persists, it develops into a left-sided SVC, visible as a straight shadow along the left mediastinum overlying the arch and proximal descending aorta. It generally drains into the coronary sinus but may drain into the left atrium and cause a right-to-left shunt. If a left SVC is present, the right SVC is present in 85% of cases but is often smaller; it is absent in 15% of cases.

BUCKLED RIGHT BRACHIOCEPHALIC ARTERY

The right brachiocephalic artery is about 5 cm long and fixed at its origin and its division. The aorta lengthens with atherosclerosis and allows the artery to buckle. It is normally not contour forming but if it is enlarged by aneurysm or tortuous and buckled, it may become visible as a smooth opacity in the right superior paramediastinal area extending upward from the arch.

AZYGOUS VEIN

The azygous vein originates at the level of the renal veins as continuation of the right subcostal vein or right ascending lumbar vein. It passes through the right side of the aortic hiatus, courses in front or to the right of T4 to T12, and at T8 or T9 the hemiazygous vein joins it. At T4 or T5, it enters the SVC. It drains the right superior and 5th through 11th intercostal veins, right subcostal vein, right bronchial veins, and superior and inferior hemiazygous veins. The superior part of the azygous vein has posterior, middle, and anterior component; the latter may be measured easily. The upper limit of normal diameter is 10 mm, except in pregnant patients, where it is at least 15 mm.

HEMIAZYGOUS VEINS

The superior hemiazygous vein is the continuation of the left fourth posterior intercostal vein and often connects to the left superior intercostal vein. It courses downward along the spine to T8-T9 then crosses retroaortic to the azygous vein. The inferior hemiazygous vein originates from the left renal vein or as a continuation of the left subcostal or ascending lumbar veins and enters the chest via the aortic hiatus behind the descending aorta; at T8 or T9, it crosses to the azygous vein.

NONVASCULAR MEDIASTINUM

THORACIC INLET

This parallels the first rib and is higher anteriorly than posteriorly. Therefore, an opacity effaced superiorly and situated at or below the clavicles must be anterior, and an opacity projecting above the clavicles is retrotracheal, the cervicothoracic sign.

THYMUS

The thymus is derived from the third pharyngeal pouches and resides in the anterosuperior mediastinum. In adults, it extends from above the manubrium to the fourth costal cartilage. It contacts the trachea, aortic arch and branches, and the ascending aortic and main-pulmonary-arterial pericardium. Most are bilobed with lobules of cortical and medullary cells. The thymus may decrease with physical stress or corticosteroid administration, then return to normal or larger size afterward, in a process called rebound. It is radiographically apparent only in infants and young children; it reaches maximum weight at 12 to 19 years of age, but is inapparent after 2 to 3 years because the body grows faster. The sail sign (only present in 5% of infants) is the right- or left-projecting triangular opacity of thymic tissue as seen on a chest radiograph. In CT, the thymus is visible in 100% of patients younger than 30 years and 17% of patients older than 49 years. Only 30% are visually bilobed, and the left lobe is generally larger than the right. In patients younger than 19 years, the thymus is as dense as or denser than muscle; in most patients older than 40 years, it approaches fat density as it regresses.

RADIOGRAPHIC LINES AND SPACES

The intermediate stem line is a vertically oriented linear opacity up to 3 mm wide because of the posterior wall of the right main and intermediate bronchi. The left retrobronchial line is formed by the left main and proximal left lower-lobe bronchial posterior walls, 3 mm thick or less, shorter, and more posterior than the intermediate stem line.

The anteromedial pleurae of both lungs contact the mediastinum in the retrosternal space, at the anterior junction line. It is composed of four pleural layers and any intervening fat, generally 1 to 3 mm thick, and in PA radiographs courses from upper right to lower left behind the sternum. The right and left superior recesses are formed by the contact of lung with retromanubrial mediastinum, forming a V-shaped anterior mediastinal triangle. Shift of the superior recesses indicates atelectasis. The anteromedial surfaces of the lungs are separated by the heart and mediastinal fat. The lung surfaces contacting this fat form the inverted-V-shaped inferior recesses.

The retrosternal stripe is formed when any mediastinal fat forms a vertical retrosternal opacity abutting the bone. The average thickness is about 3 mm, maximally 7 mm. The lung contacts the upper two-thirds of the anterior chest wall, either to the right or to the left of midline, and this contact forms the parasternal stripe. This is typically lobulated by the ribs, but can be further lobulated because of internal thoracic lymphadenopathy.

The cardiac apex and epicardial fat exclude lung from the left anteroinferior chest; this area is the cardiac incisura. Its interface with the left lung may be straight, round, or angular. The right side may have a similar process.

The aortopulmonary (AP) window is a space between the aortic arch and the left pulmonary artery, normally fat filled. The medial boundary is the ligamentum arteriosum and the lateral boundary is the left pleural surface. The aortopulmonary window interface is normally concave or straight; a convex aortopulmonary window interface suggests abnormality such as lymphadenopathy or sometimes lipomatosis. The aortopulmonary line is visible in 60% of patients as a continuous opacity with a sharp left border, extending from the arch to the left main bronchus, usually as an extension of the left heart border superiorly. If this line becomes displaced laterally, mediastinal pathology is suggested.

The two posterior pleural reflections (paraspinal lines) are about 1 mm wide, visible in thoracic spine radiographs and some chest radiographs. The left paraspinal line runs from the top or middle of the arch to T9 to T12, depending on inflation. If mediastinal fat is prominent, it may course over the arch to the apex and the subclavian artery. It is commonly parallel to the spine, anywhere medial to the lung–aorta interface. The right paraspinal line is visible less frequently, usually extending only a few vertebral levels near T8 to T12 within a few mm of the spine.

The preaortic recess is formed when the left lower lobe intrudes anterior to the descending aorta and medial to the esophagus. It is anatomically similar to the right-sided azygoesophageal recess but is usually much narrower, and may extend from the arch to the hemidiaphragm.

Contact of the supra-azygous right lung with the right lateral tracheal wall forms the right paratracheal stripe. It normally contains the pleural surface, the tracheal wall, and mediastinal fat, and should be no thicker than 4 mm. The sensitivity of paratracheal stripe widening for detection of lymphadenopathy is 30%. A left paratracheal stripe is uncommon.

The posterior tracheal stripe is formed by the posterior wall of the trachea as it abuts the right upper lobe. This can be visible along the entire length of visible trachea in a good lateral projection. It should not be over 5 mm; the most common abnormality to cause tracheoesophageal stripe thickening is esophageal cancer.

The lung apices contact the retroesophageal mediastinum anterior to T1 and T2, forming the posterior mediastinal triangle bordered by the left and right superior recesses. Anterior to T3 to T5 the lungs abut each other, and the pleural stripe thus formed is the posterior junction line. It generally projects through the trachea, and is generally straight or left convex. The inferior recesses are formed when the lungs are displaced laterally from midline by the superior intercostal veins, the azygous arch, and the aortic arch. The right inferior recess is generally larger than the left because the aortic arch is higher than the azygous arch.

The right superior esophageal stripe is formed by the right side of gas-filled superior esophagus and right upper lobe pleura. It courses obliquely from upper right to lower left, inwardly convex. The left superior esophageal stripe is formed by the left wall of gas-filled esophagus and left upper lobe pleura. It generally is parallel to the contralateral stripe though they may diverge at their ends.

The azygoesophageal recess is formed by the contact of the right lower lobe with esophagus and ascending azygous vein. It is often visible in PA radiographs as an interface extending from the diaphragm to the level of the azygous arch. Focal convexity to the right should suggest a space-occupying process, though this is not sensitive (approximately 23%). If the esophagus is gas filled, the right and (sometimes) left inferior esophagopleural stripes may be visible.

HEART

The heart shadow is essentially midline in thin people, only slightly to the left; in larger patients, it extends more to the left. The right heart border projects over the spine commonly in pectus excavatum deformity. Normal transverse heart diameter is 11.5 to 15.5 cm. On PA radiographs, a cardiothoracic ratio of 50% is typically considered upper limit of normal, but at least 10% of normal patients have ratios greater than 50%. Heart size typically changes less than 1.0 cm from diastole to systole. Lower diaphragm is associated with narrower heart shadow; elevated intrathoracic pressure decreases heart size and pulmonary vascularity; and recumbent positioning makes the heart shadow broader. Cardiophrenic recess fat pads are common. They produce obtuse angles with the diaphragm at the inferior mediastinum. Occasionally, the denser heart may be visible through them.

DIAPHRAGM

DEVELOPMENT

The diaphragm is embryologically derived from four structures: the central tendon is derived from the septum transversarium, small midlateral components are derived from pleuroperitoneal membranes, the esophageal mesentery and diaphragmatic crura are derived from body-wall mesenchyme, and the majority of the muscular diaphragm is derived from a peripheral body-wall mesenchyme.

ANATOMY

The central tendon is a broad sheet of crossing fibers, overall shaped like a chevron pointing anteriorly. The costal muscular components attach to the xiphoid process and the 7th through 12th ribs. Its posterior attachment is from the lateral margins of the right first through third and left first and second lumbar vertebrae. This crural component only lowers the diaphragm without moving the ribcage.

The phrenic arteries arise from the caudal thoracic aorta or sometimes the renal arteries to supply the posterior upper diaphragmatic surface. The musculophrenic and pericardiacophrenic arteries, distinct branches from the internal thoracic arteries, supply the anterior portion via extensive arcades and anastomoses with the intercostal arteries perfusing the peripheral portion of the diaphragm. Extensive lymphatic vessels drain to the mediastinum. Pores in the peritoneal mesothelial surface of the diaphragm allow abdominal fluid, particles, or cells to enter the pleural and mediastinal spaces directly. The phrenic nerve is the motor innervation. It has contributions from the C3, C4, and C5 spinal levels, mostly C4.

THORACIC LYMPHATIC SYSTEM

PLEURAL DRAINAGE

The pleural and pulmonary lymphatic systems are largely separate but are connected by small anastomoses. Lymphatic valves are oriented toward the pleural surface. Parietal pleural lymphatic drainage is extensive on the costal and diaphragmatic surfaces. The mediastinal pleural vessels follow the blood vessels. Visceral pleural lymphatic channels lie within the vascular layer. They are more numerous inferiorly, and form a network similar to pleural lobular boundaries, with many smaller tributaries over the pleural surface. Flow is to hilar lymph nodes.

PULMONARY PARENCHYMAL DRAINAGE

Two major pathways exist for pulmonary lymphatic drainage. Peribronchovascular lymphatic channels begin at the distal respiratory bronchioles, and drain along the bronchovascular tree to the hilum. Channels in the interlobular septa also drain eventually to the hilum. Small anastomotic channels connect the two; distension of these channels creates the Kerley A lines.

THORACIC DUCT

The right and left lumbar lymphatic trunks merge anterior to T12 to L2, forming the cisterna chyli, which continues cranially as the thoracic duct. It courses through the aortic hiatus, usually to the right of the aorta. More superiorly it crosses leftward to course posterolateral to the trachea. It continues between the esophagus and the left subclavian artery; it most commonly joins the left internal jugular vein. In most people, the thoracic duct has valves. Diameter may be up to 7 mm.

THORACIC LYMPH NODES

Parietal Nodes

The parietal nodes comprise three groups: the anterior and posterior parietal nodes and the diaphragmatic nodes. The internal mammary nodes are the anterior parietal nodes, behind the anterior intercostal spaces, draining the upper anterior abdominal wall, anterior chest wall, anterior diaphragm, and medial breast tissue. They communicate with anterior mediastinal and cervical nodes. The posterior parietal nodes are the posterior intercostal nodes and juxtavertebral nodes, draining the intercostal spaces, parietal pleura, and spine. They communicate with posterior mediastinal nodes and drain to the thoracic duct superiorly and the cisterna chyli inferiorly. The diaphragmatic nodes drain the diaphragm and anterosuperior liver: the prepericardiac group is immediately behind the xiphoid lateral to the pericardium; the juxtaphrenic group is near the phrenic nerves; and the retrocrural nodes lie behind the left and right crura.

Visceral Nodes

The visceral nodes comprise three groups: the prevascular, posterior mediastinal, and tracheobronchial groups. The anterosuperior mediastinal (prevascular) nodes are along the anterior SVC, innominate veins, and ascending aorta. They drain most of the anterior mediastinum, and drain into the thoracic or right lymphatic duct. The posterior mediastinal nodes are periesophageal and periaortic; they drain the posterior diaphragm, pericardium, the esophagus, and the lower lobes and communicate with the tracheobronchial nodes.

The tracheobronchial nodes are the most important group of visceral nodes and have several subgroups. Paratracheal nodes are anterior to and alongside the trachea. The lowermost right-sided member is the azygous node, medial to the azygous vein. These drain bronchopulmonary and tracheal–bifurcation nodes, the trachea, and the esophagus. Carinal nodes are in the precarinal and subcarinal fat, and surrounding the main bronchi; AP window nodes are a subgroup in the mediastinal fat between the left pulmonary artery and aortic arch. Carinal nodes drain the bronchopulmonary nodes, anterior and posterior mediastinal nodes, heart, pericardium, esophagus, and lungs, and drain to the paratracheal group. Bronchopulmonary or hilar nodes are located around the main bronchi and vessels and receive drainage from all lobes of the lungs. They drain to carinal and paratracheal nodes.

Suggested Reading

Cole TJ, Henry DA, Jolles H, et al. Normal and abnormal vascular structures that simulate neoplasms on chest radiographs: clues to the diagnosis. *Radiographics*. 1995;15(4):867-891.

Franquet T, Erasmus JJ, Gimenez A, et al. The retrotracheal space: normal anatomic and pathologic appearances. *Radiographics*. 2002;22(spec no):S231-S246.

Gibbs JM, Chandrasekhar CA, Ferguson EC, et al. Lines and stripes: where did they go? –From conventional radiography to CT. *Radiographics*. 2007;27(1):33-48.

Gurney JW. Cross-sectional physiology of the lung. *Radiology*. 1991;178:1-10.

Hayashi K, Aziz A, Ashizawa K, et al. Radiographic and CT appearances of the major fissures. *Radiographics*. 2001;21(4): 861-874.

Lawler LP, Corl FM, Fishman EK. Multi-detector row and volume-rendered CT of the normal and accessory flow pathways of the thoracic systemic and pulmonary veins. *Radiographics*. 2002; 22(spec no):S45-S60.

Ravin CE, Chotas HG. Chest radiography. *Radiology*. 1997;204: 593-600.

Webb RW. Thin-section CT of the secondary pulmonary lobule: anatomy and the image-the 2004 fleischner lecture. *Radiology*. 2006;239:322-338.

Woodard PK. Pulmonary arteries must be seen before they can be assessed. *Radiology*. 1997;204:11-12

QUESTIONS AND ANSWERS

1. By what gestational week is alveolar tissue always present?
   A. 30
   B. 34
   C. 36
   D. 38

   ANSWER: C. By 36 weeks of gestation, aleveolar tissue is present. It can appear as early as 30 weeks.

2. Regarding the trachea, which of the following is *true*?
   A. Normal intrathoracic trachea changes dimensions with changes in pleural pressure.
   B. Normal trachea is generally halfway between the sternum and the spine.
   C. Normal trachea has smooth wall contours.
   D. Normal trachea is seldom greater than 15 mm wide.

   ANSWER: B. The normal intrathoracic trachea does not change dimensions with pleural pressure. It is generally halfway between the sternum and the spine, but is variable. It has corrugated contour because of cartilage rings and is at most 25 mm × 27 mm in men and 21 mm × 23 mm in women.

3. In bronchopulmonary anatomy, which of the following characterizes the right upper lobe?
   A. Its bronchus arises from the bronchus intermedius.
   B. It has apicoposterior and anterior segments.
   C. Its blood supply is generally via the truncus anterioris.
   D. It is the site of the superior accessory fissure.

   ANSWER: C. The right upper lobe bronchus arises from the right main bronchus. It has apical, posterior, and anterior segments. Its blood supply is generally via the truncus anterioris. It is the site of the azygous fissure; the superior accessory fissure separates the lower lobe superior segment from the basal segments.

4. What is the smallest lung unit identifiable on HRCT?
   A. Primary lobule
   B. Secondary lobule
   C. Acinus
   D. Canals of Lambert

   ANSWER: B. Normal secondary lobules are seen with HRCT. They can only be seen with conventional radiography if there is septal thickening.

5. Regarding the relationship of pericardium to the pulmonary vessels, which of the following is *true*?
   A. Main pulmonary bifurcation is within the pericardium.
   B. Middle lobe vein generally joins the inferior pulmonary vein within the pericardium.

C. Left inferior vein often joins the superior vein outside the pericardium.
D. Right interlobar artery is intrapericardial.

ANSWER: A. The main pulmonary artery bifurcation is within the pericardium. The middle lobe vein generally flows into the base of the superior vein, but may enter separately. The left inferior vein and superior vein may enter the atrium separately, or merge within the pericardium to enter as a single vessel. The right interlobar artery is not intrapericardial.

6. Regarding lateral radiography, at what level does the carina project?
   A. T2-T3
   B. T4-T5
   C. T6-T7
   D. T8-T9

ANSWER: B. The carina projects around T4-T5. The left upper lobe is almost never more cranial than the right upper lobe bronchus and is inferior in 75% of cases. The left upper lobe bronchus is not as well-circumscribed by vessels as is the right upper lobe bronchus, so a clearly defined left upper lobe bronchus suggests a soft-tissue mass is abutting that airway. The intermediate stem line is formed by the posterior wall of the right main and intermediate bronchi.

7. What comprises the anterior junction line?
   A. Thymus and ribcage
   B. Anteromedial pleurae of both lungs
   C. Pericardium and the pulmonary ligament
   D. Visceral pleura

ANSWER:B. The anterior junction line is formed by the contact of the anteromedial pleural surfaces with each other, in the retrosternal space. The superior recess often shifts to the side of atelectasis as the other lung overinflates to compensate. The inferior recess is formed by the anteromedial surfaces of the lungs below the anterior junction line.

8. A blue dye in injected into the left posterolateral third intercostal vein. What is its most likely course?
   A. Left supreme intercostal vein, to azygous vein, to left brachiocephalic vein
   B. Left superior intercostal vein, to azygous vein, to left brachiocephalic vein
   C. Left supreme intercostal vein, to accessory hemiazygous, to left brachiocephalic vein
   D. Left superior intercostal vein, to accessory hemiazygous vein, to left brachiocephalic vein

ANSWER: D. The supreme intercostal vein generally drains the left first intercostal space; the 2nd-4th intercostal veins drain via the superior intercostal vein. The accessory hemiazygous vein drains both of these to the left brachiocephalic vein. The azygous vein drains the 5th-11th right intercostal veins and several other veins.

9. Regarding the diaphragm, which of the following is *true*?
   A. It is embryologically derived from four different structures.
   B. The septum transversarium forms the lateral muscle components.
   C. The diaphragm is not very well supplied with lymphatic drainage.
   D. The arterial supply is derived from two different arterial systems.

ANSWER: A. The diaphragm is derived from septum transversarium, pleuroperitoneal membranes, and two different body wall mesenchymes. The diaphragm is well-drained and even has pores allowing peritoneal fluid to enter the chest. The arterial supply is via the phrenic, intercostal, and internal thoracic arteries.

10. Which of the following nodal chains drains the esophagus?
    A. Internal mammary
    B. Prepericardiac
    C. Posterior mediastinal
    D. Juxtaphrenic

ANSWER: C. The internal mammary nodes are anterior parietal nodes and drain the upper anterior abdominal wall, the anterior chest wall, the anterior diaphragm, and medial breast tissue. The prepericardiac nodes drain the diaphragm and anterosuperior liver. The posterior mediastinal nodes drain the posterior diaphragm, pericardium, esophagus, and pulmonary ligaments. The juxtaphrenic group also drains the diaphragm and anterosuperior liver.

17 THORACIC IMAGING

John C. Texada and Satinder P. Singh

RADIOGRAPHIC INVESTIGATION

CONVENTIONAL RADIOGRAPHY

Conventional radiography is the cornerstone of chest diagnosis and should be the first step in establishing the presence of disease, with other modalities used to complement the radiograph.

PROJECTIONS

Posteroanterior (PA) and lateral projections are included in the most satisfactory routine examination. The patient should be standing.

Anteroposterior (AP) projection may be used if the patient cannot stand erect. It may be obtained seated or supine.

Lordotic projection can be either AP or PA. In lordotic AP projection, the patient may stand erect, and the x-ray tube is angulated 15-degrees cephalad; this is more reproducible than having the patient assume the lordotic position directly. This projection is helpful to improve the visibility of the apices, superior mediastinum, and thoracic inlet; to locate a lesion via parallax; and to identify the right minor fissure in patients who may have right middle lobe atelectasis.

Lateral decubitus projection requires the patient to lie on one side, and the beam is horizontal. The dependent hemithorax is generally the one being evaluated, so a radiolucent foam cushion or mattress should be placed under the patient's side. This projection is helpful for identification of small pleural effusions: a volume less than 100 mL may be visible in a lateral decubitus projection, whereas erect images may need a volume of 300 mL before visualization. It is also useful to demonstrate a change in an air-fluid level or determine whether part of the cavity is actually freely moving (such as a mycetoma).

Oblique projections are sometimes helpful to locate subtle nondisplaced rib fractures.

BASIC TECHNIQUES

The diagnostic accuracy of chest radiographs is partly dependent on the technical quality and reproducibility of the radiographs. Some basics like patient position are consistent across all radiographic systems (conventional, computed, or digital radiography), but others refer only to conventional imaging.

Patient positioning requires the patient to be centered and not rotated, and the scapulae rotated forward enough that they do not project over the lungs. On properly centered radiographs, the medial ends of the clavicles project equidistant from the margins of the vertebral column.

Patient respiration should be at total lung capacity and fully suspended.

Film exposure should allow faint visualization of the thoracic spine and the intervertebral discs in the PA projection and of the retrocardiac lung parenchyma. Exposure should be as short as possible so that motion is limited. Mild overexposure can be overcome with bright illumination but the decreased visibility in underexposed images cannot be compensated. PA chest radiograph skin radiation should not exceed 0.3 mGy and exposure time should not exceed 40 msec. The focal-film (source–image) distance should be at least 180 cm to minimize the effects of magnification.

Kilovoltage (kV) should be high enough to produce high-quality images. The linear–attenuation coefficients of bone and soft tissues are closer to one another at higher kV ranges, so that both bony and soft-tissue structures are both visible, and the opacity of the mediastinum is reduced so that the retrocardiac tissues and mediastinal reflections are visible. Pulmonary vessels and pulmonary nodules are more clearly visible than with low-kVp images. A range of 115 to 150 kVp is suggested for PA and lateral chest radiography.

Grids and filters help to improve image quality and/or reduce unnecessary radiation. The ACR recommends an aluminum 10:1 grid with 103 lines per inch. An air gap of 15 cm between the patient and the film reduces scatter and makes a grid unnecessary; however, a source–image distance of 10 ft should be used for this technique. A tunnel-wedge filter allows adequate exposure of the mediastinum and lung. A wedge filter equalizes the densities of the thin apical regions and the thicker basal regions and helps increase mediastinal exposure. It is constructed of copper foil to a maximum of about 0.3 mm, which also helps to reduce patient radiation exposure by about 30%. If the patient is not perfectly centered, filters may produce artifacts of attenuation.

SPECIAL TECHNIQUES

Inspiratory–expiratory radiography includes images obtained at total lung capacity and residual volume is indicated for evaluation of air trapping, whether focal or diffuse, and for suspected pneumothorax when the visceral–pleural line is not visible or when findings are equivocal.

Valsalva and Müller maneuvers forced expiration or inspiration, respectively against the closed glottis may help to determine whether a nodule is vascular or solid. The lung volumes must be about the same for the technique to be useful, usually around end of quiet inspiration. A change in size is consistent with a vessel; the absence of change does not change the differential considerations.

Bedside radiography is typically AP in positioning. It is inferior to standard radiography for many reasons, some of them uncontrollable. The patient is frequently supine; there is a short source–image distance; and many patients are unable to hold their breath or inspire to total lung capacity. In semierect or supine images, the source–image distance is often 100 to 125 cm and kVp is 80 to 100. A 6:1 or 8:1 grid significantly improves image quality but it is time consuming to properly position the grid to avoid artifact and most hospitals do not use them.

Because the patient is supine and the source–object distance is smaller, the mediastinum and heart are magnified as much as 15% to 20%, compared to the 5% magnification of PA radiographs. Similarly, technique differences alter interpretation of vascular prominence. Supine position increases pulmonary blood volume by 30%, and the normal dependence-gradient is shifted from craniocaudal to anteroposterior. Blood vessels, particularly the ones at the upper lobes, appear larger.

One study of bedside radiographs in intensive care unit patients over 2 months revealed that 65% of studies, even daily routine studies, resulted in new findings or changes affecting patient management, and 40% to 45% had at least one clinically unsuspected finding. However, unsuspected abnormalities leading to management change were present in 57% of pulmonary and unstable cardiac patients but only 3% of uncomplicated cardiac and miscellaneous groups.

DIGITAL RADIOGRAPHY

Digital radiography has several advantages over conventional screen-film systems. The exposure latitude is 10 to 100 times greater than the dynamic range of screen-film systems. The final image is almost independent on exposure levels (this may result in increased radiation dose if not monitored) and can be acquired in a much wider range of conditions. Electronic images are more easily portable and more easily manipulated. Two types are available: photostimulable storage phosphor and selenium-coated receptors.

Photostimulable Storage Phosphor Systems

These systems are known as computed radiography. The phosphor system replaces the film cassette. It has a wide dynamic range of about 1:10 000 versus 1:100 for standard films, so bedside repeat studies due to poor penetration are decreased. The phosphor retains incident x-ray energy until it is "read" by a laser and converted to visible or infrared light. This luminescence is then recorded digitally. The overall image quality of photostimulable storage phosphor (PSP) radiographs is slightly less than that of film radiographs, and the decreased quantum efficiency of the phosphor technology requires equal or greater radiation dose for the same image.

Selenium Detector Systems

These systems are known as digital radiography. The detector may be a selenium drum or a flat-plate selenium detector. The selenium detectors have greater quantum efficiency than film screen does, and the smooth selenium detector decreases intrinsic noise.

INDICATIONS FOR CHEST RADIOGRAPHY

The 1997 ACR standards for accepted medical indications (not necessarily billable but medically warranted) for chest radiography include the following: signs and symptoms related to the respiratory and cardiovascular symptoms; follow-up of previously diagnosed thoracic disease for the evaluation of improvement, resolution, or progression; staging of intrathoracic and extrathoracic tumors; preoperative assessment of patient scheduled for intrathoracic surgery; preoperative evaluation of patients with cardiac or respiratory symptoms or patients with a significant potential for thoracic pathology that may compromise the search for the result or lead to increased perioperative morbidity and mortality; and monitoring of patients with life-support devices and patients who have undergone cardiac or thoracic surgery or other interventional procedures.

INAPPROPRIATE

Cost-effectiveness analyses have determined that routine screening radiographs, obtained to satisfy admission requirements or before surgery, without medical indication or risk factor, are not cost-effective in patients younger than 20 years of age. Even in a high-risk VA population, though 36% of routine admission chest radiographs revealed abnormalities, only 4% of these changed patient management.

The 1997 ACR standards state that routine screening is not indicated in the following groups: routine screening of unselected populations, routine prenatal chest radiographs for the detection of unsuspected disease, routine radiographs solely because of hospital admission, mandated radiographs for employment, and repeated radiograph examinations on long-term facility admission.

CONVENTIONAL TOMOGRAPHY

Conventional tomography allows visualization of a particular selected depth and exclusion of structures superficial and deep to it. The x-ray tube and the film or detector moves reciprocally, causing blurring of all the structures not continuously in focus. The thin slice depth is determined by the ratio of the source–object and object–image distance. At most sites, conventional tomography has been replaced by CT.

CT

CT scanning allows planar imaging through the object of interest. The detailed mechanics and physics of CT scanning are beyond the scope of this review.

Technical Parameters

Although scanner geometry and physical requirements produce some unalterable parameters, several parameters that affect image quality are operator-dependent. Detector thickness, image slice thickness, spacing, field of view, reconstruction algorithm, and window-level settings are selectable, as are pitch, tube current, and voltage potential.

Image Thickness

The thicker the detector and/or the image slice, the more parenchyma is summed into a single image. High-resolution CT (HRCT) for evaluation of interstitial lung disease therefore uses very small detector thickness and reconstruction as low as 1 mm. Images obtained at 10-mm intervals exclude most of the lung parenchyma but allow accurate characterization of diffuse interstitial processes; with the advent of high-number multidetector row CT scanning, the entire chest may be scanned at submillimeter detector width and reconstructions obtained at 1- and 5-mm thicknesses.

Field of View

The field of view should be large enough to include the whole patient and the matrix size should be as large as possible. Using a 40-cm field of view with a 512 × 512 matrix results in a voxel size of 0.78 mm; a 25-cm FOV has voxel size of 0.49 mm.

Reconstruction Algorithm

Soft-tissue reconstruction algorithm smoothes the image and reduces image noise, but a high-spatial-frequency algorithm is required for assessment of the parenchyma; the technique sacrifices higher noise for better detection of interstitial abnormalities. The combination of a high-spatial-frequency reconstruction algorithm with thin detector width constitutes the HRCT protocol.

Window-Width and Window-Level Settings

Air has a defined HU of −1000, and water has a range of –20 to +20 HU. Lung evaluation is best at a window level of –600 to –700 HU and a window width of 1000 to 1500 HU. Window levels of 30 to 50 HU and widths of 350 to 500 HU provide good assessment of the mediastinum, hila, and pleura.

Radiation Dose

The average natural radiation exposure to a person in North America is around 3 mSv. The effective dose of a PA and lateral chest radiograph evaluation are 0.15 mSv. The effective dose of a chest CT is on the order of 8 mSv.

Technologies are variously in development, in testing, or in practice to limit radiation exposure. Rapidly varying the tube current with linear attenuation allows decreased current when the scanner is oriented more AP, because in most patients the AP dimension of the chest is less than the transverse dimension; similarly current can decrease when the radiation is penetrating mostly low-attenuation lung versus the denser mediastinum. Conventional CT is usually performed at 200 to 400 mAs, but depending on the indication image quality may be acceptable with time–current levels as low as 20 to 40 mAs. The images have increased noise but this may not necessarily reduce diagnostic quality (e.g., evaluation of metastatic lung nodules). Cardiac gating, either prospective or retrospective, significantly decreases radiation exposure without sacrificing image quality in selected studies.

Common Indications for Chest CT

Evaluation of Suspected Mediastinal Abnormalities Identified on Chest Radiograph

CT can differentiate solid from cystic, localizes masses, and can determine the tissue-type and enhancement characteristics of a lesion. CT can distinguish variable vascular anatomy from mediastinal mass.

Search for occult thymic lesions: Thymoma or thymic hyperplasia in patients with myasthenia gravis may be inapparent.

Determination of the Presence and Extent of Neoplastic Disease

Occult lung metastasis can be detected before surgery in cancers with high propensity for metastasis or when chest radiograph reveals a solitary nodule. Primary neoplasms can be detected with greater sensitivity in patients with positive sputum cytology and negative bronchoscopy. Mediastinal, pleural, osseous, muscular, and subcutaneous involvement can be detected and spinal invasion characterized.

Search for diffuse or central calcification in a pulmonary nodule: The calcification pattern in a pulmonary nodule can suggest benignity, malignancy, or indeterminance.

Diagnosis of Bronchiectasis

CT allows greater anatomic visualization of the type, course, and distribution of bronchiectasis as well as any associated abnormalities including intraluminal lesion, fibrotic parenchyma, or others.

Detection of Parenchymal Lung Disease

Patients with symptoms or pulmonary function abnormalities suggesting lung disease but normal or equivocal chest radiographic findings can be assessed with CT.

Differential Diagnosis of Diffuse Lung Disease

HRCT can assess patients whose clinical radiographic findings do not provide a confident etiologic diagnosis and in whom further radiographic evaluation is warranted. This includes chronic interstitial and airspace disease and immunocompromised patients with acute parenchymal abnormalities.

Evaluation of Acute or Chronic Cardiovascular Abnormality

CT can accurately evaluate the presence or absence of pulmonary embolism, aortic dissection or aneurysm, and in some institutions coronary–arterial disease, as well as stricture, abnormal course, malformation, or other characteristics. In some institutions, CT can serve as an adjunct to sonography or catheter angiography for evaluation of congenital or acquired heart disease.

Many Other Potential Indications Exist

Others include guidance of percutaneous biopsy; localization of loculated collections after radiographic or ultrasonic techniques prove inadequate.

MAGNETIC RESONANCE IMAGING

PHYSICAL PRINCIPLES

In quantum physical terms, an atomic nucleus has a net "spin" when it contains an unpaired proton or neutron. The spin has a magnetic moment, so when the nucleus is exposed to a magnetic field, it experiences a small torque. Its axis of spin will align with the field direction, and it will rotate at a particular resonant frequency determined by the field strength and the gyromagnetic ratio for that atom. If a pulse of radiofrequency (RF) energy is at exactly the same frequency as the resonant frequency (known as the Larmor frequency), an interaction will occur. The RF pulse changes the nucleus from an equilibrium state to an excited state that will naturally decay back to the equilibrium state with time. As the nucleus relaxes back to equilibrium, it radiates at the Larmor frequency, the energy it acquired during excitation. This energy can be detected with receiver coils. The nucleus currently used most frequently is that of hydrogen: a single proton.

RELAXATION TIMES

T1 Relaxation

T1 is the time constant corresponding to restoration of magnetization parallel to the external field, also known as spin-lattice or longitudinal relaxation time. In a pure liquid, the recovery is exponential: after three T1 periods 95% of the nuclei will have returned to equilibrium. T1 relaxation time is generally long for fluids and some proteins and shorter in fat.

T2 Relaxation

T2 is the time constant corresponding to decay of magnetization perpendicular to the external field, also known as the spin–spin relaxation time. Subtle focal field–strength variations cause the nuclei to spin at slightly different rates and become dephased, eventually with a net signal strength of zero. Nuclei are rephased for measurement. As variability of local magnetic field strength is the determinant of dephasing, T2 times are typically long for homogeneous environments like fluid, and shorter for complex tissues.

BASIC PULSE SEQUENCES

Saturation Recovery

This sequence is composed of two 90-degree pulses separated by a short time TR, shorter than T1 but longer than T2. The T1 signal is dependent on the extent of parallel relaxation that has occurred over the time TR.

Inversion Recovery

This sequence uses a 180-degree pulse to invert the net magnetization, after which the nucleus reverts to equilibrium at a rate determined by its T1 constant. The residual net magnetization can be measured after the magnetization is deflected and made coherent by a 90-degree pulse. The amplitude of the signal depends on the inversion time interval (between the 180- and 90-degree pulses) and the nucleus's T1 constant.

Spin Echo

These sequences use a 90-degree pulse to rotate the net magnetization into a plane perpendicular to the external field. The nuclei are initially phase-coherent, but begin to dephase because of local field inhomogeneities. At time TE/2, a 180-degree pulse refocuses the nuclei and generates an echo at time TE. This is used to determine T2 without contamination from field inhomogeneity effects.

T1 weighting—In spin-echo sequences, the 90-degree pulses are separated by time TR. Short repetition times allow distinction of tissues with different T1 constants, called T1-weighted sequences. A TR for a T1-weighted sequence in a 1.5 T magnet may be 600 to 1000 msec.

T2 weighting—The signal decays at a rate dependent on T2 relaxation time. To distinguish tissues with different T2 characteristics a long TE typically over 80 msec is used and to maximize T2 effects and minimize the effects of T1 relaxation, T2-weighted images have long TR intervals, perhaps 2000 to 3000 msec.

Proton density weighting—Often a double-echo sequence is obtained, in which a long TR is used with both a short TE (20 msec or less) and a long TE (80 msec or more). The short TE signal is proton density, dependent primarily on relative water content. This has the best signal-to-noise ratio but limited contrast resolution.

Other pulse sequences allow visualization of flowing blood, three-dimensional imaging, and a variety of techniques to remove signal from fat, water, or silicon. In addition, fast or turbo sequences make use of multiple echo trains per TR to increase the filling of K-space and decrease dramatically the time required per image.

ADVANTAGES OF MRI

There is no ionizing radiation. The magnetic fields may be aligned in any direction, allowing imaging along any axis (though with the advent of isovolumetric CT this advantage is reduced). Flowing blood in vessels has intrinsic contrast. Soft-tissue contrast is greatly increased.

DISADVANTAGES OF MRI FOR CHEST IMAGING

Respiratory and cardiac motion can degrade images, though with respiratory triggering and cardiac gating this is reduced. Lung parenchyma has low signal-to-noise ratio because of low parenchymal proton density. Innumerable air–water interfaces produce susceptibility gradients in inflated lung, so signal is lost by the time conventional TE = 20-msec imaging. Ultrashort TE gradient-echo sequences and short-TE (7 msec or less) spin-echo sequences can increase the signal: noise ratio in aerated lung by a factor of 3.5.

INDICATIONS

Evaluation of the Heart and Great Vessels

MR has a well-established role in evaluating congenital cardiovascular anomalies and is superior to echocardiography in evaluation of adult congenital heart disease. It is usually reserved for patients with equivocal or no diagnostic echocardiography, though. It allows excellent evaluation of central pulmonary arteries, cardiac wall motion and blood flow, valvular stenosis or insufficiency, and enhancement characteristics. MR is not as good as CT in evaluating aortic aneurysm and dissection, particularly arch–vessel involvement, though if a patient cannot receive iodinated contrast material, a MR has much higher contrast resolution even without gadolinium than an unenhanced CT.

Evaluation of the Mediastinum and Hila

MR is a good secondary modality if CT evaluation is equivocal and is superior in evaluation of cancerous invasion of the mediastinum or vessels. It can help to diagnose bronchogenic cysts if the diagnosis is in doubt after CT.

Evaluation of the Chest Wall

Primary chest wall tumors and chest wall extension of lymphoma can be well evaluated, as can extension of lung cancer. MR also is a good modality for evaluation of neurogenic tumors and paraspinal lesions since it has good tissue-characterization ability and can evaluate the extent of intraforaminal spread.

Evaluation of the Lung Parenchyma

MR has limited role in parenchymal evaluation but can be helpful in evaluation of chronic interstitial and alveolar disease, determination of lung water content, distinguishing of postobstructive atelectasis from nonobstructive atelectasis, and evaluation of mass lesions within opacified hemithorax.

BRONCHOGRAPHY

Bronchography was once used to evaluate the presence and extent of bronchiectasis, but now that CT and HRCT provide excellent information the procedure has been largely abandoned. It carried the risk of allergy to the bronchographic medium, and temporarily impaired ventilation and diffusion. A variation, fiberoptic bronchography using isosmolar nonionic contrast material, may still be useful in evaluating patients with recurrent hemoptysis in whom CT is normal or equivocal.

CATHETER ANGIOGRAPHY

Many cases that were historically evaluated with angiography of one vascular territory or another now undergo CT angiographic evaluation. However, catheter angiography still has a role to play, as the resolution of CT angiography is far inferior to catheter angiography; in most cases temporal information (such as direction of flow) is not available, and of course no intervention can be performed with CT angiography as is possible with catheter-based procedures.

PULMONARY ANGIOGRAPHY

Technique

Pulmonary angiography can be performed via arm venous injection, via catheter injection into the venous system, right heart, or main pulmonary artery, or by selective right and left pulmonary artery or branch injection; the latter is the method of choice because vascular opacification is much better.

Complications

Complications include cardiac perforation, endocardial and myocardial injury, reversible cardiac or respiratory arrest, and cardiac arrhythmia. Incidence is low, less than 1%. Minor complications include treatable arrhythmia, vasovagal syncope, chest pain, and contrast reaction.

Indications

Indications classically included detection of pulmonary vascular congenital abnormalities or investigation of thromboembolic disease. As mentioned above, CT angiography has replaced many of these cases.

AORTOGRAPHY

Technique

Direct catheterization of the thoracic aorta percutaneously via either the femoral or the brachial artery is the method of choice. Venous injection followed by digital-subtraction angiography is possible but not often used.

Complications

Complications include aortic dissection, plaque embolization, and other catheter-related problems.

Indications

Indications classically included evaluation of mediastinal injury and evaluation of congenital vascular anomalies. CT and CT angiography have greatly reduced both of those.

BRONCHIAL AND INTERCOSTAL ARTERIOGRAPHY

Technique

Only selective catheterization, usually via femoral-arterial access, allows good opacification of the small vessels. The bronchial arteries arise from the posterolateral aortic wall at around T5 or T6 in 80% of patients, so the catheter is brought to this level and selective catheterization proceeds.

Complications

Complications include damage to the artery of Adamkiewicz, which commonly arises from the aorta around T8-T12, but in 5% of cases arises from the right intercostal-bronchial trunk. Such damage can lead to spinal cord ischemia and transverse myelitis.

Indications

Indications include evaluation of hemoptysis when radiographic and CT evaluation are negative or equivocal and for percutaneous embolization of life-threatening bronchial-artery bleeding.

RADIONUCLIDE IMAGING

VENTILATION–PERFUSION SCANNING

Perfusion imaging should detect over 90% of occlusive clots in vessels over 2-mm diameter. It is sensitive but not specific, as virtually all parenchymal lung disease can cause decreased pulmonary–arterial blood flow; however, PTE causes mismatched defects, whereas many other lung diseases cause matched defects.

Technique

The perfusion and ventilation studies require different radiotracers and techniques.

Perfusion images are acquired after Tc-99m labeled human albumin microspheres (HAM) or Tc-99m-labeled macroaggregated albumin (MAA) is infused via a systemic vein over 5 to 10 respiratory cycles with the patient supine. MAA particles are 90% within 10 to 90 μm, and HAM particles are 35 to 60 μm; these pass through the pulmonary arterial system until they lodge in precapillary arterioles in proportion to the blood flow to that region.

A 2- to 4-mCi radiopharmaceutical, approximately 200 000 to 500 000 particles, is injected, enough to block about 0.1% of a patient's precapillary arterioles. The number injected should be reduced in patients with pulmonary hypertension, patients with right-to-left intracardiac or intrapulmonary shunts, children, pregnant patients, and in patients with prior pneumonectomy or single-lung transplant, but the number should not be below 60 000 particles.

When performed to evaluate pulmonary perfusion at least six views should be obtained: anterior, posterior, right lateral, left lateral, and right- and left-posterior oblique.

Ventilation images may be acquired using Xe-133 inhalation, Kr-81m, Tc-99m aerosols, or other gaseous radiotracers.

Xe-133 imaging requires that the ventilation image is obtained first, because of the radionuclide's low-energy photons. A volume of 550 to 770 Mbq (15–20 mCi) is inhaled, then a posterior wash-in image is obtained. Subsequently equilibrium images are obtained while the patient recreates the gas over 4 minutes, followed by serial washout images. Regional air trapping is visible as residual activity during washout.

Xe-127 has higher energy than Tc-99m so ventilation imaging may follow perfusion imaging; this is good because if the perfusion study is normal the ventilation study need not be performed, and if the perfusion study is abnormal the patient can be positioned to highlight the region of the abnormality in the ventilation study. It is more expensive and requires medium-energy collimation.

Kr-81m has a physical half-life of 13 seconds so only washing or breath-hold images can be acquired; however, multiple projections can be obtained. It is expensive and produced from a Rb-81 generator, which itself has a useful half-life of only 1 day. Imaging is typically obtained after perfusion imaging.

Tc-99m *aerosols* (DTPA, sulfur colloid, pyrophosphate, ethylene diphosphate, or glucohcptanate) are 0.5 to 3 μm in size. Tc-99m DTPA has a short residence time in smokers so sulfur colloid or pyrophosphate may be more useful. 30 mCi of the tracer is given via nebulizer and the patient typically acquires 1 mCi in the lungs. Images are generally done before perfusion, and multiple projections can be acquired. These agents require little patient cooperation and can be given to intubated patients; the agents may deposit in the central airways in patients with airway obstruction and most of the dose remains in the nebulizer.

Tc-99m technegas and Tc-99m pertechnegas are produced by burning Tc-99m pertechnetate at high temperature in a carbon crucible, leading to 0.02 to 0.2 μm aerosolized particles. Pertechnegas is purged in 95% argon/ 5% oxygen, whereas technegas is purged in 100% argon. Both agents distribute homogeneously according to ventilation distribution with very little central deposition even in patients with COPD. At that point, pertechnegas can easily penetrate the alveolar membrane and biologic half-life is 6 to 10 minutes; conversely, technegas has little alveolar penetration or mucociliary clearance, and the effective half-life is essentially the same as the physical half-life, about 6 hours. These agents require little patient cooperation, and require only 2 to 3 breaths to get sufficient activity into the lungs. Imaging is obtained before perfusion imaging, and multiple projections can be obtained.

INDICATIONS

Indications classically included diagnosis and follow-up of acute PTE and prediction of pulmonary function after surgery. The former has largely been supplanted by CT angiography except in certain instances, but the latter remains important. An expected postoperative FEV-1 less than 0.8 L or 35% of predicted generally precludes lung resection.

GALLIUM-67 CITRATE LUNG SCANNING

PHYSICAL PROPERTIES

This radiopharmaceutical is the agent of choice for lung inflammation and infection. Gallium is a ferric analogue that rapidly binds to the acute-phase reactant transferrin; the exact mechanism of radiotracer accumulation at sites of inflammation is uncertain, however. Ga-67 has a physical half-life of 78 hours, and the optimum time to image is after 48 to 72 hours after administration. It is taken up by normal reticuloendothelial tissues, inflammatory processes, and, notably, lacrimal glands.

GRADING

The intensity and distribution of radiotracer can be used to quantify inflammation on a 5-point system (grades 0–4): less than soft-tissue activity, equal to soft-tissue activity, more than soft-tissue but less than liver, equal to liver, and greater than liver. Multiplying the grade of uptake by the area of lung involved yields the gallium index.

IMAGING FINDINGS

In general, Ga-67 citrate radiotracer avidity is a sensitive but nonspecific indicator of inflammatory activity. Gallium-67 scan may be "hot" in conditions ranging from pneumonia to ARDS to drug reactions (such as busulfan, cyclophosphamide, amiodarone, lymphangiography contrast); pneumoconiosis; interstitial pulmonary fibrosis (IPF); sarcoidosis, uremic pneumonitis and neoplasms including lymphoma, leukemia, mesothelioma, or metastatic cancer can be radiotracer avid as well.

In sarcoid, the study produces typical findings of bilateral hilar and right paratracheal lymphadenopathy (the lambda sign), but areas of lung involvement may also be avid. This correlates with response to therapy.

In IPF, gallium imaging does not predict activity, prognosis, or response to therapy and is not recommended.

In lymphoma, high-dose Ga-67 scanning can evaluate mediastinal disease, both in Hodgkin and in non-Hodgkin types.

In immunocompromised hosts, Ga-67 is more sensitive to inflammatory processes than chest radiography. In particular, parenchymal radiotracer activity in a patient with HIV and normal chest radiograph suggests *P. carinii* pneumonia; CMV or cryptococcal infection or lymphoma may produce similar findings. Regional radiotracer uptake may be because of PCP, lymphoma, or bacterial pneumonia. Focal activity combined with regional lymph node uptake is suggestive of *M. avium-intracellulare* or *M. tuberculosis* infection. Kaposi sarcoma is not Ga-67 avid but does take up Tl-201 chloride.

POSITRON EMISSION TOMOGRAPHY

Principles

PET imaging is based on the principles of matter–antimatter annihilation. Many tracers exist, but the most common is 18-fluoro-deoxyglucose. The tracer is taken up by cells in proportion to their metabolic activity and phosphorylated; the phosphorylated FDG-6-phosphate metabolite cannot be further metabolized and cannot exit the cell. The 18-F atom decays by positron emission, and the created positron travels a short distance (1–2 mm) before it comes to rest and annihilates an electron. This event releases two 511-keV photons at nearly 180 degrees from one another, which can be detected. Images can be reconstructed from this data. Resolution in dedicated PET scanners is about 3 mm at best. Many, if not most, PET scanners are part of combined PET-CT scanners, allowing high-resolution anatomic imaging localization of metabolic activity.

Indications

Characterization of solitary pulmonary nodule is often possible; FDG-PET is 80% to 100% sensitive and 50% to 97% specific for the distinction of malignant from benign. Active inflammation, such as sarcoid, tuberculosis, or aspergillosis, can present false-positive findings.

Mediastinal staging of non–small cell lung cancer is more accurate than CT in many instances.

Differentiation of scar and recurrent tumor in patients with prior lung cancer is possible based on metabolic imaging: the sensitivity and specificity of FDG-PET for detecting tumor versus scarring are 97% and 100%, respectively.

Other indications including staging and/or restaging of multiple neoplasms that metastasize to the chest are also possible, and metabolic imaging remains an area of active inquiry.

ULTRASOUND OF THE CHEST

Principles

Ultrasonography produces images based on the transmission of high-frequency sound beams through tissue and evaluation of reflection at impedance changes. Sonography is portable, does not use ionizing radiation, and frequently provides useful information. It is most useful in evaluation of congenital and acquired heart disease, particularly valve morphology, chamber volume, wall thickness, and ejection fraction. Pericardial effusion may be easily evaluated. Transesophageal sonography can evaluate the aorta and the left atrium.

Ultrasonography can evaluate the pleura, diaphragm, and infradiaphragmatic processes, but because air and bone do not transmit sound well, parenchymal evaluation is limited to assessment of masses or consolidation abutting mediastinum, chest wall, or diaphragm.

Indications

Assessment of Pleural Effusions and Distinction of Effusion from Solid Pleural Thickening

Ultrasound is helpful; differentiating solid from liquid is difficult in a radiograph, but easy with sonography. Septations, homogeneous echogenicity, or complexity suggests exudate.

Assessment of the Diaphragm and Peridiaphragmatic Masses

Ultrasound allows evaluation of small effusions, distinction of peridiaphragmatic masses and collections, detection of right-hemidiaphragmatic tears (via transhepatic imaging), and analysis of diaphragm function. The left hemidiaphragm is often obscured by bowel gas, however.

Guidance for Needle Biopsy and Catheter Placement

Ultrasound allows reduced complications and greater positional accuracy for lesions in contact with the chest wall or diaphragm.

Suggested Reading

Bacher K, Smeets P, Bonnarens K, et al. Dose reduction in patients undergoing chest imaging: digital amorphous silicon flat-panel detector radiography versus conventional film-screen radiography and phosphor-based computed radiography. *Am J Roentgenol.* 2003;181:923-929.

Beigelman-Aubry C, Hill C, Guibal A, et al. Multi-detector row CT and postprocessing techniques in the assessment of diffuse lung disease. *Radiographics*. 2005;25:1639-1652.

Bitar R, Leung G, Perng R, et al. MR pulse sequences: what every radiologist wants to know but is afraid to ask. *Radiographics*. 2006;26:513-537.

Fink C. Hallscheidt PJ, Noeldge G, et al. Clinical comparative study with a large-area amorphous silicon flat-panel detector: image quality and visibility of anatomic structures on chest radiography. *AJR Am J Roentgenol*. 2002;178:481-486.

Fischbach F, Freund T, et al. Dual-energy chest radiography with a flat-panel digital detector: revealing calcified chest abnormalities. *AJR Am J Roentgenol*. 2003;181:15-19-15-24.

Ganten M, Radeleff B, Kampschulte A, et al. Comparing image quality of flat-panel chest radiography with storage phosphor radiography and film-screen radiography. *AJR Am J Roentgenol*. 2003;181:171-176.

Gibbs JM, Chandrasekhar CA, Ferguson EC, et al. Lines and stripes: where did they go?—from conventional radiography to CT. *Radiographics*. 2007;27:33-48.

Karabulut N, Martin DR, Yang M, et al. MR imaging of the chest using a contrast-enhanced breath-hold modified three-dimensional gradient-echo technique: comparison wtih two-dimensional gradient-echo technique and multidetector CT. *AJR Am J Roentgenol*. 2002;179:1225-1233.

Kono R, Fujimoto K, Terasaki H, et al. Dynamic MRI of solitary pulmonary nodules: comparison of enhancement patterns of malignant and benign small peripheral lung lesions. *AJR Am J Roentgenol*. 2007;188:26-36.

Kubo T, Paul Lin P, Stiller W, et al. Radiation dose reduction in chest CT: a review. *AJR Am J Roentgenol*. 2008;190:335-343.

Love C, Opoku-Agyemang P, Thomas MB, et al. Pulmonary activity on labeled leukocyte images: physiologic, pathologic, and imaging correlation. *Radiographics*. 2002;22:1385-1393.

McCollough CH, Bruesewitz MR, Kofler JM. CT dose reduction and dose management tools: overview of available options. *Radiographics*. 2006;26:503-512.

Satoh S, Kitazume Y, Ohdama S, et al. Can malignant and benign pulmonary nodules be differentiated with diffusion-weighted MRI? *AJR Am J Roentgenol*. 2008;191:464-470.

Vogt FM, Herborn CU, Hunold P, et al. HASTE MRI versus chest radiography in the detection of pulmonary nodules: comparison with MDCT. *AJR Am J Roentgenol*. 2004;183:71-78.

QUESTIONS AND ANSWERS

1. Which of the following is *true* regarding lateral decubitus projection?
   A. The patient is supine and the beam is shot laterally parallel to the floor.
   B. The patient is in Trendelenburg.
   C. It is useful for evaluating the lung apices.
   D. A pleural effusion of 150 mL would generally be visible on an adequate radiograph.

   ANSWER: D. The patient is decubitus and the beam is shot parallel to the floor. Placing the patient in slight Trendelenburg position decreases the volume required for an effusion to be visible, but this is not required. It is useful for evaluating air-fluid levels, effusions, and contents of cavitary lesions; lordotic projection would be useful for apical evaluation. Lateral–decubitus imaging may visualize an effusion as small as 100 mL.

2. What is the benefit of high over low kVp?
   A. The linear–attenuation coefficients of bone and soft tissue are more widely separated.
   B. Pulmonary vessels are more visible.
   C. Opacity of the mediastinum is increased, allowing better imaging of pleural reflections.
   D. It uses higher mAs.

   ANSWER: B. The linear–attenuation coefficients of bone and soft tissue are closer together with high kVp, so they are both visible in a single exposure. Pulmonary vessels and nodules are easier to see. The mediastinum is less opaque, allowing visualization of the retrocardiac tissues and pleural reflections. It results in less total radiation exposure and uses lower mAs.

3. Regarding the mediastinum in radiography, which of the following is *true*?
   A. AP radiography typically magnifies the heart by 15% to 20%.
   B. A longer source–object distance results in greater magnification, with all other variables constant.
   C. PA radiography does not magnify the heart.
   D. Upper lobe vessels are typically larger in PA studies than in supine AP studies.

   ANSWER: A. AP radiography uses a shorter source–object distance and places the heart further from the detector, so the heart is magnified by 15% to 20%. A longer source–object distance results in less magnification if all else is kept the same. PA radiography does magnify the heart, but much less than AP radiography, approximately 5%. Upper lobe vessels are enlarged in AP studies because supine positioning increases venous return and alters the normal gravity-dependent gradient.

4. Which of the following, on its own, is an accepted medical indication for chest radiography?
   A. Staging of extrathoracic tumors
   B. Prenatal evaluation of unsuspected disease
   C. Hospital admission
   D. Before employment

   ANSWER: A. Chest radiography is indicated for a wide variety of medical reasons including tumor staging. The ACR does not consider as medical indications the routine screening of unselected patient populations, prenatal chest radiographs for the detection of unsuspected disease, radiography solely for hospital admission, preemployment radiography, or repeat radiograph examinations on long-term facility admission.

5. How many PA and lateral chest radiograph evaluations would be required to equal the average North American background radiation exposure?
   A. 2
   B. 20
   C. 200
   D. 2000

   ANSWER: B. The average North American background radiation exposure is 3 mSv. The effective dose of a PA and lateral chest radiograph evaluation is 0.15 mSv.

6. A MR sequence uses a 180-degree pulse followed by a 90-degree pulse. What is this?
   A. Saturation–recovery
   B. Inversion–recovery
   C. Spin-echo T1
   D. Spin-echo T2

   ANSWER: B. Saturation–recovery sequences consist of two 90-degree pulses separated by a short TR. Inversion recovery sequences consist of a 180-degree pulse to invert the net magnetization, followed by a 90-degree pulse to deflect and cohere the magnetization. Spin-echo T1 uses a 90-degree pulse followed by a 180-degree pulse at TE/2, with short TE and short TR. Spin-echo T2 uses the same 90-degree and 180-degree pulses but uses long TE and long TR.

7. Which of the following is *true* regarding nuclear ventilation–perfusion imaging?
   A. The perfusion agent is typically 100 μm and blocks 4% of precapillary arterioles.
   B. Xe-133 imaging is performed before a perfusion study because of its low-energy photons.
   C. Tc-99m DTPA aerosols are specifically indicated in patients with COPD.
   D. An expected postoperative FEV-1 less than 1.5 L generally precludes resection.

   ANSWER: B. The perfusion agent is typically 10 to 90 μm (MAA) or 35 to 60 μm (HAM), and the particles occlude only about 0.1% of the patient's precapillary arterioles. Xe-133 has a low-energy photon so ventilation study with this agent must be done first; if not, down scatter from Tc-99m perfusion agent will obscure the results. Tc-99m DTPA has a short residence time in smokers and may deposit in the central airways, so sulfur colloid, pyrophosphate, technegas, or pertechnegas would be better.

8. Regarding gallium-67 citrate scintigraphy, which of the following is *true*?
   A. Imaging in interstitial pulmonary fibrosis predicts activity but not prognosis.
   B. Imaging in lymphoma is not possible with Hodgkin disease.
   C. The intensity and distribution can be quantified with the gallium index.
   D. Chest radiography is more sensitive in immunocompromised patients.

   ANSWER: C. Imaging in IPF does not predict activity, prognosis, or response to therapy and is not recommended. Gallium imaging works with both Hodgkin and non-Hodgkin lymphoma. The intensity of uptake can be graded on a five-point scale, and the intensity multiplied by the area of activity to reach the gallium index. In immunocompromised patients, Ga-67 imaging is more sensitive for the detection of inflammatory processes.

9. Regarding chest FDG-PET, which of the following is *true*?
   A. PET is 80% to 100% sensitive but 25% specific for characterization of pulmonary nodule.
   B. PET is not as accurate as CT for mediastinal staging of non–small cell lung cancer.
   C. PET sensitivity and specificity for detection of tumor versus scar are 97% and 100%.
   D. Lung parenchyma is attenuating to the 511-keV protons produced in the decay.

   ANSWER: C. PET is 80% to 100% sensitive and 50% to 97% specific for pulmonary nodule characterization and is more accurate than CT for detection of mediastinal involvement in non–small cell lung cancer. PET sensitivity and specificity for detection of tumor versus scar are 97% and 100%. Lung parenchyma is quite nonattenuating because the volume is mostly air.

10. Which of the following is *not* an indication for chest sonography?
    A. Assessment of intraparenchymal lung abscess in aerated lung
    B. Assessment of traumatic right diaphragm injury
    C. Assessment of loculated pleural effusion
    D. Guidance for biopsy of a pleural-based mass

    ANSWER: A. The sound beam cannot penetrate aerated lung so the abscess would be invisible. If the lung were collapsed or the lesion abutting the pleura it would be accessible for evaluation. The right diaphragm can be imaged via a transhepatic window. Loculated pleural effusion evaluation is a good indication for sonography: septations, homogeneous echogenicity, or complexity suggests exudates. Pleural-based masses may be imaged sonographically, reducing complications and increasing positional accuracy compared to non-image-guided biopsy.

18 CONGENITAL THORACIC ANOMALIES

John C. Texada and Satinder P. Singh

Developmental anomalies of the airways and lungs are probably caused by interference with the embryonic, pseudoglandular, and canalicular periods of lung development.

PULMONARY AGENESIS, APLASIA, AND HYPOPLASIA

In agenesis, there is no trace of bronchial, vascular, or parenchymal tissue; in aplasia, there is only a rudimentary bronchus ending in a blind pouch, with no parenchyma or vascular tissue; and in hypoplasia, the lung is grossly normal but there are fewer or smaller airways, vessels, and alveoli. The first two are closely related; the last is often associated with or the result of other anomalies. Patients may die in childhood, particularly those with agenesis, though many patients survive to adulthood. The abnormalities predispose to infection and in neonates to pneumothorax.

AGENESIS/APLASIA

Unilateral agenesis occurs in 1:10 000 people; men and women are equally affected, as are the right and left sides. It has been associated with chromosomal anomalies and with malformations of chest wall, skeleton, or ipsilateral face, suggesting genetic or arch-developmental etiologies respectively. Bilateral agenesis can be associated with tracheoesophageal anomalies, suggesting primary lung bud defect.

PRIMARY HYPOPLASIA

Primary hypoplasia (without an additional causative abnormality) occurs in 1 to 2:12 000 people. Its etiology is uncertain. A hypoplastic lung is typically smaller and less developed than a normal lung and often has 50% to 75% the normal number of airway generations, leading to alveolar count one-third normal. It is often associated with anomalies of ipsilateral pulmonary arteries and anomalous pulmonary venous drainage (hypogenetic lung syndrome).

SECONDARY HYPOPLASIA

Secondary hyperplasia may be due to decreased hemithoracic volume, pulmonary vascular hypoperfusion, decreased fetal respiratory movement, and decreased lung fluid. Other miscellaneous associations include Rh isoimmunization; anencephaly/hydranencephaly; multiple congenital syndromes including Down, Klippel-Feil, Wolcott, Rallison, Matthew-Wood, and Fryns; and other abnormalities.

Decreased hemithoracic volume is the most frequent of these. The most common cause is the presence of a space-occupying mass—often congenital diaphragmatic hernia with thoracic abdominal contents, but sometimes neuroblastoma, sequestered lung, accessory diaphragm, or pleural effusion, and occasionally large intra-abdominal masses or collections.

Decreased pulmonary vascular perfusion is proposed as a mechanism to explain unilateral hypoplasia in some patients with tetralogy of Fallot.

Decreased fetal respiratory movement such as from cord injury or phrenic nerve injury can cause hypoplasia in experimental animals and may have similar effects in people.

Decreased lung fluid such as from oligohydramnios produces hypoplasia in one of two ways. First, lung fluid exerts a positive pressure on the developing lungs. Second, Potter syndrome of renal agenesis, abnormal facial and limb development, and pulmonary hypoplasia may be caused by compression by an oligohydramniotic uterus or some other mechanism.

RADIOGRAPHIC FINDINGS

Aplasia and hypoplasia of the lung appear radiographically similar—absence or near-absence of aerated lung on one side or the other. Ipsilateral ribs are closer together, the ipsilateral diaphragm is elevated, and the mediastinum is shifted. The normal lung is generally hyperinflated and extends into the other hemithorax.

CT FINDINGS

CT can detect the bronchovascular deficiencies associated with aplasia, or conversely in hypoplasia, CT can reveal the patent bronchovascular structures and lung hypoplasia. To differentiate from Swyer-James syndrome, imaging may reveal air trapping in that syndrome but not in hypoplasia.

Main differential is pneumonectomy performed in early childhood, total atelectasis, severe bronchiectasis with collapse, and advanced fibrothorax.

BRONCHOPULMONARY SEQUESTRATION

A portion of lung tissue is detached from the normal lung and receives blood supply from a systemic artery. The abnormality may be due to anomalous systemic artery exerting traction on a bronchial bud, to failure of normal pulmonary–arterial development, to coincidence, to interference with embryonic organization, or, the favored explanation, to persistence and localized development of anomalous separate branch that retains embryonic blood supply.

The abnormality may be intralobar or extralobar, differentiated by the absence or presence, respectively, of its own visceral pleural membrane. Intralobar sequestration is typically contiguous with normal lung (in the same pleura); extralobar sequestration is generally close to normal lung but may be in or below the diaphragm.

INTRALOBAR SEQUESTRATION

Intralobar sequestration is three-fourths of all sequestrations. Arterial supply is generally the descending aorta; though abdominal aorta, branch artery, or coronary artery origins have been reported. Venous drainage is generally normal, that is, via pulmonary veins, so a left-to-left shunt forms. The anomalous artery often enters via the pulmonary ligament and is often bigger than it should be, sometimes aneurysmal; it may supply only the sequestered tissue or some normal tissue as well.

In two-thirds of cases, the sequestered tissue is in the left lower lobe posterior segment, in the paravertebral gutter. In most of the remainder, it is in the same position on the right. In the uncommon event of upper lobe sequestration, the arterial supply may be from the ascending aorta or arch vessels or their branches and cardiac anomalies are common. Intralobar sequestration is associated with other anomalies in 15% of cases, most commonly diaphragmatic hernia, but also other skeletal and cardiac anomalies.

The sequestered tissue is typically well demarcated and contains cysts resembling dilated bronchi that may contain mucus or pus. It may or may not connect to the normal bronchi; if connected, there is often infection both in the sequestration and in the adjacent lung.

RADIOGRAPHIC FINDINGS

The most common finding is a homogeneous density in a posterior basal lower lobe, usually the left, usually contiguous with the diaphragm; it may appear as a cystic mass or prominent vessels. The adjacent normal lung parenchyma's arteries and veins are displaced around the sequestration. If infected there may be air or air-fluid–containing cysts; the adjacent normal tissue is also often infected obscuring the lesion.

OTHER IMAGING FINDINGS

Calcification is rare, but visible in CT. CT may better visualize cysts, venous drainage, and other anomalies than can radiography. Catheter angiography, CT, or MR with or without angiography makes the diagnosis via imaging of the anomalous systemic arterial supply; however CT or MR may miss small vessels. HRCT may image small air-containing cysts.

EXTRALOBAR SEQUESTRATION

Extralobar sequestration, less common, than intralobar sequestration, is left sided in 90% of cases and may be beneath the left lower lobe, in or beneath the diaphragm, or in the mediastinum or retroperitoneum. The tissue will have its own pleura, generally have few airways, and may have cystic spaces. Since it has no connection to other airways, it generally does not become infected unless it communicates with the GI tract, and thus is often incidentally found during evaluation of other anomalies. It is most often discovered in newborns and often is associated with other anomalies; ipsilateral diaphragmatic paralysis or eventration is present in 60% and left diaphragmatic hernia is present in 30%. Pulmonary hypoplasia may be present if the sequestration is large.

Systemic arterial supply is commonly from the abdominal aorta or its branches; often multiple small arteries are present. Venous drainage is usually via systemic veins–vena cava, azygous or hemiazygous veins, or portal veins, resulting in a left-to-right shunt.

RADIOGRAPHIC FINDINGS

A sharply defined triangular opacity or small bump at the posterior costophrenic angle is the most common finding, usually at the left hemidiaphragm. It may appear as a mass elsewhere.

OTHER IMAGING FINDINGS

CT will reveal a homogeneous mass occasionally with cystic spaces, often with hypoattenuation in the surrounding normal lung. Conventional CT is less useful for identifying the sometimes multiple arterial feeding vessels, but CT angiography may be more useful. Aortography may be required.

BRONCHOGENIC CYSTS

There are three types of foregut cysts, based on presumed tissue derivation: paravertebral (enteric) cysts, foregut that has herniated through the notochord, often associated with spinal defects; esophageal cysts, from failure of the esophagus to canalize completely; and bronchogenic cysts, from abnormal tracheobronchial budding.

Bronchogenic cyst probably develop between days 26 and 40 of development; earlier problems lead to mediastinal cysts, while later problems lead to more peripheral lung cysts; 65% to 90% are mediastinal. Bronchogenic cysts are more commonly found in males and in Yemeni Jews. They are typically incidentally detected, though infected cysts can cause hemoptysis or typical infection symptoms, rarely pneumothorax, air embolism, or cancer can develop.

Bronchogenic cysts are generally solitary unilocular thin-walled round lesions filled with mucus or serous fluid. They generally do not connect to the tracheobronchial tree unless they become infected. The presence of cartilage, smooth muscle, and glandular tissue in the walls helps to confirm the diagnosis.

A mediastinal bronchogenic cyst may be classified as paratracheal, carinal, hilar, paraesophageal, or miscellaneous (thymic, pericardial, or vertebral body surface). Paratracheal and carinal origins are the most common. They are almost always solitary. They typically are asymptomatic but if a mediastinal bronchogenic cyst abuts an important structure, pressure effects may become apparent even if the cyst is small.

RADIOGRAPHIC FINDINGS

Typically, a bronchogenic cyst will appear as a well-circumscribed round or oval mass or nodule, usually in the medial one-third of the lungs, and more commonly in the lower lobes; right and left are affected equally. If followed radiographically, they typically do not change much with time. Since they do not connect to the airways unless infected (the presentation for 75% of cases recognized clinically), they should not contain air. Once infected they may contain air and may be surrounded by inflamed parenchyma. They may enlarge, once air filled, by a check-valve mechanism. The main differential considerations would be postabscess cavity or bulla.

A mediastinal bronchogenic cyst will appear as a clearly defined homogeneous mass, usually at the right paratracheal or right carinal region, overlapping the right hilum. Most are oval or round and some may be large. Wall calcification is uncommon. More than 90% are radiographically visible.

CT FINDINGS

The lesion may be diagnosed if it has smooth thin walls and unenhancing fluid attenuation contents. Half of intraparenchymal cases have greater attenuation contents because of proteinaceous fluid or calcium oxalate. If infected the cyst will be heterogeneous and resemble an abscess.

A mediastinal bronchogenic cyst will almost always be visible and may be diagnosed with confidence as a benign cyst in more than 50% of cases.

MR FINDINGS

T2-weighted images reveal bright homogeneous contents, with intermediate T1 signal intensity; an infected cyst would have intermediate heterogeneous T2 and T1 signal intensities. The more proteinaceous the fluid (and thus more difficult to identify as fluid on CT), the higher its T1 signal intensity will be.

BRONCHIECTASIS

Congenital bronchiectasis is rare and thought to be due to incomplete bronchial branching. Almost all bronchi in a lobe or lung are dilated, to just below the pleura. Histology reveals cartilage deficiency in the segmental and subsegmental airways. The terminating tissue is also abnormal, with few alveoli, abnormal smooth muscle, and lymphangiectasis. It may have a genetic component. Congenital bronchiectasis typically presents in childhood with cough and repeat infections.

CYSTIC ADENOMATOID MALFORMATION

Cystic adenomatoid malformation refers to a group of pathologically and possibly etiologically distinct lesions characterized by abnormal pulmonary tissue, often with cysts. When cysts are present, they often communicate with normal airways. Most of the time the arterial supply is via pulmonary arteries, but sometimes the supply is systemic. Theories of origin include localized bronchial developmental arrest, hamartoma, or bronchial obstruction. Three types are defined: cystic, intermediate, and solid (Table 18-1).

Most cases are discovered before 5 years of age and more than one-half before 1 month of age. The upper lobes are slightly more commonly involved than the lower and sometimes involvement is multilobar. They may be detected with increasing respiratory distress owing to cyst enlargement, or during evaluation of cough, fever, and recurrent infection.

RADIOGRAPHIC FINDINGS

A homogeneous opacity in a newborn becomes air filled (if type I or II) over the first few days or weeks of life. The lesion is space occupying and may enlarge and shift the mediastinum. Cysts may be visible, containing air, fluid, or air-fluid levels.

CT FINDINGS

CT reveals more fully the cystic and solid components. The lesion may displace and splay bronchovascular structures around it.

TRACHEOBRONCHIAL STENOSIS

Congenital stenosis may be due to cartilage abnormalities of the trachea or of more distal structures. Absence of tracheal cartilage leading to tracheomalacia, which may be focal, and cause expiratory airway obstruction and repeated infection. Incomplete tracheal cartilage segmentation, which may be focal or diffuse, can affect normal posterior tracheal membrane development and turn the trachea into a cartilaginous tube. This may be cylindrical or taper distally. It may cause clinically significant stenosis. It is associated with anomalous left pulmonary artery origin. Other causes include atresia, hypoplasia, and fibrous web formation. These are often associated with other anomalies, including skeletal dysplasias and neonatal lobar hyperinflation.

BRONCHIAL ATRESIA

Bronchial atresia, a rare congenital atresia or stenosis of lobar, segmental, or subsegmental bronchus, is most commonly at the apicoposterior segment of the left upper lobe; the right upper lobe, middle lobe, and lower lobes are affected with descending frequency, and lower lobe involvement is quite rare. It may be due to disconnection but subsequent normal development of a bronchial bud or a localized intrauterine bronchial–arterial disruption leading to wall ischemia and luminal obliteration.

Mucus secreted in the airways distal to the atretic segment builds up into a plug or mucocele. Air can enter via collateral pathways, leading to regional hyperinflation and expiratory air trapping. It is usually an isolated finding, found over age 15 in half of cases, and most patients are asymptomatic, though some may have repeat infections.

RADIOGRAPHIC FINDINGS

A regional pulmonary lucency is visible in 90% of cases as a result of air trapping and hypoperfusion. Normal lung nearby is compressed and displaced. A hilar mass

TABLE 18-1 Classification of Cystic Adenomatoid Malformations

Type I (50%)	Cystic	Containing large often multiloculated cysts, sometimes with smaller cysts as well; the cyst wall has smooth muscle but no cartilage	Bronchioloalveolar carcinoma may develop in type I CAMs
Type II (40%)	Intermediate	Solid areas and small cysts less than 10 mm diameter	These patients often have other pulmonary abnormalities
Type III (10%)	Solid	Grossly composed of irregular bronchiolar and alveolar tissues similar to the pseudoglandular stage of development	

is visible in 80% of cases, consisting of the branching, ovoid, or cystic dilated mucus-filled blocked distal airways. The presence of both these is found in 70% of cases.

CT FINDINGS

CT allows better visualization of the mucoid impaction and segmental abnormalities and may allow confident diagnosis.

NEONATAL LOBAR HYPERINFLATION

Neonatal lobar hyperinflation, also called congenital lobar emphysema, is defined as variably severe hyperinflation of a pulmonary lobe. It has variable causes, and is often part of a syndrome rather than an isolated process. It may be acquired. It almost always presents as infantile respiratory distress, and often requires urgent surgery; however, in some cases managed medically, the abnormalities appear to regress over time.

Half of cases have no obstructive etiology, but obstructive causes include partial airway obstruction, which may be extrinsic (anomalous vessel is most common), intramural (proposed in two-thirds of obstructive cases, often cartilaginous deficiency causing airway collapse), or intraluminal (developmental mucosal folds or bronchial stenosis, or acquired mucus plugs or bronchiolitis).

About half of patients in one study of this process also had congenital heart defects, though other studies have a lower association. It affects males 3:1; it is most common in the left upper lobe, followed by the right middle lobe and rarely the lower lobes, and is almost always unilateral.

RADIOGRAPHIC FINDINGS

Lobar hyperinflation and air trapping cause increased lobar volume and increased lucency, depressing the hemidiaphragm, and displacing the mediastinum. They may cause atelectasis of other lobes. Sometimes, in cases of impaired fluid drainage, the expanded lobe will be fluid filled and hyperattenuating for up to 2 weeks. Radiography may be diagnostic.

OTHER IMAGING FINDINGS

CT may help to confirm a diagnosis and rule out an obstructing mass. Ventilation-perfusion scan may reveal abnormalities in the affected lobe and help to evaluate the function of adjacent compressed tissue.

ANOMALOUS TRACHEOBRONCHIAL BRANCHING

Most abnormal branches are asymptomatic and of no consequence, but this may present as recurrent infection. Patients with spontaneous pneumothorax are more likely than control patients to have anomalous branching.

Abnormal number involves the duplication or less likely absence of a lobar or segmental bronchus.

Abnormal origin of a lobar or segmental bronchus may be present. The most common of these is tracheal origin of the right upper lobe, called tracheal bronchus, pig bronchus, or bronchus suis (Latin for pig, because this is a normal anatomic feature of that animal). The abnormal bronchus arises from the rightward trachea less than 2 cm from the carina. Its prevalence is 2% or less. Rarer, the apicoposterior left upper lobe bronchus may arise from the left main bronchus; this often leads to obstructive problems in that segment. A bridging bronchus may supply the right middle or lower lobe via the left main bronchus.

Cardiac bronchus is a supernumerary bronchus arising from the medial wall of the right main or intermediate bronchus opposite the origin of the right upper lobe bronchus. It is lined with bronchial mucosa and has cartilage in its wall distinguishing it from a diverticulum. It usually ends blindly though rarely associated with small abnormal pulmonary parenchyma. Most are asymptomatic. Complications may include hemoptysis caused by infection or cancer.

Isomerism, in which lobar and bronchial development is symmetric in both lungs, is often associated with cardiac defects and with heterotaxy syndromes. In left isomerism, both lungs have a left-lung pattern of two lobes and long main bronchus; in right isomerism, both lungs are three-lobed and have short main bronchi.

ANOMALOUS TRACHEOBRONCHIAL COMMUNICATIONS

TRACHEOBRONCHIAL-ESOPHAGEAL FISTULA

In 85% of cases, the esophagus ends blindly, and the trachea can communicate with either the cranial or the caudal esophageal moiety, or both. About half of patients have other congenital anomalies. Regurgitation of milk leads to aspiration and infection. Less frequently, the fistula may connect the airways to an otherwise normal esophagus. This may go undetected for longer periods, though there may be aspiration and infection. The esophageal end of the fistula is usually distal to the tracheal end, and there may be one-way valve-like membranes at the esophageal ends, which may reduce the incidence of infection.

RADIOGRAPHIC FINDINGS

Alveolar opacities from aspiration are common. "Esophageal lung" consists of total right lung opacification supplied by a rightward-deviated esophagus, with normal tracheal position; this indicates origin of the right bronchus from the esophagus. In patients without esophageal atresia, bronchiectasis from repeated infection may be visible.

BRONCHOBILIARY FISTULA

Biliary tree fistula to the carina or main bronchus has been reported a few times. Infants present with neonatal pneumonia and greenish sputum.

OTHERS

Accessory or heterotopic lung tissue is a rare finding. Occasionally a lobe or entire lung may be duplicated.

Heterotopic intrapulmonary tissue consisting of skeletal muscle, liver, thyroid, adrenal, or glial tissue may be found occasionally.

Horseshoe lung is diagnosed when a connecting band of lung tissue extends from the right lung base behind the pericardium to join the posterior-basal left lower lobe segment. This is often associated with venolobar syndrome (hypoplastic pulmonary artery, anomalous systemic pulmonary venous return, abnormal systemic arterial supply, and bronchial sequestration), more common on the right but occasionally left-sided.

DEVELOPMENTAL ANOMALIES OF THE PULMONARY VESSELS

PULMONARY ARTERIAL ANOMALIES

Absence of the Main Pulmonary Artery

The main pulmonary artery may be atretic only proximally or over its entire course; in these cases, a residual fibrous cord marks its position, and the left and right pulmonary arteries may remain in normal position, supplied by a patent ductus arteriosus (PDA).

Pulmonary atresia with ventricular septal defect (VSD) is relatively common, manifest as neonatal hypoxemia as the PDA closes. In about half of cases anywhere from one to six collateral arteries arise from the descending aorta.

Complete Absence of Main Pulmonary Artery

In persistent truncus arteriosus, a single great artery arises from a common semilunar valve, always with a VSD (see Chap. 102, Table 102-3). Pulmonary blood supply is via branches from the trunk artery.

Proximal Interruption of the Pulmonary Artery

Pulmonary arteries are usually large and patent beyond the proximal interruption. Blood supply to the lung beyond the interruption is via a systemic collateral, usually a PDA or bronchial collaterals or from a direct aortic branch. The interrupted vessel often has histologic appearance of ductus arteriosus, so this may be a physiologic response of a persistent right ductus arteriosus.

Right-sided interruption is more common and may be divided into four types: those without pulmonary hypertension, usually asymptomatic; those with PA hypertension, usually discovered in childhood; those with recurrent infection or hemoptysis, often because the lung is abnormal; and those with left PDA or congenital heart disease.

Left-sided interruption is less common and has an association with other cardiovascular anomalies, particularly tetralogy of Fallot.

Radiographic Findings

The right (or left) lung is small and hyperlucent because of hypoperfusion, and the right (or left) hilum is small. Expiratory imaging will not reveal air trapping, which helps differentiate this entity from Swyer-James syndrome. Intercostal artery enlargement may lead to rib notching.

Scintigraphic Findings

The affected lung will have no uptake in perfusion imaging (unless there is another shunt elsewhere) because its blood supply is systemic; but ventilation imaging will be normal. In Swyer-James syndrome both ventilation and perfusion are typically abnormal.

CT or MR Findings

Planar imaging may reveal the absent arterial segment, the patent intrapulmonary arteries, and possibly the systemic collateral arteries.

CONGENITAL PULMONARY ARTERY ANEURYSM

Congenital pulmonary artery aneurysms are rare and usually associated with other anomalies, particularly AVM or bronchopulmonary sequestration. Up to half are associated with congenital cardiac defects including pulmonary valve stenosis, tetralogy of Fallot, or VSD. They are present at birth and usually the result of turbulent poststenotic flow; as a result of flow dynamics they are much more common in the left pulmonary artery (so the presence of a large left PA and normal right PA should suggest pulmonary valve stenosis). They may uncommonly be isolated, in which case they usually involve the trunk and are usually fusiform.

DIRECT COMMUNICATION OF THE RIGHT PULMONARY ARTERY WITH THE LEFT ATRIUM

In this rare malformation, an anomalous right PA branch connects to the left atrium; the anomalous vessel is often aneurysmal. The right lung may be normal if the anomalous artery exists in addition to normal arteries, or the lower lobe may be aplastic or hypoplastic. Radiography may be normal or may reveal a round nodule adjacent to the left atrium in the right hemithorax.

PULMONARY VENOUS ANOMALIES

CONGENITAL VENOUS OBSTRUCTION

Congenital venous obstruction can result from compression by an intrathoracic mass or from intrinsic venous abnormalities. The intrinsic anomaly is rare, and often associated with other cardiac anomalies. It may be caused by atrial endocardial thickening, by venous muscular hypertrophy or intimal fibrosis, or occlusion by thrombus. Patients present with findings of pulmonary venous hypertension, which may be only regional in radiographs, with or without PA hypertension. Hemoptysis may be the presenting feature. Angiography would reveal small ipsilateral pulmonary artery and contrast material stasis.

PULMONARY VENOUS VARICOSITIES

Pulmonary venous varicosities, a rare abnormality, may either be congenital or acquired. The dilation is immediately preatrial, in the congenital form perhaps an abnormality in the transition from splanchnic to pulmonary-venous drainage. The vessel itself usually is structurally normal. Radiographically a round or oval lobulated opacity will often be visible in the medial third of a lung. Acquired varicosities are due to mitral valve disease, usually regurgitation; they usually are right-sided because the mitral valve plane is directed posterosuperiorly to the right. They are usually asymptomatic but can rupture.

MIXED ARTERIOVENOUS ANOMALIES

HYPOGENETIC LUNG SYNDROME

In this rare defect, with incidence 1 to 3:100 000, the right lung is hypoplastic and right lung pulmonary venous return is via portal or systemic veins. Most commonly it drains below the diaphragm via the inferior vena cava, but may drain to portal, hepatic, or azygous veins or the coronary sinus or right atrium. The right pulmonary artery is hypoplastic, and systemic arteries from the thoracic or abdominal aorta provide part or all of the blood supply of the lung. The abnormal systemic artery does not overlap territories with other pulmonary or bronchial arteries, but is responsible for all the blood flow to the lung parenchyma it supplies. Additional findings include mirror image bronchi (right isomerism), diverticula, or extension of the right lung into the left hemithorax. The syndrome is associated with other cardiovascular anomalies, with ASD present in 25% of patients and others having VSD, tetralogy of Fallot, and other anomalies. A majority of patients have symptoms of left-to-right shunt, repeated infection, or hemoptysis.

RADIOGRAPHIC FINDINGS

The abnormal vein often is visible as a large curved density descending to the diaphragm to the right of the heart. The right lung is small and hypovascular and the hilum is small. The mediastinum is shifted to the right.

CT AND MR FINDINGS

CT and MR can make definitive diagnosis if necessary, and allow identification of other abnormalities that may be present.

PULMONARY ARTERIOVENOUS MALFORMATION

Pulmonary arteriovenous malformations range from microscopic communications to complex aneurismal dilatations of multiple arteries and veins. Etiologic theories include the presence of a capillary defect allowing formation of thin-walled sacs or incomplete degeneration of vascular septa connecting the primitive arterial and venous plexuses.

They are found more commonly in the lower lobes. One-third of patients have multiple lesions in the lungs. Sixty percent of patients have extrapulmonary lesions (called hereditary hemorrhagic telangiectasia or Rendu-Osler-Weber disease; this is inherited in an autosomal dominant process). Multiple lesions may also be present in patients with Fanconi syndrome and polysplenia syndrome.

They may be asymptomatic, or may result in symptoms of right-to-left shunt. Many patients have symptoms not from their pulmonary malformations but from malformations in other organs, namely, epistaxis, hematemesis, and cerebrovascular hemorrhage. Paradoxic embolization is possible leading to stroke or transient ischemic attack. Patients may have polycythemia, though if they bleed often they may be anemic.

RADIOGRAPHIC FINDINGS

A round homogeneous mass will be well defined, most often in the medial one-third of the lung. Feeding and draining vessels are often apparent. In some cases, a heterogeneous mass representing angiomatous hyperplasia may be visible. Hemorrhage may obscure the lesion. Calcification (phlebolith formation) is sometimes evident.

Additional imaging findings and detailed evaluation are usually necessary after the radiograph, both characterize the known lesions and to find other smaller or undetected lesions. This information is necessary before surgery or embolization and is best acquired with angiography or CT angiography; the latter is much more sensitive. CT will show a homogeneous circumscribed nodule with vascular connections and serial imaging can document diminution of the lesion(s) after therapy.

Perfusion scintigraphy or echocardiography can reveal shunt physiology: in the former, some of the administered radiotracer will pass via the malformation into the systemic circulation without being stopped by the capillary bed and will be deposited in the kidneys; this deposition is detectable and quantifiable with gamma cameras.

LYMPHATIC ANOMALIES

LYMPHANGIOMA

Lymphangioma is likely the result of failure of one part of the lymphatic system to communicate with the rest of the system. Most intrathoracic lymphangiomas are in the mediastinum but they occasionally develop in the lung. Fluid accumulation may result in development of a large mass that can cause respiratory distress.

DIFFUSE PULMONARY LYMPHANGIOMATOSIS

Diffuse pulmonary lymphangiomatosis refers to lesions in which the number of lymphatic vessels is increased, leading to anastomosing pleural, interlobular-septal, and peribronchovascular lymphatic channels. It is most common in infancy and childhood, in which it accounts for up to 5% of all chronic interstitial disease. Chest radiography will reveal diffuse bilateral interstitial disease, sometimes lower lobe predominant. Chylothorax may be unilateral or bilateral and is common; chylopericardium may also occur. CT reveals interlobular septal and peribronchovascular interstitial thickening, often with pleural effusions or pleural thickening.

CONGENITAL PULMONARY LYMPHANGIECTASIA

Congenital pulmonary lymphangiectasia refers to lesions in which size of lymphatic vessels is increased, not the number or complexity. It is almost invariably fatal. Group I patients have concomitant cardiac anomaly (one-third of cases), often with pulmonary venous obstruction leading to dilated lymphatics. Group II patients do not have concomitant cardiac anomalies; it is believed that their lymphangiectasia is due to a failure of physiologically large embryonic lymph vessels to regress; these patients often have other congenital defects including polycystic kidneys and ichthyoids. Group III patients have both pulmonary lymphangiectasia and other visceral ectasia, often intestinal; pulmonary involvement in these patients is less severe.

SYSTEMIC SUPPLY TO THE LUNG

Systemic arterial supply may be congenital or acquired. Many have been described already. An additional etiology for congenital systemic arterial supply is that of a systemic artery supplying an otherwise normal lung (Pryce I malformation); this has findings similar to intralobar sequestration except that the supplied lung parenchyma is normal and is normally connected to the airways. Systemic-pulmonary fistula may be congenital or acquired after infection, trauma, or surgery.

HEREDITARY ANOMALIES OF PULMONARY CONNECTIVE TISSUE

MARFAN SYNDROME

Five to ten percent of patients may develop spontaneous pneumothorax. Patients may develop apical bullae, diffuse emphysema, bronchiectasis, or upper lobe fibrosis.

Nonpulmonary manifestations include arachnodactyly, ectopic lentis, and cardiovascular disease; cardiovascular disease is most commonly manifest as aortic aneurysm or dissection and as aortic- and mitral-valvular insufficiency and is the cause of death in 90% of patients with Marfan syndrome. The aortic abnormalities often develop in the ascending aorta. Dissection may be more common in pregnancy.

Radiographic Findings

The most common finding in Marfan syndrome is pectus excavatum; long thin chest and scoliosis are also found. Serial radiographs may reveal increasing aortic size and/or cardiomegaly, the latter from aortic valve insufficiency.

Other Imaging Findings

CT of dissection would reveal intimal flap and false lumen. While CT, transesophageal echo, and MR all have 100% sensitivity for detection of dissection, CT is more specific than the other two, 100% versus 94%.

EHLERS-DANLOS SYNDROME

This group of genetic connective tissue disorders has multiple types. Type IV is associated with fragile skin and vessel rupture, caused by a deficiency of type III fibroblast procollagen. Emphysema, often bullous, may develop and pneumothorax may occur. Connective tissue weakness may result in tracheobronchomegaly, called Mounier-Kuhn syndrome. In type IV, pulmonary artery rupture may lead to hemoptysis. Other findings may occur: pulmonary artery stenosis, bronchiectasis, thin-walled cavitary lesions, and fibrous pseudotumors.

CUTIS LAXA

Cutis laxa, also known as generalized elastolysis, is characterized by loose skin and connective tissue. It is usually transmitted in an autosomal recessive manner. In the lungs, panacinar emphysema may develop (alpha-1 antitrypsin levels will be normal) and tracheobronchomegaly (Mounier-Kuhn syndrome), bronchiectasis, and aortic aneurysm may occur.

PSEUDOXANTHOMA ELASTICUM

There is a single case of elastic tissue damage in the pulmonary vessels of a patient with pseudoxanthoma elasticum.

ALKAPTONURIA

This homogentisic acid oxidase deficiency leads to accumulation of homogentisic acid in cartilage and other connective tissues, leading to gray or black discoloration of the tracheobronchial cartilage and fibrous tissue. It has no functional pulmonary effect.

LYMPHANGIOLEIOMYOMATOSIS

Lymphangioleiomyomatosis (LAM) is predominantly peribronchovascular smooth muscle proliferation, leading to airway and vascular obstruction and cyst formation. It has pulmonary clinicopathoradiologic manifestations similar to tuberous sclerosis and may be related to that process. Both may be hamartomatous in nature; however, LAM can recur after lung transplant, so some other process must be at work.

Abnormal smooth muscle cells proliferate around bronchioles, blood and lymph vessels, and the pleura, sometimes replacing a large portion of lung parenchyma. Cysts of 2 to 20 mm develop, separated by thickened interstitium, and obstructed small vessels can lead to subclinical hemorrhage. Tiny 1- to 3-mm nodules of benign type II pneumocyte hyperplasia develop in some cases.

LAM is uncommon; it only occurs in women, generally in childbearing years. Shortness of breath is of gradual onset, unless an acute spontaneous pneumothorax develops. Patients may have cough, hemoptysis, or chest pain. Chylothorax is a common occurrence; in addition, thoracoabdominal lymph node involvement may lead to chyloperitoneum or chylopericardium. It has a generally poor prognosis, with most patients dying within 10 years of diagnosis in some studies.

Radiographic Findings

Uncommonly, the chest radiograph may be normal in patients with LAM. The most common finding is bilateral reticular interstitial lung disease, generally diffuse and uniform, but occasionally lower zone predominant. Cysts are visible in 60% of cases, and hyperinflation is often present. Thirty to forty percent of patients will develop pneumothorax and ten to twenty percent will develop effusions.

HRCT FINDINGS

Extent of disease in HRCT correlates better than that in radiographs with disease severity, correlating best with carbon monoxide diffusing capacity (DLCO). Numerous air-filled cysts are diffusely placed and surrounded by normal parenchyma; the overall size of the cysts is in general indicative of disease severity, with milder disease having smaller cysts. Sometimes there may be mild interstitial or interlobular septal thickening or ground glass attenuation from small hemorrhages. Small nodules may rarely be visible. Pneumothorax and effusion may be visible and mediastinal nodes may be enlarged.

This may be differentiated from pulmonary Langerhans cell histiocytosis in that the latter generally has upper lobe predominant cysts and spares the lower lungs, and nodules are present in most cases.

TUBEROUS SCLEROSIS

Tuberous sclerosis is a disorder of mesoderm development and an autosomal dominant disease affecting males and females equally, sometimes with positive family history. Its classic triad is mental retardation, epilepsy, and adenoma seba ceum; retinal phacoma, renal angiomyolipoma, cardiac rhabdomyoma, osseous sclerotic lesions (which must be differentiated from osteopoikilosis by their different distribution), and subungual fibromas also are common.

The disease uncommonly affects the lungs—less than 2.5% of patients will develop manifestations—and this is most commonly in women. Thin-walled cysts and small nodular foci of type II pneumocyte hyperplasia develop; there may be an increase in clear-cell tumor development.

Patients typically develop dyspnea, with hemoptysis and cough occasionally. Disease progression is variable, from stable findings to progressive dyspnea and eventual death.

IMAGING FINDINGS

Tuberous sclerosis findings are similar to those of lymphangiomyomatosis. Radiograph will reveal diffuse reticular disease with or without thin-walled cysts. HRCT will reveal thin-walled cysts throughout the lungs, sometimes with normal chest radiograph. Pneumothorax may develop in up to half of patients with tuberous sclerosis lung involvement, though chylothorax is rare.

NEUROFIBROMATOSIS

Neurofibromatosis type I is an autosomal recessive neurophacomatosis, with a gene on chromosome 17, with frequency of about 1:3000. Cutaneous cafe au lait spots and peripheral neurofibromas are the most prominent findings; patients also develop CNS gliomas, meningiomas, peripheral nerve sarcomas, pheochromocytomas, and angiosarcomas.

In the chest, intercostal nerve tumors may be associated with rib destruction, chest mass, or occasionally hemorrhage from erosion into the adjacent vessels.

Interstitial fibrosis occurs in 5% to 10% of patients; bulla formation is in up to 20% of patients. The fibrosis is pathologically an interstitial pneumonitis with fibrosis and chronic inflammation, most prominent in subpleural tissues. Macrophage aggregation is common.

Radiographic Findings

Symmetric basilar–predominant reticular interstitial lung disease is common; bullae usually are asymmetric and upper lung predominant. Cutaneous neurofibromas may be radiographically apparent. Scoliosis is nonspecific, but an acute-angle lower-thoracic curve involving five or fewer vertebrae is suggestive of neurofibromatosis. Twisted-ribbon rib deformities, scalloping of the posterior vertebral-body cortex, a sequela of dural ectasia, and lateral meningocele formation may be visible.

Intercostal neurofibromas may be visible as paraspinal masses; often these are visible running parallel to and possibly eroding the adjacent rib. As the tumors are generally benign and slow growing, the erosion is generally a remodeling process without cortical destruction. Tumors of vagus, phrenic, or sympathetic chain nerves may appear as mediastinal masses.

CT Findings

CT in the setting of neurofibromatosis will reveal reticular prominence generally in the lower lung zones, if the patient has the related fibrotic lung disease. Apical bullae are often present even if inapparent in radiographs. CT can help to distinguish a cutaneous neurofibroma from an intrathoracic nodule, if this cannot be accomplished via cutaneous marker or chest fluoroscopy, and can characterize any mass visible or suspected radiographically. A neurofibroma typically has lower attenuation than muscle, in the range 15 to 30 HU.

Suggested Reading

Berrocal T, Madrid C, Novo S, et al. Congenital anomalies of the tracheobronchial tree, lung, and mediastinum: embryology, radiology, and pathology. *Radiographics*. 2004;24(1):e17.

Lee EY, Boiselle PM, Cleveland RH. Multidetector CT evaluation of congenital lung anomalies. *Radiology*. 2008;247:632-648.

QUESTIONS AND ANSWERS

1. Regarding intralobar bronchopulmonary sequestration, which of the following is *true*?
   A. Intralobar sequestration has normal venous return but abnormal arterial supply.
   B. A left-to-right shunt is created.
   C. Swyer-James syndrome is a form of intralobar sequestration.
   D. The most common site of intralobar sequestration is right lower lobe superior segment.

   ANSWER: A. Intralobar sequestration is invested in the normal pleura and has normal venous return to pulmonary veins, but abnormal systemic arterial supply, thus creating a left-to-left shunt. Swyer-James syndrome is a syndrome of obstructive bronchiolitis. The most common site of intralobar sequestration is the posterior segment of the left lower lobe in two-thirds of cases.

2. Regarding foregut cysts, which of the following is *true*?
   A. Paratracheal bronchogenic cysts are typically symptomatic.
   B. Typically multiloculated.
   C. Esophageal cysts develop from abnormal tracheobronchial budding.
   D. Enteric cysts are associated with spinal defects.

   ANSWER: D. Paratracheal bronchogenic cysts are typically asymptomatic but can sometimes cause pressure effects on adjacent structures. All foregut cysts are typically uniloculated and single. Esophageal cysts develop from a failure of complete esophageal canalization. In enteric cysts, foregut is herniated through the notochord; it is often associated with spinal defects.

3. Regarding cystic adenomatoid malformation, which of the following is *true*?
   A. Cysts do not communicate with normal airways.
   B. Arterial supply is via pulmonary arteries.
   C. Type III is the most common.
   D. Most cases are asymptomatic.

   ANSWER: B. Cysts generally do communicate with normal airways. Most of the time the arterial supply is via pulmonary arteries, though sometimes the supply is systemic. Type I, cystic, is most common at 50% of cases. Type II is mixed solid and small cysts at 40% of cases; type III is grossly solid, but the least common type, approximately 10% of cases. Most cases are discovered before 5 years of age, and over half before 1 month of life caused by cough, fever, recurrent infection, or respiratory distress because of cyst enlargement.

4. Bronchial atresia is associated with which of the following?
   A. Atretic segment leads to focal lung collapse
   B. Most common radiographic finding is a hilar mass
   C. Apicoposterior segment of the left upper lobe is most commonly affected
   D. Defect is thought to be caused by intramural obstruction, likely cartilage collapse

   ANSWER: C. The atretic segment supplies an otherwise normal lung; hence, the alveoli of that segment are able to fill via collateral pathways. The affected parenchyma is actually generally overinflated. The most common finding is a regional pulmonary lucency, visible in 90% of cases. The presence of a hilar mass is also common, though at 80%. The apicoposterior segment of the left upper lobe is most commonly affected. The defect is thought to be due to either disconnection but subsequent normal development of a bronchial bud, or a localized intrauterine bronchial–arterial disruption leading to wall ischemia and luminal obliteration.

5. Regarding proximal interruption of the pulmonary artery, which of the following is *true*?
   A. Pulmonary arteries in the lung are generally normal.
   B. Interrupted vessel is more commonly left sided.
   C. Right-sided interruption is usually accompanied by serious heart disease.
   D. Proximal interruption and Swyer-James syndrome are indistinguishable in V-Q imaging.

   ANSWER: A. The pulmonary arteries distal to the interruption are generally normal, though their blood supply is via systemic collateral arteries. The interrupted vessel is more commonly right sided, and left-sided interruption is often associated with other heart disease, particularly tetralogy of Fallot. Proximal interruption will result in absent perfusion (because its blood supply is systemic) but normal ventilation; in Swyer-James syndrome both ventilation and perfusion are typically abnormal.

6. Which of the following is *not* a component of the hypogenetic lung syndrome?
   A. Right isomerism
   B. Pulmonary artery hypoplasia
   C. Systemic supply to lung tissue
   D. Normal venous drainage

ANSWER: D. Hypogenetic lung syndrome is composed of pulmonary hypoplasia, pulmonary arterial hypoplasia with systemic arterial supply to all or part of the lung, right isomerism, diverticula, and other cardiovascular anomalies, most commonly ASD. The venous drainage is distinctly abnormal, with the large draining vein visible as a scimitar-shaped opacity leading below the diaphragm.

7. A patient has ectopia lentis, arachnodactyly, and an aortic aneurysm. Which of the following is the most likely diagnosis?
   A. Ehlers-Danlos syndrome
   B. Cutis laxa
   C. Marfan syndrome
   D. Pseudoxanthoma elasticum

   ANSWER: C. Ehlers-Danlos syndrome is a disorder of connective tissues, with type IV caused by a deficiency of type III procollagen resulting in emphysema, tracheobronchomegaly, and pulmonary artery rupture. Cutis laxa is a recessive disorder characterized by loose skin and connective tissue, with panacinar emphysema, tracheobronchomegaly, bronchiectasis, and aortic aneurysm. Marfan syndrome is characterized by arachnodactyly, ectopia lentis, aortic disease, aortic and mitral valve insufficiency, and in the lungs apical bullae, diffuse emphysema, bronchiectasis, upper lobe fibrosis, and spontaneous pneumothorax. Pseudoxanthoma elasticum is reported to have caused pulmonary vascular damage in a single patient.

8. Regarding LAM, which of the following is *true*?
   A. Smooth muscle proliferation leads to airway and vascular obstruction.
   B. Like tuberous sclerosis, the process has a male predominance.
   C. HRCT reveals the most common abnormality to be nodules of smooth muscle.
   D. It is indistinguishable from Langerhans cell histiocytosis.

   ANSWER: A. Smooth muscle proliferation in peribronchovascular tissues leads to airway and vascular obstruction and cyst formation. It has several pulmonary manifestations in common with tuberous sclerosis, but it occurs only in women. HRCT reveals the most common abnormality to be thin-walled cysts, with the size of the cysts indicative of disease severity, with nodules only rarely visible. It can be distinguished from Langerhans cell histiocytosis because LAM is a uniform or basilar-predominant disease characterized by cysts but only rare nodules and LCH is an upper lobe predominant disease with frequent nodule formation.

9. Regarding tuberous sclerosis, which of the following is *true*?
   A. Recessive trait
   B. Classic triad of mental retardation, epilepsy, and nodular lung disease
   C. Characterized by abnormal mesoderm development
   D. It usually affects men in contrast to LAM.

   ANSWER: C. Tuberous sclerosis is an autosomal dominant trait affecting both men and women, and its classic triad is mental retardation, epilepsy, and adenoma sebaceum. It is characterized by abnormal mesoderm development leading to retinal phacoma, renal angiomyolipoma, cardiac rhabdomyoma, dense bone lesions, and subungual fibromas. Lung disease occurs in less than 2.5% of patients.

10. Regarding neurofibromatosis type I, which of the following is *true*?
    A. Most common fatal inheritable disorder.
    B. Patients develop CNS tumors.
    C. Interstitial fibrosis is a sine qua non of the disease.
    D. Intercostal neurofibromas typically produce geographic bone destruction.

    ANSWER: B. Neurofibromatosis type I is common, with a frequency of 1:3000, but cystic fibrosis is slightly more common. Patients develop CNS gliomas, meningiomas, peripheral nerve sarcomas, pheochromocytomas, and angiosarcomas, in addition to the characteristic cutaneous café-au-lait spots and peripheral neurofibromas. Interstitial fibrosis occurs in 5%–10% of patients, caused by an interstitial pneumonitis. Intercostal neurofibromas are benign neoplasms that grow slowly and cause benign-appearing bone remodeling.

19 AIRWAY DISEASES

John C. Texada and Satinder P. Singh

UPPER AIRWAY OBSTRUCTION

ACUTE UPPER AIRWAY OBSTRUCTION

Acute upper airway obstruction occurs most often in infants and children because of small and compliant airways. Acute dyspnea may be accompanied by stridor.

INFECTION

Acute pharyngitis and tonsillitis are most commonly caused by beta-hemolytic streptococci. Rarely this may cause life-threatening obstruction, particularly with Epstein-Barr virus–related mononucleosis. Acute laryngotracheitis is acute narrowing of the subglottic trachea, caused by parainfluenza or respiratory syncytial virus. Acute bacterial tracheitis is a rare but potentially life-threatening process; if caused by *Corynebacterium pseudodiphtheriticum,* it may become necrotizing. Acute epiglottitis is most often caused by *Haemophilus influenzae*, sometimes by *Staphylococcus aureus* or *Streptococcus pneumoniae*; the epiglottis, aryepiglottic folds, arytenoids, and prevertebral tissues swell. Acute retropharyngeal abscess can obstruct the airway and can extend into the mediastinum. In immunosuppressed patients, a necrotizing pseudomembranous tracheobronchitis can develop from *Aspergillus* infection.

Edema

Edema typically affects the larynx. Its causes include trauma, irritant inhalation, and angioneurotic edema. Smoke inhalation may produce enough edema to cause upper airway obstruction, as may scalding by drinking something too hot. Angioneurotic edema may be the most common cause of acute upper airway obstruction. It may be hereditary, as an adverse effect of (ACE) angio tensin converting enzyme-inhibitor therapy, or result from anaphylaxis. It is accompanied by pruritic facial, genital, and extremity swelling and sometimes urticaria. Acute reactions are mast cell reactions; subacute reactions are immune-complex reactions. If caused by ACE-I therapy, angioneurotic edema may be immediate or after prolonged use. The hereditary form is due to absence or abnormal function of C1-esterase inhibitor; resulting C1 increase leads to decreased C2 and C4.

Retropharyngeal Hemorrhage

Retropharyngeal hemorrhage may be caused by neck surgery, trauma, catheter malposition, or infectious erosion. It may be spontaneous in hematologic disorder or coagulopathy patients.

Foreign Body Aspiration

Foreign body aspiration is most often in infants and children and more commonly involves the esophagus and bronchi than the upper airway. Peanuts, coins, toys, and screws are common offenders in children; candies are hyperosmolar and can produce severe edema as they melt. Meat and bones are the most common offenders in adults. Preexisting pharyngeal disorders increase the risk of aspiration.

Faulty Intubation

Faulty intubation is more common when performed emergently. The tube should be 3 to 7 cm from the carina with neutral neck positioning. In obstruction, typically the tube enters the right main stem bronchus, and the cuff occludes the left bronchus; further down the right bronchus, the right upper lobe can be excluded as well. Collapse may take 24 hours if the lung contains air, but only a few minutes if 100% oxygen is present.

CHRONIC UPPER AIRWAY OBSTRUCTION

Dyspnea is a common symptom. Occasionally it is severe enough to result in sleep disturbance or cor pulmonale. Fixed obstruction occurs when the airway cross-sectional area does not change with changing pressures. Variable obstruction occurs when airways respond to changing pressure by changing dimensions. Intrathoracic variable obstruction leads to decreasing cross-sectional area with forced expiration and extrathoracic variable obstruction leads to decreasing cross-sectional area with forced inspiration. The most common causes of chronic upper airway obstruction are tonsillar and adenoidal hypertrophy, goiter, vocal cord paralysis, tracheal stenosis, and neoplastic disruption. Tracheomalacia may play a role in some cases.

Laryngeal Dysfunction

In inspiration, the posterior cricoarytenoid muscle dilates the larynx in expiration, sometimes the thyroarytenoid and lateral cricoarytenoid muscles narrow it. Posterior cricoarytenoid muscle paralysis leads to fixed upper airway obstruction and unopposed adductor action leads to laryngospasm. Infants may develop upper airway obstruction from laryngeal hypotonia, laryngeal hypoplasia, cleft larynx, or vocal cord paralysis. Adults may develop unopposed adductor action, sometimes via superior laryngeal nerve disruption at thyroidectomy.

Tracheal Stenosis

The extrathoracic trachea enlarges with Valsalva maneuver and decreases with Mueller maneuver (inspiration against closed upper airway). The intrathoracic trachea does not change with lung pressures but does change in proportion with lung volume. The most common etiology of stenosis is as a complication of intubation or tracheotomy: at the stoma of a tracheostomy; at the cuff; or where the tip of the tube contacts the mucosa.

Tracheal Neoplasm

Tracheal neoplasms are rare; squamous cell is responsible in the majority. Tracheal carcinoma is four times more common in men than women. Adenoid cystic carcinoma has no sex predilection. Rarely, lymphoma, leukemia, soft-tissue neoplasms, or metastasis may occur.

Other Causes of Tracheal Stenosis

A saber-sheath trachea is transversely narrowed and anteroposteriorly expanded. The entire intrathoracic trachea is narrowed, with normal extrathoracic trachea. It is more common in chronic obstructive pulmonary disease (COPD) patients than in those without and may be due to hyperinflation. Relapsing polychondritis is an uncommon autoimmune cartilage disorder affecting airway rings focally, multiply, or diffusely. The airway may become fixed-narrowed or flaccid. Relapsing polychondritis typically does not involve the membranous trachea and is commonly due to degeneration. Small nodules give affected airways a beaded appearance. In the rare disorder tracheobronchopathia osteochondroplastica cartilage and bone develop in tracheal and bronchial submucosa; this is most common in men older than 50 years. Tracheobronchomalacia is a result of cartilage weakness leading to easy collapse, most often caused by tracheal pressure necrosis from a variety of causes but occasionally primary in children. In tracheobronchomegaly, the muscular and elastic tissues are thinned and atrophied, and dilation may extend into peripheral lung tissues. It is most commonly diagnosed in young men. Its etiology is unclear. It may be acquired in patients with pulmonary fibrosis or ankylosing spondylitis.

RADIOGRAPHIC FINDINGS—UPPER AIRWAY OBSTRUCTION

Radiography plays a limited role. Lateral neck imaging excludes epiglottitis, retropharyngeal abscess, or foreign body. The upper airways are often poorly evaluated in the chest radiograph. A tracheal tumor may be visible as intraluminal nodules or as tracheal wall thickening with luminal narrowing. Relapsing polychondritis may be visible as diffuse tracheobronchial narrowing. Tracheobronchopathia osteochondroplastica commonly is seen as speckled calcification of the trachea and bronchi, better appreciated on lateral view. In tracheobronchomalacia and tracheobronchomegaly, radiography will reveal inspiratory airway dilation and premature expiratory collapse. In tracheobronchomegaly, the airways may appear corrugated owing to protruding tissues between the rings. Pulmonary edema rarely develops but indicates the presence of very negative inspiratory pressures. Cardiac enlargement suggests cor pulmonale, the result of chronic pulmonary-arterial hypertension caused by hypoxemia and acidosis.

CT AND MR FINDINGS

Planar imaging defines location and extent of disease, and any mediastinal involvement. Laryngeal paralysis may be assessed. Goiter may be clearly visible. Benign tracheal tumors such as schwannoma, leiomyoma, or neurofibroma are well-defined sessile or polypoid nodules 2 cm or less, and not extending out of the tracheal wall. Tracheal malignancies cause focal or circumferential narrowing or flat or polypoid mass, sometimes with extratracheal extension, lymphadenopathy, pulmonary nodules, or fistula. Saber-sheath trachea has the expected coronal narrowing and sagittal extension described earlier in the chapter. Relapsing polychondritis will be manifest by mild tracheobronchial circumferential thickening that may be single, multiple, or diffuse. Tracheobronchopathia osteochondroplastica is evident as nodular tracheobronchial thickening resulting in irregular narrowing, with nodular calcification often visible. Tracheobronchomalacia and tracheobronchomegaly will be visible as airways dilate with inspiration and collapse with expiration in dynamic CT. In the latter, the dilation may extend into the peripheral lung parenchyma and the large airways may appear corrugated because of tracheal diverticulosis.

OBSTRUCTIVE SLEEP APNEA

Obstructive apnea is characterized by complete closure of the upper airway for at least 10 seconds per event despite respiratory effort, present in 1% to 10% of the population. Most patients are male. The greatest risk factor for obstructive sleep apnea is obesity, particularly central or visceral obesity. Numerous neurologic, metabolic, musculoskeletal, or other factors are considered risks—anything which may decrease respiratory awareness, muscle strength, or physical ability to breathe. Family history; lower vital capacity; and the use of tobacco, alcohol, sedatives, antihistamines, or certain other drugs increase the risk. Risk also increases with advancing age.

PATHOGENESIS

Obstructive sleep apnea is caused by loss of normal upper airway muscle tone superimposed on underlying upper airway narrowing. It is likely due to a combination of anatomically narrowed airway, collapsible airway, decreased neural drive for pharyngeal abduction, decreased chemoreceptor stimulation, and uncoordinated upper airway muscular activation. Typically the soft palate gets sucked into and obstructs the hypopharynx. Neck adipose tissue is an important factor, and neck circumference is a clinically useful measurement. A structural abnormality may be readily apparent (enlarged adenoids and tonsils, macroglossia, or retro-/micrognathia) or more subtle, such as small posterior placed mandible, narrow posterior airway, inferiorly placed hyoid bone, or enlarged tongue and soft palate. Patients with obstructive sleep apnea typically have unstable collapsible pharyngeal airways. Once the airway closes, it is more difficult to reopen because of surface adhesion. Sleep deprivation and hypoxia lead to depression of normal phasic respiratory muscle activity in the pharyngeal muscles that work to dilate and stiffen the larynx.

IMAGING FINDINGS

Imaging plays a limited role. Many changes are dynamic. Lateral neck soft-tissue radiography may reveal pharyngeal or craniofacial abnormalities. CT or MR may characterize the bones and soft tissues, including airway dimensions, which is particularly helpful for surgical planning.

ASTHMA

Asthma is characterized by intermittent variable airway narrowing with airway hyperreactivity and inflammation and may lead to permanent fixed obstruction. It may be extrinsic (associated with atopy) or intrinsic. Patients with extrinsic asthma have elevated IgE levels, are more commonly male, and are typically less than 20 years old. Those with intrinsic asthma are older, are more often female, and are at increased risk of autoimmune disease and aspirin sensitivity, and they tend to respond worse to therapy. The prevalence of childhood asthma ranges from 1% to 20% and appears to be increasing. The most important factors are atopy, cigarette smoke exposure, and perhaps childhood bronchiolitis. Asthma has a genetic component, but it does not have a simple inheritance pattern.

PATHOGENESIS

There is airway wall connective tissue deposition and bronchial vascular hyperplasia. The airways and basement membranes are thickened, the soft tissues are edematous and hypervascular, and there is inflammatory cell infiltration. Elastin is degraded and smooth muscle is increased. Inflammatory polyps may form. Cellular and histamine-mediated inflammation play a major role and prostaglandin response is abnormal. Secretions produced in asthma attacks are thicker and more mucoid than normal. In addition, mucociliary clearance is slower than normal even in stable asthma. Nonspecific bronchial responsiveness is increased.

CLINICOPATHOLOGIC FINDINGS

Symptoms in controlled patients include isolated cough, caused by epithelial irritant receptor stimulation, or wheeze. There are early and late (1–8 hours) components to asthma attacks; though the physiology is similar, peripheral airway changes are more prominent late. Beta-adrenergic agonists may block the early response but are less effective for late response; corticosteroids are ineffective in early response but ameliorate the late response. Nighttime symptoms are due to a variety of causes including smaller airway caliber and abnormal inflammatory increases.

Complications are more common in children and include pneumonia, atelectasis, mucoid impaction and mucus plugging, pneumomediastinum, and arterial air embolism. Response to the first 6 hours of therapy can predict recovery time. Severe disease may require intubation; approximately 40% are subsequently extubated within 24 hours and 70% within 72 hours. Mortality for asthmatic patients requiring mechanical ventilation averages 13%.

SEVERITY CATEGORIES

Intermittent asthma means symptoms less than once a week, with brief exacerbations and less than two episodes of nighttime asthma per month. Lung function is normal (greater than 80% of predicted) between exacerbations. Mild persistent asthma means symptoms less than once per day and nighttime symptoms over twice per month, with exacerbations that may affect activity and sleep. Peak expiratory flow (PEF) or forced expiratory volume in 1 second (FEV-1) is normal, but variability is increased (20%–30%). Moderate persistent asthma means daily symptoms and nighttime asthma means symptoms once per week, with exacerbations affecting activity and sleep. Patients require daily short-acting beta-2 agonists. PEF or FEV-1 is 60% to 80% of predicted and variability is greater than 30%. Severe persistent asthma means continuous symptoms with frequent nighttime asthma and frequent exacerbations, with activities limited by symptoms. PEF or FEV-1 is less than 60% of predicted and variability is greater than 30%.

PROVOKING FACTORS

Specific extrinsic triggers include pollen or fungal spores; indoor allergens include animal dander, dust mites, and cockroaches; foods, particularly eggs, fish, shellfish, nuts, spices, and chocolate. Anaphylaxis may result from drugs, particularly penicillin, stings from *Hymenoptera*, and others including contrast material. Exercise may lead to airway narrowing, the worst usually 5 to 10 minutes after exercise and resolving within an hour. Viral upper respiratory infection and mycoplasma infection exacerbate symptoms in asthmatic patients; bacterial infection does not. Analgesic drugs particularly aspirin can provoke attacks in up to 28% of asthmatic patients. Gastroesophageal reflux may stimulate afferent pharyngoesophageal nerves or may lead to irritant aspiration. Emotional distress can trigger asthma attacks. Environmental factors include outdoor air pollution, indoor wood or gas stove, and fireplace use. Changes in pressure, temperature, and humidity have reportedly led to asthma attacks. A number of miscellaneous factors also are described: food additives; alcohol and drugs including beta-blockers, ACE inhibitors, and radiographic contrast material; perfumes and cigarette smoke; and premenstrual period.

OCCUPATIONAL ASTHMA

Occupational asthma accounts for half of occupational lung diseases. Most offending antigens are high-molecular-weight proteins, polysaccharides, or glycoproteins from living things, though some are small haptens. Cigarette smoking increases the relative risk as much as five times the normal population. The most prominent categories are animal products, grain dust, and latex. Many low-molecular-weight compounds produce symptoms similar to asthma, but may more likely be allergic. The most common of these are isocyanates used in paint, varnish, foam, plastics, adhesives, and molds.

OTHER WORKPLACE AIRWAYS DISEASES

Nonspecific occupational bronchoconstriction is characterized by work-related airway narrowing in patients who already have asthma. Reactive airways dysfunction syndrome is airway injury by acute high-concentration gaseous exposure leading to bronchial hyperresponsiveness.

RADIOGRAPHIC FINDINGS IN ASTHMA

Radiographs are often normal, even during an acute attack. Imaging serves to exclude other etiologies for symptoms and to exclude pneumothorax. The most common positive findings are hyperinflation and bronchial wall thickening. Bronchial wall thickening is visible as ring shadows or parallel linear opacities, and normally inapparent 3 to 5 mm bronchi may become visible. Radiographs may rarely reveal peripheral oligemia, central increased lung markings, and prominent hila. During an attack, the hyperinflation may be accompanied by areas of expiratory air trapping.

HRCT FINDINGS

HRCT allows quantitative evaluation. Bronchial wall thickening, bronchial luminal narrowing, bronchiectasis, air trapping, and patchy hypoattenuation may be present. The degree of abnormality correlates with disease severity; serial HRCT may document response to therapy.

CHRONIC OBSTRUCTIVE PULMONARY DISEASE

Clinical chronic bronchitis is characterized by excessive mucus production on most days for at least 3 consecutive months for not less than 2 consecutive years. Morphologic emphysema is abnormal permanent enlargement of airspaces distal to the terminal bronchioles, with wall destruction, without fibrosis. The functional description chronic obstructive pulmonary disease is persistent, largely irreversible obstruction without additional cause.

EPIDEMIOLOGY

Men are more likely to develop COPD even after controlling cigarette smoking. This is more severe in whites than non-whites. Alcoholic patients and patients with CAD have increased risk. Cigarette smoking is the largest risk factor, though only 10% to 20% of heavy smokers will develop COPD. Pipe and cigar smokers are not at as high a risk as cigarette smokers. Infants and children in the houses of smokers are at increased risk of respiratory illness and functional impairment. Air pollution in combination with cigarette smoke has additive effects. Occupational dust or fume exposure decreases lung function, though the effect is one-third to one-half that of cigarette smoking. Infection during childhood may increase the risk of COPD later, and infection in patients already with COPD may lead to more rapid decline in function. Heredity, socioeconomic factors, diet, and nutrition are factors in the development of COPD. Birth weight and weight at 1 year are risk factors for COPD development. Mucus and mucociliary clearance rate appear important. Cigarette smoke leads to delayed peripheral mucociliary clearance and heterogeneous ventilation. Leukocyte count is inversely proportional to lung function declines in smokers, nonsmokers, and former smokers alike, that is, high white blood cell count leads to greater function decline.

PROGNOSIS AND COURSE

Annual FEV-1 decline for healthy nonsmokers is 10 to 35 mL after age 30 and for smokers is 30 to 70 mL. Patients with preexisting low lung function decline more rapidly than those without. Respiratory muscle fatigue may develop due to pulmonary resistance, mechanical disadvantage, malnourishment, and possible cor pulmonale development. Patients with chronic hypoxemia may develop secondary polycythemia and hypokalemia. Resting left ventricular ejection fraction is normal in COPD patients without cor pulmonale, though exercise-induced dysfunction is common.

Prognosis is related to pulmonary vascular and right ventricular functions. Cor pulmonale may develop from long-standing pulmonary arterial hypertension. With FEV-1 more than 40% of predicted, resting pulmonary artery pressure is generally normal, but exercise leads to elevated pressure; with FEV-1 less than 40% of predicted, resting mean pulmonary artery pressure is generally more than 20 mm Hg and exercise leads to a disproportionate increase. Without therapy pulmonary artery pressure will slowly increase, at a rate correlated with loss of FEV-1. This can be prevented with chronic oxygen therapy, which has been proven to increase survival.

The mortality of acute-on-chronic respiratory failure in severe COPD is 25% per event, 50% over 1 year, and 70% over 2 years. Prognostic factors include age, PA pressure, postbronchodilator FEV-1, and percentage of ideal body weight.

EMPHYSEMA

DEVELOPMENT

There is an abnormal ratio of antielastolytic processes to elastolytic processes. Neutrophil elastase is probably the most important player, and this enzyme is increased in smokers for several reasons. Alpha-1 antitrypsin is the primary antielastolytic enzyme. It has many genetic variants, most of which lead to normal enzyme function. The phenotypes ZZ, SS, or SZ have levels much below normal and phenotypes MS and MZ have levels 60% to 80% of normal.

TABLE 19-1 Emphysema Types

Centrilobular (proximal acinar)	Most common, tobacco use, upper zone
Paraseptal (distal acinar)	Focal, peripheral
Panlobular (panacinar)	Most common nonsmokers, alpha 1- antitrypsin deficiency
Cicatricial (scar)	Most common pathologically, asymptomatic

TYPES (TABLE 19-1)

Centrilobular (proximal acinar) emphysema involves the proximal respiratory bronchioles. It is found in cigarette smokers, and is the most common form. Respiratory bronchioles dilate and alveolar septa disappear; eventually several respiratory bronchioles become confluent into a single space supplied by a terminal bronchiole, leading to relatively normal alveoli. Eventually these spaces become confluent as well. It is upper-zone predominant and heterogeneous.

Paraseptal (distal acinar) emphysema involves alveolar ducts and alveoli. It is usually focal and peripheral, and may be postinflammatory. Bullae may develop from alveolar destruction. It typically has limited extent and is asymptomatic save for occasional spontaneous pneumothorax.

Panlobular (panacinar) emphysema involves the entire acinus. This is the most common form of emphysema in nonsmokers, associated with alpha-1 antitrypsin deficiency. In severe disease the tissue may be composed only of airspaces with traversing strands of tissue and vessels. The process is lower- and anterior-zone predominant.

Cicatricial (scar) emphysema is not localized to a particular acinar site. It is fibrotic and likely postinflammatory. It is the most common form pathologically but is limited in extent and generally asymptomatic.

PATHOLOGIC FINDINGS

Tracheobronchial gland volume is correlated with degree of mucus production. Small-airway resistance increases. Emphysema is present (see the types given earlier). Larger airspaces have lower elasticity and eventually large airspaces contain essentially trapped gas. Increased vascular resistance is a product of simple vessel loss, hypoxic smooth muscle contraction, and vascular mural thickening. With severe COPD and emphysema the bronchial and pulmonary arteries will anastomose extensively.

RADIOGRAPHIC FINDINGS

Chronic bronchitis is not a radiologic diagnosis, but imaging can suggest its presence. Bronchial wall thickening may be visible as ring shadows, parallel densities, or prominent markings. Emphysema bullae and irregular lucency can be visible with very thin walls. In most cases, the findings are of hyperinflation or vascular changes: diaphragmatic flattening or concavity, increased retrosternal airspace, and increased lung height; avascular areas: vessel distortion, increased angle of branching, decreased peripheral vascularity, and hilar arterial prominence.

CT FINDINGS

HRCT detects bronchial wall thickening with greater sensitivity. In emphysema, areas of low attenuation will be present, with walls 1 mm or less thick. Centrilobular emphysema will have multiple small areas of low attenuation, typically diffuse but sometimes upper-zone predominant. Panlobular emphysema will be visible as lower-lobe predominant hypoattenuation with few vessels, sometimes with bronchiectasis. Paraseptal emphysema will be visible as subpleural hypoattenuation with intact interlobular septa. CT findings correlate well with severity of disease.

ALPHA-1 ANTITRYPSIN DEFICIENCY

Alpha-1 antitrypsin is an acute-phase reactant. It is produced mainly by the liver. There are more than 70 genetic variants. The M variant is by far the most common allele. Other variants are far less common, ranging from 0.1% to 6%. The Z variant is an autosomal recessive allele that has deficient antiproteolytic function and aggregates within the cell that produces it. ZZ homozygotes produce levels approximately 20% of normal and heterozygotes approximately 60%. The ZZ genotype is found in 1:1500 to 1:5000 births; approximately 50% to 80% of patients will develop basilar-predominant emphysema. Smoking of course increases the risk, rate, and severity—annual decline in FEV-1 is 80 mL for nonsmokers and 317 mL for smokers.

BULLOUS DISEASE

A bulla is a well-defined airspace, 1 cm or larger, with a smooth wall 1-mm thick or less, and with or without internal septa. The walls are composed of pleura, connective tissue septa, or compressed parenchyma. It may be idiopathic or associated with emphysema or prior infection. Primary disease has a familial tendency, and is increased in patients with connective tissue disorders. It is typically asymptomatic, though spontaneous pneumothorax may occur. Bullectomy may allow a healthy lung to reinflate into the space occupied by the bulla.

Vanishing lung syndrome or giant bullous emphysema is a distinct progressive clinical syndrome, characterized by large bullae in the upper lobes, often unilateral or asymmetric, often seen in young men, and mostly seen in smokers. It is often associated with several types of emphysema. The radiographic criteria for this syndrome include presence of giant bullae in one or both upper lobes, occupying at least one-third of the hemithorax and compressing the normal surrounding lung. Bullae can vary in size from 1 to 20 cm in diameter. Palliative bullectomy is often required and HRCT often is required preoperatively to determine the extent of disease and to determine the presence and severity of associated emphysema.

RADIOGRAPHIC FINDINGS

Bullae are often inapparent but may be visible as thin-walled, well-defined avascular areas. The walls are very thin and may be obscured. Large bullae may create areas of compressive atelectasis. Bullae consistently slowly enlarge with serial radiography. The presence of an air-fluid level within a bulla indicates infection, often with surrounding pneumonitis, but may be due to hemorrhage or cancer formation. Pneumothorax may develop.

CT FINDINGS

Bullae are more easily visible, and CT can define the pulmonary anatomy, lung compression, and extent of emphysema as well as help in volume calculations. CT can help to clarify whether a large airspace is a pneumothorax or a bulla, if there is doubt.

OTHER CAUSES OF EMPHYSEMA

Swyer-James syndrome may lead to emphysema. Intravenous talcosis and hypocomplementemic urticarial vasculitis produce panlobular emphysema. HIV may cause emphysema.

CYSTIC FIBROSIS

EPIDEMIOLOGY AND ASSOCIATED FINDINGS

Cystic fibrosis (CF) is the most common lethal genetic disease among patients of European descent, occurring in 1:2000 to 1:3500 births and usually diagnosed before age 5. The vas deferens may be absent; cervical mucus abnormalities in affected women also affect fertility. Ten to fifteen percent of patients will have meconium ileus obstruction as neonates, and patients may also have distal obstruction that is due to abnormal gastrointestinal fluid transport. Rectal prolapse occurs in up to one-fifth of untreated patients before age 5. Esophageal dysfunction and gastroesophageal reflux disease (GERD) are common. Hepatic steatosis and biliary cirrhosis may develop, the latter in up to 30% of patients. Gallbladder dysfunction is common. Pancreatic enzyme deficiency occurs in 90% of patients, because of duct obstruction and exocrine atrophy, and they may occasionally have acute pancreatitis.

PULMONARY SYMPTOMS AND SIGNS

Patients have recurrent chest infections and wheeze, dyspnea, productive cough, and hemoptysis. Visceral problems lead to malnutrition and hypoproteinemia. Hemoptysis is generally small but may be massive, because of bronchial-arterial hyperplasia in ectatic airways. Patients are more likely to have atopy or asthma, and often have chronic sinusitis and polyposis but infrequent symptoms. Allergic bronchopulmonary aspergillosis is more common as well.

ETIOLOGY AND PATHOGENESIS

Immune response is normal, but defense is defective because of abnormal mucociliary transport, so the long-term presence of inflammatory mediators contributes to bronchiectasis. It is due to a defect in the cystic fibrosis transmembrane receptor, a cAMP-regulated chloride channel in epithelial cells and tracheobronchial glands. In CF patients, sweat contains elevated sodium, potassium, and chloride. Pancreatic secretions become electrolyte deficient, particularly bicarbonate; major salivary gland output is normal but the products of the minor salivary glands contain elevated electrolytes (these are similar to sweat glands). Mucus contains increased glycoproteins and products of cell breakdown including DNA, and may have a factor that inhibits cilia. Respiratory infection or chronic colonization, particularly by *Pseudomonas aeruginosa* and increasingly by *Burkholderia cepacia*, increases respiratory decline.

RADIOGRAPHIC AND HRCT FINDINGS

The earliest manifestations are small subpleural opacities; thickened bronchi, hyperinflation, and hilar lymphadenopathy are less common. With progression, the bronchi and bronchial walls become larger, lung volume increases, and the peripheral opacities increase. Bronchiectasis, bronchial thickening, and mucus plugging are present in 90% to 100% of cases; cyst-like spaces visible in 25% to 30% of adults. Bronchiectasis is often diffuse but upper-zone predominant. Hilar enlargement, tracheal dilation, pneumothorax, and pneumomediastinum may develop. HRCT is the method of choice for evaluation of bronchiectasis and is particularly useful for evaluating early peripheral involvement (manifest as tree-in-bud centrilobular nodules). It is more sensitive than radiography especially for mild disease.

BRONCHIOLITIS

Bronchiolitis is inflammation of membranous and respiratory bronchioles. Radiology correlates better with histology than with etiology. It may be classified by the type of inflammation (acute or chronic) and by the type of fibrosis—called obliterative bronchiolitis when narrowing is concentric and epithelium is intact—or bronchiolitis obliterans–organizing pneumonia (BOOP) when granulation or fibroblastic tissue extends from areas of epithelial damage to narrow or obstruct the airway.

RADIOGRAPHIC FINDINGS

Radiographic findings depend on the extent of disease, chronicity, and underlying abnormality, and radiographic severity does not correlate with clinical severity. The radiographic patterns are typically limited to two categories. Hyperinflation and peripheral vascular attenuation are visible with obliterative bronchiolitis, and alveolar consolidation is visible with BOOP. Other findings of peribronchial wall thickening, perihilar linear opacities, and atelectasis are less reproducible.

HRCT FINDINGS

HRCT provides greater anatomic detail, such that this modality can suggest the histology of the process. HRCT may image several patterns of disease.

Centrilobular nodules and branching lines are due to thickening of bronchiolar walls and filling of the bronchioles with pus, mucus, or granulation tissue. This is characteristic of acute infectious bronchiolitis or diffuse panbronchiolitis, and may be accompanied by scattered ground glass or consolidation. The nodules of respiratory bronchiolitis (RB) are poorly defined, whereas the nodules of infectious bronchiolitis and panbronchiolitis are well defined.

Mosaic attenuation is due to airway closure and air trapping, with hypoxemic vasoconstriction. It is present in patients with obliterative bronchiolitis, extrinsic allergic alveolitis, asthma and bronchiectasis, and in patients with primary-vascular processes such as chronic PTE.

Consolidation is visible in BOOP, often patchy and random, because of organizing pneumonia. Centrilobular opacities may be present: granulation tissue or peribronchiolar consolidation.

Ground glass attenuation associated with respiratory bronchiolitis (RB), and RB is associated with interstitial lung disease (ILD), extrinsic allergic alveolitis, and BOOP. In RB, ground glass attenuation is bilateral and patchy or diffuse, and tends to be an upper-lung process. In extrinsic allergic alveolitis, extensive bilateral ground glass attenuation is accompanied by poorly defined centrilobular nodules, often with areas of air trapping.

ACUTE BRONCHIOLITIS

Infectious bronchiolitis is typically due to *Mycoplasma pneumoniae*, *Chlamydia* species, or viruses, most common in young children. Imaging findings include hyperinflation, reticulonodular opacities, and areas of consolidation and atelectasis. HRCT reveals centrilobular nodules or lines and focal consolidation. Noninfectious bronchiolitis may be due to acute exposure to smoke, sulfur dioxide, nitrogen oxides, or other agents. After 2 to 5 weeks, obliterative bronchiolitis develops.

CHRONIC BRONCHIOLITIS

Chronic bronchiolitis may be associated with connective tissue disease, particularly rheumatoid arthritis. Rheumatoid arthritis may lead to obliterative, follicular, lymphocytic, BOOP, or diffuse panbronchiolitis. In Sjögren syndrome, lymphocytic or follicular bronchiolitis is most common. Obliterative bronchiolitis may complicate marrow, lung, and heart-lung transplant. Swyer-James syndrome is characterized radiographically by hyperlucent lobe or lung with reduced inspiratory volume and expiratory air trapping. It is the result of decreased blood flow after bronchiolar obliteration, likely by the progression of acute viral bronchiolitis to fibrous airway obliteration.

BRONCHIOLITIS OBLITERANS–ORGANIZING PNEUMONIA (CRYPTOGENIC-ORGANIZING PNEUMONIA)

BOOP usually is subacute, progressing over several months. The process may completely resolve after corticosteroid therapy. BOOP is typically patchy, characterized by loose connective tissue plugs in distal airways and alveoli; chronic inflammation or interstitial fibrosis may be present.

Patchy airspace consolidation is the most common radiographic finding. Opacities are typically pleural based and peripheral, ranging from 3 cm to entire lobes, and can be migratory. They have indistinct margins and may contain air bronchograms. The differential considerations for this presentation include chronic eosinophilic pneumonia, bronchioloalveolar carcinoma, lymphoma, pulmonary alveolar proteinosis, and hemorrhage. Reticular or reticulonodular opacities may be isolated or associated with airspace disease. Unifocal consolidation is unusual; the differential consideration then is lung cancer, and the etiology may be unknown until after resection. Large nodules may simulate metastasis. In HRCT, most patients will have consolidation, small nodules, or both. Peripheral reticulation and ground glass opacities are less often visible.

RESPIRATORY BRONCHIOLITIS

RB is due to cigarette smoking, associated with macrophage deposition in respiratory bronchioles and alveoli, and inflammatory thickening of respiratory bronchial walls. It is called RB with ILD when symptoms are associated with added radiopathologic findings. It responds well to smoking cessation and to corticosteroids.

In simple RB, poorly defined centrilobular nodules or ground glass opacities may be diffuse or may be predominantly upper lobar; with RB-ILD ground glass opacities may be associated with fine reticular or reticulonodular opacities, with normal lung volumes.

FOLLICULAR BRONCHIOLITIS

Lymphoid tissue with prominent germinal centers develops in bronchiolar and bronchial walls, a nonspecific process found in connective tissue diseases (especially Sjögren syndrome and rheumatoid arthritis), immunodeficiency states, hypersensitivities, or infections by *M. pneumoniae* or viruses.

Diffuse reticulonodular disease will be present. Nodular opacities typically ranging from 1 to 3 mm but sometimes as large as 2 cm are mainly peribronchovascular or subpleural. Centrilobular branching opacities, bronchial thickening, and occasionally patchy hypoattenuation are present.

DIFFUSE PANBRONCHIOLITIS

Diffuse panbronchiolitis has unknown etiology but leads to chronic paranasal sinus and respiratory-bronchiolar inflammation. It responds to chronic erythromycin treatment. Most patients are 30 to 60 years old and commonly male. It may have an HLA association with a haplotype most common in Asia.

Diffuse nodules less than 5 mm are present, accompanied by mild-moderate hyperinflation. Small centrilobular nodules and branching lines, bronchiolectasis and bronchiectasis, and mosaic attenuation are present. Large cystic spaces may develop.

BRONCHIAL DISEASES

BRONCHIECTASIS

Bronchiectasis is irreversible bronchial dilation. The common factors are infection, obstruction, and peribronchial fibrosis. Inflammatory factors lead to proteolytic enzyme release. A dilated airway is commonly colonized and chronic inflammation continues the process. Chronic airway obstruction leads to mucus distension, postobstructive infection, or atelectasis, leading to radial traction. Immunologic deficiency states predispose to bronchiectasis by increasing the incidence of bronchial infection or colonization. Other causes include dyskinetic cilia syndrome, Williams-Campbell syndrome of airway cartilage deficiency leading to fourth- through sixth-generation airway bronchiectasis, and Mounier-Kuhn syndrome of tracheobronchomegaly that is due to decreased elastin and smooth muscle. Other causes are variable: measles, pertussis, latent viral infection, congenital abnormality, noxious inhalation, or necrotizing infection.

TYPES OF BRONCHIECTASIS (TABLE 19-2)

Group I, cylindrical bronchiectasis, is characterized by regular outline and peripherally normal-caliber airways, often plugged by mucus.

Group II, varicose bronchiectasis, has greater dilation and local constrictions are characterized by irregular outlines. Peripheral bronchi are more obliterated.

Group III, saccular or cystic bronchiectasis, is characterized by bronchi that continue to dilate peripherally. A mucocele may form when one of these ballooned spaces becomes filled with mucus.

TABLE 19-2 Bronchiectasis

Group I	Cylindrical
Group II	Varicose
Group III	Saccular (cystic)

RADIOGRAPHIC AND HRCT FINDINGS

The radiograph is often normal in milder disease. Parallel line opacities are due to thickened bronchial walls. Tubular opacities represent mucus-filled bronchi. Ring opacities or cystic spaces may be up to 2 cm diameter, and may contain fluid or air-fluid levels. Focal fibrosis and volume loss may occur. Oligemia may result from hypoxic vasoconstriction in severely diseased areas. The uninvolved lung may be hyperinflated.

HRCT is more sensitive and specific than radiography. There will be internal bronchial diameter greater than the adjacent pulmonary artery, lack of bronchial tapering, bronchial visualization within 1 cm of the costal pleura or abutting the mediastinal pleura, or bronchial wall thickening. Other findings such as tracheomegaly or lymphadenopathy may be better appreciated.

BRONCHOLITHIASIS

Irregular calcified or ossified material lies within the tracheobronchial lumen, ranging from submillimeter to large in size. The most common symptom is cough, sometimes hemoptysis. Erosion of calcified lymph node material into the airway is the most common etiology, usually from chronic necrotizing granulomatous lymphadenitis caused by *Mycobacterium tuberculosis*, *Histoplasma capsulatum* (most common in North America), or *Coccidioides immitis*. Broncholithiasis may manifest radiographically as a mobile calcific density or as airway obstruction. CT can generally image the broncholith.

BRONCHIAL FISTULAE

The principal causes of bronchial fistulae are infection and cancer; other causes are trauma, inflammation, or foreign body. The most common form is bronchopleural fistula, which may develop after cancer resection as a result of stump dehiscence. Dehiscence almost always develops within 90 days. Bronchoesophageal fistula may be congenital or acquired. Bronchovascular fistula results in hemoptysis. Bronchoabdominal fistula may develop with subphrenic abscess, colon cancer, or Crohn disease.

TOXIC EPIDERMAL NECROSIS

In toxic epidermal necrosis, a diffuse erythematous rash is followed by bulla formation, usually from staphylococcal infection or drug reaction. In the lungs, bronchial epithelial sloughing can cause obstruction.

PLASTIC BRONCHITIS

Plastic bronchitis results in the coughing up of debris shaped like the airway. It is most common with allergic bronchopulmonary aspergillosis, but may be seen with CF, bronchiectasis, pneumonia, alveolar proteinosis, and airway lymphoid hyperplasia. There is also an idiopathic form of plastic bronchitis.

OBLITERATIVE BRONCHITIS

Obliterative bronchitis is analogous to obliterative bronchiolitis and is often associated with it. When associated with bronchiolitis, the bronchial abnormalities are mild in comparison.

SUGGESTED READING

Lynch DA, Travis WD, Muller NL, et al. Idiopathic interstitial pneumonias: CT features. *Radiology.* 2005;236:10-21.

Muller NL, Miller RR. Diseases of the bronchioles: CT and histopathologic findings. *Radiology.* 1995;196:3-12.

Muller NL, Thurlbeck WM. Thin-section CT, emphysema, air trapping, and airway obstruction. *Radiology.* 1996;199:621-622.

Naidich DP, Harkin TJ. Airways and lung: correlation of CT with fiberoptic bronchoscopy. *Radiology.* 1995;197:1-12.

Ujita M, Renzoni EA, Veeraraghavan S, et al. Organizing pneumonia: perilobular pattern at thin-section CT. *Radiology.* 2004;232:757-761.

Wood BP. Cystic fibrosis. *Radiology.* 1997;204:1-10.

QUESTIONS AND ANSWERS

1. Regarding acute laryngotracheitis, which of the following is *true*?
   A. Causes narrowing of the supraglottic airway
   B. Caused by parainfluenza or respiratory syncytial virus
   C. Presence of stridor indicates mild disease.
   D. Associated with *H. influenzae*

   ANSWER: B. Acute laryngotracheitis causes acute subglottic tracheal narrowing, sometimes with a mucopurulent pseudomembrane requiring endoscopic removal. It is caused by parainfluenza or respiratory syncytial virus in many cases and the presence of stridor indicates immediate laryngeal visualization.

2. Regarding upper airway obstruction, which of the following is *true*?
   A. Extrathoracic variable obstruction leads to decreased area with forced inspiration.
   B. Extrathoracic variable obstruction leads to decreased area with forced expiration.
   C. Intrathoracic variable obstruction leads to decreased area with forced inspiration.
   D. Intrathoracic variable obstruction leads to increased area with forced expiration.

   ANSWER: A. An extrathoracic variable obstruction leads to decreased area with forced inspiration and an intrathoracic variable obstruction leads to decreased area with forced expiration.

3. Regarding Mounier-Kuhn syndrome, which of the following is *true*?
   A. Disorder of older women
   B. Characterized by thickened tracheobronchial muscular tissues
   C. Associated with Fanconi syndrome
   D. Eponym for tracheobronchomegaly

   ANSWER: D. Mounier-Kuhn syndrome is tracheobronchomegaly, found most commonly in young men. Muscular and elastic tissues are thin and atrophied. It is associated with Ehlers-Danlos, Kenny-Caffey, and Brachmann-de Lange syndromes and cutis laxa, but not Fanconi syndrome.

4. Which of the following is the greatest risk factor for the development of obstructive sleep apnea?
   A. Smoking
   B. Obesity
   C. Neurologic disorders
   D. Elevated circulating estrogens

   ANSWER: B. Smoking and some neurologic disorders increase the risk of obstructive sleep apnea, along with many other factors. However, obesity is the greatest risk factor, particularly central or visceral obesity. Some women with obstructive sleep apnea have higher androgen levels than women who do not.

5. A 6-year-old boy has wheezing and shortness of breath about once a day and frequently awakes from sleep gasping. His FEV-1 is 64% of predicted. Which of the following is the most likely diagnosis?
   A. Mild persistent asthma
   B. Moderate persistent asthma
   C. Intermittent asthma
   D. Severe persistent asthma

   ANSWER: B. This boy has moderate persistent asthma, which includes daily symptoms.

6. Regarding FEV-1 after age 30, which of the following is *true*?
   A. Healthy nonsmokers undergo annual FEV-1 decline of 30 to 70 mL.

B. Smokers undergo annual FEV-1 decline of 30 to 70 mL.
C. Smokers with PiZZ genotype undergo annual FEV-1 decline of 30 to 70 mL.
D. Nonsmokers with PiZZ genotype undergo annual FEV-1 decline of 30 to 70 mL.

ANSWER: B. Healthy nonsmokers undergo annual FEV-1 decline of 10 to 35 mL; healthy smokers, 30 to 70 mL. PiZZ nonsmokers undergo annual FEV-1 decline averages 80 mL; PiZZ smokers, 317 mL.

7. Which of the following is the type of emphysema commonly found in smokers without alpha-1-antitrypsin disorder?
A. Panlobular emphysema
B. Cicatricial emphysema
C. Paraseptal emphysema
D. Centrilobular emphysema

ANSWER: D. Panlobular emphysema is the most common form of emphysema in nonsmokers, associated with alpha-1 antitrypsin deficiency. Cicatricial emphysema is likely postinflammatory; it is the most common form pathologically but is limited and asymptomatic. Paraseptal emphysema leads to focal peripheral bullae and occasional spontaneous pneumothorax. Centrilobular emphysema is the emphysema of cigarette smokers.

8. Regarding associations of CF, which of the following is most common?
A. Biliary cirrhosis
B. Pancreatic enzyme deficiency
C. Meconium ileus
D. Rectal prolapse

ANSWER: B. Biliary cirrhosis occurs in up to 30% of patients. Pancreatic enzyme deficiency occurs in 90% of patients. Though meconium ileus is specific for CF, it is nonsensitive; it occurs in only 10%–15% of patients. Rectal prolapse may occur in up to 20% of untreated patients by age 5.

9. Which of the following is the etiology of mosaic attenuation on HRCT of bronchiolitis?
A. Thickening of bronchiolar walls and bronchiolar filling
B. Airway closure and air trapping with resultant arterial vasoconstriction
C. Organizing infection
D. Lymphoid aggregates

ANSWER: B. Bronchiolar thickening and filling results in centrilobular nodules and lines. Airway closure and air trapping with resultant arterial vasoconstriction leads to mosaic attenuation. Organizing infection leads to alveolar consolidation. Lymphoid aggregates lead to peribronchovascular and subpleural nodular opacities.

10. Which of the following is a radiographic sign of bronchiectasis?
A. Ground glass opacities
B. Visible right upper lobe bronchus
C. Parallel line opacities
D. Diffuse hyperinflation

ANSWER: C. Signs of bronchiectasis include parallel lines, tubular or ring opacities, or cystic spaces. Segmental increased size and decreased definition of lung markings can result from fibrosis and retained secretions. Vascular markings may be crowded from volume loss. Oligemia may result from hypoxic vasoconstriction in severely diseased areas. The uninvolved lung may be hyperinflated. The right upper lobe bronchus is visible in normal patients.

20 PULMONARY INFECTION

John C. Texada and Satinder P. Singh

GENERAL FACTS

Inhaled objects greater than 5 μm deposit on the upper airways; objects less than 0.5 μm are exhaled. Objects 1 to 2 μm land in the parenchyma. Typically many bacteria are required to cause disease but in some cases (e.g., TB), a small number is enough. Pneumonia is the number one infectious cause of death in the United States. Up to 18% of surgical patients acquire pneumonia in hospital. Ventilation carries a 1% to 3% daily infection risk. Hospital-acquired pneumonia (HAP) adds 7 to 9 days to hospital stay, with 30% to 70% mortality. Community-acquired pneumonia (CAP) is bacterial in only 2% of patients not requiring hospitalization; the remaining 98% of CAP cases treated on an outpatient basis are caused by atypical agents. Of those patients with CAP serious enough to require hospitalization, 10% have a positive blood culture: *Streptococcus pneumonia* is isolated in 35% of these; anaerobes, in 20% to 35%; and *Haemophilus influenzae,* in 2% to 8%. *Legionella* causes only 2% of CAP overall, but is more frequently encountered in patients with CAP serious enough to require hospitalization. HAP is defined as pneumonia occuring more than 48 hours after hospital admission; it is often caused by aspiration and is often polymicrobial. HAP acquired early in a hospitalization is often due to gram-positive agents; HAP acquired later in a hospitalization is often due to enteric gram-negative bacteria. Ventilator-associated pneumonia may be difficult to diagnose radiographically: the air bronchogram is the only helpful sign.

In immunocompromise, agents normally of decreased virulence have high morbidity. Combined immunodeficiency (such as severe CID, ADA deficiency, or purine nucleoside phosphorylase deficiency) causes childhood death without intervention. Antibody deficiency (for example, agammaglobulinemia, IgA or IgG deficiency, or combined-variable immunodeficiency) causes recurrent pyogenic infection. Chronic granulomatous disease predisposes to catalase-positive infection. Patients with Chediak-Higashi syndrome have defective granulocyte oxidative burst, which predisposes to skin and lung disease. Disorders leading to deficient complement predispose to repeated encapsulated organism infection. The X-linked–recessive Wiskott-Aldrich syndrome (comprising thrombocytopenic purpura, eczema, and immunodeficiency) leads to abnormal cell-mediated immunity and thus recurrent infection. The autosomal-recessive syndrome ataxia-telangiectasia (comprising cerebellar ataxia, cancer, oculocutaneous telangiectasia, and sinopulmonary infection) is associated with B- and T-cell dysfunction, with mortality via bronchiectasis and interstitial pneumonitis by the third decade of life. DiGeorge syndrome comprises thymic aplasia or hypoplasia, parathyroid aplasia, and malformations of the third and fourth branchial arches.

ROUTES OF SPREAD

Infection via vessels is usually from extrapulmonary source. Bacteria may be free, within thrombus, or directly invade the vessel wall as in TB. The individual sites of blood-borne infection are nodular: with sepsis, innumerable 1 to 5 mm nodules; with septic emboli, fewer, larger, frequently cavitary nodules. Infection via direct spread occurs with chest wound, mediastinitis, or abdominal abscess. Tracheobronchial spread may be via aspiration, inhalation, or insertion of infected sources.

AIRWAY INFECTION

Mycoplasma and viruses are most common. Bronchiolitis is more dangerous than tracheobronchitis particularly in children; respiratory syncytial vims (RSV) and parainfluenza predominate. Bacterial tracheitis is uncommon, often after viral URI, but can be serious in children. *Staphylococcus aureus* and *H. influenzae* are most common. Acute bronchitis often has normal radiograph but may have bronchial dilation, wall thickening, and peribronchial inflammation. Bacterial bronchitis occurs in patients with airway disease.

AIRSPACE INFECTION

Nonsegmental (lobar) consolidation is by *Streptococcus pneumoniae* and others. Edema develops with little purulence and spreads centrally from the periphery. Radiograph reveals homogeneous demarcated consolidation. Inflammation may expand tissue and bulge fissures. After the infection is resolved, pulmonary parenchymal architecture is typically normal since it remains intact through the infection.

Bronchopneumonia is via *S. aureus*, gram negatives, or some fungi. Exudate forms with little edema, leading to patchy opacity. Ill-defined centrilobular nodules develop and coalesce. Volume loss is common. Abscess, pneumatocele, or pulmonary gangrene may occur. Bronchopneumonia is destructive, so organization or fibrosis is typical. Interstitial pneumonia is by viruses, *Mycoplasma*, and *Pneumocystis carinii*. Interstitial exudate may be lymphocytic or have alveolar damage. Radiograph has reticular-reticulonodular opacities and septal lines. Bronchiolitis causes centrilobular opacities, bronchitis, and peribronchial thickening.

Lung abscess has smooth walls less than 15 mm (cavitated cancer has shaggy thick walls). Air-fluid level is common. Anaerobes, *S. aureus,* and *Pseudomonas aeruginosa* are common. Symptoms may be mild; hemoptysis may be fatal. Pulmonary gangrene is development of necrotic lung fragments. Small lucencies in consolidation coalesce to a cavity. Most are caused by *Klebsiella pneumoniae*. Pneumatocele is a thin-walled airspace formed when check-valve obstruction allows filling of a necrotic region. *Staphylococcus aureus* is a frequent cause with *P. carinii* also in the immunocompromised.

BACTERIAL PNEUMONIA

GRAM-POSITIVE COCCI

Streptococcus pneumoniae is an encapsulated facultative anaerobe in pairs or short chains, the most commonly isolated agent, in at least 40% of cases. Aspiration from colonized nasopharynx produces lobar consolidation. Resolution takes 2 to 4 weeks with adequate therapy; abscess, pneumatocele, or gangrene is rare. Radiograph reveals homogeneous lobar or round opacity with air bronchograms. Acutely volume loss is minimal but atelectasis may develop during resolution.

Streptococcus pyogenes is beta-hemolytic and occurs in chains. Once a common cause of serious bronchopneumonia (hemorrhage and cavitary necrosis caused rapid death), it is rare now, occasionally causing superinfection or occurring in community living sites. Radiograph reveals segmental consolidation and atelectasis. Abscess and empyema are common; pneumatocele and pyopneumothorax are absent.

Staphylococcus aureus is a clustered coagulase-producing facultative anaerobe, a cause of tracheitis or bronchopneumonia, often after influenza. It causes CAP uncommonly, but 15% of HAP. Infection can be acute hemorrhagic, acute purulent, or chronic organizing. Radiograph reveals multilobar or bilateral segmental consolidation; abscess forms in 25%. Air bronchograms are absent. Pneumatocele and effusion are common, and half the latter are empyema.

GRAM-NEGATIVE COCCI

Moraxella (Branhamella, Neisseria) catarrhalis occurs in pairs, is oxidase positive and catalase positive, and is typically intracellular. It is oral flora and may cause mild pneumonia, particularly with underlying lung disease, but is typically nonbacteremic. Most are beta-lactamase positive.

Neisseria meningitidis occurs in pairs, is oxidase positive and catalase positive, and is typically intracellular. It may cause pneumonia after viral infection often in young adults in military service. It typically forms an easily treatable bronchopneumonia, though sepsis may occur.

GRAM-POSITIVE RODS

Bacillus anthracis is a large encapsulated spore former, typically causing skin or GI infection, often in livestock workers, but may cause pneumonia or sepsis. Its toxin causes edema and hemorrhage: hemorrhagic nodes and tissues and bloody effusion are common. Radiograph reveals mediastinal widening with patchy nonsegmental opacities caused by hemorrhagic edema.

Listeria monocytogenes is a short, motile facultative intracellular organism, found in soil, water, sewage, domestic animals, and human carriers. Infection typically occurs in neonates, pregnant women, immunocompromised patients, and older patients with chronic disease.

Corynebacterium species are club shaped and cause membranous pharyngitis that can extend to the larynx, but not pneumonia. *Rhodococcus equi* is a weakly acid-fast rod or coccus that causes an often cavitary pneumonia in immunocompromised hosts. It is associated with malakoplakia.

GRAM-NEGATIVE RODS

Gram-negative rods are responsible for more than 50% of ventilator-acquired pneumonia and 25% of community-acquired pneumonias (CAP) requiring hospitalization.

The Enterobacteriaceae reduce nitrate, ferment glucose, produce endotoxin, and are oxidase negative. They cause one-third of HAP, and include *Klebsiella, Enterobacter, Serratia, Escherichia coli, Salmonella, Proteus, Morganella*, and *Yersinia*. *Klebsiella pneumoniae* pneumonia occurs typically in alcoholic patients in their fifties and often has bulging fissures; abscess, cavity, gangrene, and empyema are more likely than with pneumococcus. *Serratia marcescens* causes pseudohemoptysis of red sputum. *Proteus* and *Morganella* infect those with chronic suppurative lung disease or tracheostomy. *Yersinia pestis* is the cause of plague: in pneumonia, radiograph reveals homogeneous consolidation simulating edema or ARDS, with lymphadenopathy and occasional effusion.

The fermenting non-Enterobacteriaceae are as follows. *Aeromonas* are found in water, appear in infected wounds or GI disease, and may cause fulminant pneumonia after near drowning. *Chromobacterium violaceum* is nonmotile and catalase positive, and has caused pneumonia in patients with CGD. *Pasteurella multocida* is a nonmotile pathogen typically of animals that causes pneumonia in patients with chronic lung disease. *Vibrio* species are motile aerobic bacteria, the most common bacterium in surface water but almost never a cause of lung disease.

The nonfermenting non-Enterobacteriaceae include *Burkholderia* and *Pseudomonas*. *Burkholderia mallei* causes glanders. Acute pneumonia has abscess, empyema, and lymphadenopathy, and a chronic form similar to TB. *Burkholderia pseudomallei* causes melioidosis. Radiograph reveals consolidation or irregular coalescent cavitary 3 to 15 mm nodules. Chronic disease is similar to TB but spares the apex and rarely calcifies or retracts the hila. *Burkholderia gladioli* colonizes CF patients and can cause pneumonia. *Burkholderia cepacia* presents an opportunistic infection in CF. *Pseudomonas aeruginosa* is a motile obligate aerobe, with a mucoid matrix, a constituent of human flora. It thrives in moisture. *Pseudomonas* is the most common and lethal cause of HAP. Hemorrhagic subpleural nodules form in aspiration-prone areas and along bronchovascular bundles. *Stenotrophomonas (Xanthomonas, Pseudomonas) maltophilia*, often drug resistant, colonizes CF patients and infects the immunocompromised. *Acinetobacter*, encapsulated nonmotile aerobes, colonizes hands and catheters and may spread from person to person. Most cases are immunocompromised, severe, and bacteremic.

GRAM-NEGATIVE COCCOBACILLI

Brucella species (*B. melitensis, B. abortus, B. canis*, and *B. suis*) are small nonmotile nonencapsulated intracellular parasites that can cause human disease via skin entry; GI absorption, often via unpasteurized contaminated dairy products; or inhalation. In brucellosis, lung disease is uncommon; necrotizing granulomatous disease is similar to chronic TB.

Bordetella species cause whooping cough (*B. pertussis* and *B. parapertussis*) or rarely pneumonia (*B. bronchiseptica*). Pertussis typically occurs in patients younger than 2 years of age. The bacteria produce toxins and filamentous hemagglutinin, responsible for membrane formation.

Francisella tularensis is the nonmotile non–spore-forming cause of tularemia, a small animal disease contacted via skin entry, tick or deer fly bite, ingestion, or culture material inhalation. The disease has multiple forms, with pulmonary infection via hematogenous spread of ulceroglandular and typhoid forms: small necrotic nodules become confluent.

Haemophilus influenzae is pleomorphic non–spore forming and nonmotile, encapsulated or unencapsulated. It is responsible for 5% to 20% of cultured CAP and almost half of chronic infectious pneumonias. Encapsulated types are more virulent; unencapsulated types colonize the throat and may cause bronchitis or pneumonia. Radiograph reveals bronchopneumonia.

Legionella (particularly *L. pneumophila*) lives in water, probably in biofilms or other microbes. They prevent macrophage phagosome-lysosome fusion, preventing killing. *Legionella* causes 2% to 25% of CAP requiring hospitalization, more likely in older men. It infects via moist air drift, sometimes with liver, renal, or CNS abnormalities (Legionnaire disease). Resolution is generally slow even with therapy; radiographic improvement, slower. One-third of patients require ventilation; mortality ranges from 5% with erythromycin therapy to 20% without. Radiograph reveals nonsegmental consolidation that spreads despite appropriate therapy. Disease is often bilateral; abscess or cavitation does not occur. Pontiac fever is a nonpneumonic flu-like illness.

TREPONEMAL INFECTION

Leptospira interrogans lives in host renal convoluted tubules and is shed in urine. Infection occurs via water or soil contact. Leptospirosis is often occupational; pets also can cause it. Infection may have hepatorenal symptoms (Weil disease) or predominant lung disease. Radiograph reveals 1 to 7 mm nodules with or without consolidation, confluent consolidation, or ground glass opacities.

Treponema pallidum causes syphilis. Pulmonary syphilis occurs in congenital syphilis as pneumonia alba, usually associated with stillbirth or early death. In acquired disease, lung involvement is rare and occurs in the third stage: fibrogummatous disease involves the parenchyma and pulmonary arteritis occurs, associated with aortitis.

ANAEROBIC BACTERIA

Anaerobes cause 20% to 35% of CAP cases requiring hospitalization, often polymicrobial. Important members are gram-negative bacilli *Bacteroides*, *Fusobacterium*, *Porphyromonas*, and *Prevotella*; gram-positive bacilli *Actinomyces*, *Eubacterium*, and *Clostridium*; gram-positive cocci *Peptostreptococcus* and *Peptococcus*; and gram-negative coccus *Veillonella*. Anaerobic pneumonia is associated with poor dentition and decreased mental status, and is male predominant. Anaerobes cause necrosis, leading to abscess, cavitation, and empyema. Radiograph reveals bronchopneumonia coalescing to consolidation often with abscess, gangrene, and lymphadenopathy. Pyopneumothorax may develop with *Bacteroides fragilis* or *Clostridium perfringens*.

MYCOBACTERIAL INFECTION

Mycobacteria are slow-growing nonmotile non–spore-forming aerobes containing up to 25% lipids (helping resist degradation). They are acid-fast, as are some *Nocardia*, *Corynebacteria*, and *Legionella micdadei*. The tuberculosis complex includes *Mycobacterium tuberculosis*; *Mycobacterium bovis*, a once common infection of nodes, GI tract, and bones now uncommon with milk pasteurization; *Mycobacterium africanum*; and *Mycobacterium microti*, not a human pathogen. The nontuberculosis complex includes *Mycobacterium leprae*; photochromogens, including *Mycobacterium kansasii*; scotochromogens; nonphotochromogens, including *Mycobacterium avium-intracellulare* complex; and fast-growing species, including *Mycobacterium fortuitum* and *Mycobacterium chelonae*.

MYCOBACTERIUM TUBERCULOSIS

Infection

Up to one-third of the world population has *M. tuberculosis* infection; 3 million die annually. The U.S. rate is approximately 6 to 20:100 000. Infection increases with cough, cavity, upper airway spread, and extent of involvement, as well as ventilation, closeness and duration of contact, and susceptibility. *Mycobacterium tuberculosis* can survive and multiply within macrophages and can live within necrotic tissue for long periods of time. Virulence is related to a strain's ability to form cords, via cord factor, produce ammonia (these may inhibit lysosome-phagosome fusion), lyse phagosomes, and produce catalase.

Disease

Tuberculosis develops in 5% to 15% of infections; the risk is highest in the first 2 years. Disease may be either progressive primary TB or postprimary TB, often reactivation. There are many risk factors: socioeconomic, including malnutrition, homelessness, and population density; exposure via profession or environment; drug and alcohol use; immigration from high prevalence; and coexistent disease (immunosuppression, diabetes, renal failure, gastrectomy or jejunoileal bypass, iron overload, silicosis, and alveolar proteinosis).

Primary Pulmonary Tuberculosis

Droplets incite granuloma formation, necrosis, and coalescence surrounded by fibrous tissue. The initial site, the Ghon focus, may progress or heal and calcify. Lymph node extensions form the Ranke complex. Node enlargement may cause airway compression and atelectasis; extranodal extension may cause edema or airway ulceration; node rupture into a bronchus or vessel results in bronchopneumonia or miliary disease, respectively, or in hemoptysis if it ruptures into both. Bloodstream spread is common but miliary manifestations are not. If the disease is not controlled, it progresses to progressive primary tuberculosis, similar to postprimary disease. Most radiographs are normal. Consolidation is the most common abnormality: unilateral, dense, homogeneous, segmental or lobar, upper lobe predominant. Lymphadenopathy is visible in >90% of children and fewer adults, and may be the only finding, commonly hilar and right-sided. Atelectasis is often lobar, usually caused by nodal airway compression. Effusion is uncommon, more frequent in adults. Cavities and miliary disease occur in less than 10%.

Postprimary Tuberculosis

Postprimary tuberculosis is via reactivation of a primary focus or new acquisition. It tends to be in apical-posterior upper lobe or superior lower lobe. It is similar to primary TB except that necrosis is more rapid and infection tends to progress. Frequent airways communication allows cavitation. Infection causes vasculitis or thrombosis in adjacent vessels. Arteries near a cavity dilate in 4% of cases (Rasmussen aneurysm); death from rupture is common. TB bronchopneumonia is via endobronchial spread of necrotic material. Miliary TB occurs via lymphatic or vascular dissemination: innumerable pulmonary and pleural millet seed–sized nodules. Tracheobronchial TB may occur via luminal, miliary, or lymphatic spread, or direct extension. Cervical or supraclavicular lymphadenopathy, pericarditis, or mediastinitis may develop. Mediastinitis may lead to aortic erosion, phrenic nerve palsy, SVC syndrome, esophageal stricture or fistula, or traction diverticula. Contained infection will heal with irregular scars, emphysema, and bronchiectasis.

Imaging Findings

Consolidation suggests active disease and isolated calcification suggests inactive disease; but this is not absolute. TB localizes in apical and posterior upper lobes or superior lower lobes, often multisegmental. Consolidation often has satellite nodules. Lymphadenopathy is rarely visible; cavitation is often visible. Cavities may be single or multiple, have thick or thin walls or fluid levels, and resolve or become thin-walled cystic spaces with therapy. Hypo- or nonenhancing tuberculomas have small satellite lesions. Tree-in-bud nodules are visible in almost all patients in HRCT, the main or only manifestation in up to 25%. The 2 to 10 mm nodules of endobronchial spread are frequently visible. The 1- to 3-mm nodules of miliary tuberculosis may enlarge and coalesce with inadequate therapy. Bronchiectasis is visible in 30% to 60% of active postprimary disease via HRCT, often bilateral, and generally radiographically inapparent. Approximately 40% have concentric bronchial stenosis on CT.

THE PPD

Protein precipitates are from heat-killed bacteria. The injection is intradermal. Interpretation is on the second or third day, measuring induration. Erythema is unimportant but may suggest subcutaneous injection. Interpretation depends on patient factors. Patients are positive at 5 mm of induration if HIV or risk factors for it; recent close contact with a TB patient; or radiographs consistent with healed TB. Patients are positive at 10 mm of induration if from a high-prevalence part of the world; intravenous drug users; residents of long-term care facility; with TB-associated conditions; or treated with high-dose corticosteroids or immunosuppressive therapy. Everyone else is positive at 15 mm.

NONTUBERCULOUS MYCOBACTERIA

Patients often have COPD or other lung disease. Other risk factors are similar to those for *M. tuberculosis*. Infection by nontuberculous mycobacteria leads to identical pathologic findings and it is difficult radiologically and histologically to differentiate tuberculous from nontuberculous infection, with the possible exception of *M. avium-intracellulare*. Confident differentiation of any particular case is impossible but trends are present. *Mycobacterium avium-intracellulare* infection is bilateral in more than 60%, with endobronchial spread in more than 80% and bronchiectasis in 80% to 94% of MAI infections versus 27% in *M. tuberculosis*.

Mycobacterium avium-intracellulare bacteria are water and soil organisms. In immunocompromised patients, disease is often disseminated. Up to 50% of AIDS patients will develop it at some point. *Mycobacterium kansasii* is common in the midsouthern United States, Wales, and southern England; it is uncommon elsewhere. *Mycobacterium marinum* is acquired via contaminated water contact, commonly in fish or aquarium workers. Skin defects increase the risk. Commonly skin disease may extend to nodes. *Mycobacterium scrofulaceum* lives in natural water and raw dairy products but is absent in U.S. drinking water. Once a pediatric cervical lymphadenitis, some pneumonias have been reported with underlying lung disease. *Mycobacterium fortuitum-chelonae* complex causes pneumonia and skin disease. It favor lipids and is associated with esophageal obstruction and mineral oil aspiration.

FUNGI

HISTOPLASMOSIS

Histoplasmosis is caused by *Histoplasmosis capsulatum* and *Histoplasmosis duboisii*. *Histoplasmosis capsulatum* is a soil saprophyte, a mycelium in soil, and an yeast in animals. It prefers high nitrogen content, such as bird or bat guano. Most disease is in central and eastern North America, particularly the Ohio, Mississippi, and St. Lawrence river valleys. Inhaled microconidia become yeasts, which are engulfed by macrophages. Inflammation proceeds to granuloma formation, necrosis, and fibrosis, then to calcification. Small sites may coalesce. Lymphadenopathy is constant, more prominent than in TB, and may cause airway compression or broncholithiasis. Frequent and early dissemination leads to small visceral granulomata. Healing is rapid and clinical disease is rare.

Acute histoplasmosis is a flu-like illness, sometimes with hepatosplenomegaly, or erythema nodosum or multiforme. Most radiographs are normal; the most common finding is poorly defined migratory consolidation. Lymphadenopathy is common. With heavy exposure, disseminated nodules may appear. A histoplasmoma is a 0.5 to 3.0 cm well-defined typically lower lobe nodule often with small satellite nodules. It may be multiple; serial radiographs may reveal slow growth. It may have central or diffuse calcification, and hilar node calcification is common. Chronic pulmonary histoplasmosis is rare and appears identical to chronic pulmonary TB. Chronic mediastinal histoplasmosis from extracapsular nodal or contiguous pulmonary spread results in ill-defined necrotic tissue mass in the mediastinum. CT reveals mediastinal-hilar masses with calcifications, pericarditis, SVC or esophageal obstruction, and pulmonary artery and bronchial narrowing. If no calcification is present, the lesion should be biopsied. Disseminated histoplasmosis is rare; acute disseminated histoplasmosis has miliary nodules.

COCCIDIOIDOMYCOSIS

Coccidioidomycosis is caused by *Coccidioides immitis*, a soil fungus of the southwestern United States, northern Mexico, and parts of Central and South America. It exists in animals as spherules that divide by cleavage. Infection is common, mostly asymptomatic. "Valley fever" occurs in 5% to 20% of symptomatic patients: erythema nodosum or multiforme, arthralgia, and sometimes eosinophilia.

In primary coccidioidomycosis, arthrospores induce bronchopneumonia. Granulomata form within this inflammation. This center is generally small and resolves into scars; it may progress to nonsegmental cavitary necrosis. Lymphadenopathy is common and nodal erosion causes dissemination. Radiograph is normal or reveals unilateral, lower lobe–predominant, sometimes migratory, consolidation. Thin-walled cavities or small effusion may form. Persistent primary coccidioidomycosis, over 6 weeks, has progressive disease, with peripheral, sometimes cavitary, mid and upper lung–predominant nodules ranging from 0.5 to 5 cm. Calcification is uncommon. Chronic progressive coccidioidomycosis is less common (1%) and is due to either progression of primary disease or reactivation. It develops slowly and may produce symptoms for years. Radiograph is similar to that in chronic TB. Disseminated disease occurs in 1:6000 cases, often the immunocompromised. The CNS is involved in 30% to 50%; osteomyelitis occurs in 10% to 50%, often spinal. Miliary disease is common.

BLASTOMYCOSIS

Blastomyces dermatitidis is a soil fungus found in the central and southeastern United States that in its yeast form buds with wide-necked attachment. Infection is via spore inhalation or reactivation. Blastomycosis is male and middle age predominant and generally subclinical. It involves the urinary tract in up to 20% of cases. Initial bronchopneumonia rapidly is followed by granuloma formation and coalescence. Airway perforation, cavity formation, and ulcerative bronchitis can occur. Radiograph reveals nonspecific alveolar consolidation that may be of almost any configuration, with masses, air bronchograms, or cavitation. Lymphadenopathy is uncommon and calcification rare. Mediastinal fibrosis may lead to SVC obstruction or nerve impingement.

PARACOCCIDIOIDOMYCOSIS

Paracoccidioidomycosis is caused by the dimorphic soil fungus *Paracoccidioides brasiliensis*, which has a characteristic "pilot-wheel" pattern. It is a male-predominant disease of South and Central America. Infections are probably via inhalation. Radiographic findings are nonspecific.

CRYPTOCOCCOSIS

Cryptococcosis is often caused by *Cryptococcus neoformans*, an encapsulated yeast; heavily capsulated forms produce gelatinous disease. The variant *neoformans* is found in pigeon waste. Most patients are immunocompromised. Most cases are via inhalation. Pulmonary infection may lead to well-defined, gelatinous, or cavitary nodules; consolidation sometimes mimicking bronchioloalveolar carcinoma or pneumococcal pneumonia; miliary nodules; or interstitial proliferation without inflammation in the immunocompromised host. Radiograph reveals single or multiple nodules, 0.5 to 4 cm, typically subpleural. Cavitation and lymphadenopathy are uncommon and calcification is rare.

PNEUMOCYSTIS CARINII

Pneumocystis carinii exists as round or crescentic cysts and pleomorphic pseudopodial trophozoites. Infection, presumably via inhalation, is common but generally asymptomatic in normal patients. Trophozoites have no invasive capability, and attach to type I pneumocytes by layering in invaginations. Interstitial alveolitis is common; diffuse alveolar damage may occur. Early radiograph may be normal in 10% but often reveals bilateral perihilar lower lobe–predominant ground glass opacity, progressing to consolidation with peripheral ground glass or reticular opacity. Nodules are uncommon. Cystic spaces develop in AIDS patients. CT reveals diffuse or mosaic ground glass opacity, sometimes with interlobular septal thickening or consolidation.

CANDIDIASIS

Candida is dimorphic fungi existing as yeast in animals, common human saprophytes in normal oral, GI, and skin flora. *Candida* species are responsible for 90% of fungemias, of which 41% are caused by *Candida albicans*. Alterations of normal flora and overgrowth predispose to disease. Most cases are localized mucocutaneous infection, with pulmonary infection uncommon. The most common lung involvement is disseminated miliary disease; aspiration may produce bronchopneumonia. Effusion is uncommon; cavitation and lymphadenopathy are absent. A large acute mycetoma may form. HRCT reveals nodules sometimes with ground glass halos.

ASPERGILLOSIS

Aspergillus is ubiquitous septate uniform hyphae that branches dichotomously at 45-degree angles. The disease has several forms. (a) Saprophytic aspergillosis is noninvasive. Tracheobronchial colonization is common in CF and other lung diseases. Colony formation in a cavity or ectatic bronchus results in aspergilloma. These are often asymptomatic, but particularly mycetoma may cause hemoptysis and serve as an invasive source. (b) Extrinsic allergic alveolitis is a hypersensitivity reaction to inhaled conidia. (c) Allergic bronchopulmonary aspergillosis, a Loeffler-like syndrome, is the most common of these three. Imaging reveals proximal bronchial mucoid impaction, visible as upper lobe and central predominant finger-like opacities. Patients often have asthma or atopy. Disease may be asymptomatic or produce cough, fever, pain, or hemoptysis. Corticosteroids are helpful. The mucus may calcify, and bronchiectasis may result.

Invasive aspergillosis is a disease of the immunocompromised associated with tissue destruction. It may occur in four forms, the first two more common. Acute bronchopneumonia has a nonspecific radiograph. Angioinvasive aspergillosis manifests as sometimes cavitary well-defined nodule with hemorrhagic ground glass rim or wedge-shaped infarct from septic embolism. Hemorrhage can be massive, and chest-wall vascular involvement is possible. Pleural or chest invasion may cause effusion, fistula, or osteomyelitis. Acute tracheobronchitis is found most often in (heart) lung transplant patients. Chronic necrotizing aspergillosis is rare, most commonly occurring with underlying lung disease, characterized by slowly progressive upper lobe disease that may spread to the pleura, mediastinum, chest wall, or contralateral lung.

ZYGOMYCOSIS

Zygomycosis is caused by fungi found in decaying matter with broad, irregular, nonseptated hyphae. *Rhizopus, Mucor*, and others cause lung disease via inhalation of sporangiospores or direct invasion. Patients have underlying disease, such as lymphoproliferative-hematopoietic disorders, diabetes, or transplant. The fungi are angioinvasive. Patients have chest pain, fever, and bloody sputum. Pulmonary artery invasion may result in massive hemorrhage. Radiograph reveals homogeneous segmental or round rapidly progressing consolidation, sometimes with nodules of varying size with surrounding ground glass halos reflecting hemorrhage.

ACTINOMYCOSIS AND NOCARDIOSIS

The most important *Actinomyces* species are *Actinomyces israelii* and *Actinomyces bovis*, gram-positive nonmotile branching filamentous anaerobes or microaerophiles, composed of mycelia that fragment into bacterial-shaped forms. Actinomycetaceae are normal oral flora; infection is via aspiration or swallowing. They form sulfur granules in tissue, named for their color. The classic pulmonary disease is empyema with chest-wall sinus tracts, though this advanced form is uncommon. It occurs mostly as cervicofacial infection after tooth extraction, with GI infection second and chest infection third, frequently with other agents. Pulmonary actinomycosis has abscesses with sinus tracts, fibrous tissue, pleural fibrosis, and adhesions. Radiograph reveals lower lobe peripheral consolidation continuing to abscess without appropriate therapy or mass mimicking cancer. Wavy rib periosteal reaction may involve multiple ribs, and true bone destruction may occur.

Nocardiosis is caused commonly by *Nocardia asteroides*, aerobic gram-positive and generally acid-fast nonmotile non–spore-forming soil fungi with delicate filamentous branching hyphae. Sulfur granules are uncommon. It is often an opportunistic infection. Nocardiosis may develop as consolidation or as nodules; the most frequent radiographic finding is homogeneous nonsegmental consolidation without lower lobe predominance. Cavitation is common. Infection may extend to the pleura and cause effusion or empyema, but chest-wall extension is rare.

RNA MYXOVIRUSES

Influenza involves the upper respiratory tract, and in the old and chronically ill may cause a fulminant pneumonia. Group A is classified into hemagglutinin (H), necessary in binding and membrane penetration, and neuraminidase (N), necessary in particle release. Pneumonia is usually via group A. Disease is characterized by alveolar damage, exudates, and epithelial desquamation. Radiograph reveals coalescent lower lobe segmental opacity, similar to ARDS. Effusion is rare.

Parainfluenza causes croup and bronchiolitis and pneumonitis in infants and children. Adults get pharyngitis or coryza. Radiograph reveals nonspecific lower lobe predominant markings.

Respiratory syncytial virus causes bronchiolitis and pneumonitis in infants and young children (45% of lower airway disease), particularly with underlying disease. Adult disease is generally mild URI. Radiograph is less dramatic than symptoms and may reveal patchy consolidation and hyperinflation, with bronchial wall thickening, peribronchial infiltrates, and perihilar lines.

Measles virus can cause pneumonia; most are via superinfection. Complication risk increases in pregnancy and immunocompromise. Primary pneumonia has reticular interstitial disease and patchy consolidation, with bronchial and perihilar interstitial thickening, small nodules, and peribronchial opacities. Lymphadenopathy is common in children, uncommon in adults.

RNA PICORNAVIRUSES

Group A coxsackieviruses cause soft palate vesicles and ulcers, meningitis, and some colds. Group B viruses cause meningoencephalitis, myocarditis, pericarditis, and orchitis. Echovirus causes rash, fever, diarrhea, and meningitis; type 19 causes infantile pneumonia. Rhinovirus causes more than 50% of coryza and 40% to 50% of colds. Croup, bronchitis, bronchiolitis, and bronchopneumonia may develop. Children with bronchopulmonary dysplasia and adults with COPD have higher risk.

RNA HANTAVIRUSES

Seoul, Hantaan, Puumala, Dobrava, and Prospect Hill viruses cause hemorrhagic fever with renal syndromes, with fever, hypotension, and renal failure. The Sin Nombre, Bayou, and Black Creek Canal viruses cause a pulmonary syndrome. All are rodent borne and transmitted by excreta inhalation. Edema and interstitial lymphocyte infiltration develop; tissue damage is generally mild or absent. Pulmonary syndrome has 50% fatality.

OTHER RNA VIRUSES

Ten to fifteen percent of babies born to mothers infected with the togavirus rubella during the first trimester have teratogenic effects, often pulmonary artery stenosis, and interstitial pneumonitis. The retrovirus HTLV-I causes bronchiolitis or interstitial pneumonitis. HIV causes lymphocytic interstitial and alveolar infiltrates, lymphocytic interstitial pneumonitis, and emphysema.

DNA ADENOVIRUS

Adenovirus causes 7% of respiratory infection in infants and children. It causes hemorrhagic consolidation, atelectasis, overinflation, and necrotizing bronchitis and bronchiolitis. Pneumonia is mild. Radiograph reveals bilateral bronchopneumonia with hyperinflation and atelectasis.

DNA HERPESVIRUSES

HSV-I classically causes oral gingivostomatitis and cold sores. Lower airway infection may be common, typically ulcerating the tracheobronchial mucosa sometimes with necrotizing bronchopneumonia. Radiographs may reveal bilateral alveolar opacities, poorly defined nodular opacities, or ARDS. HSV-II classically causes genital herpes. Neonatal infection may result in hematogenous spread to the lungs. It affects the larger airways less than HSV-I and causes diffuse alveolar damage or interstitial pneumonitis. Herpesvirus 6 causes childhood roseola (exanthem subitum), and can cause interstitial pneumonitis in BMT recipients. Herpesvirus 8 is linked to Kaposi sarcoma, including of the lung, pleural lymphoma, and Castleman disease.

Varicella causes chickenpox and zoster. Pneumonia more typically develops after primary infection. The incidence of pneumonia is 15%, often in patients with preexisting disease or immune deficiency. It causes diffuse alveolar damage and giant cell pneumonia. Airway and pleural vesicles may form. Radiograph reveals 5 to 10 mm nodular opacities, well defined at the periphery but less so elsewhere, rapidly progressing to consolidation. Remote but generally adulthood chickenpox infection may in less than 2% of cases result in diffuse tiny calcified nodules.

CMV may be acquired via transplacental spread; during vaginal delivery, from infected milk or other infected infants; or via contact with secretions. Most infections are subclinical or asymptomatic. CMV pneumonia may cause scattered well-defined hemorrhagic 0.5 to 1.5 cm nodules, or diffuse alveolar damage or interstitial pneumonitis. It often is a coinfector with other agents. Radiograph reveals bilateral reticular, ground glass, and alveolar opacities.

Epstein-Barr virus infects B lymphocytes and pharyngeal and possibly lower respiratory epithelium. It can be dormant for long periods of time, and causes infectious mononucleosis, which uncommonly affects the lungs but may cause lymphadenopathy and/or interstitial pneumonitis. The most common radiographic abnormality is splenomegaly.

OTHER DNA VIRUSES

Patients with history of smallpox may have punctate pulmonary calcifications. Papillomaviruses cause laryngeal and lower respiratory papillomas; these viruses are associated with cancer in papillomatosis, and possibly with squamous cell carcinoma. Simian virus 40 may cause some mesotheliomas. Parvoviruses may cause lung disease in the immunocompromised, as part of systemic infection, and may be associated with acute chest syndrome of sickle-cell disease.

MYCOPLASMAS, CHLAMYDIAE, AND RICKETTSIAE

Mycoplasmas have some features of bacteria but they are less than 1 μm long, lack a cell wall, and have different genetic features. *Mycoplasma pneumoniae* is most important, causing 10% to 15% of all CAP cases and upto 50% of CAP cases in military recruits. Disease is most common in the young. Transmission is via droplet inhalation. Radiographs are indistinguishable from those in viral pneumonia.

Chlamydiae are obligate intracellular microbes unable to synthesize ATP and GTP. *Clamydophila pneumoniae* is a common cause of CAP, associated with lung cancer and asthma. AIDS, CF, and COPD increase risk. Radiograph reveals nonspecific alveolar or interstitial opacities. Neonates born to mothers with *Clamydophila trachomatis* have 50% conjunctivitis risk and 10% to 20% pneumonia risk. Infected patients have paroxysmal cough and tachypnea with little or no fever. Radiograph reveals bilateral diffuse interstitial and alveolar opacity with patchy overinflation and atelectasis. *Clamydophila psittaci* is a bird pathogen, with human infections via excreta. Inflammation begins at respiratory bronchioles and extends to alveoli without necrosis; inflammation resolves over weeks leaving pleural fibrosis. Radiograph reveals ground glass opacity, patchy perihilar- and basilar-predominant reticular opacities, or consolidation. Lymphadenopathy is common.

Coxiella burnetii causes Q fever, described in Queensland, Australia. It is an obligate intracellular bacterium. Its reservoir is ticks. Human infection is primarily via inhalation; it is associated with farmers, slaughterhouse and stockyard workers, and medical veterinary personnel. Radiograph reveals lower lobe–predominant multifocal large round or segmental consolidation. *Rickettsia tsutsugamushi* causes scrub typhus. *Rickettsia rickettsii* causes Rocky Mountain spotted fever; radiograph reveals congestive heart failure caused by myocardial vasculitis, nonspecific opacities, or pleural effusion. *Rickettsia conorii* causes Mediterranean spotted fever.

PROTOZOA

Entamoeba histolytica causes amebiasis. More than 95% of amebic lung abscesses are peridiaphragmatic; 75% arise from liver. Fibrous effusions are often present. Cavitation can occur.

Toxoplasmosis is caused by the obligate intracellular protozoan *Toxoplasma gondii*. Cats are definitive hosts. Infection, rarely clinically evident, is via infected stool or meat, particularly lamb. Disease is rarely pulmonary, but in immunocompromised patients pneumonitis, carditis, and hepatitis occur in addition to CNS infection. Radiograph reveals reticular opacities similar to viral pneumonia, or consolidation. Lymphadenopathy is common. In the immunocompromised, radiographs reveal bilateral reticulonodular or coarse nodules with poorly defined margins.

NEMATODES

Ascariasis is generally due to *Ascaris lumbricoides*. In a complex life cycle, larvae travel in alveoli and airways. Up to 25% of the world's population has been infected. Pulmonary disease occurs with larval passage through the lungs. Patchy consolidation may be transient and perihilar.

Strongyloidiasis is caused by *Strongyloides stercoralis* or other members of the Strongyloides genus. Its life cycle includes larval migration through the alveoli and airways. Infection is typically asymptomatic though in hyperinfection, typically in the immunocompromised, severe disease can occur. Larval alveolar migration causes hemorrhage and microabscesses but no residual damage, except in hyperinfection alveolar injury, in which sepsis and ARDS may occur. Radiographic findings are similar to that in ascariasis.

TREMATODES

Paragonimiasis is caused by flukes, usually *Paragonimus westermani*. Humans are infected by eating raw crabs or crayfish or drinking contaminated water. The life cycle is complex and leads to pulmonary larval maturation and egg deposition. Radiograph may be normal, or reveal varying opacities and thin-walled cystic lesions, with the worm sometimes visible as a crescentic or oval opacity along the cyst wall. Pleural effusion or thickening, or hydropneumothorax is common.

Schistosomiasis is commonly caused by *Schistosoma mansoni, Schistosoma japonicum,* and *Schistosoma haematobium*. The intermediate host is the snail. *Schistosoma mansoni* and *S. haematobium* are endemic in the Middle East and Africa. Schistosomes have complex life cycles; humans are infected via contaminated water. Adolescents migrate to the SMV (*S. japonicum*), IMV (*S. mansoni*), or vesical veins (*S. haematobium*). *Schistosoma haematobium* eggs released in the vesical veins embolize to lung arterioles and extrude into perivascular tissues. Inflammation leads to obliterative arteriolitis that may lead to PA hypertension if severe. Radiographs may reveal miliary or reticulonodular opacities, with areas of consolidation around dead worms and occluded arteries.

CESTODES

Echinococcus granulosus hydatid disease requires Canidae hosts. In a complex life cycle, larvae lodge in the lungs and form cysts. Most *E. granulosus* cysts are hepatic; 15% to 30% are pulmonary. The cysts are round and surrounded by inflammatory fibrous pericysts. They contain protective exocysts and germinal endocysts. Daughter cysts have poorly formed endocysts. Radiograph reveals lower lobe–predominant well-circumscribed 1 to 20 cm mass surrounded by normal lung, multiple in 20% to 30%. Rupture may produce a meniscus, air-fluid level, or floating membrane.

Echinococcus multilocularis has Canidae as definitive hosts and rodents as intermediate hosts. The life cycle and disease are similar to that in *E. granulosus*. Cysts are almost exclusively hepatic; the exocyst is poorly formed and the pericyst does not develop. Lesions are gelatinous and spongy, a series of interconnected spaces with intense inflammatory reaction and endarteritis obliterans.

ARTHROPOD INFECTION

Pentastomiasis is often via *Armillifer armillatus* or *Linguatula serrata*. Ingested eggs hatch and larvae go to the liver, intestine, mesentery, and lung. Living larvae do not cause inflammation, but with death inflammation leads to numerous 4 to 6 mm calcifications shaped like incomplete rings.

HIRUDINIASIS

Leech infestation is typically a skin disease, but internal hirudiniasis, frequently *Limnatis nilotica* can cause pulmonary disease. The nose, pharynx, larynx, or trachea may be involved. After the leech attaches and feeds on blood, it enlarges and may cause hemoptysis or airway obstruction.

SUGGESTED READING

Burrill J, Williams CJ, Bain G, et al. Tuberculosis: a radiologic review. *Radiographics.* September–October 2007;27(5):1255-1273.

Gurney JW, Conces DJ. Pulmonary histoplasmosis. *Radiology.* 1996;199:297-306.

Jeong YJ, Lee KS, Koh W, et al. Nontuberculous mycobacterial pulmonary infection in immunocompetent patients: comparison of thin-section CT and histopathologic findings. *Radiology.* 2004;231:880-886.

Kim HY, Song KS, Goo JM, et al. Thoracic sequelae and complications of tuberculosis. *Radiographics.* July–August 2001;21(4): 839-858.

Kuhlman JE. Pneumocystic infections: the radiologist's perspective. *Radiology.* 1996;198:623-635.

Logan PM, Primack SL, Miller RR, et al. Invasive aspergillosis of the airways: radiographic, CT, and pathologic findings. *Radiology.* 1994;193:383.

Miller WT. Spectrum of pulmonary nontuberculous mycobacterial infection. *Radiology.* 1994;191:343-350.

Nambu A, Saito A, Araki T, et al. *Chlamydia pneumoniae*: comparison with findings of mycoplasma pneumoniae and *Streptococcus pneumoniae* at thin-section CT. *Radiology.* 2005;238: 330-338.

Oh YW, Effmann EL, Godwin JD. Pulmonary infections in immunocompromised hosts: the importance of correlating the conventional radiologic appearance with the clinical setting. *Radiology.* 2000;217:647-656.

Tew J, Calenoff L, Berlin BS. Bacterial or nonbacterial pneumonia: accuracy of radiographic diagnosis. *Radiology.* 1977;124:607.

QUESTIONS AND ANSWERS

1. Regarding HAP, which of the following is *true*?
   A. Mechanical ventilation is associated with a 1%–3% daily risk of infection.
   B. Increases hospital stay by 2–3 days
   C. Most frequently a benign condition
   D. Infectious agent changes from gram-negative bacteria early in hospitalization to a gram-positive bacteria

   ANSWER: A. Ventilation has a 1%–3% daily risk. HAP adds an average of 7–9 days to hospital stay, and mortality is 30%–70%. It is frequently acquired via aspiration and often polymicrobial. Early HAP is often a gram-positive agent and later HAP is often an enteric gram-negative agent.

2. Which of the following is the most common cause of nonsegmental consolidation?
   A. *K. pneumoniae*
   B. *S. aureus*
   C. *S. pneumoniae*
   D. *S. stercoralis*

   ANSWER: C. Nonsegmental (lobar) consolidation is frequently caused by pneumococcus, with some cases due to *K. pneumoniae*. *Staphylococcus aureus* typically forms a bronchopneumonia. *Strongyloides stercoralis* typically produces patchy transient perihilar consolidation.

3. The radiograph of a male patient with acute-onset cough and fever reveals widened mediastinum, patchy opacities, and large effusions. Which of the following does the chest CT most likely reveal?
   A. Small cavities with peripheral densities
   B. Hemorrhagic nodes and dense effusion
   C. Apical cavitation
   D. Tree-in-bud opacities in the middle lobe

   ANSWER: B. The patient presents with acute inflammatory–widened mediastinum, suggesting pulmonary anthrax. It causes alveolar and lymph node hemorrhage and bloody effusions. Paragonimiasis causes small cavities with peripheral densities. Most causes of apical cavitation are not acute.

4. Which of the following characterizes Enterobacteriaceae?
   A. Gram-negative rods that ferment glucose and make endotoxin but are oxidase negative
   B. Gram-negative rods that cannot ferment glucose or oxidase but do make endotoxin
   C. Gram-negative rods characterized by inability to reduce nitrogen
   D. Gram-negative coccobacilli associated with ulceroglandular disease

   ANSWER: A. Enterobacteriaceae are gram-negative rods that ferment glucose, reduce nitrogen, and produce endotoxin but are oxidase negative. *Francisella tularensis* is the gram-negative coccobacillus associated with ulceroglandular disease.

5. Which of the following is *true* regarding *Legionella* species?
   A. Pneumonia caused by these bacteria is segmental.
   B. Pneumonia caused by these bacteria is benign.
   C. A cause of Pontiac fever
   D. Considered normal human flora

   ANSWER: C. *Legionella* species live in water. The infection is typically nonsegmental and rapidly progressive, and may be associated with liver, renal, or CNS abnormalities. Resolution is generally prolonged even with therapy; one-third require ventilatory support and 5% die with appropriate therapy. *Legionella* species also cause Pontiac fever, a flu-like illness without pneumonia.

6. Regarding *M. tuberculosis* virulence, which of the following is *true*?
   A. Produces a toxin against type I pneumocytes
   B. Elaborates a compound that inhibits initial phagocytosis
   C. Can form cords
   D. Can form spores

   ANSWER: C. *Mycobacterium tuberculosis* has no toxins and has no effective defense against phagocytosis. Virulence appears related to the ability of strains to form cords, via trehalose-6,6'-mycolate cord factor, and to ammonia production. Virulent strains can lyse phagosomes and produce catalase.

7. A female patient with rheumatoid arthritis controlled with an anti-TNF agent has cough and night sweats. She has no TB exposure risk factors and a normal radiograph. Which of the following would result in a positive PPD test?
   A. 5-mm indurated wheal
   B. 10-mm indurated wheal
   C. 15-mm indurated wheal
   D. Induration does not matter. It would depend on erythema

   ANSWER: B. The patient is on immunosuppression, so it would be considered positive if there is 10 mm of induration, as she is on immunosuppressive therapy (anti-TNF).

8. Which of the following is *true* regarding coccidioidomycosis?
   A. Affects CNS in acute disease
   B. Characteristic form in animal specimens is the conidium.
   C. Uncommon in the United States
   D. Progressive and disseminated forms

   ANSWER: D. Coccidioidomycosis has primary, persistent primary, chronic progressive, and disseminated forms. The disseminated phase may affect the CNS. Its characteristic form is the spherule. It occurs in the southwestern United States, northern Mexico, and parts of Central and South America.

9. Regarding allergic bronchopulmonary aspergillosis, which of the following is correct?
   A. Patients improve with corticosteroid therapy.
   B. Abnormalities are more often in the lower lobes.
   C. Bronchiectasis does not occur.
   D. It is the second most common allergic aspergillosis syndrome.

   ANSWER: A. Allergic bronchopulmonary aspergillosis is the most common allergic aspergillosis syndrome. Corticosteroid therapy is helpful. Radiographs reveal homogeneous fingerlike opacities in bronchial distribution, usually in the upper lobe. The mucus plug may calcify, and bronchiectasis is often a sequela.

10. An adult asymptomatic patient gets a chest radiograph for a new job. The radiograph reveals innumerable tiny calcified nodules. Which of the following is the patient most likely to experience?
    A. Pulmonary actinomycosis as a teenager
    B. Sore throat treated with ampicillin
    C. Remote adulthood varicella pneumonia
    D. Cytomegalovirus transplacental infection

    ANSWER: C. Actinomycosis develops into pleural and chest wall abscesses and fibrosis. CMV pneumonia can cause nodules but the findings are characteristic of remote varicella pneumonia.

21 NONINFECTIOUS INFLAMMATORY DISEASES

John C. Texada and Satinder P. Singh

CONNECTIVE TISSUE DISEASES

SYSTEMIC LUPUS ERYTHEMATOSUS

Systemic lupus erythematosus (SLE) is characterized by rash, serositis, discoid disease, photosensitivity, oral ulcers, arthritis, and renal, neurologic, hematologic, and immunologic disorders. Patients who meet four criteria may be diagnosed with lupus, others are given overlap or "lupus-like" diagnoses and tend to have good prognosis. Approximately 50% to 60% of SLE patients will have lung or pleural involvement at some point.

Women are more likely to develop lupus; mean age is around 40 years. Heredity likely plays a role: HLA-DR3 and DR2, complement deficiencies, and immunoresponse genes are associated. Environmental factors include daylight, fluorescent light, and UV light and viral infection. Drugs including hydralazine, procainamide, INH, anticonvulsants, guanidine, methyldopa, chlorpromazine, sulfasalazine, and some beta-blockers produce a lupuslike syndrome, usually lacking nephritis or cerebritis. Penicillamine chronic therapy can induce SLE-like syndrome.

Antibodies may be the cause of the syndrome or the result of tissue damage. Serum antinuclear antibodies are the primary screen but may be negative in 5% to 10% of patients. Speckled staining is most common, reflecting antibodies to nucleic ribonucleoprotein and the glycoprotein macromolecule Sm. Rim staining is specific for SLE and reflects antibodies to nuclear DNA. Double-strand DNA antibody levels often track disease status. Nucleolar staining is present in half of patients with scleroderma, rarely with SLE. Homogeneous staining reflects antibodies to nucleoproteins. Cytoplasmic and peripheral antineutrophil cytoplasm antibodies (c-ANCA and p-ANCA) can be positive in SLE but have no bearing on disease status. Antiphospholipid antibodies are associated with thrombocytopenia and thromboembolism.

Pleural fibrosis is the most common lung change, found in 80–100% of patients; effusion or thickening occurs in 70% of patients. In acute lupus pneumonitis (1%–12% of patients), characterized by fever, dyspnea, hypoxemia, and patchy diffuse opacities, there may be diffuse alveolar damage or capillaritis and alveolar hemorrhage. The "shrinking lung" syndrome of hemidiaphragm elevation and decreased vital capacity is because of muscle weakness rather than a direct SLE effect on parenchyma. Upper-airway obstruction rarely occurs with cricoarytenoid or supraglottic inflammation. Focal lung disease is common but diffuse interstitial disease and alveolar hemorrhage are uncommon (less than 5%). Bronchiolitis obliterans and separately BOOP may occur. BOOP may have presentation similar to acute lupus pneumonitis, pneumonia, pulmonary hemorrhage, or pulmonary infarct.

Antiphospholipid antibodies lead to thrombosis, fetal loss, thrombocytopenia, and livedo reticularis. Pulmonary hypertension occurs in as many as 43% of patients, though clinically important disease is rare. Two-year mortality for lupus patients with pulmonary hypertension is 50%.

Many radiographs are normal and frequently underestimate the degree of disease. Effusion is usually bilateral but small. Parenchymal disease is nonspecific; these are generally caused by infection but may be caused by BOOP. Acute lupus pneumonitis appears as patchy ground glass or alveolar opacities often with pleural effusion. Alveolar hemorrhage also appears as patchy ill-defined basilar-predominant opacities. In interstitial disease, linear opacities may be visible, usually at the bases and sometimes migratory. Nodules are rare. Pericardial effusion may enlarge the cardiac silhouette. Lupus cardiomyopathy may result in congestive failure. HRCT is more sensitive for detection of disease, particularly in patients with normal radiographs. The most common abnormalities are lower lobe predominant and include interlobular septal thickening, intralobular interstitial thickening, small nodular consolidation, and ground glass attenuation. Fibrosis is subpleural and similar to that in other connective tissue diseases.

HYPOCOMPLEMENTEMIC URTICARIAL VASCULITIS

Hypocomplementemic urticarial vasculitis is a syndrome of urticaria and leukocytoclastic vasculitis. Hypocomplementemia is caused by antibodies to C1q and probably is a result of immunocomplex deposition. Hypocomplementemic urticarial vasculitis may be associated in some patients with obstructive disease; pulmonary vasculitis has not been reported.

RHEUMATOID DISEASE

Rheumatoid arthritis (RA) is a well-known chronic inflammatory process primarily affecting joints. Tumor necrosis factor alpha appears to play a prominent role. Serum IgG rheumatoid factor is the most common antibody abnormality but 15% to 30% of patients also have ANAs. Patients with HLA-B40 are 40 times more likely than others to develop RA. RA has extra-articular manifestations in about three-fourths of patients. These are more common in men and in patients with severe articular disease, and include subcutaneous nodules, pulmonary fibrosis, vasculitis, skin ulceration, lymphadenopathy, neuropathy, splenomegaly, episcleritis, and pericarditis. Juvenile RA is a similar process, though by definition occurs in patients younger than 16 years of age. It has an acute systemic type characterized by fever, rash, lymphadenopathy, hepatosplenomegaly, and arthritis in 20% of cases, and polyarticular forms involving four or less joints in about 50% of cases. Pulmonary and pleural disease is uncommon, most commonly pleuritis and effusion.

Approximately 1% to 5% of patients have radiographic evidence of interstitial lung disease, though 40% have reduced DLCO consistent with fibrosis, and approximately 30% of asymptomatic patients have abnormal HRCT. Interstitial pneumonitis is most common in RF-positive men aged from 50 to 60 years. The appearance is the same as other interstitial pneumonitis causes, except when necrobiotic nodules are present. Serial imaging sometimes reveals decreasing lung volumes. In HRCT, reticular thickening of intralobar and interlobar septa is present, mostly subpleural and lower lung. Honeycombing will be most prominent near the diaphragm at first and spread centrally. Ground glass opacities or pleural thickening or effusion may be present.

Rheumatoid necrobiotic nodules are well-circumscribed masses usually in the subcutaneous tissues but also uncommonly in the lungs. They are typically peripheral and near pleural or interlobular septal surfaces and visible more often in CT. They may be solitary or numerous, may change size with on disease activity, and frequently cavitate with thick smooth walls. Pneumothorax is uncommon but may occur with necrobiotic nodule rupture into the pleura.

Caplan syndrome is the combination of necrobiotic nodules with pneumoconiosis. Uncommon overall, it is common in men with both RA and pneumoconiosis, up to 55%. The nodules are probably a hypersensitivity reaction to dust. A ring of necrotic-pigmented macrophages in the nodule distinguishes it pathologically from standard necrobiotic nodules. They have the same radiographic appearance as other necrobiotic nodules but tend to develop rapidly and in crops.

Pleuritis commonly manifests as chronic inflammation with rare rheumatoid nodules. Pleural fibrosis and adhesions are common autopsy findings. Effusions are typically small and unilateral but may be large or bilateral. They are typically short-lived but may persist for years.

Obliterative bronchiolitis may develop rapidly. It may be associated with penicillamine or gold therapy, though this may be coincidental. A peribronchiolar lymphocytic infiltrate develops and can grow either thickening the wall or extending into the small-airway lumen, producing constrictive or obliterative bronchiolitis, respectively. Chest radiograph is normal or hyperinflated. HRCT may reveal mosaic perfusion, subsegmental bronchiectasis, and air trapping.

BOOP associated with RA is identical to BOOP from other causes. PFT may reveal restriction or mixed restriction–obstruction. It usually improves dramatically with therapy.

Follicular bronchitis and bronchiolitis are uncommon and nonspecific and may appear in other connective tissue and nonrheumatologic conditions. They respond well to therapy. Radiograph reveals diffuse reticulonodular interstitial disease. HRCT reveals centrilobular, subpleural, and peribronchial nodules, bronchial wall thickening, and centrilobular branching opacities.

Bronchiectasis precedes joint disease in almost all cases. It may occur in up to 30% of RA patients. If the laryngeal cartilages become fixed-adducted from inflammation, airway obstruction can follow, especially when exacerbated by viral URI or laryngeal edema. Pulmonary hypertension typically occurs with diffuse interstitial fibrosis, but also with Raynaud phenomenon in which case it may be because of immunocomplex mediated arteritis. Pulmonary vasculitis is rare in RA. Hyperviscosity syndrome is a rare complication in which RF molecules conglomerate into bodies large enough to obstruct small vessels. Purplish palmar erythema, bleeding diathesis, and dyspnea are some of the symptoms.

PROGRESSIVE SYSTEMIC SCLEROSIS

Scleroderma is rare, with incidence 12:1000 000 per year. It is most common in women (3:1) and in patients aged from 30 to 60 years. Pulmonary disease is common, with up to 60% of patients having dyspnea at some point. HRCT may reveal abnormalities in 44% of patients with normal chest radiograph, and bronchoalveolar lavage detects abnormalities in 73% of these patients.

Antinuclear antibodies are common, with antibodies to topoisomerase-1 (called anti-topo-1 or Scl-70) associated with skin changes, pulmonary fibrosis, and poor prognosis. Anti-RNA-polymerase-III is less than 25% sensitive but is specific for progressive systemic sclerosis (PSS). Antihistone antibodies are associated with severe fibrosis. CREST-variant patients have anticentromere antibodies.

Interstitial disease resembles IPF and present in 20% to 65% of radiographs. Progressive radiographs reveal prominent volume loss. HRCT often reveals abnormalities in patients with normal radiographs. In up to 70% of patients, lymphadenopathy increases as disease progresses. Pleural thickening and effusion are less common than in other connective tissue disease. Pulmonary hypertension is of uncertain etiology. Cardiac involvement includes myocarditis or myocardial sclerosis leading to biventricular failure; RV failure because of pulmonary vascular disease, pericardial effusion, and constrictive pericarditis. Esophageal abnormalities (discussed elsewhere) are present in 50% of patients. Rib notching is present in 15% of patients. It is nonspecific, though, as patients with RA, SLE, and Sjogren syndrome may develop this as well.

CREST SYNDROME

CREST syndrome consists of calcinosis cutis, Raynaud phenomenon, sclerodactyly, esophageal involvement, and telangiectasias. Anticentromere antibodies are common, though only 4% to 16% of patients with these antibodies develop CREST syndrome. It typically has a more indolent course, except when complicated by pulmonary hypertension. Radiographic features are similar to those of PSS. Pulmonary hypertension is present in up to 9% of patients.

RAYNAUD PHENOMENON

Digital–arterial vasospasm leads to cyanosis. It may be idiopathic and isolated (and called Raynaud disease) or appear as an early finding of connective tissue disease.

DERMATOMYOSITIS AND POLYMYOSITIS

These are characterized by neck and proximal limb muscle weakness and pain. Approximately 50% have heliotrope rash, extensor erythema or purpura, or Gottron papules. Overall incidence is 5 to 10:1000 000. It is more common in women (2:1) and peaks in the first decade and again in the forties and fifties. Chest involvement is manifest as hypoventilation and respiratory failure from muscle weakness, interstitial pneumonitis, and aspiration pneumonia.

Anti-aminoacyl-tRNA-synthetases (the most common being Jo-1) are linked to development of interstitial lung disease. HLA-DRw52 is present in almost all patients with these antibodies. Their presence increases the incidence of ILD, arthritis, fever, disease flaring, and of scaly, hyperkeratotic-fissured hands, but they are likely a secondary finding.

The radiograph is generally abnormal. Interstitial fibrosis is identical to IPF but abnormalities may develop acutely as diffuse alveolar damage or BOOP. The appearance improves markedly with adequate therapy. Patients with respiratory–muscle weakness have small lungs with linear atelectasis; pharyngeal muscle weakness may result in aspiration pneumonia.

SJOGREN SYNDROME

This syndrome consists of keratoconjunctivitis sicca, xerostomia, and parotid swelling. It may be isolated, but in up to 59% of cases it is associated with other connective tissue disorders. Chest abnormalities include lymphocytic interstitial pneumonitis, pleuritis, and tracheobronchial gland inflammation.

Primary Sjogren syndrome is characterized by antibodies to small nuclear and cytoplasm particles; SS-A is called anti-Ro; SS-B, anti-La. The antibodies may be elicited by viral salivary damage, perhaps by prior viral infection.

Radiograph sometimes reveals reticulonodular interstitial disease that is usually basilar-predominant. This may be due in different patients to lymphoid interstitial pneumonia, interstitial fibrosis, or lymphoma development. HRCT reveals more disease and is often abnormal when the radiograph is normal. The most common findings are bronchiolectasis, poorly defined centrilobular opacities, and ground glass opacities with occasional honeycombing. A particular pattern consisting of extensive ground glass opacities with scattered thin-walled cysts has been described in the lymphoid interstitial pneumonitis of Sjogren syndrome (but also other instances of lymphoid interstitial pneumonitis); alternatively lymphoid interstitial pneumonitis may present as interlobular septal thickening with nodular bronchovascular thickening indistinguishable from lymphoma.

OVERLAP SYNDROMES AND MIXED CONNECTIVE TISSUE DISEASE

Patients who clearly have connective tissue disease but do not satisfy diagnostic criteria to fit into a particular disease fall into this category of overlap syndromes. They are female-predominant. A particular subgroup with findings of SLE, PSS, and polymyositis is called mixed connective tissue disease and is associated with antibodies to extractable nuclear antigen, anti-nRMP. These patients may develop CNS involvement in 30% to 50% of cases, and membranous glomerulonephritis in some. Pulmonary disease occurs in 20% of cases, sometimes as fatal interstitial lung disease, diffuse alveolar hemorrhage, or pulmonary hypertension. Radiographic findings include those of SLE, PSS, and polymyositis. Interstitial abnormalities are present in 85% of cases, usually basilar-predominant reticular disease that extends superiorly and develops peripheral honeycombing as disease progresses. Pleural effusion is uncommon. Pericardial effusion and myocarditis may occur, and mediastinal lymphadenopathy has been reported.

RHEUMATIC PNEUMONITIS

Patients with rheumatic fever may develop diffuse alveolar damage that can organize into alveolar fibrosis. Small-artery pulmonary vasculitis can occur. The process is usually severe and has extensive cardiac disease.

RELAPSING POLYCHONDRITIS

This disorder of cartilage inflammatory destruction is uncommon and peaks between 40 and 60 years of age. It is associated with other autoimmune disorders in up to 25% of cases, and anticartilage and anti-minor-matrix-collagen antibodies have been found in some. Complement appears activated locally. HLA-DR4 is associated with the disease. Cartilage throughout the body is attacked, fragmented, and replaced by fibrous tissue. The most common radiographic finding in the chest is tracheal stenosis, usually a few centimeters long but sometimes diffuse; bronchial stenosis may be visible as well. CT may reveal tracheal or bronchial thickening. Bronchiectasis is sometimes present, possibly because of recurrent infection from airway obstruction.

LUNG INVOLVEMENT IN INFLAMMATORY BOWEL DISEASE

Crohn disease and ulcerative colitis are not autoimmune but are immunologically mediated. Many patients have lymphocytic alveolitis but clinically significant lung disease is rare.

LUNG INVOLVEMENT IN PRIMARY BILIARY CIRRHOSIS

Some patients with primary biliary cirrhosis (PBC), often with Sjogren syndrome, have been reported to have alveolitis, bronchiolitis, BOOP, diffuse alveolar hemorrhage, and interstitial pneumonitis.

DISEASES CHARACTERIZED BY VASCULITIS

WEGENER GRANULOMATOSIS

This multisystem disease has necrotizing granulomatous inflammation of the upper- and lower-respiratory tracts, glomerulonephritis, and necrotizing vasculitis of the lungs and other tissues. Four principal criteria are: nasal or oral inflammation, abnormal chest radiograph, abnormal urinary sediment, and either biopsied granulomatous inflammation or hemoptysis. Presence of two or more is 88% sensitive and 92% specific. Its prevalence is approximately 3:100 000 and is more common in older patients. The cause may be prior respiratory infection or inhalation. It is associated with c-ANCA, specifically anti-proteinase-3, a strong but somewhat nonspecific link.

Leukocyte infiltrates aggregate into small microabscesses that become necrotic and coalesce. Small granulomata may be present. Pulmonary nodules may be 1 to 10 cm and are frequently centrally necrotic or cavitary. Alveolar hemorrhage, fibrosis, follicular bronchiolitis, and obstructive pneumonitis are usually minor. Airway granulomata are common, sometimes resulting in an obstructing granulation tissue mass. Small-to-medium pulmonary arteries are involved. Paranasal sinus involvement may cause mucosal thickening or even osseocartilaginous destruction. Upper-airway involvement may lead to hoarseness or dyspnea. Cardiac conduction abnormalities, heart failure, or pericarditis may occur but are not common.

The chest radiograph will eventually be abnormal in 85% of patients. Nodules, generally less than 10 and typically diffuse and bilateral, range less than 1 to 10 cm. They often cavitate, leaving irregular thick walls, but rarely calcify. CT reveals more nodules and inapparent cavitation in most nodules over 2 cm. There may occasionally be reticulonodular interstitial thickening. Consolidation and ground glass opacities because of hemorrhage are the second most common finding: random, peripheral wedges simulating infarct, or in peribronchovascular distribution. Bronchial narrowing is seldom radiographically apparent, but may lead to atelectasis. Pleural effusion is variable, and lymphadenopathy is visible in up to 15% of patients.

CHURG-STRAUSS SYNDROME

This syndrome includes asthma, fever, blood eosinophilia, and necrotizing vasculitis with intravascular granulomatous inflammation as well as neuropathy, nonfixed pulmonary infiltrates, paranasal sinus disease, and extravascular eosinophilia. The presence of four or more of these is 85% sensitive and almost 100% specific. It is rare, with incidence perhaps 2 to 3:1000 000. Asthma or rhinitis develops in early adulthood, with vasculitis developing later. The true causative abnormality may be a hypersensitivity reaction to an unknown agent. CSS is associated with p-ANCA, though this antibody may be found in inflammatory bowel disease, RA, SLE, autoimmune liver disease, and some infections; and with atypical ANCA. Circulating immune complexes are sometimes present.

A small-to-medium vessel vasculitis affects arteries and veins, with leukocyte infiltrates evolving into fibrinoid necrosis and granulomata. Nonvascular granulomata are more commonly extrapulmonary but may be found in the lungs; alveolar and interstitial infiltrates are more common, as are changes of chronic asthma. GI and cardiac involvement is common.

The chest radiograph is abnormal in approximately 70% of patients, usually with transient patchy consolidation that may precede systemic problems. They may be symmetric and simulate chronic eosinophilic pneumonia or may develop into nodular opacities that rarely cavitate. Interstitial thickening and hilar lymphadenopathy are uncommon. Ground glass opacities may be present in 60% of patients, either patchy or peripheral. Small centrilobular nodules, effusions, or septal thickening may occasionally be present.

POLYARTERITIS NODOSA

Polyarteritis nodosa (PAN) is a necrotizing vasculitis of the small-to-medium muscular systemic arteries without granulomata. Sites of disease are often at branch points and are aneurismal. Immunocomplex deposition may play a role. Pulmonary arterial involvement almost never occurs, though bronchial artery involvement can develop. It is associated with hepatitis-B virus infection.

MICROSCOPIC POLYANGIITIS

It is similar to PAN (formerly a subcategory of it) except it involves small arterioles, venules, and capillaries; large vessel disease may play a small role. It is associated with p-ANCA (antimyeloperoxidase) and atypical ANCA; RF and ANA may be positive. HBV infection is rare. Pulmonary vessels are affected in 15% to 30% of patients, typically manifest as hemoptysis. Pulmonary findings include alveolar hemorrhage and hemosiderin-laden macrophages. Radiographs reveal patchy opacities because of hemorrhage, occasionally with effusion or edema.

TAKAYASU ARTERITIS

This vasculitis affects the aorta and its major branches, via perivascular/intramural granulomatous inflammation. Pulmonary artery involvement is variable but can involve the main pulmonary arteries or intrapulmonary arteries. It is over 90% female-predominant, and typically develops in the age ranging from 10 to 40 years. Most cases derive from Southeast Asia. In patients from Japan, involvement is typically of the ascending aorta, arch, and arch vessels; whereas, in India, the abdominal aorta and renal arteries are commonly involved. Diagnostic criteria include onset at less than 40 years of age, extremity claudication, decreased brachial artery pulse, blood-pressure difference at least 10 mm Hg between the arms, subclavian or aortic bruit, or arteriographic abnormality. Presence of three or more is 90% sensitive and 98% specific.

Most patients have antiendothelial cell antibodies without ANCA, ANA, ENA, anti-Ro, anticardiolipin, or anti-DNA; however, it is uncertain whether these cause disease or are a response to vessel damage. Many patients have glomerulonephritis, immune-based skin reactions, or other connective tissue disease. HLA-B52 and -B39.2 are commonly encountered.

Patchy panarteritis involves adventitial fibrosis and mononuclear infiltrate. Vasa-vasorum obliteration is common. Granulomata develop in the media, and intimal fibrosis is frequent.

Contour irregularities of the aorta, including wavy or scalloped descending aortic or arch ectasia are visible in 10% to 75% of patients, and early calcification is visible in 10% to 25% of patients. Cardiomegaly may be present. Pulmonary artery involvement may be visible as focal oligemia. Rib notching may be present if the aorta is occluded. CT or MR findings include dense or calcified vessel wall, mural thickening up to 4 mm, and delayed circumferential enhancement. Descending thoracic aortic stenosis is present in 37% of patients, ascending aortic dilation, in 32% of patients. Pulmonary artery involvement is visible in 70% of patients as abnormal peripheral appearance likely because of occlusion, dilation of the pulmonary trunk is visible in 19%, and central thrombus is visible in 3% of patients.

GIANT CELL ARTERITIS

Giant cell arteritis (GCA) is one of the commonest systemic vasculitides, associated with perivascular granulomatous inflammation. It primarily affects the larger vessels of the head and neck, but the elastic and muscular pulmonary arteries may be affected. It affects patients older than 50 years and is often preceded by infection. Patients present with headache, jaw claudication, polymyalgia rheumatica, vision loss, and often focal tenderness at the involved site. ESR is elevated.

BEHCET DISEASE

This systemic disorder manifests as recurrent aphthous stomatitis, genital ulcers, skin lesions, and uveitis. Men are more frequently affected; age is typically 20 to 30 years. It has unknown etiology, possibly viral or food-induced. HLA-B5 is more common in these patients than in controls. Lung involvement is uncommon. Transmural vascular inflammation may extend into airways and erode bronchial or pulmonary vessels and cause hemoptysis. Thrombi and infarcts may occur. Pulmonary artery aneurysms are usually perihilar and may be up to 3-cm diameter.

The Hughes-Stovin syndrome of pulmonary artery and systemic venous thrombosis with fever, headache, cough, papilledema, and hemoptysis may be caused by Behcet disease. The interlobar artery is the most common to thrombose. The superior vena cava or brachiocephalic veins may thrombose and lead to mediastinal widening. Pleural effusion may develop as a sequela of pulmonary infarct.

MIXED CRYOGLOBULINEMIA

This uncommon syndrome of purpura, arthralgia, glomerulonephritis, and IgM anti-IgG cryoglobulin is sometimes associated with hepatitis C virus. Immune complex deposition may play a role. It can cause capillaritis and alveolar hemorrhage, visible as diffuse interstitial lung disease.

HENOCH-SCHONLEIN PURPURA

Purpura, abdominal pain, GI hemorrhage, arthritis or arthralgia, and glomerulonephritis constitute the syndrome. It appears most often in childhood; no specific agent is known. Immune complex deposition, typically IgA ANCA, may play a role: IgA activates the alternate complement pathway. Lung involvement is rare, usually as capillaritis and alveolar hemorrhage.

NECROTIZING SARCOID GRANULOMATOSIS

In this uncommon process, typically only detected after resection, confluent granulomata develop with necrosis and destructive vasculitis. It affects middle-aged adults, typically women. The etiology is uncertain, perhaps hypersensitivity. It responds to corticosteroid therapy and may be a variant of classic sarcoid. Radiographs reveal multiple well-defined nodules, usually 5 to 10 mm but occasionally miliary or large, usually peribronchovascular and subpleural.

SARCOIDOSIS–NONNECROTIZING GRANULOMA FORMATION

Most patients are 20-to 40-year-old when diagnosed with sarcoid. Some reports show an increased prevalence in smokers. US prevalence is approximately 10:100 000; prevalence in African American women aged 30 to 39 years is 107:100 000. About half of patients are asymptomatic at diagnosis; half of the remainder have dyspnea and the rest have extrathoracic symptoms. The cause is unknown but pulmonary parenchymal and pulmonary lymphatic involvement suggests inflammatory-immune response to an inhaled agent. Recurrence after lung transplant and transmission via bone marrow transplant suggest infectious etiology but the agent has not been cultured. There is an association with HLA-A1 and -B8. Patients often have cutaneous anergy, increased CD8:CD4 ratio, and B-cell hyperactivity.

By whatever etiology, pulmonary macrophages are activated with granuloma formation and sometimes fibrosis. The peribronchovascular, interlobular septal, and pleural interstitial tissues are dominantly involved, first as discrete granulomata but eventually coalescing into interstitial thickening. Alveolar involvement is usually minimal but can coalesce into macroscopic nodules. Pulmonary–vascular granuloma formation is common and affects vessels of all sizes. Thrombosis is rare and necrosis does not occur but they can compress the lumen. Serum angiotensin-converting enzyme and lysozyme levels are elevated, though neither of these is specific for sarcoid; and serum alkaline phosphatase is elevated in 30% to 45% of patients.

Staging is helpful for predicting outcome (Table 21-1). More than one-half and approximately one-half of patients in stages 1 and 2, respectively, will have resolution of radiographic abnormalities at follow-up. Only 20% of patients in stage 3 will undergo resolution of radiographic abnormalities. An additional 20% go on to fibrosis.

About one-half of patients will have stage 1 findings of lymphadenopathy, often in the combination of right-paratracheal (70% of cases) and bilateral hilar (95%) disease—the ("1-2-3 sign"). AP-window nodes are enlarged in 50% of cases, and subcarinal nodes are enlarged in 20% of cases. Only 5% of patients have unilateral hilar lymphadenopathy. The distribution is helpful in distinguishing sarcoid from lymphoma and tuberculous infection. Only 5% of patients have calcified nodes at presentation, typically peripheral and eggshell type, though calcification increases with progression up to 20% or more. CT will reveal more stations of lymphadenopathy than are apparent radiographically and may image radiographically occult nodal calcification. Lymphadenopathy may compress a bronchus and lead to lobar atelectasis, most commonly in the middle lobe or may lead to arterial, SVC, or innominate-venous compression.

TABLE 21-1 Staging of Sarcoidosis

STAGE	RADIOGRAPHIC FINDINGS
0 (>10%)	None
1 (50%)	Hilar, mediastinal lymph adenopathy
2 (30%)	Lymph adenopathy and pulmonary abnormalities
3 (10%)	Diffuse pulmonary abnormalities; no lymphadenopathy

Lung involvement is radiographically visible at some point in 50% to 65% of patients. Abnormalities are typically bilateral, symmetric, and mid- and upper lobe predominant. Nodular and reticulonodular disease is most common, with reticular, alveolar, or ground glass opacities less so. Cavitation is distinctly uncommon. Effusion and atelectasis are also uncommon. Nodules are typically irregular, usually less than 3 mm but as large as 1 cm, visible in HRCT as mostly peribronchovascular, peripleural, and along the interlobar and interlobular interstitium, often coalescing to nodular thickening. Reticular disease in HRCT reveals interlobular septal thickening in 20% to 90% of patients and nonseptal lines in 20% to 70%. Traction bronchiectasis is predominantly upper-lung-zone and perihilar. Honeycombing typically involves the subpleural mid-and upper-lung zones. Reticulonodular disease is likely a combination of nodules with interlobular septal or reticular thickening. Alveolar disease in HRCT is often peribronchial or less commonly peripheral. Air bronchograms are generally present, and additional interstitial findings are also generally present. Ground glass opacity is seldom radiographically apparent but visible in 20% to 60% of HRCT scans. In most cases, this is a secondary feature of nodular disease. The heart is frequently involved but the process is not often radiographically apparent. Cardiomegaly may be from cardiomyopathy, valve disease, pericardial effusion, or left-ventricular aneurysm. Pulmonary hypertension and cor pulmonale may develop late.

Approximately 20% of patients will develop pulmonary fibrosis, manifest as architectural distortion and bronchiectasis typically involving the upper lung zones, with upward retraction of the hila, bulla formation, and compensatory lower lobe hyperinflation. In HRCT, peribronchovascular opacity radiates from the hila to the upper lobes, and honeycombing is visible in 40% of cases.

Gallium-67 scan may reveal tracer-avid lymphadenopathy in a "lambda" pattern involving the para-/infrahilar and right paratracheal nodes. The "panda" pattern of elevated bilateral symmetric lacrimal and parotid uptake together with bilateral symmetric hilar lymphadenopathy or pulmonary fibrosis is also specific for the disease. (The "panda" pattern without lung disease may be seen in Sjogren syndrome, HIV, and after head–neck radiation).

LUNG TRANSPLANT-RELATED IMMUNE LUNG DISEASES

In addition to reperfusion edema, which occurs by the first postoperative day in 90% of patients and by the third day in 97% of patients, transplanted lungs are susceptible to immune-mediated disease.

Hyperacute rejection is caused by preformed alloantibodies that bind to the donor organ, and activate complement. Destruction begins within minutes. Diffuse alveolar damage, neutrophil infiltration, and IgG deposition are hallmarks. It is rare in lung transplants, and screening of blood for ABO compatibility and anti-HLA antibodies has made this complication even rarer.

Acute rejection is a T-cell anti-HLA response without B-cell or antibody response. Almost all patients will undergo acute rejection. It may be seen as early as 3 days after transplant but more typically is manifest at 1 to 2 weeks; 60% of all cases occur within 3 months, and after 4 years rejection is uncommon. A patchy mononuclear infiltrate begins in the perivascular interstitium and extends to involve endothelium and alveolar interstitium. Radiographs are abnormal in 50% to 100% of cases; they may reveal fine reticular interstitial disease, interlobular septal thickening, ground glass opacities, alveolar consolidation, and new or enlarging effusions. In the first postoperative month, HRCT findings are nonspecific and do not allow distinction between acute rejection, fluid overload, and reperfusion injury. The most common HRCT finding is ground glass opacity, more likely with higher-grade rejection. Septal lines are less common. Other findings include new or enlarged effusion, basilar consolidation, or peribronchial cuffing.

Chronic rejection may be airways-related or cause an accelerated vascular sclerosis not described here. Up to 70% of patients will develop obliterative bronchiolitis, with mortality up to 55% of affected patients. It appears immune-mediated; the development of infection, particularly CMV, is probably important as well. It may be caused by small vessel-related ischemia. It generally develops within 12 months of transplant. Membranous- and proximal-respiratory bronchiolar subepithelial connective tissues become thickened. Early disease has fibroblasts within loose connective tissue, but increasing severity leads to more fibrosis that may occlude the lumen. It may be active, accompanied by inflammatory infiltrate, or inactive. Luminal tissue deposition should suggest an alternate etiology. Bronchial dilation visible in 80% of patients, mainly segmental and subsegmental lower lobe branches. Expiratory air trapping is common and probably the most accurate indicator of obliterative bronchiolitis. Bronchial wall thickening and mosaic perfusion are less common. In seril, HRCT studies decreased lung volume, decreased peripheral vascularity, and interlobular thickening develop after 7 to 11 months. Bronchial dilation develops at a mean of 12 months; and decreased attenuation and mosaic perfusion develop at mean intervals of 16 and 21 months, respectively.

BONE MARROW TRANSPLANT-RELATED IMMUNE LUNG DISEASES

Patients may acutely develop pulmonary edema or diffuse alveolar hemorrhage, or one of several immune-related lung diseases after bone marrow transplantation (BMT). They are also at increased risk for infection.

Interstitial pneumonitis develops in 10% of patients with BMT and causes 40% of transplant-related deaths. It peaks at 14 to 80 days. Its pathogenesis is unknown; it appears immunologic but not directly related to graft-versus-host disease (GHVD). Chemotherapy and radiation therapy may influence development. Radiographic findings are nonspecific, generally bilateral interstitial thickening with ground glass opacities and small poorly defined nodules.

Obstructive small airway disease (obliterative bronchiolitis) occurs in 5% or less of patients with BMT. It does not develop in the first 3 months, and the median interval is 260 days. Mild bronchiolitis and intramural fibroblastic proliferation develop in the same process as in lung transplant disease. Radiographic findings also are similar.

Graft versus host disease occurs when donor T-cells recognize the recipient as foreign. It may be acute or chronic. Lung findings in acute GVHD are minimal, but the lungs are typically abnormal in chronic GVHD. Whether the abnormality is due directly to the immune process or to secondary causes is uncertain: patients frequently have ongoing pulmonary infection and may develop a sicca syndrome with chronic bronchitis. Some develop a lymphocytic alveolitis and fibrosis that responds well to treatment.

Lymphocytic chronic bronchitis is characterized by epithelial and submucosal lymphocyte infiltrate, with focal epithelial necrosis. It occurs in up to 25% of allogeneic BMT. It is more severe in patients with more severe GVHD and may be because of the same process.

EOSINOPHILIC LUNG DISEASE

Eosinophils contain preformed mediators, importantly major basic protein (MBP), which is toxic to some parasites but also to host cells. Other eosinophil mediators activate and enhance neutrophil response and activate platelets. Eosinophils are thus implicated in several lung diseases. Eosinophilic diseases related to drugs, parasites, and fungal infections are discussed elsewhere.

Simple pulmonary eosinophilia (Loeffler syndrome) is an uncommon disorder characterized by blood eosinophilia and patchy transient alveolar opacities. Patients are typically asymptomatic, though a history of atopy or asthma is common. Interstitial and alveolar edema is mixed with eosinophils, without immune deposits or destruction. Radiographic findings are typically of migratory and short-lived areas of consolidation, typically peripheral and homogeneous. Differential considerations include drug- and parasite-induced eosinophilic lung disease.

Acute eosinophilic pneumonia is an acute febrile illness of unknown etiology, perhaps hypersensitivity to an unknown antigen. Patients often have allergic tendencies. Radiographs early look like pulmonary edema. It progresses over hours or days to basilar-predominant interstitial and alveolar opacities, generally with small pleural effusions, and can lead to hypoxemic respiratory failure. CT reveals ground glass attenuation, septal thickening, and small effusion, occasionally with consolidation or small nodules. It responds rapidly to corticosteroid therapy, and relapse is not a feature. Patients usually do not have peripheral-blood eosinophilia.

Chronic eosinophilic pneumonia is a relapsing process usually of unknown etiology, though some cases are associated with *Aspergillus* infection, RA, or immune complex vasculitis. It affects women more than men (2:1) and the peak incidence is 30 to 39. It is associated with atopy and asthma, and IgE is elevated during relapses. It is usually insidious and patients may go several months without diagnosis. Peripheral-blood eosinophilia is usually present. It rapidly improves with corticosteroid therapy, but patients may require therapy for months or years, and relapses are common if treatment is reduced or stopped. Alveolar infiltrates containing numerous eosinophils develop and often produce microabscesses. Charcot-Leyden crystals may be visible in the airspaces and in macrophages. Interstitial infiltrates are usually present but less severe. The airways may be ulcerated and obstructive bronchiolitis may develop. The radiograph appears identical to simple pulmonary eosinophilia, except that the opacities in chronic eosinophilic pneumonia persist unchanged until corticosteroid therapy is started.

Hypereosinophilic syndrome is an uncommon multiorgan disease characterized by prolonged blood eosinophilia with eosinophilic tissue infiltrates. Mean age is 33, and there may be a male predominance. Diagnosis requires eosinophil count over 1500 for at least 6 months (unless death intervenes) without other cause and signs and symptoms of organ involvement. Radiographs reveal transient hazy opacities or consolidation that resolves spontaneously. Cardiomegaly, pulmonary edema, and pleural effusion may develop. CT may reveal reticular opacities.

GOODPASTURE SYNDROME AND IDIOPATHIC PULMONARY HEMORRHAGE

These processes have identical chest manifestation: Goodpasture syndrome is essentially idiopathic pulmonary hemorrhage with renal involvement. Both result in repeated pulmonary hemorrhage, iron deficiency anemia, and acute or chronic pulmonary insufficiency. IPH usually develops in children younger than 10 years, with no sex predominance. Goodpasture syndrome typically affects people older than 16 years, with slight male predominance. HLA-DRw15 and -DR4 are associated with Goodpasture syndrome. Antibodies to type IV collagen of glomerular and alveolar basement membranes develop. IPH may have a heritable basis, and circulating and tissue immune complexes have been found in some patients.

Hemorrhage is confined mostly to the alveoli and small airways. Much blood loss can occur before hemoptysis develops. Hemosiderin laden macrophages and free interstitial iron are present, and there is mild-to-moderate interstitial fibrosis. There may be a mild lymphocytic inflammatory component, and sometimes an acute interstitial capillaritis develops. Immunoglobulins line the basement membrane, usually IgG but sometimes IgA or IgM.

Early in either disease radiographs reveal patchy alveolar opacities, large opacities usually having air bronchograms. The opacities are typically widespread, bilateral, and asymmetric, but may be perihilar or in the mid- and lower-lung zones. Acute pulmonary hemorrhage is visible in CT as mainly dependent areas of ground glass or alveolar opacity. In MRI, the high T1 signal of blood and the low T2 signal of paramagnetic iron can provide diagnostic accuracy. Serial radiographs over the few days after an episode reveal disappearance of the alveolar opacities in 2 to 3 days to be replaced with reticulonodular opacities in the same distribution. CT reveals ill-defined 1- to 3-mm centrilobular nodules in the affected areas, sometimes with ground glass opacity and interlobular septal thickening. The radiograph usually is normal within 10 to 12 days. Repeated episodes deposit more hemosiderin in the interstitium and pulmonary fibrosis increases. A fine reticulonodular pattern in chest radiography indicates the irreversible component, visible in CT as 1- to 3-mm centrilobular nodules throughout the parenchyma.

SUGGESTED READING

Bankier AA, Kiener HP, Wiesmayr MN, et al. Discrete lung involvement in systemic lupus erythematosus: CT assessment. *Radiology.* 1995;196:835.

Desai SR, Veeraraghavan S, Hansell DM, et al. CT features of lung disease in patients with systemic sclerosis: comparison with idiopathic pulmonary fibrosis and nonspecific interstitial pneumonia. *Radiology.* 2004;232:560-567.

Hansell DM. Small-vessel diseases of the lung: CT-pathologic correlates. *Radiology.* 2002;225:639-653.

Kim EA, Lee KS, Johkoh T, et al. Interstitial lung diseases associated with collagen ascular diseases: radiologic and histophathologic findings. *Radiographics.* 2002;22:S151-S165.

Lugo-Olivifri, CH. Non-sarcoid granulomatous disease with involvement of the lungs. *Radiology.* 1996;201:784.

Mayberry JP, Primack SL, Muller NL. Thoracic manifestations of systemic autoimmune diseases: radiographic and high-resolution CT findings. *Radiographics.* 2000;20:1623-1635.

Tanaka N, Kim JS, Newell JD, et al. Rheumatoid arthritis-related lung disease: CT findings. *Radiology.* 2004;232:81-91.

QUESTIONS AND ANSWERS

1. A patient presents with serositis, photosensitivity, thrombocytopenia, and renal insufficiency. Which of these would be most specific and useful for her diagnosis?
   A. Anti-Sm
   B. Anti-ds-DNA
   C. Scl-70
   D. c-ANCA

   ANSWER: B. The patient likely has systemic lupus erythematosus. Speckled staining is most common, reflecting antibodies to nucleic ribonucleoprotein and the nonnucleic glycoprotein macromolecule Sm. Rim staining is specific for patients with SLE and reflects antibodies to nuclear DNA. The level of double-strand DNA antibodies reflects disease status in many patients. c-ANCA can be positive in SLE patients but has no bearing on disease status.

2. Regarding rheumatoid arthritis, which of the following is *true*?
   A. Extra-articular manifestations are more common in women.
   B. Approximately 1% to 5% have radiographic evidence of interstitial lung disease.
   C. Incidence of pulmonary rheumatoid nodules is about 1:50.
   D. Hyperviscosity syndrome is related to thrombocytopenia.

   ANSWER: B. RA has extra-articular manifestations in about three-fourths of patients, more common in men and in patients with severe articular disease. Approximately 1% to 5% of patients have radiographic evidence of ILD, though 40% have reduced DLCO consistent with fibrosis. Rheumatoid nodules are present in 2:1000 patients. Hyperviscosity syndrome is a rare complication of RA in which RF molecules conglomerate into bodies large enough to obstruct small vessels.

3. A 45 year-old woman with scleroderma is most likely to have which of the following?
   A. Interstitial pneumonitis
   B. Rib notching
   C. Anti-RNA-polymerase III antibodies
   D. Pleural effusion

   ANSWER: A. Interstitial pneumonitis is present in 20% to 65% of radiographs and appears similar to IPF. Rib notching is a nonspecific finding found in 15% of patients. Anti-RNA-polymerase III antibodies are specific for scleroderma but sensitivity is less than 25%. Effusion is less common than in other connective tissue diseases, radiographically apparent in 10% to 15% of patients.

4. Regarding Sjogren syndrome, which of the following is *true*?
   A. Consists of keratoconjunctivitis sicca, xerostomia, and parotid swelling
   B. An isolated syndrome in the majority of cases
   C. Associated with bullous changes in the lung apices
   D. Antibodies are developed against topoisomerase-1.

   ANSWER: A. The Sjogren syndrome consists of keratoconjunctivitis sicca, xerostomia, and parotid swelling. It is associated with other connective tissue disorders in 59% of cases. In the lungs, it is associated with lymphocytic interstitial pneumonitis, pleuritis, and tracheobronchial gland inflammation. Antibodies are developed against small nuclear and cytoplasm particles: SS-A (anti-Ro) and SS-B (anti-La). Anti-topoisomerase-1 (Scl-70) is associated with scleroderma.

5. A 55 year-old man presents with recurrent hemoptysis and renal insufficiency with abnormal urine sediment suggesting glomerulonephritis. What will the chest radiograph most likely reveal?
   A. Diffuse reticulonodular lung disease
   B. Normal study
   C. A few nodules, the largest 6 cm and cavitary, with patchy basilar predominant opacities
   D. Innumerable subcentimeter nodules with apical-predominant cysts

   ANSWER: C. The patient's hemoptysis and glomerulonephritis satisfy diagnostic criteria for Wegener granulomatosis. In such patients, the chest radiograph will eventually be abnormal in 85% of patients. Nodules, generally numbering less than 10 and typically diffuse and bilateral, range from subcentimeter to 10 cm. Consolidation and ground glass opacities because of hemorrhage are the second most common finding and are independent of nodules.

6. A chest CT angiogram obtained to rule out PTE in a 25 year-old man with hemoptysis reveals a 2.5-cm right interlobar artery aneurysm. Which of the following is *true*?
   A. His disease is associated with blood eosinophilia.
   B. Biopsy will reveal nonnecrotizing granulomas.
   C. Antibodies to myeloperoxidase are common.
   D. His disease may also manifest as aphthous stomatitis and skin lesions.

   ANSWER: D. The patient may have Behcet disease. Many inflammatory-allergic processes are associated with eosinophilia, but Behcet disease is not. The disorder is not associated with granuloma formation or with antimyeloperoxidase antibodies. Its manifestations include recurrent aphthous stomatitis, genital ulcers, skin lesions, and uveitis.

7. Chest radiographs obtained for a woman with newly diagnosed sarcoid reveal hilar lymphadenopathy and lung abnormalities. Which of the following is *true* regarding the staging and prognosis?
   A. Stage 1. Abnormalities are likely to resolve.
   B. Stage 2. Abnormalities resolve in about one-half of patients.
   C. Stage 3. Abnormalities resolve in about one-half of patients.
   D. Stage 3. Abnormalities are unlikely to resolve.

   ANSWER: B. The staging is described above. Staging is primarily helpful for predicting outcome.

8. A patient who underwent lung transplant 36 hours ago has developed shortness of breath and hypoxemia. What is the most likely diagnosis?
   A. Hyperacute rejection
   B. Acute rejection
   C. Chronic rejection
   D. Reperfusion edema

   ANSWER: D. Reperfusion edema occurs by the third postoperative day in over 97% of cases. Hyperacute rejection begins within minutes of reperfusion and is owing to preformed antibodies to ABO and HLA antigens. It should never happen with current pretransplant screening. Acute rejection is a T-cell mediated anti-HLA response, seen as soon as 3 days after transplant but more typically manifest at 1 to 2 weeks. Chronic rejection is first visible at 7 months at the earliest.

9. A 30 year-old woman with eczema presents for a prenatal screening radiograph, which reveals patchy peripheral alveolar opacities. She has no symptoms, but a CBC reveals eosinophilia. What is the most likely diagnosis?

A. Simple pulmonary eosinophilia
B. Acute eosinophilic pneumonia
C. Chronic eosinophilic pneumonia
D. Hypereosinophilic syndrome

ANSWER: A. Simple pulmonary eosinophilia has patchy transient opacities consisting of interstitial and alveolar edema and eosinophilia. Acute eosinophilic pneumonia has acute fever and does not have eosinophilia. Chronic eosinophilic pneumonia and hypereosinophilic pneumonia are associated with eosinophilia but also with long-standing symptoms.

10. Idiopathic pulmonary hemorrhage and Goodpasture syndrome are differentiated by what?
A. Artery diameter that hemorrhages and associated volume of blood loss
B. Presence of free interstitial iron
C. Demographic characteristics and sites of involvement
D. Presence of alveolar opacities

ANSWER: C. IPH usually affects children aging younger than 10 years and has no sex predominance. Goodpasture syndrome typically affects patients older than 16 years and has a slight male predominance, and it affects the kidneys as well as the lung. In both, hemorrhage is confined mostly to the alveoli and small airways. Much blood loss can occur before hemoptysis develops. Early in either disease, the radiograph may reveal patchy alveolar opacities. The alveolar opacities disappear in 2 to 3 days, replaced with reticulonodular opacities in the same distribution. The radiograph usually is normal within 10 to 12 days. A fine reticulonodular pattern in chest radiography indicates the irreversible component.

22 INTERSTITIAL LUNG DISEASE

Ian Malcolm and Satinder P. Singh

INTRODUCTION

The interstitium of the lung surrounds the central bronchovascular bundles and extends around the smaller airways and alveoli to the subpleural region. Although it is continuous, it is conveniently divided into axial and peripheral, as certain diseases have a tendency to involve either of these regions.

Interstitial lung disease (ILD) is a heterogeneous group of disorders with variable interstitial inflammation and fibrosis (Table 22-1). Idiopathic interstitial disease encompasses a group of disorders, which are syndromes rather than diseases. Their classification is determined by not only radiological findings, but also by clinical features and histology. It is impossible to determine a particular type of idiopathic interstitial pneumonia with absolute certainty on HRCT (already defined) alone.

Known causes of ILD should be considered as secondary or nonidiopathic ILD (Table 22-2).

Chest radiography and HRCT of the chest have established roles in the detection, differential diagnosis, and follow-up of patients with ILD. Chest radiograph is often abnormal in 90% of patients with diffuse lung disease although it is insensitive for early ILD. In 10% of biopsy-proven ILD, chest radiographs are normal. Therefore, a normal chest radiograph does not exclude ILD, and extensive ILD on a chest radiograph does not correlate well with physiologic impairment. Evaluation of serial radiographs provides information regarding status of disease progression or regression. By using thin section thickness (1.25 mm) and high spatial frequency reconstruction (bone algorithm), HRCT allows better visualization of fine parenchymal details such as small bronchi, branching vessels, and interlobular septa. HRCT is often performed at full inspiration in supine position. Additional prone imaging is done in patients with suspected basal ILD, which is masked or mimicked by dependent atelectasis in supine imaging. Expiratory HRCT imaging allows detection of air trapping in patients with suspected obstructed airway disease, not visible on inspiratory scans.

IDIOPATHIC PULMONARY FIBROSIS

Idiopathic pulmonary fibrosis (IPF) is the most common form of idiopathic ILD, estimated prevalence is 20 per 100 000 people.

Histology—Histological findings include heterogeneous appearance with acute, subacute, and chronic inflammation, together with fibroblastic foci and honeycombing. No other form of ILD has these heterogeneous features. These are the findings of usual interstitial pneumonitis (UIP). Approximately 70% of cases of UIP are IPF, the remainder are secondary UIP because of known causes.

Clinical—Patients are usually older than 50 years of age and present with nonproductive cough, progressive dyspnea, weight loss, and fatigue. Velcro rales may be heard in the lungs.

TABLE 22-1 Interstitial Lung Disease Histopathology

Idiopathic pulmonary fibrosis	Subpleural and basal reticulation	Honeycombing	Traction bronchiectasis	Architectural deformity	Irregular pleural, bronchial, and vascular interfaces	Minimal ground glass opacification	Commonly smokers with signs of centrilobular emphysema
Nonspecific interstitial pneumonitis	Ground glass opacities	Reticulation	Patchy consolidation	Traction bronchiectasis	Minimal or absent honeycombing	Subpleural sparing	
Cryptogenic organizing pneumonia	Subpleural and peribronchial distribution	Peripheral wedge, ground glass, or consolidation	Axial interstitial thickening	Axial interstitial nodules	Atoll sign		
Acute interstitial pneumonia	Patchy or diffuse consolidation (geographic distribution)	Patchy or diffuse ground glass opacities	Posterior lower lobe predominance	Later resolution or development of end-stage fibrosis with architectural deformity, bronchiectasis, honeycombing, etc.			
Respiratory bronchiolitis—interstitial lung disease and desquamative interstitial pneumonia							
RB-ILD	Ill-defined centrilobular nodules	Bronchial wall thickening	Air trapping (mosaic attenuation on expiration)	Upper lobe predominance (60%–75%)			
DIP	Acinar opacities (alveolitis)	Diffuse ground glass opacities	Posterior lower lobe predominance (60%–75%)	Small thin-walled cystic lucencies	Centrilobular emphysema		
Lymphocytic interstitial pneumonia	Diffuse or ground glass opacities	Ill-defined centrilobular nodules	Septal thickening (reticulation)	Small cystic lesions	Later, more diffuse cystic disease		

Pulmonary function tests—These are restrictive, with impaired gas transfer and reduced carbon monoxide diffusing capacity.

Radiographs—There are usually symmetrical, peripheral and basilar, linear, or reticular opacities, which progressively spread and coarsen. The lateral view is often more sensitive than the PA view in the detection of early disease. There is ongoing loss of volume and possibly architectural deformity. Decreased lung volumes are radiographically evident at the initial evaluation in over one-half of cases. Serial radiographs are often used to monitor disease progression and loss of lung volumes. Most patients are smokers, and if there is significant associated emphysema, lung volumes may be normal. A normal chest radiograph cannot be used to exclude UIP as over 10% of these patients have normal radiographs.

HRCT—In 70% to 95% of patients, there is a predominantly peripheral and basal interstitial reticular process because of thickening of the walls of secondary pulmonary lobules (the interlobular septa). Smaller

TABLE 22-2 Interstitial Lung Disease (Decreasing Frequency)

DISEASE	HISTOLOGY
Idiopathic pulmonary fibrosis (IPF)	Usual interstitial pneumonia (UIP)
Idiopathic nonspecific interstitial pneumonitis (NSIP)	NSIP
Cryptogenic organizing pneumonia (COP)	Organizing pneumonia
Acute interstitial pneumonia (AIP)	Acute lung injury with diffuse alveolar damage
Respiratory bronchiolitis (RB) and desquamative interstitial pneumonia (DIP)	Respiratory bronchiolitis and desquamative interstitial pneumonia
Lymphoid interstitial pneumonia (LIP)	LIP

(short) interstitial lines may also be seen because of thickening of intralobular septa, which is the interstitium within the secondary pulmonary lobule surrounding the alveoli and distal small airways. The subpleural margins and bronchial and vascular interfaces may become indistinct because of this diffuse interstitial process. There is associated architectural distortion, traction bronchiectasis, and honeycomb formation. Honeycomb cysts are characteristically similar in size, begin at the periphery, and layer progressively. Predominantly subpleural reticulation and honeycombing are present in majority of patients and fibrosis is most severe in the lower lung zones. In the remainder, all lung zones are similarly involved or mainly upper lung zones are affected. Patients with accelerated-phase disease show focal areas of consolidation, which is histologically shown to be diffuse alveolar damage and organizing pneumonia.

Management—Using clinical data and HRCT, a confident diagnosis of IPF can be made in most patients. A definite diagnosis requires open lung biopsy, but this is generally only performed if clinical management will be determined by this diagnosis. Video-assisted thoracoscopic surgery (VATS) procedure is less traumatic than open lung biopsy.

Lung carcinoma develops in 10% of cases, usually as a nodule but sometimes manifesting as focal consolidation. In the case of smokers, there may be associated emphysema and mosaic perfusion with air trapping. Adenopathy is shown in 70% of cases of IPF, but lymph nodes are unlikely to be greater than 15-mm short axis.

Treatment—Ineffective, as there is usually relentless progression of disease with death in 2 to 4 years. Five-year survival is 20%. Lung transplantation may be required for survival. The most rapid deaths occur with accelerated phase IPF. In the absence of accelerated disease, end-stage patients can also deteriorate with respiratory failure, cor pulmonale heart failure, PTE, or infection.

Secondary UIP may be caused by collagen vascular disease, asbestosis, drug toxicity, chronic hypersensitive pneumonitis (HP), and irradiation injury. These patients will often have additional findings because of the disease process itself. For example, UIP in a patient with scleroderma may also manifest with dilated atonic esophagus and aspiration pneumonia.

IDIOPATHIC NONSPECIFIC INTERSTITIAL PNEUMONITIS

Idiopathic nonspecific interstitial pneumonitis (NSIP) accounts for 14% to 35% of cases of Idiopathic ILD. This disease occurs in a younger age group than IPF (40–50 years of age).

Histology—There are no specific features to suggest UIP, DIP, OP, or AIP. In other words, this is a diagnosis of exclusion. The histology is homogeneous with thickening of alveolar walls with lymphocytes and plasma cells (cellular NSIP) or alternatively fibroblast and collagen (fibrotic NSIP). Patients with cellular disease have an excellent prognosis, whereas patients with fibrotic NSIP have a survival of only 6 to 14 years (Kim).

Clinical—Patients present with dyspnea and dry cough and have widespread basal crackles and finger clubbing (10%–35%). Average age of presentation is from 40 to 50 years.

Radiographs—There is usually bilateral patchy or confluent hazy opacification in the lungs. This predominates in the mid and lower lung zones, sometimes with reticular opacities and consolidation in the lung bases. In 15% of patients, the chest radiograph is normal.

HRCT—There is considerable overlap between the HRCT findings of NSIP and the other interstitial pneumonias. There is commonly symmetrical ground glass opacification and usually superimposed reticulation (crazy paving). Traction bronchiectasis is common. Honeycombing is unusual (10%–30%) and if present is mild, involving less than 10% of the lung parenchyma, unlike UIP and IPF. Peripheral and basal lungs are predominantly involved. In 50% of cases, there is a rim of subpleural sparing. This is also unlike IPF, which is typically most severe in the subpleural region. Patients with fibrotic NSIP have a high incidence of reticulation and traction bronchiectasis.

Honeycombing is not a feature of NSIP. Patients with cellular NSIP have predominant ground glass opacification and are more likely to improve with treatment, with better long-term prognosis. Mild mediastinal adenopathy is present in 80%. Accelerated NSIP can occur with a 1-year frequency of 3%.

Acute deterioration in NSIP can also occur with infection, PTE, pneumothorax, or right heart failure.

Secondary NSIP may occur with collagen vascular disease, chronic HP, drug toxicity, infection, and immunodeficiency. The association with collagen vascular disease is particularly common. Collagen vascular disease with interstitial fibrosis is more likely to be NSIP than UIP.

CRYPTOGENIC ORGANIZING PNEUMONIA

Cryptogenic organizing pneumonia (COP) accounts for 4% to 12% of cases of idiopathic interstitial pulmonary fibrosis. It is more common in nonsmokers and has an average age of presentation of 50 to 60 years.

Clinical—Patients present with cough and dyspnea of short duration (less than 3 months). There may be weight loss, chills, and fever. There are usually widespread lung crackles on auscultation. Patients are unresponsive to antibiotics, but usually respond well to steroids. However, recurrence is not uncommon.

Histology—Intraluminal polyps of granulation tissue distend the alveolar ducts, alveoli, and sometimes the respiratory bronchioles. There is chronic inflammation of the adjacent lung parenchyma with mononuclear cells, foamy macrophages, and organizing fibrosis. This disease has traditionally been called bronchiolitis obliterans with organizing pneumonia (BOOP), but this description unfortunately emphasizes the bronchial involvement rather than the pneumonia and is no longer favored.

Pulmonary function tests—Mild-to-moderate restrictive function is shown with decreased carbon monoxide diffusing capacity.

Radiographs—There are patchy areas of subpleural consolidation, which vary in size over time and are sometimes migratory. Margins are indistinct and air bronchograms may be seen. Nodules or masses may be seen more centrally in the lungs. There may also be small nodules or reticular markings. Small pleural effusions are seen in 20%. It is unlikely that a diagnosis of COP can be made on chest radiographs.

HRCT—Middle and lower lung zones are predominantly involved. Subpleural areas of wedge-shaped consolidation and ground glass opacification of variable size are shown in 70% of cases. These may change in distribution. Ground glass lesions may have a halo of consolidation, which is referred to as the reversed halo sign. There may be interstitial reticulation superimposed on ground glass opacities (crazy paving). Bronchovascular bundles are characteristically involved with thickening or nodules. These nodules may be of variable size and in 30% to 50% of cases are less than 10 mm. However, they may occur up to 5 cm in size or manifest as larger areas of consolidation. Reversible bronchial dilation sometimes occurs.

Secondary organizing pneumonia may occur with collagen vascular disease, inflammatory bowel disease, inhalational injury, chronic HP, drug reaction, irradiation injury, aspiration, and bronchial obstruction. Areas of organizing pneumonia are a common accompaniment of lung cancer and lung infection.

ACUTE INTERSTITIAL PNEUMONIA

Acute interstitial pneumonia (AIP) should be considered as idiopathic ARDS. It has been previously referred to as the Hamman-Rich syndrome.

Histology—This is acute lung injury with diffuse alveolar damage. In the acute exudative phase, there is sloughing of alveolar cells, intra-alveolar hemorrhage, severe interstitial inflammation, and hyaline membrane formation. The proliferative phase shows type II pneumocyte hyperplasia and early collagen formation in the interstitium. The chronic or reparative phase develops end-stage fibrosis with architectural deformity.

Clinical—Mean age is 50 years with wide age distribution. This disease usually occurs in previously healthy persons. There is often a prodromal infection with fever, chills, and myalgia for less than a week prior to diagnosis. This is followed by progressive dyspnea, hypoxia, and respiratory failure. There is a 50% death rate within 6 months of presentation.

Radiographs—There is bilateral airspace consolidation with prominent air bronchograms. This is initially patchy, but becomes more widespread and diffuse. Distribution involves the lung periphery or full thickness of both lungs, unlike cardiogenic edema, which is perihilar. There may be regional predominance in the upper or lower lung zones.

HRCT—There are geographical areas of ground glass opacification and crazy paving with uninvolved areas of normal lung interspersed with the disease process. Patchy and confluent airspace consolidation is also shown with progression to a more diffuse process over time. Air bronchograms may be very prominent. There is little, if any, pleural effusion. Heart size is usually normal. With progression to the fibroproliferative phase, ground glass opacities become diffuse and there is coalescence of the consolidation. Architectural deformity with honeycomb formation and traction bronchiectasis progressively worsens.

Pulmonary function tests—There is restrictive lung function and impaired gas exchange, with progressive hypoxemia and respiratory failure.

Management—Mechanical ventilation is required which often leads to barotrauma (pulmonary interstitial emphysema, pneumothorax, pneumomediastinum, and subcutaneous emphysema). Approximately 50% of patients die in the acute phase. Of the reminder, some recover with normal lung function and the survivors develop end-stage fibrosis.

Secondary AIP is ARDS. The cause is known. These causes include trauma, sepsis, pancreatitis, shock, aspiration, anaphylaxis, DIC, transfusion reaction, embolic disease (particularly fat embolism and amniotic fluid embolism) therapeutic or nontherapeutic drugs, ketoacidosis, and neurologic disease (head injury and cerebrovascular accident (CVA)).

LYMPHOID INTERSTITIAL PNEUMONIA

Lymphoid interstitial pneumonia (LIP) is part of a spectrum of lymphoproliferative disorders, and idiopathic LIP is extremely rare.

Histology—There is diffuse infiltration of the alveolar septa with lymphocytes and less numerous plasma cells and histiocytes. Lymphoid follicles may be present and if the small airways are predominantly involved rather than the alveoli, the condition is called follicular bronchiolitis. The histological pattern may resemble NSIP or HP.

Clinical—Average presentation is 40 to 50 years. Women are involved two times more than men. There is an insidious cough, dyspnea, and fatigue. Eighty percent of patients have dysproteinemia. Bronchoalveolar lavage shows lymphocytosis. Steroids are helpful, but one-third of patients progress to interstitial fibrosis.

Pulmonary function tests—There is a restrictive defect and reduction of total lung capacity.

Radiographs—A reticular or reticulonodular pattern may be shown in the lungs involving mainly the lower lung zones. Less commonly, there is a nodular pattern with hazy opacities or areas of consolidation.

HRCT—There are four recognized features of LIP on HRCT. Extensive ground glass opacification occurs because of diffuse lymphocytic infiltration in the alveolar walls. Poorly defined centrilobular nodules are produced by peribronchial infiltration of lymphocytes and plasma cells together with histiocytes, similar to the findings in follicular bronchiolitis. There is thickening of the central bronchovascular bundles because of interstitial cellular infiltration. Small cystic airspaces may be seen. These result from obstruction of small airways. Greater than 80% of cases of LIP show thickened peribronchovascular interstitium and septal thickening. More than 70% show cystic airspaces. Lesions have a tendency to resolve, with the exception of the cysts, which are irreversible.

Secondary LIP is much more common than idiopathic LIP. Most cases of LIP occur in patients with underlying autoimmune disease, most commonly Sjögren syndrome and dysproteinemia. Secondary LIP may also occur with AIDS, rheumatoid arthritis, lupus, Hashimoto thyroidosis, autoimmune hemolytic anemia, myasthenia gravis, pernicious anemia, chronic active hepatitis, and drug toxicity.

RESPIRATORY BRONCHIOLITIS AND DESQUAMATIVE INTERSTITIAL PNEUMONITIS

Respiratory bronchiolitis (RB) is a bronchiolitis, but is included because of its association with DIP, which is a true interstitial pneumonitis (fibrosing alveolitis). RB is localized and confined to the small airways.

Histology—Pigment-laden macrophages are shown in alveoli and respiratory bronchioles in RB. They are phagocytosed into the walls of the respiratory bronchioles with consequent inflammation and fibrosis.

Clinical—Patients remain asymptomatic for many years, but eventually develop cough, dyspnea, basal crackles, and a combined restrictive and obstructive lung pattern. At this stage, RB is classified as respiratory bronchiolitis/interstitial lung disease (RB/ILD).

Desquamative interstitial pneumonitis (DIP) may occur in association with or without RB. It is a diffuse process characterized by numerous macrophages within the alveoli, mild inflammation of the alveolar walls, and developing fibrosis. Although DIP is classified as an idiopathic disorder, more than 90% of patients are cigarette smokers.

Radiograph—In RB/ILD, there may be air trapping and peribronchial thickening. There may be linear markings because of thickened small airways peripherally resembling ILD. In DIP, 25% of radiographs are normal. The most common abnormality is ill-defined ground glass opacities in the lower lung zones.

HRCT—Ill-defined centrilobular nodules occur in over 70% because of thickened bronchiolar walls. Patchy ground glass opacities occur in 65% and are caused by alveolitis (DIP). These ground glass opacities tend to have a subpleural and lower lobe predominance. Small cystic lucencies eventually may develop within these areas of ground glass opacity. Mosaic attenuation occurs in over 75% because of air trapping. Honeycombing and septal thickening is rare.

Secondary DIP occurs in association with toxic inhalation, drug reactions, Langerhans cell histiocytosis, leukemia, asbestosis, and hard metal pneumoconiosis.

SUGGESTED READING

Hartman TE, Swensen SJ, Hansell DM, et al. Nonspecific interstitial pneumonia: variable appearance at high-resolution chest CT. *Radiology*. 2000;217:701-705.

Johkoh T, Müller NI, Pickford HA, et al. Lymphocytic interstitial pneumonia: thin section CT findings in 22 patients. *Radiology*. 1999;212:567-572.

Kawabata H, Nagal S, Hayashi M, et al. Significance of lung shrinkage on CXR as a prognostic factor in patients with idiopathic pulmonary fibrosis. *Respirology*. 2003;8:351-358.

Kim DS, Collard HR, King TE, Jr. Classification and natural history of the idiopathic interstitial pneumonias. *Proc Am Thorac Soc*. 2006;3:285-292.

Kim SJ, Lee KS, Ryu YH, et al. Reversed halo sign on high-resolution CT of cryptogenic organizing pneumonia: diagnostic implications. *AJR Am J Neuroradiol*. 2003;180:1251-1254.

King TE, Jr. Clinical advances in the diagnosis and therapy of the interstitial lung diseases. *Am J Respir Crit Care Med*. 2005; 172:268-279.

Lynch DA, Goodwin DJ, Safrin S, et al. High resolution computed tomography in idiopathic pulmonary fibrosis: diagnosis and prognosis. *Am J Resp Crit Care Med*. 2005;172:488-493.

Martinez FJ, Safrin S, Weycker D, et al. The clinical course of patients with idiopathic pulmonary fibrosis. *Ann Intern Med.* 2005;142:963-967.

Müller N, Silva I, eds. Part 8: Interstitial lung disease. *Imaging of the Chest.* Philadelphia, PA: Saunders; 2008:629-707.

Raghu G, Mageto YN, Lockhart D, et al. The accuracy of the clinical diagnosis of new-onset idiopathic pulmonary fibrosis and other interstitial lung disease: a prospective study. *Chest.* 1999;116:1168-1174.

Webb WR, Higgins CB, eds. The Ideopathic interstitial pneumonias. *Thoracic Imaging.* Philadelphia, PA: Lippincott Williams & Wilkins; 2005:406-424.

QUESTIONS AND ANSWERS

1. Concerning respiratory bronchiolitis interstitial lung disease, which of the following is *true?*
   A. Minority of cases have smoking history.
   B. Commonly shows mosaic attenuation on CT
   C. Commonly shows tree-in-bud lesions on CT
   D. Septal thickening occurs in one-half of patients.

   ANSWER: B. Respiratory bronchiolitis commonly shows a mosaic attenuation on CT. The majority of patients with respiratory bronchiolitis have a smoking history. Tree-in-bud and septal thickening are not features of acute cellular bronchiolitis.

2. Concerning interstitial lung disease, which of the following is *true?*
   A. 20% have a normal chest radiograph on initial presentation.
   B. Readily distinguishable from basal atelectasis on portable radiographs
   C. 30% show loss of volume on initial chest radiograph.
   D. Increased opacification in the lower lung zones is a helpful diagnostic feature on lateral chest radiographs.

   ANSWER: D. Lateral chest radiograph is often more sensitive for diagnosis of this disease, particularly in the early stages. Regardless, 10% still present with normal chest radiographs. Over one-half show loss of volume on initial chest radiographs. ILD can be difficult to differentiate from basal atelectasis on portable radiographs.

3. What is a prominent feature of idiopathic pulmonary fibrosis on HRCT?
   A. Honeycombing
   B. Peripheral sparing
   C. Ground glass opacification
   D. Geographic involvement of lung parenchyma interspersed with normal parenchyma

   ANSWER: A. Honeycombing is a prominent feature of IPF on HRCT. Peripheral sparing is a feature of NSIP not UIP (IPF). Ground glass opacification may be present with IPF, but is not a prominent finding. Geographic involvement of lung parenchyma interspersed with normal parenchyma describes acute interstitial pneumonia (AIP) not IPF.

4. What is a prominent feature of nonspecific interstitial pneumonitis?
   A. Traction bronchiectasis
   B. Peripheral reticulation
   C. Honeycombing
   D. Centrilobular nodules

   ANSWER: A. Traction bronchiolitis is a prominent feature of nonspecific interstitial pneumonitis. There is often peripheral sparing, unlike UIP, which has thickened interlobular septae causing reticulation extending to the lung periphery. Honeycombing can occur but is uncommon with NSIP. Centrilobular nodules are not a feature of NSIP. They occur with RB/ILD, HP, and some industrial lung diseases.

5. What is a feature of cryptogenic organizing pneumonia with HRCT?
   A. Peripheral nodules
   B. Peripheral interstitial reticulation
   C. Peripheral pleural–based ground glass, wedge–shaped lesions
   D. Mosaic attenuation

   ANSWER: C. Peripheral pleural-based ground glass, wedge-shaped lesions are a feature of nodules in COP, involve the axial interstitium, and tend to involve the perihilar or central lung regions, not the lung periphery. Reticulation is not a feature. Mosaic attenuation is a feature of a peripheral pulmonary thromboemboli and small airways disease.

6. What is a feature of acute interstitial pneumonia on CT?
   A. Cardiomegaly
   B. Pleural effusions
   C. Areas of consolidation and ground glass opacification
   D. Rapidly changing parenchymal disease

   ANSWER: C. Areas of consolidation and ground glass opacification are features of AIP. The heart size is usually normal unless the patient has an underlying cardiomyopathy. Pleural effusions are small or absent. Unlike aspiration and cardiogenic pulmonary edema, parenchymal disease changes slowly with AIP.

7. Concerning usual interstitial pneumonia, which of the following is *true?*
   A. Histologically homogenous
   B. Most common secondary interstitial lung disease associated with collagen vascular disorders
   C. 30% of cases of are idiopathic pulmonary fibrosis.
   D. Accelerated disease shows areas of organizing pneumonia and diffuse alveolar damage on histology.

   ANSWER: D. The histological pattern is characteristically heterogeneous. Nonspecific interstitial pneumonitis is the common pattern associated with collagen vascular disease. Approximately 70% of cases of usual interstitial pneumonia are IPF.

8. Concerning interstitial lung disease, which of the following is *true?*
   A. Architectural deformity and loss of volume are pathognomic.
   B. Emphysema is commonly associated.
   C. Leads to pulmonary hypertension and eventually cor pulmonale heart failure.
   D. Expected life span of 10 to 15 years

   ANSWER: C. Interstitial lung disease can lead to pulmonary hypertension and eventually cor pulmonale heart failure. Architectural deformity and loss of volume can occur with end-stage lung disease including, but not limited to, IPF. Emphysema is commonly associated with UIP (IPF), not NSIP. Patients with IPF have an expected life span of less than 5 years.

9. Concerning usual interstitial pneumonia, which of the following is *true?*
   A. Most common interstitial lung disease associated with collagen vascular disease
   B. Pathognomonic findings on HRCT
   C. Heterogeneous pattern is shown histologically.
   D. There is a 40% risk of lung cancer.

   ANSWER: C. NSIP is the most common ILD to be found in association with collagen vascular disease. A characteristic case of UIP on HRCT may prove to be some other condition such as NSIP on histology. There is a 10% lung carcinoma incidence in patients with IPF.

10. Concerning nonspecific interstitial pneumonitis (NSIP), which of the following is *true?*
    A. Patients with IPF have a better steroid response than patients with NSIP.
    B. Patients with cellular NSIP respond better than those with fibrotic NSIP.
    C. Traction bronchiectasis is uncommon.
    D. Idiopathic NSIP is more common than secondary NSIP.

    ANSWER: B. NSIP is steroid responsive, whereas UIP is not. Traction bronchiectasis is a characteristic feature. Secondary NSIP is more common than idiopathic NSIP.

23 PULMONARY NEOPLASMS

Jonathan Walter, Ian Malcolm, and Satinder P. Singh

NOMENCLATURE AND GENERAL CONSIDERATIONS

A pulmonary *nodule* may range in size from 4 mm to 3 cm and a *mass* is greater than 3 cm in size. Nodules seen in patients younger than 35 years, nonsmokers, and patients from typical endemic granulomatous disease regions (i.e., Ohio River valley) are usually felt to be benign in origin. If a pathologic specimen is not obtained, these patients may be followed at 3 to 6 months, 1 year, and 2 years after initial nodule detection. Suspicion for malignant nodules occurs in patients older than 35 years (up to 50% of noncalcified nodules in patients older than 50 years may be malignant), smokers, patients with asbestos exposure, known primary neoplasms, and large lesions. These lesions are typically not followed without obtaining a pathologic specimen unless there is clearly benign calcification, intralesional fat, or lack of growth over at least a 2-year period.

The differential diagnosis for a solitary pulmonary nodule is wide-ranging. The first consideration generally is a neoplasm—primary or metastatic. Next, an infectious process such as round pneumonia, septic embolus, abscess, and granuloma should be considered. Vascular abnormalities such as AVMs and aneurysms comprise the next general class of possibilities. Following, congenital abnormalities such as sequestration, congenital cystic adenomatoid malformation (CCAM), and bronchogenic cyst are included. Finally, and usually least likely, autoimmune disorders such as Wegner's granulomatosis and rheumatoid arthritis with necrotic nodules complete a very brief differential diagnosis.

The radiographic evaluation of a pulmonary nodule or mass may be quite extensive; however, a few general considerations should be followed. First, general radiography is felt to be largely unreliable for lesions less than 1 cm in diameter. Second, the rate of growth is an important factor in determining the nature of a lesion. A sphere has doubled in size when the diameter has increased by only 25%. Lesions such as bronchogenic carcinoma typically display a doubling time of between 1 month and 2 years; therefore, a regular follow-up schedule is vital. Third, benign lesions typically display a smooth, rounded margin. Malignant lesions are more likely to appear spiculated, notched, angulated, or lobulated. Fourth, there are benign and malignant patterns of calcification. Benign calcification generally may appear complete, central, concentric, laminated, or like popcorn. Malignant calcification may appear punctuate or eccentric. Fifth, fat within a pulmonary nodule is generally indicative of a benign lesion, such as seen with a pulmonary hamartoma. Sixth, most malignant lesions enhance by at least 15 HU (98% sensitive). Finally, PET is generally quite useful for lesions greater than 1 cm (sensitivity as high as 97%, but specificity is only upward of 78%). A lower specificity is generally seen in lesions less than 1 cm, in cases of inflammation, and with hypoactive lesions such as bronchoalveolar carcinoma and carcinoid.

Numerous primary and metastatic pulmonary neoplasms have been described in the literature and several proposed classification schemes have been introduced. Those schemes based upon neoplasm histologic origin provide a rather intuitive means for classification, and this approach will be used in this review (Table 23-1). In addition, for the sake of brevity, we shall consider only the more common primary malignant and benign lesions, followed by a brief overview of more commonly encountered metastatic lesions. More obscure pulmonary neoplasms are beyond the scope of this chapter and are likely of low yield for board examination purposes; however, suggestions for further reading will be provided at the end of this chapter.

TABLE 23-1 Overview of Common Pulmonary Neoplasms

Primary disease
Malignant
Epithelial
Bronchogenic carcinoma (>95% of all primary pulmonary neoplasms)
Adenocarcinoma
Broncioalveolar cell carcinoma
Squamous cell carcinoma
Small cell carcinoma
Large cell carcinoma
Pancoast tumor
Carcinoid
Typical carcinoid
Atypical carcinoid
Lymphoid
Hodgkin lymphoma
Non-Hodgkin lymphoma
Mesenchymal
Pulmonary blastoma
Benign
Epithelial
Squamous cell papilloma
Mesenchymal
Hamartoma
Metastatic disease
From primary lung cancer
From extra thoracic malignancies
Breast cancer
GI tract tumors
Kidney cancer
Melanoma
Sarcoma
Lymphoma and leukemia
Germ cell tumors
Ovarian cancer

MALIGNANT PULMONARY NEOPLASMS

BRONCHOGENIC CARCINOMA

The overwhelming majority (greater than 95%) of primary malignant pulmonary neoplasms fall under the general classification of bronchogenic carcinoma. These neoplasms are epithelial in origin and are derived from either bronchial or alveolar epithelium. Bronchogenic carcinoma is the leading cause of death from malignancy in the US. There are at least four broad histologic subtypes: adenocarcinoma, squamous cell carcinoma, small cell carcinoma, and large cell carcinoma. As a group, general risk factors include smoking (estimates of up to 87% of cases are related to smoking), other exposures such as asbestos (long latency, may be greater than or equal to 20 years) and radon, age greater than 40, male sex, although this association is equalizing, diffuse or localized fibrosis, and previous mediastinal lymphoma postradiation, and/or chemotherapy. In regard specifically to smoking, small cell carcinoma and squamous cell carcinoma are most closely associated with smoking in men, whereas all subtypes are fairly equally associated with cancer risk in women. The overall 5-year survival rate for patients with bronchogenic carcinoma averages about 10% to 15%.

The radiographic evaluation of the various subtypes of bronchogenic carcinoma will be discussed on an individual basis; however, there are a few general findings, which are fairly unique to this group of cancers as a whole. First, since these neoplasms are epithelial in origin, bronchial obstruction may commonly be seen. This may be observed as incomplete obstruction, analogous to a ball valve mechanism, which results in air trapping or conversely this may be seen as complete obstruction with atelectasis, obstructive pneumonitis, or even mucocele formation with mucoid impaction. Next, fairly nonspecific pleural findings may be seen such as pleural effusion or pleural thickening, and evaluation for possible chest wall invasion is critical in the evaluation process. Specifically, one may look for an obtuse angle at the point of contact with any pleural mass, greater than 3 cm of contact between the pleura and mass, pleural thickening immediately adjacent to a mass, infiltration of the extrapleural fat, and finally frank rib erosion or destruction. Other factors such as large size (typically greater than 3 cm) and malignant calcification patterns were mentioned previously. Third, mediastinal invasion must also be considered. Findings such as elevation of a hemidiaphragm may suggest invasion with compromise of the ipsilateral phrenic nerve. In addition, one must look for mediastinal widening, a mediastinal mass, which is contiguous with a pulmonary parenchymal mass, obliteration of vascular fat planes, a mass contacting more than 3 cm of the mediastinum, and a mass contacting greater than 25% of the diameter of the aorta. SVC compression may also be seen with associated SVC syndrome, with lung cancer generally considered to be the most common cause. Finally, lymphangitic carcinomatosis is a final unique consideration seen with bronchogenic carcinomatosis. As tumor invades the pulmonary lymphatics, there are interstitial deposits, interlobular septal thickening, and eventually fibrosis. More specifically, there may be linear or reticulonodular opacities, peribronchial cuffing, subpleural edema, and/or effusion, and often primarily ipsilateral hilar adenopathy.

Adenocarcinoma

This is the most common histologic subtype of bronchogenic carcinoma, comprising between 33% and 50% of cases. This is also the most common subtype seen in nonsmokers (weak association with smoking) and in women. Approximately three-fourths of these lesions are seen in the periphery of the lung, while the remaining one-fourth are central. Histologically, these masses demonstrate gland formation and mucin production, and the histochemical stain mucicarmine demonstrates both intra- and extracellular mucosubstance. With time, these lesions then typically proceed to invade the lung parenchyma and there is typically at least a mild/moderate degree of fibrosis. From a radiologic standpoint, these lesions arise from the epithelium and invade into the lung, with the early typical presentation often consisting of a peripheral subpleural nodule or mass. These lesions often become irregular/spiculated in appearance as they enlarge and pleural invasion is common. In addition, these neoplasms may grow around the lung and thus mimic a mesothelioma. These lesions may also contain air bronchograms and can thus mimic infectious processes or even atelectasis. As a group, patients with adenocarcinoma generally demonstrate a 5-year survival of approximately 17%.

Bronchioalveolar cell carcinoma (BAC) is often considered to be a subtype of adenocarcinoma. This neoplasm tends to grow along existing bronchiolar or alveolar walls without invasion or distortion. In essence, true BAC is considered to be a carcinoma in situ since there is no spread beyond the lung parenchyma. On a histologic level, since BAC is a subtype of adenocarcinoma, these lesions also typically demonstrate copious mucous production. Accordingly, with varying degrees of mucous production, these lesions may then appear as solitary pulmonary nodules, nonspecific ground glass opacities, contain air bronchograms or bubbly lucencies, or even mixed solid/ground glass attenuation. When seen diffusely throughout the lungs, BAC may produce apparent airspace opacification, which may mimic pneumonia. These lesions may also demonstrate cavitation and are the second most common type of bronchogenic carcinoma subtype to cavitate after squamous cell carcinoma.

Squamous Cell Carcinoma

This is the second most common subtype of bronchogenic carcinoma, comprising between 25% and 33% of cases. Unlike adenocarcinoma, this subtype is strongly associated with smoking and tends to be more central in location (two-thirds of cases). The remaining one-third of cases typically arise in a peripheral location. From a histologic standpoint, this subtype of carcinoma may demonstrate chronic epithelial inflammation/injury, which can then lead to squamous metaplasia. The bronchial wall invasion occurs with nest of malignant cells demonstrating abundant cytoplasm, keratin pearls, and intercellular bridges (fine lines seen extending between cells). Radiologically, these lesions appear as central/hilar polypoid masses, which grow into the bronchial lumen and invade the bronchial wall. As previously discussed, this may then result in either incomplete or complete airway obstruction. When significant obstruction has not yet occurred, this carcinoma subtype is commonly diagnosed from sputum samples (radiographically occult). Central necrosis is a common feature associated with this mass and this is also the most likely lesion to cavitate. If these lesions occur peripherally, they are typically seen as solitary pulmonary nodules or solitary masses. As an aside, squamous cell carcinoma is the first carcinoma subtype in this discussion that is known to produce a paraneoplastic syndrome. Tumors may produce a parathyroidlike substance, which results in hyperparathyroidism, manifesting most classically with hypercalcemia. The overall 5-year survival rate is reported as approximately 15%.

Small Cell Carcinoma

This is the third most common bronchogenic carcinoma subtype, comprising 15% to 25% of cases. There is a strong association with smoking and lesions are most typically found centrally (90%) arising from main or lobar bronchi. Masses arise from neuroendocrine cells embedded in the epithelium, specifically referred to as type III Kulchitsky cells. Of note, these same Kulchitsky cells (types I and II) give rise to typical and atypical carcinoid tumors, although the type III cells associated with small cell carcinoma are the most malignant. Histologically, lesions demonstrate tightly packed clusters of cells with scant cytoplasm, stippled chromatin within the nuclei, absent nucleoli, mitotic figures, and intracytoplasmic neurosecretory granules. Small cell carcinoma is also the most common bronchogenic carcinoma subtype to cause a neuroendocrine syndrome, two of which are most commonly seen. Cushing syndrome results from ectopic ACTH production and leads to fat redistribution, menstrual irregularity, HTN, DM, and osteoporosis. The syndrome of inappropriate secretion of antidiuretic hormone (SIADH) results from the secretion of an ADH-like hormone, which leads to water retention and hyponatremia. Radiologically, small cell carcinoma is a very fast growing malignancy, with early bronchial/peribronchial invasion and invasion of the submucosal/peribronchial lymphatics. These features result in early (often widespread) hematogenous dissemination, which is commonly occurring or has occurred by the time of diagnosis. There is also typically a hilar or mediastinal mass, which may extrinsically compress the airways or even vascular structures. In fact, small cell carcinoma is the most common lung tumor to result in SVC syndrome. Necrosis and hemorrhage are also common features associated with these lesions. The overall prognosis is poor, with an average 5-year survival of only 5%.

Large Cell Carcinoma

This is the least common subtype of bronchogenic carcinoma, occurring in approximately 5% to 15% of cases. There is a strong association with smoking and most masses are found peripherally. Histologically, masses demonstrate large cells (hence the name) with abundant cytoplasm, large nuclei, and prominent nucleoli. Cell clusters tend to grow in uniform sheets. There is also a histologic subtype within this family of neoplasms referred to as giant cell carcinoma. These cells are larger and appear pleomorphic, with multiple unusual shapes instead of uniform sheets. This subtype is particularly aggressive and confers a poorer prognosis. Overall, large cell carcinoma is a histologic diagnosis of exclusion and is typically defined by a non-small cell bronchogenic carcinoma, which lacks characteristics of both adenocarcinoma and squamous cell carcinoma. On radiologic evaluation, lesions arise as solitary peripheral masses, which may be quite large (greater than 3 cm). Necrosis is common seen, as lesions grow rapidly and metastasize early.

Pancoast Tumor

The Pancoast tumor is generally classified as a miscellaneous histologic bronchogenic carcinoma subtype since it may be comprised of any of the bronchogenic carcinoma subtypes, but it is most commonly adenocarcinoma or squamous cell carcinoma in origin. Lesions are seen peripherally and in the lung apices. Symptoms are often related to location, as invasion of local structures is common. Rib destruction and extrathoracic invasion are typically seen. Patients may experience arm pain, muscle atrophy, or even Horner syndrome if the sympathetic chain is invaded. In this scenario, patients may demonstrate ipsilateral ptosis (lid lag), miosis (pupillary constriction), and anhidrosis (decreased facial sweating). As an aside, a patient with metastatic thymoma may also demonstrate an apical pleural-based mass and upper extremity weakness; however, in this case, motor weakness is often secondary to the paraneoplastic effects of the disease with resultant myasthenia gravis.

CARCINOID

Aside from bronchogenic carcinoma, the other major epithelial-derived pulmonary neoplasm is the pulmonary *carcinoid*. This is a relatively uncommon malignancy seen in only 1% to 2% of all lung cancer cases, demonstrates no male/female predilection, occurs commonly in children, and is not thought to be associated with smoking. Most lesions (up to 80%) are found centrally, while peripheral lesions (20%) usually arise as solitary pulmonary nodules. Given central location, bronchoscopy is often performed. The typical appearance is that of a cherry red bronchial lesion owing to the highly vascular nature of these tumors. Biopsy should naturally be avoided secondary to the risk of hemorrhage. Carcinoid metastasizes in about 15% of cases and may be seen in the liver, bone, adrenals, and brain. Classically, patients with liver metastases develop right and often left heart disease as the carcinoid syndrome develops and serotonin levels significantly rise. This results in fibrous deposits along the endocardium, in particular the valve apparatus, with incompetency and stenosis commonly affecting at least the tricuspid and pulmonary valves. As a neuroendocrine tumor, carcinoid tumors may arise from Kulchitsky cells, neuroepithelial bodies, or pluripotential bronchial epithelial stem cells. The classic triad of symptoms includes hemoptysis (secondary to vascular nature of lesions), cough, and pneumonitis. The Carcinoid syndrome, as alluded to above, requires liver metastases. The biochemical conversion of metabolites within the liver produces flushing, diarrhea, and bronchoconstriction.

Histologically, there are two subtypes of the carcinoid tumor: typical and atypical. The typical carcinoid is more common, with uniform-appearing cells containing abundant cytoplasm arranged in sheets, trabeculae, or glandlike formations. Cells may take many forms, but can be spindle shaped or even palisading. Mitotic figures are not common. Also, since these are vascular tumors, there is a prominent fibrovascular stroma. There may be foci of dystrophic calcification, bone, or amyloid. Finally, neurosecretory granules are present which are larger and more numerous than atypical carcinoids. The other subtype of the carcinoid tumor is the atypical form. This neoplasm is less common, but more aggressive than the typical carcinoid. Histologic features are overall quite similar between the two, except the atypical carcinoid has an increased number of mitotic figures, demonstrates nuclear pleomorphism, disorganized architecture, and often areas of necrosis. On a final note, both typical and atypical carcinoids are capable of synthesizing, storing, and secreting several metabolically active compounds. Serotonin is commonly produced, with patients typically experiencing diarrhea as a consequence of rising serum levels. Cushing syndrome is also associated with carcinoid tumors, with ectopic ACTH producing symptoms as discussed with *small cell carcinoma*. Somatostatin may exert its inhibitory actions on the GI tract, pancreas, anterior pituitary gland, and nervous system. Finally, the potent vasodilator bradykinin may cause flushing.

Carcinoid tumors demonstrate multiple characteristic radiologic findings. The classic description is that of a central mass compressing the bronchus and containing calcifications. In fact, it is the typical carcinoid that is slow growing and centrally located, while the atypical subtype is rapidly growing and more commonly seen peripherally. Central lesions are usually hilar or perihilar, rarely invade the mediastinum, and typically result in external bronchial compression/obstruction. Mucoceles may develop secondary to bronchial obstruction as mucoid material accumulates and impaction occurs. When found peripherally, carcinoid tumors usually appear as rounded or lobulated solitary pulmonary nodules. Overall, carcinoids are endoluminal lesions, which may commonly appear as "iceberg" lesions since the endoluminal component may appear quite small, while the extraluminal component may be very large. Masses are generally large (averaging 2–5 cm) and typically demonstrate avid homogeneous enhancement because of their vascular composition, although some tumors may demonstrate variable or no enhancement if there is little relative vascular stroma. Eccentric calcifications are very commonly seen, but cavitation is rare. Also, pathologic adenopathy is more typically seen with atypical carcinoids. Aside from radiography, CT, and MRI, nuclear medicine is often utilized in the detection and characterization of carcinoid tumors. Since carcinoid lesions display somatostatin receptors, radionuclide-tagged octreotide may be used for tumor detection. PET is generally not useful since these neoplasms typically have a low metabolism.

Prognosis for patients with carcinoid tumors depends on the histologic subtype. Typical carcinoids usually have an excellent prognosis, often even in the presence of metastatic disease. Five-year survival rates have been reported as high as 85% to 92%. Atypical carcinoids, on the other hand, confer a worse prognosis. Five-year survival in this patient population has been reported in the range of 65% to 70%. Regardless of histologic subtype, the only effective method of treatment is surgical resection.

LYMPHOMA—HODGKIN AND NON-HODGKIN

Both Hodgkin lymphoma (HL) and non-Hodgkin lymphoma (NHL) are primarily mediastinal, hilar, or perihilar in location, although parenchymal involvement does occur and is up to three times more common with HL. Radiologically, mediastinal adenopathy is the typical finding; however, various patterns of parenchymal disease are seen. In HL, parenchymal disease may appear as linear or reticulonodular opacities extending into the lung from hilar nodes, and there is almost always associated hilar adenopathy. The parenchymal findings may produce masslike opacities and airspace consolidation, which may mimic pneumonia. Also, atelectasis is commonly seen secondary to obstructing endobronchial lesions rather than simply from extrinsic airway compression. Finally, subpleural plaques and masses may be present if tumor has invaded the lymphatics. NHL, on the other hand, occurs primarily as mediastinal adenopathy and less commonly involves the lung parenchyma. When there is parenchymal involvement, associated adenopathy may be absent (up to 50% of cases). Also, unlike HL, NHL does not typically produce coarse reticulonodular opacities. Lesions may arise as solitary pulmonary nodules, multiple masses, or as airspace opacities, which again may simulate pneumonia.

PULMONARY BLASTOMA

Pulmonary blastoma is a rare primary pulmonary neoplasm with presentation typically in the fourth and fifth decades, although a significant number of cases are seen in children. These tumors contain both epithelial and mesenchymal elements and are thought to resemble fetal lung tissue. The epithelial components are glandular, unlike squamous epithelium seen in other mixed lesions such as carcinosarcoma. In addition, pediatric lesions are thought to contain benign rests of epithelial components as opposed to frank carcinomatous elements, although these rests may become inflamed and thus differentiation from carcinoma can be difficult. Mesenchymal components range from relatively undifferentiated embryonic mesenchyma to areas of well-fibrous tissue, smooth muscle, and cartilage. The typical radiologic presentation differs in children and adults. Children may present with opacification of an entire hemithorax caused by a large parenchymal or pleural-based mass and often a large pleural effusion. Adults more commonly present with a peripheral solitary pulmonary nodule or mass. In either population, it should be noted that a clear association with benign pulmonary cysts has been established. On CT, lesions are predominantly low in attenuation and contain whorls of higher attenuation, presumably from mesenchymal components. Surgical resection is rarely curative, and chemoirradiation has been met with mixed success. Overall, prognosis is poor and metastatic disease is commonly found at autopsy.

BENIGN PULMONARY NEOPLASMS

SQUAMOUS CELL PAPILLOMA

Squamous cell papilloma is a benign, painless epithelial growth, which is caused by the human papilloma virus (HPV), typically either the HPV-6 or HPV-11 strain. Lesions are found anywhere along the oral mucosa, larynx, trachea, and bronchi. These lesions generally do not demonstrate significant growth, do not usually spread, and may appear as solitary or multiple endoluminal masses. The course is rather indolent, with regression sometimes seen by adolescence. Although therapy is not necessary since these lesions do not undergo malignant transformation, patients may elect to pursue resection or cryotherapy.

PULMONARY HAMARTOMA

Pulmonary hamartomas are benign lesions, which consist of disorganized epithelial and mesenchymal elements, typically containing cartilage surrounded by fibrous connective tissue and variable amounts of fat, smooth muscle, and mucous glands. Analogous to the pediatric pulmonary blastoma, epithelial components are felt to represent simply reactive tissue, while the mesenchymal components are felt to represent true neoplasm. The majority of tumors are found within the lung parenchyma (90%), while the remaining lesions are endobronchial (10%). Parenchymal lesions typically arise as solitary pulmonary nodules, which characteristically contain fat and often calcification/ossification, may appear lobulated, vary in size from 1 to 9 cm, and contain numerous epithelial clefts (unlike endobronchial lesions). Endobronchial lesions demonstrate similar histologic characteristics, but usually contain more fat than parenchymal lesions and may cause varying degrees of airway obstruction. As previously described, incomplete or complete airway obstruction can manifest as atelectasis, minor airway opacification, or frank consolidation. Pulmonary hamartomas are generally slow-growing lesions which can be followed over time; however, large parenchymal lesions or endobronchial lesions resulting in significant airway obstruction may be amendable to surgical resection.

LUNG CANCER STAGING

Radiologic staging is performed by utilizing the tumor, node, and metastasis (TNM) system (Table 23-2). *Clinical staging* is then based upon radiologic staging (Table

TABLE 23-2 Radiologic Staging of Pulmonary Neoplasms

Primary tumor
*T*x—malignant sputum cells without identified tumor
*T*0—no evidence of tumor
T1—tumor ≤3 cm, surrounded by parenchyma (lung, pleura), arises distal to main bronchus
T1a—tumor ≤2 cm
T1b—tumor >2 cm
T2—Tumor >3 cm, any tumor not contained by parenchyma (i.e., invading pleura), resultant atelectasis or obstructive pneumonitis of less than entire lung, greater than 2 cm from carina
T2a—tumor ≤5 cm
T2b—tumor >5 cm
T3—any tumor with more extensive invasion (chest wall, diaphragm, pericardium, mediastinal pleura) can be <2 cm from carina but cannot involve it
T4—any tumor with even more extensive invasion (mediastinum including all contained structures, vertebral bodies), separate masses in same lobe, malignant effusion
Nodal metastases
No—No nodal metastases
N1—Ipsilateral peribronchial or hilar nodes
N2—Ipsilateral mediastinal or subcarinal nodes
N3—Ipsilateral supraclavicular/neck nodes or contralateral nodes
Distant metastases
Mo—No metastases
M1—Distant metastases or separate nodules/masses in different lobes
M1a—Separate tumor nodules in a contralateral lobe or tumor with pleural nodules or malignant pleural or pericardial effusion
M1b—Distant metastases

TABLE 23-3 Clinical Staging of Pulmonary Neoplasms

Generally resectable disease (I-IIIa)
Ia—T1a or bNoMo
Ib—T2aNoMo
IIa—T1a or 2aN1Mo or T2bN0Mo
IIb—T2bN1Mo or T3N0Mo
IIIa—T1a-3N2Mo or T3N1M0 or T4N0 or 1Mo
Generally unresectable disease (IIIb-IV)
IIIb—T4N2M0 or T1a-4N3M0
IV—M1 with any other combination

23-3). It should be noted that the "resectable" versus "unresectable" designation within the stage III classification is not clearly defined and careful individual consideration must be given to these cases. For example, a tumor designated T4 would generally fall into the "unresectable" category, yet those lesions with minimal tumor invasion through the mediastinal pleura into fat are generally resectable. As another example, a tumor that has invaded the carina and the distal 3 to 4 cm of trachea (i.e., again radiologic stage T4) can sometimes be resected with pneumonectomy and sleeve bronchoplasty. Finally, small cell carcinoma staging is simplified into limited or extensive disease. *Limited small cell carcinoma* represents disease limited to one hemithorax. *Extensive small cell carcinoma* represents disease involving the contralateral lung or extending outside beyond the lung parenchyma (i.e., extrathoracic spread).

THORACIC METASTASES

Thoracic metastases are common. They develop from extrathoracic primary malignancy and also from primary malignancy arising within the thorax. Metastatic disease commonly occurs by hematogenous and lymphatic spread and also direct spread from adjacent lesions. Less commonly, aerogenic spread can occur in the acini or central airways. Occasionally, malignancies metastasize to endobronchial structures (Table 23-4).

Hematogenous spread of tumor results in deposition of malignant cells in small pulmonary arteries and arterioles. There is invasion of adjacent interstitium with the formation of nodules, which gradually increase in size.

TABLE 23-4 Endobronchial Metastasis

Breast
Colon
Rectum
Kidney
Cervix
Malignant melanoma
Sarcomas

Blockage of affected vessels occurs with prograde and retrograde growth and more peripheral embolization. Hematogenous metastases predominate in the lower lobes where pulmonary blood flow is greatest. Larger tumor deposits affecting more central pulmonary arteries can cause pulmonary thromboembolism, sometimes infarction and regional perfusion defects on CT.

Lymphatic spread may occur when hematogenous metastases invade the lymphatics in the surrounding interstitium. They also occur when blood-borne malignant deposits are carried to mediastinal, hilar, and bronchopulmonary lymph nodes. Malignant cells may reach lymph nodes directly by the thoracic duct also. There is then retrograde spread of tumor from the lymph nodes into the lymphatics of the lung and pleura.

Breast, thyroid, esophagogastric, and liver malignancies may directly spread to the pleura, lung parenchyma, and mediastinum. Chest wall lesions including primary and metastatic bone lesions, cartilaginous malignancies, neurogenic malignancies, and soft-tissue chest wall lesions such as melanoma and fibrosarcoma may also invade the intrathoracic region.

Aerogenic spread occurs within the thorax itself with BAC, where multicentric foci in the alveoli and small airways invade adjacent acinar structures while preserving the normal pulmonary architecture. Extrathoracic and intrathoracic tracheobronchial lesions such as bronchogenic carcinoma and tracheobronchial papillomatosis can also spread by direct invasion.

Primary lesions within the thorax itself, such as lung cancer, will directly invade adjacent mediastinum, pleura, and chest wall as well as spreading into surrounding extrathoracic tissue by hematogenous (arterial and venous) and lymphatic pathways. Neurogenic lesions adjacent to the spine and ribs will invade these bony structures. Mediastinal malignancy such as thymic cancer can also spread directly within the thorax.

PULMONARY NODULES

These are usually well marginated and round, although they may be irregular and sometimes have a ground glass peripheral halo. This halo sign occurs with vascular metastases such as angiosarcoma and is because of hemorrhagic necrosis around the lesion or sometimes direct malignant spread. This halo may also occur with nonmalignant nodules such as lymphoma, fungal disease, and vasculitis (Wegener's granulomatosis). Five percent of metastatic pulmonary nodules are cavitary and this is liable to occur with certain malignancies (see Table 23-5). The differential diagnosis of cavitary nodules includes fungal and mycobacterial lesions, septic emboli, and vasculitis. Less commonly, metastatic nodules can be calcific

TABLE 23-5 Cavitary Pulmonary Metastases

5% of metastatic nodules
Squamous cell carcinoma, especially head and neck and cervix lesions
Transitional cell tumors
Adenocarcinoma, especially colon
Sarcoma

(see Table 23-6). The differential diagnosis of these lesions include fungal disease, mycobacterial lesions, and hamartomas. Radiographically, small nodules are easily missed unless they are particularly numerous, which occurs with embolic spread of highly vascular peripheral lesions such as breast carcinoma (see Table 23-7). In such cases, the radiographic appearance may be similar to miliary TB. Lesions 5 mm or greater will usually be shown on good quality radiographs, but may be over looked in "blind areas" of the radiograph.

CT readily detects nodules 3 mm or greater. The sensitivity is 70% if nodules are less than 5 mm and is 95% with lesions 5 mm or greater. However, because of the common occurrence of benign nodules, specificity is limited. Common benign nodules include granulomas such as mycobacterial disease and sarcoidosis—also, fungal lesions, and intrapulmonary lymph nodes. Many of these benign lesions result from inhalational disease and affect upper lobes predominantly, unlike metastases. Follow-up CT is advisable at 6- or 12-month intervals if the lesions cannot be evaluated by bronchoscopy or percutaneous biopsy, which is usually the case with small lesions. A malignant nodule should grow slowly over several months on follow-up, whereas a benign nodule will remain stable for a 2-year period, or alternatively grow more rapidly than malignancy (weeks or months) in the case of an inflammatory mass. Solitary nodules are metastases in only 5% to 10% of cases overall. However, a solitary nodule in a patient older than 45 years of age with known primary malignancy is metastatic in 85% of cases.

Lymphangitic carcinoma may not be detected radiographically, particularly if localized. Lymphangitic spread from lung carcinoma is usually unilateral. Otherwise, unilateral and bilateral lymphangitic carcinoma occurs equally. There may be mediastinal adenopathy and pleural effusion with lymphangitic carcinoma (see

TABLE 23-6 Calcification in Pulmonary Metastases

Osteogenic sarcoma
Chondrosarcoma
Synovial sarcoma
Colon carcinoma
Ovarian carcinoma
Breast carcinoma
Thyroid carcinoma
Dystrophic calcification in other metastases following chemotherapy

TABLE 23-7 Miliary Nodular Metastasis Caused by Rapid Embolization of Highly Vascular Malignancies

Thyroid
Breast
Pancreas
Choriocarcinoma
Melanoma
Less commonly with mesothelioma and small cell lung carcinoma

Table 23-8). If lymphangitic spread originates in mediastinal nodes, there may be thickened bronchovascular (axial) interstitium and peribronchial cuffing, but these features may be absent if hematogenous deposits have originated in peripheral lung lymphatics. In most cases, there is thickened interlobular septa, and secondary pulmonary nodules may be outlined, often with a central dot because of thickened interstitium around the centrilobular duct. Associated ground glass opacification is often seen with the crazy paving appearance. Thickened septa may be smooth and resemble interstitial pulmonary edema, but are commonly nodular or beaded in appearance.

Anatomic detail provided by high resolution CT has enabled classification of pulmonary nodules into three types: centrilobular, perilymphatic, and random. Gruden has developed a simple algorithm to distinguish between these three types of nodules.

1. If there are no subpleural nodules, the type is centrilobular. Ill-defined centrilobular nodules occur with subacute hypersensitivity pneumonitis and respiratory bronchiolitis. Cellular bronchiolitis (tree-in-bud) occurs with infectious disease such as bronchitis, TB, MAI, fungal disease, and cystic fibrosis. Bronchioloalveolar carcinoma spread is also centrilobular,
2. If numerous subpleural and interlobar fissural nodules are present, the pattern is either perilymphatic or random.
   a. In the case of perilymphatic nodules, distribution will be patchy and have a bronchovascular distribution. Lymphangitic carcinoma nodules are perilymphatic. Silicosis also has perilymphatic nodules
   b. In the case of random nodules, they will either be diffuse and uniform, or predominate in the lower lobes. Hematogenous pulmonary metastases are random nodules. Disseminated fungal nodules are also random (unlike aerogenic fungal nodules)

TABLE 23-8 Key Features of Lymphangitic Carcinoma

5% unilateral and 50% bilateral
Smooth or nodular interstitial reticulation
Often thickened bronchovascular interstitium
Most common with lung, breast, stomach, and pancreatic cancer
Pleural effusion in 40%
Lymphadenopathy in 30%

PLEURAL METASTASES

These usually present as pleural effusions on radiographs and CT. There may be associated loculation, pleural thickening, nodularity, or masses. The pleural thickening may be irregular, show progressively increasing nodularity, and are likely to enhance with contrast. However, this is not specific for malignancy, as empyema will also show peripheral rim enhancement. However, nodularity would not be expected with empyema. Pleural thickening may also be seen with mesothelioma, lymphoma, and leukemia. Lung and breast carcinoma are most commonly associated with malignant pleural effusions. Pleural fluid cytology is positive in 80% to 90% of patients with malignant pleural effusions. This generally indicates unresectable disease. Those patients with lymphangitic carcinoma, which prove to have benign pleural effusions, have exudates because of lymphatic obstruction or pulmonary venous obstruction. Pleural metastatic disease results from hematogenous, lymphatic, or direct spread.

Thoracic metastases and primary malignancy evaluation with PET:

1. With pulmonary nodules greater than 1 cm, PET scanning has a sensitivity and specificity of 97% and 78% for the detection of malignancy.
2. PET scanning is indicated for the detection of metastatic disease from certain primary extrathoracic malignancies, particularly head and neck tumors, breast carcinoma, colorectal carcinoma, and melanoma.
3. Bronchioalveolar carcinoma and small cell carcinoma cannot be reliably evaluated with PET. Primary and metastatic non–small cell carcinoma and esophageal carcinoma can be reliably evaluated. PET is also routinely used in the diagnosis and staging of Hodgkin and non-Hodgkin lymphoma in the thorax.
4. Sensitivity and specificity for staging primary and metastatic non–small cell lung cancer with PET is 93% and 99%, compared with 72% and 94% with chest CT.
5. With non–small cell lung cancer, when CT is equivocal for the detection of metastatic disease, 10% of these patients are found to have metastatic disease on PET.

SUGGESTED READING

Andreoli T (Editor-in-Chief) et al. *Cecil Essentials of Medicine.* 5th ed. Philadelphia, PA: W.B. Saunders Company; 2001:553, 569-570.

Brant W, Helms C, eds. *Fundamental of Diagnostic Radiology.* 3rd ed. Philadelphia, PA: Lippincott Williams & Wilkins; 2007:433-459.

Erasmus JJ, Conolly JF, McAdams HP, et al. Solitary pulmonary nodules: part I. morphological evaluation for differentiation of benign and malignant lesions. *Radiographics.* 2000;20:43-58.

Fraser RG et al. *Diagnosis of Diseases of the Chest.* 3rd ed. Philadelphia, PA: W.B. Saunders Company; 1989:1329-1622.

Gould MK, MacLean CC, Kuschner WG, et al. Accuracy of positron emission tomography for diagnosis of pulmonary nodules and mass lesions. *JAMA.* 2001;285:914-924.

Gruden JF, Webb WR, Naidich DP, et al. Multinodular disease: anatomic localization on thin section CT—multi reader evaluation of a simple algorithm. *Radiology.* 1999;210:711-720.

Jeung MY et al. Bronchial carcinoid tumors of the thorax: spectrum of radiologic findings. *Radiographics.* 22:351-365, 2002.

Quint LE. Lung cancer: assessing resectability. *Cancer Imaging.* 2004;4(1):15-18.

Rosado-de-Christenson M et al. Bronchogenic carcinoma: radiologic-pathologic correlation. *Radiographics.* 1994;14:429-446.

Senac Melvin OS, Jr. et al. Pulmonary blastoma: a rare childhood malignancy. *Radiology.* 1991;179:743-746.

Seo JB, Im JG, Goo JM, et al. Atypical pulmonary metastases: spectrum of radiological findings. *Radiographics.* 21:403-417, 2001.

Sharma A, Fidias P, Hayman A, et al. Patterns of lymphadenopathy in thoracic malignancies. *Radiographics.* 2004;24:419-434.

Steinhert HC, Hauser M, Allemann F, et al. Non small cell lung carcinoma staging with FDG PET versus CT with correlative lymph node mapping and sampling. *Radiology.* 1997;202:441-446.

QUESTIONS AND ANSWERS

1. A patient has multiple pleural-based masses, one of which is apical, and presents with ipsilateral proximal upper extremity weakness. Which of the following is the most likely cause?
   A. Mesothelioma
   B. Bronchogenic carcinoma (i.e., Pancoast tumor)
   C. Thymoma
   D. Fibrous tumor

   ANSWER: C. Given *multiple* masses and the presence of *proximal upper extremity weakness*, thymoma with associated myasthenia gravis is the best single answer. Thymoma may commonly present with metastases to the lungs, pleura, bones, mediastinum, and local lymph nodes, and myasthenia gravis is the most common paraneoplastic disease associated with thymoma. Pancoast tumors are usually single apical lesions and patients typically present with pain and muscular atrophy secondary to brachial plexus invasion.

2. What imaging finding best characterizes lymphangitic spread?
   A. Centrilobular nodules
   B. Interlobular septal thickening
   C. Diffuse ground glass opacity

ANSWER: B. HRCT findings consistent with lymphangitic spread may include smooth or nodular interlobular septal, subpleural interstitial, or peribronchovascular interstitial thickening. In addition, there is preservation of normal lung architecture at the lobular level.

3. A patient has a 4 cm mass in the periphery of the right lung, with ipsilateral mediastinal adenopathy, no distant metastases, and a small malignant pleural effusion. What is the radiologic stage?
   A. T1bN1M0
   B. T2aN3M1a
   C. T2aN2M1a
   D. T2bN2M0

   ANSWER: C. Refer to Table 23-2. T2a represents a tumor less than or equal to 5 cm. N2 represents ipsilateral mediastinal or subcarinal nodes. M1a represents a malignant pleural effusion, malignant pericardial effusion, separates tumor nodules in a contralateral lobe, or tumor with pleural nodules.

4. An elderly man is found to have facial/upper extremity swelling and a widened mediastinum on chest radiograph. What is the most likely diagnosis?
   A. Lymphoma
   B. Mediastinitis
   C. Bronchogenic carcinoma
   D. Teratoma

   ANSWER: C. This clinical description fits the SVC syndrome. More than 50% of all cases of SVC syndrome are caused by bronchogenic carcinoma. Lymphoma is the second most common cause.

5. What is the most common presentation of bronchoalveolar cell carcinoma (BAC)?
   A. Solitary pulmonary nodule
   B. Peripheral focal infiltrate
   C. Lower lobe atelectasis
   D. Pneumonia

   ANSWER: A. The localized form of BAC is more common (60%–90% of cases) and typically presents as a solitary pulmonary nodule. The diffuse form (10%–40% of cases) may mimic any of the remaining choices.

6. Concerning bronchioalveolar cell carcinoma, which of the following is correct:
   A. Perilymphatic distribution on high resolution CT
   B. Random distribution on high resolution CT
   C. Can manifest as "*tree-in-bud*" opacities
   D. Commonly presents as interlobular septal thickening

   ANSWER: C. BAC spreads by direct spread along the alveolar walls and small airways (bronchioles). This is centrilobular spread, which occurs along the small airways and extends along the alveolar walls. Random distribution occurs with hematogeneous spread of malignancy, fungal disease, and TB (miliary). BAC does not involve the interlobular septae (walls of the secondary pulmonary make lobules).

7. Concerning pulmonary nodules, which of the following is correct:
   A. Sensitivity of detection is 95% on CT, if nodules are 5 mm or greater.
   B. Benign nodules remain stable or grow more slowly than malignant nodules.
   C. Stability for 18 months confirms a pulmonary nodule is benign.
   D. Nodules are classified into three anatomic types: centrilobular, perivascular, and random.

   ANSWER: A. Inflammatory nodules can enlarge much more rapidly than malignant nodules. However, many benign nodules do not change in size. Stability of 2 years indicates a nodule is benign. Three nodules types are centrilobular, perilymphatic, and random.

8. Concerning lymphangitic carcinoma, which of the following is correct:
   A. Bronchovascular interstitial thickening is pathognomonic.
   B. Survival time is generally less than 6 months.
   C. Nodules occur randomly or predominate in the lower lobes.
   D. Lymphadenopathy is always present.

   ANSWER: B. Bronchovascular (axial) interstitial thickening also occurs with lymphoma, sarcoidosis, and organizing pneumonia (BOOP or COP) and is not pathogenic for lymphangitic carcinomatosis. Random spread or left lower lobe predominance occurs with hematogeneous spread of malignancy and also with miliary TB and hematogeneous fungal disease. Lymphadenopathy is present in 30% of patients with lymphangitic carcinoma. The absence of subpleural nodules indicates the nodule to be centrilobular not perilymphatic.

9. Concerning PET scanning which of the following is correct:
   A. It is comparable with CT scanning in the detection of NSCLC metastases
   B. It has a sensitivity of 78% in detecting malignancy in pulmonary nodules greater than 1 cm in size
   C. It is often used to evaluate bronchioloalveolar cell carcinoma
   D. It is used routinely in lymphoma staging

   ANSWER: D. PET is superior to CT for the detection of non-small cell lung cancer metastases. Sensitivity of PET is 97% for malignancy detection in nodules 1cm or greater. Bronchiolar alveolar cell carcinoma cannot be reliably evaluated with PET scanning.

10. Which of the following is true regarding pleural disease?
    A. Nodular pleural thickening is commonly seen in empyema.
    B. Pleural fluid cytology is seldom positive in malignancy.
    C. Presence of pleural effusion in lung cancer patients indicates stage III disease.
    D. Pleural enhancement is specific for empyema,

    ANSWER: C. Presence of pleural effusion in a lung cancer patient indicates T4 disease (stage III). Nodular pleural thickening is commonly seen in malignancy rather than empyema. Pleural enhancement can be seen not only in empyema but malignancies as well. Pleural fluid cytology is positive in 85% of patients with malignant effusion.

24 PNEUMOCONIOSES

John C. Texada and Satinder P. Singh

INHALATION OF INORGANIC DUST

Inorganic dust inhalation and the resultant tissue reaction are the inciting events for pneumoconiosis. This may take the form of fibrosis, which can be focal and nodular or diffuse, and is perhaps a toxic effect of the substance on epithelium or inflammatory cells, or of aggregates of particle-laden macrophages, a reaction typically seen with inert dusts. The latter is rarely symptomatic and the former may be quite significant.

SILICA EXPOSURE

Silicon dioxide comes in three forms: crystalline, microcrystalline, and amorphous. Exposure significant enough to become radiographically apparent essentially requires occupational exposure: mining, sandblasting, stonework, foundry work, clay dye and potter's clay, and multiple other miscellaneous occupations. Silicosis is one of the most frequent types of pneumoconiosis affecting up to 3 million U.S. workers. The primary threshold is 5×10^6 particles (less than 10 μm) per cubic foot; below this exposure will not lead to silicosis. The secondary threshold is 100×10^6 particles per cubic foot: above this all patients exposed will develop silicosis. Thus the development of silicosis is concentration-dependent. The latent period does not require 10 to 20 years of exposure before radiographic abnormalities develop in most cases; in some cases of high exposure, the latent period may be only a few years.

HISTOPATHOLOGY OF SILICOSIS

The two fundamental histologic reactions to silica are silicotic nodule and silicoproteinosis.

Silicotic Nodule

Silicotic nodule is a dense concentric deposition of collagen; when severe enough to conglomerate, this becomes progressive massive fibrosis (PMF). Shortly after inhalation, activated macrophages ingest the particles, or if they penetrate the interstitium, tissue macrophages ingest them. The macrophages then interact with other inflammatory cells including neutrophils. The silica itself may be less important in pathogenesis than immune-mediated tissue damage. The earliest lesions of silicosis are typically peribronchiolar, interlobular septal, and pleural, and as they enlarge they become lamellated and more collagenous. Scattered silicate crystals may be seen in polarized microscopy or electron microscopy.

Progressive Massive Fibrosis

PMF is the conglomeration of individual nodules, composed of hyaline collagen and pigmented macrophages, often with focal central necrosis. Fibrotic nodules may be found in hilar and mediastinal lymph nodes, or less commonly in reticuloendothelial tissues.

Silicoproteinosis

Silicoproteinosis is a result of high exposure, characterized by lipoproteinaceous alveolar filling perhaps by type II alveolar cell hyperplasia as a response to type I cell damage; this is uncommon. The alveoli become diffusely filled with PAS-positive material similar to alveolar proteinosis, mixed with macrophages, membranous material, and type II cells.

ACCELERATED SILICOSIS

Accelerated silicosis is similar to acute silicosis with exudative alveolar lipoproteinosis and chronic inflammation, and is associated with fibrotic granulomas containing collagen, reticulin, and silica particles. Alveolar walls are lined with hypertrophied and hyperplastic alveolar type II epithelial cells with increased numbers of lamellar bodies.

Caplan Syndrome

Caplan syndrome is characterized by large necrobiotic nodules superposed on simple pneumoconiosis. It is a manifestation of rheumatoid lung disease (more commonly in coal workers' pneumoconiosis than in silicosis). It is significant because the progression of silicosis is faster in these patients than in those without rheumatic disease.

Other Associations

The relative risk for lung cancer is between 3 and 6 for workers with silicosis; for silica exposure without silicosis, the relative risk is 1.3. This risk is not associated with cigarette smoking. Silicosis predisposes a patient to development of tuberculosis. There is a clearly defined association between silica exposure, silicosis, and progressive systemic sclerosis (scleroderma); systemic lupus erythematosus may be linked to acute or accelerated silicosis. Any association with rheumatoid arthritis is uncertain and small if present.

RADIOGRAPHY OF SILICOSIS

Silicosis Proper

Classically silicosis will present as multiple 1- to 10-mm nodules, uniformly dense, and well-circumscribed, with an upper lobe and posterior predominance. This predominance is notable because many pneumoconioses have a basilar predominance. Calcification may occur in 10% to 20%, and reticular patterns may be visible in some cases. Accelerated silicosis has similar radiographic appearance as classic form except for earlier onset and rapid progression.

Progressive Massive Fibrosis

In PMF, large opacities more than 1 cm diameter may develop, usually upper lobe predominant, and their margins may be irregular and ill defined or smooth. They typically develop bilaterally, though they may be unilateral, at the midlung or periphery and with time shift toward the hila, leaving emphysema in their wake. They may cavitate.

Hilar Lymphadenopathy

Hilar lymphadenopathy may develop with or without lung findings. In up to 5% of cases, these nodes may undergo peripheral "eggshell" calcification, a pattern almost pathognomonic of silicosis.

CT IMAGING OF SILICOSIS

HRCT may detect smaller nodules otherwise inapparent and may allow earlier detection of confluence. PMF is visible as soft-tissue masses often with irregular margins and surrounded by emphysema and often requires evaluation of serial radiographs.

COAL AND CARBONACEOUS DUST EXPOSURE

The manifestations of carbonaceous dust exposure range from the common and insignificant, associated with low exposures, to prominent disease in patients with high exposure.

ANTHRACOSIS

Carbon dust retention is common particularly in smokers, city dwellers, and those residing near industries. Dense black particles 1 to 2 μm diameter are engulfed by macrophages in the terminal or proximal-respiratory bronchioles and in the pleura, and often deposited in bronchopulmonary, hilar, and mediastinal nodes. This exposure typically leads to minimal or no fibrosis or emphysema except when cigarette use is also present.

COAL WORKERS' PNEUMOCONIOSIS

Inhalation of large volumes of coal dust or petroleum dust is a work-exposure disease. It is prominent in coal workers, but may be found in workers involved in graphite, carbon black, and carbon-electrode trades, and may possibly be caused by fly ash inhalation. In 1969, U.S. laws required much decreased exposure, so coal workers' pneumoconiosis is decreasing; however, the current level of dust (2 mg/m^3) can still cause pneumoconiosis. Between 2% and 12% of coal miners will still develop notable disease, and 1% to 7% will develop PMF.

Development of this pneumoconiosis is clearly related to exposure, but the exact pathogenesis is unclear. Coal dust is often mixed with silica, and this may play a role. Coal dust may additionally incite a similar inflammatory response derived from alveolar macrophages. There may also be an immunologic/autoimmune mechanism, though this is unclear (remember Caplan syndrome is more common in coal workers' pneumoconiosis than in silicosis, and was originally reported in this pneumoconiosis).

HISTOPATHOLOGY OF COAL WORKERS' PNEUMOCONIOSIS

The two main manifestations of coal workers' pneumoconiosis are coal macules and PMF. Coal macules are deposits of anthracitic pigment within pigment-laden macrophages at the respiratory bronchiole, without fibrosis; these may be stellate or round, with range 1 to 5 mm. They are typically fairly uniformly distributed but are more numerous at the apices. A larger nodule, still less than 1 cm, may develop, perhaps an intermediate lesion between the coal macules and PMF. PMF in coal workers' pneumoconiosis may be unilateral or bilateral; it tends to be in the posterior upper lobe(s) or the superior lower lobe(s), often with regional emphysema and central necrosis caused by ischemia. Vascular disruption may be severe enough to cause cor pulmonale.

RADIOGRAPHY OF COAL WORKERS' PNEUMOCONIOSIS

Small nodular opacities 1 to 5 mm diameter of coal workers' pneumoconiosis tend to be less well-marginated than those of silicosis and have heterogeneous granular density rather than uniform density; however, these differences are not enough that the two are distinguishable radiographically. Nodules may calcify in 10% to 20% of cases: this begins centrally, with eggshell calcification much less common. PMF is evidenced by development of large opacities, most commonly in the upper half of the lungs, and most commonly superposed on simple pneumoconiosis. PMF may occur in 30% of patients with bilateral disease. Opacities typically start peripherally, with a well-defined lateral border and ill-defined medial border, and thicker in one direction than another (spindle-shaped). Cavitation is occasional, as are central calcifications. The opacity migrates toward the hilum leaving peripheral emphysema.

CT IMAGING OF COAL WORKERS' PNEUMOCONIOSIS

Small nodules may be present diffusely but predominant apically; similarly in silicosis, CT and HRCT are superior to radiography for detection of small nodules. Subpleural nodules are common, and these may coalesce into small linear pseudoplaques. Calcification within nodules and centrally within nodes may be visible in 30% of cases. PMF may be present.

ASBESTOS-RELATED DISEASE

Asbestos is a family of fibrous materials, in which silicic acid is mixed with magnesium, sodium, iron, and calcium. The family is subdivided into two families by fiber shape: the serpentines are curved (chrysotile is the major entity) and the amphiboles (including amosite, crocidolite, anthophyllite, tremolite, and actinolite) are straight. Of these, chrysotile, tremolite, and crocidolite are responsible for most pulmonary diseases, and crocidolite and amosite are responsible for most carcinogenic diseases. In the United States, up to 9 million people have asbestos exposure. The most common sources of exposure are asbestos mining and processing, industrial and commercial asbestos use (e.g., construction, shipbuilding and repair, boiler making and repair, railroad work, textile and plastic manufacture, gasket and brake lining manufacture, dentistry, and jewelry making), and nonoccupational or paraoccupational exposure from contaminated air or materials (such as the clothes of workers).

PATHOGENESIS OF ASBESTOS-RELATED DISEASE

Longer, thinner, and more durable fibers cause the most disease, and development of disease is dependent upon intensity and duration of exposure. Most fibers are removed by mucociliary processes, but some enter the interstitium and elicit a macrophage inflammatory response. Tissue damage is caused by inflammation and free-radical production.

Tobacco smoke increases evidence of asbestos-related disease; this is caused perhaps by increasing the inflammatory response, by retention of more short fibers, or by increasing the total fiber burden. Patient immune response also influences disease: those who develop a lymphocytic alveolitis are more prone to pleural plaques and less prone to fibrosis, perhaps by gamma-interferon elevation. Autoimmune titers are positive in 25% to 30% of workers with abnormal radiographs, but in low concentrations, raise the possibility of B-cell hyperactivity as an etiologic factor in lung disease.

Pleural manifestations are much more radiographically common than pulmonary manifestations: in one study of asbestos patients, only 11% of cases had solely parenchymal changes, whereas 48% had solely pleural disease and 41% had both. Perhaps two-thirds of asbestos patients have radiographic evidence of pleural disease.

HISTOPATHOLOGIC AND RADIOLOGIC FINDINGS OF ASBESTOS-RELATED DISEASE

Asbestos-related disease may develop in the pleura, parenchyma, lymph nodes, or airways. Manifestations are described in the following sections. Pleural disease must be differentiated from parenchymal disease, both for patient care and for medicolegal clarity.

THE ASBESTOS BODY

A central asbestos fiber is coated with iron and protein, typically 2 to 5 μm wide and 20 to 50 μm long. This is typically intramacrophage, and may be interstitial or alveolar (and because of the latter may be found in sputum); it is rarely visible in pleural plaques but may be found in hilar and mediastinal nodes and in extrapulmonary viscera. Asbestos body number is best arrived at by digestion of tissue, rather than light microscopy, as the bodies are rather rare. Noncoated fibers are between 7 and 5000 times more common than asbestos bodies, and it is likely that the former are responsible for disease. A patient with high exposure may have 20 to 100 times the number of asbestos bodies and fibers compared to that for unexposed persons and a patient with asbestosis or mesothelioma may have 100 to 1000 times more.

ASBESTOS-RELATED PLEURAL DISEASE

Pleural disease is most common, typically as parietal pleural plaques, though visceral pleural fibrosis, diffuse pleural fibrosis, and mesothelioma may develop.

PLEURAL EFFUSION

Effusions related to asbestos exposure are often organizing exudates. Biopsy may show fibrosis, nonspecific chronic inflammation, and/or mesothelial hyperplasia. The etiology is unclear, but development is dose-related. Most are small and asymptomatic. This is the most common abnormality to develop in the first 20 years after exposure.

Benign asbestos-related pleural effusion is uncommonly diagnosed, as it requires exposure history, confirmation of effusion, absence of other cause for the pleural effusion, and no cancer development in 3 years. Most effusions are small, asymptomatic, and nonrecurring (though they may recur).

PLEURAL PLAQUES

Plaques are generally not associated with other manifestations of asbestos-related disease. They are quite common, visible in 5% to 10% of autopsy patients. They are typically well-defined geographic hard collagenous plaques 2 to 5 mm thick, often with focal calcification and sometimes extensive. They typically develop along the costal and diaphragmatic parietal pleura, and generally are absent from the apices, costophrenic angles, and anterior chest wall. Plaques may calcify, typically 20 years after exposure.

Pleural plaque formation, pleural thickening, calcification, or effusion may develop. Plaques are more prominent in the caudal chest; they may be smooth or nodular, and while they are typically thin they may be up to 1 cm thick. They are most commonly visible at the dome of the diaphragm, and at the lateral and posterolateral midchest. They are typically bilateral; if unilateral, they are more commonly on the left. Radiographic plaque detection is quite specific for asbestos-related pleural disease, but not a sensitive indicator (8%–40% sensitivity). Fissural thickening, though unrelated to plaques, is found in 85% of patients with plaques and 36% of patients without plaques; it is more frequent in patients with pulmonary fibrosis. It is most frequently visible at the interlobar fissures (in 54% of patients versus 16% of controls).

Visceral Pleural Fibrosis

Discrete fibrosis is most frequently at the lateral lower lobe; in contrast to parietal pleural plaques, these areas are ill-defined and typically 1 mm or less thick. Discrete fibrosis may be associated with round atelectasis, but is otherwise generally radiographically inapparent.

Diffuse Pleural Fibrosis

Some patients develop diffuse fibrosis, typically of both the parietal and visceral pleura and associated with adhesions. This fibrosis can extend into the fissures and septa and into the mediastinum, but does not affect the lung parenchyma.

Diffuse fibrosis is defined as smooth uninterrupted pleural density over 25% or more of the chest wall. Calcification and peripheral lung fibrosis may be present, though the former is not usually prominent. It seldom involves the mediastinal pleura, which helps to differentiate benign fibrothorax from mesothelioma.

Mesothelioma

Asbestos exposure clearly increases the risk of mesothelioma.

Diffuse pleural thickening with associated volume loss is the most common appearance. Pleural effusion is common, though the mediastinum does not shift because it is fixed by malignant tissue. Mesothelioma pleural thickening is more likely than benign pleural thickening to be nodular, to be more than 1 cm thick, to spread circumferentially and/or involve the mediastinum, to involve the fissures, and to have a pleural effusion. Pleural plaques are present in 30% to 70% of patients with mesothelioma.

ASBESTOS-RELATED PULMONARY DISEASE

Lung manifestations beyond the asbestos body include peribronchiolar fibrosis, asbestosis, round atelectasis, and lung cancer.

Peribronchiolar Fibrosis

Some say that fibrosis in the walls of respiratory bronchioles is the first manifestation of disease, with peripheral spreading over time. Others believe that, because similar findings are found in other exposures, this is a nonspecific indicator of airways reaction, and term it mineral dust airway disease rather than asbestosis.

Asbestosis

Asbestosis is diffuse inhalational interstitial fibrosis, usually caused by prolonged occupational exposure. Fibrosis is most prominent in subpleural and lower lobe tissue and ranges from coarse parenchyma to honeycombing.

Radiographically this is visible as irregular small linear opacities, ranging from early fine basilar-predominant reticulation and ground glass, through prominent interstitial reticulation leading to "shaggy heart" obscuration of the heart border, through late midlung and upper lung reticulation. There is rarely radiographically apparent lymphadenopathy. Radiographs may appear normal in 10% to 20% of patients with proven asbestosis. Interestingly, gallium-67 scans are positive in people with asbestosis.

Round Atelectasis

A portion of lung tissue is collapsed and surrounded by thickened pleura. Typically small and peripheral, but possibly lobar, atelectasis is usually associated with asbestos-related visceral pleural fibrosis. This is not always asbestos related—any chronic pleural inflammatory process may lead to development of round atelectasis. The overlying pleura is fibrotic.

Atelectasis is a round or oval pleural-based opacity with volume loss and with "comet-tail" incurving of adjacent bronchovascular structures. It typically abuts an area of pleural thickening or effusion. It may be anywhere but is most typically in the posterior lower lobe. Like other findings, this is not pathognomonic for asbestos exposure—many chronic pleural diseases (hemothorax, empyema) may produce round atelectasis. They typically grow over months to years. Classically, round atelectasis is not FDG-avid.

Lung Cancer

Asbestos exposure undoubtedly increases the risk of lung cancer development, particularly in smokers, and has lower lobe predilection.

CT IMAGING OF ASBESTOS-RELATED DISEASE

CT imaging, especially HRCT, has a higher sensitivity for detection of pleural and parenchymal changes (approximately 90% sensitivity for pleural disease v. 50% for radiography, and 70% sensitivity for parenchymal disease v. 35% for radiography).

Plaques may be visible as well-defined areas of pleural thickening separated from the chest wall by a thin layer of fat. Diffuse pleural thickening is defined as thickening more than 3 mm, more than 8 cm craniocaudal, and 5 cm anteroposterior dimensions.

CT may detect asbestosis-related lymphadenopathy, and allow earlier detection and improved sensitivity for reticular changes. HRCT may detect intralobar linear opacities, irregular interlobular septal thickening, subpleural curvilinear band-like opacities parallel to the chest wall, parenchymal bands, and small rounded subpleural opacities—the latter the earliest evidence of asbestosis. Each of these is nonspecific in itself but taken together they increase the likelihood of asbestosis.

Round atelectasis enhances avidly with contrast administration, and the comet-tail bronchovascular structures are more readily apparent.

OTHER MATERIALS

TALC

Talc is magnesium silicate, used in leather, rubber, paper, textiles, ceramic tiles, and roofing, and as an additive in many consumer goods. It has low disease activity. Talc may cause pleural fibrosis, sometimes with calcification and plaque formation, nodular parenchymal fibrosis, diffuse interstitial fibrosis, and peribronchovascular opacities. Ferruginous bodies may be present. Talc plaques may involve the pericardium. Parenchymal disease may be similar to asbestosis.

MICA

Mica is one of several aluminum silicates. It is typically mixed with other compounds so disease may be related to the other agents; however, in some cases, pulmonary fibrosis indistinguishable from asbestosis or talcosis has developed from unmixed mica exposure.

FULLER'S EARTH

In the "fulling" process, clay is used to remove grease from wool. Exposure to clay may cause simple pneumoconiosis or occasionally PMF.

BERYLLIUM

Beryllium oxide is produced during beryllium extraction and alloying. Acute berylliosis is caused by exposure to high levels of dust, often accidental, and is identical to acute chemical pneumonitis: bronchitis, bronchiolitis, and diffuse alveolar damage are present without granuloma formation. Berylliosis may be fulminant or insidious, developing over weeks to months. Chronic berylliosis is more common, and is a systemic granulomatous disease caused by delayed hypersensitivity. It imitates sarcoidosis clinically and pathologically. In the lungs it produces interstitial pneumonitis, producing a finely granular haziness that often spares the apices and bases, sometimes in more severe disease developing ill-defined moderately sized nodules and lymphadenopathy. HRCT may show bronchovascular or interlobular septal well-defined nodules, similar to sarcoids.

WELDING FUMES

Welder pneumoconiosis is caused by exposure to welding fumes, with iron oxide as the principal component of inhaled dust. Welding fumes are also a risk factor for chronic bronchitis and lung cancer. Histologically the main finding is presence of iron dust and dust-laden macrophages and minimal fibrosis. Rounded ferruginous bodies are seen with black core. A ferruginous body is a mineral particle to which macrophages have added an iron-protein coat.

Chest radiograph shows small fine nodules in middle third of lungs in perihilar distribution. These nodules represent radio-opaque collection of iron particles and not fibrosis, and often resolve after the patient is removed from the exposure.

At CT these micron nodules are ill-defined and fine branching linear lines with predominant centrilobular distribution. Emphysema is often seen. The HRCT appearance mimics that of hypersensitivity pneumonitis although mosaic perfusion and GGO are less common in siderosis.

OTHERS

Numerous inorganic dusts have been associated with pulmonary disease: Kaolin, zeolites, silicates, cobalt, tungsten and silicon carbide, and numerous radiopaque dusts (aluminum, iron, silver, tin, barium, antimony, the rare earth elements). Polyvinyl chloride, titanium dioxide, volcanic dust, synthetic mineral fibers, nylon, cement dust, and zirconium also may cause disease (a single case has been identified in the case of zirconium).

SUGGESTED READING

Chong S, Lee KS, Chung MJ, Han J, Kwon OJ, and Kim TS. Pneumoconiosis: comparison of imaging and pathologic findings. *Radiographics*. 2006;26(1):59-77.

QUESTIONS AND ANSWERS

1. Which of the following is the primary threshold for silicosis development and what is its significance?
   A. 5 million particles per cubic foot. Below this number no one gets silicosis.
   B. 5 million particles per cubic foot. Above this number everyone gets silicosis.
   C. 100 million particles per cubic foot. Below this number no one gets silicosis.
   D. 100 million particles per cubic foot. Above this number everyone gets silicosis.

   ANSWER: A. The primary threshold defines the minimum exposure to develop a disease; the secondary threshold defines the level at which every exposed person will develop a disease. The primary and secondary thresholds for silicosis are 5 million particles per cubic foot and 100 million particles per square foot, respectively. This essentially means that to have radiographically apparent disease requires an occupational exposure.

2. Which of the following is *true* regarding silicoproteinosis?
   A. It is a more common finding in silicosis.
   B. It is associated with high levels of exposure.
   C. There is type I alveolar cell hyperplasia as a response to type II alveolar cell damage.
   D. The abnormal material fills the pulmonary interstitium and collapses the airways.

   ANSWER: B. Silicoproteinosis is a result of high exposure and is uncommon. It is characterized by lipoproteinaceous alveolar filling, perhaps by type II alveolar cell hyperplasia as a response to type I cell damage. The alveoli become diffusely filled with PAS-positive material similar to alveolar proteinosis, mixed with macrophages, membranous material, and type II cells.

3. Which of the following characterizes PMF?
   A. Opacities are lower lobe predominant.
   B. It is the result of coalescence of individual silicotic nodules.
   C. It is noncavitary.
   D. It typically begins as a central process, extending peripherally.

ANSWER: B. PMF is the conglomeration of individual nodules, composed of hyaline collagen and pigmented macrophages, often with focal central necrosis. In PMF, large opacities more than 1 cm diameter may develop, usually upper lobe predominant, and their margins may be irregular and ill defined or smooth. They typically develop bilaterally (though they may be unilateral) at the midlung or periphery and with time shift toward the hila, leaving emphysema in their wake. They may cavitate.

4. Which of the following characterizes the pathologic effect of anthracosis?
   A. Irreversible progressive fibrosis
   B. Moderate restrictive findings in PFT
   C. Generally minimal
   D. It is a synonym for coal workers' pneumoconiosis.

   ANSWER: C. Anthracosis is carbon dust retention. It is common particularly in smokers, city dwellers, and those residing near industries. Dense black particles 1 to 2 μm diameter are engulfed by macrophages in the terminal or proximal-respiratory bronchioles and in the pleura, and often deposited in bronchopulmonary, hilar, and mediastinal nodes. This exposure typically leads to minimal or no fibrosis or emphysema except when cigarette use is also present.

5. Coal workers' pneumoconiosis can be differentiated on the basis of which of these findings?
   A. Nodule characteristics
   B. Fibrosis characteristics
   C. Calcification characteristics
   D. Both A and C

   ANSWER: D. The small nodular opacities of coal workers' pneumoconiosis tend to be less well marginated than those of silicosis, and have heterogeneous rather than homogeneous density. Nodules may calcify in 10%–20% of cases of both silicosis and coal workers' pneumoconiosis, but when they do in the latter, they begin centrally rather than at the periphery. The same calcification patterns are found in lymph nodes. PMF has similar appearance.

6. Regarding asbestos bodies, which of the following is *true*?
   A. Most asbestos fibers undergo iron and protein coating.
   B. They make up the majority of the material in pleural plaques.
   C. They usually are free within the airways.
   D. They correlate with exposure.

   ANSWER: D. An asbestos body is an asbestos fiber coated with iron and protein, typically 2 to 5 μm wide and 20 to 50 μm long. These are typically intramacrophage. They are rarely visible in pleural plaques but may be found in hilar and mediastinal nodes and in extrapulmonary viscera. Noncoated fibers are between 7 and 5000 times more common than asbestos bodies, and it is likely that the former are responsible for disease. A patient with high exposure may have 20 to 100 times the number of asbestos bodies and fibers compared to unexposed persons and a patient with asbestosis or mesothelioma may have 100 to 1000 times more.

7. Which of the following is the most commonly encountered manifestation of asbestos-related pleural disease?
   A. Pleural effusion
   B. Pleural plaque
   C. Pleural thickening
   D. Round atelectasis

   ANSWER: B. Pleural effusion is the most common abnormality to develop in the first 20 years after exposure, and it is uncommonly diagnosed because most are small and asymptomatic. Pleural plaques are typically bilateral, caudal-predominant, well-defined, and geographic. They are visible in 5%–10% of autopsy patients. Pleural thickening is defined as smooth uninterrupted pleural density over 25% or more of the chest wall. Calcification is usually not prominent.

8. Which of the following is the pneumoconiosis most similar to sarcoid?
   A. Acute berylliosis
   B. Chronic berylliosis
   C. Fuller earth pneumoconiosis
   D. Talcosis

   ANSWER: B. Acute berylliosis is an acute chemical pneumonitis. Chronic berylliosis is a systemic granulomatous disease caused by delayed hypersensitivity. In the lungs it produces interstitial pneumonitis with bronchovascular and interlobular septal nodules. Fuller's earth may cause a simple pneumoconiosis or occasionally PMF. Talcosis causes parenchymal disease similar to asbestosis.

9. Which of the following characterizes Caplan syndrome?
   A. Large necrobiotic nodules superposed on simple pneumoconiosis
   B. Proteinaceous alveolar exudates after heavy silica exposure
   C. Round atelectasis
   D. Ferruginous bodies with splenomegaly and thrombocytopenia

ANSWER: A. This syndrome is characterized by large necrobiotic nodules superposed on simple pneumoconiosis. It is a manifestation of rheumatoid lung disease, and actually is seen more commonly in coal workers' pneumoconiosis than in silicosis. It is significant because the progression of silicosis is faster in these patients than in those without rheumatic disease. Proteinaceous alveolar exudates after heavy silica exposure are silicoproteinosis. Round atelectasis may develop after any chronic pleural inflammatory process, including asbestos-related pleural disease.

10. A radiograph of a former shipyard worker reveals basilar predominant interstitial reticulation that slightly obscures the heart border. Gallium-67 scan is positive. Which of the following is the most appropriate diagnosis?
    A. Asbestos-related pulmonary disease
    B. Asbestos exposure
    C. Asbestosis
    D. None of these

    ANSWER: C. Asbestos-related pulmonary disease is a nonspecific term that includes asbestosis, fibrosis, round atelectasis. Asbestos exposure does not necessarily lead to disease. Asbestosis is a diffuse inhalational interstitial fibrosis caused by asbestos.

25 PULMONARY EDEMA

John C. Texada and Satinder P. Singh

GENERAL FEATURES

ANATOMY

Pulmonary and Microvascular Anatomy

There is about 70 square meters of alveolar surface available for pulmonary gas and fluid exchange, generally via capillaries but also via pre- and postcapillary vessels. The alveolar septum has a thin side (0.3–0.5 μm) for gas exchange, and a thick side that serves as structural support and a medium for fluid exchange. The thin side is composed only of alveolar epithelium capillary endothelium and their fused basement membranes, whereas the thick side has interstitial tissue with connective tissue elements, myofibroblasts, and inflammatory cells. When excess water or protein develops in the septum, it does so only on the thick side. The alveolar capillaries have large fenestrations, and though they are tightly apposed to one another, there are paracellular pores through the structural proteins and their junctional complexes are not as well-developed as that of the alveolar cells. Water-soluble compounds cross the endothelium either by pinocytosis or via the paracellular pores, and the latter is probably the predominant mechanism.

A rise in pulmonary microvascular pressure has been theorized to increase the size of the gaps between the capillary cells, which increases the ease at which larger proteins can cross the pores; however, this is controversial and seems not to be correct up to pressures about 30 cm H_2O. Above this value, the high pressures can cause stress failure of the membrane, allowing hemorrhage and increased permeability edema.

Bronchial Circulation

The bronchial arteries supply the airway walls, the peribronchovascular connective tissue, the mediastinal- and diaphragmatic-surface visceral pleura, the mediastinal and hilar lymph nodes, and the vasa vasorum of the large thoracic vessels. In airway walls, there is a submucosal plexus and a peribronchial plexus; at the level of the respiratory bronchioles, bronchial capillaries mesh with the pulmonary capillary and venous system, and most bronchial artery blood (except that supplying the large airways themselves) drains to the left heart. The bronchial capillary bed may have half the surface area of the airway epithelium, allowing a large area for fluid exchange; and bronchial artery capillaries have more fenestrae than pulmonary arterial capillaries, and are more responsive to nitric oxide vasodilation as occurs in inflammation. Despite these findings, it does not appear that bronchial arteries produce much pulmonary edema.

Pulmonary Interstitium

The pulmonary interstitium is a gel of connective tissues, hydrophilic glycosaminoglycans, and cells and contains 40% of pulmonary extracellular water. This water content can double before fluid spreads into the alveoli. Much of the interstitial water is bound to proteins or glycosaminoglycans and is inaccessible or excluded, though during interstitial swelling some theorize that a portion of this excluded water may be released thereby decreasing osmotic inflow of fluid from elsewhere.

The interstitium may be divided into alveolar wall and peribronchovascular components, the latter contiguous with the pulmonary-venous, pleural, and interlobular-septal interstitium. The alveolar (parenchyma) component is much less compliant to the addition of extra fluid than is the peribronchovascular (axial) component, so interstitial edema tends to collect in the peribronchovascular tissues.

Alveolocapillary Membrane

The alveolar side of the membrane is a continuous epithelium of mostly thin processes from type I alveolar cells with a shared continuous well-defined basement membrane. As described earlier, the alveolar junctional complexes are tighter than that of the capillary endothelium, and water and small molecules like sucrose, urea, and atomic ions are the only non-lipid-soluble molecules that can cross them. The membrane is lined by a very thin fluid layer that serves to smooth the surface and provide a constant radius (via surface tension effects).

Lymphatic System

Pulmonary lymphatics have discontinuous or absent basement membranes, thin irregular endothelium, and poorly developed cellular junctions, and this structure offers no flow restriction. They begin as blind vessels at the alveolar ducts and respiratory bronchioles, bound via small filaments to the surrounding tissues so that when this tissue swells the lymphatic vessels expand. Fluid enters the vessels and is pumped centrally both passively, via respiratory motion, and actively, via smooth muscle contractions; one-way valves prevent backflow.

PHYSIOLOGY

The Starling Equation

The Starling equation relates fluid flux across a membrane to hydrostatic pressure, osmotic pressure, and permeability. In the equation below, Q is the transmembrane flow, K is the filtration coefficient, P is hydrostatic pressure, p is protein osmotic pressure, r is the osmotic reflection coefficient, and the subscripts "mv" and "PMV" refer to microvasculature and perimicrovascular interstitium respectively.

$$Q_f = K_f * [P_{mv} - P_{pmv} - r * (p_{mv} - p_{pmv})]$$

Under normal steady-state conditions, there is continuous net outward flow of fluid and protein from the pulmonary microvasculature to the interstitium, returned to circulation via lymphatics. Disruption of the balance of outflow and lymphatic return lead to pulmonary edema. Increases in microvascular pressure P_{mv} and membrane permeability K_f are the most common causes of edema.

Microvascular hydrostatic pressure is variable. There is normally a gradient in hydrostatic pressure, decreasing from the pulmonary arteries (roughly 20 cm H_2O) to the capillaries then further to the large pulmonary veins and left atrium (roughly 5 cm H_2O), with an additional physical gradient imposed by gravity of about 1 cm H_2O per cm of physical height difference. About 40% of the pressure drop takes place in the capillaries. Most pathologic conditions increase microvascular pressure by increasing outflow pressure and/or outflow resistance; that is, increasing right atrial pressure and/or pulmonary venous resistance.

Perimicrovascular interstitial hydrostatic pressure is generally about −5 to −12 cm H_2O, subpleural interstitial pressure is about −3 cm H_2O, and pericapillary interstitial pressure is even less negative (that is, closer to zero). Like microvascular hydrostatic pressure, there is probably a physical gradient because of gravity, about 0.6 cm H_2O per cm of distance; however, since this gradient is less than that of the microvascular hydrostatic pressure, the increasing pressure differences at the dependent vessels contribute to the dependent predominance of edema.

Plasma protein osmotic pressure is dependent on concentration and membrane protein permeability. It increases linearly with albumin, and nonlinearly with total protein concentration, but is constant throughout the microvasculature.

Interstitial protein osmotic pressure varies, decreasing as fluid filtration increases (i.e., in the more dependent areas, as gravity promotes filtration). Osmotic pressure is related to protein concentration in a nonlinear way, with a 50% decrease in protein concentration creating greater than 50% decrease in interstitial osmotic pressure.

The filtration coefficient is a reflection of endothelial permeability to water (mL per minute per cm H_2O of pressure per unit of lung weight). It is dependent both on endothelial permeability and surface area of membrane per unit weight, so recruiting closed capillaries to open because of increased microvascular pressure will increase the coefficient without directly affecting the permeability of any individual membrane.

The osmotic reflection coefficient reflects the fact that a solute will produce a net osmotic pressure across a membrane if the membrane is less permeable to the solute than the solvent, and if there is a solute concentration gradient across the membrane. It is thus an estimate of the effectiveness of a solute at a given concentration in producing osmotic pressure. A reflection coefficient of 1 that the membrane is completely impermeable to the solute; the values for albumin, globulin, and fibrinogen are about 0.85, 0.9, and 0.98; however, when there is endothelial damage the reflection coefficient approaches zero because the large proteins can travel via the sites of damage. This removes the most effective edema-preventing force from the Starling equation.

Alveolar Epithelial Fluid Transport

The alveolar epithelium is much less permeable than endothelium to both water and solutes. This means that solutes that exert no osmotic pressure across the endothelium because of low reflection coefficients may produce important effects at the alveolar epithelium. In the normal adult, lung surface tension in the alveolar liquid tends to exert a pressure for fluid to enter the airspaces from the interstitium, about 15 cm H_2O in normal lung because of surfactant but much higher in surfactant deficient states.

Bronchial Endothelial Fluid Transport

Many of the variables in the Starling equation are unknown for transport across the bronchial endothelium. However, the presence of large intracellular gaps, the likely much higher microvascular hydrostatic pressure because of their systemic–circulation origin, and the likely more-negative interstitial fluid pressure because of their presence in the peribronchovascular tissue, all suggest at least the possibility for important levels of fluid exchange at the bronchial endothelium.

Safety Factors

Lymphatic flow can increase 10-fold or more with acute increases in microvascular pressure or permeability before edema develops. With chronic left ventricular failure, the lymphatic vessels proliferate and enlarge. Some theorize that the limiting factor for pulmonary lymphatic drainage is not the pulmonary lymphatic vessels themselves, but the size of the thoracic and right-lymphatic ducts.

Protein sieving is a safety factor in hydrostatic (but not permeability) edema: as the interstitial fluid increases the interstitial osmotic pressure decreases, lowering the outward pressure on fluid flow.

Interstitial compliance is initially low with increasing pressure, since after the addition of only a small volume of water to the interstitial gel the interstitial pressure increases rapidly. However, at a certain point the gel expands more with only small increases in pressure, followed by a second increase in gel stiffness. It is at this second increase in stiffness (decrease in compliance) that fluid can flow into the alveoli. Notably, this increased interstitial pressure may be responsible for pulmonary vascular redistribution visible in erect chest radiographs: the increased interstitial pressure in more-edematous lung will compress the regional vessels and blood flow will be redistributed to areas with less edema. This decreases V–Q mismatch.

DEVELOPMENT AND CLEARANCE OF EDEMA

The earliest manifestation is expansion of the connective tissue space around the conducting airways and their accompanying vessels, in the interlobular septa, and in the peribronchovascular interstitium. As fluid volume increases, alveolar walls expand as fluid accumulates in the thick side of the alveolocapillary membrane, and just before alveolar edema occurs, small amounts of fluid accumulate in the alveolar corners. Alveolar edema develops after the pulmonary water content has increased 50%. An individual alveolus can only be air-filled or fluid-filled, with no halfway filling, so edema development is a rapid process for each individual alveolus. The fluid in alveolar edema has the same protein content as the interstitial, so evidently the epithelium loses its ability to sieve and allows flow of pure tissue fluid.

After normal function is restored, pulmonary lymphatics cannot clear edema as rapidly as is clinically apparent. Fluid also reenters the pulmonary microvessels, enters the tracheobronchial tree and is cleared, flows into the mediastinum, and enters the pleural space, where it is returned via pleural lymphatics. Protein clearance is probably mostly via passive diffusion, though albumin and immunoglobulin may be actively transported.

Broadly speaking, pulmonary edema can develop from increased pulmonary microvascular pressure or decreased in plasma oncotic pressure; or an increase in microvascular permeability.

HYDROSTATIC PULMONARY EDEMA

CARDIOGENIC EDEMA

The most common cause for pulmonary edema is increased pulmonary venous pressure caused by left-sided heart disease: Left ventricular failure from a wide variety of causes, mitral valve disease, left atrial myxoma or thrombus, and cor triatriatum are notable examples.

EDEMA ASSOCIATED WITH RENAL DISEASE, HYPERVOLEMIA, OR HYPOPROTEINEMIA

Both acute and chronic renal disease with or without uremia can lead to hydrostatic edema; although, left ventricular failure is likely a large component of this, decreased protein osmotic pressure, hypervolemia, and increased capillary permeability have a role. Uremic patients have constant high cardiac output from anemia and iatrogenic arterio-venous fistula, coronary artery disease, fluid overload, and left ventricular hypertrophy. Patients with renal disease caused by bilateral renal artery stenosis are prone to developing acute edema.

Fluid overload can cause pulmonary edema in otherwise healthy patients, particularly in postoperative settings and in old patients. This is perhaps attributable to temporary high-output heart failure or to decreased colloid osmotic pressure.

Patients with liver disease or prior liver transplant are more likely than others to develop edema. It is unknown whether the etiology is increased capillary pressure or endothelial permeability, or decreased plasma oncotic pressure. Development of noncardiogenic edema in a patient with end-stage chronic liver failure often is because of sepsis.

EDEMA CAUSED BY PULMONARY VENOUS ABNORMALITIES

Increased pulmonary venous pressure may rarely be caused by pulmonary venous stenosis or increased resistance, such as from congenital heart disease or pulmonary venous atresia; primary veno-occlusive disease or venous thrombosis; mediastinal mass venous invasion or compression; or chronic fibrosing mediastinitis. Type III anomalous pulmonary venous return is often associated with compression or stenosis of the abnormal infracardiac vein.

NEUROGENIC AND POSTICTAL EDEMA

Head trauma, increased intracranial pressure, and postictal state can occasionally, via a poorly understood process probably combining increased permeability and increased microvascular pressure, lead to pulmonary edema.

RADIOGRAPHIC FINDINGS

Interstitial Edema

There is generally a lag between the actual rise in pulmonary venous pressure and the development of radiographic findings. The first manifestation of increased hydrostatic pressure is pulmonary venous hypertension, described earlier, in which pulmonary vascularity is redistributed form the lower to the upper lung zones when pulmonary venous pressure rises above 10 to 14 mm Hg. This may be seen in other processes in addition to edema, including chronic venous hypertension and left-to-right shunts. This can reliably be detected only in erect images with maximal inspiration.

The normal pulmonary arteries in the upper lung zones are the same size or smaller than their companion bronchi, with flow redistribution the artery becomes larger than the accompanying bronchus.

Fluid accumulating within the perivascular interstitial tissue and the interlobular septa produce blurring of the normal sharp pulmonary vascular markings and Kerley-A and Kerley-B lines. The Kerley lines develop at pulmonary venous pressures of 17 to 20 mm Hg or higher. The presence of Kerley lines is a specific indicator of interstitial edema, but not a sensitive one compared to vascular blurring. When edema builds up in the parenchymal interstitial (the alveolar walls), the radiograph may reveal a faint predominantly lower zone or perihilar haze. Increased perihilar bronchial wall thickness and loss of sharp delimitation can be visible, with similar thickening at the large central airways. However, these findings may also be present in airways diseases such as bronchitis or asthma.

The interlobar fissures may be thickened. This is not true intrafissural fluid but rather fluid buildup in the pleural interstitium itself. Similarly, the costophrenic recesses may be thickened, by pleural interstitial edema or by small true effusions.

In cardiogenic edema, the heart is generally enlarged, though not in all cases (e.g., acute myocardial infarction). In noncardiogenic edema, conversely, the heart is typically normal-sized.

After successful therapy, edema often resolves within a few hours but may persist as long as 22 hours. Persistent interstitial thickening after adequate therapy suggests irreversible fibrosis.

Alveolar Edema

Alveolar edema may coexist with interstitial edema. Patchy or confluent bilateral alveolar opacities tend to be symmetric and to be predominantly perihilar and lower zone. Air bronchograms can occasionally be present.

Sparing of the subpleural zone creates a bat-wing pattern of opacity but is not a constant feature of alveolar edema. Several etiologies have been proposed. The peripheral pulmonary arterioles may be uniquely adapted for vasoconstriction and vasodilation, and/or the longer arterial path length to the periphery allows blunting of arterial pressures. The greater volume change of peripheral lung parenchyma with respiration may stimulate increased lymphatic flow.

Unilateral edema may exist for a variety of reasons, the most common of which is prolonged unilateral-dependent positioning. Edema will commonly develop on the same side as the abnormality in systemic–pulmonary shunts in congenital disease, bronchial obstruction, unilateral veno-occlusive disease, unilateral aspiration, pulmonary contusion, and rapid thoracentesis with reexpansion. Right-upper-lobe edema can develop in patients with mitral regurgitation, because of the valve–plane orientation. Edema can develop contralateral to the pathologic process in several processes as well: proximal pulmonary artery interruption or obstruction, Swyer-James syndrome, acute PTE, local emphysema, prior lobotomy, rapid lung reexpansion in a patient who already had left-side heart failure, systemic–pulmonary shunt, pleural disease, and unilateral sympathectomy.

A case of unilateral edema, it may be difficult to distinguish from pneumonia. Shifting the patient's position from supine to lateral decubitus may allow dependent edema to shift position, whereas pneumonia would not be expected to move. Alternatively, a trial of diuretic medication would decrease the edema but not affect the pneumonia.

Alveolar edema usually clears completely within 3 days after adequate therapy.

CT FINDINGS

Pulmonary venous hypertension is more easily defined, visible as disproportionately enlarged nondependent pulmonary vessels (the arteries by 20%; the veins by 33%). Interstitial edema is more clearly visible: the interlobular septa and the subpleural and peribronchovascular connective tissues are thickened, and ground glass attenuation is present. Pleural and pericardial effusions are more easily visualized. Mediastinal nodes may be enlarged, and the mediastinal fat may be heterogeneous.

Alveolar edema—In addition to the findings of interstitial edema, alveolar consolidation is present (though ground glass opacity is also visible in alveolar edema).

VENTILATION–PERFUSION FINDINGS

With increased pulmonary venous pressure, regional blood flow to the upper lungs rises to almost equal to that of the lower zones. Ventilation is also affected. However, the effects are that heterogeneous and V–Q mismatches occur, producing arterial hypoxemia. This is generally mild with interstitial edema but more severe with alveolar edema. V–Q mismatch and shunt can be improved by positioning the patient prone.

INCREASED-PERMEABILITY PULMONARY EDEMA

EPIDEMIOLOGY

Common causes of increased-permeability pulmonary edema (ARDS) include systemic sepsis, pulmonary infection, trauma, inhalation of noxious fumes or gases, aspiration of noxious fluids, and ingestion or injection of drugs or poisons. ARDS is a specific feature of the systemic inflammatory response syndrome characterized initially by increased microvascular permeability and subsequently by endothelial damage potentially leading to multisystem organ failure.

Mortality is over 50% overall; less if respiratory insufficiency is not accompanied by multiorgan failure, and considerably more (up to 89%) if accompanied by renal failure. Most of those who die do so within 14 days. Patients who gained weight during ARDS treatment were more likely to die than those who lost, likely a reflection of ongoing fluid accumulation or of the fact that sicker patients are likely to need more fluid resuscitation.

A wide variety of stress responses is implicated in ARDS. Endothelial and epithelial cell stimulation by endotoxins (in sepsis), by microvascular thrombosis (in hypotensive shock), or other factors lead to evolution of numerous proinflammatory cytokines, including tumor necrosis factor and interleukin-1. Active neutrophils elaborate numerous oxidative factors and also produce elastase, collagenase, and other degradative enzymes. A deficiency of surfactant develops, perhaps due to dilution by exudates, deficiency of production due to epithelial injury, or surfactant deactivation by oxidative processes. The clotting cascade is activated in one-fourth of patients with ARDS, perhaps by collagen exposure after endothelial damage, and disseminated intravascular coagulation (DIC) accompanies ARDS in a similar number of cases. The potent vasoconstrictor endothelin-1 is elevated up to seven times normal levels, and prekallikrein and bradykinin generation have been noted. The complement factor C5a, which can directly increase capillary permeability and causes mast cell histamine release, smooth muscle contraction, and leukocyte chemo taxis, may or may not play a role.

PATHOLOGIC FINDINGS

The exudative phase begins within hours after the initial insult. There is interstitial edema, capillary congestion, and consolidation by exudates and blood, but inflammatory cells are rare in the early phase. By 2 to 7 days, the edema is developing into hyaline membranes composed of cellular debris and fibrin. Type II alveolar cells proliferate. The proliferative phase runs approximately days 7 to 28. Fibroblast and my fibroblast cells proliferate, mostly within alveoli but also in the interstitium, a connective tissue matrix is formed, and lymphocytes enter the tissue. The proximal transitional airways are often spared. Bronchopneumonia development is common. The fibrotic phase occurs in some patients in whom so much collagen is produced that interstitial fibrosis develops. In less severe disease, much of proliferate changes resolve without significant residual fibrosis.

RADIOGRAPHIC FINDINGS

The exudative phase may appear normal up to 12 hours after initial respiratory failure. The earliest findings are patchy ill-defined bilateral opacities, with interstitial edema rare. The heart size is usually normal, and alveolar edema is more peripheral than in cardiogenic edema. Consolidation becomes confluent and affects the entirety of the lungs, often with air bronchograms (different from cardiogenic edema). Pleural effusions are typically not visible in AP radiographs unless superposed infection, hydrostatic edema, or infarction has developed. The proliferative and fibrotic phases are characterized by development, after about a week, of reticular or bubbly opacities probably representing ongoing fibrosis. In patients who survive, the lungs' appearance improves within the first 2 weeks; failure to improve suggests superposed pneumonia.

CT FINDINGS

Early exudative phase CT or HRCT reveals ground glass or dense consolidation, typically patchy, bilateral, and dependent. Later exudative phase findings include homogeneous and dependent opacities. The proliferative phase is characterized by decreasing overall lung density and development of interstitial reticulation. Interstitial emphysema, pneumomediastinum, pneumothorax, and subpleural air collections may be visible from barotrauma.

DIFFERENTIATING CARDIOGENIC AND PERMEABILITY EDEMA

Pulmonary vascular redistribution is visible in half of patients with cardiogenic edema, no patients with volume overload, and in 10% of patients with permeability pulmonary edema.

Homogeneous pulmonary edema is present in 90% of patients with cardiogenic edema, 30% of patients with renal failure, and 35% of patients with permeability edema.

Perihilar pulmonary edema is present in 10% of patients with cardiogenic edema, 70% of patients with renal failure, and none with permeability edema.

Peripheral-predominant pulmonary edema is present in 45% to 50% of patients with permeability edema and 13% of patients with hydrostatic edema.

Widened vascular pedicle, defined as greater than 53 mm (measured on a PA radiograph, from the crossing of the SVC and right bronchus to the left subclavian artery origin), was present in one study in 60% of patients with cardiogenic edema, 85% of patients with volume overload, and 20% of patients with permeability edema. Other studies did not find this helpful.

Septal lines are present in 30% to 43% of patients with cardiogenic or volume overload edema and in 0% to 9% of patients with ARDS.

Air bronchograms are present in 70% of patients with permeability edema and 20% to 26% of patients with hydrostatic edema.

Pleural effusion is visible in 40% of patients with cardiogenic edema and 10% of patients with permeability edema, but that number rises to 27% to 29% if decubitus, upright, or CT imaging is performed.

Cardiomegaly is present in 60% to 72% of patients with cardiogenic edema and 32% to 44% of patients with permeability edema (Table 25-1)

SPECIFIC FORMS

HIGH-ALTITUDE PULMONARY EDEMA

This symptom complex is characterized by numerous constitutional symptoms, fever, and dyspnea on exertion, with increased pulse and diastolic blood pressure. It may manifest with acute or (occasionally) chronic exposure to altitudes of 11,500 to 13,000 ft, rarely lower. It typically affects young otherwise healthy patients and appears more common in people who are returning to high altitude after a short stay at low altitude than in people reaching high altitude for the first time. Symptoms generally resolve upon returning to low altitude.

Increased capillary permeability is a factor, but the etiology is uncertain. In one theory, hypoxia causes intense inhomogeneous pulmonary arterial vasoconstriction. The unobstructed regions will experience high pressure and high flow, leading to shear stress, endothelial damage, and subsequently edema.

TABLE 25-1 Comparison of Cardiogenic and Noncardiogenic Pulmonary Edema

FACTOR	CARDIOGENIC (%)	FLUID OVERLOAD (%)	PERMEABILITY (%)
Pulmonary vascular redistribution	50	0	10
Homogeneous edema	90	30	35
Perihilar edema	10	70	0
Peripheral predominant edema	13	13	45–50
Widened vascular pedicle	60	80	20
Septal lines	30–43	30–43	0–9
Air bronchograms	20–26	20–26	70
Pleural effusion	40	—	10 (AP)
Cardiomegaly	60–72	—	44

POSTPNEUMONECTOMY PULMONARY EDEMA

This may develop in 1% of lobectomy patients and 2.5% to 5% of pneumonectomy patients. Risk factors include use of fresh-frozen plasma, high-pressure mechanical ventilation, low preoperative DLCO, and right pneumonectomy. The edema is caused by increased pulmonary permeability, perhaps because of capillary stress failure from suddenly increased arterial flow, similar to high-altitude edema. Postpneumonectomy edema has a mortality rate of over 80%.

REEXPANSION EDEMA

Edema frequently develops after rapid lung expansion, such as after thoracentesis. Typically the effusion being drained is large (over 50% of the hemithorax) and has been present at least several days. Theories for the etiology include sudden increase in negative intrapleural pressure; delay in venolymphatic return caused by stasis, reduced alveolar surfactant after long collapse, or reperfusion injury. Edema usually develops within 2 to 4 hours after lung reexpansion, with consolidation resolving within 5 to 7 days. It typically does not have severe consequences but in some instances can be fatal.

SEVERE UPPER-AIRWAY OBSTRUCTION

This occurs in lesions of the extrathoracic airway, often precipitated by laryngospasm. Edema often develops a few minutes after the obstruction is resolved, such as by reintubation.

TRANSFUSION

Transfusion-related acute lung injury is because of increased capillary permeability caused by HLA incompatibility, leukoagglutinins, or other blood factors. Patients acutely develop chills, fever, tachycardia, cough, and dyspnea, sometimes accompanied by eosinophilia. Radiograph would reveal predominantly perihilar and lower zone opacities without cardiomegaly.

PANCREATITIS

Even in patients without aspiration or sepsis, pulmonary edema can develop. The etiology is uncertain, perhaps because of pancreatic enzymes entering the blood and activating an inflammatory or thrombotic response.

FAT EMBOLISM

Permeability edema often develops with trauma, but many other factors including hypotension, sepsis, or transfusion requirement, are coexistent, so the contribution of fat embolism to ARDS is uncertain.

PHEOCHROMOCYTOMA

Some pheochromocytoma patients develop an acute transient permeability edema. The etiology may be massive sympathetic stimulation resulting in transient pulmonary micro vascular pressure.

DIABETIC KETOACIDOSIS

Noncardiogenic edema may rarely develop without any other cause. One theory is that acidosis activates the complement cascade.

PARENTERAL CONTRAST MATERIAL

Both oil- and water-based contrast materials have caused pulmonary edema. Oil-based contrast material

TABLE 25-2 Other Causes of Pulmonary Edema

Cardiogenic edema	Mitral valve disease
	Left atrial myxoma
	Cor triatriatum
	Left ventricular failure
Edema caused by abnormal volume or protein	Acute or chronic renal disease
	Hypoproteinemia
	Hypervolemia
	Liver failure
Pulmonary venous abnormalities	Venous stenosis
	Congenital heart or venous disease
	Primary veno-occlusive disease
	Venous thrombosis
	Mediastinal mass/invasion/compression
	Fibrosing mediastinitis
Neurogenic edema	Head trauma
	Increased intracranial pressure
	Postictal state
Increased-permeability edema (ARDS)	Systemic sepsis
	Pulmonary infection
	Trauma
	Inhalation of noxious fumes or gases
	Ingestion or injection of drugs or poisons

may be metabolized by esterases in the lung, releasing toxic free fatty acids. Water-based intravenous contrast material can produce pulmonary edema during anaphylactic allergic reactions, because of systemic hypotension and complement activation (Table 25-2)

SUGGESTED READING

Aberle DR, Wiener-Kronish JP, Webb WR, et al. Hydrostatic versus increased permeability pulmonary edema: diagnosis based on radiographic criteria in critically ill patients. *Radiology.* 1998;168:73.

Gluecker T, Capasso P, Schnyder P, et al. Clinical and radiologic features of pulmonary edema. *Radiographics.* 1999;19:1507-1531.

Hansell DM. Small-vessel diseases of the lung: CT-pathologic correlates. *Radiology.* 2002;225:639-653.

Herman PG, Khan A, Kallman CE, et al. Limited correlation of left ventricular end-diastolic pressure with radiographic assessment of pulmonary hemodynamics. *Radiology.* 1990;174:721.

Joynt GM, Antonio GE, Lam P, et al. Late-stage adult respiratory distress syndrome caused by severe acute respiratory syndrome: abnormal findings at thin-section CT. *Radiology.* 2004;230:339.

Paul NS, Roberts H, Butany J, et al. Radiologic pattern of disease in patients with severe acute respiratory syndrome: the toronto experience. *Radiographics.* 2004;24:553-563.

Rossi SE, Erasmus JJ, Volpacchio M, et al. "Crazy-Paving" pattern at thin-section CT of the lungs: radiologic-pathologic overview. *Radiographics.* 2003;23:1509-1519.

Slutsky RA, Brown JJ. Diagnostic radiology: chest radiographs in congestive heart failure: response to therapy in acute and chronic heart disease. *Radiology.* 1985;154:577-580.

Vock P, Fretz C, Franciolli M, et al. High-altitude pulmonary edema: findings at high-altitude chest radiography and physical examination. *Radiology.* 1989;170:661.

Westcott JL, Rudick MG. Cardiopulmonary effects of intravenous fluid overload: radiologic manifestations. *Radiology.* 1978;129:577.

QUESTIONS AND ANSWERS

1. The Starling equation relates transmembrane flow with which of these?
   A. Permeability-surface area product, protein concentration
   B. Protein osmotic pressure, hydrostatic pressure, and inflammation
   C. Protein osmotic pressure, hydrostatic pressure, and permeability
   D. Permeability-surface area product, hydrostatic pressure, blood pressure

ANSWER: C. The Starling equation relates fluid flux across a membrane to hydrostatic pressure, osmotic pressure, and permeability. In the equation below, Q is the transmembrane flow, K is the filtration coefficient, P is hydrostatic pressure, p is protein osmotic pressure, r is the osmotic reflection coefficient, and the subscripts "mv" and "pmv" refer to microvasculature and perimicrovascular interstitium respectively.

$$Q_{\mathrm{f}} = K_{\mathrm{f}} * [P_{\mathrm{mv}} - P_{\mathrm{pmv}} - r * (p_{\mathrm{mv}} - p_{\mathrm{pmv}})]$$

Under normal steady-state conditions, there is continuous net outward flow of fluid and protein from the pulmonary microvasculature to the interstitium, returned to circulation via lymphatics. Disruption of the balance of outflow and lymphatic return lead to pulmonary edema. Increases in microvascular pressure P_{mv} and membrane permeability K_{f} are the most common causes of edema.

2. By what process do most pathologic conditions increase transmembrane flow?
   A. Increasing outflow microvascular hydrostatic pressure
   B. Decreasing pulmonary venous resistance
   C. Increasing perimicrovascular interstitial hydrostatic pressure
   D. Altering membrane permeability

ANSWER: A. Most pathologic conditions increase microvascular pressure by increasing outflow pressure and/or outflow resistance; that is, increasing right atrial pressure and/or pulmonary venous resistance. Some conditions increase microvascular pressure via increasing pulmonary artery pressure or pulmonary blood flow. Processes altering membrane permeability cause the edema subtype ARDS.

3. What is the most common cause for pulmonary edema?
   A. Hypoproteinemia
   B. Left-sided heart disease
   C. Uremia
   D. Altered membrane permeability

ANSWER: B. The most common cause for edema is increased pulmonary venous pressure caused by left-sided heart disease: Left ventricular failure, mitral valve disease, left atrial myxoma or thrombus, and cor triatriatum are notable examples. Both acute and chronic renal disease with or without uremia can lead to hydrostatic edema; although, left ventricular failure is likely a large component of this.

4. What is the earliest manifestation of increased hydrostatic pressure?
   A. Pulmonary venous hypertension
   B. Kerley lines
   C. Alveolar filling
   D. Unilateral edema

   ANSWER: A. The first manifestation of increased hydrostatic pressure is pulmonary venous hypertension, in which pulmonary vascularity is redistributed form the lower to the upper lung zones when pulmonary venous pressure rises above 10 to 14 mm Hg. Fluid accumulating within the perivascular interstitial tissue and the interlobular septa produce blurring of the normal sharp pulmonary vascular markings and Kerley-A and Kerley-B lines. The Kerley lines develop at pulmonary venous pressures of 17 to 20 mm Hg or higher. Unilateral edema may exist for a variety of reasons.

5. What is the most common cause of unilateral pulmonary edema?
   A. Mitral regurgitation
   B. Unilateral veno-occlusive disease
   C. Prolonged unilateral dependent positioning
   D. Reexpansion edema

   ANSWER: C. The most common cause of unilateral edema is prolonged dependent positioning. Edema will commonly develop on the same side as the abnormality in systemic–pulmonary shunts in congenital disease, bronchial obstruction, unilateral veno-occlusive disease, unilateral aspiration, pulmonary contusion, and rapid thoracentesis with reexpansion. Right-upper-lobe edema can develop in patients with mitral regurgitation, because of the valve–plane orientation. Edema can develop contralateral to the pathologic process in several processes: proximal pulmonary artery interruption or obstruction, Swyer-James syndrome, acute PTE, local emphysema, prior lobectomy, rapid lung reexpansion in a patient who already had left-side heart failure, systemic–pulmonary shunt, pleural disease, and unilateral sympathectomy.

6. In which of the following phases of ARDS does hyaline membrane formation occur?
   A. Exudative, days 2–7
   B. Proliferative, days 7–28
   C. Fibrotic, days 28 and above
   D. Proliferative, days 2–7

   ANSWER: A. The exudative phase begins within hours after the initial insult. There is interstitial edema, capillary congestion, and consolidation by exudates and blood, but inflammatory cells are rare in the early phase. By 2 to 7 days, the edema is developing into hyaline membranes composed of cellular debris and fibrin. Type II alveolar cells proliferate. The proliferative phase runs approximately days 7 to 28. Fibroblast and myofibroblast cells proliferate, mostly within alveoli but also in the interstitium, a connective tissue matrix is formed, and lymphocytes enter the tissue. The proximal transitional airways are often spared. Bronchopneumonia development is common. The fibrotic phase occurs in some patients in whom so much collagen is produced that interstitial fibrosis develops. In less severe disease, much of the proliferate changes resolve without significant residual fibrosis.

7. Comparing patients with ARDS to patients with cardiogenic edema, which of the following is *true*?
   A. ARDS patients are more likely to have homogeneous edema and perihilar edema.
   B. ARDS patients are more likely to have visible septal lines and air bronchograms.
   C. ARDS patients are more likely to have air bronchograms and narrow vascular pedicle.
   D. ARDS patients are more likely to have pleural effusion and cardiomegaly.

   ANSWER: C. No single finding is diagnostic, but combination of findings allows accurate identification of hydrostatic edema in 80% to 90% of patients and of permeability edema in 60% to 90% of patients. ARDS patients are less likely to have pulmonary vascular redistribution, homogeneous pulmonary edema, perihilar pulmonary edema, widened vascular pedicle, septal lines, effusions, and cardiomegaly. ARDS patients are more likely to have peripheral-predominant pulmonary edema and air bronchograms.

8. Regarding reexpansion pulmonary edema, which of the following is correct?
   A. More common after removal of acutely-developed collections
   B. Edema usually develops after 1 to 2 days.
   C. More common with drainage of large collections
   D. Probably not clinically significant

   ANSWER: C. Edema frequently develops after rapid lung expansion, such as after thoracentesis. Typically, the effusion being drained is large and has been present at least several days. Edema usually develops within 2 to 4 hours after lung reexpansion, with consolidation resolving within 5 to 7 days. It typically does not have severe consequences, but in some instances can be fatal.

9. Regarding high-altitude pulmonary edema (HAPE), which of the following is *true*?
   A. Most commonly associated with chronic high-altitude exposure
   B. Associated with cardiogenic causes
   C. More common in healthy patients
   D. Not associated with constitutional symptoms

   ANSWER: C. HAPE is characterized by constitutional symptoms, fever, and dyspnea on exertion, with increased pulse and diastolic blood pressure. It may manifest with acute or occasionally chronic exposure to altitudes of 11 500 to 13 000 ft. It typically affects young otherwise healthy patients. Symptoms generally resolve upon returning to low altitude. Increased capillary permeability is a factor, but the etiology is uncertain.

10. Regarding ARDS, which of the following is correct?
   A. Mortality is over 50%.
   B. Associated with surfactant overproduction
   C. Associated with decreased endothelin-1 levels
   D. Patients who gain weight during therapy are less likely to die.

   ANSWER: A. Mortality is over 50% overall; less if respiratory insufficiency is not accompanied by MOSF, and considerably more (up to 89%) if accompanied by renal failure. Patients who gained weight during ARDS were more likely to die than those who lost, likely a reflection of fluid accumulation or of the fact that sicker patients are likely to need more fluid resuscitation. A wide variety of stress responses is implicated in ARDS. Among them, a deficiency of surfactant develops, perhaps due to dilution by exudates, deficiency of production due to epithelial injury, or surfactant deactivation by oxidative processes. The potent vasoconstrictor endothelin-1 is elevated up to seven times normal levels, and prekallikrein and bradykinin generation have been noted.

26 PULMONARY ARTERIAL HYPERTENSION

Ian Malcolm and Satinder P. Singh

PULMONARY HYPERTENSION

Normal pulmonary vascular bed is a high-flow, low-pressure, and low-resistance system with compliant thin-walled vessels and resistance less than one-tenth the resistance of systemic bed. Pulmonary vascular resistance is expressed as a quotient of the difference between pulmonary artery (PA) or inflow pressure minus pulmonary venous (PV) or outflow pressure divided by cardiac output. The normal pulmonary resistance is approximately 1 wood unit. Pulmonary arterial hypertension (PAH) is present when the PA systolic pressure is greater than 35 mm Hg or the mean PA pressure is greater than 25 mm Hg at rest or greater than 30 mm Hg with exercise. Athletes can normally have higher resting PA systolic pressure.

PATHOPHYSIOLOGY

Pulmonary blood flow is regulated by small muscular arterioles less than 1 mm in diameter, proximal to the capillary bed. Pulmonary vascular endothelium responds to changes in oxygen tension, transmural pressure, and blood flow. If these changes are prolonged and severe, endothelial damage produces structural change (Table 26-1). This change occurs earliest in the small vessels of the lung and is initially reversible (intimal proliferation and medial smooth muscle hypertrophy). However, it eventually becomes irreversible (fibrinoid necrosis, luminal thrombosis, dilation, and plexiform lesions). These latter changes are called plexogenic arteriopathy and may occur with advanced pulmonary hypertension, whatever the cause be.

In a normal individual, pulmonary vascular resistance actually decreases with increasing cardiac output, such as with exercise, because the pulmonary vasculature maintains pulmonary artery pressure (PAP) within a narrow range by its ability to fine tune the resistance

TABLE 26-1 Histologic Findings in Pulmonary Arterial Hypertension

1. Intimal hypertrophy
2. Medial hypertrophy
3. Plexiform arteriopathy

offered. The pulmonary microvasculature relaxes further when the cardiac output is increased. However, when the pulmonary vasculature is diseased with medial and smooth muscle hypertrophy, this compliance is lost and in fact vessels may actually decrease in size rather than distend, leading to increased contractile force of the right ventricle (RV) to compensate and maintain flow, which then increases pressure.

NATURAL HISTORY OF PULMONARY ARTERIAL HYPERTENSION

Decreased pulmonary vascular capacitance

⇓

Increased pulmonary arteriolar resistance (>3 wood units)

⇓

Elevated pulmonary artery pressures

⇓

Right ventricular pressure overload

⇓

Tricuspid regurgitation

⇓

RV failure, reduced cardiac output, hypotension

⇓

Myocardial ischemia

TABLE 26-2 Etilogy of Pulmonary Hypertension

Precapillary
Increased blood flow
Intracardiac shunt
Extracardiac shunt
Hyperdynamic pulmonary circulation
Small vessel disease
Idiopathic PAH
Familial PAH
Portopulmonary hypertension
Anorexigens
Connective tissue disease
HIV infection
Pulmonary thromboembolism or occlusion
Chronic PTE
Sickle cell disease
Mediastinal fibrosis (pulmonary artery occlusion)
Pleuropulmonary disease
COPD, cystic fibrosis, bronchiectasis
Interstitial lung disease
Sarcoidosis
Hypoventilation
Obstructive sleep apnea
Chest wall deformities
Neuromuscular disease
Obesity
Postcapillary
Left-sided heart failure
Mediastinal fibrosis (pulmonary vein occlusion)
Pulmonary veno-occlusive disease

PAH is classified according to the underlying etiology (Tables 26-2 and 26-3), including idiopathic, familial, connective tissue disorder, liver disease, and HIV (Table 26-4). Idiopathic PAH is uncommon with incidence of 1 to 2 per million, with median age of 40 years. It is more common in females (female-to-male ratio is 2.5:1).

Multimodality imaging plays an important role in evaluation of common symptoms including dyspnea on exertion, syncope, fatigue, dizziness, and chest pain. Classic auscultatory findings are heard in PAH (Table 26-5) and ensuing right ventricular failure (Table 26-6). It is often misdiagnosed as deconditioning, heart failure, asthma, heart rhythm disorder, coronary artery disease, and psychiatric problems. Diagnosis is often delayed up to 2 to 3 years. Chest radiographic findings include dilatation of main and central PA to pulmonary hypertension greater than 17 mm with rapid tapering, enlarged RV, and PA calcification in severe prolonged cases (Table 26-7).

Echocardiography is used as a screening tool for patients with unexplained dyspnea (Tables 26-8 and 27-9). Pulmonary pressures can be estimated, although echocardiography cannot reliably detect mild PAH. Tricuspid regurgitation is present in 90% of patients, and a tricuspid regurgitant velocity of 3 m/s corresponds with pulmonary pressures of greater than 30 mm Hg. Limitations of echocardiography include operator dependence, wide variability, under- or overestimation of severity of PAH, and missed left ventricular disease in congenital heart disease.

CT IN PULMONARY ARTERIAL HYPERTENSION

CT is used to exclude other causes of PAH, such as chronic pulmonary thromboendarterectomy (PTE), interstitial lung disease (ILD), etc. CT is more accurate in evaluation of main PA size in comparison to radiograph (Table 26-10). The ratio of transverse main pulmonary artery (MPA) diameter to that of the aortic diameter at the same level should be greater than 1. Main CT findings in pulmonary hypertension are described in Table 26-10.

TABLE 26-3 Clinical Classification of Pulmonary Hypertension*

Pulmonary arterial hypertension
Idiopathic
Familial
Collagen vascular disease
Portal hypertension
HIV infection
Drug and toxins
Pulmonary veno-occlusive disease
Persistent pulmonary hypertension of the newborn
Associated with left-sided heart disease
Associated with lung disease or hypoxemia
COPD
Interstitial lung disease
Sleep-disordered breathing
Alveolar hypoventilation
Chronic pulmonary thromboembolism
Obstruction of proximal pulmonary arteries
Obstruction of distal pulmonary arteries
Tumor, parasites, foreign material
Miscellaneous
Sarcoidosis, Langerhans cell histiocytosis, lymphangiomyomatosis, compression of pulmonary vessels

*As per World Health Organization, 2003.

MR is often used to evaluate the effect of pulmonary hypertension on RV and to establish underlying intracardiac shunt (Table 26-11). Sometimes it is performed to diagnose the presence of pulmonary hypertension when echocardiographic findings are equivocal.

Pulmonary angiography, more frequent in the past, is now done only in special circumstances, especially when other noninvasive imaging findings are equivocal or there is discrepancy in clinical suspicion and imaging results. In addition, it is also done routinely at some institutions for the evaluation of chronic thromboembolic pulmonary hypertension prior to thromboembolectomy.

Angiographic features of pulmonary hypertension include dilated PAs, abnormal tapering, and in chronic PTE the features are irregularity, webs, areas of narrowing and dilatation in PA branches. PAPs are elevated.

TABLE 26-4 Increased Risk of Developing Pulmonary Arterial Hypertension

Family history
Connective tissue disorder
Coronoary heart disease
Portal hypertension
DVT/pulmonary embolism history
Appetite suppressant drug use
HIV

TABLE 26-5 Signs of Pulmonary Arterial Hypertension

Loud P2
RV lift
Systolic murmur (TR)
Diastolic murmur (PR)
RV S4

TABLE 26-6 Signs of Right Ventricular Failure

JVD with V wave
RV S3
Hepatomegaly
Edema
Ascites

TABLE 26-7 Goal of Imaging Assessment of Pulmonary Arterial Hypertension

Determination of etiology
Cardiac (LV/valvular dysfunction): echo, MRI, +/−CT
CHD, shunts: echo, MRI, +/−CT
Lung parenchymal diseases: CXR, CT
Chronic thromboembolic diseases: CT, V/Q, MRI, PAgram
Pulmonary vascular diseases: CT, MRA, PAgram
Cardiac assessment
RV morphology and function: MRI, echo, Gated CT
Evaluation of pulmonary vasculature
Morphology/anatomy: CT, MRI, echo
Physiology (pulmonary vascular resistance): right heart catheterization, echo, MRI
Evaluation of lung parenchyma
CT

TABLE 26-8 Echocardiographic Findings in Pulmonary Arterial Hypertension

Enlarged RV and RA
Normal or small LV
Thickened and displaced interventricular septum
Quantitation of RV systolic HTN
Estimation of PA end diastolic pressure

TABLE 26-9 Poor Prognostic Echocardiographic Findings

Presence of pericardial effusion
Due to impaired lymphatic and venous drainage from RV failure
Size correlates with right atrial pressure
Inversely correlates with cardiac index and 1 y survival
RA enlargement
Septal displacement

TABLE 26-10 CT Findings in Pulmonary Hypertension

Enlarged MPA: >29 mm (sensitivity 87%, specificity 89%, PPV 97%)
Segmental artery to bronchus ratio is >1 in >3 lobes (specificity 100%)
Mosaic attenuation of lung parenchyma (common in chronic thromboembolic disease)
RV dilatation
Abnormal septal curvature and motion best seen on gated cine CTA study

TABLE 26-11 MR Features in Pulmonary Hypertension

Direct signs of PH: RV-RA enlargement, D shaped LV as a result of septal displacement, dilated IVC, loss of respiratory collapse, abnormal septal wall motion (septal bounce)
Tricuspid regurgitation
Evaluate right heart function
Cine phase contrast imaging: to determine flow velocities in PA, evaluate right to left shift
Quantitate PAH: PASP (peak velocity of TR jet, echo method)
Determine etiology of PAH

In primary PAP, V/Q scan is usually normal or may show mild heterogeneity in pulmonary perfusion. It distinguishes chronic thromboembolic pulmonary hypertension from idiopathic pulmonary hypertension with a sensitivity of 90% to 100% and a specificity of 94% to 100%. However, segmental perfusion defects occur with pulmonary veno-occlusive disease, large vessel arteritis, or encasement, compression, or occlusion of PAs in the mediastinum by fibrosing mediastinitis or invasive carcinoma in the mediastinum.

SELECTED CAUSES OF PULMONARY HYPERTENSION

CONNECTIVE TISSUE DISORDERS AND PAH

Scleroderma is the most common cause of PAH among connective tissue diseases, with one-third of patients with scleroderma and more than 50% of patients with CREST syndrome afflicted. High incidence suggests echocardiographic screening to be reasonable practice in this population. It carries a very poor prognosis. Other connective tissue disorders associated with PAH include mixed connective tissue disorder, rheumatoid arthritis, SLE, and polymyositis.

CONGENITAL HEART DISEASE

PAH can develop in adults with ASD as a result of chronic increased blood flow through its effect on the endothelium. These patients are often evaluated with echocardiography, which can show the right to left shunt on doppler in addition to the ASD itself. A bubble study can be used to differentiate intracardiac from intraparenchymal shunt: intracardiac shunt bubbles are seen within three heart beats in the left circulation while intraparenchymal bubbles are delayed up to five or more heart beats. There is often massive dilatation of PA along with cardiomegaly. PA eccentric calcification may be present and is better seen on CT.

LUNG PARENCHYMA AND CHEST WALL DISORDERS

Factors responsible for PAH include chronic alveolar hypoxia, compression of pulmonary vasculature by high lung volumes in COPD, or destruction in chronic fibrotic states leading to loss of small vessels in vascular beds, increased cardiac output, and increased viscosity from polycythemia. Development of PAH in patients with cystic fibrosis carries a grave prognosis with mean survival as short as 8 months from the time of development.

Pulmonary thromboembolism can occur following deep venous thrombosis in the legs or pelvis, venous catheter thrombus, and emboli from right atrial thrombi or endocarditis of the pulmonary and tricuspid valves. Acute PTE usually causes transient elevation of pulmonary pressures, with subsequent development of chronic thromboembolic pulmonary hypertension in less than 5% of cases. CTA shows eccentric or flattened mural thrombi in central PAs with this chronic disease, which compress or occlude the lumen. Fibrous bands or webs often develop, which also compromise the lumen. Ten percent of thrombi have calcifications. Mosaic perfusion may be present. Bronchial collateral vessels in the mediastinum enable systemic to venous shunting, and enlarged bronchial arteries (greater than 1.5-mm diameter) are a good prognostic factor, prior to thromboembolectomy. Patients may be asymptomatic for many years before developing cor pulmonale (exercise intolerance, ascites, hepatomegaly, and peripheral edema).

Role of conventional arteriography in chronic PTE is for preoperative planning before thromboendarterectomy to visualize arterial lumens, determine the presence or extent of thrombi, both acute and chronic, and provide pressure measurements. However, it is invasive and often the central embolus is not well visualized.

Thromboembolectomy is used to decrease the extent of pulmonary vascular obstruction, reduce PAP, and improve cardiac function. Patients are selected if they have

- central chronic PTE (main, lobar, or segmental arteries, more accurately seen on CTA),
- absence of concurrent disease, or
- PVR greater than 5.0 wood units.

Mortality with thromboembolectomy is 10–20%.

Drug-induced pulmonary hypertension is indistinguishable from idiopathic pulmonary hypertension. It occurs with anorexigenics, cocaine, amphetamine, and some chemotherapeutic agents. There are extensive plexogenic lesions in the pulmonary microvasculature, and parenchymal nodules are shown on high resolution CT.

Pulmonary veno-occlusive disease is a rare condition with fibrous obliteration of PVs and venules. Unlike left-sided cardiac lesions, right-sided cardiac catheterization in pulmonary veno-occlusive disease will not show elevated pressures in the left atrium. Left ventricle and left atrial size is normal. There is also absence of cephalization pulmonary venous hypertension on erect chest radiographs. Pulmonary veno-occlusive disease has been associated with pregnancy, drugs (bleomycin, carmustine, and oral contraceptives), toxic ingestion, bone marrow transplantation (GVHD), immunological disorders, and viral infection.

The rare condition, capillary hemangiomatosis or microvasculopathy, is difficult to diagnose prospectively. In fact, many patients are misdiagnosed as having heart failure.

Both pulmonary veno-occlusive disease and capillary hemangiomatosis cause similar radiographic changes including interstitial septal thickening with pleural effusion, mimicking edema but without cardiac enlargement. HRCT shows additional centrilobular ground glass opacities. Use of vasodilators in these conditions can cause fatal edema.

HIV-induced PAH affects 0.1% of the HIV population, with higher pulmonary pressures if AIDS is present. Chronic thromboembolic pulmonary hypertension is also present in a low percentage of these patients. Vasculopathy and radiographic findings are indistinguishable from idiopathic pulmonary hypertension.

Mild PAH due to associated hyperdynamic cardiac output is common in liver disease. More severe (portopulmonary) hypertension is caused by associated vasculitis. PAH occurs in up to 16% of patients referred for liver transplant assessment. Mean survival is 6 months and 10% patients have 5-year survival.

PAH secondary to left heart conditions (postcapillary pulmonary hypertension) is perhaps the most common cause of secondary PAH. Diagnosis is often made based on echocardiographic findings.

Left heart decompensation causes increased pulmonary venous pressure. Pulmonary venous hypertension is present when pulmonary venous pressure, usually approximated by capillary wedge pressure, is equal to or exceeding 18 mm Hg. This may occur with mitral stenosis (mitral valve obstruction by thrombus or myxoma), hypertension, aortic stenosis, cardiomyopathy, or constrictive pericarditis. A rise in PAP is required to maintain flow through the capillary bed, resulting in PAH.

Pulmonary veno-occlusion due to encasement of the pulmonary veins by mediastinal fibrosis, mediastinal carcinoma, or sclerotic lymphoma may also prevent forward pulmonary blood flow to the left cardiac chambers.

Treatment includes curing underlying disease (left heart disease, shunts, pulmonary parenchymal, or thrombotic processes). Pharmacotherapy includes diuretics, warfarin, O_2, digoxin, calcium channel blocker, prostanoids (Epoprostenol), endothelin receptor antagonist (Bosentan), and phosphodiesterase inhibitors.

It is important to distinguish pulmonary veno-occlusive disease from interstitial lung disease, because induced vasodilation, which is used to treat interstitial lung disease, will precipitate pulmonary edema in pulmonary veno-occlusive disease.

Surgical intervention includes atrial septostomy (palliative in precapillary PAH) and pulmonary thromboendarterectomy in chronic PTE. The survival rate in lung transplantation is 1 year for 70% to 75% patients and 5 years for 40% to 45% patients.

Suggested Reading

Bergin CJ, Rios C, King MA, et al. Accuracy of high-resolution CT in identifying chronic pulmonary thromboembolic disease. *Am J Roentgenol.* 1996;166(6):1371-1377.

Chen H, DeMarco T, Golden JA, et al. Utility of CT in predicting pulmonary hypertension in patients with parenchymal disease: similar results, different conclusion? *Chest.* 2008;133(4): 1053-1054. Author Reply 1054.

Fedullo PF, Auger WR, Channick RN, et al. Chronic thromboembolic pulmonary hypertension. *Clin Chest Med.* 2001;22:561-581.

Frazier AA, Galvin JR, Franks TJ, et al. From the archives of AFIP: pulmonary vascular— hypertension and infarction. *Radiographics.* 2000;20:491-524. Quiz: 530-532.

Gotarey MB, Reddy GP, Dawn SK, Sista A. Pulmonary arterial hypertension. In: Webb RR, Higgins CB, eds. *Thoracic Imaging.* Philadelphia, PA. Lippincott Williams & Wilkins; 2005.

Kim NH, Fesler P, Channick RN, et al. Preoperative positioning of pulmonary vascular resistance correlates with early outcome after endarterectomy for chronic thromboembolic pulmonary hypertension. *Circulation.* 2004;109:18-22.

Kuriyama K, Gamsu G, Stern RG, et al. CT-determined pulmonary artery diameters in predicting pulmonary hypertension. *Invest Radiol.* 1984;19:16-22.

McGoon M, Gutterman D, Steen U, et al. Screening, early detection, and diagnosis of pulmonary hypertension: ACC evidence-based clinical practice guidelines. *Chest.* 2004;126(suppl):14S-34S.

Mesa RA, Edell ES, Dunn WF, et al. Human immunodeficiency virus infection and pulmonary hypertension: two new cases and a review of 86 reported cases. *Mayo Clin Proc.* 1998;73:37-45.

Naidich DP, Webb WB, Müller NG, et al. eds. *Principals and Techniques of Thoracic CT and MR. CT and MR of the Thorax.* 3rd ed. New York. Lippincott-Raven; 1999.

Nikolase K, Shoenberg SO, Altenberger U, et al. Pulmonary arterial hypertension diagnosis with fast perfusion MR imaging and high-spatial-resolution MR angiography—preliminary experience. *Radiology.* 2005;236:694-703.

Resten A, Maitre S, Humbert M, et al. Pulmonary arterial hypertension: thin section CT predictors of epoprosternal therapy failure. *Radiology.* 2002;22:782-788.

Resten A, Maitre S, Humbert M, et al. Pulmonary hypertension: CT of the chest in pulmonary veno-occlusive disease. *Am J Roentgenol.* 2004;183:65-70.

Restrepo CS, Diethelm L, Lemos JN, et al. Cardiovascular complication of human immunodeficiency virus infection. *Radiographics.* 2006;26:213-231.

Robalindo BD, Moodie DS. Association between primary pulmonary hypertension and portal hypertension: analysis of its pathophysiology and clinical, laboratory, and hemodynamic manifestations. *J Am Coll Cardiol.* 1991;17:492-498.

Scharf SM, Iqbal M, Keller CC, et al. Hemodynamic characterization of patients with severe emphysema. *Am J Respir Crit Care Med.* 2002;166:314-322.

Schwickert HC, Schweden F, Schild HH, et al. Pulmonary arteries and lung parenchyma in chronic pulmonary embolism: preoperative and postoperative CT findings. *Radiology.* 1994;191:351-357.

Screaton NJ, Gopalan D. Pulmonary arterial hypertension. In: Nestor LM, Isabela SS, eds. *Imaging of the Chest.* Philadelphia, PA. Saunders; 2008.

Tan RT, Kuzo R, Goodman LR, et al.; Medical College of Wisconsin Lung Transplant Group. Utility of CT scan evaluation for predicting pulmonary hypertension in patients with parenchymal lung disease. *Chest.* 1998;113:1250-56.

QUESTIONS AND ANSWERS

1. Regarding chronic thromboembolic pulmonary hypertension, which of the following is *true*?
   A. Radionuclide scanning has only limited value in distinguishing chronic thromboembolic pulmonary hypertension from idiopathic pulmonary hypertension.
   B. Commonly develops after acute pulmonary thromboembolism
   C. Mosaic perfusion is frequently seen with CTA.
   D. Mediastinal vascular collateral circulation is a poor prognostic indicator prior to thromboembolectomy.

   ANSWER: C. V/Q scanning is the optimal method of distinguishing chronic thromboembolic pulmonary hypertension from idiopathic pulmonary hypertension. Chronic thromboembolic pulmonary hypertension develops in less than 5% of cases. Bronchial collateral circulation in the mediastinum is a good prognostic factor, prior to thromboembolectomy.

2. Regarding congenital heart disease and pulmonary hypertension, which of the following is *true?*
   A. Increased flow with shunt lesions causes pulmonary venous hypertension.
   B. Chest radiography in children is useful in the detection of shunt lesions.
   C. Lung biopsy can help determine operability and prognosis in cases that are not detected early.
   D. Patient with Eisenmenger physiology requires urgent correction of intracardiac shunt lesions.

   ANSWER: C. Increased flow with shunt lesions causes pulmonary arterial hypertension, not pulmonary venous hypertension. Chest radiographs are not useful in most cases. Echocardiography is diagnostic and also the method of choice. Surgery for cardiac lesions is required before irreversible vasculitis occurs in the lungs with Eisenmenger physiology. Lung biopsy reveals the condition of pulmonary microvasculature.

3. Regarding postcapillary hypertension, which of the following is *true*?
   A. Parenchymal sarcoidosis may be the cause.
   B. Pulmonary venous hypertension is present when pulmonary venous pressure is equal to or exceeding 14 mm Hg.
   C. Left atrial and left ventricular pressures are elevated in left ventricular failure.
   D. Mediastinal fibrosis and carcinomatous encasement of pulmonary veins can also cause elevated left atrial pressure and consequent pulmonary hypertension.

   ANSWER: C. Pulmonary arterial hypertension, secondary to left heart conditions (LA, LV, or chronic MV disease), is perhaps the most common cause of secondary PAH. Parenchymal sarcoid causes precapillary PH as a result of destruction of the capillary bed. Pulmonary venous hypertension is present when pulmonary venous pressure is equal to, or exceeds, 18 mm Hg. These conditions also cause pulmonary hypertension, but there is no elevation of left atrial pressures.

4. Regarding restrictive lung parenchymal diseases and pulmonary arterial hypertension, which of the following is *true*?
   A. If unilateral lung transplantation is being considered, radionuclide V/Q scanning may be useful to select the lung with most compromised function.
   B. CT has limited value in the evaluation of pulmonary hypertension and lung vascularity.
   C. Pulmonary hypertension occurs more commonly with collagen vascular disease than with chronic obstructive pulmonary disease (COPD).
   D. Pulmonary hypertension is readily identifiable.

   ANSWER: A. CT is useful in determining pulmonary hypertension (evaluation of right ventricle, main pulmonary artery and segmental pulmonary arteries) and is also useful for determining lung vascularity (mosaic perfusion in the case of PTE, extent of capillary bed destruction with ILD and COPD).

COPD has a higher incidence of pulmonary hypertension than ILD (including collagen vascular disease). Pulmonary hypertension may be severe yet go unrecognized until cor pulmonale develops.

5. Regarding the pathogenesis of pulmonary hypertension, which of the following is *true*?
   A. Arteriolar vasomotor tone is low in the resting state.
   B. Vasculitis in pulmonary hypertension varies with the underlying cause.
   C. Longstanding pulmonary venous hypertension results in increased arteriolar tone to facilitate pulmonary blood flow with consequent pulmonary hypertension.
   D. Increased vasomotor tone is directly responsible for dilated central pulmonary arteries in pulmonary hypertension.

   ANSWER: C. In the resting state, only a fraction of the capillary bed is active. Increased vasomotor tone enables majority of lung capillaries to be collapsed and uninvolved with gas exchange until exercise, when suitable vascular recruitment takes place as needed. The same vasculitis occurs regardless of the cause of pulmonary hypertension. Although initially reversible, it becomes irreversible as pulmonary hypertension worsens. Dilated central pulmonary arteries are a late feature of PAH and result from loss of elastic tissue in the walls following increased pressure in these vessels. This is an indirect response to the small vessel vasculitis.

6. Regarding CT imaging with pulmonary hypertension, which of the following is *true*?
   A. Measuring interlobar pulmonary arteries to evaluate pulmonary hypertension is more accurate if ratios of segmental pulmonary arteries with relation to adjacent bronchi is also performed.
   B. Ratio of main pulmonary artery diameter to ascending aortic diameter is a reliable measure of pulmonary hypertension.
   C. Evaluation of anomalous pulmonary venous return detection is unreliable with CTA.
   D. Right ventricular dilation is always present if there is right ventricular hypertrophy.

   ANSWER: A. The ascending aorta is commonly ecstatic because of atherosclerosis, cystic medial necrosis, or sometimes secondary to aortic stenosis. Consequently, the MPA/aortic ratio may be unreliable in such cases. Anomalous pulmonary venous return can reliably be detected with CT angiography. Right ventricular hypertrophy precedes right ventricular dilation and may be present without it.

7. Regarding MR imaging for pulmonary hypertension, which of the following is *true*?
   A. MRI is commonly used to detect PTE.
   B. Interventricular septal systolic dysfunction is pathognomic of PAH.
   C. MRI is often the first modality to evaluate patients with unexplained dyspnea.
   D. MRI can accurately evaluate right heart function.

   ANSWER: D. MRI is currently the gold standard for cardiac function evaluation. CTA is currently the modality of choice to evaluate PTE and echocardiography is the procedure of choice in the initial evaluation of a patient's unexplained dyspnea. Interventricular septal motion abnormality is seen in diastole and not systole.

8. Regarding pulmonary veno-occlusive disease–induced postcapillary hypertension, which of the following is *true*?
   A. Differentiation from precapillary vasculopathy is important as vasodilated therapy can lead to pulmonary edema.
   B. Pulmonary venous occlusive disease is characterized by pulmonary hypertension, radiographic features of pulmonary edema, and elevated left atrial pressure.
   C. All patients with pulmonary venous hypertension have associated pulmonary hypertension.
   D. Clinical diagnosis is easy.

   ANSWER: A. Pulmonary veno-occlusive disease is characterized by pulmonary hypertension and radiological features of pulmonary edema, but left atrial pressures are not elevated. In the case of postcapillary hypertension, pulmonary venous hypertension precedes pulmonary hypertension (pulmonary arterial hypertension) and may be present without it. In practice, a failing left heart with pulmonary venous hypertension is common, but only a few cases develop PAH. Clinical diagnosis of PVOD is difficult and often requires lung biopsy.

9. Regarding pulmonary hypertension, which of the following is *true*?
   A. In spite of newer targeted medical therapies, prognosis in patients with idiopathic pulmonary hypertension has not significantly improved.
   B. Pulmonary thromboendarectomy can temporarily improve pulmonary hemodynamics, proximal chronic thromboembolic pulmonary hypertension.
   C. Transesophageal echocardiography is very reliable in detecting mild PAH.

D. Chronic thromboembolic pulmonary hypertension is characterized by laminated internal thrombus, web stenosis, and mosaic perfusion on CT, often with dilated bronchial arteries.

ANSWER: D. Newer targeted medical therapies improve prognosis in patients with idiopathic pulmonary hypertension. Pulmonary thromboendarterectomy can permanently improve pulmonary function. Transesophageal echocardiography is not very reliable in detecting mild PAH.

10. Regarding pulmonary hypertension, which of the following is *true*?
    A. ASD and anomalous venous return are high pressure shunts, which may eventually cause Eisenmenger syndrome.
    B. Drug-induced PAH is indistinguishable from idiopathic pulmonary hypertension and may occur with anorexigenics, cocaine, amphetamines, and some chemotherapeutic agents.
    C. HIV-induced vasculopathy is commonly associated with chronic thromboembolic pulmonary hypertension.
    D. Severe portopulmonary hypertension results from associated hyperdynamic cardiac output.

ANSWER: B. ASD and anomalous venous return are low-pressure shunts, which may eventually cause Eisenmenger syndrome. HIV-induced vasculitis, in association with chronic thromboembolic pulmonary hypertension, only occurs in a small number of cases. Severe portopulmonary hypertension results from vasculitis in small pulmonary vessels.

27 RADIATION-INDUCED LUNG CHANGES

John C. Texada and Satinder P. Singh

PATHOGENESIS

Patients who develop symptomatic radiation pneumonitis most commonly have undergone irradiation for lung and breast cancer, mesothelioma, or Hodgkin lymphoma. Risk rises with total dose (seldom occurring below 30 Gray (Gy) and almost always present above 60 Gy); with daily radiation greater than 2.67 Gy; with decreasing fractionation of dose, which allows less time for repair; and with use of once-daily rather than twice-daily radiation. Prior irradiation increases the risk, as does previous or concurrent chemotherapy with actinomycin D, doxorubicin, bleomycin, busulfan, cyclophosphamide, mitomycin C, methotrexate, and vincristine. In addition, the likelihood of lung injury is proportional to the volume of lung being irradiated, thus tangential irradiation of chest wall or breast cancers is important in reducing lung toxicity.

It is believed that ion pairs and free radicals formed by photon interactions go on to damage DNA and proteins. Capillary endothelial and type I epithelial damage that characterizes acute radiation pneumonitis are the result of the accumulation of enough protein damage to impair membrane transport.

The delayed fibrotic component of radiation pneumonitis has uncertain etiology. It may be caused by disruption of the normal endothelial-fibroblast interaction: plasminogen activator secretion by the endothelial cells decreases, allowing buildup of fibrin. It may also be caused by radiation-induced cytokine production and growth factor release thus prompting increased fibroblast activity. Lung tissue outside the radiation field may be involved, perhaps via a delayed hypersensitivity reaction to a radiation-damaged antigen.

Many patients are asymptomatic. Symptoms including dry cough, exertional dyspnea, and weakness generally develop slowly, usually between 2 and 3 months. Fever and tachycardia may occur. Pulmonary function test (PFT) abnormalities are typically mild and reversible. The main abnormality is pulmonary restriction, though carbon monoxide diffusing capacity (DLCO) may decrease if a large volume of lung is involved.

PATHOLOGIC CHARACTERISTICS

Endothelial damage is one of the earliest and most consistent findings of radiation pneumonitis, evidenced by cytoplasmic swelling and vacuolization, followed by necrosis and detachment from the basement membrane. Platelet thrombi develop and can narrow or obstruct small vessels. Type I cells become necrotic soon thereafter.

Acute radiation pneumonitis is characterized by diffuse alveolar damage: proteinaceous alveolar exudates, hyaline membranes, capillary congestion, edema, and fibroblast and connective-tissue prominence without inflammatory infiltrate. Type II alveolar cells are hyperplastic and often have large bizarre nuclei.

Fibrotic radiation damage involves fibrosis of both alveoli and interstitium, with increased number of fragmented elastic fibers. Bronchiolitis obliterans and endobronchial fibrosis may be present, and venous intimae may be thickened.

CLINICAL PRESENTATION

Symptoms are proportional to the extent of the radiation-induced lung injury and pretreatment lung function of the patient. Common symptoms include cough, fever, and dyspnea and, rarely, severe respiratory failure. Late pulmonary fibrosis is usually asymptomatic though dyspnea may be present.

Symptomatic radiation-induced pneumonitis does not predict subsequent fibrosis. In acute radiation pneumonitis, patients are often more symptomatic than would be expected from the volume of lung irradiated, which is explained by hypersensitivity reaction in response to localized lung injury resulting in out-of-field radiation pneumonitis.

RADIOLOGIC FINDINGS

Acute radiation pneumonitis becomes radiographically apparent approximately 8 weeks after completion of 40-Gy dose and a week earlier for every 10 Gy higher than that. Abnormalities peak 3 to 4 months after therapy. Findings range from subtle hazy opacity to patchy or diffuse alveolar opacity, often with air bronchograms. The abnormal area often has clear, sharp margins because of the port, but does not follow anatomic or segmental margins. There is usually prominent volume loss and atelectasis. Occasionally, consolidation and ARDS or, rarely, hyperlucent lung may develop.

Chronic radiation damage typically starts after 3 to 4 months, increases gradually, and stabilizes within a year of radiotherapy completion. Findings may be as subtle as hilar elevation or pleural thickening. In more advanced cases, there is severe volume loss and normal architecture is lost. Peripheral parenchyma is often airless, replaced by fibrous tissue, and fibrotic bands extend to the hilum. Patients may develop pneumothorax or bronchopleural fistula.

CT FINDINGS

CT and HRCT reveal similar findings in acute radiation pneumonitis, but do so earlier and with slightly increased sensitivity. Homogeneous ground glass attenuation or patchy-to-diffuse consolidation involves the radiated region, with well-defined borders because of the radiation port. In chronic radiation fibrosis, CT reveals dense consolidation or stranding with volume loss and traction bronchiectasis; although often radiographically inapparent, small pleural or pericardial effusions may be visible on CT imaging.

Myocardial fibrosis, premature atherosclerosis of the aorta or coronary arteries, arterial stenosis, tracheal or bronchial stricture, and pericardial calcification may develop late. Bone demineralization, lucent areas, avascular necrosis, and fractures may develop in the radiation field, and fractures of rib or clavicle may undergo nonunion or malunion resembling osteosarcoma.

Recurrent tumor is more clearly visible in CT than in radiographs; development of a mass lesion or of a focal opacity without air bronchograms suggests recurrence.

ADDITIONAL IMAGING FINDINGS

POSITRON EMISSION TOMOGRAPHY (PET)

Acute radiation pneumonitis demonstrates increased fluorodeoxyglucose activity, which can persist for months. PET is usually done to detect local recurrence and distant metastasis and is reported to be more accurate than conventional imaging in the evaluation of recurrence after radiation therapy. Integrated CT/PET imaging with co-registration is useful for detecting local disease and allows directed biopsy, improving accuracy in diagnosis of recurrence or persistent disease.

On MRI, radiation fibrosis has T2 signal intensity lower than that of muscle, whereas recurrence often has T2 signal intensity higher than that of muscle. Persistent inflammation, infection, or hemorrhage increases T2 signal intensity as well.

Ventilation–perfusion scans are often abnormal: up to 95% of perfusion studies and up to 45% of ventilation studies. Most commonly a poorly perfused region is ventilated, sometimes similar in appearance to PTE.

Gallium-67 imaging may reveal the extent of radiation pneumonitis better than chest radiography, often detecting radiographically inapparent regions of pneumonitis.

DIFFERENTIAL DIAGNOSIS

Superimposed infection can be difficult to differentiate from radiation-induced pneumonitis because of similar clinical and radiographic presentation. Correlation with temporal relationship to radiation treatment, dose given, and technique used are helpful. Infection should be suspected if pulmonary opacities appear before completion of RT or outside the radiation port, have abrupt onset, or presence of cavitation in radiated region.

Local tumor recurrence is often difficult to diagnose with ongoing radiation-related lung changes. After stabilization of radiation-induced disease, any change in contour or density of the fibrosis should raise concern for recurrence. Endobronchial soft tissue on CT, nodules outside the port, and development of pleural effusion more than 12 months after completion of RT (ipsilateral pleural effusion, within 6 months of completion, is common and a normal phenomenon) should also be causes for concern for recurrence.

BRACHYTHERAPY

Brachytherapy is increasingly used for palliative care of obstructing lung cancer; in this process an intraluminal-endobronchial radiation source, usually iridium-192, is placed in the lesion. Changes are predominantly inflammatory at 16 weeks and predominantly fibrotic at 40 weeks. Complications include mucosal fibrosis, bronchial stenosis, localized radiation pneumonitis, bronchoesophageal fistula, and hemoptysis. In one study, stenosis was found to be developed in 12% of patients and 25% patients were found to have developed fatal hemoptysis. Large cell carcinoma, prior laser photoresection, and concurrent external-beam irradiation increase the risk of complications with brachytherapy.

SUGGESTED READING

Choi YW, Munden RF, Erasmus JJ, et al. Effects of radiation therapy on the lung: radiologic appearances and differential diagnosis. *Radiographics*. 2004;24:985-997.

Libshitz HE, Sheppard DG. Filling in of radiation therapy-induced bronchiectatic change: a reliable sign of locally recurrent lung cancer. *Radiology*. 1999;210:25.

Mesurolle B, Qanadli SD, Merad M. Unusual radiologic findings in the thorax after radiation therapy. *Radiographics*. 2000;20:67-81.

Park KJ, Chung JY, Chun MS, et al. Radiation-induced lung disease and the impact of radiation methods on imaging features. *Radiographics*. 2000;20:83-98.

QUESTIONS AND ANSWERS

1. Regarding risk of radiation-induced lung changes, which of the following is *true*?
   A. Radiation-induced pulmonary disease seldom occurs below 30 Gy.
   B. Risk is independent of radiation fractionation.
   C. Risk decreases with once- versus twice-daily radiation.
   D. Prior irradiation does not increase the risk.

   ANSWER: A. Risk for pulmonary disease from radiation rises with total dose (seldom occurring below 30 Gy and almost always present above 60 Gy), decreasing fractionation, daily radiation greater than 2.67 Gy, and use of once-daily rather than twice-daily radiation. Prior irradiation increases the risk as does previous or concurrent chemotherapy with multiple drugs.

2. Regarding pulmonary function tests and radiation-induced lung abnormalities, which is *true*?
   A. DLCO typically increases
   B. Main abnormality is pulmonary restriction.
   C. Abnormalities are usually severe.
   D. Abnormalities are usually irreversible.

   ANSWER: B. PFT abnormalities are typically mild and reversible; the main abnormality is pulmonary restriction. DLCO may decrease if a large volume of lung is involved.

3. Regarding acute radiation pneumonitis, which is *true*?
   A. Endothelial damage is not commonly encountered.
   B. Thrombosis is a minor component.
   C. Type II cells become depleted.
   D. It is characterized by diffuse alveolar damage.

   ANSWER: D. Endothelial damage is one of the earliest and most consistent findings of radiation pneumonitis. Platelet thrombi develop and can narrow or obstruct small vessels. Acute radiation pneumonitis is characterized by diffuse alveolar damage. Type II alveolar cells are hyperplastic and often have large bizarre nuclei.

4. A patient undergoing radiation for Hodgkin lymphoma receives a 60-Gy dose to the chest. Which of the following characterizes the response?
   A. Acute pneumonitis will become radiographically apparent 6 days after completion.
   B. Acute pneumonitis will become radiographically apparent 6 weeks after completion.
   C. Abnormalities will peak 6 weeks after completion.
   D. Abnormalities will resolve 6 weeks after completion.

   ANSWER: B. Acute radiation pneumonitis becomes radiographically apparent approximately 8 weeks after completion of a 40-Gy dose and a week earlier for every 10 Gy higher than that. Abnormalities peak 3 to 4 months after therapy.

5. Regarding chronic radiation change, which of the following is *true*?
   A. Usually begins after 3 to 4 months
   B. Associated with hypoinflation

C. Bronchopleural fistula is not a complication.
D. Associated with obstructive bronchiolitis

ANSWER: A. Chronic radiation damage typically starts after 3 to 4 months, increases gradually, and stabilizes within a year of radiotherapy completion. In more advanced cases, there is severe volume loss and normal architecture is lost. Patients may develop pneumothorax or bronchopleural fistula.

6. What are the CT findings in acute radiation pneumonitis?
   A. Volume loss and bronchiectasis
   B. Dense consolidation
   C. Ground glass attenuation
   D. Myocardial fibrosis

ANSWER: C. CT and HRCT reveal homogeneous ground glass attenuation or patchy-to-diffuse consolidation involving the radiated region, with well-defined borders due to the radiation port. In chronic radiation fibrosis, CT reveals dense consolidation or stranding with volume loss and traction bronchiectasis. Myocardial fibrosis, premature atherosclerosis of the aorta or coronary arteries, arterial stenosis, tracheal or bronchial stricture, and pericardial calcification may develop late.

7. Regarding ventilation–perfusion imaging, which is *true*?
   A. Study is often normal.
   B. Ventilation study is more often abnormal than the perfusion study.
   C. Can resemble PTE findings
   D. Radiation changes do not complicate evaluation of acute onset of dyspnea

ANSWER: C. Ventilation–perfusion scans are often abnormal: up to 95% of perfusion studies and up to 45% of ventilation studies. Most commonly a poorly perfused region is ventilated, sometimes similar in appearance to PTE.

8. Regarding tumor recurrence in MRI, which of the following is *true*?
   A. Pleural effusion within 6 months of radiation raises concern for tumor
   B. T2 signal intensity is higher than muscle.
   C. MRI is more sensitive than PET.
   D. Hemorrhage does not confound the appearance

ANSWER: B. In MRI radiation, fibrosis has T2 signal intensity lower than that of muscle, whereas tumor recurrence often has T2 signal intensity higher than that of muscle. Early effusion (within 6 months of treatment) is common and usually benign. Persistent inflammation, infection, or hemorrhage increases T2 signal intensity as well. PET is more accurate and sensitive than MRI in diagnosing recurrence.

9. Regarding gallium-67 imaging in radiation change, which is *true*?
   A. Less sensitive than chest radiography
   B. May detect radiographically inapparent areas of pneumonitis
   C. Radiation changes are inapparent on gallium-67 imaging.
   D. Elevated radiotracer activity is specific for radiation pneumonitis.

ANSWER: B. Gallium-67 imaging may reveal the extent of radiation pneumonitis better than chest radiography, often detecting radiographically inapparent regions of pneumonitis. Gallium-67 imaging results in nonspecific images of inflammation. The clinical history is essential.

10. Regarding brachytherapy, which is *true*?
    A. Complications include fatal hemoptysis
    B. Large cell carcinoma is associated with lower risk of therapy.
    C. Inflammatory changes peak at 40 weeks
    D. Bronchiectasis is a common complication.

ANSWER: A. Changes are predominantly inflammatory at 16 weeks and predominantly fibrotic at 40 weeks. Complications include mucosal fibrosis, bronchial stenosis, localized radiation pneumonitis, bronchoesophageal fistula, and hemoptysis. In one study, stenosis was found to be developed in 12% of patients and 25% patients were found to have developed fatal hemoptysis. Large cell carcinoma, prior laser photoresection, and concurrent external-beam irradiation increase the risk of complications with brachytherapy.

28 MEDIASTINAL MASSES

Satinder P. Singh

THYMUS

Normal thymus arises bilaterally from the third and fourth brachial pouches, which contain elements derived from all three germinal layers. Thymic lesions can occur anywhere in the anterior mediastinum and also, since thymus migrates from the third and fourth brachial

TABLE 28-1 Origin of Anterior Mediastinal Masses

Thymus
Lymph node
Thyroid
Cysts
Lymphatic
Neurogenic

pouches to the anterior mediastinum during its development, ectopic thymic tissue, or ectopic thymoma can occur anywhere along this path.

Normal thymic size in healthy infants increases up to 4 to 8 months and then decreases with age due to fatty infiltration of the thymic gland. The maximum normal thickness of the thymus perpendicular to the longest axis is 18 mm in patients younger than 20 years of age, and 13 mm in older patients. The normal thymus on CT is usually seen at the level of the aortic arch and the origin of the great vessels as a bilobed homogeneous soft-tissue attenuation structure. On MRI, in a younger patient (younger than 20 years of age), the normal thymus is homogeneous with slightly low to intermediate signal intensity on T1-weighted images (greater than that of muscle, but less than of fat). The signal intensity is slightly greater than that of muscle, but equal or slightly less than that of fat on T2-weighted images.

Thymoma and thymic carcinoma are included in the differential diagnosis of anterior mediastinal masses (Table 28-1).

THYMOMA

Thymoma is the most common primary thymic tumor of epithelial origin. It is often seen in the fifth or sixth decade of age with no gender predilection. It is often asymptomatic. In one-third of the patients, compression or invasion of surrounding structures causes signs and symptoms of cough, pain, dysphagia, hoarseness, and dyspnea.

Parathymic syndromes include myasthenia gravis, pure red cell achalasia, and hypoglobulinemia. Approximately 40% of patients with thymoma have myasthenia gravis and 10% of the patients with myasthenia gravis have thymoma. Five percent of patients with thymoma have pure red cell achalasia and 10% to 50% of patients with red blood cell achalasia have thymoma. Occasionally, it is associated with stiff person syndrome, characterized by muscle rigidity and superimposed spasm of the trunk and limbs.

Tumors are usually round or oval, encapsulated with lobulated surface. Cyst formation (40%) and focal hemorrhage and necrosis (30%) are seen.

INVASIVE THYMOMA

Invasive thymoma occurs with invasion of adjacent structure. Pleural/pericardial implantation is common; transdiaphragmatic extension and extrathoracic metastasis is often present.

Imaging Findings

In one-third of patients with thymoma, tumor is suspected incidentally on chest radiograph. As an anterior mediastinal mass, it is better seen on the lateral radiograph. CT is superior to chest radiograph in the diagnosis and determining the extent of the tumor. Thymomas on CT appear as well defined, round, or oval masses with sharp margins or lobulated contours, usually with homogeneous attenuation, though may contain hemorrhage, cysts, or necrosis causing low attenuation areas. Cystic thymomas may manifest as masses containing fluid and soft-tissue components. The CT features are suggestive of capsular invasion and extracapsular extension and include irregular margins, gross invasion of great vascular structures or chest wall, encasement of mediastinal structures, and irregular interface with the lung. Thymoma may involve the pleura or pericardium (drop metastasis). There is nodular diffuse smooth or nodular pleural thickening mimicking mesothelioma. Pericardial involvement may leave pericardial nodules, thickening, and effusion. The tumor may extend to the abdominal cavity through the diaphragmatic foraminae (gravitational metastasis).

MRI

Masses are of low to intermediate signal intensity on T1-weighted images and intermediate to high signal intensity on T2-weighted images. Areas of necrosis and cysts appear as low signal on T1-weighted and high signal intensity on T2-weighted images. Hemorrhage is seen as high signal intensity on T1-weighted and T2-weighted or may demonstrate a hemosiderin ring or fluid level on T2-weighted or gradient echo images. The tumor enhances homogeneously after contrast. MR is usually superior to CT in assessing the invasion of the capsule or extracapsular extension.

Treatment and Prognosis

Encapsulated tumors usually respond to complete surgical excision with 5-year survival after excision at 92%. Invasive thymomas often need adjuvant radiation and chemotherapy, though controversial. If resected completely, their survival is similar to encapsulated tumors.

THYMIC CARCINOMA

The two most common types of thymic carcinomas are squamous cell and neuroendocrine carcinoma. These account for 15% to 20% for all thymic epithelial tumors. They often lack capsule and demonstrate focal invasion or metastasis to mediastinal lymph nodes. These tumors are often large, lack visible septa or nodular structures, and may contain foci of necrosis and hemorrhage. Cystic changes and calcification are uncommon.

The most common clinical features include chest pain, cough, fatigue, fever, SVC syndrome, and anorexia. Not associated with myasthenia gravis or pure red cell achalasia, though paraneoplastic polymyositis has been reported. These are mostly middle-aged patients with slight female dominance. The tumor invades locally into the lungs, pericardium, and major vessels and may metastasize to lymph nodes or distantly to brain, bone, liver, or lung. These tumors have the worst prognosis in comparison to thymoma, though squamous cell carcinoma has a better prognosis in comparison to other thymic cancers.

In 25% of patients with thymic neuroendocrine tumor, there is a positive family history of multiple endocranial neoplasia (MEN) type 1 (pituitary adenoma, parathyroid adenoma, and pancreatic islet tumor). Eight percent of patients with MEN type 1 have thymic carcinoid tumor, mostly in males.

Clinical Manifestations

These are mostly local symptoms in two-thirds of the patients from SVC syndrome or compression or invasion of mediastinal structures. Carcinoid syndrome is rare (less than 1%). Cushing syndrome is the most frequent paraneoplastic syndrome; up to 30% of thymic carcinoid tumors in adults and more than 50% of childhood thymic carcinoid are associated with Cushings syndrome.

Imaging

Radiographs often show a large, poorly defined anterior mediastinal mass, better seen on CT, with areas of necrosis or cystic changes. The mass is often lobulated or irregular in contour with calcification seen in 10% to 40% of patients.

MRI

Neuroendocrine tumors have bright signal intensity on T2-weighted images, a feature that is highly suggestive of neuroendocrine tumor when present. The encasement and direct invasion adjacent mediastinal structures can be shown on MRI.

PET and Thymic Cancer

Thymic carcinoid tumors show a high uptake of FDG. Conventional bone scintigraphy and MRI are the most sensitive methods for detecting bone metastasis from carcinoid.

Treatment

Patients with thymic masses more than 3 cm should be resected. Twenty-five percent of patients after thymectomy demonstrate remission in myasthenia gravis.

GERM CELL TUMORS

These tumors occur most commonly in the gonads. Extragonadal germ cell tumors are often in midline, most commonly in the mediastinum, probably arising from the multipotential primitive germ cell misplaced along midline structures during embryogenesis (Table 28-2). Most of these are near or within the thymus and constitute 20% of all mediastinal tumor and cysts. The known risk factors for mediastinal nonseminomatous germ cell tumors are Klinefelter syndrome (47 XXY).

Teratoma is a neoplasm composed of several tissue components: with two of three embryonic layers represented. Mediastinal teratomas account for 50% to 70% of all mediastinal germ cell tumors. Teratomas are slightly more common in females, although immature teratomas occur exclusively in males. Mature teratoma is the most common type while immature teratomas are uncommon and constitute 1% of all mediastinal teratomas and are more aggressive in adults.

Clinical Features

Usually teratomas are asymptomatic; in 50% of patients, though, large tumor may compress the surrounding structures producing symptoms. Rarely, they can rupture causing trichoptysis or pleural effusion. A rupture into the mediastinum can lead to mediastinitis. Hemorrhage into the tumor can lead to rapid increase in the size with severe retrosternal pain.

Usually, lobulated, encapsulated large tumors contain hair, teeth or bone, white, yellow, brown, oily sebaceous, or gelatinous material. Most tumors are cystic, unilocular, or multilocular with focal areas of solid components.

Imaging Findings

These are sharply marginated, large, lobulated masses in the anterior mediastinum from the thoracic inlet to the diaphragm, anywhere in the mediastinum. There may be calcification in the cyst wall or tumor substance, or presence of teeth or bone. Rarely, a fat fluid level may be seen.

TABLE 28-2 Various Germ Cell Tumors

Teratoma
Seminoma
Embryonal carcinoma
Endodermal sinus tumor (yolk sac tumor)
Choriocarcinoma
Mixed germ cell tumor

CT demonstrates a large cystic mass in the prevascular space containing different variable CT attenuations corresponding to calcium, fat, fluid, and soft tissue. A mediastinal mass containing fat, calcification, and soft tissue with hair ball like opacities on CT is highly suggestive of teratoma.

MRI

The most common MRI finding of mature teratoma is a mass with markedly heterogeneous signal intensity. The masses are isointense to skeletal muscle; serous fluid shows low signal intensity on T1-weighted and high signal intensity on T2-weighted the intratumoral fat has high signal intensity on T1-weighted and relatively high signal intensity on T2-weighted images.

Treatment

Complete surgical excision has an excellent prognosis, nearly 100% 5-year survival.

SEMINOMAS (ALSO KNOWN AS GERMINOMA OR DISGERMINOMA)

These are usually seen in males in the third or fourth decade of life. One-third of patients with pure seminoma have moderately elevated serum beta-HCG levels, but normal serum AFP level.

Clinical Symptoms

These include pain, dyspnea dysphagia, hoarseness, weight loss, and fever, though the patient can be asymptomatic in one-fourth of the cases.

Imaging Findings

Large, bulky-lobulated soft-tissue anterior mediastinal masses which can grow on either side of midline. CT shows a homogenous soft-tissue attenuation lobulated mass with minimal enhancement after contrast. Necrosis and calcification are rare.

Treatment and Prognosis

Tumors are radiosensitive and radiation therapy combined with cisplatin-based chemotherapy is the treatment of choice with a survival rate at 5 years of 75% to 100%. Poor prognostic features include higher tumor stage (lymph node metastasis, hepatic metastasis, or mediastinal invasion), older patients, SVC syndrome, and pyrexia.

NONSEMINATOUS MALIGNANT GERM CELL TUMORS

Nonseminatous malignant germ cell tumors include embryonal carcinoma, endodermal sinus tumor, choriocarcinoma, and mixed germ cell tumor. These tumors are more common in males and are mostly symptomatic in 90% to 100% of patients. Associations include Kleinfelters syndrome in 20%, hematologic malignancies, elevated AFP, endodermal sinus tumor or embryonal carcinoma, elevated HCG (choriocarcinoma).

Pathologic Findings

The embryonal carcinoma is a germ cell tumor composed of large primitive cells of epithelial appearance with abundant clear or granular cytoplasm, resembling embryonal germ disc cells with tubular and acinar patterns.

ENDODERMAL SINUS TUMOR

This tumor is characterized by a pattern similar to that of yolk sac allantois and extraembryonic mesenchym with reticular pattern and multiple communicating spaces.

CHORIOCARCINOMA

This is a highly malignant neoplasm with cytotrophoblast and syncytiotrophoblast and hemorrhage. The mean age of presentation is around 27 years of age and symptoms include thoracic or shoulder pain, shortness of breath, hoarseness, cough, or SVC syndrome. These tumors frequently invade adjacent structures, mediastinal pleura, and lung and 50% have hematogenous metastasis at the lymph nodes as well as distant organs.

Imaging Findings

Large anterior mediastinal masses with smooth lobular or irregular margins are identified. At CT, there is heterogeneous attenuation of the large masses with central areas of low attenuation, peripheral enhancement. Pleural and pericardial effusions are often present. Direct tumor invasion of adjacent structures can be seen. As with other tumors, MRI is more sensitive in depicting infiltration into adjacent chest wall, mediastinal pleura, pericardium, heart, or great vessels.

Treatment and Prognosis

The treatment and prognosis carries the poorest prognosis among all germ cell tumors. Cisplatin-based chemotherapy is the therapy of choice. Serum tumor markers are helpful in assessing the response to treatment or tumor recurrence.

THYMIC CYSTS

Thymic cysts are uncommon and can be found along the embryologic course of the thymus in the mediastinum or neck. They are a congenital anomaly of the third pharyngeal pouch. They are usually seen in young patients, asymptomatic and have an excellent prognosis.

Imaging Findings

Smooth or round and may contain calcification in the cyst wall. Differential diagnosis for thymic cyst includes cystic thymoma, cystic teratoma, cystic degeneration of Hodgkins lymphoma, and other cysts.

THYMOLIPOMA

Usually found in young patients without gender predilection. It is asymptomatic in 50% of cases. A large tumor can be symptomatic.

Radiographic Findings

These lesions can be unilateral or bilateral, often in the anterior inferior mediastinum. They may conform to the shape of the heart, mimicking cardiac enlargement and may drape along a hemidiaphragm mimicking elevation of the diaphragm. They may also change in shape with change in positions. CT and MRI are useful in identification of fat within the mass.

MEDIASTINAL LYMPHOMA

Primary mediastinal lymphoma arises in the mediastinal lymph nodes or in the thymus and is relatively common. The most common type of primary mediastinal lymphomas include large B-cell lymphoma, precursor T-cell lymphoblastic lymphoma/leukemia, and classic Hodgkins lymphoma, especially the nodular sclerosing variety.

PRIMARY MEDIASTINAL LARGE B-CELL LYMPHOMA

Primary mediastinal large B-cell lymphoma accounts for approximately 2% to 3% of non-Hodgkin lymphoma. Usually found in young patients with female predominance.

PRECURSOR T-CELL LYMPHOBLASTIC LYMPHOMA/LEUKEMIA

Precursor T-cell lymphoblastic lymphoma/leukemia occurs frequently in late childhood, adolescent or young adulthood with male predominance. These tumors constitute only 2% of adult non-Hodgkin lymphoma.

HODGKINS LYMPHOMA

This is derived from B-cells in most cases. Two main varieties are nodular lymphocyte predominant Hodgkin lymphoma and classic Hodgkins lymphoma.

The nodular sclerosing Hodgkins lymphoma is a subtype of the classic Hodgkin lymphoma with collagen band surrounding the nodule and lacunar type of Hodgkin and Reed-Sternberg cell. It is especially common in higher socioeconomic groups, urban areas and industrialized countries. There is a slight female predominance and a median age of 28 years.

Clinical Presentation

These are usually because of a large bulky mediastinal mass causing superior vena cava syndrome, airway obstruction, and pleural or pericardial effusions. The precursor T-cell lymphoblast lymphoma usually presents acutely with airway compromise, SVC syndrome, and massive pleural or pericardial effusion causing cardiac tamponade.

The nodular sclerosing Hodgkins lymphoma usually presents with chest discomfort and dyspnea or may be asymptomatic with tumor discovered incidentally on chest radiography.

Imaging Findings

This usually presents as a large anterior mediastinal mass causing widening of the mediastinum and obliteration of retrosternal space on the lateral radiograph. Bulky anterior mediastinal adenopathy is the hallmark of Hodgkins lymphoma. Pleural effusion may be present, especially in one-third of patients with primary large B-cell lymphoma and is often associated with poor prognosis. In Hodgkins lymphoma, the mediastinal hilar para-aortic or deep cervical lymph nodes may be enlarged and the thymus may also be involved in up to 30% of cases. There may be mass effect on the adjacent mediastinal structures, pleura, pericardium, or chest wall. The vascular involvement is less common with Hodgkins (7%) in comparison to non-Hodgkins lymphoma (40%–60%). The lung involvement rate is higher in Hodgkins (20%) in comparison to non-Hodgkins (less than 10%). SVC syndrome can be nicely seen on contrast-enhanced CT including its collateral circulation and mediastinal edema.

MRI

Hodgkins lymphoma has a relatively homogeneous low signal intensity on T1-weighted images similar to muscle and mixed or relatively high signal intensity on T2-weighted images, equal or slightly higher than fat.

PET

Often performed to evaluate response to therapy and detect early treatment failure, as well as follow up of patients with lymphoma.

LYMPHANGIOMA

Benign, rare mesenchymal lesions in the mediastinum, typically found in children and young adults. Ninety percent are discovered by 2 years of age. The majority involves the neck or axilla and in 10% extends into the superior aspect of the anterior mediastinum.

PATHOGENESIS

Proliferation of lymph vessels sequestered from the lymphatic system in early development. Fluid accumulates in the lumen of the lymph vessels resulting from lack of communication with the lymphatic tree. When these lesions contain large cystic spaces, they are referred to as cystic hygroma. Small cystic spaces are cavernous lymphangioma.

IMAGING FINDINGS

Soft-tissue mass in the anterosuperior mediastinum may extend into the middle and posterior compartments. Cervical and axillary mass is often present. CT shows fluid density content and septations may be seen. In one-third of cases, multilocular cystic masses are present with cysts demonstrating minimal enhancement after contrast.

NEUROGENIC TUMORS

Most mediastinal and paravertebral neurogenic tumors in adults are benign. Neurogenic tumors constitute approximately 20% of all resected primary mediastinal neoplasms in adults. They constitute 75% of primary posterior mediastinal neoplasms.

SCHWANNOMA

This is the most frequent mediastinal neurogenic tumors, usually seen in the third and fourth decades of life without any sex predilection. Most patients are asymptomatic though chest pain or discomfort is most common symptom when present.

IMAGING FINDINGS

This consists of a smooth or oval, round mass. Adjacent bone changes including erosion, splaying of the ribs, or enlargement of the intervertebral foramina may be seen. CT shows a homogeneous attenuation of the large masses with a variable contrast enhancement. The masses are low to intermediate signal intensity on T1-weighted MR and have intermediate to high signal intensity on T2-weighted image with peripheral enhancement after gadolinium injection. MRI is useful in patients with suspected intraspinal tumor extension.

TABLE 28-3 Neurogenic Tumors

Arising from peripheral nerves:
Schwannoma
Neurofibroma
Malignant tumor of nerve sheath origin:
Autonomic ganglia tumors
Ganglioneuroma
Neuroblastoma
Neoplasm of paraganglia:
Paraganglioma

NEUROFIBROMA

This is the second most common neurogenic mediastinal tumor, more frequent in male than in females, usually in their twenties to forties, single or multiple, commonly associated with neurofibromatosis. The affected nerve is circumferentially compressed or diffusely penetrated by the tumor.

IMAGING FINDINGS

Smooth rounded masses of homogeneous attenuation on CT. Tumor may grow through the intervertebral foramina into the spinal canal resulting in dumb-bell or hourglass configuration.

MRI

Homogeneous low to intermediate signal intensity on T1-weighted. On T1-weighted images, the tumors have high signal intensity in the peripheral zone and a slightly lower intensity area in the center (target sign) (Table 28-3).

MALIGNANT TUMOR OF NERVE SHEATH ORIGIN

Malignant tumor of nerve sheath origin is also known as neurofibrosarcoma, and it may occur in patients with or without neurofibromatosis. Sarcomatous degeneration in neurofibromatosis is around 5%. Usually patients are young, 20 to 40 years of age, with equal sex predilection. Features favoring diagnosis of malignant nerve sheath tumor include a large size (more than 5 cm), large low attenuating areas within the primary tumor, irregular ill-defined margins, compression or destruction of the adjacent structures, pleural nodules, or effusions or presence of metastatic pulmonary nodules.

TUMORS OF SYMPATHETIC GANGLIA

These are predominantly seen in infants and children and more than 50% of malignant and include ganglioneuroma, ganglioneuroblastoma, and neuroblastoma.

GANGLIONEUROMA

These are benign and well differentiated, attached to either sympathetic or intercostal nerve. The majority occurs in patients younger than 20 years of age, in males more than females. Prognosis is excellent after surgical resection.

The most common site of tumors is the paravertebral region followed by retroperitoneum and, least common, cervical region.

IMAGING

Ganglioneuromas are elongated masses oriented in the vertical axis of the sympathetic chain. These are oval lesions with very little mass effect on surrounding soft tissue. They are low attenuating on noncontrast CT and show mild-to-moderate enhancement after intravenous contrast. Foci of calcification may be seen in 20% of patients and these calcifications are usually punctuate and discrete (rather than amorphous and coarse as in neuroblastoma). They demonstrate homogeneous intermediate signal intensity on T1-weighted and T2-weighted sequences. They may have a whorled appearance.

GANGLIONEUROBLASTOMA

These tumors contain components of malignant neuroblastoma as well as benign ganglioneuroma. Calcification is frequent and is commonly seen in younger children and rare after the age of 10. The most common site is in the abdomen, followed by mediastinum, neck, and lower extremity.

IMAGING

Similar to ganglioneuroma, they are well defined, vertically oriented soft-tissue masses with variable cystic areas.

NEUROBLASTOMA

This is the most common malignancy of early childhood. Fifty percent of patients are younger than 2 years and 90% are younger than 5 years. The most common location is the adrenal with the mediastinum the second most common location. These are neural crest origin tumors.

IMAGING

Thoracic neuroblastoma is always paravertebral and may contain calcification in up 10% and rib or vertebral erosion may also be present.

These tumors lack a capsule and have areas of inhomogeneity due to tumor necrosis. The prognosis is poor, 25% with a 2-year survival. There is a better prognosis of children younger than 1 year of age.

Tumors are paraganglionic in origin (paraganglioma), also known as chemodectoma. Rare neural tumors arise from the paraganglion cell. In the thorax, they arise near the base of the heart and great vessels, adjacent to the pericardium or heart within the interatrial septum or left atrial wall.

IMAGING

They appear as soft-tissue masses in the aortopulmonary window or paravertebral region. They show extensive enhancement after intravenous contrast, with low to intermediate signal intensity on T1-weighted images and intermediate to high signal intensity on T2-weighted images. Surgical excision can be challenging and may not be possible due to extensive collateral vascularity of these masses.

SUGGESTED READING

Kawashima A, Fishman EK, Kuhlman JE, et al. CT of posterior mediastinal masses. *Radiographics.* 1991;11(6):1045-1067.

Santana L, Givica A, Carmacho C, et al. Best cases from AFIP: thymoma. *Radiographics.* 2002;22(Spec No):S95-S102.

Whitten CR, Khan S, Munneke GJ, et al. A diagnostic approach to mediastinal abnormalities. *Radiographics.* 2007;27(3):657-671.

QUESTIONS AND ANSWERS

1. Which of the following statement is *false*?
   A. Thymus arises from fourth and fifth a brachial pouches.
   B. Normal thymic size increases in healthy infants up to 4 to 8 weeks.
   C. Normal thymus contains elements derived from all three germinal layers.
   D. In younger individuals, normal thymus has low to intermediate signal intensity on T1-weighted images.

   ANSWER: A. Normal thymus arises bilaterally from the third and fourth (and not fourth and fifth) brachial pouches, which contain elements derived from all three *germinal* layers. Normal thymic size in healthy infants increases up to 4 to 8 months and then decreases with age due to fatty infiltration of the thymic gland. On MRI, in a younger patient, younger than 20 years of age, the normal thymus is homogeneous with slightly low to intermediate signal intensity on T1-weighted images (greater than that of muscle, but less than of fat). The signal intensity is slightly greater than that of muscle, but equal or slightly less than that of fat on T2-weighted images.

2. Which of the following is *true* regarding thymoma?
   A. Most common primary thymic tumor of epithelial origin in young male adults
   B. Majority of patients are asymptomatic.
   C. 40% of myasthenia gravis patients have thymoma.
   D. 15% of thymoma have red cell aplasia.

   ANSWER: B. Thymoma is the most common primary thymic tumor of epithelial origin. It is often seen in the fifth or sixth decade of age with no gender predilection. It is typically asymptomatic; however, in one-third of the patients, compression or invasion of surrounding structures causes cough, pain, dysphagia, hoarseness, and dyspnea. Parathymic syndromes include myasthenia gravis, pure red cell aplasia, and hypoglobulinemia. Approximately 40% of patients with thymoma have myasthenia gravis and 10% of the patients with myasthenia gravis have thymoma. Five percent of patients with thymoma have pure red cell aplasia and 10% to 50% of patients with red blood cell achalasia have thymoma.

3. Regarding invasive thymoma, which of the following is *false*?
   A. Encapsulated tumors usually respond to complete surgical excision with excellent 5-year survival after excision.
   B. MR is more sensitive than CT in detecting extracapsular extension.
   C. Drop metastases are common.
   D. Chest radiography is usually abnormal.

   ANSWER: D. Thymomas with invasive of adjacent structures, pleural/pericardial implantation is common, transdiaphragmatic extension and extrathoracic metastasis is present. Only in one-third (not majority) of patients with thymoma, tumor is identified incidentally on chest radiograph. As an anterior mediastinal mass, it is better seen on the lateral radiograph. CT is superior to chest radiograph in the diagnosis and determining the extent of the tumor. Thymoma may involve the pleura or pericardium (drop metastasis). There is nodular diffuse smooth or nodular pleural thickening mimicking mesothelioma. Pericardial involvement may leave pericardial nodules, thickening, and effusion. The tumor may extend to the abdominal cavity through the diaphragmatic foramina (gravitational metastasis). MR is usually superior to CT in assessing the invasion of the capsule or extracapsular extension. Encapsulated tumors usually respond to complete surgical excision with a 5-year survival of 92%. Invasive thymomas often need adjuvant radiation and chemotherapy, though controversial. If resected completely, their survival is similar to encapsulated tumors.

4. Regarding thymic cancer, which of the following is *true*?
   A. Fifty percent patients with MEN type 1 have thymic carcinoid.
   B. Cystic changes and calcification are common.
   C. Tumor is more aggressive in patients with MEN type 1.
   D. Association with red cell aplasia is common.

   ANSWER: C. Thymic carcinoma accounts for 15% to 20% of all thymic epithelial tumors. They often lack capsule and demonstrate focal invasion or metastasis to mediastinal lymph nodes. These tumors are often large, lack visible septa or nodular structures, and may contain foci of necrosis and hemorrhage. Cystic changes and calcification are uncommon. They are not associated with myasthenia gravis or pure red cell aplasia, though paraneoplastic polymyositis has been reported. In 25% of patients with thymic neuroendocrine tumor, there is a positive family history of multiple endocrinal neoplasia (MEN) type 1 (pituitary adenoma, parathyroid adenoma, and pancreatic islet tumor). Eight percent of patients with MEN type 1 have thymic carcinoid tumor, mostly in males.

5. Which of the statements regarding germ cell tumors is *false*?
   A. Extragonadal germ cell tumors are often in midline, most commonly in the mediastinum.
   B. The known risk factor for mediastinal nonseminomatous germ cell tumors is 47XXY.
   C. Seminoma is the most common germ cell tumor.
   D. Complete surgical excision has an excellent prognosis.

   ANSWER: C. Germ cell tumors occur most commonly in the gonads. Extragonadal germ cell tumors are often in midline, most commonly in the mediastinum, probably arising from the multipotential primitive germ cell misplaced along midline structures during embryogenesis. Most of these are near or within the thymus and constitute 20% of all mediastinal tumor and cysts. Klinefelter syndrome (47XXY) is a known risk factor for mediastinal nonseminomatous germ cell tumors. Teratoma and not seminoma is the most common germ cell tumor. Complete surgical excision has an excellent prognosis, nearly 100% 5-year survival.

6. Which of the following is *true* regarding seminomatous germ cell tumors?
   A. Presence of pyrexia is a poor prognostic feature.
   B. In >80% of patients, serum AFP is elevated.
   C. Tumors are bulky with necrosis and calcification common.
   D. Tumors are radioresistant.

   ANSWER: A. Seminomas are usually seen in males in the third or fourth decade of life. One-third of patients with pure seminoma have moderately elevated serum beta-HCG levels, but normal serum AFP level (not elevated).

   Tumors are large bulky lobulated soft-tissue anterior mediastinal masses, which can grow on either side of midline. Necrosis and calcification are rare and not common. Tumors are radiosensitive, and radiation therapy combined with cisplatin-based chemotherapy is the treatment of choice with a survival rate at 5 years of 75% to 100%. Poor prognostic features include higher tumor stage (lymph node metastasis, hepatic metastasis, or mediastinal invasion), older patients, SVC syndrome, and pyrexia.

7. All of the following are nonseminatous germ cell tumors *except*:
   A. Embryonal cell carcinoma
   B. Yolk sac carcinoma
   C. Teratoma
   D. Endodermal sinus tumor

   ANSWER: C. Nonseminatous malignant germ cell tumors include embryonal carcinoma, endodermal sinus tumor, choriocarcinoma, and mixed germ cell tumor. Teratoma is the most common mediastinal germ cell tumor.

8. Which of the following regarding neurogenic tumors is *true*?
   A. Most mediastinal and paravertebral neurogenic tumors in adults are malignant.
   B. Constitute only 5% of all resected primary mediastinal neoplasms in adults.
   C. Constitute 75% of primary posterior mediastinal neoplasms.
   D. Ganglioneuroma is the most common mediastinal neurogenic tumor.

   ANSWER: C. Most mediastinal and paravertebral neurogenic tumors in adults are benign. Neurogenic tumors constitute approximately 20% of all resected primary mediastinal neoplasms in adults. They constitute 75% of primary posterior mediastinal neoplasms. Schwannoma is the most frequent mediastinal neurogenic tumors, usually seen in the third and fourth decades of life without any gender predilection.

9. Features favoring sarcomatous degeneration in neurofibroma include all *except*:
   A. Large size >5 cm
   B. High attenuating areas in tumor
   C. Irregular margins
   D. Compression or destruction of adjacent structures

   ANSWER: B. Malignant tumor of nerve sheath origin is also known as neurofibrosarcoma. May occur in patients with or without neurofibromatosis. Sarcomatous degeneration in neurofibromatosis patient is around 5%. Usually patients are young, 20 to 40 years of age, with equal gender predilection. Features favoring diagnosis of malignant nerve sheath tumor include a large size (more than 5 cm), large low (not high) attenuating areas within the primary tumor, irregular ill-defined margins, compression or destruction of the adjacent structures, pleural nodules, or effusions or presence of metastatic pulmonary nodules.

10. Which of the following is *true* regarding neurogenic tumors?
    A. Neurofibroma is the most common neurogenic mediastinal tumor.
    B. Ganglioneuroma arises from parasympathetic nerves.
    C. Ganglioneuroblastoma is usually seen before age 10.
    D. Paraganglioma commonly located in the paravertebral location in the thorax.

    ANSWER: C. Neurofibroma is the second most common neurogenic mediastinal tumor (Schwannoma is the most common). It is more frequent in males than females, usually in their twenties to forties, single or multiple, commonly associated with neurofibromatosis. Ganglioneuromas are benign and well differentiated, attached to either sympathetic or intercostal nerve (not parasympathetic nerve). The majority occurs in patients younger than 20 years of age, in males more than females. Prognosis is excellent after surgical resection. Ganglioneuroblastoma tumors contain components of malignant neuroblastoma as well as benign ganglioneuroma. Calcification is frequent and is commonly seen in younger children and rare after the age of 10. The most common site is in the abdomen, followed by mediastinum, neck, and lower extremity. Paraganglioma, also known as chemodectoma, are rare neural tumors arising from the paraganglion cell. In the thorax, they arise near the base of the heart and great vessels, adjacent to the pericardium or heart within the interatrial septum or left atrial wall (and not paravertebral location).

29 PLEURAL DISEASES

Satinder P. Singh

NORMAL PLEURAL ANATOMY

The pleura is the serous membrane of continuous surface epithelium of mesothelial cells and underlying connective tissue that covers the lung parenchyma, mediastinum, diaphragm, and the rib cage. The visceral pleura lines the lungs and fissures, and the parietal pleura lines the nonparenchymal surfaces inside of the thoracic cavities. The pleural space is a potential space containing 2 to 10 cm^3 of pleural fluid normally. Its fluid production capacity is approximately 100 cm^3/h and fluid absorption capacity is approximately 300 cm^3/h. The parietal pleura is composed of loose, irregular connective tissue covered by a single layer of mesothelial cells. Within the pleura are blood vessels, capillaries, and lymphatic lacunas. Deep to the parietal pleura is the endothoracic fascia, a band of dense irregular connective tissue composed mainly of collagen and elastin, covering the ribs and intercostal space. The visceral pleura in humans is a thick membrane composed of two layers: mesothelium and connective tissue. The connective tissue layer in the visceral pleura has two important functions: It contributes to the elastic recoil of the lung, which is important in expelling air from the lung, and it restricts the volume to which the lung can be inflated, thereby protecting the lung.

The mesothelial cells range in size from 6 to 12 μm in diameter. Under the electron microscope, the pleural surface is visible as either flattened or bumpy. Microfillae are also noted diffusely over the entire pleural surface. The most important function of microfillae is to enmesh glycoproteins rich in hyaluronic acid, especially in the lower thorax to decrease the friction between the lung and chest wall.

The mesothelial cells are active cells, but are very fragile and sensitive/responsive to various stimuli. Mesothelial cells produce type 1, type 2, type 4 collagens, elastin, fibronectin, and laminin. They also express intermediate filaments typical of both epithelial cells and fibroblasts, express coagulant activity because of a tissue factor that binds factor 7 at the cell surface. These cells also produce nitric oxide and transforming growth factor beta-1. The normal flux of fluid in the pleural space is from parietal capillaries to pleural space to visceral capillaries.

BLOOD SUPPLY OF THE PLEURA

The parietal pleura receives blood supply from systemic capillaries. Small branches of the intercostal arteries supply the costal pleura, and the pericardial phrenic artery supplies the mediastinal pleura. The diaphragmatic pleura is supplied by the superior phrenic and musculophrenic arteries. The venous drainage of the parietal pleura is primarily via the intercostal veins which drain into the inferior vena cava or brachiocephalic trunk.

The blood supply to the viscera pleura is variable; in animals with thin pleura, the blood supply is from pulmonary circulation, whereas in animals with thick pleura, the blood supply is systemic via the bronchial arteries. The venous drainage of the visceral pleura is through the pulmonary veins.

The lymphatic vessels of the costal pleura drain ventrally toward nodes along the internal thoracic artery and dorsally toward the internal intercostal lymph nodes near the head of ribs. The mediastinal pleural lymphatic vessels pass to the tracheobronchial and mediastinal nodes while the lymphatic vessels of the diaphragmatic pleura pass to the parasternal, middle phrenic, and posterior mediastinal nodes. The visceral pleura lymphatics form a plexus of intercommunicating vessels that run over the surface of the lung toward the hila and also penetrate the lung to join the bronchial lymph vessels passing in the interlobular septa. Normally, fluid from the pleural surface does not enter the lymphatics and visceral pleura in humans. The lymphatic vessels in the parietal pleura have stomas communicating with the pleural space (2–6 μm in diameter). These stomas are found mostly on the mediastinal pleura and intercostal surface. The dilated lymphatic spaces called lacinas are found in the submesothelial layer of the parietal pleura. The stomas, with their associated lacinas and lymphatic vessels, are the main pathway for the elimination of particulate matter from the pleural space. No stomas are found in the visceral pleura and the lymphatic vessels of the visceral pleura are separated from the mesothelial layer by a connective tissue layer.

Kampmeier described small milky spots in the dorsal and caudal portions of the mediastinum. Microscopically, these spots are aggregates of lymphocytes, histiocytes, plasma cells, and other mononuclear cells around the central lymphatic or vascular vessel. The high concentration of asbestosis in these foci leads to the development of pleural plaque and mesothelioma. The black spots in patients with parietal anthracosis correspond to the Kampmeier foci and the distribution of asbestosis fiber in the pleura is also concentrated in these foci.

Sensory nerve endings are present in the costal and diaphragmatic parietal pleura: intercostal nerves supply the costal and the peripheral portion of the diaphragmatic pleura. Stimulation of this area leads to pain refer to the edges and chest wall. The central portion of the diaphragm is innervated by the phrenic nerve; stimulation of this pleura causes pain in the ipsilateral shoulder. The visceral pleura contains no pain fibers. Therefore presence of pleuritic chest pain indicates inflammation or irritation of the parietal pleura.

PHYSIOLOGY OF THE PLEURAL SPACE

The pressure within the pleural space is important in cardiopulmonary physiology because this pressure plays an important role in determining the volume of three important structures: Outer surface of the lung, heart, and the inner surface of the thoracic cavity. At functional residual capacity, the opposing elastic forces of the chest wall and the lung produce a negative pressure between the visceral and parietal pleura called the pleural pressure. This pressure around the lung is the primary determinate of the volume of the lung. The pleural pressure represents the balance between the outward pull of the thoracic cavity and the inward pull of the lung. The normal pleural pressure ranges between 0.5 to 1 cm H_2O per centimeter vertical height. The pleural pressure can be safely measured indirectly via a balloon or micromanometer positioned in the esophagus. Normally, the pleural pressure is not uniform throughout the pleural space. There is often a gradient in pleural pressure with the pleural pressure being lowest and most negative in the superior aspect and highest or least negative in the inferior portion of the lungs. The factor responsible for this pleural pressure gradient includes gravity, mismatching of the shapes of the chest wall and lung, and weight of the lung and other intrathoracic structures. In an upright position, the difference in the pleural pressure between apex and the base of the lung may be 12 cm or more. Because the alveolar pressure is constant throughout the lungs, gradient in the pleural pressure results in the different parts of the lung have different distending pressures. The pleural pressure gradient causes the alveoli in the superior part of the lung to be larger than those in the inferior part of the lung. Pleural pressure gradient also accounts for the unevenness of the distribution of ventilation. Normally, the pleural pressure is a negative pressure.

Fluid in the pleural space can originate in the pleural capillary, interstitial spaces of the lungs, intrathoracic lymphatics, intrathoracic blood vessels, or the peritoneal cavity. The movement of the fluid in the pleural capillaries and pleural spaces is governed by the Starling's law.

PATHOGENESIS OF PLEURAL EFFUSION

When the rate of pleural fluid formation exceeds the rate of pleural fluid absorption, fluid accumulates in the pleural space. Normally, a small amount (0.01 mL/kg/h) of fluid constantly enters the pleural space from capillaries in the parietal pleura. Almost all of the fluid is removed by lymphatics in the parietal pleura, which has a capacity to remove at least 0.20 mL/kg/h (nearly 20 times the inflow). Fluid can accumulate because of either increased pleural fluid formation or decreased pleural fluid absorption (Table 29-1).

TABLE 29-1 Causes of Pleural Effusion

Increased pleural fluid formation
Increased interstitial fluid in the lung; heart failure, pneumonia, or PTE
Increased intravascular pressure in the pleura; right or left ventricular failure, SVC syndrome
Increased permeability of the capillaries in the pleura; pleural inflammation, increased VEGF
Increased pleural fluid protein level
Decreased pleural pressure; lung atelectasis or increased elastic recoil of the lung
Increased fluid in the peritoneal cavity; ascites or peritoneal dialysis
Disruption of the thoracic duct
Disruption of blood vessels in the thorax
Decreased pleural fluid absorption
Obstruction of the lymphatic draining the parietal pleura
Elevation of the systemic vascular pressures; SVC syndrome or right ventricular failure

VGEF: vascular endothelial growth factor

Normally there is no air in the pleural space and any movement of gas into the pleural space occurs only if the pleural pressure is less than 6 or 7 mm Hg or less than –54 mm Hg relative to atmospheric pressure. Presence of air in the pleural space indicates one of three things: communication between the alveoli and the pleural space, communication between the atmosphere and the pleural space, or presence of gas-producing organisms in the pleural space. The rate of absorption of air in the pleural space depends upon the difference between sum of the partial pressure in the pleural space and in the capillary blood. Since the sum of the partial pressure in the capillary blood is most dependent on the Po_2, this sum can be decreased by having the patient to breath supplemental oxygen which reduces the Po_2 of the capillary blood without changing the other parietal pressures. Therefore, in patients who have a small pneumothorax, administration of supplemental oxygen facilitates the resorption of the pneumothorax. The most common causes of pleural effusion in the United States is congestive heart failure (Tables 29-2 and 29-3). Pleural fluid can be transudate or exudate (Table 29-4). The number of neutrophils in the pleural fluid is correlated with the ILD-8 levels and empyemas have the highest level of ILD-8. Examination of the pleural fluid neutrophil in patients with parapneumonic effusion is useful. If pleural infection is present, the neutrophils

TABLE 29-2 Differential Diagnosis of Pleural Effusions

Transudative pleural effusion
Congestive heart failure
Cirrhosis
Nephrotic syndrome
Superior vena cava obstruction
Peritoneal dialysis
Myxedema
Hypoalbuminemia
Exudative pleural effusion
Neoplastic diseases; metastatic disease, mesothelioma, lymphoma
Infectious diseases; bacterial, tuberculosis, fungal, viral, or parasitic
PTE
GI diseases; pancreatic disease, subphrenic abscess, post-liver transplant
Heart disease; post-CABG, post-cardiac injury (Dressler syndrome), pericardial disease
OB-GYN disease; ovarian hyperstimulation syndrome, postpartum pleural effusion, Meigs syndrome, endometriosis
Collagen vascular disorder; SLE, rheumatoid arthritis, drug-induced lupus, Sjögren syndrome
Drug-induced pleural disease; nitrofutenine, methesurgide, interleukin 2, methotrexate, procarbazine
Miscellaneous; asbestosis exposure, post-lung transplant, yellow nail syndrome, sarcoidosis
Hemothorax
Chylothorax

Modified with permission from Light RW, ed. *Pleural Diseases.* 4th ed. Lippincott Williams & Wilkins; 2001;88. From Table 5.1 Differential Diagnosis of Pleural Effusions, found in Chapter 5: Approach to the Patient.

undergo a characteristic degeneration; nucleus become blurred and no longer is stained purple, cytoplasm shows toxic ventilation initially and later neutrophilic granules become indistinct and are lost. Pleural eosinophilia is present when there are more than 10% of eosinophils in the pleural fluid. The most common cause of pleural fluid eosinophilia is air in the pleural space; the mechanism responsible is unknown, probably related to IL-5. The second most common cause of pleural fluid eosinophilia is blood in the pleural space (Table 29-5). Other causes include parapneumonic effusion, malignancy, tuberculosis, asbestos-related pleural effusion, pleural effusion secondary to drug reaction (dantrolene, brocryptin, and nitrofuratonin), infections secondary to parasites (paragonimiasis, hydatidosis, amebiasis, or ascariasis) and pleural effusion associated with Churg-Strauss syndrome is eosinophilic. A low

TABLE 29-3 Common Causes of Pleural Effusion in the United States (in Decreasing Order)

Congestive heart failure
Peripneumonic effusion
Malignant pleural effusion (lung cancer, breast cancer, or lymphoma)
PTE

TABLE 29-4 Differentiating Features of Transudative and Exudative Effusions

	TRANSUDATE	EXUDATE
Pleural fluid protein divided by serum protein	Ratio less than 0.5	Ratio greater than 0.5
Pleural fluid LDH divided by serum LDH	Less than 0.6	Greater than 0.6
Pleural fluid LDH	Less than two-thirds of normal for serum LDH	Greater than two-thirds of normal of serum LDH
pH of pleural fluid	Higher than the simultaneous blood pH	Usually lower less than 7.2

pleural fluid glucose level (less than 16 mg/dL) indicates parapneumonic effusion, malignant disease, rheumatoid disease, tuberculous effusion or tuberculous pleuritis.

Pleural fluid amylase above the upper normal limit for serum amylase indicates one of three problems: pancreatic disease, malignant tumor, or esophageal rupture. Most patients with high LDH in pleural fluid have exudative effusions and those with normal protein level but high LDH are either parapneumonic or have malignant pleural disease. Pleural fluid LDH is a reliable indicator of the degree of pleural inflammation; the higher the LDH, the more inflamed the pleural surfaces. Pleural fluid from patients with mesothelioma is often abnormally viscid. This increased viscosity is due to the presence of an increased amount of hyaluronic acid (hyaluronate).

As many as 40% of hospitalized patients with bacterial pneumonia have accompanying pleural effusions and morbidity and mortality rates in patients with pneumonia and effusion is higher than that in patients with pneumonia alone. Most effusions associated with pneumonia resolve without any specific therapy directed toward the effusion; only 10% of patients require operative intervention for their resolution (Table 29-6).

Pleural fluid markers for tuberculosis include:

Pleural fluid ADA level: If pleural fluid ADA level is more than 50 U/L and the patient has predominant lymphocytes in the pleural fluid, diagnosis of tuberculosis is certainly made.

Pleural fluid interferon-gamma level: Elevated levels of interferon levels are noted in tuberculous pleuritis. Using a cutoff level of 3.7 U/mL, a sensitivity of 0.99 and specificity of 0.98 has been reported in tuberculous effusions.

TABLE 29-5 Causes of Bloody Pleural Fluid

Malignancy
Trauma
PTE

TABLE 29-6 Criteria for Intervention in Patients with Parapneumonic Effusion

Thick pus
Positive Gram stain
PH less than 7
Glucose less than 60 mg/dL
LDH more than 1000 IU

Radiographic Findings

In patients with free pleural effusion, a concave upward sloping at costophrenic angle (meniscus appearance) is commonly seen. In the presence of subpulmonic effusion, there is lateral displacement of apex of the diaphragm and flat superior surface with sharp downward slanting. Increased haziness and presence of apical cap on supine radiographs often suggest presence of effusion. Blunt posterior costophrenic angle occurs with fluid more than 75 cm^3. Blunt lateral costophrenic angle occurs with more than 200 cm^3. Fluid layering on a decubitus radiograph represents more than 5 cm^3 of fluid. Ultrasound is much more sensitive in detecting small pleural effusion and presence of echogenic or anechoic fluid with septations suggests exudate.

EMPYEMA

Empyema by definition is the presence of thick purulent pleural fluid. The differentiation of empyema from parapneumonic effusion is a subject of debate. The evolution of parapneumonic effusion has three stages:

1. Exudative stage—containing sterile pleural fluid in the pleural space with fluid likely originating from the interstitial spaces of the lung. The pleural fluid has a low WBC, low LDH, and a normal glucose level and pH.
2. Fibropurulent stage—characterized by a large effusion with many polymorphonuclear leukocytes, bacteria, and cellular debris. Fibrin is deposited as a continuous sheet with increased tendency toward loculation and formation of limiting membrane. At this stage, the pleural fluid pH and glucose levels are progressively lower and the LDH level progressively higher.
3. Organization stage—where fibroblasts grow into the exudative state producing an elastic membrane called "pleural peel." This peel encases the lung and renders it virtually functionless. The exudate is thick and if the patient remains untreated, the fluid may drain spontaneously through the chest wall (empyema necessitans) or into the lung producing a bronchopleural fistula.

Incidence of infected pleural effusion is more common in anaerobic bacterial pneumonias.

Radiographic Appearance

In the early stages, empyema appears as a free pleural effusion. In the later fibropurulent stage, more loculation appears, which can be detected on decubitus radiograph, CT, or ultrasound. An air-fluid level in the empyema can mimic lung abscess. Empyemas tend to be lenticular shaped and have different diameters on PA and lateral views, whereas abscesses are spherical and have the same diameters on PA and lateral views.

On CT, a strong enhancement of both visceral and parietal pleura separated by unenhancing fluid is useful in distinguishing empyema from lung abscess and is referred to as the split pleura sign. Development of a new air-fluid level in the empyema indicates the development of a bronchopleural fistula. Air-fluid level of empyema crosses fissures and may extend to chest wall and is longer in one view.

PLEURAL EFFUSIONS RELATED TO METASTATIC MALIGNANCIES

Carcinoma of the lung, breast cancer and lymphoma accounts for 75% of malignant pleural effusions. Metastatic ovarian cancer is the fourth leading cause of malignant effusion. Malignant pleural effusion is usually bloody and exudative in nature (Table 29-5).

CHYLOTHORAX AND PSEUDOCHYLOTHORAX

A high level of lipid accumulates in the pleural fluid in two situations: when the thoracic duct is disrupted, chyle enters the pleural space to produce a chylous pleural effusion (chylothorax), and in long-standing pleural effusions, a large amount of cholesterol or lecithin-globulin complexes accumulate in the pleural fluid to produce chyliform-like pleural effusion (pseudochylothorax).

CHYLOTHORAX

Cisternal chyli overlies the anterior surface of the second lumbar vertebra, posterior to and to the right of the aorta. Normally, one major lymphatic vessel, the thoracic duct, leaves the cistern of chyli and passes through the esophageal hiatus of the diaphragm (T-10 level) into the thoracic cavity. The thoracic duct ascends extrapleurally in the posterior mediastinum along the right side of the anterior surface of the vertebral column and lies between the azygous vein and descending thoracic aorta in close proximity to the esophagus and pericardium. At T4-6 vertebral levels, the duct crosses to the left of the vertebral column and continues cephalad to enter the superior mediastinum between the aortic arch and subclavian artery and the left side of the esophagus. More cephalad, it passes the thoracic inlet, arches 3 to 5 cm above the clavicle and passes anterior to the subclavian artery, vertebral artery, and thyrocervical trunk to terminate in the region of the left jugular and subclavian vein. Wide variation exists in the course of the thoracic duct.

Chyle is the lymph returning from the intestine to the heart drained by the thoracic duct. Chyle is a milky opalescent fluid, and approximately 1500 to 2500 mL of chyle normally empties into the venous system each day. Ingestion of fat increases the flow of lymph in the thoracic duct by 2 to 10 times the resting level. Ingestion of liquid also increases the chyle flow, but ingestion of protein or carbohydrate has little effect on the lymph flow. The protein content of the chyle is usually more than 3 g/dL and the left to right composition is similar to that of serum.

The most common cause for a chylothorax is malignancy, and lymphoma is the most common etiology in 75%. Chylothorax may be the presenting symptom of lymphoma; therefore, a nontraumatic chylothorax is an indication for a diligent search for a lymphoma. The second leading cause of chylothorax is trauma resulting from cardiovascular, pulmonary, or esophageal surgical procedure. A chylothorax is particularly frequent following an operation in which the left subclavian artery is mobilized. Penetrating trauma to the chest or neck such as a gunshot or knife wound can also injure the thoracic duct. With trauma, the spine is hyperextended or a vertebra is fractured and is most likely to cause chylothorax, especially if injury occurs after ingestion of a recent fatty meal. A chylothorax secondary to closed trauma is usually on the right side and site of rupture is most commonly in the region of T9-10 vertebrae (injuries from falls from height, or compression injury to the trunk secondary to heavy blow to the back or stomach or childbirth). Rarely, chylothorax may occur secondary to coughing, vomiting, and weight lifting. The third leading cause of a chylothorax is idiopathic. This includes congenital chylothorax. Chylothorax is the most common form of pleural effusion encountered in the first few days of life. Congenital chylothorax is more common in patients who are hydropic or who have polyhydramnios. There is also association of congenital chylothorax with Turner syndrome, Noonan's syndrome, or Down syndrome. Birth trauma causing disruption of the thoracic duct is another explanation. Other miscellaneous causes include thrombosis of the SVC or subclavian vein, fibrosing mediastinitis, radiation, mediastinal scaring, and its association with lymphangioleiomyomatosis (LAM), Gilbert syndrome, Kaposi sarcoma in AIDS patients, and Castleman disease.

Clinical Manifestations

Related to space-occupying fluid in the thoracic cavity and the usual symptom is dyspnea. Pleuritic chest pain and fever are rare, as chyle is not irritating to the pleural surface. With traumatic chylothorax, there is usually a latent period of 2 to 10 days between the trauma and the onset of pleural effusion. Lymph collects extrapleurally in the mediastinum initially after the thoracic duct disruption forming a chyloma mimicking a posterior mediastinal mass, which eventually ruptures into the pleural space. With nontraumatic chylothorax, the onset of symptoms is usually gradual.

The main threat from chylothorax is malnourishment and compromised immunologic status, since the thoracic duct carries 2500 cm^3 of fluid daily containing substantial protein, fat, electrolytes, and lymphocytes. The patient can become cachectic rapidly and develop lymphopenia if repeated chyle is removed through the chest.

Diagnosis

The diagnosis of chylothorax is usually not difficult. Chyle usually has a distinctive white, odorless milky appearance. The main differentiation is between empyema and pseudochylothorax. The milkiness of empyema is caused by suspended white blood cells, and if such fluid is centrifuged the supernatant is clear. The cloudiness in chyliform pseudochylothorax is due to high lipid level, and not cholesterol or lecithin globulin complexes. Chylus and chyliform pleural fluid remain opaque after centrifugation. It is to be noted with congenital chylothorax, the pleural fluid is initially serous and only turns chylus when milk feeding is started.

Imaging

Chylothorax mimics a pleural effusion. In the early stages, a mass may be noted in the posterior mediastinum because of chyloma. At CT, chylothorax may not be low attenuating and cannot differentiate from typical effusion. In the past, lymphangiograms have been obtained to evaluate the integrity of the thoracic duct.

PULMONARY LYMPHANGIOLEIOMYOMATOSIS

Pulmonary lymphangioleiomyomatosis (LAM) is characterized by widespread proliferation of immature smooth muscles throughout the peribronchial, perivascular, and perilymphatic regions of the lung. The perilymphatic proliferation of smooth muscle results in lymphatic obstruction and high incidence of chylothorax. The lymph nodes and the mediastinal retroperitoneal space may also be infiltrated with immature smooth muscle cells further impairing the lymphatic flow. The thoracic duct may be either dilated or obliterated. The proliferation of smooth muscles in the perivascular space may cause obstruction of the pulmonary venules and may lead to pulmonary hemorrhage, hemoptysis, and pulmonary hemosiderosis. Proliferation of peribronchial smooth muscle can partially or completely obstruct the airway to cause air trapping, cyst and bullae formation, and high incidence of pneumothorax. Approximately one-third of patients have renal angiomyolipoma.

LAM usually or exclusively occurs in women of reproductive age. Most patients have increasing shortness of breath and/or cough and, rarely, hemoptysis pneumothorax or incidentally discovered chylothorax can be the presentation. Incidence of chylothorax is approximately 30%.

GORHAM'S SYNDROME

This is a rare disease, most often found in children or young adults without sexual predilection and no inheritance pattern. Other names include hemangiomatosis, disappearing bone disease, and massive osteolysis. There is intraosseous proliferation of vascular lymphatic channels leading to disappearance of bones. There is propensity for involving maxilla, shorter girdle, and pelvis. There is a high incidence of chylothorax in these patients.

PNEUMOTHORAX

Pneumothorax is air in the pleural space (air between lung and chest wall). This can be a spontaneous pneumothorax (primary and secondary causes) without any trauma or other obvious cause, or can be traumatic, including iatrogenic injuries.

PRIMARY SPONTANEOUS PNEUMOTHORAX

Primary spontaneous pneumothorax usually occurs in an otherwise healthy individual. This can result from rupture of subpleural emphysematous blebs which are usually located in the apices of the lung. Pathogenesis of these blebs is likely related to airway inflammation and is strongly associated with the development of primary spontaneous pneumothorax in cigarette smoking which suddenly produces airway inflammation. There may be some association with broad swings in the atmospheric pressure. It is postulated that air in the apical bleb is not in free communication with the airway; therefore, when the atmospheric pressure falls, the distending pressure of the bleb may increase and result in its rupture.

Patients with primary spontaneous pneumothorax are usually taller and thinner. Since the gradient in pleural pressure is greater from the lung base to the apex in taller individuals, the alveoli at the lung apex are subjected to a greater mean distending pressure. Over a long period of time, these phenomena could lead to the formation of subpleural blebs in taller individuals.

There seems to be some familiar tendency. There is high incidence of bronchial abnormalities in nonsmoking patients with spontaneous pneumothorax. The most common abnormality is disproportionate bronchial anatomy (smaller than normal dimensions) and deviating anatomic arrangements at various locations; other abnormalities include accessory bronchus or a missing bronchus.

PATHOPHYSIOLOGY

The pressure in the pleural space is negative with reference to atmospheric pressure, and alveolus pressure is always greater than pleural pressure because of the elastic recoil of the lung. Therefore, if a communication develops between the pleural space and the alveoli, airflow will occur from the alveolus into the pleural space until the pressure gradient is equalized. The main physiologic consequences of a pneumothorax are decreased in the vital capacity and decreased in Pa_{O_2} along with increased alveolar-arterial oxygen difference. The reduction appears to be due to anatomic shunt in the areas of flow ventilation-perfusion ratio in the partially collapsed lung.

Peak age of primary spontaneous pneumothorax is in the early twenties, it rarely occurs after age 40. It usually develops while the patient is at rest with symptoms of chest pain and dyspnea. Approximately 10% to 20% of patients have an associated pleural effusion.

There is a high risk of recurrence in patients with primary spontaneous pneumothorax. Most recurrences occur within the first year.

SECONDARY SPONTANEOUS PNEUMOTHORAX

Secondary spontaneous pneumothorax occurs as a complication of underlying lung disease, most commonly COPD, and also in patients with AIDS, cystic fibrosis, LAM, or tuberculosis. Most patients with AIDS who have a spontaneous pneumothorax have a history of *Pneumocystis carinii* infection, or are on prophylactic pentamidine, and have a recurrence of their PCP infection. Pneumothorax occurs because of the presence of multiple subpleural lung cavities associated with subpleural necrosis. The bullous and cystic changes develop because of repeated episodes of inflammation and cytotoxic effects of HIV on pulmonary macrophages. Occurrence of spontaneous pneumothorax in patients with AIDS and PCP is ominous prognostically. These patients have a tendency for recurrent pneumothoraces or contralateral pneumothorax. Because of the necrotic lung surrounding the ruptured cavity, these pneumothoraces are difficult to treat.

PNEUMOTHORAX SECONDARY TO CYSTIC FIBROSIS

Sixteen to twenty percent of patients with cystic fibrosis who are older than 18 years of age will develop a pneumothorax at some time in their lives.

CATAMENIAL PNEUMOTHORAX

A catamenial pneumothorax is an unusual entity that occurs in conjunction with menstruation and is usually recurrent. Initial pneumothorax usually does not occur until the patient is in her twenties.

Classical symptoms are chest pain and sometimes dyspnea within 24 to 48 hours of onset of menstrual flow. It is usually right-sided, but left-sided or even bilateral pneumothoraces have been reported. Pathogenesis is not definitely known. Hypothesis includes air that gains access to the peritoneal cavity during menstruation and then enters the pleural cavity through a diaphragmatic defect or leakage of air from the lung into subpleural endometrial implant is a more likely explanation.

NEONATAL PNEUMOTHORAX

Spontaneous pneumothorax occurs more commonly in the newborn period than at any other age. A pneumothorax is present shortly after birth in 1% to 2% of all infants, and asymptomatic pneumothorax is present in 0.5%. Infants are usually full term or post term. The baby has a history of fetal distress requiring resuscitation or a difficult delivery with evidence of aspiration of meconium, blood, or mucous. Incidence of pneumothorax in infants with respiratory distress syndrome is high.

IATROGENIC PNEUMOTHORAX

The leading cause of iatrogenic pneumothorax is transthoracic needle aspiration of lung masses (20%–40%). The second leading cause is insertion of a central line (0%–12%). The third leading cause is thoracocentesis (5%). Mechanical ventilation is next in line as a cause of iatrogenic pneumothorax.

Other procedures associated with pneumothorax include pleural biopsy, transbronchial lung biopsy, laparoscopy, and liver biopsy. Patients who are heart/lung transplant recipients do not have an intact mediastinum and therefore iatrogenic pneumothorax in these patients may lead to life-threatening bilateral pneumothoraces.

TRAUMATIC (NONIATROGENIC) PNEUMOTHORAX

Traumatic (noniatrogenic) pneumothorax results from penetrating or nonpenetrating chest trauma. The mechanism for pneumothorax in patients without penetrating injury is caused by increased alveolar pressure from severe chest compression leading to alveolar rupture. Air then enters the interstitial space, dissects toward the visceral pleura or the mediastinum to produce mediastinal emphysema. A pneumothorax results when either the visceral or mediastinal pleura ruptures.

TRAUMATIC PNEUMOTHORAX SECONDARY TO DRUG ABUSE

There is a high incidence of traumatic pneumothorax in intravenous drug abusers. This is usually accompanied by attempted injection into the subclavian or internal jugular vein.

TENSION PNEUMOTHORAX

Tension pneumothorax is present when the intrapleural pressure exceeds atmospheric pressure throughout expiration and often during inspiration, leading to compromise of the venous return to the heart. The mechanism is related to some type of one-way valve process in which the valve is open during inspiration and closed during expiration.

Radiographs are accurate detectors of pneumothorax, although a tiny pneumothorax, especially in the supine position, may not be seen. CT is more sensitive in detecting the presence and quantifying the size of the pneumothorax. In an upright position, the pneumothorax is always at the apex, unless there are pleural adhesions. In a supine position, pneumothorax is usually more anterior and basal. Deep sulcus sign is present in the supine patient when pneumothorax has a large basilar component making the costophrenic angle steeper, sharper, and more inferior than the contralateral site. An upright expiratory radiograph is more sensitive in detecting small pneumothoraces. A tension pneumothorax is a clinical diagnosis, and radiographically is suggested as a possibility when there is a large pneumothorax with contralateral mediastinal shift.

Treatment

Supplemental oxygen used in the treatment of pneumothorax accelerates the air absorption in small pneumothoraces. Other treatments include aspiration, tube thoracostomy, tube thoracostomy with installation of sclerosing agent especially done in patients with recurrent pneumothorax, autologous blood patch for persistent air leak, intrapleural fibrin glue for persistent air leak, and VATS procedure.

Pleurodesis is done in patients with recurrent pneumothoraces or pleural effusions. The goal is to incite intense inflammatory reaction in the pleural space that would obliterate the pleural space. The commonly used sclerosing agents are talc and tetracycline. Radiographically, after pleurodesis there is diffuse pleural thickening, and on CT high attenuating material is noted along the pleura representing the talc.

Pleural Thickening

Pleural thickening due to fibrosis is the second most common pleural abnormality after pleural effusion. The thickening could be localized (apical cap, pleural plaques [Table 29-7], or rounded atelectasis) or diffuse. Most common causes of diffuse forms are from organization of recurrent effusion following collagen vascular diseases, asbestosis exposure, and drugs.

Apical Cap

Apical cap is the thickening of the pleural line at the lung apices, occasionally in the interlobar fissure usually less than 5 mm in thickness, often bilaterally and symmetric. The cause is idiopathic or commonly seen with increasing or advancing age. There is no association with tuberculosis, emphysema, or underlying lung fibrosis of any etiology. The main differential is Pancoast (superior sulcus tumor), which is often unilateral asymmetrical increased opacity, and there is often associated bone destruction from chest wall invasion. Other differentials include tuberculosis, postradiation fibrosis, and hemorrhage secondary to aortic injury or subclavian stick.

TABLE 29-7 Differences Between Diffuse Pleural Thickening and Pleural Plaque

FEATURES	DIFFUSE PLEURAL THICKENING	PLEURAL PLAQUE
Location	Visceral pleural	Parietal pleura
Involvement of costophrenic angles	Yes	No
Involvement of interlobar fissure	Typical	Rare
Loss of lung function	Typical	No loss of function

DIFFUSE PLEURAL FIBROSIS

Causes of diffuse pleural fibrosis include asbestos exposure, systemic lupus erythematosus, rheumatoid arthritis, tuberculosis, hemothorax, drugs, and CABG.

A more severe form of pleural fibrosis leads to fibrothorax with resulting decreased volume of the hemithorax, decreased intercostal spaces, and circumferential pleural thickening and sometimes calcification.

PLEURAL NEOPLASMS

Secondary pleural neoplasm is more common than primary neoplasm.

PLEURAL METASTASIS

Pleural metastasis is the most common pleural neoplasm (95%), mostly adenocarcinoma (lung, breast, ovary, stomach) or lymphoma. Pleural effusion is the most common manifestation of metastatic disease and is exudative in nature. In patients with bronchogenic carcinoma, 15% of patients have a malignant effusion at initial presentation and 50% of patients with disseminated disease have pleural effusion. Breast cancer is the second most common cause for malignant pleural effusion. Fifty percent of patients with systemic disease have malignant effusion. More common is ipsilateral (60%–80%) or could be contralateral or bilateral. Positive cytology is identified in two-thirds of these patients and carries a poor prognosis.

Etiology of pleural effusion in malignancy is either due to direct involvement of pleura or lymphatic obstruction or endobronchial obstruction/atelectasis or severe hypoproteinemia.

Ninety percent of malignant effusion is diagnosed by a combined pleural cytology and pleural biopsy. Diagnostic yield is increased with multiple thoracocentesis and multiple pleural biopsies.

SOLID PLEURAL METASTASES

Solid pleural metastases are most commonly from the peripheral adenocarcinoma of the lung, but can also be from breast, ovarian tumor, invasive thymoma, or lymphoma. There is direct pleural invasion with tumor growth along the interstitium. It can mimic diffuse

TABLE 29-8 CT Features of Malignant Pleural Thickening

Circumferential
Nodular
Pleural thickening more than 1 cm
Mediastinal pleural involvement

malignant mesothelioma or invasive thymoma. It can be bilateral. CT features suggestive of malignant pleural thickening are summarized in Table 29-8.

PRIMARY PLEURAL NEOPLASMS

Primary pleural neoplasms are less common than metastases and include diffuse malignant mesothelioma, localized fibrous tumor of the pleura, and other tumors.

MALIGNANT MESOTHELIOMA

Pleural mesothelioma is the most common primary malignant neoplasm of the pleura. Mesotheliomas derive from mesothelial cells of the pleura, pericardium, peritoneum, or tunica vaginalis of the testes. Mesothelioma develops in the parietal pleura first and then spreads to the visceral pleura, chest wall, mediastinum, diaphragm, and abdomen. Three microscopic varieties include epithelial, sarcomatous, and mixed. Epithelial type is the most common (50%).

The incidence of malignant neoplasm is higher in individuals exposed to asbestos (10%). The peak incidence is 35 to 40 years after exposure. Amphibole asbestos fibers are most tumorigenic. Incidence is highest in cities in with shipyards and asbestos plants. The male-to-female ratio is 3.6:1, and it usually is found in the sixth to eighth decade of life.

Clinical Presentation

Often there is insidious onset of symptoms of dyspnea, chest pain, cough, and weight loss. Rarely, SVC syndrome, dysphagia, vocal chord paralysis, hypertrophic pulmonary osteoarthropathy, clubbing, and Horner syndrome occur.

Radiographic findings include moderate-to-large unilateral pleural effusion, multiple pleural nodules or masses and diffuse circumferential pleural thickening involving mediastinal pleura without significant mediastinal shift (frozen mediastinum). Often the size of the hemithorax is smaller. Asbestos-related pleural disease is found in 20% to 25% of cases. CT imaging reveals nodular and circumferential pleural thickening involving the fissures associated with pleural effusions; volume loss; lung encasement; and extension into the chest wall, diaphragm, or upper abdomen (Table 29-8). MRI shows a minimally increased signal on T1-weighted images and a moderately increased signal on T2-weighted images.

TABLE 29-9 Brigham's Staging System for Malignant Mesothelioma

STAGES	FEATURES
Stage 1	Disease confined to parietal pleura: ipsilateral pleural, lung, and pericardium
Stage 2	Stage 1 with positive intrathoracic (N1 or N2) lymph nodes
Stage 3	Local extension of disease into the chest wall or mediastinum, to the heart, or through the diaphragm into the peritoneum with or without extrathoracic or contralateral (N3) lymph node enlargement.
Stage 4	Distant metastatic disease

Diagnosis

VATS is the diagnostic procedure of choice with high sensitivity. Pleural fluid cytology, fine needle aspiration and cutting needle pleural biopsy are of limited value.

STAGING OF DIFFUSE MALIGNANT MESOTHELIOMA

The TNM staging system is currently the most widely used staging system. The other most commonly used staging system is Brigham's system based on resectability (Table 29-9).

Role of PET/CT

The localized FDG uptake is significantly higher in malignant than in benign pleural diseases, such as asbestos-related pleural thickening or inflammatory/infectious pleuritis. The correlation of the T stage with PET is not significantly better than with CT or with MRI. The role of PET in nodal metastatic disease detection is also not very sensitive, perhaps because of lack of resolution of PET to distinguish tumor from contiguous mediastinal nodal metastases.

The value of PET appears to be in its ability to detect extrathoracic metastasis. PET is also very useful in the management of mesothelioma; for example, in patients with diffuse pleural thickening and only a focal area of malignancy, PET can provide information and direct biopsy to appropriate site. PET is also useful in predicting prognosis; higher FDG uptake is associated with significantly shorter survival time.

Treatment and Prognosis

The overall prognosis for mesothelioma is extremely poor, with a median survival of approximately 10 months.

The prognosis is related to the extent of local or distant tumor spread. Prognosis is better in tumors with epithelial subtype rather than sarcomatous or mixed variety types.

Often, multimodality therapy is used to improve survival and protocols include combined surgical site reduction with adjuvant radiation, chemotherapy, or both.

Sensitivity of mesothelioma to chemotherapy is only modest with a response rate in the range of 0% to 50%. Various agents which have been used include antimetabolites, platinum-based agents, such as cisplatin and carboplatin, and recent antifolate agent pemetrexed (Alimta).

Three options are available for surgical treatment: thoracoscopy with sclerosing, pleurectomy-decortication, and extrapleural pneumonectomy. Thoracoscopy with sclerosing is a palliative procedure with a success rate of more than 80%. Pleurectomy-decortication involves removal of the pericardium, visceral and parietal pleura from the apex of the lung to the diaphragm. The recurrence rate is higher, although morbidity and mortality are less than that for extrapleural pneumonectomy (1.5%–5%). Extrapleural pneumonectomy is end-block resection of the parietal and visceral pleura along with the contained lung, the pericardium, and the ipsilateral diaphragm. This procedure allows the best site of reduction and allows higher doses of radiotherapy to be delivered to the same thorax because the lung has been removed. There is, however, higher morbidity and mortality in comparison to pleurectomy decortication.

The radiosensitivity of mesothelioma is intermediate between that of non–small cell lung cancer and small cell lung cancer. The problem for radiation therapy is that a large radiation field is required to treat the entire ipsilateral pleura at high doses more than 40 mGy and association or proximity to the adjacent dose limiting structures such as lung, liver, spinal cord, heart, and esophagus. Radiotherapy has been used to prevent malignant seeding along the sites of invasive diagnostic procedures in patients with malignant pleural mesothelioma. It is also useful in palliation of symptoms, especially painful local recurrent sites. Trimodality therapy is now accepted as the only method for improved survival in a selected group of patients with mesothelioma.

LOCALIZED FIBROUS TUMOR OF THE PLEURA

Localized fibrous tumor of the pleura is also known as localized mesothelioma or pleural fibroma. This is a rare mesenchymal tumor accounting for 5% to 10% of primary tumors of the pleura. The etiology is unknown. However, occasionally tumors are recorded after chest wall irradiation. There is no known association with cigarette smoking. Usually, there is no relation to asbestosis exposure.

TABLE 29-10 Radiographic Features Suggestive of Pleural Mass

Smooth margin—best seen on tangential view
Discrepancy in margin visualization on different views
Elliptical shape, obtuse angles
May cross fissures
Osseous or soft tissue changes denote chest wall involvement

Clinical Presentation

The majority are asymptomatic. Symptoms; when present, include cough, dyspnea, and chest pain related to tumor size. There is a high incidence of clubbing of the fingers, hypertrophic osteoarthropathy, and episodic hypoglycemia. The peak age of incidence is sixth or seventh decade with equal male-to-female occurrence. It most commonly involves the visceral pleura (80%) than the parietal pleura (20%). They are encapsulated round or ovoid lobulated, pedunculated, or broad-based pleural masses (Table 29-10). Ten to twelve percent of localized fibrous tumors are malignant and range in size from 1 to 25 cm with a mean diameter of 6 cm. The presence of pedicle is associated with a lower risk of malignancy, often hypertrophied vessels are noted.

Radiographic Features

Localized fibrous tumors of the pleura classically appear as a large, round, lobulated solitary peripheral noncalcified mass. When located in the fissure, it can mimic a lung mass. The pedunculated tumor may change in position with respiration or posture. Effusion is present in 5% to 20% of cases. The tumor demonstrates contrast enhancement and calcification is rare. There is often no associated lymphadenopathy in the mediastinum or hila.

MRI

MR may better characterize the fibrous nature of the tumor with predominantly low to intermediate signal intensity on T1- and T2-weighted images. However, heterogeneous signal intensity on T2-weighted images is frequent because of associated necrosis, cystic or myxoid degeneration, and areas of increased cellularity and vascularity. A common finding on T2-weighted images is the presence of septa of low signal intensity. Intense heterogeneous enhancement after gadolinium is typical.

Treatment and Prognosis

Complete excision is the treatment of choice with a 90% cure rate. Symptoms usually resolve after surgery and only recur if there is tumor recurrence, which is seen in 10% of the patients.

MISCELLANEOUS MESENCHYMAL TUMORS

The most common mesenchymal tumor of the pleura is benign lipoma. Generally, this is detected incidentally in asymptomatic patients via pleural-based soft-tissue density which can mimic lung neoplasm. CT is diagnostic by demonstrating a fat density in the mass. Liposarcomas demonstrate a heterogeneous mixture of fat and soft-tissue attenuation and variable enhancement.

PLEURAL LYMPHOMA

Pleural lymphoma usually occurs as part of disseminated disease (secondary lymphoma). Ten percent of malignant pleural effusions are the result of pleural lymphoma. Prevalence of pleural disease in lymphoma is around 25% to 30%. There is associated mediastinal adenopathy in the majority of patients (70%).

A rare type of primary pleural lymphoma in the Japanese population is pyothorax-associated lymphoma. This is a non-Hodgkin lymphoma of large B-cell variety developing in patients with a long history of pyothorax caused by artificially induced pneumothorax done for treatment of pulmonary tuberculosis. There appears to be a link between remote tuberculous pleuritis and Ebstein-Barr virus.

Lymphoma typically involves the subpleural lymphatics in both non-Hodgkin and Hodgkin variety. The lymphomatous deposit in the lymphatic channel and lymphoid aggregate in the subpleural connective tissue below the visceral pleura are present.

Clinical presentation is variable, including usually chest pain and fever. In patients with pyothorax-associated lymphoma, chest swelling may be present. If a tumor extends into the spinal cord, there may be paralysis of the lower limbs.

IMAGING FINDINGS

Unilateral or bilateral pleural effusion with or without pleural thickening is the major finding. Effusion is more common in Hodgkin lymphoma. In non-Hodgkin lymphoma, associated lymphadenopathy is more common. CT is more sensitive in describing the extent of pleural involvement. Pleural thickening—focal or diffuse—is often nodular and typically involves the parietal pleura. Pleural effusion is easily seen. Many patients have posterior mediastinal lymphadenopathy because of the lymphatic drainage pattern of parietal pleura and chest wall. Lymphomatous pleural effusion may be chyliform. Pyothorax-associated lymphoma appears as a large inhomogeneous soft tissue masses often extending into the chest wall with associated rib destruction.

SUGGESTED READING

Roach HD, Davies GJ, Attanoos R, Crane M, Adams H, Phillips S. Asbestos: when the dust settles – An imaging review of asbestos-related disease. *Radiographics*. 2002;22:S167-S184.

Rosado-de-Christenson ML, Abbott GF, McAdams HP, Franks TJ, Galvin JR. From the Archives of the AFIP: Localized fibrous tumors of the heart. *Radiographics*. 2003;23:759-783.

Tyszko SM, Marano GD, Tallaksen RJ, Gyure KA. Best Cases from the AFIP: Malignant mesothelioma. *Radiographics*. 2007;27:259-264.

QUESTIONS AND ANSWERS

1. Which of the following is *false* regarding pleura?
   A. Visceral pleura consists of mesothelium and connective tissue.
   B. Visceral layer contributes to the elastic recoil of the lung.
   C. Parietal pleura is supplied by systemic circulation.
   D. Venous drainage of visceral pleura is via intercostals veins.

   ANSWER: D. The visceral pleura in humans is a thick membrane composed of two layers: mesothelium and connective tissue. The connective tissue layer in the visceral pleura has two important functions: it contributes to the elastic recoil of the lung, which is important in expelling air from the lung, and it restricts the volume to which the lung can be inflated, thereby protecting the lung. The parietal pleura receives its blood supply from the systemic capillaries. The venous drainage of the parietal pleura is primarily via the intercostal veins which drain into the inferior vena cava or brachiocephalic trunk. The blood supply to the viscera pleura is from pulmonary circulation and the venous drainage is through the pulmonary veins.

2. Regarding pleural pressure, which of the following is *false*?
   A. Normal pleural pressure is negative.
   B. Pleural pressure is lowest and most negative in the lung bases.
   C. Alveoli in the lung apices are larger than in the lung bases because of pressure gradient.
   D. Primary determinate of the volume of the lung

   ANSWER: B. At functional residual capacity, the opposing elastic forces of the chest wall and the lung produce a negative pressure between the visceral and parietal pleura called the pleural pressure.

This pressure around the lung is the primary determinate of the volume of the lung. The pleural pressure represents the balance between the outward pull of the thoracic cavity and the inward pull of the lung. Normally, the pleural pressure is not uniform throughout the pleural space. There is often a gradient in pleural pressure with the pleural pressure being lowest and most negative in the superior aspect and highest or least negative in the inferior portion of the lungs. The normal pleural pressure ranges 0.5 to 1 cm H_2O per centimeter vertical height. The pleural pressure gradient causes the alveoli in the superior part of the lung to be larger than those in the inferior part of the lung. Pleural pressure gradient also accounts for the unevenness of the distribution of ventilation.

3. Regarding pleural effusion, which of the following is *true*?
   A. Most of the fluid produced is removed by lymphatics in the visceral pleura.
   B. Pleural eosinophilia is present when there are > 25% eosinophils in the pleural fluid.
   C. Most common cause of pleural effusion in the United States is metastatic disease.
   D. In the presence of infections, pleural neutrophils undergo degeneration with toxic vacuolation with blurred nucleus.

   ANSWER: D. Normally, a small amount (0.01 mL/kg/h) of fluid constantly enters the pleural space from capillaries in the parietal pleura. Almost all of the fluid is removed by lymphatics in the parietal (and not visceral) pleura, which has a capacity to remove at least 0.20 mL/kg/h (nearly 20 times the inflow). The most common cause of pleural effusion in the United States is congestive heart failure (not metastatic disease). Examination of the pleural fluid neutrophil in patients with parapneumonic effusion is useful. If pleural infection is present, the neutrophils undergo a characteristic degeneration, the nucleus become blurred and no longer is stained purple, the cytoplasm shows toxic vacuolation initially, and later neutrophilic granules become indistinct and are lost. Pleural eosinophilia is present when there are more than 10% (and not >25%) of eosinophils in the pleural fluid.

4. Common causes of pleural eosinophilia include all *except:*
   A. Asbestosis
   B. Drugs
   C. Parasite infection
   D. Pyothorax

   ANSWER: D. The most common cause of pleural fluid eosinophilia is air in the pleural space. The second most common cause of pleural fluid eosinophilia is blood in the pleural space. Other causes include parapneumonic effusion, malignancy, tuberculosis, asbestos-related pleural effusion, pleural effusion secondary to drug reaction (dantrolene, brocryptin, and nitrofuratonin), infections secondary to parasites (paragonimiasis, hydatidosis, amebiasis, or ascariasis), and pleural effusion associated with Churg-Strauss syndrome is eosinophilic. Pyothorax is associated with increased neutrophil (and not eosinophil) counts and characteristic degeneration of the neutrophils.

5. Low pleural glucose level is seen in all *except:*
   A. TB
   B. Pneumonia
   C. Pancreatitis
   D. Rheumatoid arthritis

   ANSWER: C. A low pleural fluid glucose level (less than 16 mg/dL) indicates parapneumonic effusion, malignant disease, rheumatoid disease, tuberculous effusion, or tuberculous pleuritis. In pancreatitis, pleural glucose levels are normal though amylase level is high.

6. Regarding pleural effusions, which of the following statement is *true*?
   A. Pleural fluid LDH is a reliable indicator of the degree of pleural inflammation.
   B. Pleural fluid from patients with mesothelioma is often abnormally viscid.
   C. Esophageal rupture leads to elevated pleural amylase level.
   D. Elevated pleural fluid interferon-gamma levels are seen in rheumatoid arthritis.

   ANSWER: D. If pleural fluid ADA level is more than 50 U/L and the patient has predominant lymphocytes in the pleural fluid, diagnosis of tuberculosis is certainly made. Elevated levels of interferon levels are noted in tuberculous pleuritis (and not RA). Using a cutoff level of 3.7 U/mL, a sensitivity of 0.99 and specificity of 0.98 has been reported in tuberculous effusions. Most patients with high LDH in pleural fluid have exudative effusions and those with normal protein level but high LDH are either parapneumonic or malignant pleural disease. Pleural fluid LDH is a reliable indicator of the degree of pleural inflammation; the higher the LDH, the more inflamed the pleural surfaces. Pleural fluid amylase above the upper normal limit for serum amylase indicates one of three problems:

pancreatic disease, malignant tumor, or esophageal rupture.

7. Transudative pleural effusion is seen in all *except:*
   A. CHF
   B. Cirrhosis
   C. PTE
   D. Nephrotic syndrome

   ANSWER: C. Causes of transudative pleural effusion include congestive heart failure, cirrhosis, nephrotic syndrome, superior vena cava obstruction, peritoneal dialysis, myxedema, and hypoalbuminemia. PTE usually leads to exudative effusion.

8. Which of the following statement is *false* regarding transudative pleural effusion?
   A. Pleural fluid protein to serum protein ratio of <0.5
   B. Pleural fluid LDH less than two-thirds of normal for serum LDH
   C. pH <7.2
   D. Pleural fluid LDH divided by serum LDH ratio <0.6

   ANSWER: C. pH of pleural fluid <7.2 is seen in exudative effusion and not transudation. All other statements are correct for transudate effusion.

9. Which of the following parameters suggests intervention in a patient with parapneumonic effusion?
   A. Negative Gram stain
   B. LDH <1000 IU
   C. pH <7.0
   D. Glucose >60 mg/dL

   ANSWER: C. Criteria for intervention in patients with parapneumonic effusion include presence of thick pus, positive (not negative) Gram stain, pH less than 7.0, glucose less (not more) than 60 mg/dL, LDH more (not less) than 1000 IU.

10. The radiographic features suggesting pleural origin of a mass include all of the following *except:*
    A. Irregular margin
    B. Cross fissure
    C. Elliptical shape
    D. Margins are not well seen on different views.

    ANSWER: A. Radiographic features of a pleural mass include elliptical shape with obtuse margins, smooth (not irregular) margins. Discrepancy in margin visualization on different views may cross fissures and osseous or soft tissue changes denote chest wall involvement.

30 ATELECTASIS

Satinder P. Singh

Atelectasis is defined as incomplete expansion of all or part of the lung with corresponding decreased lung volume. The term "collapse" is usually reserved for complete atelectasis.

MECHANISMS OF ATELECTASIS

There are different mechanisms of atelectasis (Table 30-1). Obstructive atelectasis is secondary to airway obstruction with resorption of oxygen, leading to decreased alveoli volume. The partial pressure of nitrogen and carbon dioxide in the alveoli increases relative to capillary blood, leading to diffusion of both of these gasses into the blood thus further decreasing in alveolar volume. Airway obstruction leads to distal volume loss either at lobar or entire lung, depending on the location of the obstruction. It often takes approximately 24 hours for atelectasis to develop in a normal person with central airway obstruction. A patient on 100% oxygen develops atelectasis within a few hours.

Passive atelectasis is the collapse of the lung because of pneumothorax. Pleural effusion can also cause passive atelectasis, although some consider it as compressive. The proportion of atelectasis of lung is usually proportional to the amount of air in the pleural space without any adhesions.

Compressive atelectasis results from a space-occupying lesion compressing the lung, usually a large pleural effusion, a neoplasm, emphysematous bulla, or cyst.

Adhesive atelectasis occurs in part as a result of deficiency of surfactant, commonly seen in radiation pneumonitis, acute respiratory distress syndrome, pulmonary thromboembolism, as well as hyaline membrane disease in the newborn. The function of the surfactant is to reduce the surface tension of the alveoli as their surface area or volume decreases, and therefore the critical closing pressure of alveoli occurs at a lower volume and distending pressure, thereby effectively protecting against collapse.

Cicatrization atelectasis results in volume loss, secondary to pulmonary fibrosis, regardless of underlying

TABLE 30-1 Mechanisms of Atelectasis

Obstructive (resorbed)
Passive
Compressive
Adhesive
Cicatricial (scar)

etiology. The fibrotic process undergoes retraction and results in loss of volume of the affected portion of the lung. The fibrosis can be localized as seen in healed granulomatous infection, such as histoplasmosis, tuberculosis, and radiation fibrosis, or could be diffuse as seen in idiopathic pulmonary fibrosis. The bronchi within the affected lungs are usually dilated because of the increased elastic recoil from surrounding pulmonary fibrosis and traction bronchiectasis.

PATTERNS OF ATELECTASIS

Depending on the site of obstruction, atelectasis could be complete lung, lobar, segmental, or subsegmental.

COMPLETE LUNG COLLAPSE

This is usually secondary to main bronchial occlusion: central bronchogenic carcinoma in adult and elderly, carcinoid in young females, mucous plugging in patients with asthma, or foreign body in children.

Radiographic findings include complete opacification of hemithorax with ipsilateral mediastinal shift (Table 30-2). The hemidiaphragm is elevated and apparent on the left side as seen from displaced stomach bubble. In the chronic state, there is crowding of the intercostal spaces. Often, the overexpanded contralateral lung crosses the midline, an unusual lucency projected over the mediastinum. Complete atelectasis may be seen with tension pneumothorax, where the loss of volume may occur with slightly increased radiodensity of the collapsed lung around the hila.

LOBAR ATELECTASIS

Right Upper Lobe Atelectasis

In right upper lobe atelectasis, the minor fissure and the upper major fissure are displaced upward and forward, respectively. In complete atelectasis, there is increased density of the collapsed lung along the right superior mediastinum; on the lateral view, the collapsed lung may appear as an indistinct triangular shadow with its base contiguous with the pleura, just posterior to the apex of the hemithorax, and its apex at the hila.

TABLE 30-2 Radiographic Findings of Atelectasis

Direct signs
Displacement of interlobar fissure
Crowding of vessels and bronchi
Indirect signs
Local increase in opacity
Elevation of the ipsilateral hemidiaphragm
Displacement of the mediastinum
Compensatory overinflation of remaining lung and displacement of the hila

The "S" sign of Golden is seen with central obstructing mass. The superior curve is the displaced minor fissure, while the inferior portion is the curved surface of the tumor itself. Juxtaphrenic sign is a triangular, sharply defined opacity that projects upward from the medial half of the diaphragm, at or near the highest point of the dome. It results from upward retraction of the portion of the visceral pleura that protrudes into the recess of the basal segment of the lung near the inferior pulmonary ligament. In majority of the cases, the juxtaphrenic peak is related to an inferior accessory fissure.

Left Upper Lobe Atelectasis

The major difference between the right and left upper lobe is due to absence of minor fissure on the left; therefore, all lung tissue anterior to the major fissure is involved. The oblique fissure is more vertical than the major fissure on the right, is displaced forward in a plane parallel to the anterior chest wall, and is better seen on the lateral view. The collapsed lobe obliterates the left cardiac border in the frontal view (silhouette sign). With hyperexpansion of the lower lobe, especially the superior segment of the lower lobe, the aerated lung is interposed between the aortic arch and collapsed left upper lobe, therefore maintaining a sharp interface of the arch (known as air crescent or Luftsichel sign).

Right Middle Lobe Atelectasis

This is easily recognized on the lateral view, but is difficult on frontal radiographs. The minor fissure and caudle portion of the major fissure approximate, resulting in a triangular pancake of tissue, which has an apex at the hila and base approximately contiguous with the parietal pleura over the anterolateral thorax, best seen on the lateral view. The right cardiac margin is not well seen on the frontal view (silhouette sign). Because of the obliquity of the atelectatic lobe, the right middle lobe atelectasis may not be well seen on the frontal view but can be detected on a lordotic or lateral view. On CT, a triangular opacity is seen with the apex toward the hila, the minor fissure moves downward, while the major fissure moves upward and forward.

Lower Lobe Atelectasis

Right and left lower lobe atelectasis has a similar appearance with collapse medially toward the mediastinum. Their contact with the hemidiaphragm is maintained, leading to diaphragmatic indistinctness (silhouette sign). On the frontal view, the hila and interlobar arteries are displaced downward and medially and the hemidiaphragm is not well seen. On the lateral view, the oblique fissure is displaced posteriorly and downward. On the frontal view, the collapsed lung is also seen as a triangular opacity with a sharp lateral margin because of displaced oblique fissure.

COMBINED LOBAR ATELECTASIS

Atelectasis of two lobes simultaneously produces a very distinctive radiographic pattern only in the right lung.

Combined Right Middle and Lower Lobe Atelectasis

This is due to obstruction of the bronchus intermedius. On the frontal view, the collapsed lower lobe obscures the right hemidiaphragm and the collapsed middle lobe obscures the right heart margin. Both major and minor fissures are displaced downward and backward so that the opacity occupies the posteroinferior portion of the right hemithorax. CT nicely demarcates the right middle and lower lobe atelectasis, which usually abuts the right cardiac border and right hemidiaphragm.

Combined Right Upper and Middle Lobe Atelectasis

This is uncommon, but may occur usually as a result of lung cancer, carcinoid, inflammatory processes, or mucus plugging. The radiographic findings are similar to that of left upper lobe atelectasis. On the frontal view, an opacity obscures the outline of the mediastinum and indistinctly fades laterally. There is displacement of the hilar vessels along with obscuration of the right cardiac margin. On the lateral view, the major fissure is displaced anteriorly, while the minor fissure may be straight, convex anteriorly, or convex posteriorly.

MIGRATING LOBAR ATELECTASIS

Atelectasis with fluid, pneumonic consolidation, or tumor may migrate within the hemithorax with change in body position. Migrating atelectasis may occupy a dependent position on erect radiograph and lateral view and mimic hilar or mediastinal mass.

SEGMENTAL ATELECTASIS

Segmental atelectasis results from bronchial obstruction and is associated with obstructive pneumonitis. The homogeneous opacity is noted in the distribution of the bronchopulmonary segment; usually no air bronchogram is seen. The radiographic appearance depends on the original volume of lung parenchyma as well as the volume of inflammatory tissue within the segmental atelectasis.

LINEAR OR DISCOID OR PLATE-LIKE ATELECTASIS

These are linear soft tissue opacities ranging from 1 to 3 mm in thickness and 4 to 10 cm in length, usually in the mid and lower lungs, unilateral or bilateral, single or multiple. It commonly occurs in the setting of restricted inspiratory effort, such as rib fracture or chest pain from any etiology, intra-abdominal surgery, or inflammatory process near the diaphragm.

ROUND ATELECTASIS

This is a distinct form of atelectasis associated with focal pleural thickening. It appears as a homogenous round or oval or wedge-shaped mass in the periphery of the lung, adjacent to the thickened pleura. It is variable in size, ranging from 3 to 6 cm, and is associated with loss of volume of the affected lobe. The bronchi and vessels in the adjacent lung are displaced in a curvilinear fashion (comet tail sign); this finding is best seen on CT. It is most commonly found in the lower lobes. Air bronchograms are seen in approximately 60% of the cases. Subpleural fat may be seen within the mass suggesting its chronicity. The mass may be mistaken for malignancy. MR reveals signal intensity higher than muscle and lower than fat on T1-weighted images and similar to or lower than fat on T2-weighted images. There is uniform enhancement of the atelectatic lung after administration of gadolinium. FDG PET usually shows little or no uptake and is quite helpful in distinguishing round atelectasis from cancer. It is usually seen in patients exposed to asbestosis, but can also be seen in chronic pleural effusion from tuberculosis, malignancies, pulmonary infarct.

Suggested Reading

Feung MY, Gasser B, Gangi A, et al. Bronchial carcinoid tumors of the thorax: spectrum of radiologic findings.*Radiographics.* 2002;22:351-365.

Hayashi, K, Aziz A, Ashizawa K, Hayashi H, Nagaoki K, Otsuji H. Radiographic and CT appearances of the major fissures. *Radiographics.* 2001;21:861-874.

Rosado de Christenson M, Abbott GF, Kirejczyk WM, Galvin JR, Travis WD. Thoracic carcinoids: radiologic-pathologic correlation. *Radiographics.* 1999;19:707-736

QUESTIONS AND ANSWERS

1. How long does it take for atelectasis to develop in a normal person with central airway obstruction?
   A. 2 hours
   B. 12 hours
   C. 24 hours
   D. 2 days

   ANSWER: C. It takes approximately 24 hours to develop, but significantly less time for patients dependent on oxygen.

2. What is the underlying cause of adhesive atelectasis?
   A. Deficiency of surfactant
   B. Large bulla
   C. Pneumothorax
   D. Mucus plug

   ANSWER: A. Adhesive atelectasis is caused by decreased surfactant occurring with radiation pneumonitis, ARDS, PTE, and hyaline membrane disease.

3. Luftsichel sign suggests what diagnosis?
   A. RUL atelectasis
   B. RLL atelectasis
   C. LUL atelectasis
   D. LLL atelectasis

   ANSWER: C. Luftsichel (air crescent) sign is the strip of hyperinflated superior segment of the lower lobe between the aortic arch and the collapsed left upper lobe.

31 DIAPHRAGMATIC DISEASES

John C. Texada and Satinder P. Singh

ABNORMALITIES OF DIAPHRAGMATIC POSITION AND MOTION

Diaphragmatic motion accounts for 60% to 75% of vital capacity, with excursion from expiration to inspiration highly variable but approximately 3 to 7 cm and slightly greater on the right.

Diaphragmatic motion is best visualized fluoroscopically. Imaging should be obtained PA and at multiple obliquities, and should include evaluation during tidal breathing, deep rapid breathing, and sniffing. Sniffing may reveal otherwise inapparent restriction or paradoxic motion; however, in some normal people, sniffing may produce paradoxic motion of one hemidiaphragm and so this should be considered pathologic only if greater than 2 cm and involving the entire hemidiaphragm. Sonography of the diaphragm may reveal additional abnormalities not visible fluoroscopically and may evaluate thickness, configuration, and relationships to other structures.

UNILATERAL DIAPHRAGMATIC PARALYSIS

Patients with unilateral diaphragmatic paralysis are often asymptomatic, though some may have dyspnea on exertion, or orthopnea. Pulmonary function tests show mild restriction.

ETIOLOGY

This is usually caused by phrenic nerve interruption from any of a variety of causes: cancer, injury (section such as during coronary artery bypass surgery, stretching, cooling, venipuncture, birth injury, cervical manipulation), neuritis (brachial neuritis [Parsonage-Turner syndrome], herpes zoster, mononeuritis multiplex), CNS or cord abnormalities (stroke, multiple sclerosis, rhizotomy, amyotrophic), nerve compression (spondylosis, mediastinal lymphadenopathy, goiter), or others including diabetes, carbon monoxide poisoning, or upper abdominal surgery. The latter is a temporary response to inhibitory nerve stimulation in the diaphragm, most severe at 8 hours post-procedure. Malignant invasion is most common, with the most common cancer being lung cancer. "Unknown" is the second most-common etiology; this idiopathic form is encountered almost always on the right side and in males, and may be due to a viral neuritis.

RADIOGRAPHIC FINDINGS

Radiographically, the paralyzed hemidiaphragm is elevated and the dome is accentuated. The costophrenic and costovertebral sulci are deep and narrow. If left-sided, the stomach and colon will rise and the stomach may undergo mesenteroaxial volvulus (in which the stomach rotates along its mesenteric axis such that the greater curve lies superior to the lesser curve). Motion will be diminished, absent, or paradoxic, with paradoxic motion during sniffing; the mediastinum will swing laterally with respiration.

The most reliable test is sniffing evaluation. Normally both hemidiaphragms descend sharply; a paralyzed hemidiaphragm will rise. False positives are 5%, and false negatives may be produced if the patient uses abdominal muscles.

BILATERAL DIAPHRAGMATIC PARALYSIS

EPIDEMIOLOGY

Patients with bilateral diaphragmatic paralysis are severely short of breath; bilateral paresis will produce milder symptoms. Most patients with paralysis will develop ventilatory failure and hypercapnia; some may develop cor pulmonale. Severe restriction will be found with pulmonary function tests. In addition to the causes listed previously, sympathetic or muscular dystrophy may produce diaphragmatic weakness and a number of CNS and cord abnormalities may be considered.

Radiographic Findings

Both hemidiaphragms will be elevated, and basilar atelectasis may be present. Both hemidiaphragms will rise paradoxically during sniffing; this, accompanied by outward chest motion and inward abdominal motion, is called thoracoabdominal paradox.

EVENTRATION

Etiology

Eventration is the congenital failure of muscle development, in part or whole of the diaphragm. Partial eventration is most often at the anteromedial right hemidiaphragm. Complete hemidiaphragm eventration is called Petit's eventration; this is almost exclusively left-sided (in contrast to the almost exclusively right-sided idiopathic unilateral paralysis).

Radiographic Findings

Eventration appears radiographically same as paralysis, though on fluoroscopy and ultrasound, the affected area will move with the normal portions of the hemidiaphragm (it may have a slight inspiratory lag).

OTHER ABNORMALITIES OF DIAPHRAGMATIC MOTION

Numerous diseases, not directly affecting the diaphragm, may restrict diaphragmatic motion, for example, Emphysema or severe acute asthma produces hyperinflation and air trapping, which prevents normal motion. Localized infectious inflammatory processes may produce splinting of the hemidiaphragm. Tonic contraction may be due to tetany, tetanus, rabies, strychnine poisoning, and Coxsackie B infection. Respiratory myoclonus may produce diaphragmatic flutter. Hiccups are a notable example as well.

DIAPHRAGMATIC HERNIAS

Normal Diaphragmatic Openings and Weak Points

The aortic aperture lies behind the left median arcuate ligament at the T12 level; it contains the aorta, the thoracic duct, and other lymphatic, azygous, and hemiazygos veins. The esophageal aperture splits the medial fibers of the right diaphragmatic crus usually at T10; it contains the esophagus, the vagal nerves, and the gastric vessels. The inferior vena cava aperture lies at T8 between the central tendon and the costal muscle portion of the right hemidiaphragm. The foramen of Morgagni (the parasternal hiatus) and the foramen of Bochdalek (pleuroperitoneal hiatus) lie inferiorly and posteromedially, respectively.

Esophageal Hiatal Hernia

This is the most common nontraumatic hernia. It is largely acquired, with the most important factors being obesity and pregnancy. In one study, the prevalence of hiatal hernia increased from 5% in patients older than 40 years to 65% in patients aged 60 to 79 years. The stomach is the most common structure to herniate.

Radiographically, a herniated stomach will appear as a retrocardiac mass, often with an air–fluid level; diagnosis may require barium evaluation or CT. If large, the stomach may undergo volvulus in the chest or become incarcerated or strangulated.

Pleuroperitoneal Hiatal Hernia (Through the Foramen of Bochdalek)

This is the most common and most serious hernia in infancy, with an incidence of 1:2200 and 75% to 90% being left-sided. They may be so large that the hemidiaphragm is almost absent and much of the abdomen lies in the chest. Mortality rate for large hernias is 30% even after surgical correction, and this is due to pulmonary hyperplasia and pulmonary artery hypertension. In adults, small pleuroperitoneal hiatal hernias are generally asymptomatic and usually fat-containing; their incidence increases with age. Prevalence may be 6% to 12%, mostly left-sided. Peritoneal lining is generally not present.

Radiographically, a Bochdalek hernia may appear as a focal diaphragmatic bulge or a posteromedial basilar mass; it is often less attenuating than soft tissue because of internal fat. It is easily defined with CT.

Parasternal Hiatal Hernia (Through the Foramen of Morgagni)

Also called retrosternal hernia, this is mostly a right-sided process, as the left parasternal hiatus abuts the heart. The defect is developmental but the hernia is associated with obesity, severe effort, and increased intra-abdominal pressure. Most patients are obese, middle-aged women. Most are asymptomatic, though epigastric or sternal pressure and discomfort may be described. Peritoneal lining is often retained; the hernia may contain omentum or less likely liver, bowel, or other structures; strangulation and obstruction can occur.

Radiographically, a Morgagni hernia is a well-defined right cardiophrenic angle mass. Other differential diagnoses for a CP angle mass include epicardial fat, pericardial cyst, lymphoma, and thymoma. If bilateral (a rare occurrence), abdominal organs will herniate in the midline. CT or MR can easily image the lesion.

DIAPHRAGMATIC NEOPLASMS

PRIMARY NEOPLASMS

Primary diaphragmatic tumors are rare, more than 50% are benign and mostly from the tendinous or anterior muscular portion. Lipoma is the most common tumor, though angiofibroma, neurofibromatosis, leiomyoma, teratoma, and other tumors may develop. The most common malignant neoplasm is fibrosarcoma, though malignant fibrous histocytoma, hemangiopericytoma, germ cell tumors, and others may be found. Benign diaphragmatic neoplasms are most often asymptomatic, but patients with a diaphragmatic cancer may complain of chest or abdominal pain, cough, or dyspnea.

Most of these tumors present radiographically as round or lobulated masses extending into the lung base, mimicking unilateral elevation of diaphragm. Malignant tumors often involve much of the hemidiaphragm and often have associated pleural effusions.

SECONDARY NEOPLASMS

The most common secondary neoplasm of the diaphragm is the direct extension of lung cancer or mesothelioma; other hepatic, peritoneal, or lung tumors may spread by extension. Ovarian cancer is a likely site of origin for metastasis of peritoneal origin. Distinct hematogenous or lymphatic nodular metastasis is uncommon.

OTHER DIAPHRAGMATIC ABNORMALITIES

ACCESSORY DIAPHRAGM

In this rare process, the right hemidiaphragm is divided by a musculotendinous membrane; 30 cases had been reported by 1995. The accessory tissue is usually in the oblique fissure and attaches to the pericardium, diaphragm, and chest wall.

DIAPHRAGMATIC DEFECTS

Defects may be too small to allow true herniation, but allow passage of fluid in Meigs syndrome or cirrhotic ascites.

INTRADIAPHRAGMATIC CYSTS

These are rare and are usually formed by extralobar sequestration, and are almost always left-sided. A chronic diaphragmatic hematoma may evolve into a cyst.

SUGGESTED READING

Panicek DM, Benson CB, Gottlieb RH, et al. The diaphragm: anatomic, pathologic, and radiologic considerations. *Radiographics*. 1988;8(3):385-425.

QUESTIONS AND ANSWERS

1. Regarding unilateral diaphragmatic paralysis, which of the following is *true*?
   A. Etiology is typically related to nerve damage.
   B. Etiology is uncommonly tumor invasion.
   C. Paralyzed hemidiaphragm is lower than the normal one.
   D. Most reliable test is Valsalva maneuver.

   ANSWER: A. This is usually caused by phrenic nerve interruption from any of a variety of causes: cancer, injury, neuritis, CNS or cord abnormalities, diabetes, carbon monoxide poisoning, or upper abdominal surgery. Malignant invasion is most common, with the most common cancer being lung cancer. Radiographically, the paralyzed hemidiaphragm is elevated and the dome is accentuated. The most reliable test is sniffing evaluation.

2. Regarding diaphragmatic eventration, which of the following is *true*?
   A. Etiology is unknown.
   B. Ultrasound may be helpful in diagnosis.
   C. Petit eventration is usually right-sided.
   D. Associated with severe restriction in PFT.

   ANSWER: B. Eventration is congenital failure of muscle development, in part or whole of the diaphragm. Complete hemidiaphragm eventration is called Petit eventration; this is almost exclusively left-sided, in contrast to the almost exclusively right-sided idiopathic unilateral paralysis. Eventration appears radiographically similar to paralysis, though on fluoroscopy and ultrasound the affected area will move with the normal portions of the hemidiaphragm (it may have a slight inspiratory lag).

3. Strychnine poisoning produces which of the following in the diaphragm?
   A. Respiratory myoclonus
   B. Splinting
   C. Air-trapping
   D. Tonic contraction

   ANSWER: D. Emphysema or severe acute asthma produces hyperinflation and air trapping that prevents normal motion. Localized infectious inflammatory processes may produce splinting of the hemidiaphragm. Tonic contraction may be due to tetany, tetanus, rabies, strychnine poisoning, and Coxsackie B infection. Respiratory myoclonus may produce diaphragmatic flutter.

4. What type of hernia contains peritoneum?
   A. Parasternal hiatus
   B. Bochdalek
   C. A congenital diaphragmatic hernia causing pulmonary hypoplasia
   D. Pleuroperitoneal hiatus

   ANSWER: A. The Morgagni hernia of the parasternal hiatus generally retains peritoneal lining. The Bochdalek hernia typically does not.

5. The radiograph of an obese, 50-year-old woman reveals a well-defined right cardiophrenic angle mass. Of these, which is most likely?
   A. Parasternal hiatal hernia
   B. Bochdalek hernia
   C. Diaphragmatic cancer
   D. Accessory diaphragm

   ANSWER: A. Radiographically, a Morgagni hernia is a well-defined right cardiophrenic angle mass. The defect is developmental but the hernia is associated with obesity, severe effort, and increased intra-abdominal pressure. Most patients are obese, middle-aged women. Radiographically, a Bochdalek hernia may appear as a focal diaphragmatic bulge or a posteromedial basilar mass. Primary diaphragmatic tumors are rare. Accessory diaphragm is rare and is not a mass-like entity.

6. What is the most common cause of intradiaphragmatic cyst?
   A. Hematoma
   B. Cystic adenomatoid malformation
   C. Extralobar sequestration
   D. Degenerated myoma

   ANSWER: C. Intradiaphragmatic cysts are rare and are usually formed by extralobar sequestration, and are almost always left-sided. A chronic diaphragmatic hematoma may evolve into a cyst.

7. Regarding diaphragmatic neoplasms in general, which is *true*?
   A. Primary tumors arise mostly from the posterior muscular portion.
   B. Primary tumors are more common than secondary tumors.
   C. Secondary neoplasms arise by hematogenous seeding.
   D. Ovarian cancer is a common etiology.

   ANSWER: D. Primary diaphragmatic tumors are rare, mostly from the tendinous or anterior muscular portion. The most common secondary neoplasm of the diaphragm is the direct extension of lung cancer or mesothelioma; other hepatic, peritoneal, or lung tumors may spread by extension. Ovarian cancer is a likely site of origin for metastasis of peritoneal origin. Distinct hematogenous or lymphatic nodular metastasis is uncommon.

8. What is the most common primary tumor of the diaphragm?
   A. Angiofibroma
   B. Lipoma
   C. Leiomyoma
   D. Fibrosarcoma

   ANSWER: B. Lipoma is the most common tumor, though angiofibroma, neurofibromatosis, leiomyoma, teratoma, and other tumors may develop. The most common malignant neoplasm is fibrosarcoma, though malignant fibrous histocystoma, hemangiopericytoma, germ cell tumors, and others may be found.

9. A 25-year-old man presents after an upper respiratory infection with shortness of breath. If the etiology is related to the diaphragm, which of these is *true*?
   A. More likely a right-sided process
   B. Associated with a depressed hemidiaphragm
   C. Bacterial in origin
   D. Motion will be normal.

   ANSWER: A. Idiopathic hemidiaphragm paralysis is almost always right-sided, and in males, perhaps a viral neuritis. Radiographically, the paralyzed hemidiaphragm is elevated and the dome is accentuated. Motion will be diminished, absent, or paradoxic, with paradoxic motion during sniffing; and the mediastinum will swing laterally with respiration.

10. Regarding bilateral diaphragmatic paralysis, which is *true*?
    A. Severe obstruction is visible with pulmonary function tests.
    B. Hypercapnia is an uncommon complication.
    C. Associated with thoracoabdominal paradox
    D. Petit eventration

    ANSWER: C. Patients with bilateral diaphragmatic paralysis are severely short of breath; bilateral paresis will produce milder symptoms. Most patients with paralysis will develop ventilatory failure and hypercapnia; some may develop cor pulmonale. Severe restriction will be found with pulmonary function test. Both hemidiaphragms will rise paradoxically during sniffing; this, accompanied by outward chest motion and inward abdominal motion, is called thoracoabdominal paradox. Petit eventration is complete hemidiaphragm eventration.

32 CHEST TRAUMA

Ian Malcolm and Satinder P. Singh

INTRODUCTION

Thoracic trauma is a common cause of significant morbidity and mortality. Most thoracic injuries in developed countries result from motor vehicle crashes (MVC) and other causes are falls or blow from blunt objects. Thoracic injuries account for 25% of trauma-related deaths. Imaging of patients with thoracic trauma must be accurate and timely to avoid preventable death.

Imaging usually starts with conventional radiography, often followed by CT imaging depending on severity of injury. Anteroposterior radiographic technique, poor inspiratory effort, patient rotation, aortic tortuosity, congenital arch anomalies, and mediastinal lipomatosis can simulate mediastinal widening because of traumatic hematoma, and mediastinal trauma is difficult to evaluate in children secondary to normal thymus. Also, 60% of patients with traumatic aortic injury do not have clinical signs on physical examination. Although the negative predictive value of a normal chest radiograph in trauma setting is quite high (98%), it is not specific, and in patients with abnormal chest radiograph, only 10% to 20% have positive angiographic findings.

CT of the chest is the modality of choice for initial evaluation of trauma. It has high sensitivity and negative predictive value and its specificity is good. CT study has false-positive rate of 0% to 39% and very low false-negative rate of 1% to 2%. The use of CT should be determined by the level of trauma, rather than the radiological signs and clinical findings. Trauma CT should be contrast-enhanced and CT angiography is preferable for the evaluation of aortic injury. Reformatted coronal and sagittal images improve diagnostic accuracy. Commonly observed artifacts that are due to aortic or cardiac pulsation may require CT angiography to exclude injury. These artifacts may resemble focal dissection or pseudoaneurysm and often occur on the medial aspect of the ascending aorta and can be overcome by using gated CT study.

TRAUMATIC AORTIC INJURY

Thoracic aortic injury accounts for up to 15% of deaths in MVC in the United States (Table 32-1). Between 85% and 90% of patients die before reaching the hospital, and approximately 50% of those who initially survive may die within 1 week in the absence of appropriate treatment. Rapid deceleration results in an intimal tear of the thoracic aorta, typically at the sites of aortic attachments, including (in descending order of frequency) the proximal descending aorta near the ductus, aortic root, and distal descending aorta at the aortic hiatus. Transsection with subsequent rupture results in rapid exsanguination. Sixty percent of aortic tears involve the intima and media, with intact adventitia. Seventy percent of severe aortic injuries cause death at the injury scene. There are three sites of relative aortic fixation where compression and shear forces cause traumatic aortic injury. The predominant site of injury is at the isthmus between the left subclavian artery and the ligamentum arteriosum. The second site is the ascending aorta, which is involved in 5% of clinically observed cases. The incidence of injury at this site, on autopsy series, approximates 20%. In this region, aortic injury may be accompanied by hemopericardium, possible tamponade, and intracardiac valve injury. The final site involves less than 2% of cases and is at the level of the aortic diaphragmatic hiatus. Hemopericardium and mediastinal hematoma are not specific for aortic trauma. Hemopericardium more commonly occurs with cardiac contusion, without aortic injury. Mediastinal hematoma commonly occurs with sternal and costochondral fractures, which injure the internal mammary and intercostal vessels. Mediastinal venous injury and aortic arch branch vessel injury also may cause mediastinal hematoma.

There are often associated severe injuries elsewhere. The patient may be in hemorrhagic shock with upper body hypertension, interscapular pain, rarely paraplegia, and lower body and leg ischemia.

Imaging features of aortic injury are summarized in Tables 32-1 and 32-2. A normal aorta on CT with no

TABLE 32-1 Traumatic Aortic Injury

1%–2% of all blunt trauma
18% of deaths in MVC
Poor prognosis: 80%–90% die before reaching a hospital, 50% of the survivals die in 24 hr, 80% of the treated live
2%–5% of the untreated survive and develop pseudoaneurysm (PSA)
Location (sites of fixation)
Ligamentum arteriosum, isthmus (most common)
Sinus of valsalva within pericardium (5%)
Diaphragmatic hiatus (2%)
Mechanism of injury: shear, torque, pinching, and compression at attachment sites cause intimal rupture. Pressure for rupture: 2500 mm Hg

TABLE 32-2 Types of Traumatic Aortic Injury

Transsection: transverse tear, which may be complete or incomplete (intact adventitia)
Dissection: intimal tear with leakage of contrast into the media; this may remain localized or create a channel in the media, which connects more distally with the lumen via a second intimal tear
Pseudoaneurysm: focal bulge of the weakened aortic wall following a traumatic defect of the intima and media

mediastinal hematoma excludes traumatic aortic injury. A periaortic hematoma typically accompanies thoracic aortic injury and is believed to represent bleeding from small veins in the area or from the vasa vasorum of the aorta itself. A periaortic hematoma may be seen at chest radiography as a mediastinal abnormality such as mediastinal widening, blurring of the aortic contour, or thickening of the paratracheal stripe. The presence of a mediastinal abnormality at chest radiography has a diagnostic sensitivity of 90% to 95% for a thoracic aortic injury but a poor specificity of only 5% to 10% (Table 32-3). Anteroposterior radiographic technique, poor inspiratory effort, patient rotation, aortic tortuosity, congenital arch anomalies, and mediastinal lipomatosis can simulate mediastinal widening as a result of traumatic hematoma.

CT is considered the modality of choice for detecting and characterizing aortic injury especially with its multireformat capabilities. Intramural hematoma in the aortic wall can occur in a trauma setting with no visible flap. Intramural hematoma demonstrates high attenuation soft tissue in thickened aortic wall and appears hypodense on a contrast-enhanced CT (Table 32-4).

Arterial and venous injury may occur not only in the superior mediastinum but also in branch vessels of the axilla, thoracic inlet, and base of the neck. When the aorta is involved, the most common arch branch vessel involved is the brachiocephalic artery. In the absence of aortic injury, all arch branch arteries are equally involved. The injured vessel may be detected on the initial contrast CT, but follow-up angiography or CT

TABLE 32-3 Radiographic Signs of Traumatic Aortic Injury

Wide mediastinum (>8 cm)
Aortic contour abnormality
AP window opacification
Wide left paratracheal stripe
Depressed left bronchus
Right tracheal/esophageal deviation
Left pleural cap
First rib fracture

Chest radiographs have only a 15% positive predictive factor for mediastinal hematoma.

TABLE 32-4 CT Signs of Aortic Injury

Direct: irregular contour, change in caliber, presence of intimal flap
Indirect: mediastinal hematoma
False positive: thymus, atelectasis, motion, volume averaging, normal adjacent structures

angiogram is often required prior to surgical repair (Table 32-5). CT angiographic detail now approaches that of angiography, which remains the reference standard. Optimal bolus timing is required, and the patient is positioned appropriately to evaluate the injured artery or vein. The venous injection is made in the arm away from the injured vessel to avoid volume-averaging artifact, which results from intense contrast agent in the injected vein.

Transesophageal echocardiography (TEE) is a bedside examination that is very useful in evaluating an unstable patient, especially when other imaging findings are equivocal. However, it is technically inadequate in 15% patients and is minimally invasive with a complication rate of 2% to 3%. Findings suggestive of aortic injury include detection of intimal flap, pseudoaneurysm, or aortic wall hematoma. False-positive results can occur as a result of atherosclerotic disease. MRI has no role in an acute trauma setting, though it can be used to follow traumatic aortic injury and pseudoaneurysm.

Cardiac and pericardial injuries include contusion, chamber rupture, arrhythmia, coronary artery injury, pneumo- and hemopericardium, and tamponade. Electrocardiographic (EKG) changes in trauma setting indicate traumatic cardiac injury. Bedside echocardiography is a commonly used initial modality. Hemopericardium can be missed on echodiography (Table 32-6).

Prehospital deaths because of cardiac injury are common, according to autopsy findings. Hemopericardium often occurs as a result of ruptured pericardial vessels and less commonly because of aortic or myocardial rupture. Pneumopericardium occurs secondary to pneumomediastinum, some cases of which result from tracheobronchial and esophageal injury. Pericardial rupture occurs rarely and may result in herniation of myocardium through the defect with impaired myocardial contractility.

TABLE 32-5 Contrast-Enhanced CT Signs of Nonaortic Arterial and Venous Injury

Intimal tear
Dissection
Vessel disruption
Extraluminal contrast extravasation
Absent vascular enhancement
Decreased vascular enhancement

TABLE 32-6 Hemopericardial Tamponade Clinical Presentation

Classic triad
Tachycardia
Muffled heart sounds
Elevated jugular venous pressure
Anxious, short of breath, diaphoretic
Echocardiography is diagnostic
Treatment includes pericardiocentesis, pericardial window

TABLE 32-8 CT Signs of Pulmonary Laceration

Focal consolidation without air bronchograms.
Linear or bubbly air collections within the lung parenchyma on CT. These must be distinguished from loculated hydropneumothorax.
Hematomas. These are circumscribed round or oval lung lesions.
Pneumatoceles. These are round, usually thin-walled air collections, sometimes with air fluid levels. These may or may not develop following contusion and are generally present on follow-up CT examination.
Pneumatoceles may persist as lung cysts. Hematomas may persist for months or years as pulmonary nodules. These progressively decrease in size and organize into fibrous lesions or parenchymal scars.

LUNG INJURY

- *Contusion*: common, hemorrhage in alveoli, appears quickly and clears in a few days
- *Laceration*: tear in lung leading to hematoma cyst formation; takes longer to resolve
- Other causes of consolidation in trauma: aspiration, atelectasis from mucous plug or splinting, and cardiac and noncardiac edema

PULMONARY CONTUSION AND LACERATION

Pulmonary contusion and laceration injury occur in up to 70% of cases of chest trauma and have a mortality of 10% to 25%. The patient may be hypoxic and have dyspnea and hemoptysis. Acute respiratory failure or ARDS may develop. There may be signs of aspiration as well as contusion (Table 32-7). Contusion is alveolar distention with blood from injured blood vessels. Air bronchograms are less frequent than with other forms of consolidation (pneumonia, pulmonary edema), likely because the airways are often also distended with blood. Contusion resolves completely with no residual injury. Laceration is a parenchymal tear resulting from shear forces or laceration by an adjacent displaced rib fracture. In the latter case, a pneumothorax and subcutaneous air is usually seen (Tables 32-8 and 32-9). These signs are more difficult to detect radiographically. The distribution of pulmonary contusion and laceration depends on the site and severity of blunt trauma. Aspiration at the time of, or subsequent to, injury may be distinguished from contusion by "tree-in-bud" lesions. If more than 20% of the lungs are involved with contusion, there is an 80% chance of developing ARDS. In some patients, consolidation occurring because of pulmonary contusion does not resolve but stabilizes or progressively worsens because of the development of other parenchymal disease.

TABLE 32-7 Radiographic Signs of Pulmonary Contusion

Patchy nonsegmental airspace consolidation
Air bronchograms are usually not present
May take up to 6 hours to develop
Opacification reaches its maximum in 1–3 d
Resolves in 1–2 wk, unless associated laceration is present
Must be distinguished from aspiration, pulmonary edema, pneumonia, or ARDS on subsequent radiographs

ASPIRATION

Opacities caused by aspiration develop in the dependent portions of the lungs, variable with patient positioning. In a supine patient, the posterior segments of upper lobes and superior segments of lower lobes tend to be involved. Hospitalized patients frequently develop perihilar opacities because of aspiration in the lower lobe superior segments, which can be mistaken for pulmonary edema. Because of gastric acid, opacities may develop and change more rapidly than pulmonary contusion or pneumonic consolidation. There is likely to be cellular bronchiolitis (tree-in-bud and centrilobular nodules) because of aspiration into terminal and respiratory bronchioles. Aspirated food particles may block large- and medium-sized airways with lobar, segmental, or subsegmental collapse or alternatively air trapping.

ACUTE RESPIRATORY DISTRESS SYNDROME (ARDS)

ARDS is secondary to increased-permeability pulmonary edema caused by alveolar epithelial or capillary endothelial damage. ARDS commonly develops as a result of acute lung injury; however, there are many other causes including shock and sepsis. Patients have refractory hypoxemia with dyspnea, parenchymal consolidation, and no evidence of left heart failure. There is an acute hemorrhagic phase with epithelial cell sloughing, hemorrhagic alveolar filling, hyaline membrane formation, and intense interstitial inflammation. A subsequent fibroproliferative phase results from granulation tissue

TABLE 32-9 Radiographic Signs of Tracheobronchial Injury

Pneumomediastinum
Lower lobe collapse
Endotracheal tube outside the airway lumen
Overinflated endotracheal cuff
Double wall sign
Occasionally pneumothorax and subcutaneous emphysema

formation in the interstitium and subsequent development of fibrous tissue. Because of intractable hypoxemia and poor lung compliance (stiff lungs), assisted ventilation is required with common development of barotrauma. Approximately 30% to 50% of patients die in the acute phase and the remaining ones recover or develop pulmonary fibrosis and end-stage lung disease. Radiographically, there is patchy consolidation in both lungs, which becomes progressively more diffuse over time. A coarse reticular pattern develops in the fibroproliferative phase with progressive loss of lung volumes. CT abnormalities develop within 12 hours. There are extensive ground glass opacities, with or without airspace consolidation, in a geographical pattern with interspersed areas of normal lung. Interstitial reticulation may be superimposed on the ground glass opacities thus causing the crazy paving pattern. Consolidation worsens and becomes gravitational dependent with prominent air bronchograms. In the fibroproliferative phase, there is coarse reticulation, traction bronchiectasis, and honeycomb cystic change.

AIRWAYS INJURY

Tracheal injury is uncommon because of shear or crush injury (Table 32-10). There is usually pneumomediastinum, but pneumothorax, deep cervical and subcutaneous emphysema, and also retroperitoneal air in the abdomen may occur. Bronchial fracture may cause delayed lower lobe collapse or, rarely, the fallen lung sign. In the latter case, the lung collapses dependently below the hilum, rather than inferomedially. Air may track along the bronchial wall causing the double wall sign. Injuries to the right lower lobe bronchus occur more commonly than left lower lobe bronchial or tracheal injuries. Injuries predominate within 2 cm of the carina. The endotracheal cuff may appear hyperinflated and the endotracheal tube itself may be visualized outside the tracheal lumen. Bronchoscopy is used to detect these injuries and also complications such as bronchostenosis, bronchopleural fistula, bronchiectasis, and postobstructive pneumonia. These lesions are treated by direct surgical repair of the airway or by lobectomy or pneumonectomy in severe cases.

TABLE 32-10 Traumatic Airway Injury

1.5% of blunt chest trauma
Often not recognized, delayed diagnosis
Associated fractures: 1–3 ribs, scapula, clavicle, sternum in up to 40%
Bronchial fractures within 2.5 cm of carina

PNEUMOTHORAX

CT readily shows extremely small pneumothoraces, but the detection of pneumothoraces is more challenging on radiographs. Displaced rib fractures may tear the parietal pleura. Pneumomediastinum may rupture through the parietal pleura and cause pneumothorax. Direct trauma may force air from the alveolar spaces into the alveolar interstitium. This may subsequently rupture the visceral pleura and cause pneumothorax. Alternatively, air may track medially into the bronchovascular interstitium (pulmonary interstitial emphysema) and subsequently into the mediastinum. Thirty percent of pneumothoraces are missed on supine or semierect radiographs. Rib fractures, together with subcutaneous air, indicate that pneumothorax is present even though it may not be visualized radiographically. The mediastinum may be more sharply defined than normal, with small pneumothoraces. A deep costophrenic sulcus may be seen if the air is situated inferomedially. Contralateral mediastinal shift indicates tension requiring chest tube decompression.

PNEUMOMEDIASTINUM

Small pneumothoraces and small collections of mediastinal air are readily identified with CT. There is direct air leakage if tracheobronchial structures are injured. Pneumomediastinum may also arise from extension of subcutaneous or deep cervical emphysema or direct extension of retroperitoneal air. Direct trauma or assisted ventilation may cause pulmonary interstitial emphysema, with subsequent pneumomediastinum. This commonly occurs with ARDS, where the lungs have loss of compliance and positive pressure is required to improve hypoxemia. On chest radiographs, pneumomediastinum reveals as vertical streaks in the mediastinum, which may extend into the cervical soft tissues. The air may surround vessels ("ring around the artery" and "tubular artery signs") or around the airway ("double bronchus sign"). A peripheral lucency may be present along one or both sides of the mediastinum with surrounding parietal pleural line. Alternatively, lucency may outline the heart with surrounding pericardium (pneumopericardium).

Air posterior to the pericardium may show the continuous diaphragm sign, where the entire upper margin of the diaphragm is outlined by air. Pneumomediastinum should resolve. If this does not occur, tracheal injury should be ruled out with bronchoscopy.

HEMOTHORAX

Fifty percent of cases with blunt trauma show hemothorax. The blood may arise from pulmonary, intercostal, phrenic, or internal mammary vessels and may also be seen with traumatic aortic injury. Small hemothoraces are readily seen on CT. On radiographs, small- and medium-sized hemothoraces may be missed, particularly on portable examinations taken in erect or semierect positions. Supine radiographs may show an apical cap of pleural fluid or mild opacification of the affected side because of blood layering posteriorly in the pleural space. Some 200 to 500 mL of pleural fluid is required to cause blunting of the costophrenic recesses on erect radiographs, but lateral decubitus films may show collections as small as 5 mL. CT detects small collections and can differentiate blood from serous fluid by high attenuation values (35–70 HU). Aortic bleeding can occasionally be detected by contrast extravasation into the pleural space. Loculation is inclined to develop and fibrothorax may result if chest tube drainage of the blood is not carried out.

TRAUMATIC DIAPHRAGMATIC INJURY

Penetrating trauma (10%) is the most common cause of traumatic diaphragmatic injury and is usually small. In 3% to 6% of major blunt trauma, the diaphragm can be injured and this is usually a large-size injury. Majority of diaphragmatic injuries (70%) are initially missed because of associated lung injury, pleural effusion, and mechanical ventilation. Left-sided injury is more common (77%–95%) with liver protecting the diaphragm from right-sided injury. More than three-fourths of patients have other visceral injuries. Radiographic diagnosis is often difficult. Associated pulmonary contusion, hemothorax, and lacerations of the liver and spleen may conceal the area of interest.

The mechanism of injury for diaphragmatic injury is increased intrathoracic pressure and shearing forces. The most common site of injury is the posterolateral portion of the diaphragm at the junction of central tendon and posterior leaves because of congenital weakness of fusion of costal and lumbar muscular attachments.

Chest radiographs are abnormal in 77% patients, though injury is suspected only in 50% patients. The most reliable radiographic signs are intrathoracic bowel and enteric tube tip in the thorax. Other signs are elevation of the diaphragm, indistinct diaphragm, or contralateral mediastinal shift. CT has a sensitivity of up to 90% in the detection of tears, and the confidence of interpretation is helped by reformatted coronal and sagittal images (Table 32-11). False-positive diagnosis is often due to splenic injury and peridiaphragmatic hematoma. False-negative diagnosis is due to associated lower lobe consolidation or pleural effusion. Treatment is by direct surgical repair or synthetic graft repair. Mortality from diaphragmatic rupture is 30% and delayed diagnosis results in bowel strangulation.

TABLE 32-11 CT Signs of Diaphragmatic Tear

Diaphragmatic defect
Diaphragmatic thickening
Nonvisualized portion of the diaphragm
Elevated hemidiaphragm
Intrathoracic viscera. This may be bowel, liver, spleen, or mesenteric fat. The amount of herniated viscera is dependent upon the size of the tear.
Dependent viscera sign: upper third liver abutting posterior ribs, or stomach/bowel lay in contact with posterior ribs, in 90%, may be an early indicator before visceral herniation.
Nasogastric tube tip within the thorax
Contralateral mediastinal shift
Collar sign: waistlike constriction of the displaced intrathoracic; sensitivity 67% for left, and 50% for right, specificity 100%.

SKELETAL TRAUMA

Rib fractures without displacement have no serious consequences. Displaced fractures may cause pneumothorax, hemothorax, and subcutaneous emphysema. Individual ribs with multiple fractures may result in flail chest with impaired ventilation (Table 32-12). An unusually large extrapleural hematoma on chest radiographs, in association with rib fractures, should raise the suspicion of flail chest. Elderly patients have osteopenic ribs and vertebrae that fracture more readily. Children have flexible ribs that fracture less readily and consequently, childhood rib fractures are associated with higher mortality. Certain rib fractures have common associated injuries. First through third rib fractures

TABLE 32-12 Flail Chest

Fractures of 4 consecutive ribs in >2 places or >3 segmental rib fractures (multiple rib fractures)
Significant kinetic force injury
Diagnosis: physical examination, paradoxical chest wall motion, chest radiograph findings, physiologic derangement
Usually associated with lung contusion

commonly occur with aortic, great vessel, and tracheobronchial injury. Tenth through twelfth rib fractures are associated with hepatic, splenic, and renal injuries.

Sternal fractures may be associated with bleeding and consequent mediastinal hematoma or hemothorax. They are often associated with cardiac, aortic arch, and great vessel injury. Posterior sternoclavicular dislocations cause penetrating injury, which may involve the trachea, esophagus, and mediastinal great vessels.

Scapula fractures indicate significant trauma also. Patients with scapula fractures commonly have a pneumothorax and there is an 11% chance of ipsilateral subclavian, axillary, or brachial artery injury. Ipsilateral subclavian axillary or brachial artery injury should be searched for when scapula fractures are identified.

Suggested Reading

Alkadhi H, Wilderworth S, Desboilles L, et al. Vascular emergencies of the thorax after blunt and iatrogenic trauma: multidetector ROW CT and 3 dimensional imaging. *Radiographics.* 2004;24:1239-1255.

Collins J. Chest wall trauma. *J Thorac Imaging.* 2000;15:112-119.

Costantino M, Grosselin MO, Primak SL. The ABC's of thoracic trauma imaging. *Semin Roentgenol.* 2006;41:209-225.

Creasey J et al. Overview of traumatic injury of the thoracic aorta. *Radiographics.* 1997;17:27-45.

Groskin S. Selected topics in chest trauma. *Semin Ultrasound CT MR.* 1996;17:119-141.

Kuhlman JE, Posniak MA, Collins J, Knisely BL. Radiographic and CT findings of blunt chest trauma: aortic injuries and looking beyond them. *Radiographics. 1998;* 18:1085-1106.

Mayberry J. Imaging in thoracic trauma: the trauma surgeon's perspective. *J Thorac Imaging.* 2000;15:76-85.

Miller LA. Chest wall, lung and pleural space trauma. *Radiol Clin North Am.* 2006;44:213-224.

Miller PR, Corce MA, Bee TK, et al. ARDS after pulmonary contusion: accurate measurement of contusion volume indicates high risk patients. *J Trauma.* 2001;51:223-230.

Müller NL, and Silva CIC. *Imaging of the Chest.* Philadelphia, PA. Saunders Elsevier; 2008.

Shackleton KL, Stewart ET, Taylor AJ. Traumatic diaphragmatic injury: spectrum of radiographic findings. *Radiographics.* 1998;18:49-59.

Stark P. *Radiology of Thoracic Trauma.* Boston, MA: Andover Medical Publishers; 1993.

Van Hise ML, Primack SL, Israel RS, et al. CT in blunt chest trauma: indications and limitations. *Radiographics.* 1998;18:1071-1084.

Wintermark M, Schnyder P. The Macklin effect. *Chest.* 2001;120:543-547.

Zylak CM, Standen JR, Barnes GR, Zylak CJ. Pneumomediastinum revisited. *Radiographics.*2000;20:1043-1057.

QUESTIONS AND ANSWERS

1. Concerning CT evaluation of aortic injury, which of the following is *true*?
   A. Aortic injury is excluded if the aorta is normal and no mediastinal hematoma is identified.
   B. Clinical evaluation of the patient determines whether HRCT is indicated.
   C. Hemopericardium indicates ascending aortic injury.
   D. Aortic arch branch vessel injury is common.

   ANSWER: A. The level of trauma, not the clinical examination, should determine whether CT is indicated. Hemopericardium occurs more commonly with cardiac injury than ascending aortic injury. Aortic branch vessel injury occurs much less commonly than aortic injury.

2. Concerning aortic injury, which of the following is *true*?
   A. Majority of patients with aortic trauma have clinical signs when examined.
   B. Traumatic dissection is most likely to occur in the ascending aorta.
   C. Aortic transsection usually results in death before surgery can be initiated.
   D. Chest radiography has a 25% positive predictive factor for mediastinal hematoma.

   ANSWER: C. Sixty percent of patients have no clinical signs on initial examination, when aortic injury is present. Traumatic dissection predominantly occurs at the isthmus. Chest radiography has only a 15% positive predictive factor for mediastinal hematoma.

3. Concerning pulmonary contusion, which of the following is *true*?
   A. Readily distinguished from pulmonary laceration on initial radiographs
   B. May progressively worsen on radiographs for the first 3 days
   C. Forty percent of the lungs must be involved before ARDS subsequently develops.
   D. Air bronchograms are usually present.

   ANSWER: B. Pulmonary contusion and laceration cannot usually be differentiated on initial radiographs. If 20% of the lungs are involved, there is an 80% chance of subsequent ARDS. Air bronchograms are not usually seen.

4. Concerning pulmonary laceration, which of the following is *true*?
   A. Lucent round, oval, or linear areas are shown on initial chest radiographs.
   B. Lacerations must be distinguished from hydropneumothorax on CT.
   C. Penetrating injury is required for pulmonary laceration to develop.
   D. Injuries severe enough to cause pulmonary lacerations are likely to have associated aortic injury.

   ANSWER: B. Initially, only consolidation is seen on radiographs. Laceration may also occur due to shear forces associated with blunt chest trauma. Pulmonary laceration occurs more commonly than aortic injury. Aortic injury involves more severe trauma than is required for pulmonary laceration to occur.

5. Concerning tracheobronchial injury, which of the following is *true*?
   A. Left lower lobe bronchus is more readily involved than the trachea or right lower lobe bronchus.
   B. Tracheobronchial injury is the most common cause of traumatic pneumomediastinum.
   C. The endotracheal tube may be identified outside the tracheal lumen.
   D. Tracheobronchial injury is commonly associated with pneumothorax.

   ANSWER: C. Right lower lobe bronchus is most commonly involved. Tracheobronchial injury is not common and consequently is not a common cause of pneumomediastinum. Pneumothorax is only occasionally found in association with tracheobronchial injury.

6. Concerning traumatic diaphragmatic injury, which of the following is *true*?
   A. Sensitivity of detection with CT is 50% to 70%.
   B. Diaphragmatic injury may initially be obscured by other injuries.
   C. Common cause of mediastinal shift.
   D. Bronchopleural fistula is a common complication.

   ANSWER: B. Sensitivity of detection with CT is 70% to 90%. Mediastinal shift occurs much more commonly than diaphragmatic injury because of a variety of causes such as pneumothorax and hemothorax. Bronchopleural fistula is an unrelated injury.

7. Concerning sternal fractures, which of the following is *true*?
   A. Displaced sternal fractures and mediastinal hematoma indicate traumatic aortic injury.
   B. May be associated with cardiac contusion and hemopericardium
   C. Anterior sternoclavicular joint dislocations may result in injury to the trachea and esophagus.
   D. Pulmonary contusion occurs in less than 10% of cases.

   ANSWER: B. Both sternal fractures and mediastinal hematoma are commonly seen in the absence of aortic injury. Posterior sternoclavicular dislocation is liable to cause trauma injury to the trachea and esophagus. Pulmonary contusion occurs in up to 70% of cases of chest trauma.

8. Concerning branch vessel injury, when the aorta remains intact
   A. Arch branch vascular injury should be searched for in the case of first rib fractures
   B. Brachiocephalic artery is the arch branch usually injured
   C. Hematoma is often identified in the pretracheal and AP window regions
   D. Angiography is required prior to surgical repair

   ANSWER: A. Arch branch vessels are involved equally if there is no aortic injury. Hematoma is usually in the anterior mediastinum. It also occurs less commonly in the posterior mediastinum with injuries of the descending aorta or spinal injury. Pretracheal hematoma may occur with tracheal injury that is much less common. Good quality CT angiography provides adequate information in many cases and avoids the delay caused by angiography if surgery is urgently required.

9. Concerning aspiration with chest trauma, which of the following is *true*?
   A. Aspiration is invariable with severe chest trauma.
   B. Rib fractures should be expected if aspiration is present.
   C. Aspiration can simulate pulmonary edema with rapidly developing and rapidly resolving opacities in the perihilar region.
   D. Aspiration is seldom severe enough to precipitate ARDS.

   ANSWER: C. Aspiration can occur, but usually does not. No known relationship between rib fracture and aspiration has been described. The level of consciousness and the severity of trauma would be expected to correlate with the severity of aspiration. Severe aspiration may cause ARDS and is more likely to occur with head injury with loss of consciousness in a patient who has recent food or fluid ingestion, prior to the chest trauma.

33 DRUG-INDUCED LUNG TOXICITY

John C. Texada and Satinder P. Singh

INTRODUCTION

Drug reactions are quite common and must always be considered as the etiology for a patient's new symptoms. They may be categorized into one or more of six types: bronchospasm, systemic lupus erythrematosis–like syndrome, responses from illicit drug abuse, eosinophilic reactions, interstitial or airspace pneumonitis, or pulmonary edema from increased permeability.

CHEMOTHERAPEUTIC AND IMMUNOSUPPRESSIVE DRUGS

BLEOMYCIN

Bleomycin is an antibiotic isolated from *Streptomyces verticillus*. Although bleomycin does not produce myelosuppression like many other chemotherapeutic agents, many patients will develop dose-related lung toxicity—overall incidence is 3% to 5%, but above 450 units of drug incidence is 13% to 17%. The risk of developing toxicity rises in old people, smokers, and people receiving combined chemotherapy, oxygen, or radiation therapy. Radiographic changes are more common than symptoms, and CT changes are still more common.

Histopathologic Findings

The compound gets concentrated in lung and skin, and these tissues do not have much of the enzyme necessary to degrade it. Once within cells, it can cleave DNA. Alveolar macrophage recruitment is an early response, followed by inflammatory cell recruitment, tissue injury, and fibrosis. Diffuse alveolar damage (DAD) is characteristic. BOOP, eosinophilic pneumonia and pleuritis, and venoocclusive disease may occur.

Radiographic Findings

Findings develop 6 to 12 weeks after beginning therapy; they may resolve after therapy is stopped, or may persist. Bilateral basilar reticular/reticulonodular/nodular opacities are often peripheral, and often involve or are confined to the costophrenic angles. More severe disease extends upward in the lungs or evolves to airspace consolidation.

CT Findings

CT detects parenchymal abnormalities in 38% of patients as against 15% from the radiography. CT or HRCT may reveal focal consolidation or dense irregular lines; in mild disease, as in radiography, the findings are subpleural and posterior, with disease spreading with increasing severity.

OTHERS

Mitomycin

Mitomycin is an antibiotic derived from *Sporobolus caespitosus*. It may cause lung disease in 3% to 7% of patients, via an uncertain mechanism perhaps related to its alkylating properties. It causes endothelial damage, type I cell damage and type II cell proliferation, and interstitial fibrosis. It may be associated with a hemolytic-uremic syndrome.

Busulfan

Busulfan is used in myeloproliferative disorders and in bone-marrow transplant preparation. It produces clinically apparent lung disease in 5% of patients, but 50% of patients have pathologic evidence of damage. The former is associated with long-term use, at least of several months, and symptoms are insidious. Large atypical mononuclear cells (altered type II cells) are present, and fibroblasts and collagen deposition increase leading to fibrosis that may be diffuse or basilar-predominant. Mean survival after fibrosis develops is 5 months.

Cyclophosphamide

Cyclophosphamide is an alkylating agent. Its pulmonary toxicity is probably less than 1%; fibrosis may develop after a dose of as little as 150 mg, but the risk increases with higher doses. There is DAD and atypical alveolar cells, with chronic pneumonitis, fibrosis, and less commonly BOOP. Basilar reticular opacities, often with consolidation, are visible; pleural thickening also is commonly present. The presentation is often acute or subacute, but may be chronic. Steroids help prevent and reverse toxicity.

Chlorambucil

Chlorambucil is an alkylating agent useful in blood malignancy. It rarely causes lung toxicity. When chlorambucil does lead to pulmonary toxicity, it usually manifests as interstitial pneumonitis and fibrosis. Bilateral basilar reticular opacities are present. Onset may be delayed. Mortality can be high, though drug cessation and steroid therapy may help.

Others drugs, including melphalan (a phenylalanine derivative of nitrogen mustard gas useful in multiple myeloma), nitrosoureas (alkylating agents that interfere with DNA repair and synthesis), the anti-androgen nilutamide, and the vinca alkaloids, may produce similar toxicity syndromes.

Tamoxifen may increase the risk of thrombotic events. Cyclosporine may cause acute respiratory distress syndrome (ARDS). Procarbazine may cause acute allergic reaction.

ANTIMETABOLIC DRUGS

METHOTREXATE

Methotrexate is a folic acid analogue that creates acute deficiency of intracellular folate coenzymes and thereby inhibits cell reproduction. It is used both in cancers and as disease-modifying therapy in several autoimmune diseases. The incidence of reaction is estimated at 2% to 5% for low-dose therapy as with rheumatoid arthritis. Frequency, dose, and duration are risk factors as is preexisting lung disease.

Pathologic Findings

Unlike many other agents, methotrexate-induced lung disease is often reversible; it is generally a hypersensitivity reaction, evidenced by eosinophilia and pulmonary granuloma or eosinophil infiltration. It can, though, induce chronic interstitial fibrosis occasionally. Interstitial pneumonitis or fibrosis are the most common findings, with occasionally DAD or rarely BOOP.

Radiographic Findings

The radiographic appearance is characteristic. Initially a basilar or diffuse reticular or ground glass opacity develops, which in turn rapidly develops into patchy consolidation before reverting to interstitial opacity and then resolves. Nodules or lymphadenopathy may also develop.

OTHERS

Cytosine arabinoside (an inhibitor of DNA synthesis) may cause lung disease in 15% to 30% of patients treated with high IV doses, often in treatment for leukemia; DAD or a proteinaceous acellular alveolar exudates may develop. Gemcitabine is similar to cytosine arabinoside. Azathioprine (an interferon of purine synthesis) has been reported to rarely cause lung disease, in a dose-related manner. Fludarabine may cause interstitial pneumonitis or DAD. L-Asparaginase increases the risk of thrombotic events.

BIOLOGIC RESPONSE MODIFIERS

Interleukin-2 is believed to increase capillary permeability, and thereby may cause a syndrome of cardiopulmonary failure with edema, hypotension, and weight gain. Radiographic manifestations range from mild-to-severe edema, often with pleural effusions. Tumor necrosis factor may cause asymptomatic noncardiogenic edema, or rarely DAD. Granulocyte–macrophage colony stimulating factor produces a capillary leak syndrome and may produce acute eosinophilic pneumonia, pleural and pericardial effusions, and PTE. Interferon has been shown to produce interstitial pneumonitis and BOOP, and may spur development of antiphospholipid antibody and thus increase risk of thrombosis.

ANTIMICROBIAL DRUGS

NITROFURANTOIN

This drug may rarely cause lung disease, and severe disease is still rarer. Two presentations occur with nitrofurantoin toxicity: (1) an acute reaction, almost certainly due to hypersensitivity, as evidenced by abrupt onset and peripheral eosinophilia and (2) a less common chronic reaction developing after weeks to years of therapy, likely due to oxidant tissue damage.

Pathologic Findings

Interstitial pneumonitis and fibrosis are indistinguishable from IPF. Rare cases of other findings may occur.

Radiographic Findings

In acute reaction, a diffuse basilar-predominant reticular pattern develops, sometimes with septal lines; the pattern resembles interstitial edema. Pleural effusions often occur, sometimes without other findings. Some patients developed ARDS. In chronic toxicity, a bilateral lower lung predominant reticular interstitial pattern develops; HRCT reveals subpleural and peribronchovascular consolidation and fibrosis. In chronic toxicity, effusions are uncommon.

OTHERS

Sulfasalazine may occasionally produce an acute migratory opacity and peripheral eosinophilia, almost certainly due to hypersensitivity. Biopsy may reveal BOOP or interstitial pneumonitis and fibrosis. Radiographs may reveal poorly defined peripheral and upper-lung (not lower-lung) predominant consolidation.

Tetracycline and minocycline produce pulmonary eosinophilia, likely due to hypersensitivity; sulfonamides, penicillin, *para*-aminosalicylic acid, ethambutol, ampicillin, maloprim, cephalosporins, and other agents may cause pulmonary hypersensitivity reactions.

ANTIARRHYTHMIC DRUGS

AMIODARONE

Amiodarone HCl is an iodinated benzofuran derivative used in arrhythmia therapy. The drug accumulates in various organs but is most concentrated in the lungs—up to seven times more concentrated than in other body tissues. Up to 5% to 7% of patients on amiodarone develop lung toxicity, and of those 5% to 10% will die. Its pathogenicity is uncertain; it is, though, dose related. The drug causes inhibition of phospholipids degradation, so phospholipids accumulate, and this may be one etiology for damage; the drug itself may also directly cause cell damage; or an immune-inflammatory response may cause the damage. Damage onset is generally months after initiation of therapy in patients taking dosages greater than 400 mg/d, although lung injury has been reported with treatment for periods as short as 3 weeks and with dosage as low as 200 mg/d. Treatment with drug removal and steroids is very effective.

Pathologic Findings

There is often chronic inflammation and septal fibrosis, type II hyperplasia, and foamy macrophage accumulation with characteristic lysosomal inclusions probably containing the drug or a metabolite (though the presence of these inclusions is not diagnostic of drug toxicity). Less commonly, DAD, BOOP, necrotizing bronchiolitis, or necrotizing pneumonia may develop.

Clinical Presentation

Chronic interstitial pneumonitis is the most common presentation, characterized by insidious onset of cough, dyspnea, and weight loss.

ARDS is rare but potentially fatal form of lung toxicity, with fulminant course and typically seen in patients who undergo surgery or pulmonary angiography. It is hypothesized that amiodarone may sensitize susceptible individuals to either high concentrations of inspired oxygen or to iodinated contrast media.

Radiographic Findings

Radiographs often show diffuse bilateral reticular or alveolar opacities, often peripheral and often upper-lung predominant, resembling chronic eosinophilic pneumonia. Focal consolidation, nodule development, and pleural thickening have been described.

CT Findings

Because amiodarone contains iodine, dense liver and spleen are common; dense lung lesions are also common; dense myocardium has been reported but is uncommon. Consolidation, (often wedge shaped and pleural based), reticular interstitial disease, atelectasis, or round consolidation may be present. Effusions are visible in 50% of cases. Gallium-67 imaging will be positive in amiodarone-induced lung disease.

OTHERS

Lidocaine, tocainide, verapamil, procainamide, and sotalol have caused lung toxicity or edema in a few cases.

ANTICONVULSANT DRUGS

DIPHENYLHYDANTOIN

This antiseizure medication acts as a membrane stabilizer. It may produce an acute hypersensitivity reaction with peripheral eosinophilia and diffuse reticulonodular interstitial disease that resolves within 2 weeks of discontinuing therapy. Mediastinal lymphadenopathy may develop, often reactive, though incidence of lymphoma in patients on this drug is increased up to ten times. Rarely airspace consolidation or miliary nodules may develop.

CARBAMAZEPINE

Twelve cases of carbamazepine-induced lung toxicity have been reported, manifested by pneumonia, eosinophilia, and skin rash; radiograph appearance may be of reticular or reticulonodular interstitial disease or alveolar opacity, occasionally with lymphadenopathy. In addition, patients may also develop decreased diffusion capacity of the lung for carbon monoxide (DLCO) but have normal radiographs.

ANALGESIC DRUGS

Aspirin can produce acute pulmonary edema, particularly in middle-age and elderly patients taking large doses. Younger people often do not develop edema in aspirin overdose. The edema is the result of increased capillary permeability, perhaps from increased intracranial pressure causing neurogenic edema, or from inhibition of prostaglandin productions leading to vasodilation and permeability.

Nonsteroidal anti-inflammatory drugs (NSAIDs) may rarely produce lung toxicity; there are scattered reports describing acute development of pulmonary alveolar opacities and eosinophilia in patients taking naproxen or other NSAIDs.

ANTIRHEUMATIC DRUGS

PENICILLAMINE

This penicillin derivative can chelate metals and is used to treat lead poisoning, Wilson disease (abnormal copper deposition), cystinuria, and connective tissue diseases. It may produce a wide variety of lung diseases, including lupus-like disease, myasthenia-like disease, alveolitis, obliterative bronchiolitis, and DAD. The risk is quite low and is not dose related. The reactions are probably type I and/or type III immune reactions. Acute hypersensitivity has a good prognosis; however, patients who develop pulmonary–renal syndrome or obliterative bronchiolitis often die. Radiographs may reveal one of the following three patterns: (1) reticular/reticulonodular interstitial disease with or without limited alveolar opacity; (2) overinflation, associated with advanced obliterative bronchiolitis; and (3) diffuse alveolar consolidation in patients with DAD. HRCT findings in patients with obliterative bronchiolitis include areas of mosaic attenuation and bronchial dilation.

GOLD

Gold therapy causes lung disease in less than 1% of patients, in a non–dose-dependent manner that may be associated with certain major histocompatibility complex antigens. The reaction is believed to be a hypersensitivity reaction, with perhaps a cell-mediated immune component. Pathology reveals interstitial pneumonitis and fibrosis, or occasionally BOOP or obliterative bronchiolitis. Chest radiograph may reveal interstitial and alveolar opacities.

SYMPATHOMIMETIC DRUGS

Beta-Agonist medicines terbutaline, ritodrine, and isoxsuprine suppress preterm labor; they can rarely produce a hyperpermeability pulmonary edema.

ILLICIT DRUGS

SEDATIVE-NARCOTIC DRUGS

The opiates can produce pulmonary edema, as often as 50% to 75% of cases of heroin overdose and also reported with multiple other sedative-narcotic drugs. The presence of high protein concentrations in the developed fluid indicates a capillary hyperpermeability state, perhaps from endothelial damage caused by hypoventilatory acidosis. Bronchiectasis may be found in patients with opiate-induced edema, but this is likely a sequela of prior infections from aspiration. Pneumothorax may develop from attempts at venous access.

Cocaine

Crack cocaine causes a variety of lung toxicities. Users often report cough, black sputum production, chest pain, shortness of breath, or hemoptysis. Pulmonary edema may develop, perhaps from endothelial damage, or perhaps from cardiac dysfunction. Pulmonary hemorrhage is an important manifestation of "crack lung," characterized by acute respiratory failure and diffuse consolidation in radiography. Thermal injury may be complicated by tracheal stenosis or reactive airway disease. BOOP, pneumothorax, pneumomediastinum, and pneumoperitoneum have been reported. Chronic use may lead to reduced DLCO by an uncertain mechanism.

Marijuana

Marijuana users may develop acute and chronic bronchitis similar to tobacco smokers. Because marijuana often contains *Aspergillus*, its users may develop allergic bronchopulmonary aspergillosis and immunocompromised smokers may develop *Aspergillus* infection. Long-term use may lead to reduced DLCO.

OTHER DRUGS

Antidepressants and antipsychotic drugs have been reported to cause occasional lung toxicity, most often ARDS but occasionally hypersensitivity or BOOP.

Ethiodol used in lymphangiography and hysterosalpingography may produce a subacute ARDS picture similar to fat embolism.

Water-soluble contrast material can cause pulmonary edema if aspirated, likely because it is quite hyperosmolar.

Ionic contrast material produces acute reactions in 5% to 15% of injections, though 0.05% to 0.1% are life threatening. Nonionic contrast material produces fewer reactions, on the order of 3%.

ACE inhibitors cause a chronic nonproductive cough in up to 44% of patients, probably closer to 10%. It often begins after months of therapy, but may happen after the first dose or as late as a year. It disappears within 10 days of drug cessation. These drugs may also cause asthma, angioedema, and peripheral eosinophilia.

Hydrochlorothiazide may rarely cause hyperpermeability edema. Beta-blockers can produce a lupus-like syndrome, and importantly may produce bronchospasm. A large number of other drugs have been reported to cause lung toxicity in rare or individual cases.

POISONS

ORGANOPHOSPHATES

Organophosphate pesticide poisoning occurs commonly in farm workers during or after spraying of crops; it occurs occasionally in industry workers and in accidents and suicide attempts. Parathion and malathion may be absorbed through the skin and are converted in the liver to metabolites that inhibit nerve-ending acetyl cholinesterase. This results in initial hyperstimulation and subsequent inhibition of nerve transmission, and symptoms develop within 5 minutes to 24 hours depending on dose. The nerve action leads to miosis, diaphoresis, salivation, bronchorrhea, bronchoconstriction, bradycardia, and hyperperistalsis. Neurogenic muscle fasciculations lead to paralysis, including of the diaphragm. CNS cholinergic receptor stimulation and subsequent inhibition leads to depression and coma.

PARAQUAT

This bipyridylium herbicide (Gramoxone, Weedol, Orthoparaquat, Orthodualparaquat, and Ortho-spot) may be ingested in accidents or suicide attempts, or absorbed through the skin. It may produce respiratory failure from acute exposure, and prolonged absorption of low concentrations may produce lung damage. Its mechanism is believed to be oxidative damage, and it primarily affects type I alveolar cells and largely spares the endothelium. Pulmonary edema and hemorrhage develop, and may result in rapid death. Those who do not die may go on to develop DAD and fibrosis, which may be progressive.

OTHERS

Carbamate insecticides may cause asthma. Propoxur, a carbamylester agent, binds acetyl cholinesterase and produces symptoms similar to organophosphate toxicity. Toxaphene is a chlorinated camphene agent that is 68% chlorine. Inhalation causes allergic bronchopneumonia.

HYDROCARBONS

Five percent of childhood poisonings are hydrocarbon based, often kerosene. Although fairly common, the process is generally mild, but can uncommonly have progressive disease. Some believe that the hydrocarbon is absorbed from the GI tract and transported to the pulmonary capillaries; others believe the hydrocarbon arrives via emesis and aspiration. Regardless of its route, once in the lungs hydrocarbon produces hemorrhagic edema, necrosis, and acute inflammation. Radiographs are typically abnormal within an hour of kerosene ingestion but abnormalities may take longer to develop with other hydrocarbons. Patchy alveolar opacities, predominantly basilar, may develop, and the pulmonary hila may become indistinct. Resolution tends to be a slow process that lags clinical improvement; pneumatocele formation is a common sequela.

INHALED SUBSTANCES

Many gases, fumes, and aerosols provoke pulmonary irritation and/or damage. Most of the time capillary damage results in pulmonary edema, but in some cases the bronchi and bronchioles are the site of chemical damage. After the acute insult obliterative bronchiolitis may develop.

OXYGEN, OZONE, AND NITROGEN DIOXIDE

These oxidants produce reactive oxygen species that damage lipids, DNA, and proteins. Hyperoxia (including iatrogenic oxygen administration) provokes intracellular oxygen free radical production, and the cellular damage produces bronchoconstriction, mucus secretion, decreased surfactant function, and increased permeability. Changes may appear within 24 hours: Type I cells may be swell or desquamate, and type II cells proliferate. After prolonged administration macrophage function and intrapulmonary immune defense are impaired.

The oxygen concentration that leads to toxicity is unknown, but FIO_2 of 50% can be tolerated for long periods without irreversible damage.

Ozone does not cause a serious acute response, but chronic exposure to even low levels of ozone (which is a major constituent of smog) produces toxicity: cilia swell and mat; collagen production increases; epithelial hyperplasia and macrophage aggregation occur; and reversible fibroblast and macrophage accumulation occur.

Nitrogen dioxide exposure is responsible for silo-filler disease; fresh material in newly filled silos produces nitric oxide that oxidizes to form nitrogen dioxide. Early injury is characterized by abrupt onset of cough, dyspnea, and a choking feeling; pathologically, there is bronchiolitis and peribronchiolitis, occasionally with alveolar damage. Pulmonary edema can develop but usually clears without permanent damage if the patient survives. In the subacute phase, which lasts 2 to 5 weeks, constitutional symptoms and shortness of breath may persist, and the chest radiograph is normal. In the late phase, after 5 weeks, obliterative bronchiolitis may develop, characterized by development of multiple nodular opacities of varying size.

SULFUR DIOXIDE

On exposure to moist tissues, sulfur dioxide becomes sulfuric acid, which causes direct mucosal injury. In addition to its presence as an environmental pollutant, high accidental exposures may be found in pulp and paper factories, refrigeration plants, and fruit-preserving factories. Exposure may produce a similar triphasic response to nitrogen dioxide.

HYDROGEN SULFIDE

Sulfide ions act as direct cytotoxins by binding to mitochondrial cytochrome oxidase and inhibiting electron transport. This compound is responsible for a rotten-eggs odor at 0.2 ppm. At 250 ppm the compound produces keratoconjunctivitis, bronchitis, and pulmonary edema, and at higher concentrations it affects the CNS. Several people have died from acute exposures to high concentrations produced by decaying organic matter; if the patient survives pulmonary sequelae are not usual.

AMMONIA

Inhalation of ammonia leads to serosanguineous and purulent secretion production, and inflammation and desquamation of large bronchi. Bronchiectasis and obliterative bronchiolitis may develop after the acute exposure. Even household ammonia is strong enough to cause esophageal necrosis and ARDS if ingested.

CHLORINE

Acute exposure to high concentration causes pulmonary edema, epithelial necrosis, and bronchial inflammation.

PHOSGENE

Carbon oxychloride is a colorless dense gas that when inhaled splits into hydrochloric acid and carbon dioxide. The acid then produces necrosis of the epithelium and pulmonary edema. There is often a delay of several hours after exposure before dyspnea develops, but pulmonary edema can kill the patient within 24 hours.

FORMALDEHYDE

Formaldehyde compounds are used in wood adhesives and foam housing insulation. Exposure may produce upper-respiratory symptoms, but no acute or chronic respiratory impairment has been found.

METAL FUMES

Fumes of mercury, zinc, manganese, cadmium, nickel, and vanadium can cause acute tracheobronchitis, ARDS, interstitial pneumonitis, and "fume fever" characterized by thirst, metallic taste, substantial tightness, headache, fever, chills, muscle aches, increased BAL TNF, and neutrophilic alveolitis. Symptoms usually appear within 12 hours, and resolve within 24, without sequelae.

BURNS

Pulmonary complication incidence is directly proportional to burn severity. Direct heat trauma may severely damage the upper respiratory mucosa, with symptoms developing particularly in the first 24 hours. Cyanide and hydrochloric acid cause tissue damage. Patients may develop edema after 12 to 48 hour latency; and may develop intravascular fibrin thrombi and intra-alveolar hemorrhage. After 2 to 5 days atelectasis, edema, and pneumonia may develop, and later than that, PTE and ARDS may develop.

SUGGESTED READING

Akira M, Ishikawa H, Yamamoto S. Drug-induced pneumonitis: thin-section CT findings in 60 patients [published online ahead of print]. *Radiology.* 2002;224:852-860. doi:10.1148/radiol.2243011236.

Hagan IG, Burney K. Radiology of recreational drug abuse. *Radiographics.* 2007;27:919-940.

Johkoh T, Müller NL, Akira M, et al. Eosinophilic lung diseases: diagnostic accuracy of thin-section CT in 111 patients. *Radiology.* 2000;216:773.

Restrepo CS, Carrillo JA, Martínez S, et al. Pulmonary complications from cocaine and cocaine-based substances: imaging manifestations. *Radiographics.* 2007;27:941-956.

Rossi SE, Erasmus JJ, Page McAdams H, et al. Pulmonary drug toxicity: radiologic and pathologic manifestations. *Radiographics.* 2000;20:1245-1259.

QUESTIONS AND ANSWERS

1. Which of the following is *not* a type of pulmonary drug reaction?
   A. Bronchospasm
   B. SLE-like syndrome
   C. Scleroderma-like syndrome
   D. Interstitial pneumonitis

   ANSWER: C. Drug reactions may be categorized into one or more of six types: bronchospasm, SLE-like syndrome, responses from illicit drug abuse, eosinophilic reactions, interstitial or airspace pneumonitis, or pulmonary edema from increased permeability.

2. Regarding bleomycin toxicity, which of the following is *true*?
   A. It produces myelosuppression.
   B. It produces a dose-related lung toxicity.
   C. Radiographic changes are less common than symptoms.
   D. It produces a dose-unrelated lung toxicity.

   ANSWER: B. Although bleomycin does not produce myelosuppression like many other chemotherapeutic agents, many patients will develop dose-related lung toxicity. Overall incidence is 3% to 5%, but above 450 units of drug incidence is 13% to 17%. Radiographic changes are more common than symptoms, and CT changes are more common still.

3. What is the most common form of pulmonary bleomycin toxicity?
   A. Central and superior ground glass opacity.
   B. Subpleural and posterior predominant findings.
   C. Apical-predominant reticulonodular disease.
   D. It is inapparent.

   ANSWER: B. Bilateral basilar reticular/reticulonodular/nodular opacities are often peripheral and often involve or are confined to the costophrenic angles. More severe disease extends upward in the lungs or evolves to airspace consolidation. CT or HRCT may reveal focal consolidation or dense irregular lines; in mild disease, as in radiography, the findings are subpleural and posterior, with disease spreading with increasing severity.

4. Regarding amiodarone toxicity, which of the following is *true*?
   A. Most concentrated in the liver
   B. Unrelated to dose
   C. Associated with chronic inflammation
   D. Radiograph may reveal dense nodules

   ANSWER: C. Amiodarone accumulates in various organs but is most concentrated in the lungs—up to seven times more concentrated than in other body tissues. Up to 5% to 7% of patients taking amiodarone develop lung toxicity, and of those, 5% to 10% will die. Its pathogenicity is uncertain; it is, though, dose related. There is often chronic inflammation and septal fibrosis, type II hyperplasia, and macrophage accumulation. Radiographs often show diffuse bilateral reticular or alveolar opacities, often peripheral and often upper-lung predominant, resembling chronic eosinophilic pneumonia.

5. Regarding organophosphate poisoning, which of the following is *true*?
   A. Results from acetyl cholinesterase inhibition
   B. Most commonly occurs as childhood poisoning
   C. Associated with reactive oxygen species
   D. Related to direct mucosal injury by a metabolite

   ANSWER: A. Organophosphate pesticide poisoning occurs commonly in farm workers during or after spraying of crops; it occurs occasionally in industry workers, and in accidents and suicide attempts. Parathion and malathion may be absorbed through the skin, and are converted in the liver to metabolites that inhibit nerve-ending acetyl cholinesterase. This results in initial hyperstimulation and subsequent inhibition of nerve transmission, and symptoms develop within 5 minutes to 24 hours depending on dose. Neurogenic muscle fasciculations lead to paralysis, including of the diaphragm. CNS cholinergic receptor stimulation and subsequent inhibition leads to depression and coma.

6. Which of the following is responsible for silo-filler disease?
   A. Nitrogen dioxide
   B. Sulfur dioxide
   C. Ozone
   D. Hydrogen sulfide

   ANSWER: A. Nitrogen dioxide exposure is responsible for silo-filler disease: fresh material in newly filled silos produces nitric oxide that oxidizes to form nitrogen dioxide. Sulfur dioxide is an environmental pollutant and may produce accidental exposures in some industries. Ozone does not cause a serious acute response.

7. What is the latency of pulmonary edema in burn patients?
   A. Immediate
   B. 2–5 days

C. 12–48 hours
D. There is no edema

ANSWER: C. Direct heat trauma may severely damage the upper respiratory mucosa, with symptoms developing particularly in the first 24 hours. Patients may develop edema after 12 to 48 hour latency; and may develop intravascular fibrin thrombi and intra-alveolar hemorrhage. After 2 to 5 days atelectasis, edema, and pneumonia may develop, and later than that, PTE and ARDS may develop.

8. Regarding hydrocarbon poisoning, which of the following is *true*?
   A. Generally a mild process.
   B. Radiographic resolution is rapid.
   C. Produces chronic inflammation and fibrosis.
   D. Radiographic abnormality is more delayed with kerosene than other hydrocarbons.

   ANSWER: A. Although fairly common, hydrocarbon poisoning is generally mild. Once in the lungs, hydrocarbon produces hemorrhagic edema, necrosis, and acute inflammation. Radiographs are typically abnormal within an hour of kerosene ingestion but abnormalities may take longer to develop with other hydrocarbons. Patchy alveolar opacities, predominantly basilar, may develop, and the pulmonary hila may become indistinct. Resolution tends to be a slow process that lags clinical improvement; pneumatocele formation is a common sequela.

9. Concerning lung toxicity secondary to diphenylhydantoin, which of the following is the best descriptor?
   A. Pathognomonic radiographic appearance
   B. Disorder of membrane deposition
   C. Associated with mesothelioma
   D. An acute hypersensitivity reaction

   ANSWER: D. Diphenylhydantoin may produce an acute hypersensitivity reaction with peripheral eosinophilia and diffuse reticulonodular interstitial disease that resolves within 2 weeks of stopping therapy. Mediastinal lymphadenopathy may develop; though this is often reactive, the incidence of lymphoma in patients on this drug is increased up to ten times. Rarely airspace consolidation or miliary nodules may develop.

10. Regarding methotrexate therapy, which of the following is *true*?
    A. Incidence of lung toxicity is 2% to 5% for low-dose therapy.
    B. Duration of therapy is not a risk factor for lung toxicity development.
    C. Lung toxicity is generally irreversible.
    D. Radiographic appearance is nonspecific.

    ANSWER: A. Methotrexate is used both in cancers and as disease-modifying therapy in several autoimmune diseases. The incidence of reaction is estimated at 2% to 5% for low-dose therapy as with rheumatoid arthritis. Frequency, dose, and duration are risk factors, as is preexisting lung disease. Unlike many other agents, methotrexate-induced lung disease is often reversible; it is generally a hypersensitivity reaction, evidenced by eosinophilia and pulmonary granuloma or eosinophil infiltration. The radiographic appearance is characteristic. Initially a basilar or diffuse reticular or ground glass opacity develops, which develops rapidly into patchy consolidation before reverting to interstitial opacity and then resolves.

Section 3
CARDIAC

34 CARDIAC MRI TECHNIQUE

Satinder P. Singh

INTRODUCTION

Cardiac MR imaging has evolved over the last decade from traditional spin echo sequences to spoiled gradient echo and balanced steady-state free precession sequences obtained during breath-hold. These developments allow evaluation of ventricle function, perfusion and viability, flow quantification, coronary MR angiography, and better morphologic assessment of the heart. Various cardiac MR sequences are listed in Table 34-1.

TABLE 34-1 Cardiac MR Sequences and Their Use

TECHNIQUE	USES
ECG-gated spin echo	Morphology
Cine GRE	Morphology, cardiac dimensions and volumes, global and regional functions of left and right ventricles
Fast (turbo) GRE	Regional myocardial (relative) perfusion, rapid imaging of great vessels
Segmented fast (turbo) GRE	Morphology (including coronary arteries), cardiac dimensions and volumes, global and regional functions of left and right ventricles
Velocity-encoded cine GRE	Valvular function (quantification of regurgitation, estimation of peak valvular gradient), measurement of stroke volume and cardiac output of both ventricles, quantification of shunts, measurement of differential flow in right and left pulmonary arteries, quantification of gradients of stenosis or coarctation of great arteries
Echoplanar	Global and regional function of left and right ventricles, quantification of regional myocardial blood volume and perfusion

DARK OR BLACK BLOOD TECHNIQUE

Fast flow blood is black or of low-signal intensity in these sequences and provides excellent anatomic delineation of blood vessel lumen and cardiac chambers. Examples of such technique include conventional spin echo, breath-hold turbo, or fast spin echo (TSE, FSE) and half Fourier turbo spin echo sequence with double inversion recovery (IR) pulses to suppress blood signal (HASTE, double–IR TSE-FSE).

BRIGHT BLOOD TECHNIQUE

Flowing blood is white or of high-signal intensity in gradient recalled echo sequence (GRE). Examples of such technique include fast low-angled shot (Turbo FLASH), fast spoiled gradient recalled echo, turbo field echo, and fast field echo. Cine GRE sequences produce a motion picture loop through various phases of the cardiac cycle.

Newer, fast, short TE GRE sequences with completely refocused gradients provide excellent contrast between the myocardium and blood flow. Examples of such sequences include true FISP, balanced fast field echo, or FIESTA. The true FISP type sequences are very useful for segmenting the myocardium from the blood flow and are excellent for the functional assessment of the myocardium. Standard GRE sequence should be used in the assessment of cardiac valves or when attempting to identify intracardiac shunts.

VELOCITY-ENCODED CINE MR IMAGING

Velocity-encoded cine (VEC) MR imaging is used for the quantitative assessment of flow dynamics across valves and in congenital heart disease. This is a phase-contrast sequence, which is used to assess the vessel of interest in a plane perpendicular to the flow vector. Magnitude and phase VEC images are obtained in a plane perpendicular to the direction of flow in the vessel. To determine flow volume across a vessel lumen, spatial mean velocity of the vessel of interest is multiplied by the cross-sectional area of the vessel. The pressure gradient is estimated with the modified Bernoulli equation: $P = 4v^2$, where v = peak flow velocity in m/s and P = peak pressure gradient in mm Hg.

CARDIAC IMAGING PLANES

The three standard orthogonal planes used for cardiac imaging are axial, sagittal, and coronal. Two additional imaging planes parallel or orthogonal to the cardiac axes are the short and the long axis of the heart.

Examination usually begins with a dark blood anatomic survey examination in one or more planes: axial, sagittal, and coronal.

1. Scout images are done on the axial plane and display normal anatomy of the heart and great vessels, which is especially useful in evaluating congenital heart disease.
2. The coronal and sagittal planes are useful for viewing the aortic valve, the entrance of pulmonary veins into the left atrium, and the extension of pericardium, and so on. Double oblique (oblique sagittal) planes through the pulmonary trunk and aorta are useful for demonstrating pulmonary and aortic valve and their respective outflow tracks.
3. The vertical long-axis plane (two-chamber view) is used to evaluate the left heart structures including mitral valve. This plane is prescribed from an axial image.
4. The horizontal long-axis plane (four-chamber view) displays the relationship of the four cardiac chambers to each other on a single image. A cine GRE image in this plane demonstrates mitral, tricuspid, and aortic valve functions as well as right and left ventricular contraction. This image plane can be prescribed from the left ventricular long-axis or two-chamber view as well as oblique transverse imaging through a short-axis scout.
5. The short-axis plane demonstrates the true cross-sectional dimensions of the cardiac chambers, with the initial chamber viewed through the papillary muscle and subsequent views toward the heart apex and base. Cine GRE images allow quantification of systolic myocardial wall thickening. This plane is also used for quantifying left and right ventricular volume and mass and ventricular ejection fraction.
6. The long-axis view through aortic and mitral valve is usually prescribed from a coronal image. This plane demonstrates both the aortic and mitral valves and demonstrates or displays portions of the left ventricle, right ventricle, left atrium, right atrium, and ascending aorta. Therefore, it is sometimes known as the five-chamber view or LVOT view.

MYOCARDIAL PERFUSION AND VIABILITY

Imaging to determine myocardial perfusion and viability is performed using first-pass myocardial turbo flash type sequences with rapidly establishing T1 contrast for multiple slices with high-temporal resolution. Depending on the "RR" interval, 3 to 5 slice positions can be obtained over multiple phases. Underperfused myocardium is seen as a low-signal area due to either ischemia or infarction.

Single-slice inversion recovery turbo flash, true FISP, or newer three-dimensional IR prepared sequences are used for delayed imaging, usually 10 to 15 minutes after contrast injection. An infarcted area shows delayed contrast enhancement on T1-weighted images.

With these sequences, selection of the IR pulse is the key to suppress (null) the signal from the normal myocardium. Usually, between 200 and 300 milliseconds, the optimal IR pulse is dependent upon the dose of contrast given and the length of delay after contrast injection.

TAGGED MYOCARDIAL IMAGING FOR WALL MOTION ABNORMALITY OR CONSTRICTIVE PERICARDITIS

Saturated tagged sequences are obtained in short-axis as well as long-axis views. The saturation bands appear as dark lines that deform during ventricular muscle contraction. An area of nondeformation suggests lack of muscle contraction or pericardial adhesions from constrictive pericarditis.

SUGGESTED READING

Finn JP, Nael K, Deshpande V, Ratib O, Laub G. Cardiac MR imaging: State of the technology. *Radiology.* 2006;241(2): 338–354.

Hom JF, Ordovas K, Reddy GP. Coarctation: functional assessment of hemodynamic events. *RadioGraphics.* 2008;28: 407–416.

Kellenberger CF, Yoo SF, Valsangiacomo B. Cardiovascular MR imaging in neonates and infants with congenital heart disease. *RadioGraphics.* 2007;27:5–18.

Pons-Lado, G. Assessment of cardiac function by CMR. *Eur Radiol Suppl.* 2005;15(2):B23–B32.

Saremi F, Grizzard JD, Kim RF. Optimizing cardiac MR imaging: practical remedies for artifacts. *RadioGraphics.* 2008;28: 1161–1187.

QUESTIONS AND ANSWERS

1. Which of the following is used for quantifying ventricular function?
   A. Vertical long axis
   B. Short axis
   C. Horizontal long axis
   D. Sagittal plane

   ANSWER: B. Vertical long-axis plane (two-chamber view) is used to evaluate the left heart structures including the mitral valve. Horizontal long-axis plane (four-chamber view) displays the relationships of four cardiac chambers to each other on a single image. A cine GRE image in this plane demonstrates mitral, tricuspid, and aortic valve functions as well as right and left ventricular contraction. Short-axis plane shows the true cross-sectional dimensions of the cardiac chambers. Cine GRE images allow quantification of systolic myocardial wall thickening, and this plane is also used for quantifying left and right ventricular volume and mass and ventricular ejection fraction. Coronal and sagittal planes are useful for evaluating the aortic valve, the entrance of pulmonary veins into the left atrium, and the extension of pericardium.

2. If the myocardium demonstrates decreased signal on fast turbo first-pass GRE and no enhancement on delayed single-slice inversion recovery turbo flash images, what is the diagnosis?
   A. Ischemia
   B. Infarction
   C. Normal
   D. Myocarditis

   ANSWER: A. Underperfused myocardium is seen as a low-signal area because of either ischemia or infarction in the first-pass imaging. Single-slice inversion recovery turbo flash, true FISP, or newer three-dimensional IR prepared sequences are used for delayed imaging, usually 10 to 15 minutes after contrast injection. Infarcted areas show delayed contrast enhancement on T1-weighted images, and the ischemic region will be isointense with the rest of the myocardium. Myocarditis shows regions of patchy hyperenhancement of the myocardium but usually shows no perfusion abnormality in the first-pass images.

3. Which of the following is used to determine the pressure gradient across stenosis?
   A. Fast spin echo
   B. Turbo FLASH
   C. Velocity-encoded cine MR imaging
   D. Tagged myocardial imaging

   ANSWER: C. Fast spin echo is an example of a dark blood spin-echo sequence where fast flow blood appears as black or of low-signal intensity. It provides excellent anatomic delineation of blood vessel lumen and cardiac chambers. In the bright blood technique, the flowing blood is "white" or of high-signal intensity. Cine GRE sequences produce a motion picture loop through various phases of the cardiac cycle. Examples include fast low-angled shot (Turbo FLASH), fast spoiled gradient recalled echo, turbo field echo, and fast field echo. For quantitative assessment of flow dynamics across valves and in CHD, velocity-encoded cine MR imaging is used. This is a phase-contrast sequence used to assess the vessel of interest in a plane perpendicular to the flow vector. In tagged myocardial imaging, saturated tagged sequences are obtained in short-axis as well as long-axis views. The saturation bands appear as dark lines that deform during ventricular muscle contraction. An area of nondeformation suggests a lack of muscle contraction or pericardial adhesions from constrictive pericarditis.

35 CYANOTIC CONGENITAL HEART DISEASE

Satinder P. Singh

INTRODUCTION

Cyanotic heart disease is a heart defect, present at birth (congenital), that results in low blood oxygen levels. The defect affects the structure or function of the heart or vessels, and there may be more than one defect (Tables 35-1 and 35-2).

TABLE 35-1 Cyanotic Congenital Heart Disease with Decreased Pulmonary Vascularity

Tetralogy of Fallot
Tricuspid atresia
Pulmonary atresia
Pulmonary stenosis and atrial septic defect
Ebstein anomaly

TABLE 35-2 Cyanotic Congenital Heart Disease with Increased Pulmonary Vascularity

Total anomalous pulmonary venous connection (TAPVC)
Truncus arteriosus
Transposition of great arteries
Single ventricle
Double outlet right ventricle

TETRALOGY OF FALLOT

Tetralogy of Fallot (TOF) is the most common cyanotic congenital heart malformation (beyond *neonatal* period) and accounts for 6% to 10% cases of congenital heart disease (CHD). The most common neonatal cyanotic CHD is transposition of the great arteries. Four anatomic features of TOF include a right ventricular outflow track obstruction, ventricular septal defect (VSD), aorta overriding VSD communicating with left ventricle (LV) and right ventricle (RV), and right ventricular hypertrophy.

A failure of the conal septum to fuse with the septal band leads to anatomic malformation. The infundibular septum deviates anteriorly and cephalad from its normal position. The most common type of VSD in TOF is perimembranous; the next most common is muscular VSD, and the least common VSD is within the ventricular outlet.

The pulmonary trunk is usually smaller than normal, and there is a variable degree of stenosis involving the trunk and the right and left pulmonary arteries. Often hypoplasia of the right and left pulmonary arteries is present. Left pulmonary artery stenosis is more common than right.

Common anomalies associated with TOF include patent ductus arteriosus (PDA), multiple VSDs, atrial septal defect/patent foramina ovale (pentalogy of Fallot), and the presence of left superior venous cava (SVC) and anomalous origin of the left common artery from the right coronary artery. Associated extracardiac anomalies include DiGeorge syndrome, Klippel-Feil syndrome, and VACTERL and CHARGE associations.

Pulmonary atresia with VSD is a variant of TOF in which the communication between the RV and the pulmonary artery is lost; this condition is often called pseudotruncus arteriosus or truncus arteriosus type IV. The VSD is usually juxta-aortic, and the RV is hypertrophied. Although the patients usually appear normal at birth, the infant becomes cyanotic after several hours because of closure of the ductus arteriosus.

CLINICAL PRESENTATION

Patients with TOF present with cyanosis, depending on the degree of pulmonary stenosis present. In the milder form, cyanosis develops only with exertion, resulting in a delay of symptoms and therefore delayed presentation later in childhood. Patients with severe stenosis or pulmonary atresia are severely cyanotic after the closure of the ductus and are dependent on aortopulmonary collaterals.

On examination there is a moderate systolic ejection murmur, which disappears during a hypoxic spell. Patients with aortopulmonary collaterals have continuous murmurs. Associated polycythemia and clubbing occurs, usually in older children.

RADIOGRAPHY

Depending on the degree of pulmonary stenosis, the heart size may be normal or slightly enlarged with right ventricular enlargement visible on chest radiography. The pulmonary trunk is not obvious, and central pulmonary arteries are usually small. Decreased and asymmetric pulmonary vascularity are common, are often due to system-pulmonary collaterals from peripheral pulmonary artery stenosis, or are due to prior palliative shunt. A right aortic arch is seen in 25% to 50% of the patients. However, the natural history is determined by the severity of the right ventricular outflow track; 25% of untreated infants die in the first year of life.

TREATMENT

Very young infants with a complicated morphology can be managed with a staged shunt (usually modified Blalock-Taussig) procedure. Progressive hypoxemia and recurrent spells are common indications for elective repair. Patients with TOF and pulmonary stenosis without symptoms and uncomplicated morphology usually undergo elective repair between 3 and 24 months of age.

The goal of surgery for TOF with pulmonary atresia is to repair the defect and provide blood flow from the RV to as many pulmonary segments as possible. Surgical options include shunting and second-stage repair to relieve RVOD obstruction and to leave the VSD open. Residual VSD can be closed after further development of pulmonary vasculature. Ligation of the aortopulmonary collateral is required.

Risk factors for early death from TOF include very young age of diagnosis, severity of annular hypoplasia, small size of pulmonary arteries, high peak RV–LV pressure ratios, multiple VSDs, and coexisting cardiac anomalies. Survival rate at the age of 5 years is about 90%. A 25-year survival rate of 90% or better is common with complete correction of TOF. Late complications usually occur from pulmonary valve insufficiency and right ventricular dysfunction.

TRANSPOSITION OF GREAT ARTERIES (D-TGA)

Complete TGA is a combination of concordant atrioventricular and discordant ventriculoarterial connections. This is the most common cyanotic heart disease in the newborn. The aorta is anterior and slightly rightward. The left and right ventricular outflow tracks are parallel. (Normally they cross each other diagonally.) A significant VSD is present in approximately 30% of patients.

The right and left coronary arteries arise from the right and left posterior cusp facing the pulmonary artery. If the VSD is small, or the septum is intact, the newborn is intensely cyanotic and often needs balloon atrial septostomy (Rashkind procedure). If a large VSD is present, cyanosis is usually less intense, but early heart failure occurs.

RADIOGRAPHY

In a newborn with TGA and an intact ventricular septum, the heart size is normal with mild plethora and an egg-shaped cardiac silhouette on a narrow vascular pedicle (Table 35-3). The pedicle is narrowed because of the posterior medial location of the pulmonary trunk.

If a large VSD is present, the heart is often dilated with increased pulmonary shunt vascularity (Table 35-4). In patients with left ventricular outflow tract (LVOT) obstruction, the pulmonary vascularity is decreased.

Two-dimensional echocardiography can provide most of the important information to evaluate cases of TGA. However, coronary arteries may need further evaluation with selective angiography, which is also needed to determine other associated cardiovascular anomalies.

TABLE 35-3 Imaging Signs of Various Congenital Heart Defects

ANOMALIES	INDICATING SIGN
Transposition of great arteries	Egg-on-a-string sign
TAPVR	Snowman sign
Partial anomalous pulmonary venous return	Scimitar sign
Endocardial cushion defect	Gooseneck sign at left ventricular angiography
Tetralogy of Fallot	Boot-shaped heart
Aortic coarctation	Figure of 3 and reverse figure of 3, (indentation on esophagus filled with barium)
Ebstein anomaly	Box-shaped heart

TABLE 35-4 Cyanosis with Shunt Vascularity ("T Lesions")

Transposition of great arteries (most common)
Truncus arteriosus
TAPVC
Tingles (single ventricle or atrium)
Tricuspid atresia without RVOT obstruction

SURGICAL TREATMENT

Palliative procedures for treating TGA include the creation of an atrial septal defect (ASD), to ensure adequate admixture of blood, and pulmonary artery banding in patients with VSD and TGA where surgical correction early in life is not possible. Banding is performed to reduce the pressure in the pulmonary circulation to prevent development of obstructive pulmonary vascular disease.

Complete repair of TGA includes performing Senning-Mustard, Rastelli, and Jantene procedures. The atrial switch operation (Senning-Mustard procedure) involves rerouting of the systemic venous return to the left atrium through a surgically created channel after resection of the atrial septum. The pulmonary venous return is directed to the right atrium. Complications of atrial switch operation include stenosis of the connection of the inferior or superior vena cava to the left atrium or right pulmonary vein to the right atrium. Transventricular rerouting of the left ventricular outflow (Rastelli procedure) is possible in patients with VSD without LVOT obstruction. VSD is closed by a patch so that the LV is joined to the right ventricular outflow and to the aorta. The pulmonary trunk is ligated and divided, and an external conduit is put in place between the RV and the pulmonary trunk.

In the three-stage arterial switch procedure (Jantene procedure), the great arteries are transected above the sinus of Valsalva, the aorta is reconnected to the pulmonary root, and the pulmonary artery is reconnected to the original aortic root. The coronary arteries are then detached from the aortic root with a cuff and translocated to a new arterial trunk.

Late complications of the arterial switch operation include stenosis in the right ventricular outflow track, stenosis in the pulmonary trunk, stenosis in the middle portion of the ascending aorta, and stenosis of the coronary arteries.

CONGENITALLY CORRECTED TRANSPOSITION (L-TGA)

Congenital correction of TGA consists of a discordant ventriculoarterial connection and a discordant atrioventricular connection. The aorta is anterior and to the left of pulmonary artery. The ventricles are inverted. The LV with its mitral valve lies to the right, posteriorly and inferiorly to the RV. Both ventricular outflow tracks are side by side and do not cross each other. Cardiac apex is mostly on the left. In 25% of cases of L-TGA, there is dextrocardia. Associated anomalies include VSD, which is present in 80% of hearts with perimembranous defects most common, and often the defect is large. The tricuspid left-sided valve is abnormal in the majority of hearts. The most common anomaly is leaflet dysplasia and the least common is Ebstein anomaly. Other important associated conditions include coarctation, interruption of the aortic arch, PDA, and pulmonary outflow track obstruction.

The coronary arteries arise from the posterior cusp. The right-sided coronary artery has morphology of the normal left coronary artery with LAD and circumflex branches, and the left-sided right coronary artery arises from the left cusp and distributes over the RV. Clinical presentation depends on the pulmonary blood flow and the associated intracardiac anomaly. Diagnosis is made by echo and catheterization.

TREATMENT

Treatment includes a double switch procedure: atrial switch (Senning or Mustard) and arterial switch or Rastelli repair.

TOTAL ANOMALOUS PULMONARY VENOUS CONNECTION

All pulmonary veins drain into the right atrium, either directly or via tributaries, in cases of total anomalous pulmonary venous connection (TAPVC). A patent foramen ovale or an ASD is present and necessary for postnatal survival. Four major types of TAPVC include supracardiac (45%) to the SVC or tributaries; cardiac (25%) to the coronary sinus or right atrium; infracardiac (25%) to portal vein, ductus venosus, or a tributary; and mixed (5%) anomalous connection to multiple sites.

The infracardiac TAPVC is frequently associated with pulmonary venous obstruction (Table 35-5), which could be due to high resistance of hepatic parenchymal circulation, physiologic compression at the esophageal hiatus due to diaphragmatic contraction or during swallowing, or area of stenosis within the common vein or its junction with the portal vein.

TABLE 35-5 Pulmonary Edema in Newborn

Total anomalous pulmonary venous return with obstruction
Left hypoplastic heart
Transient tachypnea of the newborn

TABLE 35-6 Atrial Isomerism

FEATURES	RIGHT-SIDEDNESS	LEFT-SIDEDNESS
Spleen	Asplenia	Polysplenia
Systemic venous anomalies	Uncommon	Azygous continuation of IVC interruption, bilateral SVCs
Pulmonary venous anomalies	TAPVC	Rare
Ventriculoarterial connections	Discordant, DORV 30%	DORV 35%
ASD/VSD	AVSD	AVSD
Pulmonary outflow	Obstructed in majority	Less common obstruction

In supracardiac TAPVC, the vertical vein connecting the common pulmonary vein to the left innominate vein can pass anterior to the pulmonary artery or between the left main bronchus and left pulmonary artery or left main pulmonary artery resulting in obstruction to the pulmonary venous flow.

Intracardiac TAPVC is frequently associated with atrial isomerism (polysplenia or asplenia syndrome) (Table 35-6).

RADIOGRAPHIC APPEARANCE

- When there is no pulmonary venous obstruction (usually supracardiac and cardiac variety), the heart is enlarged and there is increased pulmonary shunt vascularity. In supracardiac TAPVC, dilated systemic veins (vertical vein, innominate vein, and dilated right SVC) form part of the head of the snowman configuration, the body being formed by enlarged cardiac mass (Table 35-3). The intracardiac TAPVC mimics left-to-right shunt at the atrial level with cyanosis.
- In patients with pulmonary venous obstruction (usually the infracardiac variety), the heart is of normal size. Pulmonary venous hypertension and pulmonary edema are present. The differential diagnosis for these findings include noncardiac diseases such as aspiration, transient tachypnea of the newborn, and respiratory distress syndrome. In patients with severe obstructions, the infant will be critically ill with tachypnea, hypoxemia, and metabolic acidosis.

Echocardiography can trace all pulmonary venous connections. Chest CTA can also nicely demonstrate the anomalous pulmonary venous connections. However, catheterization will delineate the exact anatomy, evaluate the degree of pulmonary venous obstruction and hypertension, and identify other associated structural intracardiac abnormalities.

TREATMENT

Obstructed TAPVC is a surgical emergency. Nonobstructed TAPVC requires prompt repair to prevent rapid deterioration, sequelae of cyanosis, and volume overload of the heart and lungs. The corrective procedure is reconnection of pulmonary vein to the left atrium. The surgical death rate is greatest for the infradiaphragmatic type.

TRICUSPID ATRESIA

In cases of tricuspid atresia (TA), the right atrioventricular valve is atretic with obligatory admixture in the left atrium. The RV is small and the chamber is incomplete (missing inlet portion). A VSD is present in the majority (60%) of cases and is located in the trabecular septum. Patients with large VSDs have increased pulmonary shunt vascularity.

Patients are usually cyanotic from birth due to atrial right-to-left shunt and decreased pulmonary blood flow due to right ventricular outflow tract (RVOT) obstruction or restrictive VSD. Patients with TA and large VSDs are usually asymptomatic at birth and develop increased shunt vascularity progressing to heart failure in later life.

RADIOGRAPHY

The radiographic appearance of TA is quite variable. It may resemble TOF or occasionally the radiograph is normal. In patients with TA and concordant ventriculoarterial connections, pulmonary vascularity is decreased with hypoplasia of RVOT. In patients with discordant ventriculoarterial connections, pulmonary plethora is present along with cardiomegaly and a narrow pedicle.

Left juxtaposition of the atrial appendages is a common association and appears as a bulge in the left midcardiac silhouette simulating enlarged left atrial appendage. CT and MRI reveal no right atrioventricular connections, hypoplastic RV, large LV, or ASD.

TREATMENT

Surgical repair procedures include the Glenn, bidirectional Glenn, and Fontan-Kreutzer procedures (atriopulmonary connection).

EBSTEIN MALFORMATION

Ebstein malformation is a congenital anomaly of the tricuspid valve leaflet with septal leaflet displacement downward and toward the apex. There is physiologic atrialization of the right ventricular inlet segment with thinning of the atrialized myocardium. The right AV orifice and right atria are enlarged. Usually, the posterior and septal leaflets are displaced with a variable degree of valvular dysplasia commonly associated with tricuspid insufficiency due to dilatation of the tricuspid annulus and RV. There is dilatation of the right atrium as well as atrialized portion of the RV, which may pulsate paradoxically in ventricular systole. The left atrium and LVs are usually normal.

The most commonly associated anomalies are pulmonary stenosis, atresia, patent foramen ovale or ASD, and Wolff-Parkinson-White syndrome. There is a high incidence of this anomaly in patients with a history of ingesting lithium during early pregnancy.

RADIOGRAPHY

A chest radiograph will reveal a box-shaped heart with a narrow pedicle (Table 35-7). The predominant feature is dilatation of the right atrium and right ventricular outflow track. In a cyanotic patient, pulmonary vascularity is decreased because of atrial right-to-left shunt. Differential diagnosis includes Uhl anomaly, which is a rare, focal, or complete absence of RV myocardium.

TRUNCUS ARTERIOSUS

Truncus arteriosus is a conotruncal anomaly in which a single common trunk arises from the heart through a single arterial valve and can give rise to aortic, pulmonary and coronary arteries. The typical morphologic abnormalities are single truncal valve, juxta-arterial VSD, and partial or complete deficiency of aortopulmonary septum. The truncal semilunar valve has a posterior and inferior location and annulus is usually in continuity with the mitral valve. The valve has three leaflets in the majority of patients; in the remaining patients, there are four cusps. The origin of pulmonary arteries from the truncus is variable. In type 1, a short pulmonary trunk arises from the truncus and then divides into right and left pulmonary artery. In type 2, the pulmonary trunk is absent; therefore, right and left pulmonary arteries arise directly from the truncus from the posterior aspect. In type 3, the right

TABLE 35-7 Massive Cardiac Silhouette Enlargement in Newborn

Ebstein anomaly
Uhl disease (right ventricular myocardial thinning)
Tricuspid atresia
Massive pericardial effusion
Diaphragmatic herniation into the pericardial sac

and left posterior pulmonary arteries arise separately from the lateral wall of the truncus. Type 4 is not considered as truncus but rather TOF with pulmonary atresia and origin of branch pulmonary arteries from collaterals (see Table 102-3).

The VSD of the truncus arteriosus is located in the outlet septum, immediately below the truncal valve. The aortopulmonary septum is absent or deficient. The ventricular mass is usually formed by two ventricles. Right ventricular hypertrophy is present, but the LV is usually normal unless severe truncal valve insufficiency is present. Coronary arteries arise from the sinus of Valsalva above the truncal leaflets.

RADIOGRAPHY

The heart is usually enlarged with right ventricular prominence visible on chest radiography, and pulmonary vascularity is usually increased. The vascular pedicle is narrow. The main pulmonary artery silhouette is usually absent, and the left pulmonary artery projects higher than usual. The aortic arch is right-sided in 30% to 50% of cases, usually with mirror image branching. A chest radiograph demonstrating pulmonary plethora, right aortic arch, and a high position of the left pulmonary artery in a patient with cyanosis is strongly suggestive of truncus arteriosus.

HYPOPLASTIC LEFT HEART SYNDROME

Hypoplastic left heart syndrome is characterized by hypoplasia or atresia of the ascending aorta, aortic valve, LV, and mitral valve. This is usually associated with patent ductus arteriosus and juxtaductal coarctation.

HEMODYNAMICS

Hypoplastic left heart is a ductus-dependent lesion with severe outflow obstruction and systemic hypoperfusion. Cranial and coronary perfusion is via retrograde flow from PDA into hypoplastic arch and ascending aorta. There is left-to-right shunt and admixture in the right atrium leading to severe cyanosis.

CLINICAL PRESENTATION

The clinical presentation of hypoplastic left heart syndrome involves congestive heart failure with severe cyanosis and hypoxia (Table 35-8). Poor systemic perfusion leads to metabolic acidosis, renal failure, and necrotizing enterocolitis. Death occurs within days or weeks if the patient is not treated.

TABLE 35-8 Differential Diagnosis of Congenital Heart Disease Based on Patient Age at Presentation

AGE	DIAGNOSIS
0–2 days	Hypoplastic left heart, aortic atresia, obstructed total anomalous pulmonary venous return
7–14 days	Aortic stenosis, coarctation
Infants	VSD or PDA
Adults	ASD

IMAGING

Chest radiograph will show cardiac enlargement with pulmonary venous hypertension and edema. The mediastinum is narrow due to thymic atrophy. Echocardiogram is useful for prenatal as well as postnatal diagnosis and is sufficient for treatment planning. CTA or MR is occasionally performed after staged Norwood or Stanzel procedures.

TREATMENT

Prostaglandin E-1 is initially administered in order to keep the PDA open. Rashkind balloon atrial septostomy is performed in patients with restricted foramen ovale.

Palliative procedure includes Norwood procedure, which is atrial septectomy and reconstruction of the aorta from the pulmonary artery, and a Blaylock-Taussig shunt is placed for pulmonary perfusion. The Damus-Kaye-Stanzel procedure is a variation of the Norwood procedure with side-to-side anastomosis between the pulmonary artery and the hypoplastic ascending aorta. Conversion to Hemi-Fontan (connection between SVC and right pulmonary artery) is performed at 4 to 6 months. When the patient is approximately 2 years of age, a Fontan procedure is performed to create a fenestrated venous conduit through the right atrium connecting the inferior caval flow to the right pulmonary artery.

SUGGESTED READING

Bardo DME, Frankel DG, Applegate KE, Murphy DF, Saneto DO. Hypoplastic left heart syndrome. *RadioGraphics.* 2001; 21:705-717.

Ferguson EC, Krishnamurthy RK, Oldham SAA. Classic imaging signs of congenital cardiovascular abnormalities. *RadioGraphics.* 2007;27:1323-1334.

Goo HW, Park I-S, Ko FK, et al. CT of congenital heart disease: normal anatomy and typical pathological conditions. *RadioGraphics*. 2003;23:S147-S165.

Varaprasathan GA, Araoz PA, Higgins CB, Reddy GP. Quantification of flow dynamics in congenital heart disease: applications of velocity-encoded cine MR imaging. *RadioGraphics*. 2002;22:895-906.

QUESTIONS AND ANSWERS

1. Regarding tetralogy of Fallot, which of the following is *true*?
   A. Most common neonatal cyanotic congenital heart malformation.
   B. Embryological basis is anomaly of sinus venosus.
   C. Auscultation may reveal continuous murmurs.
   D. Symptoms depend upon size of VSD.

   ANSWER: C. Tetralogy of Fallot is the most common cyanotic congenital heart malformation beyond the neonatal period. The most common neonatal cyanotic congenital heart disease is transposition. The failure of conal septum fusion with the septal band leads to two anatomic malformations and deviation of infundibular septum anteriorly and cephalad from its normal position. The clinical presentation depends upon the degree of pulmonary stenosis not the size of VSD. Patients with severe stenosis or pulmonary atresia are severely cyanotic after the closure of the ductus. Patients often develop aortopulmonary collaterals, which produce continuous murmur on auscultation.

2. Regarding treatment and prognosis of tetralogy of Fallot, which of the following is *incorrect*?
   A. Progressive hypoxemia and occurrence of spells are indications for elective repair.
   B. Presence of aortopulmonary collaterals is contraindication for surgery.
   C. Risk factor for early death include multiple VSDs and coexisting cardiac anomalies.
   D. Twenty-five-year survival rate of 90% or more is common after complete correction of tetralogy of Fallot.

   ANSWER: B. Patients with tetralogy of Fallot and pulmonary stenosis without symptoms and uncomplicated morphology usually undergo elective repair between 3 and 24 months of age. Many young infants with a complicated morphology are managed with a staged shunt procedure. However, progressive hypoxemia and occurrence of spells are common indication for early elective repair. Risk factors for early death include very young age, severity of annular hypoplasia, small size of pulmonary arteries, high peak RV–LV pressure ratios, multiple VSDs, and coexisting cardiac anomalies. A 25-year survival rate of 90% or more is quite common after complete correction of tetralogy of Fallot.

3. Which of the following is *true* regarding D-TGA?
   A. There is atrioventricular concordance and ventriculoarterial discordance.
   B. It is considered congenitally corrected transposition.
   C. The aorta is anterior and slightly leftward to pulmonary artery.
   D. Newborns are asymptomatic if the ventricular septum is intact.

   ANSWER: A. D-TGA or complete transposition of great arteries is a combination of concordant atrioventricular and discordant ventriculoarterial connections. The left and right ventricle outflow tracts are parallel with the aorta anterior and slightly rightward of the pulmonary trunk. For survival, an intracardiac defect at the ventricular or atrial septum level is a must. Newborns with intact ventricular septum are intensely cyanotic and often need emergent balloon atrial septostomy to live.

4. Regarding L-TGA, which of the following is *true*?
   A. Aorta lies to the right and anterior of pulmonary trunk.
   B. Coronary arteries arise from anterior cusps.
   C. Large muscular VSD is a common association.
   D. There is ventriculoarterial and atrioventricular discordance.

   ANSWER: D. L-TGA is congenitally corrected transposition and consists of discordant ventriculoarterial and atrioventricular connection. The aorta is anterior and to the left of the pulmonary arteries and ventricles are inverted. VSD is present in 80% of heart diseases with perimembranous defect most common. The coronary arteries arise from the posterior (not anterior) cusps; the right-sided coronary artery has morphology of the normal left coronary artery with LAD and circumflex branches, and the left-sided right coronary artery arises from the left cusp and distributes over the right ventricle.

5. What is the most common type of total anomalous pulmonary venous connection?
   A. Supracardiac
   B. Cardiac
   C. Infracardiac
   D. Mixed

   ANSWER: A. Supracardiac TAPVC is the most common type (45%) draining into SVC or its tributaries. Cardiac (25%) TAPVC connects to the coronary sinus or right atrium, and intracardiac (25%) TAPVC drains into the portal vein, ductus venosus, or a tributary. Mixed type is the least common (5%).

6. Regarding total anomalous pulmonary venous connection, which of the following is *incorrect*?
   A. Atrial isomerism is frequently associated with infracardiac TAPVC.
   B. Intracardiac TAPVC is frequently associated with pulmonary venous hypertension and edema.
   C. In patients with pulmonary venous obstruction, the heart is enlarged.
   D. Patent foremen of ovale or ASD is often present.

   ANSWER: C. Patent foramen ovale or ASD is present in TAPVC and is necessary for postnatal survival. The intracardiac TAPVC is frequently associated with pulmonary venous obstruction leading to pulmonary venous hypertension and edema on radiograph. The intracardiac TAPVC is frequently associated with atrial isomerism (polysplenia or asplenia syndrome). When there is no pulmonary venous obstruction, heart is enlarged and there is increased shunt vascularity. A patient with pulmonary venous obstruction has a normal-sized heart with pulmonary venous hypertension and edema.

7. Regarding atrial isomerism, which of the following is *true*?
   A. Asplenia is not commonly associated with systemic venous anomalies.
   B. Polysplenia is associated midpulmonary venous anomaly.
   C. Bilateral right-sided bronchial anatomy is seen in polysplenia.
   D. Bilateral left-sided bronchial anatomy is seen in asplenia.

   ANSWER: A. Asplenia is associated with right-sided bronchial anatomy and has common pulmonary venous anomalies such as TAPVC. The systemic venous anomalies such as azygous continuation of IVC interruption is common in polysplenia, which is associated with bilateral left-sided bronchial anatomy.

8. Which of the following is *not* a common cause for pulmonary edema in the newborn?
   A. Obstructed TAPVC
   B. Hypoplastic left heart syndrome
   C. Transposition of great arteries
   D. Transient tachypnea of the newborn

   ANSWER: C. Transposition of great artery is the most common cyanotic neonatal CHD and radiographic appearance depends upon the presence of VSD. A patient with large VSD presents with increased pulmonary shunt vascularity and those with intact ventricular septum have normal to mild plethora. Pulmonary edema is not a presentation for transposition but the common presentation for obstructive TAPVC, hypoplastic left heart syndrome, and transient tachypnea of the newborn.

9. Regarding radiographic signs of congenital cardiac anomalies, which of the following is *incorrect*?
   A. Gooseneck sign at left ventricular angiography is seen in endocardial cushion defect.
   B. Egg-on-a-string sign is seen in Epstein anomaly.
   C. Snowman sign is seen in supracardiac TAPVR.
   D. Boot-shaped heart is associated with tetralogy of Fallot.

   ANSWER: B. Egg-on-a-string sign is commonly seen in transposition of great arteries due to a narrow vascular pedicle from posterior and medial location of the pulmonary trunk. Boot-shaped heart is due to right ventricular enlargement and shift of apex upward and outward, commonly seen in tetralogy of Fallot. In the supracardiac TAPVC, the vertical vein connecting the common pulmonary vein to the left innominate vein, innominate vein, and dilated right SVC form the head of the snowman configuration, the body being formed by an enlarged cardiac mass. Gooseneck sign on ventriculography is pathognomic of AVSD (endocardial cushion defect) and is due to elongation of the left ventricular outflow track caused by the absence of AV septum and apically displaced atrioventricular valves.

10. Regarding Epstein malformation all of the following are *true,* except:
    A. Right cusp leaflets are dysplastic.
    B. Posterior and septal leaflet are displaced toward the apex.
    C. Tricuspid stenosis is present.
    D. Right atrium dilatation is present.

    ANSWER: C. Ebstein malformation is a congenital anomaly of the tricuspid valve leaflet with septal leaflet displacement downward and toward the apex with physiologic atrialization of the right ventricular inlet segment. The right AV orifice and right atria are enlarged and there is associated tricuspid insufficiency (not stenosis) due to dilatation of the tricuspid annulus and right ventricle.

36 ACYANOTIC CONGENITAL HEART DISEASE

Satinder P. Singh

INTRODUCTION

Congenital heart defects are the most common type of birth defect, affecting 6 to 8 of every 1,000 newborns. Each year, more than 35,000 babies in the United States are born with congenital heart defects. Acyanotic congenital lesions account for 70% of all cases of congenital heart disease. Acyanotic heart diseases can be further categorized as those with left-to-right shunt and the resultant increased pulmonary shunt vascularity or those without any shunt and normal pulmonary vascularity (Tables 36-1 and 36-2).

Management of patients with CHD heavily relies on imaging. Echocardiography is often the first line of investigation due to its easy to use, portability, and inexpensiveness. However, echo is limited in evaluating vessels beyond the heart and is user dependent especially in patients with poor acoustic windows. More detailed anatomical and functional information is usually acquired from cardiac catheterization, which however is invasive, and does not provide any three-dimensional information. More recently cardiac MRI and MDCT have evolved as important noninvasive modalities for diagnosis and follow-up of patients with CHD.

PERSISTENT LEFT SUPERIOR VENA CAVA

Persistent left superior vena cava (SVC) is present in 0.3% of the general population and in approximately 4% of hearts with congenital cardiac malformation. In the majority of cases, the left SVC drains through the coronary sinus into the right atrium. Coronary sinuses are invariably larger than normal. In 80% of patients, a right SVC is present. Rarely, the SVC may be connected directly to the right atrium or it may drain into the left atrium through unroofed coronary sinus. Usually it is detected incidentally and is easily recognized on CT or MRI.

TABLE 36-1 Acyanotic Congenital Heart Disease with Increased Pulmonary Vascularity

Atrial septal defect
Ventricular septal defect
Patent ductus arteriosus
Endocardial cushion defect
Partial anomalous pulmonary venous collection (PAPVC)
A-P Window
Sinus of Valsalva aneurysm rupturing into RA or RV
Coronary artery fistulas to right circulation

TABLE 36-2 Acyanotic Congenital Heart Disease with Normal Pulmonary Vascularity

Coarctation of the aorta
Aortic stenosis
Pulmonary stenosis
Corrected transposition of great arteries (LTGA)

ANOMALOUS PULMONARY VENOUS CONNECTION

Anomalous pulmonary venous connection (APVC) can be total or partial. In cases of total anomalous pulmonary venous connection, the entire pulmonary venous drainage is connected to the right atrium or tributary (a cyanotic condition and discussed under cyanotic heart diseases). In partial anomalous pulmonary venous drainage, one or both lungs connect to right atria or its tributary (a noncyanotic anomaly).

In partial anomalous pulmonary venous connection, the abnormal connection may be to the left SVC, innominate vein, right SVC, interior vena cava (IVC), right atrium, or the coronary sinus. It is usually associated with an atrial septal defect (ASD).

Right pulmonary vein connection to SVC is associated with sinus venosus ASD. Sometimes, the anomalous vein can be seen on chest radiograph, connected to the SVC, or if drainage is into the azygous vein, chest radiographs will show an enlarged right vascular pedicle and dilated azygous vein.

Right pulmonary vein connection to the IVC usually involves the entire right lung drainage into the IVC. Occasionally, only the middle or lower lobe is involved. The anomalous vein descends to the diaphragm with a crescent shape and then sharply curves to the left, toward the IVC. The anomalous vein is usually anterior to the hila of the right lung, and the entrance to the IVC is just superior to the hepatic vein orifices. In most instances, this anomaly is part of the scimitar syndrome, which includes right lung hypoplasia with marked mediastinal shift and dextroposition of the heart, hypoplastic right pulmonary artery, and systemic vascular blood supply from descending thoracic and abdominal aorta.

ATRIAL SEPTAL DEFECT

Atrial septal defect (ASD) is the most common type of congenital cardiac malformation. The four anatomic types are as follows: fossa ovalis or ostium secundum (most common), ostium primum, sinus venosus, and coronary sinus.

Ostium primum ASD is due to absence of atrioventricular septum located in the inferior aspect of the atrial septum near the mitral valve, associated with partial or complete AV canal defect. Sinus venosus defect is located immediately below the orifice of the SVC and is often (80%) associated with right upper lobe pulmonary venous anomalous connection to the SVC or azygous vein. The coronary sinus ASD is part of the unroofed coronary sinus syndrome. The association of mitral stenosis and hemodynamically significant ASD is called Lutembacher syndrome.

CLINICAl FEATURES

The clinical features of patients with ASD are largely due to left-to-right shunt. The typical symptoms in an adult patient include exertional dyspnea and recurrent respiratory tract infections. Volume overload leading to atrial dilatation predisposes the patient to arrhythmias, and ASD is also a risk factor for paradoxical thromboembolic stroke. In patients with chronic long-standing ASD, especially those in the third and fourth decades of life, pulmonary arterial hypertension may develop, and it is usually due to thrombosis in the dilated pulmonary arteries with secondary changes in intima and media. Older patients may present with congestive heart failure. Infants may present with large left-to-right shunt across the atrial septal defect, especially in the presence of partial anomalous venous connection, and may also present with congestive heart failure and tachypnea.

RADIOGRAPHIC FINDINGS

Patients with significant left-to-right shunt demonstrate cardiomegaly with right atrial and right ventricular enlargement. The pulmonary trunk is enlarged with dilated central, right and left pulmonary arteries. Increased pulmonary shunt vascularity is noted in both lungs. The left atrium is typically normal in size. The left ventricle is not enlarged, but may be displaced by a dilated right ventricle. The aortic arch is small because of decreased systemic blood flow. If the QP/QS ratio is less than 1.5, the patients are asymptomatic and no radiographic findings are noted on chest radiograph. In patients with associated mitral stenosis, the left atrial dilatation is present.

In the typical evaluation of ASD, the following information is needed: type and location of defect, quantification of the shunt, detection of any intra-atrial thrombus, assessment of right ventricular function, and detection of any associated pulmonary venous anomaly.

Echocardiography is the main imaging technique to assess ASD. However, it cannot adequately quantify the shunt and is not good at detecting small ostium secundum and sinus venosus defects or associated pulmonary venous anomalies. Cardiovascular MRI is often used in equivocal cases as well as to determine the functional significance of ASD by calculating the shunt (QP/QS ratio).

TREATMENT

Options include closure of ASD via transcatheter ASD mechanical occluding devices or open surgical repair, especially for large defects greater than 40 mm in size.

ATRIOVENTRICULAR SEPTAL DEFECT

Atrioventricular septal defect (AVSD) is a complex cardiac anomaly with deficiency of the atrioventricular septum resulting in ostium primum ASD above the atrioventricular (AV) valve and defect in the inlet portion of the ventricular septum beneath the AV valve. This is also known as endocardial cushion defect, or AV canal defect.

AVSDs are classified as partial or complete, depending on the presence or absence of interventricular communication. In partial defects, there are two AV valves, while in complete defects, only one AV valve is found. The AV septum separates the right atrium from the left ventricle in normal hearts, with concordant atrioventricular connections.

There is a high association of atrioventricular septal defect in patients with Down syndrome (trisomy 21) (Table 36-3). Down syndrome is present in 75% of patients with complete forms of AVSD. Other associated anomalies are noted in 25% of patients with AVSD and include PDA, TOF, and double outlet right ventricle.

CLINICAL FEATURES

Clinical features of AVSD are due to left-to-right shunt. In partial form, features are similar to other types of

TABLE 36-3 Syndromes Associated with Congenital Heart Disease

Down syndrome: hypersegmented manubrium, eleven ribs in one-fourth, AVSD, duodenal atresia (double bubble)
Holt-Oram syndrome: absence of radius, bowing of ulna, hypoplasia of thumb, absence of thumb or triphalangeal thumb, ASD or VSD
Turner syndrome: coarctation of aorta
Noonan syndrome: dysplastic PV stenosis
Cornellia de Lange syndrome: common atrium

ASD. If there is associated AV valve incompetence, the atrial shunt is increased, leading to early heart failure. In cases of complete AVSD, there are large shunts at the atrial and ventricular levels, leading to biventricular failure early in life.

RADIOGRAPHIC FINDINGS

Complete AVSD usually presents in infancy at around 6 to 8 weeks of age; large atrial ventricular shunts are present with dilatation of both ventricles and a globular heart. In patients with Down syndrome, multiple ossification centers for the manubrium are found. Because of the absence of AV septum, the atrioventricular valves are displaced apically, elevating the location of the aortic valve and elongating the left ventricular outflow track, resulting in a characteristic angiographic appearance during left ventriculography. This is known as the "goose-neck deformity," which is pathognomic of AVSD. Echo, MRI, and CT studies all show defects in the atrial and ventricular septum and abnormal AV valves.

VENTRICULAR SEPTAL DEFECT

Ventricular septal defect (VSD) is the most common congenital heart lesion. It is an isolated anomaly in 20% of cases and associated with other anomalies in 5% of cases.

VSD is classified based on the location in the septum and its borders.

A. Perimembranous defects (most common, 80%) are located in the confluence of the inlet, trabecular, and outlet portions of the left ventricle and involve the membranous septum. The superior border of such VSD is formed by the junction of the right and noncoronary cusp of the aortic valve.
B. Muscular defects (10%) are completely surrounded by the muscular septum and can be multiple. When multiple small ventricular septal defects exist they produce a Swiss cheese septum appearance.
C. Juxta-arterial defects are subpulmonary or supracrystal and are situated in the right ventricular outflow track, higher than the perimembranous defect. The superior rim in these defects is formed by valve tissue of both the aortic and pulmonary valve. The infundibular septum, which separates the aortic valve and the right ventricular outflow track, is hypoplastic or absent and the aortic and pulmonary valves are at about the same level instead of the pulmonary valve being higher. It is more commonly associated with prolapse of the right cusp of the aortic valve through the VSD resulting in aortic insufficiency and is more common among Japanese and other Asian populations.

CLINICAL FEATURES

The clinical features depend on the magnitude of intracardiac shunt, depending on the size of the defect and pulmonary vascular resistance. As the pulmonary vascular resistance decreases, the left-to-right shunt increases and both ventricles dilate. Patients with a large VSD can develop heart failure as well as hyperinflation of the lungs from compression of the bronchi from distended pulmonary arteries.

On physical examination there is wheezing, precardial pan systolic murmur, hyperactive heart, and apical diastolic murmur from large flow across the mitral valve.

About 80% of patients with large VSD are seen at 1 month of age, 60% at 3 months, 50% at 6 months, and 25% at 12 months close completely.

IMAGING FINDINGS

Echocardiogram is the first modality for evaluation and is quite accurate. Cases of VSD with QP/QS ratio of less than two are often not detected on chest radiograph. There is often left ventricular enlargement in patients with a large defect. Right and left ventricle enlargement, as well as pulmonary hypertension, may develop. The aortic arch is often small at angiography, so the long axial oblique view is most useful in detecting various types of VSD. Fifty percent of patients with VSD have associated additional cardiac anomalies; aortic stenosis and coarctation of the aorta are common associations.

TREATMENT

Indications for surgery include a large VSD, a patient younger than 3 months of age with heart failure, and QP/QS ratio of 2:1 or more. Elective repair is usually done at 6 months of age if the patient's pulmonary vascular resistance is less than 8.0 units, or if there is the presence of endocarditis, aortic insufficiency, or supracrystal VSD of any size.

PATENT DUCTUS ARTERIOSUS

The ductus arteriosus connects the descending aorta to the pulmonary artery. After birth, the ductus closure is mediated by the release of vasoactive substance (acetylcholine, bradykinin), variation in pH, oxygen tension, and prostaglandins. Increasing oxygen tension constricts the ductus musculature, while prostaglandin relaxes it. Complete ductus closure occurs by 8 weeks of age in the majority of people. Associated anomalies include severe pulmonary stenosis or pulmonary atresia, aortic atresia, or interruption of the aortic arch.

In the left aortic arch, ductus arteriosus joins the descending aorta just beyond the origin of the left subclavian artery and the junction of the left pulmonary artery and pulmonary trunk. In patients with a right aortic arch, the ductus usually arises from the origin of the left innominate artery or the aberrant left subclavian artery.

CLINICAL FEATURES

The clinical features depend on the size of the PDA. With a large ductus, there is a large left-to-right shunt, ultimately leading to pulmonary hypertension and congestive heart failure. In a smaller ductus, symptoms are not present, though typically a murmur can be heard.

RADIOGRAPHIC FINDINGS

On chest radiograph, there is shunt vascularity in the lungs and the heart is enlarged with left ventricular and left atrial enlargement. The aortic arch is enlarged as well. In patients with increased pulmonary vascular resistance, the pulmonary trunk is dilated.

TREATMENT

PDA can be closed percutaneously or via left thoracotomy.

COR TRIATRIATUM

Cor triatriatum is an uncommon cardiac anomaly, mostly involving the left atrium, in which pulmonary veins enter a proximal left atrial chamber that is separated from the distal chamber that contains the atrial appendage and the mitral valve. The proximal chamber is often larger. Associated anomalies include persistent left SVC, ASD or partial anomalous pulmonary venous connection, unroofed coronary sinus, VSD, AV septal defect, and coarctation of the aorta.

Clinical features are due to pulmonary venous obstruction (Tables 36-4 and 36-5). The heart size is normal or slightly enlarged with a normal left atrium. The pulmonary vascularity is prominent due to a combination of pulmonary venous hypertension and a variable left-to-right shunt through the fossa ovalis. Diagnosis is often made with two-dimensional echocardiography. CT or MR can clearly show the accessory chamber and its connections.

TABLE 36-4 Congenital Heart Disease with Congestive Heart Failure in Neonate

Hypoplastic left heart
Critical aortic stenosis
Coarctation of the aorta
Obstructed total anomalous pulmonary venous connection
Congenital severe mitral stenosis
Cor triatriatum

CONGENITAL MITRAL STENOSIS

Congenital mitral stenosis is a rare cardiac anomaly that includes commissural fusion, parachute mitral valve, mitral archade, and supravalvular stenosing ring of the left atrium. Parachute mitral valve may be associated with Shone syndrome (coexistent supravalvular stenosing ring of the left atrium, subaortic stenosis, and coarctation of the aorta).

PULMONARY VALVE STENOSIS

This is a critical stenosis of the pulmonary valve with a pin hole opening usually with shortened, thickened rigid leaflet tissue (pulmonary valvar dysplasia). The dysplastic pulmonary valve is often seen with Noonan syndrome. This abnormality usually presents in neonates who are critically ill, irritable, tachypnic, and severely hypoxic. Echocardiography is often diagnostic.

CLINICAL FEATURES

In a milder form of stenosis, only partial commissural fusion and thickening of the free edges of the valve are present. Many patients are asymptomatic. Dyspnea on exertion is the most common symptom, with a harsh systolic murmur ejection click and right ventricular heave. In a neonate with critical pulmonary stenosis, marked tricuspid insufficiency is usually present.

TABLE 36-5 Differential Diagnosis of Acyanotic Neonate with Normal Heart Size and PVH

Cor triatrium
Pulmonary vein atresia
Congenital MS

RADIOGRAPHY

In the neonate with severe congestive heart failure, the heart is enlarged with marked dilatation of the right atrium and pulmonary oligemia. In adults, the heart size is normal or mildly enlarged, with right ventricular prominence; pulmonary trunk and left pulmonary arteries are dilated (in 70%) and pulmonary vascularity is usually normal. At angiography, the leaflets are moderately thick and fused at the level of the commissures, creating a dome appearance during systole.

TREATMENT

Balloon valvuloplasty is the treatment of choice for isolated pulmonary valvar stenosis.

RIGHT VENTRICULAR INFUNDIBULAR STENOSIS

The ventricular and infundibular fold and the infundibular septum form the crista supraventricularis in normal hearts. The discrete form of infundibular stenosis is most frequently associated with other conditions such as tetralogy of Fallot. Most hearts with right ventricular outflow stenosis also have VSD.

AORTIC STENOSIS

Aortic stenosis obstruction can be at the level of the valve (valvar stenosis), beneath the valve (subaortic stenosis), or above the valve (supravalvar stenosis) (Table 36-6).

VALVULAR AORTIC STENOSIS

This is the most common (75%) type of aortic stenosis. *Severe valvular stenosis* in the neonatal period is from hypoplasia of the annulus or dysplastic, myxomatous thick valve leaflets to commissural fusion. The most common abnormality, however, is bicuspid aortic valve. This is estimated to occur in 2% to 3% of all live births. These valves, however, are not stenotic in infancy, but during adult years become stenotic from early degenerative calcifications.

TABLE 36-6 Types of Aortic Stenosis

Valvular (75%)
Subvalvular (discrete or in association with IHSS)
Supravalvular (associated with William syndrome)

Left coronary arterial dominance is present in 20% to 50% of patients with bicuspid aortic valves. Of all patients with congenital valvular aortic stenosis, 5% to 30% have associated cardiac anomalies such as coarctation of the aorta, congenital mitral stenosis, and PDA.

CLINICAL FEATURES

Infants with aortic stenosis usually develop congestive heart failure (Table 36-7). The bicuspid aortic valve becomes stenotic in adolescent or adult life with presenting symptoms of dyspnea on exertion, angina, or even syncope. Bicuspid aortic valve is a risk factor for aortic dissection.

IMAGING FEATURES

Two-dimensional echo is fairly accurate is diagnosing stenotic aortic valve. Cardiac MR can determine the severity of aortic stenosis as well as the aortic valve area for surgical planning.

SUPRAVALVAR AORTIC STENOSIS

A supravalvar aortic stenosis is due to localized or diffuse narrowing of the aorta above the valve. The localized variety is more common. Abnormality of the aortic valve is uncommon. Coronary artery ostia may be involved. The most commonly associated anomaly is multiple stenoses in the peripheral pulmonary arteries, which when familial are known as Williams syndrome.

SUBVALVAR AORTIC STENOSIS

Subvalvar aortic stenosis is due to obstruction of the left ventricular outflow track below the aortic valve. There may be a thin, fibrous membrane below the valve annulus and often attached to the anterior mitral leaflet, producing mitral regurgitation. Subvalvar stenosis frequently coexists with other congenital cardiac defects such as VSD and Shone syndrome.

TABLE 36-7 Differential Diagnosis of Acyanotic Neonate with Cardiomegaly and PVH/Edema

Coarctation of aorta (most common in second and third week)
Critical AS (4–6 weeks)
Interruption of aortic arch
Cardiomyopathy/myocarditis
Anomalous origin of left coronary from pulmonary artery
Noncardiac causes: hydrops fetalis, peripheral A-V fistula, chorioangioma of placenta

PERIPHERAL PULMONARY ARTERY STENOSIS

Congenital pulmonary artery stenosis is often associated with other congenital cardiac anomalies such as pulmonary atresia TOF or tricuspid atresia. Peripheral pulmonary artery stenosis may be associated with Ehlers-Danlos syndrome, Takayasus disease, congenital rubella syndrome, or part of a genetic disorder such as Bouillaud syndrome.

SINUS OF VALSALVA ANEURYSM

Sinus of Valsalva is a potential space between the semilunar valve cusp and the adjacent lateral wall of the great artery. This aneurysm can be congenital or acquired (from bacterial endocarditis, inflammatory and degenerative diseases of the aortic wall such as syphilis or Marfan syndrome, or may be associated with VSD).

Congenital sinus of Valsalva aneurysms most commonly involves the right sinus followed by noncoronary sinus. Because of congenital weakness in the aortic wall, there is a protrusion of the sinuses into the underlying cardiac chamber. The aneurysm progressively enlarges and eventually ruptures into the chamber. The site of rupture is most commonly into the right ventricle followed by the right atrium.

CORONARY ARTERIOVENOUS FISTULAS

There can be a direct communication between a coronary artery and one of four cardiac chambers, coronary sinus, vena cava, or pulmonary artery. The right coronary artery or its branches are involved in 50% to 55% of cases. The left coronary artery is involved in 45% of cases and more than 90% of fistulas open into the right heart chamber or its connecting vessels. The involved coronary artery is usually dilated and tortuous due to increased flow through the vessel; rarely coronary artery aneurysms are noted.

Clinically, symptoms include exertional dyspnea or angina due to coronary steal. Continuous murmur from the fistula is heard commonly. The diagnosis is confirmed by selective coronary angiography. CT can also demonstrate the dilated coronary arteries and its fistulous communications.

Suggested Reading

Cascade PN. Adult Congenital Heart Disease: the Blues. Society of Thoracic Radiology, 2008.

Goo HW, Park I-S, Ko JK, et al. CT of congenital heart disease: normal anatomy and typical pathologic conditions. *RadioGraphics.* 2003;23:S147-S165.

Leschka S, Oechslin E, Husmann L, et al. Evaluation of congenital heart disease in children and adults with 64 section CT. *RadioGraphics.* 2007;27:829-846.

QUESTIONS AND ANSWERS

1. Regarding persistent left SVC, which one of the following is *correct*?
   A. Commonly associated with congenital cardiac malformation.
   B. Directly drains into the right atrium.
   C. In less than 50%, a right-sided SVC is present.
   D. Incidence is 0.3% in general population.

   ANSWER: D. Persistent left SVC is present in 0.3% of the general population and in only 4% of hearts with congenital cardiac malformation. In the majority of cases, the left SVC drains through the coronary sinus into the right atrium. In 80% of cases, right SVC is present.

2. Regarding anomalous pulmonary venous connection, which one of the following is *correct*?
   A. Total anomalous pulmonary venous connection is an acyanotic condition.
   B. Partial anomalous pulmonary venous connection is often associated with ostium primum ASD.
   C. Scimitar syndrome includes anomalous right pulmonary venous connection, right lung and pulmonary artery aplasia, and systemic blood supply from the descending thoracic and abdominal aorta.
   D. Partial anomalous primary venous connection is an acyanotic condition.

   ANSWER: D. Partial anomalous pulmonary venous drainage is an acyanotic congenital anomaly, whereas the total anomalous pulmonary venous connection is a cyanotic condition. The most common association of partial anomalous pulmonary venous connection is sinus venosus type ASD. Scimitar syndrome includes anomalous right pulmonary venous collection to IVC, right lung and pulmonary artery hypoplasia (not aplasia), and systemic blood supply from descending thoracic and abdominal aorta.

3. Which of the following is *correct* for ASD?
   A. Ostium primum type of ASD is most common.
   B. Left atrium is commonly enlarged.
   C. Aortic arch is dilated.
   D. Patient becomes symptomatic when QP/QS ratio is more than 1.5.

   ANSWER: D. Ostium secundum is the most common type of ASD. If the QP/QS ratio is less than

1.5, patients are often asymptomatic and no radiographic findings are noted on chest radiograph. Left atrial enlargement is not present in ASD unless there is associated mitral valve disease. Because of decreased systemic blood flow, the aortic arch is smaller than normal.

4. Which of the following is *correct* regarding atrioventricular septal defects?
   A. Atrioventricular septum separates the left atrium from right ventricle.
   B. Common association of atrioventricular septal defect is Trisomy 21.
   C. Clinical features are due to right-to-left shunting.
   D. Left ventricular outflow tract is shortened.

   ANSWER: B. The normal AV ventricle septum separates the right atrium from the left ventricle. Because of the absence of AV septum, the atrioventricular valves are displaced apically, elevate the location of aortic valves, and elongate the left ventricular outflow track, resulting in a characteristic angiographic appearance during left ventriculography, the goose-neck deformity pathognomic of AVSD. The clinical features are due to left to right shunting and the most common association of AVSD is Down syndrome (trisomy 21).

5. Indication for surgery for VSD include all *except*:
   A. Large VSD
   B. QP/QS ratio of 2 or more
   C. Severe pulmonary vascular disease
   D. Patients with supracristal defect

   ANSWER: C. Surgical closure of VSD is indicated for patients of any age with large VSD in whom clinical symptoms and failure to thrive cannot be controlled medically and in infants 6 to 12 months of age who have large defects associated with pulmonary hypertension, even if symptoms are controlled by medication. Patients older than 24 months with a QP/QS ratio greater than 2 and patients with supracristal VSD of any size are usually referred for surgery because of the high risk of aortic valve regurgitation. Severe pulmonary vascular disease is a contraindication to surgical closure of a VSD.

6. Which of the following is the most common site for sinus of Valsalva aneurysm rupture?
   A. RA
   B. RV
   C. LA
   D. LV

   ANSWER: B. The most common site of rupture of sinus of Valsalva aneurysm is the right ventricle followed by the right atrium.

7. Which of the following statements is *correct*?
   A. Congenital sinus of Valsalva aneurysm most commonly involves left sinus followed by the right and noncoronary sinus.
   B. Coronary artery fistula involves the left circulation more commonly than right.
   C. Coronary artery fistulas are most commonly communicated with right cardiac chambers.
   D. Sinus of Valsalva aneurysm is a common cause of acyanotic congenital heart disease with decreased pulmonary vascularity.

   ANSWER: C. Congenital sinus of Valsalva aneurysm is a rare cause of acyanotic congenital heart disease with increased (not decreased) pulmonary vascularity. It most commonly involves the right sinus followed by noncoronary and rarely the left sinus. The direct communication between a coronary artery and cardiac chamber most commonly involves right coronary circulation and more than 90% of fistulas open into the right heart chamber or its connecting vessels.

8. Regarding aortic stenosis, which of the following is *incorrect*?
   A. Valvular stenosis is the most common form of aortic stenosis.
   B. Diffuse variety of supravalvular stenosis is more common than the localized type
   C. Common association of valvular aortic stenosis is Williams syndrome.
   D. Shone syndrome is frequently associated with supravalvar aortic stenosis.

   ANSWER: A. Stenosis at the valvular level is the most common form of aortic stenosis resulting from hypoplasia of the annulus or dysplastic myxomatous thick valve leaflets to commissural fusion. Supravalvar aortic stenosis is more commonly localized rather than diffuse and may be associated with multiple peripheral pulmonary artery stenosis, which is commonly known as Williams syndrome. Shone syndrome is frequently associated with subvalvar stenosis, which is due to obstruction of the left ventricle outflow tract below the aortic valve.

9. What is the most common type of ventricular septal defect?
   A. Muscular
   B. Perimembranous
   C. Juxta-arterial
   D. Mixed

   ANSWER: B. The classification of ventricular septal defect is based on the location in the septum and its borders. Perimembranous location is the most common form of VSD (80%). It is located in the confluence of the inlet, trabecular, and outlet portions of the left ventricle, and it involves the membranous septum. The muscular defect (10%) is completely surrounded by muscular septum and can be multiple. The least common variety is juxta-arterial situated in the right ventricle outflow tract higher than the perimembranous defect.

10. Which of the following statements is *true* for ventricular septal defect?
    A. Majority close spontaneously
    B. Chest radiograph may be normal in patients with QP/QS ratio of 3.
    C. Associated cardiac anomalies are uncommon.
    D. Perimembranous VSD is often associated with aortic insufficiency.

    ANSWER: A. The most common natural outcome of the VSD is spontaneous complete closure. QP/QS ratio of more than 2 is often associated with chest radiographic abnormalities, commonly left ventricular enlargement, right ventricle enlargement, and pulmonary hypertension features. Of all cases of VSD, 50% have associated additional cardiac anomalies; coarctation of aorta and aortic stenosis are the most common associations. The juxta-arterial VSD, which is situated higher than the perimembranous defect, is commonly associated with prolapse of the right cusp of the aortic valve through the VSD, leading to aortic insufficiency.

37 VALVULAR HEART DISEASE

Satinder P. Singh

INTRODUCTION

In developed countries, acquired valve heart disease is now most commonly due to degenerative diseases rather than rheumatic and infectious causes. There is an increasing prevalence of mitral regurgitation and aortic stenosis compared to a higher incidence of mitral stenosis and aortic insufficiency. Patients are presenting at advanced age, and many disease processes have few radiographic findings because of early detection with echocardiography.

MITRAL VALVE DISEASE

World-wide rheumatic heart disease still remains a prevalent condition. Nonrheumatic mitral valve disease is now the most common mitral valve (MV) abnormality in the Western world. Nonrheumatic disease is usually manifested as mitral regurgitation, and mitral stenosis is extremely rare.

A normal MV has two leaflets (bicuspid) with surface area of 4 to 6 cm^2. The larger anterior leaflet is contiguous with the aortic valve while the posterior smaller, scalloped leaflet extends more than 50% of mitral annulus circumference.

MITRAL REGURGITATION

Mitral regurgitation (MR) can result from either abnormality of the leaflets such as in mitral valve prolapse (MVP), bacterial endocarditis, mitral commissurotomy, prosthetic valve leaks, SLE, and mucopolysaccharidosis or due to abnormality of the supporting structures such as dilatation of MV annulus, chordae tendineae rupture, mitral annulus calcification, papillary muscle rupture as a complication of myocardial infarction and atrial myxoma.

MITRAL VALVE PROLAPSE

MVP most commonly occurs in isolation, but can be associated with atrial septal defect and Marfan syndrome. Myxomatous degeneration of the valve leaflet and elongation of chordae tendineae allows prolapse of MV leaflet back into the left atrium in ventricular systole. Its diagnosis requires more than 2.5 mm prolapse into the left atrium. It may be associated with chest pain and EKG changes suggesting ischemic heart disease.

CHORDAE TENDINEAE RUPTURE

Chordal rupture leading to mitral regurgitation can be seen in bacterial endocarditis and, less frequently, in connective tissue diseases and myocardial infarction. There is improper coaptation of the leaflets in systole, producing severe mitral regurgitation. On auscultation, the murmur is usually mid-to-late systolic in onset. If chordal rupture occurs suddenly, as in myocardial infarction, it can lead to acute pulmonary edema with normal heart size.

Functional mitral regurgitation due to dilatation of left ventricle or mitral annulus dilatation as occurs in dilated cardiomyopathy or ischemic heart failure. The resulting mitral regurgitation is usually mild-to-moderate.

MITRAL ANNULUS CALCIFICATION

It occurs in the angle between the left ventricular wall and MV cusp and is seen as a "C"-shaped ring on chest radiographs. Calcification occurs more frequently in women and in the elderly. It is usually benign, but may be associated with transient ischemic attacks due to emboli and atrioventricular conduction disturbances. The risk of infective endocarditis also increases in the presence of calcification. Mitral annular calcification is another marker for atherosclerosis and premature calcification is seen in patients with end-stage renal disease.

IMAGING FINDINGS

The chest radiographic appearance depends on the duration and severity of mitral regurgitation and associated heart disease. Acute severe nonrheumatic mitral regurgitation may present with acute edema with normal heart size. In chronic states, the heart usually enlarges with left ventricular dilatation. Left atrium enlargement is variable and left atrial appendage is usually not enlarged. The severity of mitral regurgitation can be estimated with cardiac MR and echocardiography. On cardiac MR, mitral regurgitation is seen as signal loss jet due to turbulent regurgitant flow into the left atrium during systole. Intraoperative transesophageal ultrasound is commonly used to determine the functional status of MV repair by detecting and quantifying regurgitation during the repair.

RHEUMATIC MITRAL VALVE DISEASE

Rheumatic fever is a systemic inflammatory disease occurring in response to group A beta-hemolytic streptococcal infection due to immune response injury to heart. The majority of patients are between 5 and 15 years of age; 30% of patients develop RHD after the first attack of rheumatic fever, 50% have only MV involvement, and 20% to 50% have MV and aortic valve (AV) involvement. Tricuspid valve involvement is less common and PV is rarely affected.

In the early acute rheumatic carditis, mitral regurgitation is present due to myocarditis. This mitral regurgitation is often transient and reversible. Chronic rheumatic MV disease usually results in mitral stenosis due to fusion of the commissures, thickening and shortening of the chordae tendineae, and fibrosis of the papillary muscles. This most commonly results in a mixture of mitral stenosis and regurgitation. Valve replacement or valvuloplasty is indicated for severe stenosis with a valve area of 0.8 to 1.2 cm^2. There is usually an increased left atrial pressure, which is transmitted back to the pulmonary veins, thus ultimately leading to interstitial and then alveolar pulmonary edema. In chronic MV disease, lung parenchymal changes of hemosiderosis and intraparenchymal ossification may be seen. The patient can develop secondary pulmonary artery hypertension, leading to right ventricular dysfunction and functional tricuspid regurgitation. Left atrial fibrillation can be complicated by thrombi, which can result in systemic embolization.

IMAGING FEATURES

The classic radiographic feature of rheumatic MV disease is left atrial enlargement and left atrial appendage enlargement. Left atrial enlargement on chest radiograph is seen as double density through the heart. Displacement of the left main bronchus, and occasionally the esophagus posteriorly, is best seen on lateral radiographs. Left ventricular enlargement is seen in significant mitral regurgitation but is not common in pure mitral stenosis. Curvilinear calcification in the wall of the left atrium or the thrombus lining the atrial wall can be seen in long-standing MV disease. MV calcification, if present, strongly suggests rheumatic etiology, and there is a variable degree of pulmonary venous hypertension. Echocardiography is the best method for the assessment of MV disease. Cardiac MR shows restricted opening of the MV and thickening of the leaflets in mitral stenosis.

TRICUSPID VALVE DISEASE

Normal tricuspid valve usually has three leaflets (tricuspid): anterior, septal, and one or two posterior leaflets.

TRICUSPID INSUFFICIENCY

Tricuspid regurgitation can be due to rheumatic diseases, functional from right ventricular dilatation, due to endocarditis (a frequent cause among intravenous drug abusers), and is rarely due to trauma. Tricuspid valve abnormality is also seen in congenital heart disease, corrected transposition of the great arteries, and Ebstein anomaly. Severe tricuspid regurgitation can also occur in endomyocardial fibrosis and carcinoid syndrome.

TRICUSPID STENOSIS

Tricuspid stenosis is usually caused by rheumatic heart disease, and carcinoid syndrome is the second most common cause. The majority of patients also have MV disease, and common clinical presentation includes long-standing fatigue and edema. Its treatment includes balloon valvuloplasty or surgical replacement.

Clinically, presence of pulsating, enlarged liver and high venous pressure with big *v* wave suggest tricuspid regurgitation. A slow *y* descent in neck vein pulsation indicates presence of tricuspid stenosis

IMAGING FEATURES

There is enlargement of the right atrium which shows bulging to the right with increased curvature of the right heart border. Presence of prominent right atrium in rheumatic heart disease patients always suggests tricuspid valve involvement. Ultrasound is the definitive modality to diagnose tricuspid disease. In severe regurgitation, the pressure drop across the valve is low and may not be recognized immediately on ultrasound or cardiac MR.

AORTIC STENOSIS

The most common cause of aortic stenosis in the Western countries is degenerative calcific disease in middle-aged or elderly patients. Calcium deposition on the aortic cusp causes obstruction to the outflow as well as stiffening of the cusp, leading to stenosis (see Table 36-6). Aortic stenosis in adults is also commonly seen in a congenitally deformed bicuspid valve (Table 37-1). Other causes of aortic stenosis include rheumatic heart disease as well as degeneration of normal tricuspid trileaflet aortic valve.

The clinical presentation includes chest pain, syncope, or shortness of breath. Left ventricular hypertrophy is noted on the ECG. There is systolic ejection murmur on auscultation. Echocardiography easily recognizes the severity of aortic stenosis. Severe aortic stenosis is present when aortic valve area decreases below 0.5 cm^2 (normal aortic area is 2.5 cm^2).

IMAGING FEATURES

Chest radiograph demonstrates left ventricular hypertrophy and, in chronic stages, LV dilatation. Ascending aorta may be dilated. Aortic valve calcification can be seen on the lateral chest radiograph, although best documented by fluoroscopy or now by MDCT. Cardiac MR can show impaired aortic valve opening, assess stenosis, and determine morphology of the valve. There is systolic flow defacing in the aortic root. Associated regurgitation is seen as diastolic flow defacing in the left ventricular outflow track.

Rheumatic aortic stenosis is usually associated with MV involvement. Clinically, dyspnea is pronounced due to associated mitral disease. On chest radiography, there is often left atrial enlargement due to associated MV disease. Poststenotic dilatation of the aorta is rare in rheumatic aortic stenosis and gross aortic valve calcification is also uncommon. Ultrasound is often required to determine the severity of aortic and MV disease in rheumatic heart disease.

TABLE 37-1 Etiology of Aortic Stenosis

Degenerative
Rheumatic
Congenital: unicuspid, bicuspid, tricuspid (5%)

AORTIC REGURGITATION

Aortic regurgitation can be due to disease of the aortic wall or disease of the cusp, such as bacterial endocarditis, trauma, or aortic dissection (Table 37-2). Chronic aortic regurgitation may also been seen from congenital bicuspid aortic valve or subarterial ventricular septal defect. Aneurysm of the ascending aorta causes dilatation of the valve link, leading to aortic regurgitation. The most common cause of acquired chronic aortic regurgitation is the complication of congenital deformity of the valve or rheumatic heart disease.

IMAGING FEATURES

The chest radiograph shows left ventricular dilatation, although the patient may remain asymptomatic until cardiac

TABLE 37-2 Aortic Regurgitation

Degenerative
Congenital
Rheumatic
Bacterial endocarditis
Dissection
Marfan syndrome
Takayasu arteritis
Ehlers-Danlos syndrome
Ankylosing spondylitis
Rheumatoid arthritis
Syphilis
Trauma
Balloon valvuloplasty

failure develops. The entire thoracic aorta may be moderately dilated. When MV disease is present, left atrial enlargement may dominate. Ultrasound is the primary modality for aortic valve disease evaluation. Aortic root diseases such as annuloaortic ectasia or dissection are best evaluated by CT angiography or cardiac MR. Complications of endocarditis with paravalvar abscess are best seen on cardiac MR or contrast-enhanced CT angiography.

Marfan syndrome and syphilis are two conditions that can involve the ascending aorta and cause aortic aneurysm formation. In Marfan syndrome, the aneurysm involves the aortic sinuses and aortic calcification is rarely seen, whereas in patients with syphilitic aortitis, the aortic sinuses are spared and aortic calcification is seen commonly.

Suggested Reading

Carabello BA, Crawford FA Jr. Aortic stenosis [published correction appears in *New Eng J Med.* 1997;337:1474; *New Eng J Med.* 1997;507a; and *New Eng J Med.* 2001;345:1652]. *New Eng J Med.* 1997;337(1):32-41.

Sebastia C, Quiroga S, Boye R, Perez-Lafuente M, Castella E, Alvarez-Castells A. Aortic stenosis: spectrum of diseases depicted at multi-section CT. *RadioGraphics.* 2003;23:S78-S91.

Vogel-Claussen J, Pannu H, Spevak PJ, Fishman EK, Bluemke DA. Cardiac valve assessment with MR imaging and 64-Sectin multi-detector row CT. *RadioGraphics.* 2006;26:1769-1784.

Woolley K, Stark P. Pulmonary parenchymal manifestations of mitral valve disease. *RadioGraphics.* 1999;19:965-972.

QUESTIONS AND ANSWERS

1. What is the most common cause of valvular heart disease in the United States?
   A. Rheumatic
   B. Infective endocarditis
   C. Degenerative
   D. Congenital

   ANSWER: C. In developed countries, acquired valve heart disease is now most commonly due to degenerative diseases rather than rheumatic and infective causes. There is an increasing prevalence of mitral regurgitation and aortic stenosis compared to a higher incidence of mitral stenosis and aortic insufficiency.

2. Which of the following is *false* regarding mitral valve?
   A. World-wide rheumatic heart disease is the most common cause of mitral valve disease.
   B. In the Western world, nonrheumatic mitral stenosis is the most common mitral valve abnormality.
   C. The anterior leaflet is the largest and is contiguous with the aortic valve.
   D. Mitral valve prolapse can occur in Marfan syndrome.

   ANSWER: B. World-wide rheumatic heart disease still remains a prevalent condition. Nonrheumatic mitral valve disease is now the most common mitral valve abnormality in the Western world. Nonrheumatic disease is usually manifested as mitral regurgitation, mitral stenosis is extremely rare. The mitral valve is bicuspid with larger anterior leaflet which is in fibrous continuity with aortic valve, in comparison to tricuspid valve which is separated from the pulmonary valve by muscular infundibulum. Mitral valve prolapse most commonly occurs alone, but can be associated with atrial septal defect and Marfan syndrome. Myxomatous degeneration of the valve leaflet and elongation of chordae tendineae allows prolapse of mitral valve leaflet back into the left atrium in ventricular systole.

3. Regarding rheumatic heart disease, which of the following is *true*?
   A. Injury to heart is caused by immune response to group B beta-hemolytic *Streptococcus* infection.
   B. In the majority, both mitral and aortic valves are involved.
   C. In early stages of myocarditis, mitral stenosis is common, transient, and reversible.
   D. Left ventricle enlargement is seen more commonly in mitral regurgitation than in pure mitral stenosis.

   ANSWER: B. Rheumatic fever is a systemic inflammatory disease in response to group A beta-hemolytic streptococcal infection with immune response injury to heart. The majority of patients are between 5 and 15 years of age; 30% of patients develop RHD after the first attack of rheumatic fever, 50% have only MV involvement, and 20% to 50% have MV and AV involvement. TV involvement is less common and PV is rarely affected. In the early acute rheumatic carditis, mitral regurgitation is present due to myocarditis. This mitral regurgitation is often transient and reversible. Chronic rheumatic mitral valve disease usually results in mitral stenosis due to effusion of the commissures, thickening and shortening of the chordae tendineae, and fibrosis of the papillary muscles. This most commonly results in a mixture of mitral stenosis and regurgitation.

4. Which of the following is *false* regarding tricuspid valvular disease?
   A. Tricuspid stenosis is most commonly caused by carcinoid syndrome.
   B. Tricuspid insufficiency is commonly due to right heart failure.
   C. Pulsatile large liver suggest tricuspid insufficiency.
   D. Echo is the definitive modality for diagnosing tricuspid valve diseases.

   ANSWER: A. Tricuspid stenosis is usually caused by rheumatic heart disease, and carcinoid syndrome is the second most common cause. Pulsating, enlarged liver and high venous pressure with big *v* wave suggest tricuspid regurgitation. A slow *y* descent in neck vein pulsation suggests tricuspid stenosis. TR is most commonly due to right heart failure of any etiology (PS, primary PAH, or MV disease). Other causes include Ebstein anomaly, carcinoid syndrome, rheumatic heart disease, and infective endocarditis.

5. Regarding aortic stenosis, which of the following is *false*?
   A. Most common cause in Western world is degenerative disease.
   B. At CMRI, there is diastolic flow dephasing.
   C. Rheumatic aortic stenosis is often associated with mitral valve disease.
   D. Poststenotic dilatation is not commonly seen in rheumatic aortic stenosis.

   ANSWER: B. The most common cause of aortic stenosis in the Western countries is degenerative calcific disease in middle-aged or elderly patients. Calcium deposition on the aortic cusp causes obstruction to the outflow as well as stiffening of the cusp, leading to stenosis. Aortic stenosis in adults is also commonly seen as a congenitally deformed bicuspid valve. Cardiac MR can show impaired aortic valve opening, assess stenosis, and determine morphology of the valve. There is systolic (and not diastolic) flow defacing in the aortic root. Associated regurgitation is seen as diastolic flow defacing in the left ventricular outflow track. Rheumatic aortic stenosis is usually associated with mitral valve involvement and chest radiography often shows associated mitral left atrial enlargement. Poststenotic dilatation of the aorta is rare in rheumatic aortic stenosis. Gross aortic valve calcification is also uncommon in rheumatic disease.

38 ISCHEMIC HEART DISEASE

Satinder P. Singh

INTRODUCTION

Myocardial ischemia results from an imbalance between myocardial oxygen demand and myocardial blood flow. This imbalance typically occurs due to a decreased blood flow resulting from atherosclerotic disease of the coronary arteries, but can also result from excessive oxygen demand such as that occurring in severe hypertension, severe aortic stenosis, or hyperdynamic states (Table 38-1).

The primary clinical presentation of ischemia is angina and infarction. This may lead to ventricular failure, mitral regurgitation, ventricular aneurysm formation, ventricular rupture, or arrhythmias.

CORONARY ARTERY ANATOMY

Two coronary arteries, the right and the left, originate from the right and left sinuses of Valsalva, respectively. In the majority of people, the left coronary artery (LCA) supplies the majority of the left ventricle (LV) and the right coronary artery (RCA) supplies the inferior portion of the LV as well as the entire right ventricle.

RIGHT CORONARY ARTERY

The RCA arises from the right coronary cusp at a slightly higher location in comparison to the LCA. The first branch of the RCA is usually the conal artery branch, which supplies the right ventricle outflow tract. (In up to 50% of cases, the conus branch may arise from the sinus itself and therefore has been referred to as the third coronary artery.) The RCA courses under the right atrial appendage to the right atrioventricular groove. In

TABLE 38-1 Causes of Myocardial Ischemia

Decreased oxygen supply
Decreased coronary blood flow, which could be due to atherosclerosis, thrombosis, coronary artery spasm, dissection, or malignant anomalous coronary artery compression
Severe anemia
Hypoxemia
Increased oxygen demand from increased after-load
Increased preload
Metabolic disturbances such as hyperthyroidism

more than 50% of patients, a sinoatrial nodal artery arises from the proximal RCA, coursing backward toward the junction of the SVC and right atrium. The free anterior wall of the right ventricle is supplied by acute marginal branches, which are an important source of collateral blood flow to both the distal RCA as well as the left anterior descending (LAD) coronary artery. After the crux, the RCA gives rise to the posterior descending artery (PDA), which runs along the inferior surface of the heart in the posteroinferior interventricular groove supplying the inferoposterior third of the interventricular septum. This vessel is usually accompanied by the middle cardiac vein, which serves as an identifying marker for PDA on cardiac computed tomography (CT). The atrioventricular (AV) nodal branch often originates at the crux and marks the beginning of the posterolateral segmental branch (PLB), which supplies the posterolateral wall of the LV. The PLB courses to a variable distance in the posterior (AV groove, depending on the length of the left circumflex artery (LCX)). In patients with left dominance circulation, both PDA and posterolateral branches arise from the LCX in addition to LAD wrap at the LV apex. In codominant circulation, the PLB branches arise from the circumflex artery, while the PDA comes from the RCA.

LEFT CORONARY ARTERY

The LCA arises from the left coronary sinus and divides into two or sometimes three branches shortly after its origin. The major branches are LAD and LCX. In patients with trifurcation of LCA, the ramus intermedius branch supplies the anterolateral wall of LV.

The LAD runs in the anterior interventricular groove toward the apex and sometimes wraps at the apex extending into the inferior interventricular groove, especially in patients with a small PDA or codominance. It supplies the anterolateral wall of the LV with diagonal branches and supplies the anterior two-thirds of the interventricular septum with multiple septal perforator branches.

The circumflex artery runs in the posterior or left AV groove and gives off branches to the left atrium and lateral LV free wall (known as obtuse marginal branches). In 45% of patients, the SA nodal branch arises from the proximal circumflex artery.

CORONARY ARTERY DISEASE

Coronary artery disease begins as fatty streaks in the coronary arteries and other arterial beds quite early in life. The development of atherosclerosis appears to follow a complex pathway including endothelial dysfunction (caused by a number of factors such as hypertension, hyperlipidemia, cigarette smoking, etc.) and infiltration of leukocytes, lipids, and macrophages within the intimal layer of the artery followed by inflammation (lipid-rich foam cells form as macrophages ingest LDL particles), leading to proliferation and migration of smooth muscle cells from the medial layer to form a fibrous cap over the lipid-rich lesion (proliferation of vasovasorum provides the blood supply to the lesion). Further plaque progression causes growth and necrosis of lipid core calcifications, hemorrhage in the plaque, and surface erosions leading to formation of nonobstructive clots. Thinning and weakening of the fibrous caps may cause acute plaque rupture. Plaques that are less than 70% obstructed appear to be more likely to undergo rupture due to their higher lipid content, thin fibrous cap and more irregular configuration, and the presence of shear forces at the edges of the plaques.

PREVALENCE AND INCIDENCE OF CORONARY HEART DISEASE

The incidence of coronary heart disease death from myocardial infarction (MI) is approximately 1.2 million cases per year with a prevalence of 13.2 million cases in the United States. The risk factors for coronary heart disease can be differentiated into three types: nonmodifiable factors, which include male sex, age, and family history of premature coronary heart disease; major modifiable risk factors, which include low HDL cholesterol, elevated LDL cholesterol, diabetes, and hypertension; and the minor risk factors, which include lack of regular exercise, psychological stress, and obesity.

The normal coronary artery is a smooth, gently tapering structure. Atheromatous disease leads to irregularity and progresses to stenosis. A greater than 60% decrease in the diameter of the artery can be flow limiting. In the initial stages of atherosclerosis, the atheromatous burden in the wall is eccentric and bulges outward from the artery lumen, which remains unchanged in diameter (known as the Glagov effect or positive remodeling). Therefore, catheter coronary angiography performed at this stage is often normal. However, coronary CT angiography (CTA) has a distinct advantage over catheter angiography since it can provide information about the coronary artery wall in addition to coronary lumen status.

The collateral flow between adjacent coronary arteries is responsible for variable presentation of CAD. Angiographically, collateral pathways are identified as tortuous vessels, which are usually smaller than native arteries, though, occasionally, these can be quite large. The common collateral pathways between LAD and RCA are conus artery, septal perforators, marginal branches, and PLB to diagonal branches. And those between LAD and circumflex artery include diagonal to obtuse marginal branches, distal LAD to obtuse marginal branches, and septal to left PDA branches. The common collateral pathway between LCX and RCA is PLB to obtuse marginal branches. Anastomosis between the atrial branch of LCX and AV nodal artery is known as the Kugel artery. The collateral flow between the conus artery (arising from RCA) and proximal LAD forms the ring of Vieussens.

CORONARY THROMBOSIS

Coronary thrombosis most frequently occurs in conjunction with atherosclerotic disease in a moderate-grade stenosis from plaque rupture due to activation of platelets. Less common causes include high hematocrit, which occurs in cases of polycythemia vera and tetralogy of Fallot. A clot can also be seen following severe coronary artery spasm.

CORONARY ARTERY SPASM

Coronary artery spasm can occur in both normal and atherosclerotic arteries. The classic description is Prinzmetal angina where chest pain occurs at rest and is accompanied by ST segment elevation. If coronary angiograms are performed, they are usually normal. Spasm is often confirmed by pharmacological provocation with acetylcholine or ergonovine.

CORONARY ARTERY DISSECTION

Coronary artery dissection occurs most frequently during interventional procedures (percutaneous transluminal coronary angioplasty [PTCA]), but occasionally can also be seen in otherwise healthy patients, especially young pregnant women. In patients with type A aortic dissection, the dissecting flap can extend into the coronary artery and in these patients the origin of the RCA is most commonly compromised.

MYOCARDIAL INFARCTION

Following a critical imbalance between oxygen supply and myocardial demand, there is a rapid development of myocardial necrosis. The most common cause of MI is narrowing of the epicardial blood vessels due to atherosclerotic plaques. Irreversible myocardial damage occurs if the total occlusion of the vessel persists for more than 4 to 6 hours; therefore, reperfusion within this period can salvage significant myocardium, thereby reducing morbidity and mortality. It is now well known that the infarct-causing lesion is not the most stenosing lesion. In fact, in the majority of patients, MI is caused by plaque rupture from a lesion, which causes less than 50% diameter stenosis.

The nonatherosclerotic causes of MI include coronary vasospasm (Prinzmetal angina), use of cocaine and amphetamine, vasculitis, embolization from infected valve, and rarely trauma.

CLINICAL PRESENTATION OF MI

The clinical manifestations of plaque rupture known as acute coronary syndrome include acute MI, unstable angina, and sudden death due to ventricular fibrillation. Other manifestations include stable angina and ischemic cardiomyopathy. Chest pain (radiating to jaw, neck, and arm), dyspnea, anxiety, diaphoresis, and wheezing are common symptoms. A silent MI can occur in patients who are diabetic, in female patients, in patients with dementia, and in patients with heart failure.

Diagnostic Evaluation of MI

The initial diagnostic evaluation of a suspected MI includes serial cardiac enzymes (troponin, creatinine kinase [CK], and myoglobin) and serial EKGs. Chest radiography is often done to assess the heart size and detect the presence of edema and to exclude other diseases causing chest pain (such as pneumonia, pneumothorax, etc.). Echocardiography is useful to detect regional wall motion abnormality and to detect complications of MI such as acute mitral valve regurgitation from papillary muscle rupture, myocardial rupture, or presence of pericardial effusion. Myocardial perfusion imaging is done to assess the viability and extent of ischemic damage.

Serum troponin levels start increasing within 3 to 12 hours, peak at 24 to 48 hours, and then gradually return to the baseline in 1 to 2 weeks. According to the ACC/AHA consensus statement, troponin levels are now the criterion standard in defining and diagnosing MI. CK levels increase within 3 to 12 hours of chest pain, peak at 24 hours, and return to the baseline in 2 to 3 days. CK levels have high sensitivity and specificity, though less than that of troponin. The three subtypes of CK are CK-MM (found in skeletal muscle), CK-BB (found in the brain), and CK-MB (found mainly in the heart). Myoglobulin levels can rise within 1 to 4 hours of chest pain and are highly sensitive in early detection of MI but may not be specific.

Ventricular function can be evaluated with echocardiography, radionuclide imaging, MDCT, CMR, and conventional ventriculography. CMRI is perhaps the most accurate and widely used method to evaluate ventricular function. The ejection fraction is calculated as stroke volume divided by end diastolic volume. Impaired wall motion abnormalities can be designated as reduced motion (hypokinesia), absent wall motion (akinesia), or paradoxical wall motion (dyskinesia). Normal LVEF is greater than 50%. Regional wall motion abnormalities can be seen in patients with ischemia as well as scarring. Reversible wall motion abnormalities can be seen in patients with stress-induced ischemia. Severity of LV dysfunction is an important prognostic factor that plays a role in outcome after MI.

The role of cardiac CT in evaluating acute chest pain is evolving. Because of its high negative predictive value, it is extremely useful in excluding significant coronary artery disease. CT can also help effective and quick triage, thereby reducing health care cost by avoiding unnecessary further expensive testing.

Coronary angiography is often performed in patients with typical chest pain occurring due to atherosclerotic disease or unstable angina. It is performed to guide management by providing anatomic assessment of disease severity. Percutaneous coronary intervention (PCI) or coronary artery bypass graft (CABG) is indicated for severe coronary artery disease not responding to medical treatment, life-threatening left main coronary artery disease, positive stress test with severe disease in corresponding artery, and acute MI to salvage myocardium.

Myocardial stunning refers to temporary prolonged myocardial dysfunction following an ischemic episode. The myocardium is viable and has contractile reserve. The key elements of a stunned myocardium are (a) short-term total or near total reduction in the coronary blood flow, (b) reestablishment of the coronary blood flow, and (c) subsequent temporary LV dysfunction. Acute, coronary occlusion causes a rapid decline (within seconds) in ventricular performance. If the coronary flow is reestablished, ventricular function will slowly return to normal. The duration of reduced performance (myocardial stunning) depends on the duration of the preceding ischemia. Stunning is completely reversible, and therefore there is no permanent damage to the myocardium. The stunned myocardium, however, is less responsive to inotropic drugs and cardiogenic shock may occur. Stunning may occur following coronary angioplasty, thrombolysis, coronary vasospasm, and cardiopulmonary bypass.

Myocardial hibernation is a term used to describe the condition in which regional cardiac function is depressed due to chronic ischemia. Restoration of the normal coronary flow (e.g., by coronary bypass) will restore normal function in the affected region. Myocardial hibernation can occur in chronic stable or unstable angina, acute MI, heart failure with and without severe LV dysfunction, and in patients with an anomalous coronary artery. The pathophysiology of myocardial hibernation is characterized by reduced regional contractile function distal to a coronary artery stenosis that recovers after removal of the coronary stenosis. It is estimated that 20% to 50% of patients with ischemic LV dysfunction have a significant viable hibernating myocardium, which has the potential for improvement after revascularization. In summary,

- a transient postischemic LV dysfunction is called "stunned" myocardium.
- a chronic but potentially reversible ischemic dysfunction due to a stenosed coronary artery is called "hibernating" myocardium.

Although the mechanism of stunning and hibernation are not completely known, evidence suggests that impaired calcium handling by the sarcoplasmic reticulum as well as damage by oxygen free radicals may play an important role.

Complications of MI include arrhythmias, cardiac rupture, papillary muscle rupture leading to acute mitral valve regurgitation, left ventricle aneurysm, and thrombus formation.

Post-MI mitral valve regurgitation usually occurs due to posterior papillary muscle rupture after inferior MI. A chest radiograph in this situation may show alveolar consolidation due to atypical acute edema, which is often localized to the right upper lobe because of the direction of regurgitant jet passing into the right upper lobe pulmonary vein mimicking air space pneumonia. Often, the cardiac size is normal unless there is long-standing hypertension. A systolic murmur is heard on examination and echo may show the disrupted mitral apparatus and LV inferior wall motion abnormality.

ISCHEMIC CARDIOMYOPATHY

Ischemic cardiomyopathy is a result of coronary artery disease with impaired left ventricular function and decreased left ventricular ejection fraction (LVEF), usually occurring after a transmural infarct with LV remodeling. Diffuse LV involvement usually due to three-vessel coronary artery disease results in a dilated hypokinetic LV.

IMAGING FINDINGS

A chest radiograph may demonstrate enlarged heart with evidence of failure. PET is considered to be the gold standard for myocardial viability assessment, although MR is evolving and may even be superior to PET.

MR IMAGING

First-pass MR perfusion may show hypoperfusion (subendocardial or transmural). Delayed contrast enhancement obtained 10 to 15 minutes after bolus of 0.1 mL/kg of gadolinium may reveal the infarct. Scar tissue appears as a bright, hyperenhanced region, and viable myocardium appears black.

DRESSLER SYNDROME

Dressler syndrome occurs 10 to 30 days after MI or cardiac surgery. It may remit and relapse over weeks or months and is characterized by pleuritis, pneumonitis, and pericarditis. Aspirin or steroids provide good symptomatic response.

CARDIAC MDCT

Current indications of cardiac CTA include evaluation for suspected CAD, atypical chest pain, patient with equivocal stress tests or discrepancies between imaging and clinical assessment, graft or coronary stent evaluation, anomalous coronary artery evaluation, and coronary vein and pulmonary venous mapping.

Recent advances in MDCT technology with high temporal and spatial resolution and submillimeter slice collimation allow evaluation of coronary arteries in a single breath-hold. A coronary CTA is highly accurate in excluding significant (greater than 50% luminal narrowing) stenosis with very high negative predictive value of 97% to 100%. MDCT can detect calcified and noncalcified plaques in coronary arteries and has good correlation with intravascular ultrasound. The most important parameter in obtaining a good quality coronary CTA study is a low heart rate of preferably less than 60 bpm.

There are two ways to gate cardiac CT to EKG: prospective and retrospective gating. In prospective gating, the scanning begins at a predetermined time interval from the R wave usually in late diastole, followed by table movement, and then repetition in a "step and shoot" axial scanning protocol. Axial image thickness is greater than 2 mm. This is commonly used for noncontrast coronary calcium scoring. Recently, however, different manufacturers are now offering a prospective gated coronary CTA with contrast images obtained at thin collimation (0.625 mm) with significant reduction in radiation dose (often less than 3 mSv). This prospective gated CTA is possible only in patients with a heart rate of less than 65 bpm and in some vendors is limited by patient weight (weighing less than 250 lb). Since imaging is performed in one phase of cardiac cycle, no functional information can be obtained from a prospective scan.

Retrospective gating is commonly used for all coronary CTA examinations wherein continuous helical scanning is obtained in a single breath-hold. The data is reconstructed in different phases of cardiac cycle, which is used to obtain ventricular functional information as well as anatomic information.

ANOMALOUS CORONARY ARTERIES

Coronary arteries anomalies are rare, potentially life-threatening anatomic variants with an incidence of 1%. The anomalous origin and course of coronary artery is categorized as benign (retroaortic or prepulmonic), malignant (between aorta and pulmonary artery), and transseptal (below the interarterial space). The latter is considered less malignant. The most common anomalous coronary artery is LCX originating from RCA with retroaortic course, a benign incidental finding.

MALIGNANT INTERARTERIAL COURSE OF LCA ARISING FROM THE RIGHT SINUS OF VALSALVA OR RCA

This anomaly is found in approximately 1.3% of all coronary anomalies. The most common signs and symptoms in an infant or young patient are due to MI, heart failure or ventricular arrhythmias, or in a young adult compression of the LCA, immediately after exercise, may cause MI and is a well-known cause of sudden death in young athletes.

The anatomical features of symptomatic interarterial course of the LCA arising from RCA or right cusp are the following: vessel lumen is slitlike near its origin, acute angle of origin, intramural course of anomalous vessel, and interarterial path.

Treatment for this condition is reimplantation or unroofing procedure, and prognosis is excellent with early treatment.

BLAND WHITE GARLAND SYNDROME

Bland White Garland syndrome is also known as ALCAPA (anomalous LCA origin from the pulmonary artery). The majority of patients present in infancy with heart failure. Rarely these patients survive into adulthood and present with angina, MI, or heart failure.

The best noninvasive diagnostic test for ALCAPA is the coronary CTA. Imaging findings show a large LCA arising from the pulmonary artery, multiple collateral vessels, and dilated RCA with left-to-right shunt from right coronary to left coronary to the pulmonary artery. This syndrome is treated by direct reimplantation of the anomalous coronary artery into the aorta.

CORONARY FISTULAS

Coronary-cameral fistulas are abnormal communications between the coronary artery and the cardiac chamber. Vessels are often large and tortuous and may have aneurysmal dilatation. This condition may be associated with coronary steal phenomena via collateral pathways if draining into low-pressure system.

MYOCARDIAL BRIDGE

Myocardial bridge is a congenital variant in which a segment of the epicardial coronary artery has an intramyocardial course. The condition most commonly involves midsegment of the LAD, the LCX, and less likely the RCA. Most patients are asymptomatic, although some may develop ischemia. Myocardial bridge is easily demonstrated on a cardiac CT. There are scattered reports of increased predisposition to atherosclerosis in patients with deep myocardial bridges.

CORONARY ARTERY ANEURYSM

Coronary artery aneurysm is present when the diameter of the coronary artery is more than 1.5 times the normal adjacent segments. There are many causative factors including atherosclerosis, Kawasaki disease, congenital, trauma, iatrogenic, mycotic, and connective tissue disorder (Table 38-2).

Treatment includes anticoagulants/deep platelet therapy, bypass and exclusion of aneurysm, and covered stent graft placement.

KAWASAKI DISEASE (MUCOCUTANEOUS LYMPH NODE SYNDROME)

Kawasaki disease is an idiopathic febrile multisystem disease in children, and its symptoms include fever and cervical lymphadenopathy with accompanying rashes on palms and soles. Coronary artery aneurysms are present in 25% of patients, often multiple, usually in the proximal segments. Transient gallbladder hydrops can also occur. Treatment for Kawasaki disease includes aspirin and gamma-globulin.

TABLE 38-2 Etiologies of Coronary Artery Aneurysm

Atherosclerosis	Most common in the United States
Kawasaki disease	Most common worldwide
Congenital, trauma, iatrogenic, mycotic, connective tissue disorder	

SUGGESTED READING

Hoffman U, Pena AF, Cury RC, et al. Cardiac CT in emergency department patients with acute chest pain. *RadioGraphics*. 2006;26:963-980.

Kim SY, Seo FB, Do K-H, et al. Coronary artery anomalies: classification and ECG-gated multi-detector row CT findings with angiographic correlation. *RadioGraphics*. 2006;26:317-334.

O'Brien JPO, Srichai MB, Hecht EM, Kim DC, Jacobs JE. Anatomy of the heart at multidetector CT: what the radiologist needs to know. *RadioGraphics*. 2007;27:1569-1582.

Pannu HK, Flohr TG, Corl FM, Fishman EK. Current concepts in multi-detector row CT evaluation of the coronary arteries: principles, techniques, and anatomy. *RadioGraphics*. 2003;23:S1111-1125.

Reeder SB, Du YP, Lima JAC, Bluemke DA. Advanced cardiac MR imaging of ischemic heart disease. *RadioGraphics*. 2001;21:1047-1074.

Vogel-Claussen F, Rochitte CE, Wu KC, et al. Delayed enhancement MR imaging: utility in myocardial assessment. *RadioGraphics*. 2006;26:795-810.

QUESTIONS AND ANSWERS

1. Which of the following is *correct* regarding coronary circulation?
   A. Obtuse marginal branch arises from the RCA.
   B. Acute marginal branch supply left ventricular lateral wall.
   C. Majority of the interventricular septum is supplied by LAD.
   D. In a codominant circulation, PLB comes from the RCA and PDA branches arise from the circumflex.

   ANSWER: C. The obtuse marginal artery is a branch of the circumflex and not the RCA. The acute marginal artery is a branch of the RCA and supplies the right ventricular free wall and not the left ventricle. The LAD supplies anterior two-thirds of the interventricular septum via multiple septal perforators. The posterior one-third of the septum is supplied by the PDA. In a codominant circulation, PDA arises from the RCA and PLB comes from the circumflex.

2. Which of the following is *correct* regarding coronary artery disease?
   A. Positive remodeling can be easily diagnosed with conventional catheter angiography.

B. The ring of Vieussens is a common collateral pathway between RCA and circumflex arteries.
C. The majority of the culprit lesions in acute coronary syndrome are significant stenotic lesions.
D. Collateral circulation is difficult to evaluate by coronary CT angiography.

ANSWER: D. Collateral vessels are usually smaller and more tortuous than native vessels and are commonly seen in patients with significant coronary artery disease, and are commonly seen on a catheter angiography in patients with coronary artery disease. These collaterals are difficult to identify by a coronary CTA because of limited spatial resolution and the nondynamic nature of CT. Positive remodeling refers to outward expansion of the vessel wall because of atheromatous plaque deposition without compromising the lumen. Therefore, it is not often seen on conventional catheter angiography. However, CT can nicely demonstrate the wall abnormalities and remodeling. The ring of Vieussens is a common collateral pathway between RCA and LAD (not circumflex). The majority of the culprit lesions in acute coronary syndromes are due to less than 50% diameter stenotic lesions.

3. Which of the following is *incorrect* regarding myocardial infarction?
   A. Earliest cardiac marker to rise is myoglobin level.
   B. Troponin levels are the diagnostic defining criteria for myocardial infarction.
   C. Creatinine kinase levels peak at 24 hours and return to the baseline in 2 to 3 days.
   D. Coronary CT has high positive predictive value and low negative predictive value in evaluating chest pain.

ANSWER: D. The coronary CTA has a very high negative predictive value and therefore is extremely useful in excluding coronary artery disease in patients with chest pain. The troponin levels are the criterion standard in defining and diagnosing myocardial infarction: they start increasing in 3 to 12 hours, peak at 24 to 48 hours, and then gradually return to the baseline in 1 to 2 weeks. CK levels increase within 3 to 12 hours of chest pain, peak at 24 hours, and return to the baseline in 2 to 3 days. Myoglobin levels can rise within 1 to 4 hours of chest pain and are highly sensitive in the early detection of MI, but are not specific.

4. Which of the following is *correct*?
   A. Post-myocardial infarction MR is due to anterior papillary muscle rupture.
   B. Myocardium can be salvaged by PCI if performed within 48 hours.
   C. Presence of delayed enhancement on cardiac MRI indicates reversible ischemia.
   D. Dressler syndrome responds well to steroids.

ANSWER: D. Dressler syndrome occurs 10 to 30 days after myocardial infarction or cardiac surgery and responds well to aspirin or steroids. Postmyocardial infarction MR is usually due to posterior papillary muscle rupture from inferior myocardial infarction leading to severe acute MR. Irreversible myocardial damage occurs if the total occlusion of the vessel persists for more than 4 to 6 hours and therefore reperfusion within the period (not within 48 hours) can salvage significant myocardium. The presence of delayed enhancement on cardiac MR indicates scar due to irreversible ischemia/infarction.

5. Which of the following is *correct* regarding cardiac MDCT?
   A. Cardiac function is routinely evaluated on prospective gaited CTA.
   B. Radiation dose is higher in prospective gating than retrospective gating.
   C. The most important parameter in obtaining good quality studies is a low heart rate.
   D. Dose modulation technique is very useful to decrease radiation dose, especially in patients with a high heart rate.

ANSWER: C. In prospective gating, only one phase of the cardiac cycle, usually late diastole, is imaged and therefore cardiac function cannot be evaluated. Retrospective gating, on the other hand, obtains images through the cardiac cycle, and therefore cardiac function is routinely evaluated. Since the x-ray exposure is continuous throughout the helical retrospective imaging, radiation dose is much higher for retrospective gated study and lower for prospective gated imaging. The most important parameter in obtaining a good quality CTA is a low heart rate of less than 60 bpm.

6. Regarding coronary artery anomalies, which is *correct*?
   A. Most coronary artery anomalies are benign.
   B. ALCAPA commonly presents in adults.
   C. Coronary artery aneurysms are commonly congenital in origin.
   D. Coronary-cameral fistula is a common cause for sudden death.

ANSWER: A. Most coronary artery anomalies of origin and course are benign and are usually detected incidentally on conventional angiography. Anomalous LCA origin from the pulmonary artery

(ALCAPA) is most commonly found in infancy with heart failure as the presenting feature. Rarely, patients surviving into adulthood may present with angina, myocardial infarction, or heart failure. The most common cause of coronary artery aneurysm is atherosclerosis in the United States and Kawasaki disease worldwide. Coronary-cameral fistulas are abnormal communications between the coronary artery and cardiac chambers and may be associated with coronary steal phenomena via collaterals if draining into a low-pressure system. It is not a common cause for sudden death.

7. Which of the following is *incorrect* regarding Kawasaki disease?
   A. Coronary artery aneurysms are commonly in the distal segments.
   B. Treatment includes surgical resection.
   C. Symptoms include fever, lymphadenopathy, and rash on the palms and soles.
   D. Associated with gallbladder hydrops.

   ANSWER: D. Transient gallbladder hydrops can occur in Kawasaki disease, an idiopathic febrile multisystem disease in children with typical symptoms of fever, cervical lymphadenopathy, and rashes on palms and soles. Coronary artery aneurysms are present in 25% of patients, are often multiple, and usually occur in the proximal segments (not distal segments). Treatment usually includes aspirin and gamma-globulin and not surgical intervention.

8. Regarding LV aneurysm, which of the following is *correct*?
   A. True LV aneurysm has a narrow neck.
   B. True LV aneurysms are more likely to rupture.
   C. LV pseudoaneurysm has a broad neck.
   D. LV pseudoaneurysms typically occur in the basal, inferior, and lateral LV segments.

   ANSWER: D. True LV aneurysms can involve all walls of the myocardium, have a broad neck, usually occur in the LV apex, and are less likely to rupture. Pseudoaneurysms are surrounded by pericardium or organized clot, have a narrow neck, typically occur in the basal, inferior, or lateral LV segment, and are more likely to rupture (Table 38-3).

TABLE 38-3 Left Ventricular Aneurysm

TRUE LEFT VENTRICULAR ANEURYSM	PSEUDOANEURYSM
Usually in the LV apex from LAD disease	Typically basal inferior or lateral LV segment
Involves all walls of the myocardium	Often surrounded by pericardium or organized clot
Broad neck	Narrow neck
Less likely to rupture	Increased risk of rupture

9. Which of the following is *incorrect*?
   A. Malignant interarterial course of the LCA can cause sudden death in young athletes.
   B. Cardiac CT is the gold standard to evaluate anomalous coronary artery.
   C. Cardiac MDCT has a high temporal resolution in comparison to cardiac MRI.
   D. Cardiac MR has a better spatial resolution than cardiac CT.

   ANSWER: C. Cardiac MDCT has high spatial resolution in comparison to MR, while its temporal resolution is lower than that of cardiac MR. Cardiac MDCT is the gold standard to evaluate anomalous coronary artery origin and course. Common causes of sudden death in a young athlete include malignant interarterial course of the LCA, hypertrophic cardiomyopathy, and ARVD.

10. Which of the following is *correct*?
    A. First branch of the RCA is usually the SA nodal branch.
    B. Conus artery is also known as the third coronary artery.
    C. Right ventricle is supplied by the acute marginal branches.
    D. Circumflex artery supplies the inferior and posterior wall of the left ventricle.

    ANSWER: B. In 50% of the patients, conus artery is the first branch of the RCA and in the rest, it arises separately from the right coronary cusp and that is why it is also known as the third coronary artery. The circumflex artery supplies the lateral wall of the left ventricle, whereas the inferior and posterior walls are supplied by the PDA and PLD branches of the RCA.

39 CARDIAC AND PERICARDIAL TUMORS

Satinder P. Singh

CARDIAC TUMORS

Metastatic tumors to the heart and pericardium are 20 to 40 times more common than primary heart tumors. Primary tumors of the heart account for less than 5% of all cardiac tumors and the remaining 95% are metastatic. Among primary cardiac tumors, benign tumors are more common than malignancies. The most common primary cardiac tumors in adults are myxomas followed by lipomas and fibroelastomas. The most common cardiac tumor in children is rhabdomyxoma.

METASTASIS

The heart can be involved by metastasis in three ways: direct mediastinal infiltration by lung cancer, breast cancer, or lymphoma; hematogenesis metastasis from malignant melanoma, lymphoma, leukemia, or sarcoma; and transvenous spread from inferior vena cava (renal, hepatic, or adrenal tumors) or via the pulmonary veins or superior vena cava from lung cancer. Pericardial metastasis presenting with pericarditis is the most common symptom of metastatic heart disease (Table 39-1). Less common is asymptomatic pericardial effusion detected incidentally on chest radiograph or echocardiography. Myocardial metastasis may be asymptomatic or may present with arrhythmia, heart block, or myocardial dysfunction. Echocardiography is the most commonly used modality in suspected cardiac metastasis but CT and MR are complementary modalities. Pericardiocentesis allows the diagnosis of pericardial metastasis in 70% to 80% of patients.

CT features that suggest a malignant nature of a cardiac neoplasm are wide attachment to the all of the heart, destruction of the cardiac chamber wall, involvement of more than one cardiac chamber, invasion of the pericardium, extension into the pulmonary artery, pulmonary vein, or vena cava, and involvement beyond the pericardium, lung or mediastinum. CT is not an accurate technique to detect direct invasion of the mediastinum and cardiovascular structures by lung cancer.

PRIMARY CARDIAC TUMORS

Primary cardiac tumors are rare and a great majority are benign (Table 39-2). Myxoma is the most common benign tumor followed by rhabdomyoma and fibroma. The most common malignant tumor is sarcoma.

TABLE 39-1 Causes of Neoplastic Pericarditis

Lung cancer
Breast cancer
Hodgkin disease, leukemia, lymphoma
Melanoma
Sarcomas
Others

TABLE 39-2 Common Primary Tumors of the Heart

Benign (75%)
Myxoma
Rhabdomyxoma
Fibroma
Lipoma and lipomatous hypertrophy of atrial septum
Papillary fibroelastoma
Hemangioma
Malignant (25%)
Angiosarcoma
Rhabdomyosarcoma
Fibrosarcoma

PRIMARY BENIGN TUMORS OF THE HEART

Cardiac Myxoma

Cardiac myxoma commonly arises in the left atrium (75%) or right atrium (20%) and the rest in either ventricle. Myxomas tend to be solitary, pedunculated, or polypoid masses. These are more common in women and are attached to the interatrial septum near the fossa ovales in the majority of cases. Familial myxomas are uncommon (less than 10% of all myxomas), tend to present at an earlier age, are more likely to have multiple myxomas at atypical locations, and tend to develop recurrent tumors. These are also associated with other dermatological and endocrine abnormalities (*Carney complex*) (Table 39-3).

Clinical Features

Patient may be asymptomatic or may demonstrate peripheral embolic phenomena, signs and symptoms of mitral valve obstruction, and other constitutional symptoms of fever, anemia, elevated ESR, and sometimes clubbing, mimicking infective endocarditis. Systemic symptoms are largely due to the secretion of interleukin-6 by myxomas. Right atrial myxomas may mimic Ebstein anomaly, ASD, or constrictive pericarditis.

TABLE 39-3 Familial Cardiac Tumors (10%)

Carney syndrome:
Cardiac myxoma
Noncardiac myxoma in breast or skin
Pigmentation of skin
Endocrine tumors (pituitary adenomas, adrenocortical disease, or testicular tumors)
NAME syndrome:
Nevi
Atrial myxoma
Myoid neurofibromas
Ephelides
LAMB syndrome:
Lentigines
Atrial myxoma
Blue nevi

Imaging Findings

Heart is commonly enlarged and there is evidence of left atrial enlargement; although rare, the left atrial appendage is also enlarged. Depending on the severity and duration, pulmonary venous hypertension, edema, or even secondary pulmonary artery hypertension may be present. Rarely, these tumors can calcify, which can be detected on CT or fluoroscopy. Myxomas are of intermediate signal intensity on spin-echo MR images, similar to that of myocardium, have low signal intensity on gradient echo images because of partial calcification, and demonstrate higher signal intensity on T2-weighted images. Intratumoral hemorrhage can produce high signal intensity on both T1- and T2-weighted images and contrast enhancement is often seen after gadolinium-enhanced MR. Both cine MRI and echocardiography can show mobility of the tumor often prolapsing through the mitral orifice in ventricular diastole.

Differential for atrial myxoma includes left atrial thrombus and valvular vegetations in endocarditis. The distinguishing features for thrombi are as follows: these usually occur in an enlarged chamber, atrial appendage is the most common site, and atrial fibrillation is often present. Thrombi are usually sessile and do not demonstrate contrast enhancement. Myxomas can be sessile or pedunculated and commonly attach to the interatrial septum. Clinical features help in distinguishing myxomas from endocarditis and vegetations are always related to a cardiac valve.

Rhabdomyxomas

Rhabdomyxomas is the most common pediatric primary cardiac tumor. It is associated with tubular sclerosis in up to 50% of cases, manifesting in the neonatal period. It usually is intramural and starts in the intraventricular septum; arrhythmia is the main presenting feature. These tumors are often inoperable because of their deep location, poor demarcation, and multiplicity.

Fibromas

Fibromas usually involve the left ventricular wall and are resectable. These tumors can calcify, which may suggest the specific diagnosis. Fibromas are more common in children (85%) than in adolescents and adults (15%) and present with heart failure, arrhythmia, or sudden death. Fibromas are reported in associations with Gorlin syndrome. Fibromas are iso- to hyperintense on T1-weighted spin-echo images and low signal intensity relative to myocardium on T1- and T2-weighted spin-echo images due to the short T2 relaxation time of the fibrous tissue.

Lipomas

Lipomas can occur in the septa or myocardial free wall. These are best and easily identified on CT as low-density masses. Lipomatous hypertrophy of the interatrial septum is often found incidentally on routine chest CT and classically spares the fossa ovalis. Lipomas are usually asymptomatic but may be associated with supraventricular arrhythmia. A large right atrial lipoma may present with obstructive symptoms and exertional dyspnea, necessitating surgical resection. Lipoma has high signal intensity on MRI because of its short T1 and long T2 relaxation and loses signal on fat suppression sequences (help differentiating it from melanoma metastasis).

Papillary Fibroelastoma

Papillary fibroelastoma is a collection of avascular fronds of dense connective tissue lined by endothelium. Majority of patients with these tumors are asymptomatic, although symptoms can arise due to embolization from thrombi that collect on the tumor. The majority occur on valve surfaces and the most common valve involved is aortic, followed by mitral, and then pulmonary and tricuspid. Fibroelastomas are easily detected at echocardiography as small mobile masses attached to valves by a short pedicle. Because of their small size, they are not well seen at CT or MR imaging. They may appear as elongated strandlike projection or may have a well-defined head. Surgical excision and leaflet repair is curative.

PRIMARY MALIGNANT TUMORS OF THE HEART

Sarcomas

Angiosarcoma is the most common malignant tumor of the heart, with a male predominance and presentation in early childhood. The right atrium and then the right ventricle are the most commonly affected chambers. Tumors are infiltrating and intramural, usually presenting with intractable arrhythmias, heart failure, caval obstruction, or valvular obstruction. Angiosarcoma often involves the pericardium leading to hemorrhagic pericardial effusion. Echocardiography is the initial primary noninvasive test, which can show the mass as well as the pericardial effusion.

Lymphoma

Primary cardiac lymphoma is rare, usually non-Hodgkin, and more common in HIV-positive population. Secondary cardiac lymphoma is more common in patients with known lymphoma. Pericardium is frequently the common site of involvement. Lymphomas may involve myocardium, mimicking hypertrophic cardiomyopathy, or intracavitary masses.

Paraganglioma

Paraganglioma are tumors that arise from the paraganglia, clusters of neuroendocrine cells in adrenal medulla, carotid, vagal, and para-aortic bodies, and groups of several associated bed sympathetic ganglia. Typical age of presentation is young adults in their thirties and forties, most patients presenting with hypertension and biochemical evidence of catecholamine overproduction. The tumors are easily localized to the heart with nuclear medicine imaging with I-131 or I-123 MIBG. These tumors are highly vascular and tend to involve adjacent structures, including coronary arteries, making surgical resection difficult. The majority of the cardiac paragangliomas are sporadic. The tumors occur in the distribution of the cardiac paraganglia: most arise from the visceral paraganglia in the left atrium, in the posterior wall of the left atrium or left atrial roof. They may also arise from interatrial septum or paraganglia along the coronary arteries. At echocardiography, paraganglia appear as echogenic large left atrial masses. Unlike myxoma, paraganglioma have a broad base of attachment and are firmer than myxoma. At CT, these masses appear as heterogeneous circumscribed low attenuation with extracardiac extension and infiltrative borders and demonstrate intense enhancement after contrast administration. At MR, primary cardiac paraganglioma have markedly increased signal intensity on T2-weighted images and iso- to hypointense signal intensity relative to myocardium on T1-weighted images. Intense contrast enhancement is noted after gadolinium with central nonenhancing areas because of tumor necrosis.

Suggested Reading

Araoz PA, Mulvagh SL, Tazelaar HD, Fulsrud PR, Breen JF. CT and MR imaging of benign primary cardiac neoplasms with echocardiographic correlation. *RadioGraphics.* 2000;20: 1303-1319.

Best AK, Dobson RL, Ahmad AR. Best cases from the AFIP: cardiac angiosarcoma. *RadioGraphics.* 2003;23:S141-S145.

Chiles C, Woodward PK, Gutierrez FR, Link KM. Metastatic involvement of the heart and pericardium: CT and MR imaging. *RadioGraphics* 2001;21:439-449.

Grebenc ML, Rosado-de-Christenson ML, Burke AP, Green CE, Galvin JR. Primary cardiac pericardial neoplasms: radiology-pathologic correlation. *RadioGraphics* 2000;20:1072-1103.

Grebenc ML, Rosado-de-Christenson ML, Green CE, Burke AP, Galvin JR. From the archives of the AFIP: Cardiac myxoma: imaging features in 83 patients. *RadioGraphics.* 2002; 22:673-689.

Sparrow PF, Kurian JB, Jones TR, Sivananthan MU. MR Imaging of cardiac tumors. *RadioGraphics.* 2005;25:1255-1276.

QUESTIONS AND ANSWERS

1. Which of the following is *true* regarding cardiac neoplasm?
   A. Primary tumors constitute 20% of all cardiac tumors.
   B. Among primary neoplasms, benign tumors are more common than malignant tumors.
   C. Most common cardiac tumor in children is angiosarcoma.
   D. Pericardiocentesis is always diagnostic in cardiac malignancies.

   ANSWER: B. Metastatic tumors to the heart and pericardium are 20 to 40 times more common than primary heart tumors. Primary tumors of the heart account for less than 5% of all cardiac tumors and the remaining 95% are metastatic. Among primary cardiac tumors, benign tumors are more common than malignancies. The most common primary cardiac tumors in adults are myxomas, followed by lipomas and fibroelastomas. The most common cardiac tumor in children is rhabdomyxoma. Pericardiocentesis allows the diagnosis of pericardial metastasis in 70% to 80% of patients.

2. All of the following CT features suggest malignant nature of a cardiac neoplasm *except*:
   A. Involvement of multiple cardiac chambers
   B. Invasion of pericardium
   C. Narrow attachment to the heart
   D. Extension into pulmonary artery

   ANSWER: C. CT features that suggest a malignant nature of a cardiac neoplasm are wide (not narrow) attachment to the heart, destruction of the cardiac chamber wall, involvement of more than one cardiac chamber, invasion of the pericardium, extension into the pulmonary artery, pulmonary vein, or vena cava, and involvement beyond the pericardium lung or mediastinum.

3. Regarding cardiac myxoma, which of the following is *true*?
   A. Most common site is right atrium.
   B. Majority are multiple.
   C. Familial myxomas present at an early age.
   D. Demonstrate low signal intensity on T2-weighted images.

   ANSWER: C. Cardiac myxoma commonly arises in the left atrium (75%) or right atrium (20%) and the rest in either ventricle. Myxomas tend to be solitary, pedunculated, or polypoid masses. These are more common in women and are attached to the interatrial septum near the fossa ovalis in the majority of cases. Familial myxomas are uncommon (less than 10% of all myxomas), tend to present at an earlier age, are more likely to have multiple myxomas at atypical locations, and tend to develop recurrent tumors. These are also associated with other dermatological and endocrine abnormalities (Carney complex). Myxomas are of intermediate signal intensity on spin-echo MR images, similar to that of myocardium, have low signal intensity on gradient echo images because of partial calcification, and demonstrate higher signal intensity on T2-weighted images.

4. Which of the following is *true* regarding cardiac thrombus?
   A. Often pedunculated
   B. Most common site is right ventricle.
   C. Atrial fibrillation is often present.
   D. Enhance after contrast injection

   ANSWER: C. Cardiac thrombus usually occurs in an enlarged chamber, atrial appendage is the most common site, and atrial fibrillation is often present. Thrombi are usually sessile and do not demonstrate contrast enhancement.

5. Which of the following is *true*?
   A. Primary cardiac lymphoma is common in HIV patients.
   B. Papillary fibroelastoma most commonly involve mitral valve.
   C. Angiosarcoma is the most common malignant tumor of heart.
   D. Fibromas usually involve right ventricle.

   ANSWER: C. Fibromas usually involve the left ventricular wall and are resectable. These tumors can calcify, which may suggest the specific diagnosis. Fibromas are most common in children (85%) than in adolescents and adults (15%). Angiosarcoma is the most common malignant tumor of the heart, with male predominance and presentation in early childhood. The right atrium and then the right ventricle are the most commonly affected chambers. Papillary fibroelastoma are mostly asymptomatic, and symptoms can arise due to embolization from thrombi that collect on the tumor. The majority occur on valve surfaces. The most common valve involved is aortic, followed by mitral, and then pulmonary and tricuspid. Primary cardiac lymphoma is rare, usually non-Hodgkin, and more common in HIV-positive population. Secondary cardiac lymphoma is more common in patients with known lymphoma.

40 PERICARDIAL DISEASE

Satinder P. Singh

INTRODUCTION

The pericardium consists of two layers: outer fibrous and inner visceral. The wall thickness of the inner layer is 0.05 to 1 mm, slightly thicker along the right ventricle free wall. The mesothelial cells lining the outer layer produce serous fluid; approximately 20 to 25 cc of serous fluid is present under normal physiologic conditions. The pericardial sac encloses the heart, proximal ascending aorta, pulmonary trunk, and short segments of the pulmonary veins.

The transverse sinuses of the pericardium are seen located between the ascending aorta and the pulmonary trunk as well as between the superior vena cava and the left atrium. Fluid collection in these sinuses may be misinterpreted as lymphadenopathy. The oblique sinus of the pericardium is a blind pouch confined laterally by the pulmonary veins, cranially and anteriorly by the left atrium, and posteriorly by the esophagus. In CT and MR, the normal pericardium is visualized as a pencil-thin line, especially in front and along the right atrioventricular groove and right ventricle separated from the right ventricular myocardium by a connective fat tissue. The normal pericardium thickness on the right side is less than 2 mm. The pericardium line is thinner along the left ventricle and the amount of subepicardial fat is narrower; therefore, the pericardium frequently may not be visualized along the left myocardial wall, although it can be seen in front of the left atrioventricular groove.

Echocardiography is the imaging modality most often used for the initial evaluation of suspected pericardial disease, especially effusion or tamponade. Restricted acoustic window, loculated effusions in unusual locations, and the inability to accurately detect pericardial thickening are the limitations of echocardiography. CT or MR imaging is often used when findings at echocardiography are nondiagnostic or difficult to interpret. CT and MR imaging also help in further characterization of pericardial masses.

PERICARDIAL EFFUSION

The common causes of pericardial effusion include heart failure, renal insufficiency, infection (bacterial, viral, or tuberculous), neoplasm (carcinoma of the lung or breast or lymphoma), and injury (trauma or myocardial infarction). A pericardial effusion with CT attenuation close to that of water is likely simple effusion. Effusion with CT attenuation greater than that of water suggests exudative effusion from malignancy, infection, and hemopericardium or effusion associated with hypothyroidism. Chylopericardium demonstrates low attenuation with negative CT HU. Nonhemorrhagic fluid has a low signal intensity on T1-weighted spin-echo images and higher intensity on gradient-echo cine images. Hemorrhagic fluid demonstrates high signal intensity on T1-weighted spin-echo images and low intensity on gradient-echo cine images. Nodular, irregular thickening of the pericardium suggests malignancy.

With inflammatory pericarditis, the patient usually has effusion and pericardial thickening. Pericardial effusion originates due to the obstruction of the venous or lymphatic drainage from the heart. MRI is superior to CT in differentiating fluid from thickened pericardium.

PERICARDIAL CYSTS

Pericardial cysts are remnants of defective embryological development of the pericardium. They are most often asymptomatic and discovered incidentally on chest radiographs or CT. The typical location of pericardial cysts is the pericardiophrenic angle, much more common on the right but can be located throughout the mediastinum. On CT, these cysts are seen as nonenhancing well-circumscribed ovoid, fluid density masses adjacent to the pericardium. On T1-weighted MR images, pericardial cysts demonstrate low signal intensity and high and homogeneous intensity on T2-weighted images because of low protein concentration and nonhemorrhagic fluid. On short T1 inversion recovery images, the water content of the cyst shows high signal intensity. If the cystic fluid is proteinogenous, the signal intensity on T1-weighted images is high. The tendency to change in size or shape with respiration or body position is a discriminating feature of pericardial cyst.

PERICARDIAL DEFECTS

The majority of pericardial defects are congenital but can also result from surgery or trauma. Congenital pericardial defect is due to premature atrophy of the left duct of the Cuvier (Cardinal vein) and failure of nourishment of left pleural pericardial membrane, leading to failure of the pericardium to develop. These defects are more common in men and may be detected at any age, usually in the twenties. These may be associated with bronchogenic cysts, diaphragmatic hernia, pulmonary sequestration, VSD, PDA, and mitral stenosis. Clinically, most pericardial defects are asymptomatic and rarely may have tachycardia, palpitation, right bundle branch block, positional discomfort, or chest pain, especially when lying on the left side. The chest radiograph may show a focal bulge in the area of the main pulmonary artery and left atrial appendage. On the lateral radiograph, there is an increased distance between the sternum and the heart because of the absence of the sternal pericardial ligament. On CT or MR, the cardiac axis is rotated to the left and lung interposes between the aorta and pulmonary artery. If these patients develop left pneumothorax, there is an automatic pneumopericardium owing to the absence of the pericardium. Pericardial defect can be partial or complete. Herniation and strangulation of the left atrial appendage can be symptomatic and may require surgical treatment.

CONSTRICTIVE PERICARDITIS

Patients with constrictive pericarditis frequently present with symptoms of heart failure such as dyspnea, orthopnea, and fatigue, and occasionally with liver enlargement and ascites (Table 40-1). The most frequent cause of constrictive pericarditis is cardiac surgery and radiation therapy; other causes include infection (viral or tuberculous or fungal), connective tissue diseases, uremia, neoplasm, or idiopathic.

Difficult to differentiate clinically, both constrictive pericarditis and restrictive cardiomyopathy have similar manifestations and findings at cardiac catheterization and echocardiography. In both conditions, ventricular filling is restricted, leading to increased diastolic pressures in all the four cardiac chambers and equalization of atrial and ventricular pressures. The diagnosis of constrictive pericarditis is aided by CT and MR imaging. Pericardial thickness of 4 mm or more indicates abnormal thickening, and when accompanied by clinical findings of heart failure, it is highly suggestive of constrictive pericarditis. CT is also good at demonstrating

TABLE 40-1 Clinical Features of Constrictive Pericarditis

Symptoms (>75% of patients)
Dyspnea
Edema
Abdominal swelling
Pleural effusions
Severe fatigue
Signs
Present in > 95%
Increased JVP
Hepatomegaly
Present in < 25%
Pulsus paradoxus
Pericardial knock
Present in <5%
Clubbing

pericardial calcification, although neither pericardial thickening nor calcification is diagnostic of constrictive pericarditis, unless the patient has symptoms of physiologic constriction or restriction. The right ventricle has a reduced volume and narrow tubular configuration. The interventricular septum has an abnormal contour with a prominent leftward convexity and abnormal septal bounce which is quite suggestive of constrictive physiology. Systemic venous dilatation, especially of the vena cava, coronary sinus, hepatomegaly, and ascites are also frequently present.

ACUTE TAMPONADE

Pericardial pressure is normally subatmospheric and becomes more negative during inspiration. Transpericardial pressure is highest at end-diastole when the ventricular volume is greatest. The pressure–volume curve for the pericardium rises steeply after a certain volume is exceeded, so removal of a small amount of fluid will result in a significant reduction in pressure. A rapid increase in intrapericardial fluid can produce acute tamponade with pressure reaching 20 to 30 mm Hg. Systemic venous pressure increases, heart volumes are reduced, and systemic arterial pressures fall (Beck triad). Compression also causes pulsus paradoxus (decrease in the arterial pressure of more than 10 mm Hg during inspiration). The *x* descent is accentuated while the *y* descent is flattened or absent as cardiac filling is severely restricted during diastole (Table 40-2).

CHRONIC CONSTRICTIVE PERICARDITIS

The fibrous envelop reduces end-diastolic volume and causes inadequate preload. The right ventricular pulse wave during diastole demonstrates an early drop followed by a high plateau (square root sign). Mean venous pressure is elevated and *x* and *y* descents are steep and deep. Pulsus paradoxus is infrequent and especially difficult to detect in the setting of atrial fibrillation. Systolic left ventricular function is preserved, but the heart may still have impaired contractility.

TABLE 40-2 Cardiac Tamponade Versus Constrictive Pericarditis

	TAMPONADE	CONSTRICTIVE PERICARDITIS
Pulsus paradoxus	Present	May be present
Kussmaul sign	Absent	May be present
Pericardial knock	Absent	May be present
JVP	Large *x* descent	Normal *x* descent
	Small or absent *y* descent	Large *y* descent

RESTRICTION VERSUS CONSTRICTION

Clinical and hemodynamic profiles are similar in both of these conditions. Both are caused primarily by diastolic filling abnormalities, with preserved global systolic function. The diastolic dysfunction in restrictive cardiomyopathy results from a stiff and noncompliant ventricular myocardium, whereas it is due to a thickened noncompliant pericardium in constrictive pericarditis. Both conditions result in restricted diastolic filling, leading to diastolic heart failure. Pericardium is thickened in constriction but is normal in restriction.

PERICARDIAL HEMATOMA

Acute hematomas show homogeneous high signal intensity; subacute hematomas of 1 to 4 weeks old typically show heterogeneous signal intensity with areas of high signal intensity on both T1- and T2-weighted images. Chronic organized hematomas show peripheral dark rim and low-intensity internal foci because of calcification, fibrosis, or hemosiderin deposition on T1-weighted and gradient-echo images. High-signal-intensity areas on T1- or T2-weighted images often correspond to hemorrhagic fluid.

Coronary or ventricular pseudoaneurysm or neoplasm may resemble hematoma on MR images. Hematomas do not enhance on postcontrast MRI and do not show internal flow on velocity-encoded cine MR images.

PERICARDIAL NEOPLASMS

Pericardial metastases are much more common than primary pericardial tumors. Breast and lung cancer are the most common sources of metastasis in the pericardium followed by lymphoma and melanoma. At CT, there is presence of pericardial effusion and irregular thickening of the pericardium or presence of pericardial masses. Most neoplasms have low signal intensity on T1-weighted images and high signal intensity on T2-weighted images; metastatic melanoma is an exception and has high signal intensity on T1-weighted images because of the paramagnetic metals bound by melanin. There is usually enhancement of the pericardial metastatic masses after contrast administration.

Primary neoplasms of the pericardium are rare. Benign pericardial tumors include lipoma, teratoma, fibroma, and hemangioma; malignant pericardial tumors include mesothelioma, lymphoma, sarcoma, and liposarcoma. Lipoma has a low attenuation on CT images and high signal intensity on T1 spin-echo MR images. Presence of calcium or fat in a pericardial mass at CT suggests teratoma. Pericardial fibroma statistically has low signal intensity on T2-weighted images and often shows either no enhancement or heterogeneous enhancement because of poor vascularization. Primary malignant mesothelioma is rare and manifests as pericardial effusion with or without pericardial nodules or plaques. Lymphoma, sarcoma, and liposarcoma typically appear as large heterogeneous enhancing masses associated with exudative pericardial effusion.

SUGGESTED READING

Truong MT, Erasmus JJ, Gladish GQ, et al. Anatomy of pericardial recesses on multidetector CT: implications for oncologic imaging. *AJR Am J Roentgenol*. 2003;181:1109-1113.

Wang ZJ, Reddy GP, Gotway MB, Yeh BM, Hetts SW, Higgins CB. CT and MR imaging of pericardial disease. *RadioGraphics*. 2003;23:S167-S180.

QUESTIONS AND ANSWERS

1. Regarding oblique pericardial sinus, which of the following is *false*?
   A. Bounded anteriorly by ascending aorta.
   B. Left atrium lies superior to the oblique sinus.
   C. Esophagus is posterior to the oblique sinus.
   D. It is a blind pouch.

   ANSWER: A. The oblique sinus of the pericardium is a blind pouch confined laterally by the pulmonary veins, cranially and anteriorly by the left atrium, and posteriorly by the esophagus. Localized fluid collection in this area can sometimes mimic subcarinal adenopathy.

2. Regarding pericardial defects, which of the following is not *true*?
   A. Mostly asymptomatic and detected incidentally.
   B. Result from atrophy of the right duct of the Cuvier (Cardinal vein) and failure of nourishment of right pleural pericardial membrane.
   C. On cross-sectional imaging, there is interposition of the lung between aorta and pulmonary artery.
   D. Herniation and strangulation of the left atrial appendage may be symptomatic and need surgical intervention.

   ANSWER: B. The majority of pericardial defects are congenital but can also result from surgery or trauma. Congenital pericardial defect is due to premature atrophy of the left (and not right) duct of the Cuvier (Cardinal vein) and failure of nourishment of left pleural pericardial membrane, leading to failure of the pericardium to develop. Clinically, most pericardial defects are asymptomatic and rarely may have tachycardia, palpitation, right bundle branch block, positional discomfort, or chest pain, especially when lying on the left side. The chest radiograph may show a focal bulge in the area of the main pulmonary artery and left atrial appendage. Herniation and strangulation of the left atrial appendage can be symptomatic and may require surgical treatment. On CT or MR, the cardiac axis is rotated to the left and lung interposes between the aorta and pulmonary artery.

3. Regarding cardiac tamponade, which of the following is *true*?
   A. Tamponade can occur when a small amount of pericardial fluid develops rapidly.
   B. Pericardial pressure is normally positive and becomes negative during inspiration.
   C. Transpericardial pressure is highest at end-systole.
   D. Systemic venous pressure increases, heart volumes are reduced, and systemic arterial pressures rises.

   ANSWER: A. Pericardial pressure is normally subatmospheric (not positive) and becomes more negative during inspiration. Transpericardial pressure is highest at end-diastole (and not end-systole) when ventricular volume is greatest. The pressure–volume curve for the pericardium rises steeply after a certain volume is exceeded, so removal of a small amount of fluid will result in a significant reduction in pressure. A rapid increase in intrapericardial fluid can produce acute tamponade with pressure reaching 20 to 30 mm Hg. Systemic venous pressure increases, heart volumes are reduced, and systemic arterial pressures fall (not rise), also known as Beck triad.

4. Regarding chronic constrictive pericarditis, which of the following is *true*?
   A. Caused by a systolic abnormality
   B. Pulsus paradoxus is commonly present.
   C. Large x and small y descents.
   D. Hepatomegaly is commonly present.

   ANSWER: D. Patients with constrictive pericarditis frequently present with symptoms of heart failure such as dyspnea, orthopnea, and fatigue, and occasionally with liver enlargement and ascites. Mean venous pressure is elevated and x and y descents are steep and deep (and not large x and small y descent). Pulsus paradoxus is infrequent (not common) and especially difficult to detect in the setting of atrial fibrillation. Systolic left ventricular function is preserved, but the heart may still have impaired contractility. It is caused primarily by diastolic filling abnormalities (not systolic abnormality), with preserved global systolic function.

5. Which of the following statement is *false*?
   A. Nodular pericardial thickening is suspicious for malignancy.
   B. Pericardium is easily seen along the left ventricle lateral wall.
   C. MR is superior to CT in distinguishing fluid from thickening.
   D. Mesothelial cells lining the outer layer produce the serous fluid.

   ANSWER: B. The pericardium consists of two layers: outer fibrous and inner visceral. The wall thickness of the inner layer is 0.05 to 1 mm, slightly thicker along the right ventricle free wall. The mesothelial cells lining the outer layer produce serous fluid; approximately 20 to 25 cc of serous fluid is present under normal physiologic conditions. In CT and MR, the normal pericardium is visualized as a pencil-thin line, especially in front and along the right atrioventricular groove and right ventricle separated from the right ventricular myocardium by a connective fat tissue. CT or MR imaging is often used when findings at echocardiography are nondiagnostic or difficult to interpret. CT and MR imaging also help in further characterization of pericardial masses. The normal pericardium thickness on the right side is less than 2 mm. The pericardium line is thinner along the left ventricle and the amount of subepicardial fat is narrower; therefore, the pericardium frequently may not be visualized along the left myocardial wall. Nodular, irregular thickening of the pericardium suggests malignancy. MRI is superior to CT in differentiating fluid from thickened pericardium.

41 CARDIOMYOPATHY

Satinder P. Singh

INTRODUCTION

Cardiomyopathies are a heterogeneous group of disorders (Tables 41-1, 41-2, and 41-3) with the dominant feature being diseased cardiac muscle itself, ultimately leading to cardiac dysfunction.

TABLE 41-1 WHO Classification of Cardiomyopathies

Dilated cardiomyopathy
Hypertrophic cardiomyopathy
Restrictive cardiomyopathy
Arrhythmogenic right ventricular dysplasia
Unclassified
Specific cardiomyopathy associated with specific diseases or systemic disorders

DILATED CARDIOMYOPATHY

Dilated cardiomyopathy is the most common type with global impairment of contractility and dilatation of all chambers, and is the most common indication for cardiac transplantation (Table 41-4).

CLINICAL FEATURES

Presenting symptoms are usually due to congestive heart failure, and patients can have an acute influenza-like illness. Chest pain is unusual. Differential diagnoses of dilated cardiomyopathy include alcoholic heart disease, diffuse silent ischemic disease, and critical aortic stenosis.

IMAGING FEATURES

Chest radiographs demonstrate enlarged heart due to left ventricular dilatation or enlargement of all chambers, and there is often associated pulmonary venous hypertension with variable degrees of edema. There is often associated mitral regurgitation due to dilatation of the mitral ring. Pericardial effusion may be present, but is without tamponade. Echocardiography, radionuclide ventriculography, and MRI reveal regional or global hypokinesis; regional wall thickening is best seen in short axis views. Gadolinium-enhanced cardiac MR is the best imaging method to categorize various forms of cardiomyopathies and to specifically distinguish the far more common ischemic myocardial disease. In patients with dilated cardiomyopathy secondary to myocarditis, delayed enhancement (DE) may be seen with patchy distribution and

TABLE 41-2 American Heart Association Classification of Cardiomyopathies (Based on Predominant Organ Involved)

Primary cardiomyopathy: genetic, nongenetic or acquired, predominantly confined to heart
Secondary cardiomyopathy: part of systemic multiorgan disorder (specific cardiomyopathy in WHO classification)

TABLE 41-3 Specific Cardiomyopathies

Ischemic
Valvular
Hypertensive
Inflammatory
Metabolic
Muscular dystrophy
Toxic reactions
Postpartum

normal perfusion imaging. The aortic valve must be examined to exclude end-stage aortic stenosis because both can have similar clinical presentations and aortic stenosis responds favorably to valve replacement.

HYPERTROPHIC CARDIOMYOPATHY

Hypertrophic cardiomyopathy is often familial with autosomal dominant inheritance. The majority of mutations involve proteins of cardiac sarcomere, leading to altered sarcomere function and ultimately to hypertrophy and fibrosis. Hypertrophic cardiomyopathy is less common that dilated cardiomyopathy and is characterized by excessive hypertrophy of the left ventricular myocardium. This hypertrophy is symmetrical in the majority of patients, although in approximately 25% of patients; the upper interventricular septum is most affected, resulting in subvalvular obstruction idiopathic hypertrophic subaortic stenosis (IHSS). A rare variant of hypertrophic cardiomyopathy, commonly seen in the Japanese population, affects only the apex of the left ventricle. The complex pathophysiology of hypertrophic cardiomyopathy is due to left ventricular diastolic dysfunction, myocardial ischemia, arrthymias, left ventricular outflow tract obstruction, mitral regurgitation, and autonomic dysfunction. The left ventricular contractility is often hyperdynamic and leads to small end-systolic left ventricular volume. Systolic anterior motion of the mitral valve (SAM) contributes to left ventricular outflow obstruction.

CLINICAL FEATURES

The clinical presentation of hypertrophic cardiomyopathy is quite variable, ranging from asymptomatic with diagnosis made based on heart murmur or abnormal screening, EKG, to sudden death. The typical triad in symptomatic patients includes the following:

1. Dyspnea on exertion (due to increased left atrial pressure).
2. Angina (abnormal oxygen supply/demand mismatch due to left ventricular hypertrophy, increased arteriolar compressive wall tension due to diastolic relaxation abnormality, and endothelial dysfunction).
3. Presyncope or syncope (due to arrhythmia or sudden increase in outflow tract obstruction).

TABLE 41-4 Common Causes of Dilated Cardiomyopathy

Postchemotherapy cardiac toxicity (Doxorubin)
Peripartum
Alcohol abuse
AIDS

IMAGING FEATURES

Chest radiograph may show a normal-sized heart to a variable degree of left ventricular enlargement, and the left atrium may also be enlarged. Echocardiography often is diagnostic and nicely shows the hypertrophy as well as systolic anterior motion of the mitral valve. Cardiac MR can demonstrate the left ventricular wall hypertrophy (greater than 15 mm), assess the left ventricular mass and mitral regurgitation, and often diagnose hypertrophic cardiomyopathy when echocardiography results are negative or equivocal, especially in patients with anterolateral wall hypertrophy.

Serial follow-up evaluation of the left ventricular mass is best done with cardiac MRI. Patchy DE can be seen on delayed postcontrast cardiac MR images and, if present, is associated with increased risk for certain cardiac death. Catheter angiography can be dangerous due to induced arrhythmias. Selective coronary angiography usually shows no arterial disease; coronary arteries are enlarged with prominent septal perforators demonstrating compression during ventricular systole. Left ventriculography reveals a normal size left ventricular cavity in diastole and narrowing of the left ventricular cavity with typical curved shape, like a banana, in patients with severe septal hypertrophy. Ventricular trabeculations are usually coarse.

RESTRICTIVE CARDIOMYOPATHY

Restrictive cardiomyopathy may be idiopathic, secondary to infiltrative and storage diseases (such as amyloidosis and sarcoidosis) or associated with myocardial disorders such as hypereosinophilic syndromes. It is characterized by reduced ventricular filling and diastolic volume, leading to atrial dilatation and venous stasis, usually with preserved systolic function.

Cardiac MR is a fundamental diagnostic tool and helps to differentiate between restrictive cardiomyopathy and constrictive pericarditis as both demonstrate reduced ventricular filling and diastolic volumes. Pericardial thickening of more than 4 mm is typical for constrictive pericarditis, best assessed with morphologic T2-weighted "black blood" images. In restrictive cardiomyopathy, the septal convexity is maintained in all respiratory phases, whereas in constrictive pericarditis, septal flattening and bounce can be observed in early inspiration.

AMYLOID HEART DISEASE

Amyloid heart disease is a classic example of low compliance restrictive cardiomyopathy. There are three general categories. Immunoglobulin light-chain (AL) amyloidosis (previously called primary amyloidosis) is due to light chain immunoglobulin produced by monoclonal plasma cells. It is the most severe form and the most common type encountered in the United States. It can involve the kidneys, liver, heart, and peripheral nerves. Familial amyloidosis (ATTR amyloidosis) is an uncommon autosomal dominant disease resulting from production of unstable variant of the serum protein transerithritin). It can involve the heart and central nervous system. Senile systemic amyloidosis is secondary to deposition of wild-type transthyretin and is exclusively limited to the heart.

Patients with amyloid heart disease present with low output cardiac failure without murmur. EKG is often low voltage. Echocardiography is the noninvasive test of choice, but lacks specificity, especially when other comorbid conditions such as hypertension are present. Gadolinium-enhanced cardiac MRI is more specific and demonstrates decreased T1 of the myocardium and global and/or subendocardial DE.

SARCOIDOSIS

Only 5% of patients with systemic sarcoid have clinical evidence of cardiac involvement, though the incidence is higher (20%–30%) at autopsy. These patients may present with cardiac arrhythmia as well as restrictive cardiomyopathy. Rarely, papillary muscle involvement leads to mitral regurgitation. Cardiac MR can identify sarcoid granulomas as high signal areas on T2-weighted images with fat suppression or areas of hyperenhancement after gadolinium administration. Myocardial biopsy can be falsely negative due to patchy involvement of the myocardium, and cardiac MR can direct endomyocardial biopsy, as well as monitor the results of therapy.

HEMOCHROMATOSIS

Hemachromatosis can be primary, an inherited autosomal recessive disease with iron deposition in liver, heart, and pancreas or secondary due to repeated blood transfusion and less commonly from long-term hemodialysis and alcohol abuse. It involves both the liver and spleen; however, iron deposition in primary hemochromatosis spares the spleen. Since iron reduces T1 and T2 relaxation rates, hemochromatosis can be diagnosed by cardiac MR. The amount of signal decrease on T2-weighted images correlates well with the iron level in the tissue and therefore cardiac MR can be used to monitor the results of treatment.

ANDERSON-SABRY DISEASE

Anderson-Sabry disease is an X-linked disorder characterized by alpha-galactosidase enzyme deficiency leading to abnormal accumulation of sphingolipids catabolites in various organs including the heart. This abnormal accumulation can lead to arrhythmia, valvulopathy, myocardial infiltration with secondary restrictive cardiomyopathy, and myocardial hypertrophy. MR shows symmetric myocardial wall thickening with increased left ventricle ejection fraction and reduced volume. There is late enhancement due to expression of both intramyocyte accumulation of sphingolipids and interstitial expansion due to fibrosis and collagen deposition. This DE has a specific location (midbasal, lateral left ventricle wall) and distribution pattern (subepicardial and mesocardial) in patients with cardiac symmetric hypertrophy helping in differentiation from hypertropic cardiomyopathy.

LEFT VENTRICULAR NONCOMPACTION

Left ventricular noncompaction is a rare form of congenital cardiomyopathy resulting from arrest of normal intrauterine developmental progression of loose myocardial fiber network. It can be an isolated finding that is increasingly recognized in adults, or a nonisolated form associated with other congenital heart disease such as hypoplastic left ventricle and ventricular septal defect. The left ventricle is typically involved and has a spongy appearance with increase trabeculations and deep intertrabecular recesses. The clinical presentation ranges from cardiac arrhythmias, embolic events, or premature heart failure at a young age. Diagnosis of left ventricular noncompaction is based on ratio of trabeculations in the ventricular apex and thickness of the left ventricular free wall in end-diastole; all of these features can be seen on echo, CT, and cardiac MRI. A ratio of more than 2.5 to 3.0 is considered abnormal and specific.

TABLE 41-5 Arrhythmogenic Right Ventricular Dysplasia Diagnostic Criteria

Major criteria	Right ventricular dysfunction: severe dilatation and reduction of RV ejection fraction with little or no LV impairment, localized RV aneurysms, severe segmental dilatation of the RV
	Fibrofatty replacement of myocardium on endomyocardial biopsy
	Conduction abnormalities: epsilon waves in V1 to V3, localized prolongation (>110 ms) of QRS in V1 to V3
	Family history: disease confirmed on autopsy or surgery
Minor criteria	Right ventricular dysfunction: mild global RV dilatation and/or reduced ejection fraction with normal LV, mild segmental dilatation of the RV, regional RV hypokinesis
	Fibro fatty RV wall replacement
	Conduction abnormalities: inverted T waves in V2 and V3 in an individual older than 12 years in the absence of a right bundle branch block (RBBB), ventricular tachycardia with a left bundle branch block (LBBB) morphology, frequent PVCs (>1000 PVCs/24 h)
	Family history of sudden cardiac death before age 35 or family history of ARVD

*Diagnosis depends on two major and two minor criteria or four minor criteria.

ARRHYTHMOGENIC RIGHT VENTRICULAR DYSPLASIA

Arrhythmogenic right ventricular dysplasia (ARVD) is characterized by fibrofatty degeneration of the right ventricle leading to arrhythmias and sudden cardiac death. Diagnosis of ARVD is based on strict criteria (Table 41-5) and is present if one of the following is met:

- Two major criteria are present or
- One major and two minor criteria are present or
- Four minor criteria are present

Clinical presentation includes syncope, ventricular arrhythmias (left bundle branch block), or sudden death, especially in young athletes, and heart failure. EKG reveals epsilon waves, small depolarization at the beginning of ST segment. T-wave inversion is present in early leads. MR is the modality of choice for evaluating right ventricular morphology, volume, and intramyocardial fatty infiltration. To optimize demonstration of fat, imaging in systole is preferred.

TAKOTSUBO CARDIOMYOPATHY

Takotsubo cardiomyopathy is also known as transient left ventricular apical balloon syndrome, resulting in sudden onset of transient akinesia or dyskinesia of the left ventricular apex without significant coronary artery stenosis. It often follows periods of severe emotional or physical stress often in postmenopausal women. Clinical presentation is acute chest pain with reversible ST segment abnormalities and abnormal cardiac biomarkers. It is named because the left ventricle resembles a Japanese octopus pot, which has a narrow mouth and large round base. Akinesia and ballooning are typically seen in the left ventricle apex, and this dysfunctional myocardium distribution does not correspond to perfusion territory of single epicardial coronary vessel. The best imaging tool is cardiac MR, which demonstrates the morphology and left ventricle functional abnormality. In comparison to acute myocardial infarction, there is no evidence of delayed hyperenhancement. The differential diagnosis includes acute myocardial infarction, acute myocarditis, and coronary vasospasm. Rapid and prompt aggressive pharmacologic and hemodynamic support can result in rapid reversal of left ventricle dysfunction.

SUGGESTED READING

Belloni E, De Cobelli F, Esposito A, et al. MRI of cardiomyopathy. *AJR Am J Roentgenol.* 2008;191:1702-1710.

Kayser HWM, van de Wall EE, Sivanantnan MU, Plein S, Bloomre TN, de Roos A. Diagnosis of arrhythmogenic right ventricular dysplasia: a review. *RadioGraphics.* 2002;22: 639-650.

Kimura F, Sakai F, Sakomura Y, et al. Helical CT features of arrhythmogenic right ventricular cardiomyopathy. *RadioGraphics.* 2002;22:1111-1124.

QUESTIONS AND ANSWERS

1. Which of the following is *not true* regarding dilated cardiomyopathy?
   A. It is the most common type of cardiomyopathy.
   B. Chest pain is a common presentation.
   C. It is the most frequent reason for cardiac transplantation.
   D. It can mimic severe aortic stenosis.

   ANSWER: B. Dilated cardiomyopathy is the most common type of cardiomyopathy and is the most common reason for cardiac transplantation. The presenting symptoms are usually due to congestive heart failure, and sometimes patients may have acute influenzalike illness, but chest pain is unusual. The aortic valve must be examined to exclude end-stage aortic stenosis, which has a similar clinical presentation as dilated cardiomyopathy.

2. The typical clinical presenting triad in hypertrophic cardiomyopathy include all *except*:
   A. Dyspnea on exertion
   B. Syncope
   C. Lower extremity swelling
   D. Angina

   ANSWER: C. The typical triad in symptomatic hypertrophic cardiomyopathy patients include dyspnea on exertion due to increased left atrial pressure, syncope from arrhythmia or sudden increase in outflow tract obstruction and angina due to abnormal oxygen supply/demand mismatch, increased arteriolar compressive wall tension, and endothelial dysfunction.

3. Regarding hypertrophic cardiomyopathy, which of the following is *true*?
   A. It can cause sudden death.
   B. Catheter angiography is often required for diagnosis.
   C. Chest radiographs are always abnormal.
   D. Ventricular hypertrophy is asymmetric in the majority of patients.

   ANSWER: A. Hypertrophic cardiomyopathy is one of the causes for sudden death. The chest radiographs may be normal or may show left atrial enlargement and a variable degree of left ventricular configuration. In the majority of patients, the ventricular hypertrophy is symmetrical, and in approximately 25% of patients only the upper intraventricular septum is most affected. Catheter angiography can be dangerous due to induced arrhythmia and usually is not required for diagnosing hypertrophic cardiomyopathy.

4. Which of the following is *true* for restrictive cardiomyopathy?
   A. It is characterized by systolic dysfunction and reduced ventricular diastolic volume.
   B. Cardiac MR is the diagnostic tool commonly used to differentiate restrictive cardiomyopathy and restrictive pericarditis.
   C. Septal bounce is commonly present.
   D. HIV infection leads to restrictive cardiomyopathy.

   ANSWER: B. Restrictive cardiomyopathy is characterized by reduced ventricular filling and diastolic volume, leading to atrial dilatation and venous stasis, but usually with reserved systolic function. Septal wall motion abnormality and bounce is typically seen in constrictive pericarditis and not in restrictive cardiomyopathy. HIV infection is a common cause for dilated cardiomyopathy and not restrictive cardiomyopathy.

5. Which of the following is *true* regarding cardiomyopathy?
   A. In 25% of patients with systemic sarcoid, the heart is involved.
   B. Most cases of hypertrophic cardiomyopathy are familial.
   C. Primary hemochromatosis commonly involves the heart, pancreas, and spleen.
   D. Regional wall thickening is best seen in horizontal long-axis view.

   ANSWER: B. Only 5% of patients with systemic sarcoid have clinical evidence of cardiac involvement, though the incidence is higher at 20% to 30% at autopsy. Hypertrophic cardiomyopathy is often familial (autosomal dominant) and the majority of mutations involve proteins of cardiac sarcomere causing altered sarcomere function leading to hypertrophy and fibrosis. Secondary hemochromatosis results from repeated blood transfusions, long-term hemodialysis, and alcohol abuse and involves both liver and spleen, whereas primary inherited autosomal recessive hemochromatosis is characterized by island deposition in the liver, heart, pancreas, and spares spleen. Regional wall thickening on echocardiography or cardiac MRI is best evaluated in short-axis views and not horizontal long-axis views.

6. Regarding ARVD, which of the following is *incorrect*?
   A. It can cause sudden cardiac death.
   B. Family history of ARVD diagnosed clinically is a major criterion for ARVD diagnosis.
   C. Left bundle branch block is a common arrhythmia.
   D. The left ventricle can be involved.

   ANSWER: B. ARVD is characterized by fibrofatty degeneration of the right ventricle leading to arrhythmia including sudden cardiac death. Sustained left bundle branch block type of ventricular arrhythmia is considered a major criterion. Family history of ARVD diagnosed clinically is a minor, and not major, criterion. ARVD most commonly involves the right ventricle, though left ventricular involvement has been reported.

7. Which one of the following is the most likely diagnosis in a young postmenopausal female presenting with sudden onset of acute chest pain following severe emotional stress and LV apex dysfunction?
   A. Left ventricular noncompaction
   B. Cardiac amyloid
   C. Takotsubo cardiomyopathy
   D. Alcohol-induced dilated cardiomyopathy

   ANSWER: C. Takotsubo cardiomyopathy typically occurs in postmenopausal females with acute sudden onset chest pain and reversible ST segment abnormalities following severe emotional or physical stress. The dysfunctional myocardium at the LV apex leads to akenesis and ballooning, which often responds rapidly to aggressive pharmacologic and hemodynamic support (that is why it is also known as transient left ventricular apical balloon syndrome). LV noncompaction is a rare congenital cardiomyopathy with clinical presentation of cardiac arrhythmia, embolic events, or premature heart failure at a younger age. At imaging, the left ventricle is typically involved and has a spongy appearance with increased trabeculations. Cardiac amyloid is an example of low compliance restrictive cardiomyopathy and presents clinically as low output failure without murmur. Alcohol-induced dilated cardiomyopathy presents with features of congestive heart failure, and chest pain is unusual.

8. Regarding ARVD, which of the following is *not* a major diagnostic criteria?
   A. Severe dilatation and reduction in the right ventricular ejection fraction.
   B. Regional right ventricular hypokinesia
   C. Localized right ventricular aneurysms
   D. Familial disease confirmed at surgery

   ANSWER: B. Severe dilatation and reduction in the right ventricular ejection fraction and localized right ventricular aneurysm are considered major criteria, whereas regional right ventricular hypokinesia or mild segmental dilatation of the right ventricle, or minor global right ventricular dilatation or ejection fraction reduction are minor criteria. Familial disease confirmed at necropsy or surgery is a major criterion, whereas a family history of premature sudden death caused by ARVD or family history diagnosed clinically based on current criteria are considered minor.

9. Which one of the following is *not* a type of restrictive cardiomyopathy?
   A. Anderson-Sabry disease
   B. Hypereosinophilic syndrome
   C. Postchemotherapy cardiac toxicity
   D. Amyloidosis

   ANSWER: C. Postchemotherapy cardiac toxicity (usually from doxorubin) is a common cause of dilated cardiomyopathy. Restrictive cardiomyopathy may be idiopathic, secondary to infiltrative and storage disorders such as amyloidosis, sarcoidosis, Anderson-Sabry disease, hemochromatosis, or associated with myocardial disorders such as hypereosinophilic syndrome.

10. Which of the following statements is *correct*?
   A. Delayed contrast hyperenhancement is commonly seen in Takotsubo cardiomyopathy.
   B. Echocardiography is the modality of choice to diagnose ARVD.
   C. A ratio of more than 3 for LV apex trabeculations and thickness of LV free wall at end-systole is diagnostic for LV noncompaction.
   D. Hemochromatosis can be diagnosed by cardiac MRI.

   ANSWER: D. Since iron reduces T1 and T2 relaxation rates, hemochromatosis can be diagnosed by cardiac MR. The amount of signal decrease in T2-weighted images correlate well with iron level in the tissue. In Takotsubo cardiomyopathy, there is no delayed contrast hyperenhancement on cardiac MRI in comparison to acute myocardial infarction. CMRI is the modality of choice for evaluating ARVD. A ratio of more than 3 for LV apex trabeculations and thickness of LV free wall at end-diastole and not systole is diagnostic for LV noncompaction.

42 CARDIAC SURGERIES

Satinder P. Singh

INTRODUCTION

Congenital heart disease (CHD) affects 1% of newborns. Of these, the majority are minor lesions that do not require surgery. However, some are serious and may result in significant morbidity. CHD remains the largest cause of neonatal mortality second to prematurity. Advances in pediatric heart surgery over the past few decades have led to increasing numbers of long-term survivors from both palliative and corrective surgery. Currently 80% to 85% of patients born with congenital heart disease can expect to reach adulthood. Over the past several years, the indications for and timings of palliative procedures have also changed. Common palliative procedures done for CHD are listed in Table 42.1. See Table 42-2 for a list of surgical approaches for congenital and acquired heart disease repair and Table 42-3 for a list of congenital heart lesions suitable for catheter intervention.

CLASSIC BLAYLOCK-TAUSSIG SHUNT

This shunt is created between the subclavian and the pulmonary artery and is constructed on the opposite side

TABLE 42-1 Common Cardiac Surgical Procedures used for CHD

To increase the pulmonary blood flow (aortopulmonary shunt)
Classic Blalock-Taussig shunt: subclavian to pulmonary artery, constructed on opposite side from arch
Modified Blaylock-Taussig shunt: Gortex subclavian to pulmonary artery shunt, constructed on same side as arch
Central shunt: Gortex ascending aorta to main pulmonary artery
Waterson: ascending aorta to right pulmonary artery
Pott procedure: descending aorta to left pulmonary artery
Brock procedure: pulmonary valvotomy closed with or without infundibular dilatation or resection
To decrease the pulmonary blood flow
Pulmonary artery banding; Muller-Dammann procedure
To improve mixing of blood
Blalock-Hanlon septectomy: clamps placed behind right pulmonary veins and across a portion of both atria. The lateral portion of the atrial septum is excised
Rashkind balloon septostomy (palliative treatment for TGA)
Park-Blade septostomy at catheterization: used for thicker septum or when large interatrial communication is desired
Open atrial septectomy: most commonly performed during repair of hypoplastic left heart
To reduce ventricular function
Bidirectional Glenn: SVC to pulmonary artery, end-to-side anastomosis
Classic Glenn: SVC to right pulmonary artery, end-to-end anastomosis

from the arch. The orifice of subclavian artery controls flow. This procedure is technically challenging, often leading to pulmonary artery distortion. Reported complications include arm ischemia and decreased growth,

TABLE 42-2 Surgical Approach for Congenital and Acquired Heart Disease Repair

Median sternotomy
ASD/VSD repair
AV stenosis
PV stenosis
Central shunt creation
Repair of TGA, TOF
Placement of adjustable PA band
Aortic dissection
CABG
Left thoracotomy
PDA closure
Coarctation repair
Left Blaylock-Taussig shunt
Mitral commissurotomy
PA banding
Right thoracotomy
Mitral commissurotomy
Right Blaylock-Taussig shunt
Waterson shunt
Glenn shunt

TABLE 42-3 Congenital Heart Lesions Suitable for Catheter Intervention

Septal communications
ASD
Patent ovale foramen
Postoperative fenestrations
Baffle leaks after atrial switch procedure
Luminal communications
PDA
Coronary artery fistula
Aortopulmonary collaterals
Dilatation of valvular lesions
Pulmonary valve stenosis
Aortic valve stenosis
Vessel or conduit
Coarctation of aorta
Pulmonary artery stenosis
Conduit stenosis
Venous baffle stenosis

phrenic nerve injury, Horner syndrome, chylothorax, and endocarditis.

MODIFIED BLAYLOCK-TAUSSIG SHUNT

This Gore-Tex shunt is created between the subclavian and the pulmonary artery and is constructed on the same side as the arch. This procedure is reproducible, has less pulmonary artery distortion and better pulmonary artery growth, and it can be done left or right or the same side of the aortic arch. However, the modified shunt is less durable than the classic Blalock-Taussig shunt. Complications include shunt stenosis or thrombosis.

PULMONARY ARTERY BANDING

The goal of pulmonary artery banding is to reduce pulmonary artery pressure to one-third of systemic pressure. Selecting the correct band diameter is important for good results.

The most common general indication for banding is congestive heart failure in infancy with anticipated delayed repair. The single ventricle is the most common lesion requiring banding to protect the pulmonary bed for future Fontan conversion.

Mortality from these procedures is 5% to 20% and is increased in younger infants with complex lesions. Complications include pulmonary artery distortion, malpositioned band resulting in supravalvular pulmonary stenosis, or a more distal band disrupting the pulmonary bifurcation.

CLASSIC GLENN SHUNT

The classic Glenn procedure is done to reduce ventricle work by creating a shunt between the SVC and the right pulmonary artery with end-to-end anastomosis. It divides pulmonary circulation and diverts all venous return to the larger right lung, so that subsequent Fontan procedure can only use the smaller left lung. Arterial venous fistula is a late complication.

BIDIRECTIONAL GLENN SHUNT

The bidirectional Glenn procedure is done by creating an end-to-side anastomosis between the SVC and the pulmonary artery . It reduces the ventricular work, decreases Fontan mortality, allows blood flow to both lungs, and can be done as preparation for future Fontan conversion or in combination with Fontan procedure. This procedure is less likely to cause right heart failure from overcirculation as seen with aortopulmonary shunts. As pulmonary vascular resistance gradually increases, the shunt flow decreases over time.

FONTAN OPERATION

The original Fontan operation consists of classic Glenn anastomosis between the superior vena cava and the right pulmonary artery, closure of the atrial septal defect, insertion of a homograft valve in the inferior vena cava, and placement of a homograft valve conduit between the right atrium and the left pulmonary artery. Various modifications of this procedure were developed because of late morbidity from valve conduits. The operation basically bypasses the right ventricle and, via a surgically constructed atriopulmonary connection and atrial separation, conducts blood into the lung without the benefit of pulsatile ventricular flow.

Late complications after the Fontan procedure include right atriomegaly and hepatic dysfunction, narrowing and/or leak in the Fontan pathway, dilatation of the coronary sinus, myocardial dysfunction and failure, recanalization of ligated main pulmonary trunk, systemic venous collateralization, plastic bronchitis, protein-losing anteropathy, sinus node dysfunction, and pulmonary arteriovenous malformations.

ATRIAL SWITCH REPAIR FOR TRANSPOSITION OF GREAT ARTERIES

The Mustard and Senning operations are the definitive operations for transposition of great arteries to correct the physiologic abnormalities of the transposed great arteries by forming a baffle within the atria in order to switch the flow of blood at in-flow level. This results in a reversion of the normal flow of blood with the heart and lungs being in series, with the left ventricle becoming the pulmonary ventricle and the right ventricle the systemic ventricle. In the Senning operation, the baffle is created from the right atrial wall and atrial septal tissue without the use of extrinsic material, whereas the Mustard operation involves resection of the atrial septum and the creation of a baffle from the pericardium or synthetic material. These operations are performed at varying stages of life, but usually when the patient is between 1 month and 1 year of age.

RASTELLI OPERATION

The Rastelli operation is the most frequently used procedure for patients with transposition of great arteries, pulmonary outflow track obstruction, and VSD. It involves placement of a baffle within the right ventricle, directing blood from the VSD to the aorta, and utilizes the VSD as part of the left ventricular outflow track. The pulmonary valve or subpulmonic region is oversewn and the conduit is inserted between the right ventricle and pulmonary artery. The main advantage of this operation is that the left ventricle becomes the systemic ventricle. An important limitation in this procedure is that the patient is committed to further operations, as the conduit is likely to be replaced several times during the patient's life.

ARTERIAL SWITCH OPERATION (JATENE PROCEDURE)

The arterial switch operation involves transsection of the aorta and pulmonary artery above the valve sinuses; coronary arteries are detached from the aorta with a surrounding button of aortic wall and sutured into place into the neoaorta. The pulmonary trunk is moved forward into the new position anterior to the aorta, and the switched great arteries are sutured into place. This is a technically challenging operation performed within the first 2 weeks of life and should be undertaken, at the latest, by 4 to 6 weeks of life. Its advantage over the Mustard or Senning procedure is that the left ventricle becomes the systemic ventricle.

NORWOOD PROCEDURE

The Norwood procedure is used for repair of hypoplastic let heart. It is a two-stage procedure: in stage I the aorta origin is widened, the PA is transected and closed, and then followed by a modified right BT shunt and atrial septectomy; in stage II a modified Fontan procedure is performed when cyanosis is increased.

PERCUTANEOUS OCCLUSION OF ASD

Early closure of ASD in asymptomatic adults with enlargement of the right ventricle is performed to reduce the risk of atrial arrhythmias, for symptoms of right ventricular failure, and at onset of pulmonary vascular disease.

Device closure is not appropriate for sinus venosus defects, atrioventricular septal defects, or secundum defects greater than 40 mm in size. Two common devices used are the Amplatz septal occluder and the CardioSEAL implant. Anatomic consideration for device closure includes detailed anatomic study typically with transesophageal echocardiography, especially to evaluate the pulmonary veins, right upper lobe pulmonary vein, mitral and tricuspid valves, coronary sinus, and vena cava. The presence of anomalous pulmonary venous drainage or close proximity of the defect to these structures preclude the use of device closure.

QUESTIONS AND ANSWERS

1. For what congenital cardiac defect is pulmonary banding used?
   A. ASD in infants
   B. TOF
   C. Single ventricle
   D. TGA

   ANSWER: C. Pulmonary artery banding is done in patients with excessive pulmonary blood flow causing CHF in infants who get definitive repair later in life. The single ventricle is the most common lesion requiring banding in order to protect the pulmonary bed for future Fontan conversion. In ASD usually a definitive repair with a septal patch or percutaneous occlusion is done. TOF patients have decreased blood flow therefore need a shunt procedure to increase blood flow and not banding. In TGA the repair is either done by switching the atria (Senning/Mustard procedure) or arteries (Jatene procedure).

2. Regarding percutaneous atrial septal occlusion, which of the following is *false*?
   A. Early closure in asymptomatic adults is often done to decrease atrial fibrillation.
   B. The onset of pulmonary vascular disease is decreased.
   C. It is ideal for sinus venosus defects.
   D. Defects must be <40 mm.

   ANSWER: C. Early closure of ASD in asymptomatic adults with enlargement of the right ventricle is done to reduce the risk of atrial arrhythmias, symptoms of right ventricular failure, and onset of pulmonary vascular disease. Device closure is not appropriate for sinus venosus defects, atrioventricular septal defects, or secundum defects greater than 40 mm in size.

3. Regarding the Fontan procedure, which of the following is *false*?
   A. It bypasses the right ventricle.
   B. It includes Glenn anastomosis between the aorta and pulmonary artery.
   C. Blood flow to the lungs is nonpulsatile.
   D. Protein losing enteropathy is a known complication.

   ANSWER: B. The original Fontan procedure consists of classic Glenn anastomosis between the superior vena cava and the right pulmonary artery (not aorta and PA), closure of the atrial septal defect, insertion of a homograft valve in the inferior vena cava, and placement of a homograft valve conduit between the right atrium and the left pulmonary artery. Various modifications of this procedure were done because of late morbidity from valve conduits. The operation basically bypasses the right ventricle and, via a surgically constructed atriopulmonary connection and atrial separation, conducts blood into the lung without the benefit of pulsatile ventricular flow. Protein losing enteropathy is a known late complication of this procedure.

4. The following surgical procedures are done in transposition of great arteries, *except*:
   A. The Rastelli procedure
   B. The Norwood procedure
   C. The Senning procedure
   D. The Jatene procedure

   ANSWER: B. The Norwood operation is done in cases of hypoplastic left heart syndrome and is a two-stage procedure: in stage I the aorta origin is widened, the PA is transected and closed, and then followed by a modified right BT shunt and atrial septectomy; in stage II a modified Fontan procedure is performed when cyanosis is increased.

   The Rastelli procedure involves placement of a baffle within the right ventricle, directing blood from the VSD to the aorta, and utilizes the VSD as part of the left ventricular outflow track. The pulmonary valve or subpulmonic region is oversewn, and the conduit is inserted between the right ventricle and pulmonary artery. It is most frequently used for patients with TGA, pulmonary outflow track obstruction, and VSD. Jatene or arterial switch operation involves transsection of the aorta and pulmonary artery at the level above the valve sinuses, detaching the coronary arteries from the aorta with a surrounding button of aortic wall, and suturing into place into the neoaorta. The pulmonary trunk is moved forward into the new position anterior to the aorta, and the switched great arteries are sutured into place. The Senning procedure (atrial switch operation) involves forming a baffle within the atria in order to switch the flow of blood at in-flow level. In the Senning operation, the baffle is created from the right atrial wall and atrial septal tissue without the use of extrinsic material, whereas the Mustard operation involves resection of the atrial septum and the creation of a baffle from the pericardium or synthetic material.

5. What is the shunt between the ascending aorta to right pulmonary artery known as?
   A. The Pott procedure
   B. The Blalock-Taussig procedure
   C. The Waterson procedure
   D. The Brock procedure

   ANSWER: C. The Waterson procedure involves a shunt between the ascending aorta to the right pulmonary artery; the Pott procedure involves connecting the descending aorta to the left pulmonary artery; the classic Blalock-Taussig procedure involves a shunt between the subclavian to the pulmonary artery, constructed on the opposite side from the arch; the Brock procedure includes a pulmonary valvotomy closed with or without infundibular dilatation or resection.

43 AORTIC DISEASES

Satinder P. Singh

ACQUIRED AORTIC DISEASES

THORACIC AORTIC ANEURYSM

Thoracic aortic aneurysm is defined as localized or diffuse dilatation of more than 50% of the normal diameter of the thoracic aorta. In the thoracic aorta, more than 4.5 cm is considered aneurysmal. More than 6 cm is considered to present a significant risk of rupture. They are mostly fusiform (80%) and less common saccular (20%). Aneurysms of the descending aorta are most common, followed by those of the ascending aorta, and least commonly involve the arch. Thoracic aortic aneurysms are less common than the abdominal aorta aneurysm. Although atherosclerosis is the most common cause of aortic aneurysms, there are numerous other etiologies (Table 43-1), which are dependent on location (Tables 43-2, 43-3, and 43-4). Thoracic aneurysms are often associated with an abdominal aneurysm. They are more common in men (2.5:1).

The lifetime probability of rupture of thoracic and thoracoabdominal aneurysms is 75% to 80%, with 5-year untreated survival rates of 10% to 20%.

TABLE 43-1 Etiology of Thoracic Aortic Aneurysm

Atherosclerosis (most common)
Trauma
Infection
Cystic medial necrosis (Marfan, Ehler-Danlos syndrome)
Hypertension
Bicuspid aortic valve
Inflammatory (Takayasu, giant cell arthritis)

CLINICAL FEATURES

Clinical presentation of aortic aneurysms includes the following:

- Asymptomatic (40%), often discovered incidentally on physical examination or chest radiography.
- Chest pain.
- Peripheral embolization (bowel or extremity ischemia, TIA).
- Systemic symptoms in inflammatory or mycotic aneurysms (Table 43-5).

COMPLICATIONS OF THORACIC AORTIC ANEURYSM

Complications of thoracic aneurysm include expansion, rupture, and dissection. Thoracic aortic aneurysms expand at a rate of 0.43 cm/y (faster in aneurysms greater than 5 cm). Rupture of thoracic aortic aneurysms is more frequent than abdominal aortic ruptures. Patients may be asymptomatic, though they are more often symptomatic and these symptomatic patients have poor prognosis. There is dramatic onset of excruciating pain,

TABLE 43-2 Causes of Ascending Aortic Aneurysm

Marfan syndrome
Syphilis
Atherosclerosis (rare)

TABLE 43-3 Etiology of Aortic Arch Aneurysm

Takayasu arteritis
Atherosclerosis

and rupture commonly occurs into the left pleural space. Intrapericardial rupture leads to hypotension or even tamponade.

Imaging Features

CT is a common and reliable modality performed for initial diagnosis of aneurysm, preoperative assessment, and postoperative surveillance. Transesophageal echocardiogram (TEE) is not accurate for diagnosing thoracic aneurysm though it is quite accurate in diagnosing dissection and can be done bedside if the patient is unstable. TEE is excellent in documenting pericardial effusion and aortic regurgitation. MRI is particularly useful for long-term serial follow-up and in those with coexisting aortic valve disease.

Treatment

Treatment for thoracic aneurysm includes surgical or endostent repair or a combined staged approach. Indications for repair of aortic aneurysm include the following:

- Growth rate > 1 cm/y.
- Symptomatic aneurysm.
- Size > 5.5 cm ascending and > 6.5 descending aorta. (In familial and Marfan syndrome cases, surgery is performed sooner.)

Prior to endostent repair, preoperative assessment is performed with CTA with multiplanar reformatting. It is important to describe any branch vessel involvement, any angulation of the aorta, diameter and length of the aneurysm, and presence and extent of aortic wall calcification. Typically greater than 1 cm of normal aortic wall is required adjacent to the abnormal aneurysm wall, and there should be 40 to 42 mm or less diameter of proximal and distal aortic necks, 9 mm or larger size of femoral and iliac arteries, and no severe tortuosity. Follow-up after stent placement is also performed with CTA at 3-, 6-, and 12-month intervals and yearly thereafter.

TABLE 43-4 Syphilitic Aneurysm

Typically involves the ascending aorta
Spares the sinuses (sinuses in Marfan)
Calcification is common (tree bark appearance)

TABLE 43-5 Key Features of Mycotic Aneurysm

Etiology
Bacterial aortitis (usually *Salmonella* or *Staphylococcus aureus*)
Syphilitic aortitis (ascending aorta sparing sinuses)
Rapid eccentric saccular aneurysmal growth
Periaortic soft tissue stranding, edema, fluid or gas, lobular outline, enhancement of periaortic soft tissue
Major branching points
Increased risk in
Bacterial endocarditis
Immunocompromised status
Prosthetic vascular devices
Intravenous drug abuser
Treatment
Surgical resection and grafting following antibiotic therapy
In some cases, endovascular stent repair with antibiotic therapy

Complications of endostent treatment include endoleak (see Table 66-1 in Chapter 66), stent migration, pseudoaneurysm formation, dissection, perforation, thrombosis, kinking, coverage of visceral branch, and spinal ischemia. Type I endoleak is the most common in the thoracic aorta, but type II is the most common endoleak in the abdomen. Both types I and III have an increased risk of rupture; type IV endoleak is usually transient.

POSTTRAUMATIC PSEUDOANEURYSM

Posttraumatic pseudoaneurysm is typically located at the isthmus with or without typical eccentric peripheral calcification. A saccular pseudoaneurysm is contained by adventitia and does not contain normal aortic wall. Following initial trauma, 2.5% of patients develop chronic posttraumatic pseudoaneurysm. It is usually asymptomatic with an increased tendency to rupture if larger than 6 cm. It is treated with endovascular stent graft or open surgical repair.

INTRAMURAL HEMATOMA

Intramural hematoma, also known as noncommunicating aortic dissection, is part of the acute aortic syndrome. It is secondary to hemorrhage within the aortic wall due to rupture of the vasa vasorum with typical absence of intimal tear. Classification and treatment are similar to aortic dissection: type A (ascending aorta involved) and type B (descending aorta only) (Table 43-6). Most patients are hypertensive and present with acute chest pain.

TABLE 43-6 Aortic Dissection Classification

Stanford classification
Type A: Involves ascending aorta, descending aorta may or may not be involved, surgical treatment
Type B: Limited to descending aorta, medical management
DeBakey classification
Type 1: Involves ascending aorta, aortic arch, and descending aorta
Type 2: Ascending aorta
Type 3: Descending aorta distal to the left subclavian artery

Natural history of intramural hematoma includes complete resolution (30%), progression to dissection or aneurysm, and subsequent rupture.

Imaging Features

CT is the primary modality of choice for diagnosis and reveals crescentic hyperdense aortic wall thickening on noncontrast examination. Hypodense aortic wall with elliptical aortic lumen with well-defined margins, but without intimal flap, is identified on contrast-enhanced CT.

MR reveals high signal in the aortic wall on T1-weighted images. There is low signal on postcontrast T1-weighted images. Postcontrast images show lack of contrast in the intramural hematoma.

PENETRATING AORTIC ULCER

Ulcerated atherosclerotic lesions penetrate the elastic lamina into the media with associated aortic wall hematoma. The most common location is the descending aorta (more than 90%) followed by the ascending aorta. In 10%, multiple ulcers are present.

Pathological findings include focal outpouching of the aortic wall and irregular edges with associated extensive aortic atheroma. The risk of aortic rupture is high. The most common signs and symptoms are similar to those of aortic dissection. Sometimes the patient may be asymptomatic. It is commonly seen in elderly men more than in women. Treatment includes medical therapy to decrease blood pressure or surgical repair, especially if the ascending aorta is involved. Lately, endovascular endostent treatment is used.

AORTIC DISSECTION

Etiology

Many diseases predispose to aortic dissection: atherosclerosis, hypertension (most common), collagen disorders, Marfan and Ehlers-Danlos syndrome, collagen vascular diseases, pregnancy, and congenital disorders (bicuspid aortic valve or aortic coarctation).

Iatrogenic causes include cardiac surgery, valve replacement, coronary artery bypass, or percutaneous catheter placement. Other rare causes include crack cocaine abuse and syphilitic aortitis.

Imaging Features

Chest radiography may be normal or may show a widened mediastinum of more than 8 cm with an ill-defined large aortic knob with medially displaced intimal calcification when compared with prior radiographs. If there is rupture, hemothorax, left apical cap, tracheal deviation, depression of left main bronchus, esophageal deviation, pericardial effusion, or loss of peritracheal stripe may be visible.

Contrast-enhanced CT will demonstrate the site and extent of dissection, involvement of great vessels in the thorax, and extension and involvement of abdominal aortic branches. Complications such as rupture into the pericardial space or formation of intramural thrombus or rupture of dissecting aneurysm may occur.

CT is recommended for acute presentation. MR is good for follow-up, and transesophageal echo is often obtained in unstable patients at bedside.

Treatment

Treatment is surgical for type A and medical for type B dissections. Medical control of hypertension is employed, and surgery is reserved for complicated cases of type B dissection (such as those with mesenteric or extremity ischemia, renal artery involvement or rupture, or aneurysmal enlargement of false lumen). More recently, percutaneous endostent treatment has been used for type B dissection.

TRAUMATIC AORTIC LACERATION

Traumatic aortic laceration is usually secondary to sudden deacceleration injury to the thorax (motor ventricle collision or fall from height). Typical location is the aortic isthmus, followed by the aortic arch, descending thoracic aorta, and ascending aorta cranial to the aortic valve.

Imaging Features

Chest radiography demonstrates mediastinal widening of greater than 8 cm. Other supportive findings include indistinct aortic outline, increased paratracheal soft tissue density, left apical cap, associated first or second rib fractures, and tracheal and downward left mainstem bronchus displacement. Contrast-enhanced CT is the best modality for diagnosis. Laceration must be differentiated from ductus diverticulum and penetrating atherosclerotic ulcer. Ductus diverticulum, which is located at the aortic isthmus, has a smooth contour with obtuse margins and broad-based outpouching. However, no intimal flap or tear is identifiable. Multiplanar reconstruction helps in diagnosis. On the other hand, a penetrating ulcer is located not at the inner aspect of the aortic isthmus, but rather at the descending thoracic aorta and is associated with extensive calcified atherosclerotic plaques.

Treatment

The mainstay of treatment is surgical repair with left thoracotomy and placement of interposition graft or anastomosis. Endovascular stent grafting with or without associated open thoracotomy approach is increasingly used.

With surgery, a 60% to 70% survival rate is expected. However, without intervention, 80% of patients die within 1 hour, 85% within 24 hours, and 98% in 10 weeks. Long-term outcome if the patient survives the initial period includes chronic posttraumatic pseudoaneurysm.

TAKAYASU ARTERITIS

Takayasu arteritis is a granulomatous inflammatory vasculitis, affecting medial and large vessel walls, especially the aorta and its branches. It is most common in Asian countries. There is patchy thickening of the large- and medium-sized vessels.

Early in the inflammatory (nonobstructive) phase patients have nonspecific symptoms with elevated ESR. The late (occlusive phase) is also considered the "pulseless phase" because of vascular stenoses. Takayasu arteritis usually presents in younger patients, more commonly in women rather than men.

Imaging Features

Chest radiograph may show premature calcification of the aorta. CT or MR are the diagnostic modalities most commonly used. There is concentric wall thickening, which may be enhanced with contrast. The left subclavian artery is the most common site of involvement, followed by other main branches and the aorta. Occasionally, the pulmonary artery is involved. Stenosis or ostial arch vessel occlusion is common.

Treatment

Treatment includes corticosteroids with angioplasty or surgical bypass for narrowing or occlusion. However, stenting has a high failure rate.

GIANT CELL ARTERITIS

Giant cell arteritis is a rare occurrence in patients younger than 50 years (in comparison with Takayasu arteritis, which is common in younger patients). Otherwise, there is a similar appearance to Takayasu arteritis with mural inflammation, vessel wall thickening, and enhancement. The most common location is the extracranial carotid vessel with a propensity for a superficial temporal artery. It rarely involves the thoracic or abdominal aorta. Like Takayasu arteritis, it is treated with steroids.

CONGENITAL AORTIC DISEASES

COARCTATION OF THE AORTA

Coarctation of the aorta is caused by congenital narrowing of the proximal descending thoracic aorta opposite the origin of the ductus arteriosus (postductal being most common). Less commonly, coarctation occurs proximally between the left subclavian artery and the left common carotid artery, which is more common in infants and neonates. Coarctation accounts for 6.5% of cases of congenital heart disease.

Collateral circulation is present, proximal and distal to the coarctation and usually involves branches of the subclavian artery, especially the internal mammary, vertebral, costocervical, and thyrocervical trunks. The most common anomaly associated with coarctation is the bicuspid aortic valve (27%–46%).

Associated abnormalities of the subclavian artery can significantly alter collateral pathways. Stenosis of the left subclavian artery or anomalous origin of the right subclavian artery (if coexisting with coarctation of the aorta) restricts collateral circulation on the affected side, leading to unilateral rib notching.

Clinical Features

The age of presentation depends on the severity of the coarctation and associated anomalies. Severe coarctation usually presents during the first week of life, soon after closure of the ductus arteriosus; patients present with heart failure and acidosis from hyperprofusion of the lower body. Less severe forms usually present in patients at a later age with manifestations of systemic hypertension.

Imaging Features

In the neonatal period, the heart is invariably enlarged with signs of heart failure. Abnormality of the aortic contour and rib notching is not evident at this age. In older patients, left ventricular hypertrophy is present. Rib notching is more commonly identified after patients are 8 years of age and is usually due to dilatation of the posterior intercostal arteries and is seen along the medial half of the inferior rib margins of the fourth through eighth posterior ribs. The aortic arch is less prominent due to hypoplasia of the arch with increased prominence of the left subclavian artery. At the site of coarctation, the contour of the descending aorta becomes discontinuous followed by dilatation of the descending aorta (poststenotic dilatation), resembling the number "3." A reverse "3" sign is seen from the impression on the barium-filled esophagus from coarctation.

Imaging is required to establish the location and degree of stenosis, length of stenotic segment, associated aortic arch abnormalities, and collateral pathways.

Echocardiography is used for diagnosis in the neonatal period, whereas MR and CT are used in later life to establish diagnosis as well as for follow-up evaluation after treatment.

Treatment

Surgery is the treatment of choice for most coarctations. Balloon angioplasty also has a high success rate. Recently, endostent treatment following angioplasty has shown excellent results.

PSEUDOCOARCTATION

Pseudocoarctation is an uncommon condition where the aortic arch is unusually high and the descending thoracic aorta buckles at the level of the aortic isthmus. There is no hemodynamic obstruction, and no collateral flow is present. Often radiographic abnormality is detected incidentally, mimicking paramediastinal mass or aortic aneurysm.

VASCULAR RING

Vascular ring is an anomalous configuration of the aortic arch and/or associated vessels creating a complete ring around the trachea or esophagus.

This anomaly, associated with deletion of chromosome region 22q11 occurs early in embryologic development and occurs in many forms. Vascular ring results from incomplete regression of first of the six embryonic brachial arches. Early in development, a dorsal and ventral aortic arch is present. Six embryonic brachial arches connect the two arches. The third, fourth, and sixth arches are crucial in the development of the aortic arch, its major branches, the ductus arteriosus, and the pulmonary artery. In normal development, each arch develops into a vascular structure or involutes in the following manner:

- Right and left first and second arches develop into a portion of the arterial supply of the face.
- The third arch forms the carotid arteries.
- The dorsal aorta between the third and fourth arches involutes.
- The fourth arch is the main contributors to the aortic arch. The proximal right fourth arch develops into the right subclavian artery. The left fourth arch remains as the aortic arch.
- The fifth arch involutes bilaterally.
- The ventral sixth arch develops into the proximal right pulmonary artery. The ventral left sixth arch develops into the left pulmonary artery, while the dorsal portion becomes the ductus arteriosus.
- The seventh segmental arterial branches of the dorsal aorta form the left subclavian artery and the distal right subclavian artery.

DOUBLE AORTIC ARCH

The double aortic arch is due to the persistence of both left and right fourth aortic arches, and it is the most common *symptomatic* vascular ring. The majority of cases are dominant right arch with left descending aorta (75%). In 20% of cases, it is dominant right arch with right descending aorta. The most common symptom is inspiratory strider worsening with feeding. The trachea is deviated from the dominant arch and right arch and is often larger and more superior than the left arch. As a result, severe tracheal compression may occur.

Imaging Features

CT or MRI can identify both arches and their branches. Each arch gives rise to a vertebrocarotid and dorsal subclavian artery ("four artery sign").

Echocardiogram, (suprasternal) notch view, is most helpful in demonstrating two separate arches giving rise to separate carotid and subclavian arteries without brachiocephalic trunks. Echo is inadequate to demonstrate airway compression. On the lateral chest radiograph, the anterior and posterior compression of the trachea may be seen at the level of the arch. (In the left pulmonary sling, there is compression on the anterior aspect of the esophagus and posterior aspect of the trachea.)

Treatment

Treatment includes thoracotomy on the side of the smaller aortic arch with division of the smaller of the arch, the atretic segment, and ligamentum arteriosum. Complications of surgery include aortoesophageal fistula, persistent airway compression, and symptoms leading to tracheobronchomalacia.

RIGHT AORTIC ARCH

Right arch with mirror image branching is associated with cyanotic congenital heart disease, whereas right arch with aberrant left subclavian artery is not. There may be dilatation of the origin of the left aberrant subclavian artery (diverticulum of Kommerell). The presence of left ligamentum arteriosum may lead to complete vascular ring and may be associated with airway compression. A right arch is the most common congenital anomaly of the aortic arch in asymptomatic patients. Commonly associated congenital anomalies (10%–15% of cases) include tetralogy of Fallot, pulmonary atresia with VSD (25%), and truncus arteriosus (30%). Tetralogy of Fallot is the most likely diagnosis in the setting of a cyanotic heart lesion with right aortic arch.

PULMONARY SLING

Anomalous origin of the left pulmonary artery from the proximal right pulmonary artery forms a sling around the distal trachea, passing in between the trachea and esophagus. This is the only vascular ring coursing between the trachea and esophagus and, therefore, the only vascular ring associated with asymmetric lung inflation and aeration. The most common clinical presentation is severe strider, hypoxia, and ventilator dependency. This vascular anomaly is secondary to agenesis or obliteration of the left sixth arch, which normally forms the left pulmonary artery branch.

Lateral chest radiograph reveals soft tissue density between the distal trachea and esophagus with posterior compression of the trachea. On frontal radiographs, the left hilum is lower in position. Barium esophagography reveals anterior indentation on the esophagus. Imaging diagnosis can be made from echo, CT, or MR.

SUGGESTED READING

Batra P, Bigoni B, Manning J, et al. Pitfalls in the diagnosis of thoracic aortic dissection at CT angiography. *RadioGraphics.* 2000;20:309-320.

Bean MJ, Johnson PT, Roseborough GS, Black JH, Fishman EK. Thoracic aortic stent-grafts: utility of multidetector CT for pre- and postprocedure evaluation. *RadioGraphics.* 2008;28: 1835-1851.

Castaner E, Andreu M, Gallardo X, Mata JM, Cabezuelo MA, Pallardo Y. CT in nontraumatic acute thoracic aortic disease: typical and atypical features and complications. *RadioGraphics.* 2003;23:S93-S110.

Eisenbud L, Francis IR, Williams DM, Monaghan HM, Deeb GM. Synthetic interposition grafts of the thoracic aorta: postoperative appearance on serial CT studies. *Radiology.* 1999; 211:317-324.

Hayashi H, Matsuoka Y, Sakamoto I, et al. Atheroslerotic ulcer of the aorta: imaging features and disease concept. *RadioGraphics.* 2000;20:995-1005.

Liu Q, Lu JP, Wang F, Wang L, Tian JM. Three-dimensional contrast-enhanced MR angiography of aortic dissection: a pictorial essay. *RadioGraphics.* 2007;27:1311-1321.

Sundaram B, Quint LE, Patel HJ, Deeb M. CT findings following thoracic aortic surgery. *RadioGraphics.* 2007;27:1583-1594.

Stavropoulos SW, Clark TWI, Carpenter JP, et al. Use of CT angiography to classify endoleaks after endovascular repair of abdominal aortic aneurysms. *J Vas Interv Radiol.* 2005;16: 663-667.

QUESTIONS AND ANSWERS

1. Regarding thoracic aortic aneurysms, which of the following is *true*?
   A. Thoracic aortic aneurysm is more common than abdominal aneurysm.
   B. Thorax aneurysm most frequently involves the aortic arch.
   C. Abdominal aortic aneurysm rupture is more frequent than thoracic rupture.
   D. In a patient with known aneurysm, sudden onset excruciating pain usually indicates rupture.

   ANSWER: D. Abdominal aortic aneurysm is more common than thoracic aneurysm, but thoracic aortic aneurysms rupture more frequently than abdominal aortic aneurysms. Sudden pain in a patient with known aortic aneurysm often indicates rupture, which most commonly occurs into the left pleural cavity. Descending thoracic aorta is the most common site for aneurysm in the chest.

2. Which of the following is *not* an indication for repair of thoracic aortic aneurysm?
   A. Symptomatic aneurysm
   B. Growth rate more than 1 cm/y
   C. Involvement of the ascending aorta
   D. Size more than 6.5 cm

   ANSWER: C. Involvement of the ascending aorta is indication for repair for aortic dissection and not aortic aneurysm. Repair is indicated if the aneurysm increases more than 5.5 cm in size for ascending aorta and >6.5 cm for descending aorta. Most aortic aneurysms grow at rate of 0.43 cm/y; if growth rate is faster (>1 cm/y), then surgery should be considered. The presence of symptoms in patients with aneurysm is also an indication for surgical repair.

3. Regarding endoleak, which of following is *correct*?
   A. Type II is the most common type of endoleak in the thoracic aorta.
   B. There is increased risk of rupture for type III endoleak
   C. Type IV endoleak is related to graft failure.
   D. Retrograde perfusion of patent aortic branches is the most common cause for endoleak.

   ANSWER: B. Type I endoleak is the most common type of endoleak in the thoracic aorta. Type II is secondary to retrograde perfusion of patent aortic branches, but it does not carry an increased risk of rupture. Type I endoleak usually occurs at the proximal or distal stent attachment site, and there is increased risk of rupture for type I and type III endoleak. Type III endoleak is due to graft-related failures, and type IV endoleak is due to graft wall porosity, a transient phenomenon.

4. Concerning mycotic aneurysm, which of following is *incorrect*?
   A. Show rapid fusiform growth
   B. Often caused by bacterial infection
   C. Usually occurs at branching points
   D. High incidence in intravenous drug abusers

   ANSWER: A. Mycotic aneurysms are usually caused by bacterial infections, *Salmonella* or *Staphylococcus aureus,* and occur at branching points with high incidence in patients with immunocompromised status, intravenous drug abuse, bacterial endocarditis, or prostatic vascular devices. The mycotic aneurysms show rapid eccentric saccular growth, not fusiform growth.

5. Regarding aortic dissection, which is *true*?
   A. The most common site of dissection is the aortic root followed by the proximal descending aorta, and aortic diaphragmatic hiatus.
   B. Type A dissections are managed medically and type B dissections surgically.
   C. Iatrogenic cause is common.
   D. Chest radiograph can be normal.

   ANSWER: D. The most common site of aortic dissection is proximal descending thoracic aorta near the ductus ligament attachment, followed by aortic root and aortic diaphragmatic hiatus. Type B dissections involve only descending thoracic aorta and are managed medically. Type A dissections involve ascending aorta and are treated surgically. Chest radiograph may be normal in a patient with aortic dissection, and CT angiography is the modality of choice for diagnosis in an acute setting.

6. Which of the following is *correct* regarding aortic aneurysm?
   A. In Marfan syndrome, ascending aortic aneurysm spares the sinus of Valsalva.
   B. Tree bark appearance is commonly described for mycotic aneurysm.
   C. The most common site of rupture for an ascending aorta is the right pleural space.
   D. Posttraumatic pseudoaneurysm is typically located at the isthmus.

   ANSWER: D. Ascending aortic aneurysm can be due to atherosclerosis, Marfan syndrome, or syphilis. The aortic sinus is spared in syphilis but is involved in Marfan syndrome. Tree bark appearance refers to the calcification of the syphilitic ascending aortic aneurysm. The ascending aortic aneurysm usually ruptures into the pericardial space and can lead to tamponade. The descending thoracic aortic rupture is usually into the left pleural space. Posttraumatic aneurysm is commonly located at the isthmus and occurs only in 2.5% of patients following initial trauma.

7. Which of following is *correct* for acute aortic syndrome?
   A. Penetrating aortic ulcers are common in young women.
   B. Descending thoracic aorta is the most common site.
   C. The majority of patients are asymptomatic.
   D. Intramural hemorrhage is commonly due to blunt trauma.

   ANSWER: B. Penetrating aortic ulcers are most commonly seen in the descending aorta in elderly men who have extensive atherosclerotic aortic disease. The most common presentation is chest pain similar to dissection, and only occasionally there are no symptoms. Intramural hemorrhage occurs due to hemorrhage into the aortic wall from rupture of the vasa vasorum. It is often seen in patients with hypertension and is less commonly due to trauma.

8. Regarding aortic arch development, which of the following is *correct*?
   A. The second and third arches are the main contributors to aortic arch.
   B. Double aortic arch is due to persistence of dorsal and ventral third arches.
   C. The proximal right fourth arch develops into the right subclavian artery.
   D. Pulmonary sling is due to obliteration of left fifth aortic arch.

ANSWER: C. Aortic arch is mainly formed from the left fourth arch and double aortic arch forms from persistent right and left fourth arches. Normally, the right fourth arch forms the proximal right subclavian artery. The left pulmonary artery develops from the left ventral sixth arch, and obliteration of the latter leads to formation of pulmonary sling.

9. Regarding coarctation, which of the following is *correct*?
   A. Coarctation of aorta is most commonly located between the left subclavian and left common carotid arteries.
   B. Patients with postductal coarctation present with upper extremity cyanosis.
   C. The most common associated anomaly is atrial septal defect.
   D. There is no hemodynamic gradient in pseudocoarctation.

ANSWER: D. The most common location of coarctation is postductal beyond the origin of the left subclavian artery. Most patients with postductal coarctation present with systemic hypertension during young adolescence, while those with severe coarctation present in infancy after ductus closure with heart failure, severe acidosis, and lower extremity hypoperfusion. Bicuspid valve is the most common associated anomaly (27%–43%). Pseudocoarctation is due to an unusual high arch with buckling of descending aorta detected incidentally on radiograph mimicking aneurysm or coarctation. It is differentiated from coarctation based on the absence of hemodynamic gradient and collateral flow.

10. Regarding aortic dissection, which is *correct*?
   A. The majority of patients survive aortic transsection.
   B. Chest radiographs are often abnormal.
   C. Surgical repair is done via right thoracotomy.
   D. In 40% of patients, a chronic pseudoaneurysm develops after initial trauma.

ANSWER: B. The majority of aortic transaction patients die before reaching the hospital due to exsanguination. With surgery, a 60% to 70% survival rate is expected; without intervention, 80% die within 1 hour, 85% die within 24 hours, and 98% die within 10 weeks. Chronic posttraumatic pseudoaneurysm can develop but only in a minority of patients (fewer than 5%). Since the most common location of aortic traumatic injury is near the isthmus, a left and not right thoracotomy is required for repair. Chest radiographs are abnormal in the majority of patients who make it to the hospital.

Section 4
GASTROINTESTINAL TRACT

44 GI TRACT CONTRAST AND TECHNIQUE

Cheri L. Canon

There are two general categories of contrast agents used in gastrointestinal (GI) tract fluoroscopy: barium sulfate-based and iodine-based agents. The type of contrast prescribed is determined by the clinical indication for the examination.

Although relatively few, there are risks associated with barium contrast fluoroscopy. Barium sulfate is relatively inert but can incite inflammatory response if spilled into the mediastinum or peritoneal cavity, particularly if spilled with infected bowel contents. For this reason, a water-soluble agent is preferred if perforation is suspected. Some patients may have a hypersensitivity to the additives or the latex in the rectal tube or balloon. Aspiration of small quantities of barium is not a significant danger; however, as with all types of liquids, there is increased risk of respiratory failure with large-volume aspiration, particularly in patients with compromised pulmonary function.

Barium contrast must be used cautiously when performing diagnostic enema examinations in patients suspected of having mechanical obstruction of the colon, because of the danger of barium becoming inspissated above the site of obstruction. In general, if barium flows freely in a retrograde fashion across a strictured region, in all likelihood it will pass without difficulty. Additionally, rectal balloons should be employed with caution and only inflated with fluoroscopic visualization after the rectum has been distended with contrast to ensure normal compliance. Its use is contraindicated in patients with proctitis or with history of prior pelvic radiation, most commonly for prostate cancer in men and cervical cancer in women. Small bowel obstruction is not a contraindication to the oral administration of barium, but CT is a better method to evaluate this clinical condition. As with all studies that incorporate ionizing radiation, pregnancy status must be determined before beginning any fluoroscopy examination in women of childbearing age.

Barium agents come in various densities. They are measured by weight per volume (total number of grams of barium sulfate present in 100 mL of the barium solution) or weight per weight (total number of grams of barium sulfate in each 100 g of dry product). "Thin-barium" suspensions for the upper GI tract usually range from 35% to 80% w/v. These solutions, usually used in the single-contrast examinations, provide good luminal distension and can be used for assessment of emptying and motility. High-density or "thick-barium" solutions, usually 210% to 250% w/v, are used in the double-contrast portion of the upper GI examination. They provide good mucosal relief when an effervescent agent is used for distension. Small bowel studies typically use 46% to 60% w/v solution with a minimum volume of 500 mL of the barium solution. Double-contrast barium enema examination uses a solution of 60% to 120% w/v, and 12% to 15% w/v is used for single-contrast enema examinations.

Barium swallow and upper GI studies are typically biphasic in nature, containing both elements of single- and double-contrast examinations. Therefore, assessment for stricture, motility, and mucosal pathology is completed with one study. Double-contrast, or air-contrast, examination indicates that both air and high-density barium are used to delineate a mucosal surface. Single-contrast examination incorporates a full column of usually slightly less dense medium to distend the GI tract. Prone, single-contrast views of the stomach and duodenum may incorporate the use of a compression paddle to displace the dense pool of barium, allowing for a more see-through view. Collapsed views of the esophagus are helpful for the diagnosis of varices which tend to fill (distend) in this view and are effaced with esophageal distension.

Diatrizoate meglumine (Gastrografin) and diatrizoate sodium (MD-Gastroview) solutions are iodine-based water-soluble contrast agents for enteric use. They have high osmolality and can cause severe bronchospasm, flash pulmonary edema, pneumonitis, and even death if aspirated. As a result, they are contraindicated in patients at risk for aspiration or with a tracheoesophageal fistula. Additionally, because of their high osmolarity (1940 mOsm/kg H_2O, 2000 mOsm/kg H_2O, respectively. Remember, plasma is approximately 300 mOsm/kg H_2O), they are limited in volume that can be administered orally, ranging from 30 to 120 mL (up to 4 oz). Volumes higher than this can drastically alter fluid balance by drawing fluid into the bowel lumen. This becomes a particular concern with infants and elderly patients, particularly if dehydrated, because of risk of aspiration and large volume shifts using the hyperosmolar enteric contrast agents. There has been a significant shift to use low-osmolar agents (Omnipaque, Isovue) typically administered intravenously for contrast-enhanced CT examinations. The typical enteric dose ranges from 50 to 500 mL.

As with intravenous iodinated agents, there is a small risk for anaphylactoid reactions. Theoretically, small quantities of luminal contrast agent can be absorbed across the mucosa and enter into the bloodstream. Since these types of reactions are not volume dependent, even a small amount may lead to mild reactions of urticaria to life-threatening reactions including laryngospasm, bronchospasm, arrhythmia, hypotension, and death. Therefore, a history of a severe anaphylactoid reaction to iodinated agents is a contraindication to their administration enterally as well as parenterally.

Glucagon is the most common antispasmodic agent used in the United States. It can be given intravenously, submucosally, or intramuscularly (Table 44-1). It increases the concentration of blood glucose and is used in the treatment of hypoglycemia. It also relaxes the smooth muscle of the stomach, duodenum, small bowel, ileocecal valve, and colon. However, its effect on the esophagus is less apparent. Dosages typically range from 0.1 to 1 mg. Smaller dosages can be used in the upper GI tract, but 1 to 2 mg dosages are need to induce colonic hypotonia. It is contraindicated in patients who have known hypersensitivity, usually to one of the additives and not glucagon itself. Additionally, in patients who have an insulinoma or pheochromocytoma, it can result in severe subsequent hypoglycemia because of the release of insulin or catecholamines, respectively.

TABLE 44-1 Glucagon Pharmacokinetics

DOSE	ROUTE	ONSET	DURATION
0.5 mg	IV	1 min	9–17 min
1.0 mg	IV	1 min	22–25 min
	IM	8–10 min	12–27 min

IM, intramuscular; IV, intravenous.

Suggested Reading

ACR Contrast Media Manual, Version 6.0. May 2008.

Skucas J. Contrast media. In: Gore RM, Levine MS, Laufer I, eds. *Textbook of Gastrointestinal Radiology*. Vol. 1. Philadelphia, PA: W.B. Saunders; 1994;190: 709-714.

QUESTIONS AND ANSWERS

1. Which of the following is the typical density of barium contrast used in the air-contrast portion of biphasic esophagography?
   A. 15% w/v
   B. 35% w/v
   C. 60% w/v
   D. 250% w/v

   ANSWER: D. Air-contrast views typically use 210%–250% w/v density barium agents (thick barium).

2. Which of the following is the dose of glucagon used to induce colonic hypotonia?
   A. 0.5 mg
   B. 0.75 mg
   C. 1.0 mg
   D. >5 mg

   ANSWER: C. Typical dose range for glucagon for barium enema examination is 1–2 mg, 0.5–1.0 mg for upper GI tract.

45 ESOPHAGUS

Cheri L. Canon and Sanjiv K. Bajaj

NORMAL ANATOMY

PHARYNX

The pharynx is divided into three sections: nasopharynx, oropharynx, and hypopharynx. The soft palate separates the naso- and oropharynx. Radiographically, the boundary between the oro- and hypopharynx is the hyoid bone. The anatomic boundary, not well-visualized on contrast studies, is the pharyngoepiglottic fold overlying the stylopharyngeal muscle.

ESOPHAGUS

The esophagus originates at the cricopharyngeus, the upper esophageal sphincter (UES); courses through the posterior mediastinum; and terminates after 23 to 25 cm at the lower esophageal sphincter (LES). It has three segments: cervical, thoracic, and abdominal. The wall, 3 mm thick when normally distended, is composed of layers common to the gastrointestinal (GI) tract: mucosa, submucosa, muscularis propria with inner circular and outer longitudinal layers, and adventitia. However, unlike the remainder of the GI tract, there is no serosal layer allowing rapid dissemination of infection and tumor. The mucosa is composed of squamous, not columnar epithelium. The muscularis comprises striated muscle in the upper one-third portion and smooth muscle in the remaining portion. Contrast esophagography visualizes three normal extrinsic compressions: aortic arch, left main stem bronchus, and left atrium.

Identification of normal anatomy at the gastroesophageal junction (GEJ) avoids misdiagnosis of pathology (Fig. 45-1). The phrenic ampulla (or esophageal vestibule) represents normal relaxed LES, and its mild dilation should not be confused with a hiatal hernia. The A ring delineates the superior aspect of the phrenic ampulla, which is a muscular boundary, and the upper component of the LES. The B line, a mucosal boundary that occurs at the squamocolumnar junction (also known as the Z line) and the GEJ, migrates superiorly in the abnormal setting of Barrett metaplasia. The LES (measuring 2–4 cm) lacks mucosal delineation and requires manometric identification. Its normal resting pressure is approximately 15 to 45 mm Hg.

A hiatal hernia is diagnosed when the GEJ, identified by the termination of the gastric folds, lies more than 1.5 cm above the diaphragmatic hiatus. The hiatus can be identified as the "pinched" area through which the esophagus or fundus courses. The level of the GEJ is not static; it moves with positioning, respiration, and swallowing.

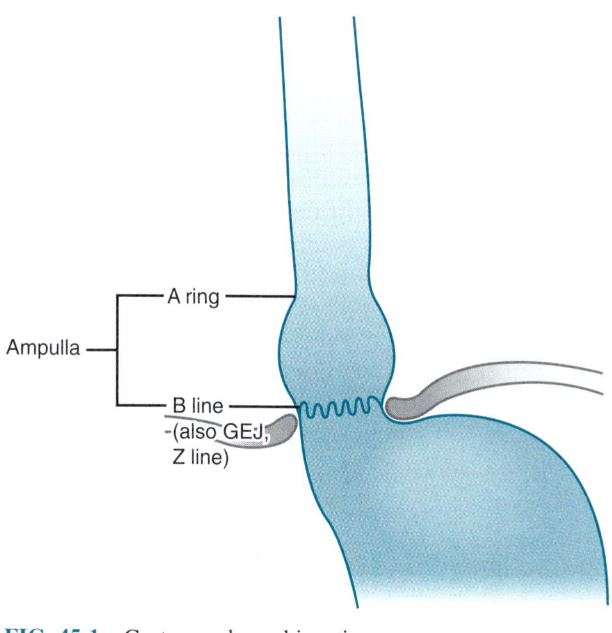

FIG. 45-1 Gastroesophageal junction.

PATHOLOGY

PHARYNX

DIVERTICULA

Pharyngeal pouches and diverticula occur in areas of anatomic weakness, most commonly at the level of the thyrohyoid membrane, where the superior laryngeal vessels and the accompanying branch of the superior laryngeal nerve perforate the alimentary tract. Less commonly, these protrusions occur from the tonsillar fossa. Pouches are transient, usually bilateral, and almost always asymptomatic. Diverticula occur in the setting of significantly increased pharyngeal pressure, classically in glass blowers, are persistent, and may be symptomatic depending upon their size. Both pharyngeal pouches and diverticula increase with age. A laryngocele is a focal dilatation of the laryngeal ventricle, not the pharynx; therefore, it is not typically identified on esophagography, except as an air-filled sac.

Zenker diverticulum is a posterior, midline diverticulum arising from the hypopharynx at Killian dehiscence (not the cervical esophagus)—an inherent weakness at the junction of the inferior pharyngeal constrictors and oblique and horizontal fibers of the cricopharyngeus. It is associated with both cricopharyngeal achalasia and reflux disease. Patients present with pharyngeal dysphagia, chronic halitosis, and symptoms of aspiration (cough, hoarseness, pneumonia, etc.). Radiographically, Zenker diverticulum appears as a posterior outpouching from the hypopharynx, extending downward to the level of the cervical esophagus where it can cause extrinsic compression. There is an entity called a pseudo-Zenker (or pre-Zenker) diverticulum, which is a small, asymptomatic collection of barium in the same region as a Zenker diverticulum. However, it is significantly smaller, does not extend beyond the normal contour of the posterior pharyngeal wall, and completely disappears after pharyngeal peristalsis discontinues.

Killian-Jamieson diverticulum (or pouch) arises from the Killian-Jamieson space, an area of weakness in the anterolateral cervical esophagus. It is more common than a Zenker diverticulum and is usually asymptomatic. Lateral pharyngeal views best detect a Zenker diverticulum, while frontal views best demonstrate a Killian-Jamieson diverticulum (Table 45-3).

WEBS

Webs in the hypopharynx and cervical esophagus appear as 1 to 2 mm shelflike filling defects. These should

TABLE 45-1 Etiology of Cervical Esophageal Webs

Congenital/idiopathic
Epidermolysis bullosa dystrophica
Benign mucus membrane pemphigoid
Pemphigus vulgaris
GERD
Plummer-Vinson Syndrome

not be confused with the "postcricoid defect"—a region of redundant mucosa along the anterior wall of the hypopharynx at the level of the cricoid cartilage, which at one time was incorrectly thought to represent a venous plexus. A web is likely clinically significant when there is a "jet effect," proximal ballooning, and proximal retained contrast. It is most commonly congenital/idiopathic and asymptomatic (Table 45-1). Diseases associated with cervical esophageal webs include epidermolysis bullosa dystrophica, benign mucous membrane pemphigoid, pemphigus vulgaris, and reflux disease. Plummer-Vinson (or Paterson-Kelly) syndrome is a cervical esophageal web in the setting of iron deficiency anemia. In some countries, it is considered premalignant for pharyngeal and esophageal carcinoma, although this is not true in the United States.

Neoplasia

True benign neoplasms of the pharynx are rare (lipoma, neurofibroma, hamartoma). Retention cysts are the most common benign lesions, but they are not neoplastic. Radiographically, these entities present as smooth, round filling defects, most commonly arising from the vallecuae or aryepiglottic folds.

Squamous cell carcinoma, the most common malignant tumor of the pharynx, carries a slightly better prognosis than esophageal cancer. Patients with pharyngeal cancer should have their esophagus screened because of the increased risk of a synchronous or metachronous esophageal cancer. Lymphoma (non-Hodgkin type) accounts for 10% of pharyngeal cancers and usually occurs in the palatine tonsil. Lymphoid hyperplasia of the lingual tonsil must be differentiated from lymphoma. Both present with nodules extending from the tongue base into the vallecula. Lymphomatous nodules tend to be larger, and therefore masslike, and asymmetric.

ESOPHAGUS

Normal Motility and Motility Disorders

The swallowing process has three phases: oral, pharyngeal, and esophageal. There are three types of peristalsis in the esophagus: primary, secondary, and tertiary. Primary esophageal peristalsis is initiated by swallowing. Its initial inhibitory wave, deglutitive inhibition, precedes a continuous wave of contraction that courses through the entire length of the esophagus, cephalad to caudal. LES relaxation quickly follows the UES relaxation. Secondary peristalsis resembles primary in its propagation. It is initiated by distention at the level of a retained bolus and extends downward. Secondary contractions occur only when the initial wave does not clear the esophagus. Tertiary contractions are uncoordinated, nonperistaltic segmental contractions, usually involving the smooth muscle portion of the esophagus, and are always abnormal. Peristaltic evaluation requires horizontal positioning to eliminate effects of gravity. Additionally, single swallows should be observed from UES to LES. Deglutitive inhibition with a second swallow interrupts prior peristalsis.

Achalasia is defined as failure of LES relaxation along with loss of esophageal peristalsis (Table 45-2). The etiology is unknown, but thought to be neurogenic. Barium fluoroscopy demonstrates a dilated esophagus with "bird beak" tapering at the hypertonic LES. The LES intermittently opens, but never to a normal caliber. Primary and secondary peristalsis are absent, although tertiary waves may occur (vigorous achalasia). The LES remains tightly closed, giving a persistent air–fluid level in the upright position. Additionally, the esophagus often contains retained food and saliva. A gastric bubble is usually absent. Longstanding achalasia leads to marked dilatation, referred to as megaesophagus (or sigmoid esophagus when it becomes elongated). It carries an increased risk of esophageal cancer. Chagas disease, caused by destruction of the myenteric plexus after infection with the protozoan *Trypanosoma cruzi*, appears identical to achalasia both radiographically and manometrically. Unlike achalasia, Chagas disease can affect the entire GI tract.

The appearance of the LES helps differentiate achalasia from other dysmotility disorders, including pseudoachalasia and scleroderma. Pseudoachalasia is narrowing of the distal esophagus secondary to carcinoma of the GEJ or gastric cardia. (Often, esophageal or gastric origin of cancer is impossible to determine.) Patients have irregular distal tapering extending into the gastric cardia. Tumor spread occasionally causes smooth

TABLE 45-2 Esophageal Hypomotility

GERD (no tertiary contractions)
Presbyesophagus (tertiary contractions)
Achalasia (bird beak deformity)
Pseudoachalasia (fixed, irregular beaking)
Scleroderma/mixed connective tissue disorders (patulous LES, can be strictured)
Diabetes
Chagas disease (other GI tract abnormalities)

tapering of the LES as seen in achalasia. However, in pseudoachalasia, the LES remains fixed and does not intermittently open.

On the other hand, scleroderma, or progressive systemic sclerosis, presents with a patulous LES and aperistalsis. Severe reflux esophagitis often causes distal stricture that mimics achalasia. Patients may even retain an air–fluid level in the upright position along with a dilated esophagus. However, opening of the LES is absent, and the stricture in scleroderma is fixed. Findings of diffuse interstitial lung disease and asymptomatic esophageal dilatation on cross-sectional imaging strongly suggest the diagnosis. Other collagen vascular diseases present with similar hypomotility: dermatomyositis, polymyositis, systemic lupus erythematosus, and mixed connective tissue disease.

Patients with diffuse esophageal spasm (DES) present with chest pain and dysphagia. Radiographically, severe tertiary contractions give a "corkscrew" appearance. However, there is intermittent normal primary and secondary peristalsis. DES involves the smooth muscle of the distal two-thirds of the esophagus. Radiographically and manometrically, DES and vigorous achalasia appear similar. On CT, DES presents as circumferential thickening of the distal two-thirds of the esophagus and achalasia has a dilated esophagus with a normal wall thickness.

Patients with nutcracker esophagus also present with chest pain and dysphagia. This manometric diagnosis typically has normal radiographic findings with occasional pathologic nonperistaltic contractions. Manometrically, one finds normal peristalsis with distal high-amplitude, prolonged contractions. Some feel that nutcracker esophagus is an early form of DES.

There are many nonspecific dysmotilities. Presbyesophagus occurs in the elderly and radiographically appears as decreased primary and secondary peristalsis with scattered tertiary contractions. Reflux often causes dysmotility with decreased primary and secondary peristalsis that improves with treatment. Unlike presbyesophagus, reflux dysmotility does not have tertiary contractions. Alcoholism and diabetes also cause nonspecific dysmotility similar to presbyesophagus.

Congenital Abnormalities

Although esophageal duplication cysts are rare, they are the second most common duplication of the GI tract after ileal duplications. These cysts occur more commonly in men and are often diagnosed in childhood. These usually occur in the distal right lateral esophagus and do not communicate with the lumen. These cysts are composed of mucosa and muscularis propria and can contain ectopic gastric or pancreatic tissue. In contrast, esophageal retention cysts are acquired (postinflammatory) and are less common. They represent dilated submucosal glands, occur in the distal esophagus, are usually smaller, and can be multiple.

TABLE 45-3 Pharyngeal and Esophageal Diverticula

Zenker diverticula	Hypopharynx, pulsion, posterior midline
Killian-Jamieson diverticula	Cervical esophagus, pulsion, anterolateral
Traction	Mid esophagus, granulomatous disease, angular borders
Pulsion	Distal esophagus (epiphrenic), dysmotility or stricture
EIPD	Pseudodiverticula, GERD

In the esophagus, ectopic gastric mucosa is most commonly seen in the postcricoid region, at or below the UES. This "inlet patch" is a normally asymptomatic congenital abnormality containing columnar epithelium. It carries the same risk of carcinoma as the stomach. Esophagography demonstrates a flat lesion with a marginal indentation around a raised border, giving an oval ring shadow.

Diverticula

Two types of diverticula, neither of which is congenital, present in the esophagus: traction and pulsion (Table 45-3). Traction diverticula develop in the midthoracic esophagus adjacent to calcified mediastinal lymph nodes. They arise secondary to scarring and retraction from granulomatous disease and tend to be more angular. In contrast, pulsion diverticula are round and occur in the distal esophagus (epiphrenic diverticulum) in the setting of DES, achalasia, or less frequently proximal to a stricture. Zenker diverticula are considered pulsion diverticula.

Esophageal intramural pseudodiverticulosis (EIPD) represents pathologically dilated submucosal mucous glands. It occurs most commonly with gastroesophageal reflux disease (GERD) but is also associated with candidiasis, diabetes, and esophageal cancer. Contrast fluoroscopy detects numerous flask-shaped outpouchings along the course of the esophagus, easily confused with tiny ulcerations seen in infectious esophagitis such as herpes. The pseudodiverticula can appear to "float" outside the lumen of the esophagus when the communicating duct is not filled with barium. Linear intramural tracking between pseudodiverticula arises secondary to acute inflammation and contained rupture with healing and fibrosis, similar to the tracking that occurs in colonic diverticular disease. EIPD is not premalignant or symptomatic.

Inflammation and Infection

Gastroesophageal Reflux Disease (GERD)

GERD is the most common inflammatory condition in the esophagus. Its presentations range from retrosternal burning and dysphagia to asthma, chronic cough, and hoarseness. Transient inappropriate intermittent relaxation of the LES is the primary pathology in most patients with mild-to-moderate reflux. Those with severe reflux typically have decreased resting LES pressure. The severity of reflux is determined by its frequency, duration of acid contact time with the esophagus, and the acid content of the refluxate. Therefore, patients with scleroderma (without LES pressure and peristalsis to clear acid) and Zollinger-Ellison syndrome have significantly worse esophagitis and stricture.

Double-contrast esophagography findings in reflux esophagitis include granular mucosa (mucosal edema) and linear erosions; severe cases have nodularity, which is difficult to differentiate from candidiasis (Table 45-4). Transient contractions of the muscularis mucosa, feline esophagus, occur in addition to nonspecific dysmotility.

Several types of strictures occur in GERD. Most occur in the distal esophagus, proximal to or at the GEJ. Strictures can be tapered or focal and ringlike. Strictures greater than 20 mm in caliber are usually asymptomatic. Strictures less than 13 mm are almost always symptomatic. Schatzki ring is a focal symptomatic ringlike stricture at the GEJ. Prone positioning facilitates viewing. GERD can also cause longitudinal stricturing thus shortening the esophagus with increasing hiatal hernia. Diagnosis of short esophagus before antireflux surgery is imperative for success because an esophageal lengthening procedure (Collis gastroplasty) provides better outcome.

The esophagogastric polyp is not neoplastic; a rugal fold enlarges secondary to chronic inflammation and granulation from GERD and extends into the distal esophagus. It can appear as a pedunculated polyp, but careful radiographic examination reveals continuity with the rugae in the gastric fundus.

TABLE 45-4 Esophagitis

DISEASE	LOCATION	APPEARANCE
GERD	Distal	Granular mucosa, nodularity, linear erosions, stricture
Pill	Mid (arch or left mainstem bronchus)	Focal erosions
NGT & Alendronate sodium	Distal	Severe, long segment stricture and ulceration; worse than with GERD
Eosinophilic	Proximal & mid	Long segment stricture with multiple rings or diffusely small caliber esophagus; resolves with oral liquid steroids
Radiation	Limited to radiation port	Ulceration (acute), focal stricture (chronic)
Candida	Mid	Linear plaques, ulceration, "shaggy"
Herpes	Diffuse	Multiple small ulcers, rarely large ulcer
CMV & HIV	Mid	Large, solitary or few flat ulcer(s)
TB & Crohn	Diffuse	Severe ulceration and fistula

Barrett esophagus occurs secondary to metaplastic esophageal healing in the setting of chronic reflux. It is a premalignant condition occurring in approximately 10% of patients with GERD. Classic findings of Barrett esophagus include a mid-to-high esophageal stricture or ulceration with focal reticular mucosa. However, the reticular pattern is often absent.

The incidence of hiatal hernia increases with aging due to laxity of the phrenoesophageal ligaments anchoring the esophagus to the diaphragmatic hiatus. The hiatal hernia is not the primary cause of GERD (*remember*: abnormal, intermittent relaxation of the LES) but the result of chronic reflux. There are four types of hiatal hernia: Type I, the most common, is a sliding hiatal hernia where the GEJ lies above the level of the diaphragmatic hiatus. Type II is a true paraesophageal hernia, a rare phenomenon where the GEJ retains its normal position below the diaphragmatic hiatus and a portion of the fundus herniates above the diaphragm in a paraesophageal location. Type III hernia combines type I and type II hernia, where the GEJ lies above the hiatus, and there is an associated paraesophageal component. This occurs more commonly than type II hernia. Type IV hernia, the rarest type, presents with a gaping hiatus and intrathoracic stomach with herniation into the chest of other organs, such as colon, omentum, and small bowel. Types II, III, and IV can be large enough to have an intrathoracic stomach, which most commonly rotates in an organoaxial, along the long axis, fashion. Mesoaxial, perpendicular to the long axis, rotation is less common, usually seen in a type II hernia. These gastric rotations are secondary to ligamentous laxity and should not be confused with gastric volvulus, which is an emergency and indicates obstruction with vascular compromise (strangulation).

Esophagitis

Noninfectious: Drug-induced ("pill") esophagitis (Table 45-4) presents at the level of an extrinsic esophageal compression, most commonly at the aortic arch or left main stem bronchus. Antibiotics (tetracycline and doxycycline) and vitamin C pills most often cause the etiologic contact esophagitis. NSAIDs and aspirin have also been implicated. Radiographically, focal ulcers appear at the level of the aortic arch or left main stem bronchus. There may be focal fold thickening, but the remainder of the esophagus is normal.

Alendronate sodium (Fosamax), a bisphosphonate used to treat osteoporosis and Paget disease, causes a radiologically distinct "pill" esophagitis. It presents as changes of severe GERD with a long segment of distal stricturing and acute ulceration similar to nasogastric tube (NGT) esophagitis. Patients must take this medication with plenty of water and remain erect for at least 30 minutes to prevent these complications.

Severe strictures of the esophagus occur in several other conditions. NGT intubation can rapidly cause long strictures of the distal esophagus, secondary to GERD from stenting of the LES by the tube. Caustic esophagitis can present with a long segment stricture, but it is typically more proximal. Lye is the most common etiologic agent and causes severe pharyngeal abnormality with aspiration. Importantly, lye strictures have an increased risk of squamous cell carcinoma.

Eosinophilic esophagitis usually presents in young men with an allergic history, particularly food allergies. In addition to the dysphagia found in most esophagitis, patients present with peripheral eosinophilia. Radiographically, long-segment stricture can appear anywhere in the esophagus. These strictures are unique, with a stacked ring appearance resembling the cartilaginous rings in the trachea. Their length is shorter when they present in the distal esophagus. However in other patients, the only radiographic finding may be a diffusely small caliber esophagus, once thought to be congenital. After satisfactory treatment with swallowed liquid steroids, these strictures typically resolve and the esophagus looks completely normal.

Radiation esophagitis with stricture occurs more focally, predictably within the radiation field. The dose must exceed 5000 rads and is potentiated by Adriamycin. An acute phase of 1 to 4 weeks precedes a chronic phase. The acute phase has mucosal edema and ulceration. The chronic phase demonstrates smooth strictures which can progress for years.

Crohn disease can occur anywhere from the mouth to the anus, including the esophagus. As in the remainder of the GI tract, it can present with aphthous ulcers, strictures, or fistulae. Esophageal involvement is the most uncommon form and does not occur in isolation. Behçet disease, a chronic inflammatory vasculitis characterized by oral and genital ulceration and uveitis, presents with distal esophageal ulceration similar to that found in Crohn disease.

Esophagitis

Infectious: Candida is the most common infectious agent in esophagitis. It usually presents in patients who are immunocompromised. However, it also occurs in patients undergoing radiation therapy and even rarely in those with normal immune function. Early *Candida* esophagitis presents with focal mucosal plaques. These plaques are discreet with surrounding normal mucosa and have a similar appearance to glycogenic acanthosis—a benign, degenerative condition seen in older patients in which glycogen accumulates in plaques in the squamous epithelial mucosa. Candidal plaques are linear and less well-defined, whereas glycogenic acanthotic plaques are round. However, symptomatology provides optimal differentiation between these entities. Glycogenic acanthosis is asymptomatic, whereas candidiasis typically presents with odynophagia. As *Candida* progresses, plaque and pseudomembrane formation increase, and ulceration develops as membranes slough. When barium insinuates around the plaques and pseudomembranes, one visualizes the advanced "shaggy" esophagus (a common finding in AIDS).

Herpes esophagitis, the second most common infectious type, also presents with ulcers, which are small and numerous. As with other infectious esophagitis, patients with herpes esophagitis present with odynophagia. The early stage of vesicle formation does not appear on barium swallow. Once the vesicles rupture, characteristic punctate ulceration suggests the diagnosis. Advanced herpes can mimic candidal plaques and nodularity secondary to reflux esophagitis. In rare occurrences, herpes esophagitis can present with a solitary or a few large ulcers.

Cytomegalovirus (CMV) and human immunodeficiency virus (HIV) esophagitis have radiologically indistinguishable appearances. Typically, one or a few large ulcers occupy the mid esophagus. Endoscopic brush biopsies must evaluate for the Cowdry intranuclear inclusion bodies of CMV. If not present, the patient is treated for HIV esophagitis. The two treatments vary drastically: CMV is treated with antiviral agents, whereas HIV esophagitis is treated with oral steroids.

Tuberculous involvement of the esophagus is typically secondary to spread from regional lymph nodes. There can be ulceration with sinus tracts and fistulous connections to adjacent nodes. The ulceration is deeper than that seen in other infectious esophagitis, and cross-sectional imaging reveals marked mediastinal lymphadenopathy, which may be low in density.

In general, patients with odynophagia should be evaluated with endoscopy, which allows biopsy necessary for therapy. Although barium esophagography can identify these lesions and often suggest an etiology, the diversity of treatments requires microbial confirmation.

NEOPLASIA

Radiographically, one must identify esophageal lesions as mucosal or intramural in origin (Table 45-5). Mucosal lesions tend to form acute angles with the adjacent mucosa; intramural lesions have more obtuse angles and normal overlying mucosa.

Benign Tumors

Benign tumors of the esophagus are rare, representing less than 1% of all esophageal neoplasms. The leiomyoma, an intramural lesion arising from the circular layer of muscularis propria, comprises approximately two-thirds of benign tumors and usually presents distally.

TABLE 45-5 Benign Esophageal Lesions

MUCOSAL	SUBMUCOSAL
Papilloma (most common benign *mucosal* lesion)	Leiomyoma (most common overall)
Adenoma	Fibrovascular polyp (pedunculated)
Glycogenic acanthosis (degenerative, not neoplastic)	Granular cell tumor
Esophagogastric polyp (inflammatory, not neoplastic)	Duplication cyst (congenital, not neoplastic)

TABLE 45-6 Malignant Esophageal Tumors

Adenocarcinoma (most common in western countries)
Squamous cell carcinoma (most common worldwide)
Spindle cell (carcinosarcoma)
Leiomyosarcoma (GIST rare, unlike remainder of GI tract)
Lymphoma (usually Hodgkin, non-Hodgkin in AIDS)
Small cell
Melanoma (primary tumor more common than metastatic tumor)
Metastases (lung, breast, stomach)

Multiple leiomyomata, a condition referred to leiomyomatosis, is associated with Alport syndrome and visceral leiomyomatosis. Leiomyomata are usually asymptomatic and small. Larger lesions result in dysphagia, ulceration, and bleeding. On esophagography, they present as intramural lesions with normal, smooth overlying mucosa. On CT, they are round, well-circumscribed intramural masses with soft tissue density. Malignant degeneration is exceedingly rare, obviating the need for surgical enucleation. The diffuse proliferation of smooth muscle in leiomyomatosis does not present as a discreet mass but as a long tapered stricture. When occurring at the GEJ, it can mimic achalasia.

Fibrovascular polyps contain both fibrovascular and adipose elements and include tumors previously referred to as fibromas, fibrolipomas, myxofibromas, lipomas, and angiolipomas. They arise in the cervical esophagus but are attached by a long pedicle such that the head of the polyp typically lies in the midthoracic esophagus. Classically, patients present with a mass that has been regurgitated into the oral cavity. More commonly, they have dysphagia. The CT and MR imaging appearances are variable, depending upon the adipose and vascular content of the specific tumor.

Granular cell tumors arise from Schwann cells and radiographically appear like leiomyomata but can be multiple. They are resected only if symptomatic.

Esophageal lipomatosis is fatty deposition in the esophageal wall in patients with a long history of steroid use. Cross-sectional imaging demonstrates a "double-ring" appearance of the esophageal wall from the low-density intramural fat.

The most common benign mucosal lesion of the esophagus is a papilloma, which is composed of hyperplastic squamous epithelium. Multiple lesions are called papillomatosis. Adenomas can occur in the esophagus in the setting of Barrett esophagus but are rare. Like colonic adenomas, these premalignant lesions require resection.

Malignant Tumors

There are two major esophageal mucosal malignancies: squamous cell carcinoma and adenocarcinoma (Table 45-6). Recently, the incidence of adenocarcinoma has surpassed squamous cell carcinoma in western countries and has the fastest growing incidence rate of all cancers in the United States, and this increase is attributed to GERD. Worldwide, squamous cell carcinoma remains more common.

Esophageal adenocarcinoma occurs with GERD and usually arises in Barrett esophagus. This disease typically presents in middle-aged and older white male patients. Prior research reported that the risk of developing adenocarcinoma in the setting of Barrett esophagus was 125 times greater than the general population; however, more recent studies have suggested a lesser risk.

Etiologic factors for squamous cell carcinoma include alcohol and tobacco use, which have a synergistic effect, environmental toxins including asbestos, petroleum contaminants, thermal injury, and diet. There is also an increased incidence secondary to radiation injury, lye ingestion, achalasia, tylosis, celiac disease, and Plummer-Vinson syndrome. Squamous cell carcinoma most commonly presents in older African American male patients. Unlike adenocarcinoma, it has a predilection for the proximal and mid esophagus.

Several terms describe the pathologic and radiographic findings in esophageal cancer. *Early* esophageal cancer is limited to the mucosa or submucosa and does not involve lymph nodes, whereas *superficial* cancers are also mucosal or submucosal but have positive nodes. *Small* cancers are less than 3.5 cm regardless of nodal status. Advanced carcinomas are described as infiltrating (stricture), ulcerating (flat with ulcer), or varicoid (submucosal spread resembling varices).

Both types of esophageal cancer carry a poor prognosis because of the advanced stage at diagnosis and also because the lack of serosa results in rapid local extension. Both cancers also spread via lymphatic and hematogenous metastases. Lymph node involvement occurs locally in the mediastinum with extension to neck lymphatics for proximal and mid tumors. Spread to the celiac nodal group commonly occurs with more distal cancers. Hematogenous metastases include lung and liver, which have a significantly worse prognosis than with abdominal lymphadenopathy alone. The extent of primary tumor invasion and nodal and distant metastases determine stage, treatment, and prognosis. Cross-sectional imaging is somewhat handicapped in the staging of esophageal cancer, particularly in nodal staging. The incorporation of PET and endoscopic ultrasound (EUS) with fine needle aspiration (FNA) has improved staging. Except for the absence of serosa in the esophagus, the entire gut has a similar sonographic appearance. Proceeding from the lumen outward, there is a hypoechoic mucosa, hyperechoic submucosa, hypoechoic muscularis propria, and hyperechoic serosa and adventitia.

Leiomyosarcoma is relatively rare in the esophagus but has a better prognosis than other esophageal cancer. It typically presents with a large ulcerating mass. Leiomyosarcomas are more common than gastrointestinal stromal tumors in the esophagus, although the latter are more common in the remainder of the GI tract. Leiomyosarcoma arises de novo and not from malignant degeneration of a leiomyoma.

The esophagus is the most uncommon site in the GI tract for primary lymphoma. It is most commonly Hodgkin pathology in young men. Non-Hodgkin type occurs in AIDS. Both types of lymphoma can extend to the esophagus from adjacent mediastinal adenopathy. The radiographic appearance of lymphoma varies, but it commonly presents as a bulky, nonobstructing mass.

Spindle cell carcinoma, previously referred to as carcinosarcoma, is a rare cancer of the esophagus and carries a very poor prognosis. It presents as a large nonobstructing mass. Small cell carcinoma of the esophagus is even rarer with a worse prognosis. On imaging, it appears similar to squamous cell and adenocarcinoma. Unlike the latter, it typically presents with significant mediastinal lymphadenopathy.

Gastric adenocarcinoma is the most common metastatic lesion in the esophagus, secondary to direct extension from cardia tumors. These patients can present with an appearance of pseudoachalasia, but as mentioned before, the thickening of the LES is usually asymmetric and irregular. Breast carcinoma and melanoma demonstrate hematogenous spread to the esophagus, although esophageal melanoma is more commonly seen as a primary tumor than a metastatic lesion. Local extension to the esophagus occurs in lung cancer. Kaposi sarcoma also involves the esophagus.

Miscellaneous Conditions

There are two types of esophageal varices: uphill and downhill. The more common uphill varices, seen in the setting of cirrhosis with portal hypertension (hepatofugal flow, away from the liver), occur secondary to reversal of flow in the coronary vein. The distal esophageal plexus dilates and drains systemically into the azygous vein. Downhill varices occur when there is an obstruction of the superior vena cava. These varices drain into the azygous system if the obstruction is superior to the azygous vein or into the portal venous system via the coronary vein if the obstruction occludes the azygous vein. Uphill varices occur in the lower esophagus, while downhill varices occur in the upper portion with a patent azygous system or throughout the entire esophagus if the azygous vein is obstructed. On esophagography, varices present as serpentine structures that change in appearance during fluoroscopy. Classically, the collapsed view of the esophagus reveals enlargement of these structures, while the distended air-contrast view effaces the dilated veins. On CT and MR, varices are well seen with contrast enhancement as tubular structures in the paraesophageal region. Differential diagnosis includes varicoid carcinoma, which typically has a fixed appearance during fluoroscopy.

Most commonly, esophageal perforation is secondary to iatrogenic trauma sustained during endoscopy. These types of tears usually occur in the posterior hypopharynx or cervical esophagus. Distal esophageal tears can occur during vomiting (known as Boerhaave syndrome). Perforations in the distal esophagus tend to result in left-sided pleural effusions, while right-sided effusions usually occur in the setting of mid esophageal perforations. Classically, esophageal perforation is a surgical emergency. Cross-sectional imaging evaluates for paraesophageal fluid and mediastinitis, directing clinical care; many perforations are amenable to conservative treatment. Mallory-Weiss tears are limited to the mucosa and have normal radiographic findings in most cases.

Esophageal intramural hematoma occurs secondary to bleeding within the wall. It presents spontaneously in anticoagulation or after a mucosal tear in trauma or sclerotherapy. Cross-sectional imaging reveals an oval intramural mass that does not enhance. On CT, there is increased density, consistent with hemorrhage. Depending on the stage of evolution, MR has a variable appearance.

Esophagogastrectomy with gastric pull-up is commonly performed for primary esophageal cancer. Two surgical approaches are commonly employed. The Ivor-Lewis procedure includes a laparotomy for gastric mobilization and right thoracotomy for esophageal resection and gastric pull-up. The esophagogastric anastomosis lies in the upper thorax or neck. The pylorus sits at the level of the esophageal hiatus, and a pyloromyotomy or pyloroplasty can help gastric emptying, which is poor as a result of denervation of the mobilized stomach. A transhiatal esophagectomy is performed less often. Postoperative recovery is more rapid as there is no thoracotomy, but only a laparotomy and left neck incision. The incidence of postoperative leaks is higher, but overall morbidity is lower because leaks tend to occur in the neck instead of the more devastating mediastinal location. In this approach, the esophagus is resected transhiatally through the abdominal incision, and the anastomosis is more cranial, near the thoracic inlet. In the immediate postoperative period, contrast fluoroscopy evaluates leak and obstruction. Abscess appears on contrast-enhanced CT. For more remote patients, CT helps identify recurrent and metastatic disease.

Fundoplication is a common treatment for reflux disease. A Nissen fundoplication is a complete 360-degree wrap, while the Toupet fundoplication is a partial 270-degree posterior wrap. For the wrap to be clinically successful, it must encircle the LES for a length of 2 to 3 cm and be situated below the diaphragmatic hiatus. Collis gastroplasty, an esophageal lengthening technique where a segment of neoesophagus is made distal to the GEJ from the gastric cardia, is performed in the setting of short esophagus. Preoperative failure to identify a short esophagus is the most common cause of wrap failure. Contrast fluoroscopy excludes leak postoperatively. CT readily assesses abscess formation.

SUGGESTED READING

Abbara S, Kalan MMH, Lewicki AM. Intrathoracic stomach revisited. *AJR Am J Roentgenol.* 2003;181:403-414.

Canon CL, Morgan DE, Einstein DM, et al. Surgical approach to gastroesophageal reflux disease: what the radiologist needs to know. *Radiographics.* 2005;25:1485-1499.

Jang KM, Lee KS, Lee SJ, et al. The spectrum of benign esophageal lesions: imaging findings. *Korean J Radiol.* 2002; 3(3):199-210.

Karasick S, Lev-Toaff AS. Esophageal strictures: findings on barium radiographs. *AJR Am J Roentgenol.* 1995;165:561-565.

Kim TJ, Lee KH, Kim YH, et al. Postoperative imaging of esophageal cancer: what chest radiologists need to know. *Radiographics.* 2007;27:409-429.

Levine MS. Esophageal cancer: radiologic diagnosis. *Radiol Clin North Am.* 1997;35(2):265-279.

Levine MS. Benign tumors of the esophagus: radiologic evaluation. *Semin Thorac Cardiovasc Surg.* 2003;15(1):9-19.

Levine MS, Rubesin SE. Diseases of the esophagus: diagnosis with esophagography. *Radiology.* 2005;237:414-427.

Luedtke P, Levine MS, Rubesin SE, et al. Radiologic diagnosis of benign esophageal strictures: a pattern approach. *Radiographics.* 2003;23:897-909.

Noh HM, Fishman EK, Forastiere AA, et al. CT of the esophagus: spectrum of disease with emphasis on esophageal carcinoma. *Radiographics.* 1995;15:1113-1134.

Zimmerman SL, Levine MS, Rubesin SE, et al. Idiopathic eosinophilic esophagitis in adults: the ringed esophagus. *Radiology.* 2005;236(1):159-165.

QUESTIONS AND ANSWERS

1. Where is the origin of Zenker diverticula?
   A. Vallecula
   B. Piriform sinus
   C. Hypopharynx
   D. Cervical esophagus

   ANSWER: C. Zenker diverticulum arises from the inferior hypopharynx, just superior to the cricopharyngeus from an anatomic area of weakness called Killian dehiscence. This occurs at the junction of the oblique and horizontal fibers of the cricopharyngeus. (Not to be confused with Killian-Jamieson diverticulum, which arises from the Killian-Jamieson space.)

2. What is the typical finding of HIV esophagitis on esophagography?
   A. Shaggy mucosa
   B. Giant, shallow ulcer
   C. Multiple punctate ulcers
   D. Intramural pseudodiverticulosis

   ANSWER: B. HIV esophagitis is radiographically indistinguishable from CMV esophagitis. Both present with large, shallow ulcers, which are often solitary. Shaggy mucosa is classically seen in *Candida* esophagitis, although it can be seen in severe *herpes* esophagitis. Intramural pseudodiverticulosis is most commonly associated with reflux disease. However, it was originally described in esophageal candidiasis.

3. Regarding secondary esophageal peristalsis, which of the following is true?
   A. Occurs directly preceding the primary peristalsis
   B. Usually abnormal
   C. Begins at the upper esophageal sphincter and spreads distally
   D. Initiated by local distension

   ANSWER: D. Primary peristalsis begins at the upper esophageal sphincter and spreads in a systematic fashion distally. Secondary peristalsis does not occur with every swallow and is initiated locally by a retained portion of the bolus. It is not abnormal.

4. Which of the following is an anterolateral cervical diverticulum?
   A. Killian-Jamieson diverticulum
   B. Zenker diverticulum
   C. Traction diverticulum
   D. Congenital diverticulum

   ANSWER: A. Killian-Jamieson diverticulum occurs in the cervical esophagus, arising from a region of anatomic weakness, the Killian-Jamieson space. By comparison, a Zenker diverticulum arises in the posterior midline of the hypopharynx above the cricopharyngeus from another anatomic region of weakness, Killian dehiscence.

5. Regarding esophagitis in an immunocompromised patient, what is the most likely etiology for small punctate ulcers?
   A. Candida
   B. CMV
   C. Herpes
   D. HIV

   ANSWER: C. *Herpes* typically presents with small punctate ulcers, although it rarely can have a giant ulcer. CMV and HIV esophagitis more typically have solitary, large flat ulcers, and candidiasis presents with multiple plaques, often progressing to a shaggy esophagus in an immunocompromised patient. EIPD can mimic small ulcers when seen en face.

6. Which of the following is most helpful in differentiating achalasia from pseudoachalasia?
   A. Degree of dilatation of the esophagus
   B. Absent primary peristalsis
   C. Presence of reflux
   D. Appearance of the LES

   ANSWER: D. Achalasia presents with smooth tapering of the lower esophageal sphincter ("bird beak appearance"). Pseudoachalasia presents with narrowing, but it is more typically irregular with nodular folds extending from the gastric cardia. Additionally, the sphincter is fixed in pseudoachalasia, whereas it may intermittently open during true achalasia.

7. Regarding esophageal varices, which of the following is true?
   A. On esophagography, carcinoma is included in the differential diagnosis
   B. Downhill varices are more common
   C. Systemic drainage for downhill varices is via the brachiocephalic vein
   D. Air-contrast view of the esophagus is the best method for radiographic diagnosis

   ANSWER: A. Varicoid carcinoma is included in the differential diagnosis of varices on esophagography. However, varicoid carcinoma is fixed, while varices tend to fill and empty with peristalsis. Uphill varices are more common than downhill varices, and both can empty into the azygous system; and downhill varices can also empty into the portal system through the coronary vein.

8. Regarding esophageal leiomyosarcoma, which of the following is true?
   A. Worse prognosis than adenocarcinoma
   B. Presents with an annular mass
   C. More common in the esophagus than GIST
   D. Arises from malignant degeneration of leiomyoma

   ANSWER: C. Leiomyosarcomas have a better prognosis than other esophageal cancers and typically present as a large ulcerating mass. GISTs of the esophagus are very rare, unlike those in the remainder of the GI tract. Leiomyosarcomas typically arise de novo and not from malignant degeneration of their benign counterparts. They are usually solitary.

9. What is the most common benign mucosal tumor of the esophagus?
   A. Papilloma
   B. Adenoma
   C. Fibrovascular polyp
   D. Leiomyoma

   ANSWER: A. Papilloma is the most common benign esophageal mucosal tumor. Adenomas are rare and occur in the setting of Barrett esophagus. Fibrovascular polyps, although intraluminal, are actually submucosal lesions. Leiomyomas are the most common tumor of the esophagus but are not mucosal; they are intramural.

10. Regarding the cricopharyngeus, which of the following is true?
    A. Also considered upper sphincter
    B. Not normally identified on barium studies
    C. Located above a Zenker diverticulum
    D. Not affected by GERD

    ANSWER: A. The cricopharyngeous is the UES and is implicated in the formation of the more superior Zenker diverticulum. It is normally identified on contrast studies, but is more prominent (fails to relax) with cricopharyngeal achalasia. Its dysfunction can also be seen in GERD.

46 STOMACH

Sanjiv K. Bajaj and Cheri L. Canon

NORMAL ANATOMY

The stomach begins at the distal end of the esophagus and extends to the pyloric sphincter. It varies considerably in size. Its unfixed intraperitoneal length contains five parts: cardia, fundus, body, antrum, and the pyloric sphincter. The cardia is a histologically defined region where the esophagus enters the stomach. The fundus projects as a dome immediately adjacent to the cardia and superior to it, related to the left hemidiaphragm, and extending to the fifth intercostal space in most people. Radiologically, the gastric bubble appears in this region in upright radiographs. The largest portion of the stomach, the body, extends to the incisura angularis on the lesser curvature. The antrum occupies the region between the incisura angularis and the pyloric sphincter. This 1-cm-long distal sphincter composed of circular muscle controls the rate of gastric emptying. The lesser curvature comprises the superior outline of the stomach, and the greater curvature appears as the inferior outline. In the nondistended stomach, one sees rugae, the longitudinal mucosal folds. The anterior gastric wall abuts the diaphragm, the left lobe of the liver, and the anterior abdominal wall. The posterior aspect forms the major portion of the anterior wall of the omental bursa, also referred to as lesser sac, and relates to the pancreas.

Double-contrast examination of the stomach can reveal the areae gastricae, the normal polygonal mucosal pattern, representing tiny mucosal crevices. It can be seen throughout the stomach, but most commonly seen in the body and antrum. Increase in the size of the areae gastricae can be seen with normal aging or with *Helicobacter pylori* infection. Areae gastricae are notably absent in atrophic gastritis.

Lymph from the superior two-thirds of the stomach drains to the gastric nodes, and the superior body and fundus additionally feed the pancreaticosplenic nodes. The right two-thirds and inferior third of the stomach empty into the pyloric nodes, while lymph from the left third of the greater curvature enters the pancreaticoduodenal nodes.

PATHOLOGY

CONGENITAL ABNORMALITIES

Congenital hypertrophic pyloric stenosis arises from hypertrophy of the pylorus's circular muscles with extension to the antrum, creating a tight sphincter and gastric outlet obstruction. The disorder usually presents in the first 2 to 6 weeks of life with nonbilious, projectile vomiting. Physical examination demonstrates an "olive" in the epigastric region representing the hypertrophied pylorus. Ultrasound is the preferred diagnostic imaging modality. It reveals a thickened muscular wall (>4 mm), a pyloric canal greater than 14-mm long, hyperactive gastric peristaltic waves, and absent gastric emptying. Upper GI examination also demonstrates the condition, showing the string sign (contrast in a narrowed, elongated pylorus), Kirklin sign (shouldering by the pylorus in the duodenal bulb), crowded mucosa with multiple ridges, and pyloric channel elongation. This diagnosis necessitates surgery, most often a pyloromyotomy. Pyloric stenosis can present in the adult population when the process is less severe. Intermittent nausea and vomiting may be the only symptoms, and upper GI examination will demonstrate the abnormality.

Ectopic pancreatic tissue (pancreatic rest) presents most commonly in the stomach after a fragment of the pancreas implants in the gastric wall during embryologic development. Functional tissue can produce local ulceration and subsequent bleeding as enzymes erode the mucosal surface. It appears radiographically as a small filling defect, sometimes with central depression representing a duct, in the distal stomach along the greater curvature. Rarely, this tissue undergoes neoplastic change into malignant pancreatic adenocarcinoma. Lesions causing obstruction or other symptoms usually yield to endoscopic removal.

Gastric diverticula are rare compared to their colonic counterparts. Most of them are true diverticula in that all layers of bowel wall protrude, and they most commonly present in the posterior fundus. Upper GI examination demonstrates a barium filled defect with normal mucosal pattern usually found near the gastroesophageal junction (GEJ). It changes in size and with peristalsis. On CT, these can be confused with a low density left adrenal adenoma, but the presence of an air bubble or gastric contrast excludes this diagnosis. A gastric intramural diverticulum is a pseudodiverticulum occurring along the greater curvature of the antrum secondary to a small invagination of mucosa between the muscular layers. It can mimic an ulcer, although it is not fixed, changes configuration with peristalsis, and has no adjacent fold thickening.

Situs describes the heart and visceral anatomic relationships to the midline. Situs solitus is the normal position. Situs inversus is a rare disorder characterized by abnormal location of the body's organs in mirror image to situs solitus. It occurs more commonly with dextrocardia, in which case it carries a 5% incidence of congenital heart disease, or levocardia, which is rare and almost always complicated by congenital heart disease. Thoracic imaging demonstrates inversion of the lungs, cardiac silhouette, and great vessels. The stomach likewise presents on the right side, with the liver occupying the left. Many patients have Kartagener syndrome, characterized by situs inversus and immotile cilia resulting in pulmonary disease. Some patients present with incomplete situs inversus, known as situs ambiguous. Situs ambiguous can occur with polysplenia, bilateral left sidedness; and asplenia, bilateral right sidedness. Almost all individuals with asplenia have congenital heart disease that is often more severe than in other situs anomalies.

INFLAMMATION AND INFECTION

Peptic ulcer disease most commonly arises secondary to *H. pylori* infection and nonsteroidal anti-inflammatory drugs (NSAIDs). Other contributors include alcohol, autoimmune diseases, sepsis, and severe physiologic compromise. Radiologically, one finds thickened rugal folds, erosions, and frank ulceration. Most gastric ulcers are benign erosions into the submucosa. The majority occur along the lesser curve or posterior wall of the gastric body or antrum. Ulcers in older patients tend to be more proximal, particularly along the lesser curve. Contrast studies reveal a smooth oval rimmed defect through the muscularis mucosa with a swollen lip and gastric folds radiating to its border. These lesions are fixed and, unlike diverticula, do not change with peristalsis. Ulcer extension into the submucosa creates Hampton line, a thin line of barium near the ulcer's most superficial edge. Multiple gastric ulcers or association with enlarged rugae suggests Zollinger-Ellison syndrome (gastrinoma). Ulcers can lead to adhesions, allowing a fistulous tract between the antrum and duodenum that mimics a second pylorus ("double barrel pylorus"). Webs occasionally appear in the gastric antrum, often in association with ulcers. They present as a thin band proximal to the pylorus, sometimes giving the appearance of a second duodenal bulb.

Approximately 95% of gastric ulcers are benign. Double-contrast radiography can demonstrate features suggesting malignancy (Table 46-1). Benign ulcer craters can have various shapes including circular, ovoid, or even linear, but the borders are smooth. Malignant ulcer crater borders are more irregular. Size and multiplicity have no implication regarding malignancy.

Atrophic gastritis is classified based upon etiology. Type A is autoimmune related with mucosal atrophy in the body and fundus. Decreased synthesis of intrinsic factor causes B_{12} malabsorption and pernicious anemia, and these patients are at an increased risk for gastric adenocarcinoma. Direct mucosal injury to the antrum by alcohol, bile acids, or other caustic agents results in type B atrophic gastritis. Atrophic gastritis on barium examination presents with a smooth tubular stomach that is nondistensible. Rugal folds and areae gastricae are absent.

TABLE 46-1 Benign Versus Malignant Gastric Ulcer

BENIGN	MALIGNANT
Crater projects beyond lumen	Crater projects within lumen (Carman meniscus sign)
Folds symmetric, smooth, extend to crater edge	Folds asymmetric, nodular, and end proximal to edge
Less common in fundus	More common in fundus
Adjacent areae gastricae may be enlarged	Areae gastricae obliterated

Chronic alkaline gastritis and esophagitis can result from postsurgical bile reflux through an incompetent pyloric sphincter or anastomotic connection (Billroth I, II). Mucosal protecting agents or further surgery with a Roux limb revision provide amelioration.

There are several etiologies of granulomatous gastritis. Crohn disease can involve any portion of the GI tract, and like elsewhere, presents in the stomach with aphthous ulcers, strictures, and fistulae. The normal pyloric channel becomes patulous, resembling a primary gastroduodenostomy (Billroth I). Tuberculosis, sarcoid, and syphilis sometimes present as gastritis. One generally finds marked architectural distortion with deep ulceration and fistulae, commonly with extraintestinal manifestations such as lymphadenopathy. Gastric tuberculosis is very uncommon and presents with pyloric fibrosis and gastric outlet obstruction. It can be difficult to differentiate from cancer. The stomach is the most common portion of the gut affected by sarcoid, but most patients are asymptomatic. Eosinophilic gastritis presents with eosinophilic infiltrate and gastric outlet obstruction and is associated with food allergy. Steroids resolve the primary process.

CMV also causes a diffuse gastritis with thick gastric folds, especially in immunocompromised patients. There is commonly small bowel and colonic involvement with skip lesions. Ulceration can be superficial but is more often very deep.

Emphysematous gastritis is most commonly secondary to caustic ingestion and alcohol abuse. It can also occur in the setting of trauma and gastric ischemia/infarction, and with superimposed phlegmonous (bacterial) gastritis, especially with *Staphylococcus aureus, Escherichia coli,* streptococci, and clostridia. It can lead to stenosis, gastric rupture, and sinus tracts and progresses rapidly to death. Radiologic studies demonstrate gastric pneumatosis with marked fold thickening. CT demonstrates thickening as very low density. This must be distinguished from benign gastric emphysema often seen in the setting of COPD, endoscopy, and violent retching. Fold thickening is notably absent in benign emphysema.

NEOPLASIA

BENIGN TUMORS

Hyperplastic polyps are composed of gastric epithelium and glandular tissue with inflammatory infiltrate. They are usually small (<2 cm) and sessile with a well-demarcated smooth border. They are the most common polyp found in the stomach, can arise anywhere (most commonly in fundus or body), and have no malignant potential, as they are not neoplastic.

Commonly found in the antrum, gastric adenomas contain cells with nuclear atypia and intestinal metaplasia. They present a true malignant potential, like their colonic counterparts. However, most gastric cancers arise de novo and not from adenomas. In the stomach, unlike the colon, adenomas are significantly less common than hyperplastic polyps, except in patients with polyposis syndromes. They are generally broad based and large (>2 cm) with an irregular or lobulated border.

Lipomas are submucosal lesions that are radiographically indistinguishable from other mesenchymal neoplasms. They are benign but can ulcerate and are typically solitary. Identification of fat content on CT is diagnostic. Neurogenic tumors occasionally present in the stomach. Neurofibromas are most often benign, solitary lesions (multiple in neurofibromatosis) that sometimes undergo malignant transformation. Barium studies demonstrate well-demarcated small submucosal masses with occasional central ulceration. CT additionally shows their extragastric portion. Schwannomas, the most common neurogenic tumors in the stomach, present as benign, well-demarcated submucosal tumors covered by normal mucosa with ulceration. Endoscopic biopsy provides a diagnosis of these slow growing neoplasms. Although glomus tumors are rare in the stomach, they are the most common gastric vascular tumor. They are usually solitary, arising in the antrum. Lymphangiomas are even rarer and develop as aberrant lymphatic tissue not possessing normal lymphatic drainage. Unlike glomus tumors, they do not demonstrate arterial enhancement on imaging studies and appear cystic, mimicking duplication cysts.

MALIGNANT TUMORS

Adenocarcinoma ("gastric cancer") comprises the majority of cases of malignant gastric neoplasms (Table 46-2). It has declined in incidence and mortality in the United States, although it remains the fourth most common cancer worldwide with a death rate exceeded only by lung cancer. It is now the third most common GI malignancy. There are several predisposing conditions associated with gastric adenocarcinoma: *H. pylori* infection, adenomas, polyposis syndromes, pernicious anemia, atrophic gastritis, and partial gastrectomy (Billroth II > I). In fact, *H. pylori* is now classified as a type I carcinogen by the World Health Organization. Diets high in nitrates, nitroso compounds, red meat, and alcohol are also risk factors for development of gastric cancer. It is more common in Asia and twice more common in men than women. Patients present with GI bleeding, weight loss, and often pain. Physical examination sometimes demonstrates a swollen left supraclavicular lymph node (Virchow node) in metastatic cases. This cancer infiltrates early and commonly ulcerates, with size correlated to prognosis and aggressiveness. Barium studies show an ulcerated filling defect with irregular borders and deranged mucosa. Malignant ulcers more commonly appear on the greater curvature or fundus and differ from their benign counterparts in their irregular borders that do not penetrate into the submucosa, associated irregular mass, and fused surrounding folds. Barium studies can elicit the Carman meniscus sign, the convexity of the crater oriented toward the lumen. This type of ulcer commonly comes to attention with failure to respond to pharmacologic therapy. Diagnosis is confirmed by endoscopic biopsy. CT can demonstrate the primary gastric tumor, metastases (hepatic and peritoneal most commonly), and lymphadenopathy. Mucinous calcification may be present. Metastatic involvement of the ovaries, the Krukenberg tumor, can also be detected by CT.

TABLE 46-2 Malignant Gastric Neoplasms

Adenocarcinoma (most common), >90%
Lymphoma
MALT lymphoma
GIST
Leiomyosarcoma
Carcinoid
Small cell carcinoma
Metastases: lung, breast, melanoma, colon, prostate, pancreas

Linitis plastica is most commonly seen with primary gastric adenocarcinoma, but lymphoma and metastases can produce this morphology (Table 46-3). Breast cancer is the most common metastasis giving rise to this appearance, but local extension from pancreatic and colon carcinoma is also implicated. Infiltrative carcinomas can spread through the wall of the stomach. Upper GI examination demonstrates fixed luminal narrowing and fold effacement, usually with a primary mass. CT shows the thick wall and effacement of rugae. Prognosis is especially poor for this form of malignancy.

The stomach is the most common GI site for primary extranodal lymphoma, almost always non-Hodgkin type. The small bowel is the next most common site, with the esophagus being the least common location in the GI

TABLE 46-3 Tumors Causing Linitis Plastica

Adenocarcinoma (most common)
Metastatic breast cancer
Lymphoma
Crohn disease
Local invasion by colon or pancreatic cancer
Gastritis (severe)

TABLE 46-4 Risk Factors for Gastric Non-Hodgkin Lymphoma

H. pylori infection
HIV infection
Immunosuppression
Inflammatory bowel disease
Celiac disease

tract. Multiple risk factors for the development of gastric lymphoma have been implicated (Table 46-4). They often present as filling defects on upper GI studies but can evidence gastric wall thickening (>1 cm) or large, lobulated masses. The wall thickening in lymphoma tends to be greater than that in adenocarcinoma, and it is more homogeneous. Preservation of the perigastric fat plane is more often seen in lymphoma than in gastric adenocarcinoma. Both tend to have nodal disease, but adenopathy in lymphoma often extends below the renal veins. As mentioned above, lymphoma can also present as linitus plastica. Lymphoma is more likely than adenocarcinoma to spread across the pylorus into the duodenum; however, since adenocarcinoma is significantly more common overall, spread from the stomach to the duodenum is usually in the setting of adenocarcinoma.

Most mucosal-associated lymphoid tissue lymphomas (MALTomas or MALT lymphomas) arise in the stomach. B cells comprise these normally indolent non-Hodgkin neoplams commonly associated with *H. pylori* infection. Upper GI series can demonstrate wall thickening, discrete nodules, or a mass. CT and MRI facilitate determination of tumor extent and extranodal disease, but they cannot assess malignant potential. Endoscopic biopsy allows histologic determination of grade and invasiveness. Treatment of underlying infection with antibiotics and proton pump inhibitors induces remission in the overwhelming majority of cases. Chemotherapy may be necessary for less common nonresponders.

Gastrointestinal stromal tumors (GISTs) are the most common mesenchymal tumors of the GI tact and arise from the pacemaker cell (interstitial cell of Cajal) in the smooth muscle. They are distinctly different from smooth muscle tumors (leiomyoma and leiomyosarcoma), as evidenced by their positive immunohistochemical staining to KIT, a tyrosine kinase growth factor. The stomach is the most common organ involved, but they can arise anywhere in the GI tract, even primarily in the mesentery or omentum. They are considered intramural in origin yet appear as a large exophytic mass. They have a predilection for ulceration, and thus usually present at an earlier stage with bleeding. The majority are benign, with the few malignant ones having a high mitotic index, central necrosis, larger mass, local invasion, or metastases. Radiographically, it is impossible to differential benign from malignant tumor, but larger lesions have a greater risk of malignancy. Upper GI studies detect filling defects or ulceration. Most intraluminal GISTs present at around 6 cm in diameter while extraluminal ones often grow to 12 cm or more before discovery. CT usually discovers these small, round, or larger lobulated masses. They heterogeneously enhance with intravenous contrast and occasionally calcify.

The stomach is the most common gastrointestinal site for leiomyosarcomas. These lesions frequently come to clinical attention at a large size and with visceral metastases, commonly as incidental findings or after bleeding into the lumen or peritoneum. Barium findings vary from large ulcerated intraluminal mass to extrinsic compression from an extragastric mass. CT shows a heterogenous mass containing enhancing solid portions alternating with multiple areas of hemorrhage and necrosis. Carney triad involves this neoplasm, pulmonary hamartomas or nodules, and extragastric paraganglioma.

Carcinoid tumors arise from the enterochromaffin cells of Kulchitzky, and there are three classes of gastric carcinoid tumors, all relatively uncommon. Type I, the most common type, develops in the setting of autoimmune-related chronic atrophic gastritis and less commonly pernicious anemia. These tumors are generally benign, arise in the fundus, and can be multiple. Type II tumors are the least common and develop in the setting of Zollinger-Ellison syndrome in patients with multiple endocrine neoplasia type I. Lymph node metastasis is common, but hepatic metastasis with carcinoid syndrome is rare. Type III tumors are sporadic and are large solitary masses. Hepatic metastases can result in carcinoid syndrome, and prognosis is poor.

Gastric small cell carcinoma carries the aggressive characteristics and poor prognosis of its pulmonary counterpart. It presents radiographically as a poorly enhancing large exophytic mass, frequently with metastases at the time of diagnosis.

Kaposi sarcoma of the stomach presents with bleeding and multiple submucosal masses with a bull's eye appearance. Skin lesions are always present. The infiltrating form is rare.

The stomach is a common site for tumor metastases, with melanoma, breast, and lung being frequent offenders. Studies commonly show nodules, either solitary or multiple. Melanoma usually has multiple umbilicated lesions, while breast cancer often causes linitis plastica morphology. Pancreatic cancer sometimes directly spreads to the stomach, creating a filling defect. Additionally, pancreatic pseudocysts can compress the stomach, and surgeons will sometimes drain them into the stomach via direct fistula, cystogastrostomy.

MISCELLANEOUS CONDITIONS

Portal venous hypertension, most commonly from hepatic cirrhosis, results in increased portal pressure leading to increased flow and dilatation of the coronary vein and subsequently the esophageal venous plexus. The systemic shunt is via the azygous vein. Most gastric varices arise from hepatic cirrhosis secondary to alcohol abuse or viral hepatitis. However, one sees isolated gastric varices in splenic vein thrombosis, which can occur in the setting of pancreatitis or pancreatic carcinoma. Short gastric venous dilation creates masslike fundal varices in both situations. In gastric varices secondary to portal venous hypertension, upper GI series demonstrates tortuous and scalloped-appearing filling defects in the esophagus and stomach representing dilated veins. In splenomegaly, one often sees the outline of the enlarged vasculature on the greater curvature of the stomach. Additionally, CT may demonstrate retroperitoneal varices. Portal hypertensive gastropathy has nonspecific findings of gastric wall edema that may have transient perfusion defects on arterial imaging.

The stomach contains fixed ends and a mobile length. Significant twisting causes torsion and vascular compromise. Acute onset results in nausea, vomiting, and severe epigastric pain. Organoaxial volvulus involves rotation along the long axis, a line from the pylorus to the GEJ. The greater curve is displaced superior and to the right of the lesser curve. It is the more common pattern and rarely results in significant permanent morbidity. Mesenteroaxial volvulus occurs along the short axis extending between the greater and lesser curves, resulting in superior displacement of the antrum relative to the fundus, with switching of the pylorus and GEJ. It is less common than organoaxial rotation but represents a more serious threat for ischemia. Radiographic studies demonstrate absent filling of part of the stomach with an acute angle transition point or show two portions of the stomach, both with contrast and with air.

Menetrier disease presents with hypoproteinemia and hypochlorhydria secondary to parietal cell loss. Rugae are typically markedly hypertrophied with antral sparing. Patients complain of pain, nausea, vomiting, and weight loss. Many develop a protein losing enteropathy, and endoscopy with biopsy is indicated for diagnosis. After resolution, one carefully monitors patients secondary to the increased risk of gastric adenocarcinoma.

Bezoars represent agglomerated undigested material. They present in the stomach with a mottled appearance and ulceration and sometimes can obstruct the flow of food. The most common types are trichobezoars (hair), which form in the setting of Rapunzel syndrome, and phytobezoars (vegetable matter). Upper GI study shows an unattached filling defect or mass floating in a pool of contrast. Obstruction also clues to the diagnosis.

Amyloidosis results in extracellular deposition of amorphous fibrillar protein and can affect any portion of the gut. It usually occurs in the setting of chronic infection, inflammation, or hemodialysis. Radiographically, it has a protean appearance with fold thickening, mucosal nodules, or even mass.

In the past, antrectomy with vagotomy was commonly performed for the treatment of ulcer disease. There were several methods developed for reconnecting the stomach to the small bowel. Billroth I, a primary gastroduodenostomy, was abandoned because of severe alkaline gastritis and esophagitis. Billroth II (Fig. 46-1), an end-to-side gastrojejunostomy, provided some improvement from alkaline gastritis, although not complete. Additionally, these patients were at an increased risk for gastric carcinoma, greater than the risk seen with Billroth I patients. Patients who have undergone Billroth II procedure may present with afferent obstruction leading to dilation and pain secondary to retained secretions, afferent limb syndrome. They complain of early satiety and pain relieved by bilious vomiting. Distention with rupture is the most severe complication, requiring strict monitoring. Upper GI examination often does not fill the fluid-filled, dilated afferent loop. CT demonstrates biliary obstruction and a fluid-filled

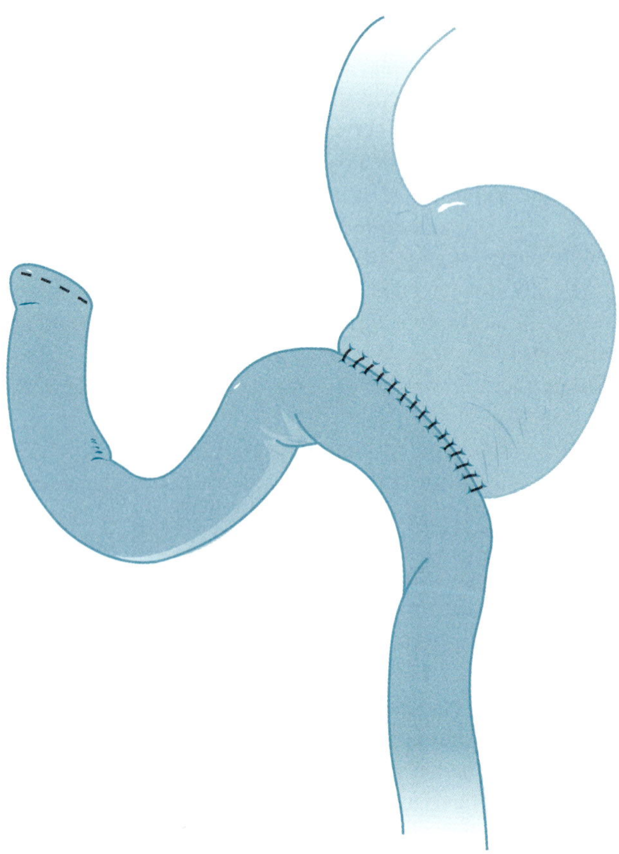

FIG. 46-1 Partial gastrectomy with Billroth II gastrojejunostomy. SOURCE: Courtesy of Anthony F. Zagar, UAB, Department of Radiology, Birmingham, Alabama.

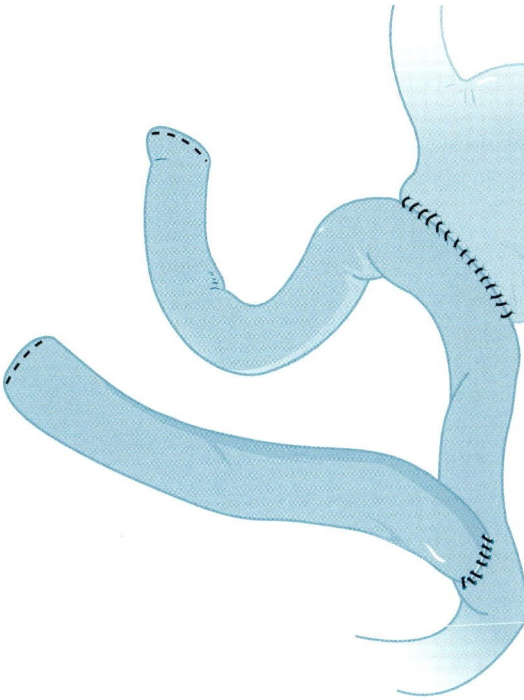

FIG. 46-2 Partial gastrectomy with Roux-en-Y gastrojejunostomy.

afferent limb. Patients with Billroth II anastomosis can also experienced severe dumping syndrome.

A Roux-en-y configuration (Fig. 46-2) was developed to address the issues of alkaline reflux, and this is

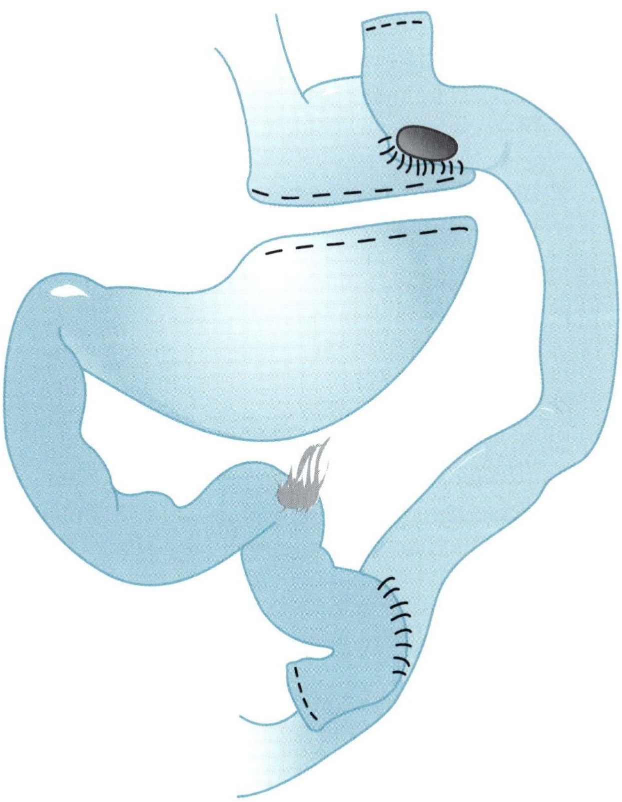

FIG. 46-3 Roux-en-Y gastric bypass.

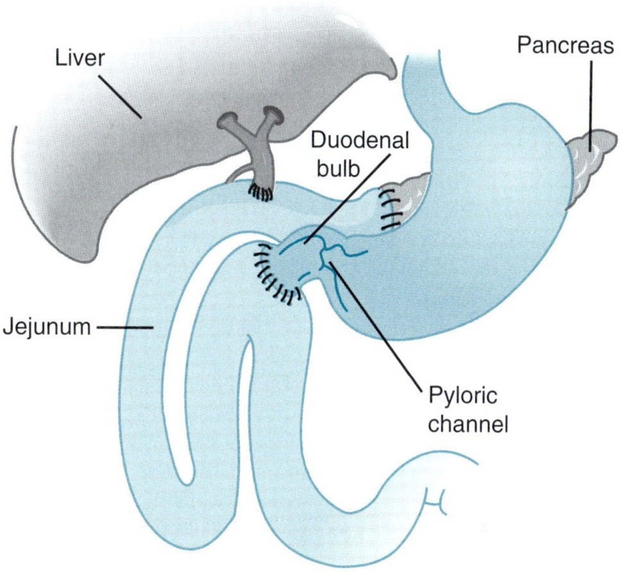

FIG. 46-4 Pylorus—preserving pancreaticoduodenectomy (Whipple procedure) with duodenojejunostomy, hepaticojejunostomy, and pancreaticojejunostomy.

the surgery commonly used today. Because of improved medical therapy, surgeries are rarely performed for peptic ulcer disease. Roux limb reconstruction is commonly used gastric bypass (Fig. 46-3) surgery. Laparoscopic gastric bypass is now the most commonly performed bariatric surgery procedure, and these patients are at an increased risk of internal hernia. In the past, congenital paraduodenal hernias were the most common internal hernia. Now, postsurgical mesenteric hernias are most common. Gastric bypass patients are at increased risk because of the loss of their mesenteric fat during weight loss, making obstruction more likely.

The pancreaticoduodenectomy, Whipple procedure (Fig. 46-4), involves resection of the head or all of the pancreas, the adjacent duodenum, and the distal common bile duct. Reconstruction is via Roux-en-y or loop hepaticojejunostomy and pancreaticojejunostomy. There is also a gastrojejunostomy or a duodenojejunostomy if it is pylorus preserving.

SUGGESTED READING

Ba-Ssalamah A, Prokop M, Uffmann M, et al. Dedicated multidetector CT of the stomach: spectrum of diseases. *Radiographics.* 2003;23:625-644.

Blachar A, Federle MP, Pealer KM, et al. Gastrointestinal complications of laparoscopic Roux-en-Y gastric bypass surgery: clinical and imaging findings. *Radiology.* 2002;223(3):625-632.

Chandler RC, Srinivas G, Chintapalli KN, et al. Imaging in bariatric surgery: a guide to postsurgical anatomy and common complications. *AJR Am J Roentgenol.* 2007;190:122-125.

Choi D, Lim HK, Lee SJ, et al. Gastric mucosa-associated lymphoid tissue lymphoma: helical CT findings and pathologic correlation. *AJR Am J Roentgenol.* 2002;178:1117-1122.

Fulcher AS, Truner MA. Abdominal manifestations of situs anomalies in adults. *Radiographics.* 2002;22:1439-1456.

Ghai S, Pattison J, Ghai S, et al. Primary gastrointestinal lymphoma: spectrum of imaging findings with pathologic correlation. *Radiographics.* 2007;27:1371-1388.

Grayson DE, Abbott RM, Levy AD, et al. Emphysematous infections of the abdomen and pelvis: a pictorial review. *Radiographics.* 2002;22:543-561.

Horton KM, Fishman EK. Current role of CT in imaging of the stomach. *Radiographics.* 2003;23:75-87.

Kim KW, Choi BI, Han JK, et al. Postoperative anatomic and pathologic findings at CT following gastrectomy. *Radiographics.* 2002;22:323-336.

Kim SH, Han JK, Lee KH, et al. Abdominal amyloidosis: spectrum of radiological findings. *Clin Radiol.* 2003;58(8):610-620.

Lepanto L, Gianfelice D, Dery R, et al. Postoperative changes, complications, and recurrent disease after Whipple's operation: CT features. *AJR Am J Roentgenol.* 1994;163:841-846.

Levy AD, Remotti HE, Thompson WM, et al. From the archives of the AFIP: gastrointestinal stromal tumors: radiologic features with pathologic correlation. *Radiographics.* 2003;23:283-304.

Levy AD, Sobin LH. From the archives of the AFIP, gastrointestinal carcinoids: imaging features with clinicopathologic comparison. *Radiographics.* 2007;27:237-257.

Park SH, Han JK, Kim TK, et al. Unusual gastric tumors: radiologic-pathologic correlation. *Radiographics.* 1999;19:1435-1446.

Smith C, Deziel DJ, Kubicka RA. Evaluation of the postoperative stomach and duodenum. *Radiographics.* 1994;14:67-86.

QUESTIONS AND ANSWERS

1. Which of the following features is most commonly seen with a malignant gastric ulcer?
   A. Large crater
   B. Ovoid-shaped crater
   C. Truncated rugal folds ending before the crater
   D. Enlargement of the areae gastricae
   E. Multiplicity

   ANSWER: C. Malignant ulcers typically present with truncated, nodular folds that are somewhat asymmetric. The crater is irregular, but size or shape does not help differentiate benign from malignant. The crater typically does not extend beyond the gastric lumen, as it does in benign ulcer disease. They are typically solitary.

2. In which of the following conditions does one see isolated gastric varices?
   A. Portal hypertension
   B. Budd-Chiari
   C. Pancreatic carcinoma
   D. Post-TIPS
   E. Splenic infarction

   ANSWER: C. Splenic vein thrombosis results in isolated gastric varices. This commonly occurs in the setting of pancreatic cancer or pancreatitis. Portal venous hypertension typically presents with esophageal, gastric, splenic, and other mesenteric varices. Budd-Chiari presents with absent hepatic veins and absent or occluded inferior vena cava.

3. Which of the following is associated with enlarged areae gastricae?
   A. Peptic ulcer disease
   B. Young age
   C. Gastric adenocarcinoma
   D. Atrophic gastritis
   E. Linitus plastica

   ANSWER: A. Areae gastricae are commonly enlarged in the elderly and in patients with *H. pylori* infection. Focal enlargement can be seen adjacent to ulcers. Areae gastricae are usually obliterated with gastric carcinoma and completely absent in the setting of atrophic gastritis and linitus plastica.

4. What is the most common etiology for multiple small gastric polyps?
   A. Hyperplastic polyps
   B. Metastatic melanoma
   C. Primary adenocarcinoma
   D. Lymphoma
   E. Adenomas

   ANSWER: A. Statistically, multiple small polyps almost always represent benign hyperplasia, as gastric adenomas are much less common. Melanoma typically presents with multiple target mucosal lesions. Adenocarcinoma is usually a primary mucosal mass. Lymphoma can have various appearances, including marked fold nodularity, but focal polyps are atypical.

5. What is the most common GI tract location for primary extranodal lymphoma?
   A. Esophagus
   B. Stomach
   C. Small bowel
   D. Colon
   E. Rectum

   ANSWER: B. The most common site for extranodal lymphoma is the stomach, usually non-Hodgkin type.

6. Concerning situs anomalies, which of the following presents with more serious congenital heart disease?
   A. Situs solitus
   B. Situs inversus with dextrocardia
   C. Situs inversus with levocardia
   D. Situs ambiguous with polysplenia
   E. Situs ambiguous with asplenia

ANSWER: E. Congenital heart disease occurs in almost all individuals with a splenia and is more severe than any of the situs anomalies.

7. Concerning gastric carcinoid tumors, which of the following is true?
   A. Associated with Zollinger-Ellison syndrome
   B. Associated with multiple endocrine neoplasia type II
   C. Metastasize early
   D. Typically present with carcinoid syndrome
   E. Increased risk for adenocarcinoma

   ANSWER: A. Carcinoid tumors are associated with multiple endocrine neoplasia type I and Zollinger-Ellison syndrome. They seldom metastasize or produce carcinoid syndrome. There is no increased risk for carcinoma.

8. Concerning gastric leiomyosarcomas, what is the most common cross-sectional imaging appearance?
   A. Ulcerating mucosal plaque
   B. Mural necrotic mass
   C. Mucosal nodule
   D. Multiple target lesions
   E. Linitus plastica

   ANSWER: B. Gastric leiomyosarcoma is typically a large, necrotic mural tumor. It is often exophytic but has ulceration. Radiographically, it cannot be distinguished from GIST. Multiple target lesions are classically seen with metastatic melanoma.

9. Concerning gastric diverticula, which of the following is true?
   A. Most commonly occur in the greater curvature
   B. Can mimic an adrenal adenoma
   C. Intramural diverticula are true diverticula.
   D. Intramural diverticula typically occur in the fundus.
   E. Cannot be distinguished from an ulcer

   ANSWER: B. Gastric diverticula most commonly arise from the posterior fundus and can mimic a left adrenal adenoma on cross-sectional imaging. Intramural pseudodiverticula represent an invagination of the mucosa through the muscular layer along the greater curve in the antrum. They change shape during peristalsis and do not have adjacent fold thickening, differentiating them from ulcers.

10. What is the most common type of internal hernia?
    A. Left paraduodenal
    B. Right paraduodenal
    C. Congenital
    D. Transomental
    E. Transmesenteric

    ANSWER: E. Postoperative, transmesenteric hernias are now the most common internal hernia.

47 SMALL BOWEL

Sanjiv K. Bajaj and Cheri L. Canon

NORMAL ANATOMY

The small intestine extends from the pylorus to the ileocecal valve in three parts: duodenum, jejunum, and ileum. Its smaller caliber and valvulae conniventes (fine circumferential folds also referred to as plica circularis) distinguish it from the large bowel. The duodenum is the short initial small bowel segment that forms a C loop encompassing the head of the pancreas. Its segment proximal to the major papilla derives from the foregut, while the remainder arises from the midgut. It lies retroperitoneally except in its first 2 cm (the duodenal cap or bulb of the superior segment). The first (superior) segment of the duodenum courses transversely for 5 cm at the L1 vertebral level. It lies immediately anterior to the portal vein, bile duct, and inferior vena cava. As the first portion turns posterior and downward, a flexural pseudotumor is created on double-contrast duodenography representing the redundant mucosa along the inner angle of the superior flexure. The second (descending) segment of the duodenum encircles the head of the pancreas in its 7 cm inferior course. The main pancreatic duct empties here at the major papilla (ampulla of Vater). The third (inferior) part crosses the L3 vertebral body anterior to the inferior vena cava and aorta during its 6 cm. The superior mesenteric artery's (SMA) passage anterior to it creates a possible sight of compression. The fourth (ascending) part courses superiorly for 5 cm and joins the jejunum at the duodenojejunal junction, an angulated area suspended by the ligament of Treitz. The celiac trunk sends the gastroduodenal artery's superior pancreaticoduodenal branch to the foregut derivatives, while the SMA feeds the midgut portion via the inferior pancreaticoduodenal artery. The veins follow the arteries. The lymphatic channels drain via the pyloric lymph nodes to the superior mesenteric group.

The jejunum and ileum comprise 40% and 60% of the small bowel's 7 m length, respectively. The jejunum primarily occupies the left upper quadrant while the ileum resides in the right lower quadrant. One distinguishes the two based on appearance; the jejunum grossly possesses deeper color, thicker wall, greater vascularity involving long vasa rectae without complicated arcades, less mesenteric fat, fewer Peyer patches, and many valvulae conniventes. Imaging demonstrates its feathery mucosal pattern. Both segments derive their blood supply from terminal branches of the SMA and drain into the superior mesenteric vein. Lymphatics drain to the superior mesenteric group except in the terminal ileum, where they drain to the ileocolic area.

PATHOLOGY

CONGENITAL ABNORMALITIES

Meckel diverticulum, the most common congenital anomaly of the GI tract, derives from persistence of a portion of the embryonic yolk stalk (the omphalomesenteric duct). It presents as a 2-in long outpouching containing all three bowel layers (including a muscular layer), 2 ft proximal to the ileocecal junction in 2% of people. Half of these lesions contain heterotopic (gastric or pancreatic) mucosa. Bleeding, discomfort, and rare perforation initiate investigation. The invaginated diverticulum serves as a leading edge, causing intussusception in children. Radiographs may demonstrate a focally dilated sentinel loop. Fluoroscopy finds contrast filling the diverticulum with other manifestations of disease, such as intussusception or an ulcer. Meckel diverticulitis is readily identified on CT. Technetium-99 concentrates in gastric mucosa, and nuclear medicine scanning localizes the abnormality when these cells are present.

Small polygonal filling defects can be seen in the duodenal bulb with contrast fluoroscopy. These represent heterotopic gastric mucosa with surrounding normal duodenal mucosa. It is important not to confuse this incidental (clinically insignificant) finding with real pathology. Prolapsing gastric mucosa can protrude into the duodenal bulb, creating a transient, mass-like filling defect. This too is an incidental finding. Like in the stomach, ectopic pancreatic rests can also occur in the duodenal bulb.

Atresia, failure of canalization of the bowel lumen, most commonly occurs in the duodenum secondary to intrauterine insults during bowel development in the first trimester of life. This disorder presents neonatally with obstruction causing bilious emesis and absent stool. Patients have a history of fetal polyhydramnios that is due to inability to swallow amniotic fluid. Many have Down syndrome or associated cardiac or urinary defects. Conventional radiographs demonstrate the "double bubble" sign, representing dilated stomach and duodenum separated by the pylorus. Treatment involves support with nasogastric tube decompression and (intravenous) fluids followed by surgery to excise the atretic segment and reanastomose the bowel.

Annular pancreas presents similarly to atresia, but its emesis is nonbilious because of more proximal obstruction. The pancreas begins as two separate lobes flanking the duodenum, the ventral and dorsal enlarge. Normally, the left lobe circles the bowel and its remnant atrophies. In this disorder, a ring of pancreatic tissue remains surrounding the descending segment of the duodenum. CT demonstrates the pancreatic ring. Treatment involves supportive stabilization followed by surgery.

Diverticula arise from points of mural weakness in the intestinal tract. Duodenal diverticula commonly appear on upper GI series and CT but are mostly asymptomatic. Duodenal diverticula are usually acquired, containing only mucosa and submucosa, and extend toward the pancreas from the second or third portions of the duodenum; they occasionally cause ampullary obstruction. Because of their close proximity to the pancreas, they can be confused with a cystic pancreatic neoplasm, and care should be taken to identify gas or oral contrast in these collections. Intraluminal duodenal diverticula, usually diagnosed during infancy, give the classic windsock deformity on barium studies and CT. Small bowel diverticula other than Meckel diverticula rarely occur; they can cause bleeding, diverticulitis, and perforation. Malabsorption secondary to bacterial overgrowth is seen only in extensive diverticulosis. Jejunal diverticula are larger and more common than their ileal counterparts.

Duodenal and small bowel duplication is rare. Like other locations in the gut, these cystic lesions seldom communicate with the lumen.

Congenital intestinal lymphangiectasia is a rare congenital condition diagnosed in the young. Dilated small bowel lymphatics result in a protein-losing enteropathy. CT findings are nonspecific, with diffuse mural edema.

OBSTRUCTION

Mechanical obstruction presents with waxing and waning crampy abdominal pain, high-pitched bowel sounds, vomiting, constipation, and distention. Patients most commonly have adhesions secondary to surgery, but tumor, hernia, nonsteroidal anti-inflammatory drug (NSAID)-related stricture, foreign body, and intussusception can also cause obstruction (Table 47-1). Upright radiographs show dilated proximal bowel with multiple air-fluid levels and collapsed distal bowel, and supine films depict stacked bowel loops. In cases involving dilated, fluid-filled small bowel and a paucity of small bowel gas, air-fluid levels may be replaced by the appearance of string of pearls representing air bubbles

TABLE 47-1 Small Bowel Obstruction

Adhesions (most common)
Hernia (inguinal, ventral, internal)
Tumor
Intussusception (usually lead point in setting of obstruction)
IBD
NSAID stricture
Foreign body
Gallstone ileus (uncommon)

trapped between the valvulae conniventes. CT shows the transition point by demonstrating dilated proximal loops and collapsed distal ones. It commonly delineates the cause of obstruction as well. Therapy involves bowel rest with nasogastric tube decompression and fluid and electrolyte stabilization. Surgery treats cases failing conservative therapy.

There are several hernia types. External hernias include inguinal hernias, more common in men, femoral hernias, more common in women, and abdominal wall protrusions. Richter hernia is a partial hernia involving only one side of the bowel wall, and Spigelian hernia is a protrusion through the linea semilunaris at the lateral margin of the rectus abdominis, midway between the umbilicus and symphysis pubis. Obturator hernias are rare.

Intussusception involves telescoping of bowel loops, with the proximal intussusceptum telescoping into the distal intussuscipiens. It occurs most commonly in children, although adults with mass lesions are also at risk, and presents with intermittent crampy abdominal pain secondary to obstruction. Vomiting and bloody stools with currant jelly appearance classically accompany these symptoms. Radiographs occasionally demonstrate a paucity of gas in the right abdomen. Barium enema examination shows a coiled spring appearance representing contrast between the concentric bowel loops. CT and ultrasound depict telescoped loops as the target sign with mesenteric vessels surrounded by mesenteric fat. Longitudinal section demonstrates a sandwich appearance. On the other hand, small jejunal intussusceptions are typically fleeting and of no consequence in the adult. They commonly occur around intestinal tubes or surgical anastomoses. Multiple, recurrent intussusceptions suggest sprue. However, ileocolonic or colocolonic intussusceptions in the adult are almost always associated with a pathologic lead point, typically adenocarcinoma but also possibly lipomas.

Complicated obstruction can occur in the setting of appendicitis, Crohn disease, diverticulitis, and ischemia to name a few. CT is the imaging modality choice for diagnosis. Strangulation of small bowel most commonly occurs in the setting of closed loop obstruction and is secondary to the interruption of blood flow. Adhesion and internal hernia are usually implicated in closed loop obstruction. CT remains the modality of choice, although this entity can be difficult to diagnose on this modality. Internal hernias are now most commonly seen in the postoperative patient with transmesenteric obstruction. CT findings included small bowel loops clustered along the anterior abdominal wall, often in a “c” or “u” shape. There may be a swirled appearance to the mesentery.

Volvulus involves torsion of an intestinal segment about its mesenteric stalk. Midgut volvulus most commonly occurs in children congenitally afflicted with malrotation of the intestine. It classically presents in the first month of life with proximal obstruction, bilious emesis, and abdominal pain. Interruption of the vascular supply to the affected area often results in ischemia progressing to infarction, and mortality approaches 20%. Radiographs evidence partial duodenal obstruction or a gasless abdomen. Barium studies show a corkscrew duodenum, an abnormal location of an intestinal segment, and a duodenojejunal junction displaced inferiorly to the right. Emergent surgery minimizes morbidity and mortality.

Adynamic ileus represents a paralytic lack of coordinated intestinal movement with resultant functional obstruction. It presents with abdominal distention and decreased bowel sounds in the setting of surgery, electrolyte imbalance, inflammation, and systemic illness. Radiographs show diffuse small and large bowel dilatation, typically with air-fluid levels on the same level and air in the rectum. It can appear radiographically indistinguishable from obstruction and sometimes evidence a transition point. Real-time fluoroscopy shows absent bowel peristalsis. Treatment involves bowel rest and nasogastric tube decompression. Focal inflammatory lesions such as pancreatitis, appendicitis, diverticulitis, and abscess can cause adynamic ileus in adjacent single loops of small bowel, referred to as sentinel ileus.

VASCULAR ABNORMALITIES

Mesenteric ischemia arises from inadequate blood flow to the intestines, usually secondary to thromboembolic disease or in the setting of closed loop obstruction. The acute form generally follows systemic hypoperfusion or thromboembolic phenomena and presents with pain out of proportion to physical findings. Radiographs are usually unremarkable or demonstrate an ileus. CT demonstrates the ileus, which is often focal mural edema, and sometimes directly visualizes the embolus. Focal enhancement defect in the small bowel wall indicates ischemia or even infarction. Prompt diagnosis improves mortality.

TABLE 47-2 Small Bowel Pneumatosis

MALIGNANT	BENIGN
Ischemia/infarction	Surgery/trauma
Typhlitis	Endoscopy
Obstruction	Enteric tube
	COPD
	Immunosuppression (AIDS, chemotherapy, transplant, steroid use)

Pneumatosis and portal venous gas in the setting of bowel ischemia are ominous. However, there are many other causes of benign pneumatosis (Table 47-2), and clinical correlation with serum lactic acid level is the most important predictor of morbidity and mortality.

Chronic mesenteric ischemia arises from atherosclerosis in two of the three major intestinal vessels (celiac trunk, SMA, IMA) and presents as weight loss with nonspecific intestinal pain shortly after meals. Radiographs may be unremarkable. CT and MR angiography can demonstrate the diseased visceral vessels. Vascular surgery ameliorates symptoms.

Shock bowel results from severe ischemic injury to the intestine after systemic hypoperfusion. It usually arises in cases with significant acute blood loss, as in traumatic bleeding. Hyperenhancement of the mucosa coupled with low density of mural edema give the bowel a cerebriform appearance on CT. Other findings of shock, collapsed inferior vena cava, hyperenhancing adrenal glands, splenic hypoperfusion are typically present. Shock bowel is reversible and seldom progresses to infarction.

Vasculitis results in focal transient ischemia. Like in other causes of ischemia, CT demonstrates mural edema, but it is focal and may be multisegmental. The latter helps distinguish it from thromboembolic ischemia. Systemic lupus erythematosus and polyarteritis nodosa can affect any portion of the GI tract.

Radiation enteritis is another form of vasculitis and causes bowel wall edema in the setting of radiation, leading to smooth fold thickening on imaging. It usually resolves spontaneously. The chronic form presents after history of radiation with nausea, vomiting, diarrhea, and abdominal pain. Microangiopathy causes chronic ischemia resulting in fibrosis, stricture formation, and fistulae in addition to mural edema and fold effacement.

INFLAMMATION AND INFECTION

Duodenitis can be seen in multiple conditions: peptic ulcer disease, Zollinger-Ellison syndrome, uremia in the setting of hemodialysis, Crohn disease, and infection. Findings are nonspecific and include mural edema. Uremic duodenitis tends to present with worse, more nodular fold thickening.

Small intestinal ulceration most commonly occurs in the proximal duodenum secondary to *Helicobacter pylori* infection; smoking and chronic NSAID and steroid consumption confer increased risk. This lesion presents with occult bleeding and epigastric pain improved by meals. It sometimes progresses to perforation into the peritoneum or pancreas. Barium studies show pooled contrast as a discrete radioopaque lesion. Conventional radiographs and CT find complications such as free air and abscess. Treatment involves cessation of the offending agent and triple therapy when applicable with bismuth salt, proton pump inhibitor, and antibiotic active against *H. pylori*.

Multiple ulcers or ulceration in distal duodenum raise suspicion for etiologies such as Zollinger-Ellison syndrome, characterized by gastric acid hypersecretion, secondary to a gastrinoma. The disease presents sporadically or as part of multiple endocrine neoplasia syndromes with ulceration, GI bleed, diarrhea, and abdominal pain. Fluoroscopy demonstrates the ulceration, and conventional radiographs evaluate for perforation. Nuclear medicine studies for somatostatin receptors visualize the etiologic neoplasm, with CT finding larger tumors. Serum gastrin diagnoses the abnormality. Amelioration comes with proton pump inhibitors and H2 receptor antagonists, and cure comes with surgical resection or total gastrectomy.

Crohn disease involves transmural inflammation with ulceration. It manifests most commonly in the distal ileum but can appear anywhere in the GI tract. It presents bimodally in young and middle-aged patients as colicky lower abdominal pain, diarrhea, obstruction, fever, weight loss, peripheral rash, and arthritis. Fistulae, adhesions, and strictures are common late sequelae. Barium studies demonstrate classic skip lesions with long-strictured segments and deep ulceration in addition to fold thickening and solitary ulcers. CT finds mural edema, mesenteric inflammation, abscesses, and other late manifestations and detects malignancy. Fibrofatty proliferation, secondary to the protective creeping fat, is well seen on CT. Congestion of the mesenteric vasa recta, the "comb" sign, suggests active disease, although there continues to be somewhat poor correlation with radiologic findings and clinical presentation. Colonoscopy allows biopsy of cobblestoned mucosa when it can be visualized. Treatment involves sulfasalazine and vitamin replacement in addition to immunosuppression using steroids, TNF receptor antibodies, methotrexate, and other agents. Surgery treats complications but is largely ineffective in ameliorating the primary process, as the disease tends to recur. Cancer, most commonly adenocarcinoma, occurs at increased rates decades after diagnosis.

Celiac disease (sprue) results from an intestinal hypersensitivity reaction to gluten, a protein found in many grains. It presents with malabsorptive fatty diarrhea, weight loss, bloating, and iron-deficiency anemia. It sometimes regresses after appearance in childhood and reappears later in life. Barium studies demonstrate pooling or flocculation of contrast material in the dilated bowel lumen secondary to secreted fluid, the moulage sign. Folds are decreased in the jejunum and increased in the ileum (jejunization of the ileum), causing the areas to appear similar. As the process progresses, there may be reversal of the fold pattern. The duodenum may have a bubbly or frankly shaggy appearance. There may be multiple transient intussusceptions. Dermatitis herpetiformis, lymphadenopathy, and hyposplenism are associated with sprue. Antibody tests suggest the disorder, but diagnosis requires small bowel biopsy demonstrating villous atrophy with infiltrating inflammatory cells and crypt hyperplasia. Treatment involves avoidance of gluten. Small bowel adenocarcinoma and lymphoma, esophageal cancer, and melanoma risks are increased. Hypogammaglobulinemia mimics sprue. The lymphoid hyperplasia in this setting results in nodular filling defects along small bowel folds.

Graft-versus-host disease is most common in the setting of bone marrow transplantation and results when the transplanted cells reject the host. It can affect any portion of the gut, most commonly the small bowel. Imaging reveals nonspecific mural thickening with a tubular appearance of the small bowel, nicely depicted on small bowel series.

Infectious enteritides rarely benefit from radiographic imaging. They present with fold thickening, mural edema, and ulceration. Findings are generally nonspecific. *Giardia lamblia* and *Strongyloides stercoralis* involve the duodenum and proximal small bowel, while *Mycobacterium tuberculosis* and *Yersinia enterocolitica* involve the terminal ileum and cecum, mimicking Crohn disease. CMV produces skip lesions with deep ulceration, typically in immunocompromised patients.

Whipple disease is a systemic infectious disorder that is due to a gram-positive bacillus causing watery diarrhea, lymphadenopathy, splenomegaly, arthralgias, and CNS and cardiac pathology. Barium studies demonstrate intestinal fold thickening with small nodules and with flocculation of contrast. CT reveals low density, bulky lymphadenopathy. Diagnosis requires biopsy with PAS stain. A year-long course of ampicillin and tetracycline provides an effective cure.

NEOPLASIA

Benign Tumors

Brunner gland hyperplasia occurs in the setting of an immunologic disorder, such as hypogammaglobulinemia, and presents with multiple small, round filling defects in the duodenal bulb. These should not be confused with heterotopic gastric mucosa.

Both hyperplastic and adenomatous polyps are seen in the duodenum. Villous tumors have a predilection for the duodenum, usually near the ampulla, and can be seen in the setting of familial adenomatous polyposis syndrome (FAPS).

Gastrointestinal stromal tumors (GISTs), arising from mesenchymal cells, are the most common benign tumor of the small bowel. These distinctly differ from leiomyoma and leiomyosarcoma and are diagnosed by staining for cKIT. They are rarely malignant, vary greatly in size, and can be either intraluminal or extraluminal. Malignancy is based on histology and metastasis. Tumors mostly spread via local extension, and they commonly recur after resection. Distant spread often involves the liver and peritoneum. Their predisposition to necrosis leads to hemorrhage and perforation, which are common presenting signs in addition to obstruction and abdominal pain. Fluoroscopic and CT studies demonstrate appearance similar to GISTs in the remainder of the GI tract: large, heterogeneous, necrotic tumors.

Other benign tumors of the small bowel include adenomas, lipomas, leiomyomas, and hemangiomas. Hamartomas arise most commonly in Peutz-Jeghers syndrome. Neurofibromas are single except in patients with neurofibromatosis type I, von Recklinghausen disease. Lesions are smooth and well demarcated without extension and rarely hemorrhage. Most patients are asymptomatic, although bleeding, obstruction, and intussusception occur in a minority.

Malignant Tumors

Adenocarcinoma is the most common duodenal malignancy, but occurs rarely in the remainder of the small bowel. It is more common in the distal duodenum. It usually presents with obstruction and can be annular or polypoid. Malignant small intestinal tumors occur less frequently than in other bowel areas and often present in settings such as Crohn disease and ulcerative colitis. Tumor syndromes such as FAPS and hereditary nonpolyposis colon cancer syndrome (HNPCC) also predispose to these lesions.

Carcinoid tumors, the most prevalent primary small bowel neoplasms, generally arise in the distal ileum from enterochromaffin cells. They are usually malignant when in the small bowel. Most of these tumors are slow growing, asymptomatic neoplasms producing substances including serotonin. Liver metastases lead to carcinoid syndrome, characterized by flushing, diarrhea, bronchoconstriction, and right-sided cardiac valvular disease. Barium studies may demonstrate the primary lesion as a rounded intraluminal filling defect.

Arterial phase CT imaging allows better delineation because of its hypervascular nature. Nodal metastases to the mesentery appear as large stellate calcified masses with adjacent desmoplastic reaction and small bowel thickening secondary to secreted vasoactive amines and lymphatic obstruction. CT allows evaluation of extraluminal masses and metastases. However, the primary tumor is often never identified. The differential diagnosis includes sclerosing mesenteritis, treated lymphoma, and lymphadenopathy secondary to *M. tuberculosis*.

Intestinal lymphoma presents with fevers, diarrhea, and abdominal pain, often with lymphadenopathy and hepatosplenomegaly on physical examination. It generally occurs in the distal ileum and appendix, usually non-Hodgkin type (B cells more common). Burkitt lymphoma arises intestinally in children secondary to Epstein-Barr virus infection and follows an aggressive course. Small bowel follow-through demonstrates fold thickening, diffuse nodular masses, luminal narrowing from intrinsic or extrinsic lesions, filling defects, and ulceration. CT reveals retroperitoneal lymphadenopathy, sometimes with intestinal lymphadenopathy, and can visualize the mass. The pathognomonic finding of aneurysmal dilatation is due to internal ulceration and sloughing of the mucosa. Unlike adenocarcinoma, lymphoma does not usually obstruct. Treatment involves resection with radiotherapy.

Leiomyosarcomas are also seen in the small bowel but less commonly than GISTs. They appear similar to leiomyosarcomas and GISTs in the remainder of the gut.

Metastases to the small bowel arise from nearly any source (Table 47-3), most commonly lung carcinoma and melanoma through hematogenous spread or gastric, pancreatic, and colon cancer through local spread or peritoneal implants. Ovarian and breast cancer can also cause peritoneal carcinomatosis with serosal implants. They are often multiple and appear as filling defects or extraluminal compression along the antimesenteric border. CT demonstrates the lesions and sometimes elucidates the primary.

TABLE 47-3 Metastases to Small Bowel

Peritoneal
Ovarian
Colon
Stomach
Pancreas
Hematogenous (antimesenteric border)
Lung (squamous cell most common)
Breast
Melanoma
Kaposi sarcoma

MISCELLANEOUS CONDITIONS

SMA syndrome is obstruction of the third portion of the duodenum by the SMA as the duodenum crosses midline. It is typically seen in patients after rapid weight loss because of loss of mesenteric fat, decreasing the angle between the aorta and SMA.

Amyloidosis can occur anywhere throughout the GI tract and has a protean appearance. It classically presents with smooth fold thickening throughout the small bowel.

Traumatic injury to the small bowel is best evaluated with CT. The duodenum is particularly susceptible to traumatic compression against the vertebral bodies and may present with intramural hematoma, perforation, or transection. Small bowel hematomas can also occur in the setting of over-anticoagulation and in Henoch-Schönlein purpura. On CT, there is circumferential thickening, which is often high density on noncontrast imaging. Obstruction may occur.

Angioedema occurs secondary to increased capillary permeability and can involve any mucosal surface. It can occur with the use of angiotensin-converting enzyme (ACE) inhibitors. In this case, onset is usually within a week of initiation of medication, but can also be more remote and resolve within 2 days of discontinuation. CT shows nonspecific mural edema which may be focal or multisegmental. It also has been reported secondary to intravenous iodinated contrast.

Scleroderma (progressive systemic sclerosis) is vasculitis that results in fibrosis. Scleroderma results in small bowel dilatation and decreased peristalsis without fold thickening. Fibrosis of the inner circular muscular layer results in shortening of the bowel, a stack-of-coins appearance. Wide-mouth sacculations along the mesenteric border may be present.

Mastocytosis is a mast cell proliferation that presents with multiple small bowel nodules, numerous sclerotic bone lesions, and organomegaly. Waldenström macroglobulinemia also presents with innumerable sand-like small bowel nodules.

Evaluation of the small bowel lumen and fold pattern (Table 47-4) in conjunction with the clinical presentation is helpful in determining the diagnosis. There is significant overlap in the imaging appearance of small bowel disease, so differential diagnoses may be lengthy. Clinical data are imperative.

In general, CT is the imaging modality of choice for the evaluation of the postoperative small bowel. Exceptions include contrast fluoroscopy in the immediate postoperative period to evaluate for leak. Many patients with ulcerative colitis and FAPS undergo prophylactic total proctocolectomy to prevent colon carcinoma. Ileal pouch-anal anastomosis (j-pouch) provides a continent reservoir for these patients, thus eliminating the need for a permanent

TABLE 47-4 Pattern Approach to Small Bowel Disease

Smooth fold thickening
- Hypoproteinemia (cirrhosis, sprue, nephrotic syndrome, Cronkhite-Canada syndrome)
- Amyloidosis
- Radiation enteritis
- Hemorrhage
- Eosinophilic gastroenteritis

Nodular fold thickening
- Crohn disease
- Lymphoma
- Lymphangiectasia
- Hypogammaglobulinemia
- Tumor
- Amyloidosis
- TB
- CMV

Nodules
- Mastocytosis
- Lymphoma
- Whipple disease (micronodules)
- Waldenström macroglobulinemia (micronodules)
- Lymphangiectasia (micronodules)

Dilatation
- Obstruction
- Scleroderma
- Sprue

Fluid-filled
- Obstruction
- Sprue
- Zollinger-Ellison syndrome
- Lymphangiectasia

ostomy. A j-shaped pouch is created from ileum and anastomosed to the dentate line. After 6 to 8 weeks, patients typically undergo a water-soluble "enema" (pouchogram) to evaluate for leak and obstruction before reversal of the diverting ileostomy. It is imperative that a digital rectal examination is *not* performed and a small rectal tube (red rubber catheter or soft pediatric enema tube) is used to prevent disruption of the anal anastomosis. Leak most commonly occurs from this distal anastomosis along the inner surface of the external anal sphincter. Leak can also occur at the stump or pouch anastomosis.

SUGGESTED READING

Alfisher MM, Scholz FJ, Roberts PL, et al. Radiology of ileal pouch-anal anastomosis: normal findings, examination pitfalls, and complications. *Radiographics.* 1997;17:81-98.

Bennett GL, Birnbaum BA, Balthazar EJ. CT of Meckel's diverticulitis in 11 patients. *AJR Am J Roentgenol.* 2004;182(3): 625-629.

Blachar A, Federle MP, Dodson SF. Internal hernia: clinical and imaging findings in 17 patients with emphasis on CT criteria. *Radiology.* 2001;218:68-74.

Boudiaf M, Soyer P, Terem C, et al. CT evaluation of small bowel obstruction. *Radiographics.* 2001;21:6613-6662.

Buckley JA, Fishman EK. CT evaluation of small bowel neoplasms: spectrum of disease. *Radiographics.* 1998;18(2):379-392.

Chou CK. CT manifestations of bowel ischemia. *AJR Am J Roentgenol.* 2002;178:87-91.

De Backer AI, Schepper AM, Vandvenne JE, et al. CT of angioedema of the small bowel. *AJR Am J Roentgenol.* 2001;176:649-652.

Elsayes KM, Menias CO, Harvin HJ, et al. Imaging manifestations of Meckel's diverticulum. *AJR Am J Roentgenol.* 2007; 189:81-88.

Fletcher JG, Barlow JM, Thomas CW, et al. Crohn's disease: playing by new rules. *Appl Radiol.* November 2003;11:11-21.

Gore RM, Balthazar EJ, Ghahremani GG, et al. CT features of ulcerative colitis and Crohn's disease. *AJR Am J Roentgenol.* 1996;167:3-15.

Ho LM, Paulson EK, Thompson WM. Pneumatosis intestinalis in the adult: benign to life-threatening causes. *AJR Am J Roentgenol.* 2007;188:1604-1613.

Horton KM, Fishman EK. Uncommon inflammatory diseases of the small bowel: CT findings. *AJR Am J Roentgenol.* 1998;17(2): 385-388.

Jayaraman MV, Mayo-Smith WW, Movson JS, et al. CT of the duodenum: an overlooked segment gets its due. *Radiographics.* 2001;21:S147-S160.

Kim SH, Cho JY, Lim HK. CT findings of isolated small bowel angioedema due to iodinated radiographic contrast medium reaction. *Abdom Imaging.* 1999;24:117-119.

Lappas JC. Imaging of the postsurgical small bowel. *Radiol Clin North Am.* 2003;41(2):305-326.

Lee SS, Ha HK, Yang SK, et al. CT of prominent pericolic or perienteric vasculature in patients with Crohn's disease: correlation with clinical disease activity and findings on barium studies. *AJR Am J Roentgenol.* 2002;179:1029-1036.

Levy AD, Hobbs CM. From the archives of AFIP: Meckel diverticulum: radiologic features with pathologic correlation. *Radiographics.* 2004;24:565-587.

Levy AD, Sobin LH. From the archives of AFIP: Gastrointestinal carcinoids: imaging features with clinicopathologic comparison. *Radiographics.* 2007;27:237-257.

Macari M, Chandarana H, Balthazar E, et al. Intestinal ischemia versus intramural hemorrhage: CT evaluation. *AJR Am J Roentgenol.* 2003;180:177-184.

Macari M, Megibow AJ, Balthazar EJ. A pattern approach to the abnormal small bowel: observations at MDCT and CT enterography. *AJR.* 2007;188:1344-1355.

Miller PA, Mezwa DG, Feczko PJ, et al. Imaging of abdominal hernias. *Radiographics.* 1995;15:333-347.

Rha SE, Ha HK, Lee AH, et al. CT and MR imagining findings of bowel ischemia from various primary causes. *Radiographics.* 2000;20:29-42.

Sebastia C, Quiroga S, Espin E, et al. Portomesenteric vein gas: pathologic mechanisms, CT findings, and prognosis. *Radiographics*. 2000;20:1213-1224.

Seggerman RE, Chen MY, Waters GS, et al. Radiology of ileal pouch-anal anastomosis surgery. *AJR Am J Roentgenol*. 2003;180:999-1002.

Wiesner W, Mortele KJ, Glickman JN, et al. Pneumatosis intestinalis and portomesenteric venous gas in intestinal ischemia: correlation of CT findings with severity of ischemia and clinical outcome. *AJR Am J Roentgenol*. 2001;177:1319-1323.

Zalev AH. Radiographic diagnosis of diseases of the small intestine by pattern analysis. *Appl Radiol*. October 1994;20-26.

QUESTIONS AND ANSWERS

1. Which of the following is the most common congenital abnormality of the GI tract?
   A. Pancreatic rest
   B. Duodenal pseudotumor
   C. Ectopic gastric mucosa
   D. Meckel diverticulum
   E. Atresia

   ANSWER: D. Meckel diverticulum is the most common GI tract anomaly.

2. Which of the following is a true small bowel diverticulum?
   A. Meckel diverticulum
   B. Duodenal diverticulum
   C. Jejunal diverticulum
   D. Ileal diverticulum
   E. Scleroderma sacculations

   ANSWER: A. All of the other diverticula are acquired. Diverticula of the duodenum and small bowel typically do not include the muscular layer of the GI tract.

3. Which of the following is the most common cause of small bowel obstruction?
   A. NSAID stricture
   B. Adhesions
   C. Tumor
   D. Intussusception
   E. Hernia

   ANSWER: B. More than 80% of small bowel obstructions are the result of adhesive disease. All other responses can result in small bowel obstruction, although significantly less frequently.

4. Which of the following types of hernia involves only one side of the bowel wall?
   A. Spigelian
   B. Obturator
   C. Richter
   D. Internal
   E. External

   ANSWER: C. Richter hernia is a partial hernia involving only one side of the bowel wall. It can involve colon or small bowel. Spigelian hernia is a herniation through the linea semilunaris along the lateral margin of the rectus abdominus muscle, halfway between the umbilicus and synthesis pubis. Obturator hernias occur through the obturator canal and are extremely rare.

5. Which of the following is *not* a cause of complicated small bowel obstruction?
   A. Appendicitis
   B. Crohn disease
   C. Scleroderma
   D. Diverticulitis
   E. Strangulation

   ANSWER: C. Scleroderma can present as pseudoobstruction with dilatation of small bowel and slow transit time. However, there is no frank mechanical obstruction.

6. Which of the following is a form of vasculitis?
   A. Scleroderma
   B. Lymphangiectasia
   C. Crohn disease
   D. Mastocytosis
   E. Whipple disease

   ANSWER: A. Scleroderma is the only one that represents a true vasculitis.

7. Which of the following is the most common benign tumor of the small bowel?
   A. Lipoma
   B. Adenoma
   C. GISTs
   D. Leiomyoma
   E. Neurofibroma

   ANSWER: C. GISTs are the most common benign tumor of the small bowel. They are rarely malignant.

8. Which of the following is the most common malignant tumor of the duodenum?
   A. Adenocarcinoma
   B. GISTs
   C. Lymphoma
   D. Carcinoid
   E. Small cell

   ANSWER: A. Adenocarcinoma is the most common malignancy of the duodenum, but is fairly rare in the remainder of the GI tract.

9. Which of the following is the most common malignant tumor of the small bowel?
   A. Adenocarcinoma
   B. GISTs
   C. Lymphoma
   D. Carcinoid
   E. Small cell

   ANSWER: D. Carcinoid is the most common small bowel neoplasm, typically arises in the distal ileum, and is usually malignant.

10. Which of the following causes nodular fold thickening?
   A. Cirrhosis
   B. Sprue
   C. Amyloid
   D. Radiation enteritis
   E. Hemorrhage

   ANSWER: C. Amyloidosis has a protean in appearance. Classically, it presents with smooth fold thickening, but can also have nodularity or even a focal mass. All other responses demonstrate smooth fold thickening.

48 COLON AND RECTUM

Sanjiv K. Bajaj and Cheri L. Canon

COLON AND RECTUM

NORMAL ANATOMY

The colon begins at the cecum and extends to the anus. It differs from the small intestine in appearance and function. The wall of the colon is less than 4 mm in thickness when normally distended; it contains the four layers seen in the remainder of the gut: mucosa, submucosa, muscularis propria, and serosa. The teniae coli, three thickened bands of the incomplete outer longitudinal muscularis propria, gird it longitudinally from the base of the appendix to the rectosigmoid junction. They fuse in the rectum. The taeniae's restriction of large intestinal length creates the saccular haustra. The colonic caliber greatly exceeds that of the small intestine. While the small intestine largely functions in resorption of nutrients, the large intestine resorbs fluid. In the past, diffuse fatty infiltration of the colonic wall was thought to be secondary to inflammatory bowel disease (IBD). We now know that this can be seen in normal patients, and IBD should only be considered if there are other findings such as wall thickening, stranding changes in the mesentery, abscess, or fistula.

The first colonic division, the ascending colon, rises retroperitoneally from the level of the ileocecal valve to the right lobe of the liver. It is slightly narrower than the cecum and is covered by peritoneum anteriorly and laterally, with the right paracolic gutter at its lateral aspect. The cecum is the portion extending inferiorly from the level of the ileocecal valve. The transverse colon lies intraperitoneally; it begins its horizontal course at the termination of the ascending colon, the hepatic flexure, and extends to the splenic flexure. The descending colon immediately turns caudally at this juncture, taking a retroperitoneal course with the left paracolic gutter abutting it laterally. The S-shaped sigmoid colon follows from the iliac fossa to the third sacral ligament, where it joins the rectum. It has a long mesentery that contributes to its mobility.

The rectum continues inferiorly where the sigmoid terminates at the S3 vertebral level. It transforms to the anal canal at the anorectal flexure, an 80-degree bend maintained by the puborectalis muscle. The terminal dilation of the rectum, the rectal ampulla, holds feces in preparation for defecation. The flexure and ampulla, with their support by the levator ani muscles, are crucial mechanisms enabling fecal continence. Peritoneum covers the anterolateral superior rectum and anterior middle rectum. The male rectum is separated from the bladder by a peritoneal reflection, creating the rectovesical pouch. In females, the vagina lies between the bladder and the rectum, and a similar peritoneal reflection here forms the rectouterine pouch of Douglas, or cul-de-sac. This is the most dependent portion of the peritoneal cavity in upright individuals.

The superior mesenteric artery supplies the ascending colon and proximal two-thirds of the transverse colon through the right and middle colic arteries, respectively. The inferior mesenteric artery supplies the distal third of the transverse colon, the descending colon, and the sigmoid through the left colic artery and superior sigmoid arteries. The junction of these two vessels occurs at the marginal artery of Drummond, an anastomotic vessel located approximately two-thirds across the transverse colon; this area, Griffith point, proves extremely vulnerable to watershed ischemic injury in low-perfusion states. The other watershed region, the point of Sudek, is located at the rectosigmoid colon, at the junction of the inferior mesenteric artery and internal iliac artery. The superior and inferior mesenteric veins drain their respective tributaries into the portal circulation. The lymphatic drainage passes through the paracolic, epicolic, and intermediate colic areas to the right colic area and then to the superior mesenteric group. The intermediate colic nodes drain to the inferior mesenteric group. The neuronal supply to all parts of the colon includes vagal parasympathetic and lumbar sympathetic innervation via the mesenteric plexi.

The proximal rectum derives its arterial supply from the superior rectal artery, a branch of the inferior mesenteric artery. The middle and inferior rectum derive their supplies from the middle rectal arteries of the inferior vesicle distribution. The inferior rectal artery, arising from the internal pudendal artery, supplies the anal canal. The sympathetic system innervates the rectum via lumbar branches of the sympathetic trunk, and the parasympathetics traverse the pelvic splanchnic nerves.

The superior rectal veins drain the superior rectum into the inferior mesenteric vein of the portal circulation. The middle and inferior rectal veins drain the middle and inferior rectum and anal canal into the systemic circulation. Anastomoses between these drainages in the rectal venous plexus provide a common site for portosystemic shunting. In conditions like cirrhosis, portal hypertension forces retrograde flow through these vessels, dilating these channels.

PATHOLOGY

Congenital Abnormalities

Hirschsprung disease arises from a congenital defect in neural crest cell migration. Dilation of the colon requires these cells' presence; their absence creates a tonically contracted internal anal sphincter and varied length of contracted rectum and sigmoid. This obstruction to fecal flow dilates the normal bowel proximal to the defect. Neonates classically present in the first 48 hours of life with the absence of meconium, although less severe cases can go unrecognized as chronic constipation for weeks or years. Infants evidence refusal to eat, vomiting, constipation, and failure to thrive. Physical examination finds a distended abdomen. Abdominal radiography demonstrates colonic distention and absence of air in the rectum. Barium enema shows the proximal dilation with distal narrowing representing obstruction. Rectal biopsy demonstrates the lack of ganglion cells, confirming the etiology. Treatment involves surgical excision of the affected segment with eventual anastomosis of the colon to the distal normal anorectal segment.

Nonrotation of the bowel is the most common rotational anomaly. The entire colon is located in the left abdomen. There are various degrees of malrotation, resulting from a failure of the fetal bowel's extracorporeal 270-degree rotation during the first trimester of pregnancy. The proximal large intestine thus lies above the level of the duodenum and distal stomach, with Ladd bands in place of a peritoneal cover. These conditions predispose to volvulus and resultant ischemia secondary to irregular attachments and decreased length of mesenteric base. Intussusception, Hirschsprung disease, and abdominal wall defects also occur with greater frequency in this setting.

Duplication presents as either communicating or noncommunicating cysts in the colon and rectum. Unlike the remainder of the gastrointestinal (GI) tract, colonic duplication cysts usually communicate with the lumen. Colonic duplications warrant removal for fear of complications such as obstruction and volvulus, and rectal cysts are always removed because of malignant potential.

Inflammation and Infection

Two major pathophysiologic patterns comprise IBD: Crohn disease (granulomatous colitis) and ulcerative colitis (UC). UC involves colonic inflammation, worse distally than proximally, especially in the rectum. It presents with microabscesses of the crypts of Lieberkuhn and produces bloody diarrhea, weight loss, fever, and cramping left lower abdominal pain. The pathology involves contiguous distal inflammation limited to the mucosa. Radiologic studies find large ulcerations alongside contiguous shallow lesions that appear as fine serrations. Granular mucosa represents mucosal edema, and pseudopolyps represent normal mucosal islands among erosions. Thumbprinting evidences mural edema secondary to inflammation. UC often associates with other HLA/B27-positive diseases, such as ankylosing spondylitis, and increases the risk of primary sclerosing cholangitis. Acute flares are treated with bowel rest and intravenous fluid. These patients are at significantly increased risk for colonic adenocarcinoma. Total proctocolectomy provides a cure for the primary process and prophylaxes against cancer.

Ulcerative proctitis is a localized form of UC with only rectal involvement. Patients present with diarrhea, tenesmus, and bleeding. Diagnosis and treatment are the same as for UC, but only approximately 20% of cases progress to the diffuse form of the disease. Because carcinoma risk is relatively low, prophylactic bowel resection is rarely indicated.

Crohn disease, on the other hand, most commonly involves chronic granulomatous inflammation of the terminal ileum, although the entire GI tract can be involved. It presents with colicky lower abdominal pain, diarrhea, protein loss, weight loss, malaise, obstruction, and fistulous tracts. Pathology demonstrates noncaseating granulomas with transmural inflammation and mural edema. Lesions classically skip areas of bowel. Ulcerations are deeper than with UC, and patients additionally often have long strictures. Barium enema examination demonstrates bowel wall edema, cobblestoning representing deep fissures, strictures, stenoses, fistulous tracts, stranding of mesenteric fat, and aphthous ulcers. CT demonstrates fibrofatty proliferation, "creeping fat," and congested mesenteric vasa recta, the "comb sign." The latter is thought to be one of the more accurate indicators of acute inflammation. MR is the study of choice for evaluation of perianal disease. The fistulous tracts can be identified relative to the levator muscles, described using the Parks classification and allowing determination of the surgical approach. Severe sequelae include toxic megacolon and adenocarcinoma, although the latter is more common in UC. Surgical intervention is warranted for abscess, severe bleeding, cancer, and severe obstruction secondary to stricture. Disease commonly recurs following surgery. Medical management consists of 5-aminosalicylic acid, immunosuppressants, and steroids.

UC, and to a lesser degree Crohn disease, is the primary cause of toxic megacolon. Other causes included ischemic colitis, pseudomembranous colitis, and amebiasis. This disorder involves extreme acute dilation of the bowel to a diameter of at least 6 cm with loss of tone and function. Patients present with severe abdominal distention, pain, fever, and leukocytosis. Pathology most often occurs in the transverse colon. Radiography demonstrates extreme dilation with mucosal edema and loss of haustral markings. CT shows the thin flimsy bowel wall and massive dilation. Physicians must avoid barium studies in this disorder because of the risk of perforation. Treatment involves conservative medical therapy for 48 to 72 hours. Total colectomy is necessary for failed cases.

Behçet disease occurs in young males, and presents with oral and genital ulceration as well as ulceration of the entire GI tract. Radiographically, it mimics Crohn disease.

Diversion colitis involves bacterial overgrowth in a blind loop through which stool no longer courses. The radiographic appearance often mimics UC, and differentiation of the processes can be difficult, especially when bowel loops are diverted in a patient with IBD. Surgical treatment replaces the loop into continuity with the remainder of the bowel.

Diverticula present in older patients with a history of low-fiber diet as colonic outpouchings of the mucosa and muscularis mucosa where the vasa recta perforate the muscular layer. Most bleed to some degree, although the amount is generally small. Symptomatic left-sided lesions produce bright red blood per rectum, and right-sided pathology presents with dark, tarry schools (melena). The sigmoid colon holds the majority of lesions, with most of the remainder in the ascending segment. Patients can experience significant blood loss. Barium studies demonstrate the outpouchings as barium or air-filled lesions approximately 1 cm in diameter.

Diverticulitis complicates 25% of cases of diverticulosis. It usually manifests as a peridiverticular abscess secondary to microperforation and presents with fever, chills, constipation, and left lower quadrant pain, sometimes greater to rebound than pressure. Barium enema shows the outpouching, abscess, and contrast leakage into the abdomen. CT, the imaging modality of choice, demonstrates the abscess, diverticula, and mesenteric inflammation. Gas within the bladder suggests colovesical fistula; however, secondary signs of inflammation of the bladder (wall thickening) and no history of recent bladder catheterization should be determined before confirming this diagnosis. Differentiating between diverticulitis and colorectal carcinoma can be difficult, particularly with severe thickening. Regional lymphadenopathy suggests a malignancy, while a low-density "halo sign" (mural stratification) suggests benign disease.

Right-sided diverticulitis is less common but has similar imaging findings. The patient population is generally younger and Asian, and the disease process may be difficult to differentiate from appendicitis. CT findings of circumferential thickening and adjacent diverticula versus inflammation centered on the appendix help with this dilemma. Surgical indications include frank perforation, toxicity, and instability from severe bleeding.

The epiploic appendages along the serosal surface of the colon can torse, resulting in epiploic appendagitis. Patients present with severe focal abdominal pain. It is most commonly left-sided, and patients may present with mild elevation of white count, mimicking diverticulitis. On CT, a fat-containing mass with increase density rim and surrounding stranding changes are present. There is often a central dot thought to represent thrombosed vessels. Unlike diverticulitis, there is not typically concentric bowel wall thickening. Omental infarction is typically a larger mass with a more ovoid shape and more internal soft-tissue density. It is more commonly anterior to the transverse colon or right-sided and not as intimately associated with the colon. Both diagnoses are self-limiting.

Ischemic colitis results from thrombotic or embolic occlusion, systemic hypoperfusion, and iatrogenic complications from surgery. It classically presents with pain out of proportion to physical findings in patients at risk. The marginal artery of Drummond is especially vulnerable. Findings include fever, abdominal tenderness, and heme-positive stools. Radiography demonstrates mucosal edema or thumbprinting, classically in the splenic flexure watershed area. CT is the imaging study of choice and demonstrates segmental mural thickening. Pneumatosis in this setting suggests infarction. Flexible sigmoidoscopy shows edematous, friable mucosa with ulceration. Conservative measures optimizing perfusion provide the best outcome; surgery removes obstructing or necrotic bowel. Healing can result in an annular stricture. Unlike adenocarcinoma, the narrowing is smooth, without shouldering.

Acute radiation colitis presents with mural enema localized to the region of the treatment port. During the chronic phase, there is luminal narrowing and increased pericolonic and perirectal fat. The use of a rectal balloon is contraindicated in patients having prior radiation to the rectum, most commonly for prostate and cervical cancer.

Thickening of the entire GI tract can occur in the setting of cirrhosis. It most commonly is seen in the ascending colon secondary to portal hypertension, but can occur anywhere in the GI tract. These patients are also at risk for hypoproteinemia, further increasing diffuse mural edema.

Colitis cystica profunda occurs in young adults. Radiographically, there are multiple mucous-filled cysts in the rectal wall. It is associated with solitary rectal ulcer syndrome and rectal prolapse.

Several infectious diseases target the colon specifically or substantially involve it. The protozoan *Entamoeba histolytica* causes bloody dysentery with frequent bloody mucoid stools, tenesmus, and fever. Patients often have history of foreign travel. Ingested cysts release the organism, which travels to the colon. From there it may spread and cause abscesses in the liver ("anchovy paste–" filled cysts), spleen, and brain, and can lead to toxic megacolon. Diagnosis requires stool studies for the parasite, endoscopic colonic biopsy showing flask-shaped ulcers, or aspiration of cysts with examination of the fluid. Imaging is generally not used. Barium enema reveals ulcerated mucosa representing the flask-shaped invasions and the classic "coned cecum." CT shows generalized inflammation and abscesses. Metronidazole provides the cure.

Some amoebic infections remain localized to the rectum, especially in homosexual men. These cases tend to present with bloody dysentery, most commonly without the systemic manifestations mentioned earlier. Diagnosis and treatment are as with generalized infection.

Colonic tuberculosis involves the terminal ileum and right colon. There are ulcers and focal areas of stenosis with a coned cecum. Fleischner sign, with enlarged, gaping ileocecal valve, is present; Stierlin sign is seen with narrowing of the terminal ileum.

CMV colitis occurs in patients with immunosuppression, diabetes, and IBD. Cases present with bleeding and abdominal pain; perforation is the most severe complication. Barium enema examination and CT suggest the entity by showing deep ulceration in patients with predisposing history. Diagnosis requires endoscopic biopsy demonstrating Cowdry type A intranuclear inclusion bodies. Ganciclovir effectively controls the infection.

Pseudomembranous colitis arises from infection with the gram-positive bacillus *Clostridium difficile*. Antibiotic use, most commonly clindamycin and beta-lactams, depletes resident colonic flora, predisposing to infection with this agent, which presents 3 to 4 weeks after treatment. *Clostridium difficile* enterotoxin necroses colonic mucosal cells, and their sloughed mass comprises the pseudomembranes. Patients present with watery diarrhea, crampy abdominal pain, fever, and tenderness. Radiography demonstrates increased colonic caliber and mural thickening. Barium enema examination shows thumbprinting, ulceration, and irregularity. CT finds wall thickening, ascites, and the "accordion sign," representing contrast trapped within edematous mucosal folds. Diagnosis requires stool assay for *C. difficile* toxin, and in some cases, CT may be normal. Metronidazole is the first line of treatment, with vancomycin and bacitracin reserved for resistant cases. Toxic megacolon and perforation are rare but severe sequelae may require colectomy.

Neutropenic colitis, more specifically typhlitis when limited to the cecum, occurs in the setting of severe neutropenia. The neutropenia, via an unclear mechanism, allows the breach of colonic flora across the mucosal barrier. This causes mural thickening and typically more pericolonic ascites than seen with other colitides. Graft-versus-host disease can occur throughout the GI tract, resulting in luminal narrowing and typically less thickening than neutropenic colitis. Graft-versus-host disease involves significantly longer segments of bowel, particularly ileum and colon. It occurs after allogenic bone marrow transplantation and is secondary to rejection of the host by the transplanted cells.

Lymphogranuloma venereum (LGV) is proctitis secondary to *Clamydia trachomatis* infection. It presents with stricture, sinus tract formation, and fistula, resembling Crohn disease. Gonococcal proctitis can also be seen in HIV-positive and AIDS patients.

NEOPLASIA

Benign Tumors

Polyps are discrete mucosal projections into the bowel lumen. They can be hyperplastic, containing focal cell proliferation with normal nuclear and architectural features, or adenomatous, representing a premalignant state. Hyperplastic polyps are round, well circumscribed, sessile, and usually small. They are more common than adenomas, particularly in the rectum, but are not true neoplasms.

Adenoma is the most common benign tumor of the colon and rectum (Table 48-1). Adenomatous polyps are larger than hyperplastic polyps; can have irregularity; possess a larger base; and can be sessile or pedunculated

TABLE 48-1 Colonic Neoplasms

BENIGN	MALIGNANT
Hyperplastic polyp (most common "polyp"; not true neoplasm)	Adenocarcinoma
Adenoma (most common benign tumor)	Squamous cell carcinoma (anus)
Lipoma (second most common)	Lymphoma
GIST	GIST
Hemangioma	Carcinoid
	Cloacogenic carcinoma

with villous, tubular, or tubulovillous histology. Large, sessile, villous adenomas harbor the greatest risk for malignancy. Endoscopy and barium enema have been the traditional methods to screen and diagnose colonic polyps. CT colonography is the newest modality in the colorectal cancer screening armamentarium and is showing great promise.

Many polyposis syndromes are associated with adenomatous polyps (Table 48-2). Familial polyposis is an autosomal dominant condition involving mutations in the APC gene. It presents with hundreds of adenomatous polyps in the colon, as well as the remainder of the gut, and frequently carcinoma near the ampulla of Vater. Epidermoid cysts, desmoid tumors, and osteomas occur with colonic polyps in the Gardner syndrome variant of this disease. Turcot syndrome is an autosomal recessive polyposis syndrome with central nervous system glioblastoma. Patients with polyposis require subtotal colectomy by age 30 with close monitoring, as the majority will otherwise develop cancer by age 40.

Hamartomatous polyps are normal colonic mucosal cells organized atypically; they represent developmentally abnormal tissue and not a neoplastic process. They may arise anywhere in the GI tract and can lead to bleeding. Peutz-Jeghers syndrome is autosomal dominant and involves mucocutaneous pigmentation and GI tract hamartomas. Negligible malignant potential of the colonic polyps obviates the need for removal except with clinically significant bleeding. However, these patients are at an increased risk of breast, ovarian, and pancreatic carcinoma.

Lipomas are the second most common tumor in the colon. They are submucosal and easily identified by their fat density on CT. GISTs occur throughout the colon but are more common in the anorectum. As in the remainder of the GI tract, they are typically large, exophytic masses and may be ulcerated. They can be benign or malignant, but no imaging findings reliably determine malignant potential.

Cavernous hemangioma usually occurs in the rectum in the setting of congenital anomalies and syndromes, including Klippel-Trenaunay-Weber and blue rubber bleb syndromes and VATER complex. These present as multiple rectal mural nodules or large pelvic masses. They may or may not enhance, depending upon if they are thrombosed. Phleboliths may be identified.

MALIGNANT TUMORS

Adenocarcinoma of the colon causes more deaths than any malignancy, except lung cancer. Risk factors include diets high in animal fat, low in calcium and antioxidants, and advancing age, in addition to IBD, polyposis, and nonpolyposis syndromes. Right-sided lesions (25%) present with iron-deficiency anemia secondary to occult blood loss or with melena. Left-sided pathology includes obstruction and decreased stool caliber. Metastases usually involve the liver, lung, brain, or bone. Barium enema examination demonstrates a mass fungating into the intestinal lumen or a narrowing representing a circumferential, "apple-core" lesion. CT

TABLE 48-2 Polyposis Syndromes

Adenomatous	Inheritance Pattern	
FAPS	AD	Most common; gastric hyperplastic polyps and GI tract and adenomas; ampullary carcinoma
Gardner syndrome	AD	Epidermoid cysts, desmoid, osteoid osteoma
Turcot syndrome	AD	CNS glioblastoma
Hamartomatous		
Peutz-Jeghers syndrome	AD	GI hamartomas, pigmented mucous membrane lesions
Juvenile polyposis	AD	GI hamartomas
Infantile polyposis	AR	Congenital anomalies, ganglioneuroma
Cronkhite-Canada syndrome	Sporadic	Skin hyperpigmentation, alopecia, onychodystrophy, malabsorption, 60% mortality
Cowden disease (multiple hamartoma syndrome)	AD	Only one to involve esophagus

shows lymphadenopathy, distant metastases, and the lesion, often directly extending into pericolonic tissues. Transrectal ultrasound provides staging and allows biopsy of the primary tumor and regional lymph nodes. Colonoscopy provides direct visualization of the lesion with concurrent biopsy. Treatment combines surgery, radiation, and chemotherapy. Stage I and II lesions are limited to the bowel wall while stages III and IV extend to the lymph nodes or possess metastases. Prognosis correlates most closely with stage.

Hereditary nonpolyposis colon cancer (HNPCC) syndrome involves mutations of genes regulating cell growth. HNPCC type I presents in young patients with adenocarcinoma, most commonly in the ascending colon. HNPCC type II presents with cancers of the colon, endometrium, ovary, pancreas, kidney, stomach, and liver. Patients require vigilant monitoring for early treatment of malignancies.

Lymphoma of the colon has a protean appearance. It can have multiple nodules, a large mass, or diffuse thickening. Classically, it is a soft tumor that does not cause obstruction.

Squamous cell carcinoma occasionally arises in the anus and presents much like adenocarcinoma of this region. Digital rectal examination suggests the diagnosis, and CT characterizes the extent of disease to assess resectability. Treatment is with surgery and chemotherapy.

Carcinoid occurs most commonly in the rectum but can occur throughout the remainder of the colon. Patients typically present with a calcified mesenteric metastatic nodal mass, and the primary tumor is often not found.

Cloacogenic carcinomas are tumors arising from the pectinate line. They have variable histologic types and present most commonly with bleeding, decreased caliber of stools, and tenesmus. Barium studies show the narrowed lumen, and CT assesses the extent of the tumor for determination of resectability. Treatment involves surgery and radiation.

The colon serves as a potential site for metastases via the intraperitoneal and occasionally vascular routes. Peritoneal seeding most commonly occurs with ovarian carcinoma. These present with eccentric serosal masses with varying degrees of obstruction. Because of their dependent location, the rectouterine pouch in females, the rectovesical space in males, the rectal shelf, and the ileocolonic junction are common sites for peritoneal spread. Hematogenous metastases usually occur in the setting of lung or breast cancer.

MISCELLANEOUS CONDITIONS

Obstruction complicates many processes, including adhesions, stricture, cancer, intussusception, volvulus, fecaliths, and incarcerated hernia. Patients present with vomiting, abdominal distention, and cramping abdominal pain. Physical examination includes abdominal distention and high-pitched, tinkling bowel sounds. Radiographs show dilated proximal bowel loops with a distinct transition point and collapsed distal bowel. Air-fluid levels are prominent in upright films. CT shows the transition point and delineates the cause.

Intussusception represents telescoping of a segment of bowel, sometimes secondary to a mass lesion that functions as a lead point. It most often occurs in the distal ileal/cecal area, but also occurs in the colon. It presents most commonly in children with intermittent crampy abdominal pain, bloody stools, and sometimes fever. In this setting, there is typically no lead point. Adults usually have less severe presentations, and there is more commonly a lead point when it involves the colon, either ileocolonic or colocolonic intussusception. Radiography demonstrates the associated mass, small bowel obstruction, and the "crescent sign" representing shouldering on an air-filled segment of bowel. CT visualizes the telescoped bowel loops, demonstrating fat inside the bowel lumen. Ultrasound shows concentric rings, the "target sign." Barium enema examination evidences the string sign, representing barium contrast passing through the narrowed lumen of the inner loop.

Colonic volvulus involves intestinal twisting about its mesenteric stalk, creating an obstruction and often interrupting the blood supply, leading to ischemia. The sigmoid colon is the most common site for adult volvulus, which usually occurs in debilitated patients after stroke or nursing home placement; younger patients more often present with cecal pathology. Cases not involving the vascular supply present with years of intermittent obstructive attacks. In sigmoid volvulus, radiography demonstrates distention with obstruction, a paucity of haustra, and a coffee bean-shaped bowel loop representing the twisted segment, usually directed toward the right hemidiaphragm and often above the transverse colon. Barium studies show the classic beaking of the twisted segment. Initial conservative therapy with rectal tube placement resolves most cases. Some can be reduced endoscopically. Surgery ameliorates refractory cases or situations with vascular interruption. Cecal volvulus results in small bowel obstruction. There is a large gas collection, the dilated cecum, usually projecting in the left upper quadrant, and the remainder of the colon is collapsed. Cecal volvulus is much less common than sigmoid volvulus.

Angiodysplasia refers to vascular abnormalities, most commonly seen in older patients in the ascending colon and cecum. Patients present with painless lower GI bleeds, often in the setting of cardiac valvular or renal diseases. Angiography or technetium scanning localizes the lesion. Colonoscopy provides the potential for diagnosis and cure. There is no role for barium studies.

SUGGESTED READING

Chintapalli KN, Chopra S, Ghiatas AA, et al. Diverticulitis versus colon cancer: differentiation with helical CT findings. *Radiology.* 1999;210:429-435.

Gore RM, Balthazar EJ, Ghahremani GG, et al. CT features of ulcerative colitis and Crohn's disease. *AJR Am J Roentgenol.* 1996;167:3-15.

Harisinghani MG, Wittenberg J, Blake MA, et al. Halo sign: useful CT sign for differentiating benign from malignant colonic disease. *Clin Radiol.* 2003;58:306-310.

Harisinghani MG, Wittenberg J, Lee W, et al. Bowel wall fat halo sign in patients without intestinal disease. *AJR Am J Roentgenol.* 2003;181:781-784.

Horton KM, Corl FM, Fishman EK. CT evaluation of the colon: inflammatory disease. *Radiographics.* 2000;20:399-418.

Kawamoto S, Horton KM, Fishman EK. Pseudomembranous colitis: spectrum of imaging findings with clinical and pathologic correlation. *Radiographics.* 1999;19:887-897.

Lee SS, Ha HK, Yang S, et al. CT of prominent pericolic or perienteric vasculature in patients with Crohn's disease: correlation with clinical disease activity and findings on barium studies. *AJR Am J Roentgenol.* 2002;179:1029-1036.

Long FR, Kramer SS, Markowitz RI, et al. Radiographic patterns of intestinal malrotation in children. *Radiographics.* 1996;16:547-556.

Singh AK, Gervais DA, Hahn PF, Rhea J, Mueller PR. CT appearance of acute appendagitis. *AJR Am J Roentgenol.* 2004;183(5):1303-1307.

Szucs RA, Turner MA. Gastrointestinal tract involvement by gynecologic diseases. *Radiographics.* 1996;16:1251-1270.

QUESTIONS AND ANSWERS

1. Which of the following is a benign colonic neoplasm?
   A. Adenocarcinoma
   B. GIST
   C. Cavernous hemangioma
   D. Carcinoid
   E. Hyperplastic polyp

   ANSWER: C. Hyperplastic polyps are not true neoplastic tumors. Adenocarcinoma and carcinoid are malignant tumors. GIST can be benign or malignant.

2. Which of the following disease processes is strictly extracolonic?
   A. Crohn disease
   B. Diverticulitis
   C. Behçet disease
   D. Epiploic appendagitis
   E. Tuberculosis

   ANSWER: D. Epiploic appendagitis occurs secondary to torsion of an epiploic appendage and is not a primary colonic process. All other responses primarily involve the colon and may or may not have extracolonic extension.

3. Which of the following polyposis syndromes presents with epidermoid cysts, desmoid tumors, and osteomas?
   A. Gardner syndrome
   B. Turcot syndrome
   C. Familial polyposis
   D. HNPCC
   E. Cowden disease

   ANSWER: A. Turcot syndrome has CNS glioblastomas. Cowden disease is a hamartomatous condition that can involve the esophagus.

4. Which of the following groups should begin screening for colorectal carcinoma at age 50?
   A. Patients with polyposis syndrome
   B. Patients with family history of colon cancer
   C. Asymptomatic patients with no known risk factors
   D. Patients with prior history of colon cancer
   E. Patients with heme-positive stools

   ANSWER: C. High-risk patients begin screening at age 40 or when symptomatic.

5. Which of the following findings suggests colon cancer rather than diverticulitis?
   A. Regional lymphadenopathy
   B. Halo sign
   C. Pericolonic inflammatory change
   D. Ascites
   E. Mural thickening

   ANSWER: A. Regional lymphadenopathy is more commonly seen with cancer than with diverticulitis. Halo sign is indicative of diverticulitis, and mural thickening and pericolonic inflammatory change can be seen in both cancer and diverticulitis. Ascites is not a discriminator.

6. Which is *not* predominantly an ileocolonic disease?
   A. Tuberculosis
   B. Campylobacter
   C. Crohn Disease
   D. Giardia
   E. Typhlitis

   ANSWER: D. Giardia more commonly involves the duodenum and jejunum.

7. What is the most common colonic polyp?
   A. Hyperplastic polyp
   B. Adenoma
   C. Lipoma
   D. Hemangioma
   E. Lymphangioma

   ANSWER: A. An adenoma is the most common neoplasm, while hyperplastic polyps are the most common polyps and are not neoplastic.

8. Which of the following is classically seen with sigmoid volvulus?
   A. U-shaped sigmoid
   B. Dilated sigmoid directed toward right hemidiaphragm
   C. Twisted appearance of ileo-cecal region
   D. Decompressed small bowel
   E. Transverse colon cranial to sigmoid colon

   ANSWER: B. Sigmoid volvulus typically presents with a markedly dilated sigmoid colon in the shape of an inverted "U" or coffee bean directed toward the right hemidiaphragm and often projecting above the transverse colon. A beaked appearance of the twisted rectosigmoid is often seen with barium enema examination, with proximal obstruction of colon and small bowel. Many cases are treated endoscopically, although surgery may be required for recurrent volvulus.

9. In the United States, what segment of the colon is most commonly involved with diverticulitis?
   A. Cecum
   B. Ascending
   C. Transverse
   D. Sigmoid
   E. Rectum

   ANSWER: D. The sigmoid colon is the most common segment involved with diverticulitis. Right-sided diverticulitis (ascending colon and cecum) typically occurs in younger patients, with increased propensity for the Asian population.

10. What is the most common cause of colon obstruction?
    A. Adhesion
    B. Malignancy
    C. Hernia
    D. Gall stone
    E. Volvulus

    ANSWER: B. Although all of these can cause colonic obstruction, malignancy is the most common.

49 APPENDIX

Camden L. Hebson and Cheri L. Canon

APPENDIX

NORMAL ANATOMY

The appendix arises at the junction of the taeniae coli, at the posteromedial base of the cecum. It is directed toward the side of the ileocecal valve. There is a wide range of normal locations of the appendix. The ileocolic artery from the superior mesenteric artery provides the blood supply via the appendicular artery branch. The appendix contains the four layers as seen elsewhere in the gastrointestinal tract and is rich with lymphoid tissue.

PATHOLOGY

INFLAMMATION AND INFECTION

Inflammation of the appendix is the most common abdominal surgical emergency and is usually secondary to obstruction (50%–75% of cases) by a fecolith. Other causes include gallstones, lymphoid hyperplasia, stricture, parasite, foreign body, and tumor. Diagnosis is often made based on history, physical examination, and laboratory assessment. Cross-sectional imaging is usually used to confirm the diagnosis. The goal in treatment is surgical resection before appendiceal rupture.

The sequence of events in acute appendicitis is well documented. As mentioned, the inciting event is usually obstruction, with fecolith impaction or reactive hyperplasia of lymphoid tissue. Mucinous fluid continues to be produced in the obstructed lumen, leading to increased intraluminal pressure and collapse of venous drainage. Subsequent ischemia provides a supportive environment for bacterial proliferation, which further increases local inflammation. Inflammation is tied to perception of pain, as the early periumbilical pain is due to increased intraluminal pressure, which stimulates visceral nerve fibers. The classic shift to severe right lower quadrant pain comes after inflamed appendiceal serosa contacts the parietal peritoneum, thus allowing the patient to accurately localize the inflammation. Perforation can result if left untreated, as persistent ischemia leads to transmural infarction.

Appendicitis is most common in adolescents and young adults, but can occur in any age group. Signs and symptoms include tenderness to palpation over the abdomen, fever, leukocytosis, possible nausea and vomiting, and the classic pain pattern: periumbilical pain shifting to the right lower quadrant. This classic presentation, however, is often absent. Deviations include tenderness in atypical locations, right flank or pelvic pain that is due to a retrocecal appendix, and left upper quadrant pain that is due to malrotation of the colon. These presentations are more common in the very young and old. The differential diagnosis includes epiploic appendicitis, right-sided diverticulitis, mesenteric lymphadenitis, viral infection, inflammatory bowel disease, pelvic inflammatory disease, ectopic pregnancy, cystic fibrosis, and Meckel diverticulitis.

On CT, there is dilatation of the lumen, greater than 6 mm, mural thickening and increased enhancement, and periappendiceal inflammatory change. In early appendicitis, surrounding inflammation may be absent. Appendicoliths may be present, but can be obscured by luminal contrast if bone window settings are not used.

Complicated appendicitis includes perforation, abscess, and small bowel obstruction. CT findings indicating perforation include moderate or severe periappendiceal inflammation, focal defect in enhancing appendiceal wall, extraluminal air, and extraluminal appendicolith.

Chronic appendicitis appears like acute appendicitis on imaging studies, although may have less periappendiceal inflammation. Chronic processes include granulomatous appendicitis, lymphoid hyperplasia, fibrosis, and nonspecific chronic inflammation. Granulomatous appendicitis typically does not progress to Crohn disease in the remainder of the gastrointestinal tract. Chronically inflammed appendices are larger than in simple appendicitis with notable absence of definable wall, and it can be difficult differentiating this entity from neoplasm. Crohn disease of the terminal ileum and cecum can secondarily involve the appendix.

The appendix can contain diverticula and therefore develop diverticulitis. It is not possible to differentiate between acute appendicitis and appendiceal diverticulitis unless the offending diverticulum is identified on CT.

NEOPLASIA

Almost half of patients with appendiceal tumors will present with signs and symptoms of appendicitis. Tumor can mimic appendicitis and should be considered if the diameter is greater than 15 mm. Of all appendiceal tumors, carcinoid is the most common (Table 49-1). Carcinoids arise from neural crest cells of the gastrointestinal tract, which normally function to generate bioactive compounds (peptide hormones) that help coordinate gut function. On gross inspection of the tumors, they are often described as firm, rubbery yellow nodules that often grow through the muscularis mucosa into the mesentery. Histological examination reveals cell structure similar to adenocarcinoma, but without such aggressive metastatic tendency.

TABLE 49-1 Tumors of the Appendix

Tumors of the Appendix
Carcinoid (most common neoplasm)
Mucocele (not neoplastic)
Mucinous cystadenoma
Mucinous cystadenocarcinoma
Non-Hodgkin lymphoma
Leiomyoma
Leiomyosarcoma

Often, carcinoid is an incidental diagnosis at the time of appendectomy for appendicitis. The distal tip of the appendix is the most common location where the tumor will be present as a solitary nodule a few centimeters in diameter. Although transmural extension can occur, appendiceal carcinoids rarely metastasize and follow a benign course as a rule.

Less common than carcinoids in the appendix are mucinous tumors, which range from benign retention mucoceles to neoplastic cystadenomas and mucin-secreting cystadenocarcinomas. Mucoceles are often found incidentally: inspection will reveal appendiceal dilation secondary to mucinous secretion (globular enlargement), and eventual atrophy of mucosal cells secondary to distension. Mucoceles are for the most part asymptomatic. On CT, they appear as dilated tubular structures and may have thin mural calcification.

Mucinous cystadenomas are the most common mucinous tumors of the appendix. Distension can lead to perforation in 15% to 20% of cases, allowing mucus into the peritoneal cavity. Histological examination, however, reveals no malignant cells. This is not the case with mucin-secreting adenocarcinomas, which are less common but more worrisome than the cystadenomas because of propensity to disseminate to the peritoneum. Cystadenocarcinomas produce mucinous dilatation of the appendix identical to cystadenomas, but the invasive cells also spread locally and implant into the peritoneum, which can sometimes lead to mucinous ascites, a condition called pseudomyxoma peritonei. Poorly differentiated adenocarcinoma cells can be found on cytologic examination, distinguishing this more malignant process from other mucin-producing conditions. CT findings include cystic dilatation of the appendix with a nodular enhancing wall. Pseudomyxoma peritonei presents with complicated ascites with areas of attenuation greater than that of water. There is mass effect on adjacent bowel and solid organs, producing a scalloped appearance on the liver and spleen. Repeated debulking procedures have been used to keep this condition in check, but a fatal course is often the rule. There is no way to accurately differentiate benign mucoceles from their malignant counterpart, so all should be resected.

Lymphoma, non-Hodgkin type, can involve the appendix and even present with symptoms of acute appendicitis. On CT, lymphomatous appendix is usually larger than one with acute inflammation, typically 2.5 cm or greater. Aneurysmal dilatation seen in small bowel lymphoma can also be seen in the appendix.

Leiomyoma and leiomyosarcoma rarely occur in the appendix, more commonly the benign form.

Suggested Reading

Alobaidi M, Shirkhoda A. Value of bone window settings on CT for revealing appendicoliths in patients with appendicitis. *AJR Am J Roentgenol.* 2004;180:201-205.

Checkoff JL, Wechsler RJ, Nararian LN. Chronic inflammatory appendiceal conditions that mimic acute appendicitis on helical CT. *AJR Am J Roentgenol.* 2002;179:731-734.

Foley TA, Earnest IVF, Nathan MA, et al. Differentiation of nonperforated from perforated appendicitis: accuracy of CT diagnosis and relationship of CT findings to length of hospital stay. *Radiology.* 2005;235:89-86.

Hoeffel C, Crema MD, Belkacem A, et al. Multi-detector row CT: spectrum of diseases involving the ileocecal area. *Radiographics.* 2006;26(5):1373-1390, .

Honnef I, Moschopulos M, Roeren T. Appendiceal mucinous cystadenoma. *Radiographics.* 2008;28(5):1527-1527.

Horrow MM, White DS, Horrow JC. Differentiation of perforated from nonperforated appendicitis at CT. *Radiology.* 2003;227:46-51.

Lim HK, Lee WJ, Kim SH, et al. Primary mucinous cystadenocarcinoma of the appendix: CT findings. *AJR Am J Roentgenol.* 1999;173(4):1071-1074.

Pickhardt PJ, Levy AD, Rohrmann CA, et al. Non-Hodgkin's lymphoma of the appendix: clinical and CT findings with pathologic correlation. *AJR Am J Roentgenol.* 2002;178:1123-1127.

Pickhardt PJ, Levy AD, Rohrmann CA, et al. Primary neoplasms of the appendix manifesting as acute appendicitis: CT findings with pathologic comparison. *Radiology.* 2002;224:775-781.

See TC, Ng CS, Watson CJE, et al. Appendicitis: spectrum of appearances on helical CT. *Br J Radiol.* 2002;75:775–781.

Walensky RP, Venbrux AC, Prescott CA, et al. Pseudomyxoma peritonei. *AJR Am J Roentgenol.* 1996;167:471-474.

Zissin R, Gayer J, Bernheim J, et al. Granulomatous appendicitis presenting as right lower quadrant pain: CT findings. *Abdom Imaging.* 2003;28:280-283.

QUESTIONS AND ANSWERS

1. Which of the following is the most common tumor of the appendix?
   A. Carcinoid
   B. Mucinous cystadenoma
   C. Mucinous cystadenocarcinoma
   D. Mucocele
   E. Leiomyoma

   ANSWER: A. Carcinoid is the most common tumor of the appendix. Mucinous cystadenoma and cystadenocarcinoma are less common. Mucoceles are fairly common, but are not a frank neoplastic process. Leiomyomas are exceedingly rare.

2. Which of the following helps differentiate granulomatous appendicitis from acute appendicitis?
   A. Appendicolith
   B. Extraluminal gas
   C. Mural enhancement
   D. Small bowel obstruction
   E. No definable wall

   ANSWER: E. All other responses can be seen in acute appendicitis. Lack of definable wall with large soft-tissue component suggests granulomatous appendicitis.

3. Concerning the appendix, which of the following is *true*?
   A. Contains taeniae coli
   B. Most commonly retrocecal
   C. Directed toward the side of the ileocecal valve
   D. Supplied by branch of the inferior mesenteric artery
   E. Does not contain a serosal layer

   ANSWER: C. The appendix arises at the junction of the taenia coli. Although it can be located posterior to the cecum, this is not the most common presentation. Its vascular supply is from the appendicular artery branch of the superior mesenteric artery. It is covered in serosa.

4. Which of the following suggests perforated appendicitis?
   A. Periappendiceal inflammation
   B. Mural thickening
   C. Increased mural enhancement
   D. Focal defect in enhancing appendiceal wall
   E. Appendicolith

   ANSWER: D. Focal defect in the enhancing appendiceal wall and severe periappendiceal inflammatory change both suggest perforated appendicitis. All other findings are seen in uncomplicated appendicitis.

5. Which of the following suggests malignant mucinous tumor of the appendix?
   A. Globular dilatation of the appendix
   B. Thin mural calcification

C. Nodular mural enhancement
D. Periappendiceal inflammation
E. Small bowel obstruction

ANSWER: C. Enhancing nodularity indicates mucinous cystadenocarcinoma. All other findings can be seen in mucoceles as well as mucinous cystadenomas.

50 IMAGING OF THE LIVER

Allen B. Groves and Lincoln L. Berland

INTRODUCTION

The liver's primary functions include detoxification, glycogen storage, plasma protein synthesis, bile production, and decomposition of red blood cells.

EMBRYOLOGY AND ANATOMY

In the fetus, the hepatic diverticulum eventually becomes the biliary tree and the ventral pancreas. Initially, the liver grows in the ventral mesentery, which later involutes leaving behind the falciform ligament and the lesser omentum. Fetal circulation involves the liver in a critical way. The umbilical vein reaches the liver along the inferior aspect of the falciform ligament. At approximately 8 to 12 weeks gestation, the left branch of the umbilical vein becomes the ductus venosus, which bypasses the liver and carries oxygenated blood from the maternal circulation to the heart of the fetus. After birth, the umbilical vein becomes the ligamentum teres in the inferior edge of the falciform ligament, and the ductus venosus becomes the ligamentum venosum.

The liver in the adult is covered by visceral peritoneum except at the porta hepatis, bare area, and the gallbladder fossa. The liver is attached to the posterior abdominal wall and diaphragm by the triangular and coronary ligaments. The liver is connected to the anterior abdominal wall and diaphragm by the falciform ligament. Classically, the liver is divided into five segments, two in each of the right and left hepatic lobes and the fifth being the entire caudate lobe. The falciform ligament divides the medial and lateral segments of the left hepatic lobe, and the right hepatic vein divides the right hepatic lobe into anteroposterior segments. The middle hepatic vein divides the liver into right and left hepatic lobes and defines a plane that extends from the inferior vena cava to the gallbladder fossa.

Functional division of the liver into multiple individual portions is defined by the Couinaud system (Fig. 50-1). These are functionally independent and defined by individual branches of the hepatic artery, bile duct, and portal vein. These are bound by branches of the hepatic veins. Blood supply to the liver is dominated by the portal vein, which drains the intestines and spleen but is supplemented by systemic arterial blood in the form of the hepatic artery. Outflow of blood from the liver is by hepatic veins, which drain into the inferior vena cava. These eight segments are numbered in a clockwise direction beginning with the caudate lobe. The following is a list describing the position of the Couinaud segments in relation to conventional segmental hepatic anatomy:

I) Caudate lobe
II) Left posterolateral segment
III) Left anterolateral segment
IVa) Left superomedial segment
IVb) Left inferomedial segment
V) Right anteroinferior segment
VI) Right posteroinferior segment
VII) Right posterosuperior segment
VIII) Right anterosuperior segment

The caudate lobe has a direct connection to the inferior vena cava through hepatic veins, which do not communicate with the primary hepatic veins. The caudate lobe may also be supplied by branches of both the right and left portal veins. This is important in many disease

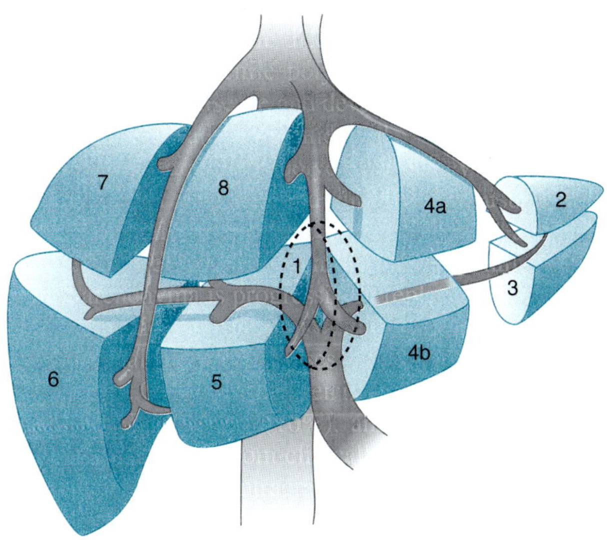

FIG. 50-1 Hepatic (Couinaud) segments.
SOURCE: Courtesy of Anthony F. Zagar, UAB, Department of Radiology, Birmingham, Alabama.

states, which may spare and even hypertrophy the caudate lobe, when there is loss of normal remaining hepatic parenchyma such as in Budd-Chiari. Although rare, there can be congenital absence of one or more hepatic segments.

The vascular anatomy of the liver has many common variations. One of the more frequently encountered vascular variants is the replaced right hepatic artery arising from the superior mesenteric artery, occurring in approximately 11% of patients. The left hepatic artery can also be "replaced" from the normal branching pattern from the proper hepatic artery and arise from the left gastric artery. With regard to portal venous anatomy, the most common variation is a trifurcation at the porta hepatis (rather than a bifurcation) into a left branch and two branches to the right hepatic lobe. Finally, hepatic venous variation is less constant but typically involves small branch vessel drainage directly into the inferior vena cava from the posterior right hepatic lobe rather than passing into either the right, middle, or left hepatic veins which classically drain the liver into the inferior vena cava. Clearly, these vascular variations are important in patients undergoing liver surgery including partial hepatectomy, liver transplant, and so on.

PATHOLOGY

CONGENITAL

Perhaps because of its size and complex operations, the liver is subject to many congenital disorders and mass lesions. Autosomal dominant and recessive polycystic kidney disease can also affect the liver resulting in numerous cysts and fibrosis, respectively. The liver is also subject to hamartomas and congenital mass lesions including hepatoblastomas and infantile hemangioendotheliomas.

Hemangioendothelioma is the most commonly encountered benign liver tumor in the infant. An infant with congestive heart failure should undergo imaging of the liver to exclude this tumor, as it is associated with high-output congestive heart failure. Hemangioendothelioma is also associated with cutaneous hemangiomas approximately 40% of the time. Because of platelet sequestration in these vascular tumors, patients can also present with disseminated intravascular coagulation (DIC) or thrombocytopenia.

Hepatoblastoma is the most common primary hepatic malignancy in children. These typically present as large hepatic masses. There are associations with Beckwith-Wiedeman, hemihypertrophy, and familial adenomatous polyposis syndrome.

Mesenchymal hamartoma is an uncommon benign tumor, most frequently encountered in children. It is typically cystic and solitary and may contain thin septae and intervening nodules (Table 50-1).

INFECTION

Infectious diseases affecting the liver can be subdivided: viral, abscess (pyogenic and amoebic), fungal, parasitic, and granulomatous—with the three former categories representing the most common hepatic infections. Dual blood supply to the liver means that hematogenous dissemination is a cause for hepatic infection. Ascending cholangitis is another common route for spread of infection to the liver. Finally, penetrating trauma can directly inoculate the liver.

Viral infection of the liver can be caused by hepatitis A, B, C, D, and E. In acute hepatitis, the liver is often enlarged. On US, the liver may appear more hypoechoic with relative increased echogenicity of the portal triads resulting in the "starry sky" appearance. Chronic infection may occur with hepatitis B and C and may lead to cirrhosis and increased risk of hepatocellular carcinoma.

Pyogenic abscesses may mimic cysts. Solitary lesions are often caused by *Klebsiella* species, whereas multiple lesions are most commonly associated with *Escherichia coli* One of the more common appearances on CT is the "double target" sign, consisting of a central hypodense abscess cavity surrounded by an enhancing rim and an outer hypodense zone. Of course, the presence of gas in the lesion is highly suggestive of a pyogenic abscess, but history of percutaneous intervention must be excluded.

TABLE 50-1 Congenital Hepatic Lesions and Associations

INFANTILE HEMANGIOENDOTHELIOMA	HEPATOBLASTOMA	ANGIOMYOLIPOMA	HEPATIC CYSTS OR CYSTLIKE LESIONS
High-output congestive heart failure	Beckwith-Wiedeman, hemihypertrophy	Female > Male	ADPKD
		Tuberous sclerosis	Caroli disease
Most common benign tumor in infancy	Familial adenomatous polyposis syndrome		Biliary hamartomas (von Meyenberg complexes)
			Infection
			Metastases
			Mesenchymal hamartoma

TABLE 50-2 Hepatic Infections and Classic Imaging Findings

VIRAL HEPATITIS	PYOGENIC ABSCESS	CANDIDA INFECTION	AMOEBIC ABSCESS	HYDATID DISEASE	SCHISTOSOMIASIS	TUBERCULOSIS/ HISTOPLASMOSIS
Starry sky appearance (US)	Double target sign (CECT)	Bull's eye appearance (US)	Extrahepatic extension	Hydatid sand snow storm sign (US)	Tortoise shell appearance (CECT)	Calcified granulomata
			Enhancing wall with peripheral edema (CECT)	Water-lily sign (US)		

Fungal infection is most commonly caused by *Candida* infection, typically in immunocompromised patients. The lesions are multiple and less than 10 mm in size. Ultrasound (US) may show a "bull's eye" appearance with an echogenic nidus and hypoechoic rim in the acute phase. Contrast-enhanced CT shows numerous low attenuation lesions, which may have central enhancement.

Finally, secondary inflammation of the liver capsule and diaphragm or perihepatitis related to extrapelvic manifestation of pelvic inflammatory disease (PID) is known as Fitz-Hugh-Curtis syndrome. *Chlamydia* and *Neisseria gonorrhoeae* are the typical causative organisms. One may see an enhancing liver capsule on CT or MRI with this syndrome.

Amoebic abscess accounts for the most common hepatic abscess worldwide and is caused by *Entamoeba histolytica*, although these are rare in the US. Patients are usually younger than those with pyogenic abscess and present acutely ill with fever and right upper quadrant abdominal pain. These typically appear as complex, peripherally enhancing cystic lesions with septae on CT and can be associated with extrahepatic extension.

One of the most common parasitic infections to affect the liver is hydatid disease from the larval stage of the *Echinococcus* tapeworm. Patients are commonly from, or have traveled to, the Mediterranean region, Africa, South America, the Middle East, Australia, or New Zealand. Therefore, patients suspected of having a hydatid cyst should be questioned about foreign travel. The mature hydatid cyst consists of three layers: the outer layer (pericyst), a thick fibrous capsule, the middle membrane (ectocyst), and the germinal layer (endocyst). The middle layer is secreted by the inner layer. Scolices can be present in cyst fluid as a sediment and is known as hydatid sand. This can be appreciated occasionally on US as echogenic foci falling dependently with changes in position during the examination known as the "snowstorm" sign. Floating membranes within the cyst caused by detachment of the endocyst have been termed the "water-lily" sign.

Schistosomiasis may also affect the liver with the three most common species being *Schistosoma japonicum, Schistosoma haematobium, and Schistosoma mansoni.* Schistosomes live in the bowel and lay eggs in mesenteric veins that embolize to the portal vein. Subsequent inflammation and even chronic granuloma formation and cirrhosis can occur. Calcification in periportal areas and along the hepatic capsule in the fibrotic liver gives rise to a "tortoise shell" appearance on CT. Left untreated, cirrhosis is common, and there is an increased risk of developing hepatocellular carcinoma.

Tuberculosis (TB) is fairly uncommon, but liver disease is seen in 80% to 90% of autopsy patients with disseminated pulmonary disease. In endemic populations, focal calcifications in the liver are commonly the result of healed granulomas or foci of prior TB, histoplasmosis, or other granulomatous disease (Table 50-2).

BENIGN LIVER TUMORS

Hepatic cysts are the most frequently encountered liver masses in imaging. True cysts are felt to arise from hamartomatous tissue and can be seen with autosomal dominant polycystic kidney disease (ADPKD). Rarely, multiple hepatic cysts can exist as a separate genetic entity isolated to the liver. In both of these conditions, the size and number of cysts generally progresses with time and can occasionally lead to hepatic dysfunction and symptoms requiring intervention and, rarely, transplantation. Some of the above-described infections can also present as predominantly cystic masses. Finally, congenital abnormalities such as Caroli disease or biliary hamartomas (von Meyenberg complexes) can result in numerous cystic masses.

Biliary cystadenoma is a potentially premalignant tumor, which can appear cystlike. It will generally present as a multiloculated cystic mass with septation and nodularity; the locules of fluid will contain varying amounts of debris and be of varying consistency. Contents may include blood products, bile, mucinous substances, or serous fluid. Differentiating biliary cystadenomas from simple cysts may be difficult, but true, simple cysts are typically of water density and have no septations, internal debris, peripheral or central enhancement, perceptible wall, or mural nodularity.

HEMANGIOMA

The most common benign solid liver mass is the cavernous hemangioma. These may be multiple in up to 50% of cases and are rarely associated with calcification. Typical hemangiomas are 2 to 10 cm in size and demonstrate early, peripheral, nodular, discontinuous enhancement with centripetal filling on delayed imaging. Because these lesions reflect vascular filling, they also have virtually identical attenuation to the blood attenuation at all phases. Therefore, a lesion with "washed out" attenuation lower than the hepatic veins does not represent hemangioma.

This tumor is also typically hyperintense on T2-weighted images. On US, hemangiomas are classically well-defined homogeneous echogenic lesions with no significant Color Doppler flow. It occasionally demonstrates acoustic enhancement. In the background of hepatic steatosis, the echogenic texture of hemangioma is difficult to recognize. Tc-99m-labeled RBC scan with SPECT shows a focal defect or less uptake on early dynamic scan and persistent filling over 30 to 50 minutes on delayed scans.

FOCAL NODULAR HYPERPLASIA

Focal nodular hyperplasia (FNH) is also a common benign neoplasm of the liver, reported in 3% to 5% of the population and usually discovered incidentally in young women. Because of its association with other benign vascular neoplasms, many believe that FNH is caused by a "hyperplastic response to a localized vascular abnormality." On contrast-enhanced imaging, FNH is homogeneously hyperattenuating in the arterial phase and isoattenuating to liver on delayed and unenhanced phases. In lesions larger than 3 cm, 65% will have a fibrous central scar that is initially hypoattenuating and subsequently enhances on 5 to 10 minutes delay series. The central scar is usually hyperintense on T2-weighted images. Because FNH has Kupffer cells, there is normal or increased uptake on Tc-99m-sulfur colloid scanning. There is also prolonged enhancement in roughly 80% on Tc-99m-HIDA imaging because of the presence of bile ductules. Septations radiating from the central scar to the periphery of the lesion are common and can result in surface nodularity. Multiple lesions have been reported in up to 25% of cases.

HEPATIC ADENOMA

Hepatic adenoma is a fairly uncommon benign liver tumor most often seen in young women with a history of oral contraceptive use. Another group of patients who may have hepatic adenomas are those with type I glycogen storage disease. Anabolic androgenic steroids also increase the risk of adenoma development. The classic clinical manifestation of the tumor is rupture or hemorrhage resulting in acute onset of pain or, rarely, even death because of exsanguination. Unlike FNH, adenomas have only a few, nonfunctioning Kupffer cells and no bile ductules. Therefore, there is often absent or reduced uptake on Tc-99m-sulfur colloid scanning. Adenomas do contain large hepatocytes, glycogen, and lipid. This can manifest as macroscopic fat on occasion. The presence of hemorrhage can complicate imaging diagnosis. Adenomas, particularly small ones, are usually hyperattenuating compared to normal liver on CT and demonstrate rapid homogeneous enhancement. On MR and CT imaging, particularly of larger lesions, there is often heterogeneity. On MRI, heterogeneity may appear on both T1- and T2-weighted images because of the presence of old or new blood products, microscopic or macroscopic fat, cystic spaces, and occasionally calcification. Adenomas have also been reported to undergo malignant transformation to hepatocellular carcinoma.

HEPATIC ANGIOMYOLIPOMA

Hepatic angiomyolipoma is a rare benign lesion with macroscopic fat and is usually seen in patients with tuberous sclerosis. There is a marked female predominance for this lesion (Table 50-3).

TABLE 50-3 Cross-Sectional Imaging Characteristics of Benign Hepatic Lesions

HEPATIC HEMANGIOMA	FOCAL NODULAR HYPERPLASIA	HEPATIC ADENOMA	BILIARY CYSTADENOMA (PREMALIGNANT)	HEPATIC ANGIOMYOLIPOMA
Early, peripheral, nodular, discontinuous enhancement and subsequent centripetal filling	Homogeneous early enhancement	Hemorrhage	Rare	Female > Males
	Delayed enhancement of central scar	Higher attenuation than liver	Multilocular cystic lesion	Rare gross macroscopic fat
	Central scar T2 hyperintense	Occasional fat content		Multiple in patients with tuberous sclerosis
		Rapid homogeneous enhancement		

MALIGNANT LIVER TUMORS

HEPATOCELLULAR CARCINOMA

Hepatocellular carcinoma (HCC) is the most common primary malignant tumor of the liver. Worldwide, it is the eighth most common malignancy. There is an increased incidence in the Far East, Southeast Asia, and sub-Saharan Africa, and it continues to increase in the US. Risk factors include hepatitis B and C, toxins, certain medications, and other chronic liver diseases. The most common sites of metastatic disease include regional lymph nodes, lung, and skeleton. Imaging is important in the detection of HCC because symptoms of the disease are often masked by the chronic conditions leading to the malignancy. Various methods of surveillance are used to monitor patients at risk for HCC, but even the best tests detect only about 70% of cases. HCC can appear as a solitary mass, multiple nodules, or be diffusely infiltrative. The most common appearance on US is that of a hypoechoic mass, but US is not as sensitive as contrast-enhanced MR or CT. On contrast-enhanced, cross-sectional imaging, HCC enhances maximally during the hepatic arterial phase. Classically, in the portal venous phase of imaging, the tumor will be hypoattenuating to normal hepatic parenchyma. Sometimes, lesions are only clearly visible as hypoattenuating lesions on delayed phase. HCC has a broad range of appearances. With MR imaging, the most important sequences for the diagnosis of HCC are the dynamic gadolinium-enhanced images . Usually, the tumors are hypointense on T1 precontrast and slightly hyperintense on T2-weighted images. Hepatocellular carcinoma is also well-known to invade the portal venous system with "enhancing" thrombus.

FIBROLAMELLAR HEPATOCELLULAR CARCINOMA

Fibrolamellar hepatocellular carcinoma is an uncommon hepatocellular malignancy different from classic HCC. This is a slow-growing tumor that occurs in an otherwise normal liver in younger patients. It most often presents as large lobulated hepatic mass with a central scar. An important differentiating feature from benign lesions such as FNH is the appearance of the central scar on MR imaging; it is hypointense on T2-weighted sequences. Another feature is lack of enhancement of the central scar on delayed contrast-enhanced series with either CT or MR. Calcifications, necrosis, and a more disorganized appearance than hepatic adenoma or FNH are common.

INTRAHEPATIC CHOLANGIOCARCINOMA

Intrahepatic or peripheral cholangiocarcinoma has a poor prognosis and is most often seen in patients aging from 50 to 60 years. Contributing factors to the development of this tumor include primary sclerosing cholangitis, other forms of chronic or recurrent cholangitis (including parasitic disease), congenital cystic disease of the liver, and prior thorotrast administration. On contrast-enhanced imaging, the classic appearance of cholangiocarcinoma is that of a diffusely infiltrative tumor with associated capsular retraction. However, it may appear as ill-defined hypoattenuating lesion that may cause intrahepatic biliary obstruction. Delayed enhancement 10 to 20 minutes after the administration of intravenous contrast material is associated with cholangiocarcinoma, related to late enhancement of the fibrous component. However, this finding is seen in a minority of cases.

ANGIOSARCOMA, EPITHELIOID HEMANGIOENDOTHELIOMA, AND LYMPHOMA

Primary hepatic angiosarcoma and epithelioid hemangioendothelioma are rare tumors. Angiosarcoma is aggressive and has been linked to environmental and industrial toxins. These tumors contain numerous vascular spaces and may demonstrate peripheral or unusual enhancement patterns that progress with delayed enhanced series.

Epithelioid hemangioendothelioma is a low-grade primary vascular hepatic malignancy. It may demonstrate targetlike enhancement with nonenhancing center, enhancing tissue surrounding the center, and avascular peripheral zone. This should not be confused with infantile hemangioendothelioma. In contradistinction to that disease, epithelioid hemangioendothelioma is a disease of adults (average age 45 years), primarily women.

While primary hepatic lymphoma is rare, secondary lymphoma in the liver is much more common, especially in the setting of HIV disease. Both are typically hypoattenuating on CT without significant enhancement on contrast studies. Both are usually hypointense on T1-weighted images and hyperintense on T2 weighted images. Hepatic involvement with lymphoma typically enlarges the liver because of diffuse infiltration. However, discrete masses may occasionally be seen (Table 50-4).

HEPATIC METASTASES

Metastases to the liver far outnumber primary hepatic malignancies. This may be secondary to the dual blood supply, but is also likely related to the presence of humoral factors, which promote cell growth. Metastases to the liver can originate virtually anywhere in the body but most commonly arise from the colon, stomach, pancreas, breast, and lung. Renal cell carcinoma metastases

TABLE 50-4 Primary Hepatic Malignancies

HEPATOCELLULAR CARCINOMA	FIBROLAMELLAR HEPATOCELLUAR CARCINOMA	INTRAHEPATIC CHOLANGIOCARCINOMA
Early enhancing tumor	No enhancement of central scar	Infiltrative tumor
Portal vein invasion	Low T2 signal in central scar	Occasional delayed enhancement (5–20 min)

and metastatic melanoma are also relatively common in the liver. Some metastases are vascular and have fairly avid enhancement on contrast imaging. These include metastases from breast and renal carcinoma, islet cell tumor, carcinoid, melanoma, choriocarcinoma, thyroid carcinoma, pheochromocytoma, and sarcomas. Many metastatic lesions in the liver are hypovascular on imaging. These are some of the most common metastatic tumors to the liver including lung cancer, gastrointestinal adenocarcinomas, and some ovarian malignancies. However, although these are typical patterns, some commonly hypervascular lesions may be hypoenhancing and vice versa. Other metastatic lesions in the liver may be classified according to features such as calcification or a cystic appearance.

Large metastases tend to outgrow their blood supply and will present with regions of central necrosis. Other metastatic lesions may incite a fibrous or sclerosing reaction around tumor acini leading to scar formation; these include breast and pancreatic metastases. Patients with widespread liver metastases from breast cancer, which respond to treatment, may develop an appearance of "pseudocirrhosis" secondary to the fibrotic reaction. These patients can develop portal venous hypertension and secondary associated findings.

Imaging features of metastases to the liver are often nonspecific. With US, a hypoechoic halo around a well-defined lesion is usually indicative of aggressive behavior. With any modality, the appearance of metastatic lesions will vary depending on the presence or absence of enhancement, cystic regions, calcifications, and necrosis. Posttreatment-related changes are also quite variable. With the advent of some recent chemotherapy agents, such as Gleevec used for gastrointestinal stromal tumors, some metastatic lesions may necrose quickly and develop a cystic appearance (Table 50-5).

MISCELLANEOUS DISEASES/ CONDITIONS OF THE LIVER

CIRRHOSIS

Cirrhosis is a chronic liver disease resulting from damage to hepatocytes and subsequent regenerative nodule formation, fibrosis, parenchymal necrosis, and often fatty change. Because cirrhosis is the end-stage of chronic hepatocyte injury, its causes are numerous. Exposure to toxic agents including ethanol, chronic viral hepatitides, nonalcoholic steatohepatitis (NASH), other chronic infection, autoimmune disease, and hemachromatosis are some of the causes of hepatic cirrhosis.

Because of the unusual vascular supply of the liver previously described, one of the gross morphologic features of cirrhosis is relative enlargement of the lateral segment of the left hepatic lobe and caudate lobe. This is felt to be on the basis of regenerative change rather than solely on the basis of fibrosis of the right hepatic lobe and medial segment of the left hepatic lobe. The caudate-to-right-lobe ratio is a reasonably sensitive indicator of cirrhosis. A ratio of a horizontal line extending from the medial edge of the caudate lobe to the lateral aspect of the bifurcation of the right portal vein is divided by the distance from the latter point to the lateral extent of the right lobe. A value greater than 0.9 should lead to the suspicion of cirrhosis. Worthy of note,

TABLE 50-5 Classification of Hepatic Metastases

VASCULAR METASTASES	HYPOVASCULAR METASTASES	CALCIFIED METASTASES	CYSTIC METASTASES
Breast	Lung	Mucinous adenocarcinoma	Mucinous adenocarcinoma
Renal	GI adenocarcinoma	Leiomyosarcoma	Serous adenocarcinoma
Islet cell	GI stromal tumor	Carcinoid	*Any rapidly growing tumor with cystic degeneration including*
Carcinoid	Some ovarian	Endocrine pancreas	Sarcomas
Melanoma	Some pancreas	Medullary thyroid	Neuroendocrine
Choriocarcinoma		Osteosarcoma	Melanoma
Thyroid		Neuroblastoma	Some lung
Pheochromocytoma		Renal cell carcinoma	Some breast
Sarcomas		Testicular	
		Lung	
		Treated carcinoma	

cirrhosis associated with Budd-Chiari or hepatic veno-occlusive disease is associated with a massively enlarged caudate lobe, which is occasionally confused with neoplasm.

On US, CT, and MRI, the contour of the liver is nodular in patients with cirrhosis. As the disease progresses and fibrosis predominates, vascular flow in the liver changes. Portal hypertension develops and is often manifest by a large main portal vein, splanchnic collaterals, and enlargement of the spleen. Flow in the portal vein slows and eventually reverses. When there is portal thrombosis, numerous collaterals may form in the porta hepatis and are referred to as cavernous transformation. Hepatic arteries slowly enlarge and become tortuous. Hepatic venous flow, usually triphasic, becomes monophasic as the "stiffness" of the liver increases. Because of the portal hypertension, spontaneous portosystemic shunts may occur. Iatrogenic shunts (TIPS) or surgical portacaval or splenorenal shunts may be created to reduce portal hypertension and help control secondary features such as variceal bleeding and recalcitrant ascites.

Other secondary effects of portal hypertension include increased thickness of the walls of the stomach and bowel and mesenteric edema. This can affect bowel motility and function and result in the so-called portal enteropathy. The progressive loss of liver function can result in a host of abnormalities in the patient including decreased serum protein synthesis, decreased coagulant synthesis, and inability to metabolize and/or catabolize toxins.

Imaging of patients with cirrhosis is often performed to screen for hepatocellular carcinoma for which these patients are at increased risk. Imaging is also used to evaluate the primary and secondary effects of cirrhosis on the liver and mesenteric vasculature. US with Doppler can evaluate intra- and extrahepatic vasculature to monitor disease progression. US, CT, and MR can also define the presence of varices, spontaneous shunts, ascites, portal enteropathy, and other secondary features. Contrast-enhanced series are important to screen for HCC for reasons delineated in the section concerning this malignancy. Pre- and postcontrast series are also useful to help distinguish siderotic regenerative nodules that contain increased amounts of iron and are hyperattenuating on noncontrast CT and hypointense on T1- and T2-weighted MR sequences. Siderotic nodules in the spleen are referred to as Gamna Gandy bodies and are markedly hypointense on MR imaging.

HEPATIC STEATOSIS

Fatty liver is commonly encountered in imaging. It ranges from diffuse to focal and can be associated with a number of disease conditions or represent an isolated abnormality. Fatty liver or steatosis is characterized by the presence of triglyceride accumulation in the cytoplasm of hepatocytes. Fatty liver is seen in alcoholic liver disease and insulin resistance most commonly. It is also seen with obesity, hyperlipidemia, viral infection, drug use including chemotherapeutic agents, surgery, metabolic disorders including storage disorders, and many other conditions.

On US, fatty liver is manifest by increased echogenicity exceeding that of the spleen and renal cortex. There is decreased penetration of the sound beam and poor definition of intrahepatic architecture. On unenhanced CT, fatty liver can be diagnosed if attenuation of the liver is at least 10 HU less than that of the spleen or if the absolute attenuation is less than 40 HU. With MR imaging, fatty liver is manifest by signal loss on opposed-phase imaging compared with in-phase images. A variant of fatty infiltration of liver is focal or geographic rather than diffuse. Small foci of fatty infiltration are commonly seen adjacent to the falciform ligament, porta hepatis, and in the gallbladder fossa. However, these are secondary to common anomalies of embryologic vascular supply to these areas and do not reflect an abnormal condition. Atypical forms of fatty infiltration can be distinguished from mass lesions by the lack of mass effect on vessels, geographic configuration, and normal enhancement.

BUDD-CHIARI SYNDROME

This syndrome is an unusual condition, representing the result of hepatic venous outflow obstruction at any level, regardless of the cause of obstruction. It is referred to as primary when venous outflow obstruction is the result of an endoluminal venous lesion such as thrombus. It is referred to as secondary when obstruction is either extravascular or related to substance in the lumen of the vessel not originating from the venous system. Budd-Chiari syndrome is more common in women.

Acutely, the disease is manifest by decreased enhancement of the hepatic periphery and increased central enhancement (specifically the caudate lobe). Large ascites is common. In the more chronic setting, portosystemic and intrahepatic collaterals are noted. Intrahepatic collaterals have been described as "comma-shaped" on US and MR imaging. On US with Doppler, vascular flow may mimic that seen with cirrhosis; that is, monophasic or no flow in hepatic veins and slow hepatofugal flow in the portal vein. Regenerative nodules in Budd-Chiari are typically large, differentiating themselves from the small nodules associated with alcoholic cirrhosis. Angiographic finding with venacavography is that of a "spiderweb" pattern of collateral vessels, which is pathognomonic.

TABLE 50-6 Diffuse Hepatic Diseases

CIRRHOSIS	STEATOSIS	BUDD-CHIARI	HEMACHROMATOSIS
Nodular contour	10 HU less than the spleen on noncontrast CT	Early decreased peripheral enhancement and increased central and caudate enhancement	Early primary disease manifest by low signal in the liver on MR
Caudate and lateral segment left hepatic lobe enlargement	Absolute HU value less than 40	Intrahepatic comma-shaped collateral vessels	Secondary disease manifest by low signal in the liver and spleen on MR
Right hepatic lobe and medial segment left hepatic lobe fibrosis	Loss of signal on opposed phase MR		Increased attenuation of liver on unenhanced CT (up to 75–135 HU; normal liver is 45–65 HU)
Widening of fissures	Increased echogenicity > spleen or renal cortex on US		

HEMOCHROMATOSIS

Primary hemochromatosis is an autosomal recessive disease of iron metabolism affecting men much more commonly than women. There is increased intestinal absorption of iron and subsequent deposition in the liver, pancreas, myocardium, endocrine glands, joints, and skin. Secondary hemochromatosis is the result of reticuloendothelial deposition of iron in patients who require numerous blood transfusions, have increased iron intake, or have chronic liver disease and/or portacaval shunts. Important imaging characteristics include increased attenuation of the liver on unenhanced CT (up to 75–135 HU, when it is usually 45–65 HU). On MR, with early primary disease, there is signal loss in the liver. With secondary disease, there is signal loss in the liver and spleen. T2*GRE may be the most sensitive MR sequence for the disease (Table 50-6).

SUGGESTED READING

Awaya H, Mitchell D, Kamishima T, et al. Cirrhosis: modified caudate-right lobe ratio. *Radiology*. 2002;224:769-774.

Brancatelli G, Vilgrain V, Federle MP, et al. Budd-chiari syndrome: spectrum of imaging findings. *AJR Am J Roentgenol.* 2007;188:W168-W176.

Brant WE, Helms CA. *Fundamentals of Diagnostic Radiology*. 2nd ed. Philadelphia, PA: Lippincott Williams & Wilkins; 1999.

Doyle DJ, Hanbidge AE, O'Malley ME. Imaging of hepatic infections. *Clin Radiol*. 2006;61:737-748.

Federle, MP, Jeffrey RB, Desser TS, et al. *Diagnostic Imaging Abdomen*. Salt Lake City, UT: Amirsys Inc; 2008.

Gabata T, Kadoya M, Matsui O, et al. Dynamic CT of hepatic abscesses. *AJR Am J Roentgenol*. 2001;176:675-679.

Grazioli L, Federle MP, Brancatelli G, et al. Hepatic adenomas: imaging and pathologic findings. *Radiographics*. 2001;21:877-894.

Hamer OW, Aguirre DA, Casola G, et al. Fatty liver: imaging patterns and pitfalls. *Radiographics*. 2006;26:1637-1653.

Kamel IR, Liapi E, Fishman, EK. Focal nodular hyperplasia: lesion evaluation using 16-MDCT and 3D CT angiography. *AJR Am J Roentgenol*. 2006;186:1587-1596.

Kim S, Kim TU, Lee JW, et al. The perihepatic space: comprehensive anatomy and CT features of pathologic conditions. *Radiographics*. 2007;27:129-143.

Mergo PJ, Ros PR, Buetow PC, et al. Diffuse disease of the liver: radiologic-pathologic correlation. *Radiographics*. 1994;14:1291-1307.

Morgan DE, Lockhart M, Canon C, et al. Polycystic liver disease: multimodality imaging for complications and transplant evaluation. *Radiographics*. 2006;26:1655-1668.

Szklaruk J, Silverman PM, Charnsangavej C. Pictorial review: imaging in the diagnosis, staging, treatment, and surveillance of hepatocellular carcinoma. *AJR Am J Roentgenol.* 2003;180:441-454.

QUESTIONS AND ANSWERS

1. Which of the following is *true* regarding contrast-enhanced MR imaging of fibrolamellar hepatocellular carcinoma?
   A. Central scar is T1 hyperintense and enhances on delayed postgadolinium sequences.
   B. Central scar is T2 hypointense and does not enhance.
   C. Central scar is T2 hyperintense and enhance.
   D. Central scar is T1 hypointense and does not enhance.

   ANSWER: B. In fibrolamellar hepatocellular carcinoma, the central scar is hypointense on T2 and does not enhance on delayed postgadolinium sequences. In FNH, if there is a central scar, it will be hyperintense on T2-weighted images and does typically enhance on delayed postgadolinium sequences.

2. Which of the following conditions increases risk for hepatic adenomas?
   A. von Hippel-Lindau disease
   B. Hereditary hemorrhagic telangiectasia syndrome

C. Type I glycogen storage disease
D. Multiple endocrine neoplasia IIa

ANSWER: C. Patients with type I glycogen storage disease may have multiple hepatic adenomas.

3. The presence of which of the following imaging features is suggestive of hepatic amoebic abscess in patients with an appropriate clinical history?
A. The "water-lily" sign
B. Hepatic artery thrombosis
C. Capsular retraction
D. Extrahepatic extension

ANSWER: D. Extrahepatic extension can be seen with amoebic abscess and can be a helpful distinguishing feature from pyogenic or other abscess. "Water-lily" sign is secondary to floating membranes within the hydatid cysts.

4. Which of the following is an imaging feature suggestive of focal nodular hyperplasia (FNH)?
A. Intratumoral hemorrhage
B. Delayed activity on Tc-99m-HIDA scan
C. "Cold spot" on Tc-99m-sulfur colloid scan
D. Hyperintense on T1 because of the presence of fat

ANSWER: B. Delayed activity in a lesion on Tc-99m-HIDA scan is suggestive of FNH because of the presence of bile ductules in the mass.

5. A large infiltrative hepatic mass demonstrating early enhancement and portal vein invasion is most consistent with which of the following?
A. Cholangiocarcinoma
B. Biliary cystadenoma
C. Primary hepatic lymphoma
D. Hepatocellular carcinoma

ANSWER: D. While hepatocellular carcinoma can have a varied appearance, it does usually show early (arterial) enhancement and can be associated with portal vein invasion.

6. What portion of the liver is not covered by visceral peritoneum?
A. Porta hepatis, caudal right hepatic lobe, and the bare area
B. Bare area, porta hepatis, and the gallbladder bed
C. Bare area, hepatic dome, and lateral segment
D. Porta hepatis, hepatic dome, and gallbladder bed

ANSWER: B. The adult liver is covered by visceral peritoneum except at the bare area, the porta hepatis, and the gallbladder bed.

7. Concerning MR imaging features (with T2-weighting) of primary and secondary hemochromatosis, which of the following is *true*?
A. Liver and spleen are hypointense in early primary hemochromatosis.
B. Liver is hyperintense in secondary hemochromatosis.
C. Liver and spleen are hypointense in secondary hemochromatosis.
D. Spleen is hypointense in early primary hemochromatosis.

ANSWER: C. In early primary hemochromatosis, the liver is hypointense. In secondary hemochromatosis, both the liver and spleen are hypointense on T2.

8. All of the following are considered vascular metastases on liver imaging, *except*:
A. Choriocarcinoma
B. Pheochromocytoma
C. Renal cell carcinoma
D. Lung carcinoma

ANSWER: D. Lung carcinoma is usually associated with hypovascular metastases to the liver.

9. Which of the following is the most common primary hepatic malignancy in children?
A. Hepatocellular carcinoma
B. Neuroblastoma
C. Hepatoblastoma
D. Infantile hemangioendothelioma

ANSWER: C. Hepatoblastoma is the most common primary hepatic malignancy in children.

10. A solitary infiltrative hepatic mass demonstrates capsular retraction and delayed enhancement on contrast enhanced CT. What is the most likely diagnosis.
A. Metastatic thyroid carcinoma
B. Atypical siderotic nodule
C. Hepatocellular adenoma
D. Peripheral cholangiocarcinoma

ANSWER: D. Peripheral cholangiocarcinoma.

51 BILIARY SYSTEM

Desiree E. Morgan

NORMAL ANATOMY AND CONGENITAL ABNORMALITIES

The biliary system arises from the hepatic diverticulum on the ventral aspect of the developing gut in the embryo. In general, the intrahepatic bile ducts run parallel to the portal veins within the liver. The right hepatic duct drains segments 5 through 8 and has two major branches, the posterior duct that drains segments 6 and 7, and the anterior duct that drains segments 5 and 8. The left hepatic duct is formed from segments 2 through 4. The common hepatic duct (CHD) is formed by the confluence of the right and left hepatic ducts, and the cystic duct joins the common hepatic duct (CHD) to form the common bile duct (CBD). Approximately 60% of individuals have this "normal" biliary anatomy. The most common anomalous drainage of the biliary system is drainage of the right posterior duct into the left hepatic duct above its confluence with the right anterior duct. Another common variant is a triple confluence of simultaneous emptying of the right posterior duct, right anterior duct, and left hepatic duct to form the CHD.

The gallbladder is the repository for bile produced in the liver. The gallbladder is composed of the fundus, usually projecting below the inferior border of the liver, the body, and the neck. Typically measuring 2.5 cm in width and 7 to 10 cm in length, normal gallbladder wall thickness is less than 3 mm and the average volume of the gallbladder is 30 to 50 mL. When a patient is fasting, there is concentration of bile in the gallbladder. On MRI, during fasting, the concentration of cholesterol and bile salts increases, leading to shortened T1 relaxation time and brighter signal on T1-weighted images, often with a layered appearance.

Cystic duct insertion into the CHD may also vary, with the most common variants being a low cystic duct insertion (9%), medial cystic duct insertion (10%–17%), or common channel for greater than 2 cm (up to 25%). Small ducts from the hepatic parenchyma (ducts of Luschka) may empty directly into the gallbladder lumen. In general, there may be an increased incidence of bile duct variant configurations in patients who also have portal vein variation.

Anomalous biliary pancreatic duct union occurs when there is fusion of the main pancreatic duct and CBD outside the duodenal wall, with a long common channel (greater than 15 mm) from the papillary orifice to the branch point. In anomalous biliary pancreatic duct union, the bile duct inserts at a 90-degree angle onto the pancreatic duct. This may allow reflux of pancreatic secretions into the biliary system. This anomaly is associated with choledochal web or choledochal cyst (Todani type 1).

Choledochal cysts are rare congenital anomalies of the biliary tree characterized by varying configurations and distribution of duct dilatation. Most choledochal cysts are diagnosed in childhood, however up to 20% of patients will not present until adulthood. The most common clinical presentation of a patient with a choledochal cyst is the constellation of abdominal pain, right upper quadrant mass, and jaundice. The Todani classification is used to discuss the varying types of cysts (Table 51-1).

TABLE 51-1 Todani Classificaton of Choledochal Cysts

Type I	Extrahepatic bile duct
Type Ia	Diffuse cyst formation along the extrahepatic duct
Type Ib	Focal cyst along the extrahepatic bile duct
Type Ic	Fusiform dilation of the extrahepatic bile duct (80%–90% of cases)
Type II	True diverticulum of the extrahepatic bile duct
Type III	Focal dilation of the common bile within the intramural portion of the duodenum; may be associated with biliary colic or pancreatitis (choledochocele)
Type IV	Multiple cysts
Type IVa	Involving both extra- and intrahepatic bile ducts
Type IVb	Which involves only the extrahepatic bile ducts with multiple sacculations
Type V	Dilatation of the intrahepatic bile ducts (Caroli disease)

Type V (Caroli disease) involves a defect in the embryonic plate that results in varying levels of intrahepatic bile cyst formation versus hepatic fibrosis. When both are present, the condition is known as Caroli syndrome, and it is inherited by an autosomal recessive pathway. One imaging feature of Caroli disease is the "central dot sign," representing a portal vein branch surrounded by cystic dilation of the intrahepatic bile duct. Patients with Caroli disease may have intraluminal biliary calculi.

STONE DISEASE

Bile may become supersaturated with cholesterol leading to crystal deposition and gallstone formation. Cholesterol stones account for approximately 80% of all gallstones present in the US population. Cholesterol stones are composed of at least 50% cholesterol. Pigment stones on the other hand contain lesser amounts of cholesterol and higher percentages of calcium bilirubinate and glycoproteins. Because of their different makeup, gallstones may be distinguished on MR imaging. Pigmented stones are hypointense on T2-weighted sequences and have increased signal intensity on T1-weighted images, whereas cholesterol stones tend to be hypointense on both T1- and T2-weighted images. Gallstones are found in about 10% of the general population, are twice as common in women as in men, and become more prevalent with increasing age. Risk factors include pregnancy, estrogens, obesity, and rapid weight loss. Most patients with cholelithiasis, however, remain asymptomatic throughout life.

INFLAMMATION

Acute cholecystitis is the most common acute complication of gallstone disease, with clinical presentation characterized by right upper quadrant abdominal pain, fever, and elevated white cell count. In most cases (90%), the cause of acute cholecystitis is impaction of a gallstone in the gallbladder neck region or cystic duct with obstruction. Ultrasound is the modality of choice for diagnosing acute cholecystitis, with findings described in other chapters. Because sonographic evaluation may be limited in patients with a large body habitus, CT and MRI are being utilized more frequently to evaluate patients with equivocal findings or suboptimal ultrasound examinations. On MRI, the gallbladder wall may show increased signal intensity and thickening, edema of the adjacent liver tissue, and pericholecystic fluid. The signal intensity of bile in the setting of acute cholecystitis is variable because of an inflammation-related increase in bile protein. However, signal within bile is usually markedly hypointense on T1-weighted images because of impairment of gallbladder concentrating ability in the acutely inflamed state. On intravenous, gadolinium-contrast-enhanced, fat-suppressed T1-weighted images, enhancement of the gallbladder wall, adjacent fat, and surrounding hepatic parenchyma may be noted. When there is patchy enhancement of gallbladder mucosa, this is referred to as the "interrupted rim sign" and represents areas of necrosis in gangrenous acute cholecystitis. Other findings of gangrenous cholecystitis on MRI include asymmetric gallbladder wall thickening, intramural hemorrhage, and complex pericholecystic fluid. These latter findings may also be seen on contrast-enhanced CT in patients with acute cholecystitis.

Mirizzi syndrome, defined as impaction of a gallstone within the gallbladder neck or cystic duct leading to extrinsic CHD compression and biliary obstruction, may occur in patients with an intact gallbladder or in patients after cholecystectomy, when there is a stone lodged within the cystic duct remnant. Magnetic resonance cholangiopancreatography (MRCP) is particularly helpful in this condition as it can noninvasively identify the impacted gallstone in the cystic duct or gallbladder neck, the upstream biliary dilation, and the configuration of the cystic duct insertion into the CHD. Patients with low insertion of the cystic duct or long parallel cystic and CHD channels are at increased risk for this condition.

Approximately 10% of patients with acute cholecystitis have no stones. This condition is known as acute acalculus cholecystitis, is usually seen in more acutely ill patients, and carries a higher morbidity and mortality than typical gallstone-induced acute cholecystitis.

Emphysematous cholecystitis is caused by gas-forming bacteria that infect the gallbladder wall, is typically seen in diabetic patients, and is usually not associated with gallstones. Ischemia caused by cystic artery atherosclerosis may also produce emphysematous cholecystitis.

Chronic cholecystitis is invariably associated with gallstones and is the most common form of the symptomatic gallbladder disease. Typically, the gallbladder is small and contracted, with irregular and thickened walls. Presenting symptoms are vague upper abdominal pain. The diagnosis is usually confirmed using a physiologic test such as HIDA scan.

Xanthogranulomatous cholecystitis is an uncommon inflammatory disease of the gallbladder characterized by focal or diffuse inflammation of the gallbladder wall by foamy histiocytes or xanthoma cells admixed with fibrosis. It is hypothesized that this condition results from cystic duct obstruction leading to mucosal injury, macrophage recruitment, and subsequent phagocytosis of insoluble bile lipids and cholesterol which in turn leads to lipogranuloma formation and fibrosis. Most patients have gallstones and many are diabetic. The inflammatory process may extend to the adjacent colon and duodenum with fistula or abscess formation. On imaging, this condition may resemble gallbladder carcinoma with focal or diffuse wall thickening, heterogeneous enhancement, and intramural nodules. On MRI, the intramural nodules have markedly elevated T2 signal intensity. This may help distinguish this condition from gallbladder carcinoma.

Acute cholangitis is a life-threatening complication of incomplete biliary obstruction. Human bile is normally sterile, but may become infected in the presence of gallbladder and/or CBD stones with ascending infection. The triad of jaundice, fever, and right upper quadrant pain, originally described by Charcot, is the classic presentation of cholangitis; however, this constellation of symptoms usually occurs late in the disease. In most patients, biliary sepsis resolves with conservative treatment including fluid resuscitation and administration of broad-spectrum antibiotics (gram-positive and gram-negative organism coverage). The spectrum of bacteria varies between reported series (depending on underlying etiologies and practice profile of the reporting center), but in patients with choledocholithiasis, the most frequent organisms are gram-negative: *Escherichia coli, Klebsiella, Proteus,* and *Pseudomonas aeruginosa.* Fungal infections are more prevalent in patients who have had previous biliary surgery or nonoperative (endoscopic/radiological) biliary interventions. Those patients with cholangitis who do not respond to conservative therapy require biliary decompression, usually performed endoscopically with endoscopic papillotomy with or without stone extraction, and placement of biliary stents. When patients are extremely ill, stent placement without stone removal is preferred, as excessive manipulation in attempts to remove large stones may result in worsened septicemia. Patients not responding to endoscopic biliary drainage and appropriate antibiotics should be investigated for malfunction of the biliary drainage system (stent occlusion or migration), associated gallbladder empyema, associated cholangitic abscesses, or additional undrained hepatic segments. When endoscopic drainage fails, or if the cholangitis is because of intrahepatic stones or hilar cholangiocarcinoma, transhepatic biliary drainage is indicated. Whatever method of drainage is used, injection of contrast medium under pressure should be avoided as much as possible, as this may lead to cholangio-venous reflux and exacerbation of septicemia as well. Identification of the underlying cause and level of biliary obstruction with multidetector CT or MRCP is important, with definitive treatment attempted after the patients respond to initial antibiotics or biliary decompression. Choledocholithiasis remains the commonest cause of cholangitis.

Oriental cholangiohepatitis, also known as recurrent pyogenic cholangitis, is most commonly seen among patients from Southeast Asia and is associated with bacterial infection and intrahepatic stones. Endoscopic decompression is less successful in this clinical scenario, and often, surgical drainage is required.

PRIMARY SCLEROSING CHOLANGITIS

Primary sclerosing cholangitis (PSC) is a chronic cholestatic liver disease of unknown etiology that is characterized by progressive inflammation and fibrosis of the bile ducts. It appears to be caused by complex interaction between deregulated immune mechanisms in genetically predisposed individuals, also potentially affected by environmental factors and infectious agents. The disease often results in secondary biliary cirrhosis and is associated with a high risk of cholangiocarcinoma. Most patients are young (mean age 40 years) at the age of diagnosis and there is a male-to-female predominance. Concomitant inflammatory bowel disease may be found in 62% to 72% of patients. Ulcerative colitis is much more common (80%), however there is an association with Crohn disease in up to 14% of all PSC patients. Conversely, up to 4% of patients with inflammatory bowel disease have PSC. Clinically, these patients are often asymptomatic at presentation with isolated biliary enzyme abnormalities; over time, they suffer from recurrent episodes of cholangitis with jaundice, pruritus, and fever, resulting ultimately in end-stage liver disease. The main causes of death in patients with PSC are cholangiocarcinoma and liver failure. Liver transplantation is the only therapeutic option with a cure potential.

PSC is a disease mainly of large bile ducts. On imaging, patients with PSC have characteristic localized or multifocal strictures of the intra- and/or extrahepatic bile ducts, with intervening segments of normal or dilated ducts. Short segment strictures, pseudosacculation, and serrated bile duct margins are best depicted with cholangiography. While endoscopic retrograde cholangiography (ERC) is the goal standard for visualization of duct abnormalities in patients with PSC, MRC has a high sensitivity and specificity, with the added advantage of visualizing bile ducts proximal to points of complete bile duct obstruction. Conversely, because of inferior spatial resolution, areas of marked stenoses may be mistaken for complete occlusion with MRC and wall irregularity overestimated.

Patients with small-bile-duct PSC present with similar biochemical and histologic features as typical PSC but have a normal cholangiogram. Formerly, this condition was known as "pericholangitis." Only 3% to 17% of patients with small duct PSC disease or undergo liver transplantation, compared to 42% to 47% in patients with typical large duct PSC. Histologic findings in PSC include portal fibrosis (onionskin pattern), portal lymphocyte infiltration, and cirrhosis.

Cholangiocarcinoma may arise at any stage of PSC. The frequency of hepato biliary cancer in patients with PSC is 1.5% per year, corresponding to a 161-fold increased risk. Cholangiocarcinomas occur as mass lesions in the liver in 15% of patients, lesions in the distal CBD in 20% of patients, and tumors in the hilar region in 65% of PSC patients. Effective surveillance strategies for PSC patients are challenging. Tumor development may be heralded by elevation of CEA or CA-19-9. ERC alone has a low sensitivity and specificity to discriminate between benign and malignant bile duct stenoses in PSC patients; however, any increase in cholestasis should trigger ERC with brush cytology of suspicious strictures as this yields high specificity despite low sensitivity for cholangiocarcinoma detection.

Selecting the appropriate time for liver transplantation is difficult in patients with PSC, as even those with advanced destructive cholangiopathy may exhibit only mild signs of liver failure, based upon findings of portal hypertension or abnormal coagulation and hypoalbuminemia. The difficulty of screening the high-risk PSC patients for cholangiocarcinoma only compounds the transplant timing conundrum. Compared to patients with nonmalignant diseases, patients with PSC-associated cholangiocarcinoma have a worse prognosis after liver transplantation; thus, it is important to identify these cancers beforehand. In some centers, transplantation following neoadjuvant therapy has shown some benefit, but curative treatment is not possible in the majority of cases.

PRIMARY BILIARY CIRRHOSIS

Primary biliary cirrhosis is an autoimmune disease that results in destruction of small intralobular bile ducts and cholestasis. The cholestasis produces direct liver injury, causing inflammation and necrosis and ultimately leading to progressive scarring and fibrosis. The condition primarily affects middle-aged women and most patients are asymptomatic at presentation. These asymptomatic patients are identified when routine health examinations reveal elevation of serum alkaline phosphatase (ALP), and gamma-glutamyl transpeptidase (GGT), total serum cholesterol, or positive antimitochondrial antibody (specifically subtype M2 AMA) titers. Occasionally (10%), patients with PBC are AMA negative and must distinguished from patients with other cholestatic liver pathologies (PSC, sarcoidosis, nonalcoholic fatty liver disease). Primary biliary cirrhosis may be associated with other autoimmune conditions as well as complications of cholestasis such as osteoporosis and hypercholesterolemia. Physical examination is generally normal but hepatomegaly may be present in 4% to 31% and splenomegaly in 5% to 25%. If symptomatic, patients most commonly complain of fatigue (11%–81%) and pruritus (18%–41%). The onset of pruritus typically precedes onset of jaundice, a finding that occurs only in the late stages of the disease. Diagnosis is confirmed with liver histology; the characteristic lesion of PBC is destruction of the intralobular bile ducts.

The role of imaging in patients with PBC is not to diagnose the disease, but to distinguish this cholestatic liver disease from others, particularly when the AMA is negative. MRC demonstrates normal bile ducts in early stages of disease helping to distinguish PBC from primary sclerosing cholangitis. In early stages, cross-sectional imaging may show only an enlarged liver with lacelike fibrosis and few regenerative nodules. Adenopathy, ascites, and varices may occasionally be present. In late stages, there is irregular dilation and a truncated appearance of the intrahepatic bile ducts on MRC or ERC, with normal extrahepatic bile ducts. CT and MRI findings in advanced PBC are similar to those seen in other forms of cirrhosis. On T2-weighted MRI, when parenchymal lacelike fibrosis and rounded, low signal intensity lesions surrounding portal vein branches (periportal halo sign) are seen together, the sensitivity for PBC detection is 69%; thus, the imaging findings may support the clinical and laboratory findings of PBC even in the early stages. Patients with PBC are at risk for developing hepatocellular carcinoma when the disease is advanced. In the past, the most common cause of death in patients with primary biliary cirrhosis was liver failure and PBC was a leading indication for liver transplantation, but now there is effective medical therapy using ursodeoxycholic acid. This is particularly effective when the patient is diagnosed with early stage disease and with this therapy, survival for patients with PBC may approach normal life span.

TABLE 51-2 AIDS Cholangiopathy Pathogens

Cryptosporidium
Microsporidia
Cyclospora
Isospora
Cytomegalovirus
Mycobacterium avium-intracellulare complex
Candida
Other bowel pathogens

AIDS CHOLANGIOPATHY

AIDS cholangiopathy represents one of the hepatobiliary diseases in patients with AIDS. Clinical presentation includes fever, right upper quadrant pain, and marked elevation of serum ALP. Jaundice is usually absent. Many patients are asymptomatic or have only mild elevation of liver serum enzyme tests. As many as 30% of patients with chronic AIDS-related diarrhea have AIDS cholangiopathy. Infection of the biliary epithelium is the cause of ductal disease in most patients. *Cryptosporidium* is the single most common identifiable pathogen (Table 51-2).

These infections cause severe inflammatory changes resulting in an irregularly narrowed duct appearance. The most common imaging findings are intrahepatic and/or extrahepatic changes mimicking sclerosing cholangitis, often associated with papillary stenosis (50%–60% of patients). The left ductal system is disproportionally more severely involved. Focal strictures of the extrahepatic bile duct may be greater than 2 cm in length. This latter feature may help distinguish AIDS cholangiopathy from PSC as the extrahepatic strictures in PSC rarely exceed 4 to 5 mm. Another distinguishing feature is the absence of saccular deformities of the ducts, seen more commonly in PSC compared to AIDS cholangiopathy. Treatment of symptomatic patients with AIDS cholangiopathy consists of endoscopic papillotomy in those with papillary stenosis. While this often results in pain relief, the intrahepatic sclerosing cholangitis tends to progress after papillotomy and is associated with a further rise in serum ALP. If a patient has a dominant extrahepatic stricture, endoscopic stent placement may help, although risk of long-term bacterial infection is not known. Although AIDS cholangiopathy is infectious in etiology, medical therapies are not typically effective. The prognosis in patients with AIDS cholangiopathy is poor (median survival approximately 10 months), not because of the biliary inflammation but because opportunistic infection of the biliary tree occurs only in patients with severe immunodeficiency (CD4 counts less than 50/mm^3).

Other diseases of the biliary tract in patients with AIDS include acalculous cholecystitis, lymphoma,

Kaposi sarcoma, and gallstones. The most common manifestation of gallbladder disease in an HIV-infected patient is acalculous cholecystitis. Gallstones may be the cause of cholecystitis in up to 25% of AIDS patients. Treatment for these gallbladder conditions is similar to that in patients with normal immunity.

PARASITIC DISEASE

The most common parasites affecting the biliary tree include *Clonorchis sinensis, Opisthorchis viverrini, Opisthorchis felinus,* and *Fasciola hepatica.* Patients are often asymptomatic unless they are heavily infected. In addition, *Ascaris lumbricoides* may migrate from the small bowel into the bile duct through the papilla, causing obstructive jaundice and biliary colic. The first three parasites are trematodes that vary in geographic distribution. All are flat, elongated worms ranging from 8 to 15 mm in length and may persist for 20 years or more within the medium-size and small intrahepatic bile ducts. Occasionally, they enter the extrahepatic duct, gallbladder, or pancreatic duct resulting in mechanical obstruction, inflammatory reaction, adenomatous hyperplasia, and periductal fibrosis. Adult flukes within the bile ducts are usually difficult visualize sonographically or with CT, but are easily identified within the gallbladder. *F. hepatica* is a trematode that infects cattle and sheep but interacts with humans as an accidental host when there is ingestion of contaminated water or aquatic plants. The metacercariae penetrate the intestinal wall and migrate through the peritoneal cavity to the liver where they pass through Glisson's capsule and track through the liver parenchyma to enter the bile ducts and gallbladder. Adult flukes may measure 20 to 40 mm long and appear as clusters of microabscesses in subcapsular portions of the liver. Filling defects that represent the flukes may be identifiable on cholangiogram. *A. lumbricoides* adult worms are 15 to 30 cm long and if present in the biliary tree may produce obstruction, cholangitis, or pancreatitis. Sonographically, these flukes are nonshadowing echogenic tubular structures visible within the bile ducts.

OTHER CHRONIC CONDITIONS

Adenomyomatosis is a very common noninflammatory benign condition that is more often seen in women than men and clinically presents with right upper quadrant pain associated with gallstones. There is proliferation of surface epithelium with invagination through Rokitansky-Aschoff sinuses into the thickened tunica muscularis. When diffuse, the entire gallbladder wall is thickened with luminal narrowing. Focal circumferential thickening in the midportion of the gallbladder is seen in the segmental form, producing an hourglass configuration. Localized adenomyomatosis is typically found in the fundus and may mimic an early gallbladder cancer. Dysplasia and carcinoma may arise from adenomyomatosis but this is usually related more to gallstones and chronic inflammation than the adenomyomatosis itself.

NEOPLASM

GALLBLADDER CARCINOMA

Gallbladder carcinoma is the most common biliary tree malignancy and is the fifth most common malignancy of the GI tract, with common risk factors being gallstones, chronic cholecystitis, porcelain gallbladder, and primary sclerosing cholangitis. There is a slight female-to-male predominance. Additional risk factors include choledochal cyst, anomalous biliary pancreatic duct union, and gallbladder polyps. Gallbladder cancers may be infiltrative, papillary, or colloid subtypes. Infiltrative forms more strongly assisted with gallstones. Most gallbladder cancers originate in the fundus. Three patterns of presentation are seen with imaging: focal or diffuse wall thickening, intraluminal polypoid mass, or subhepatic mass replacing or obliterating gallbladder and invading the adjacent liver (Table 51-3).

The management of gallbladder carcinoma is surgical. Because the extent of surgery is determined by the extent of local tumor spread, accurate staging is important. The overall accuracy for MDCT in T-stage assessment is 83.9%; the addition of multiplanar reformations to the axial CT dataset improves accuracy. The most common imaging presentation of gallbladder cancer is a gallbladder fossa mass that is difficult to separate from the liver. Because there is no serosa at the attachment of the gallbladder to the liver, the connective tissue of the gallbladder is contiguous with that of the liver, providing a ready path of spread. When there is replacement of the gallbladder by tumor, the mass often appears centrally necrotic with

TABLE 51-3 Staging of Gallbladder Cancer

TX	Primary tumor cannot be assessed
T0	No evidence of primary tumor
Tis	Carcinoma in situ
T1	Tumor invades lamina propria or muscle layer
T2	Tumor made to a muscular connective tissue does not extend through the serosa or into liver
T3	Tumor perforates serosa, directly invades an adjacent organ, or both (extension into the liver less than 2 cm)
T4	Tumor extends more than 2 cm into the liver, or into to or greater adjacent organs

irregular contrast enhancement. If tumor invades the liver, resection of segments 4, 5, and 6, or the entire right lobe, or right lobe plus segment 4 may be necessary for complete resection. Contraindications to surgical resection include multiple bilobar liver, peritoneal, or distant metastatic disease. Portal vein occlusion or encasement, or involvement of left hepatic artery preclude resection attempt if the right hepatic lobe is involved. Partial colonic and duodenal resections may be employed for complete resection. Prognosis is poor, with less than 5% overall 5-year survival, and overall mean survival of 6 months.

CHOLANGIOCARCINOMA

The majority of cholangiocarcinomas arise from the epithelium of the bile ducts. The tumors may be located within the intrahepatic ducts, the perihilar region (Klatskin tumor), or the distal extrahepatic bile duct. Anatomically, the upper third of the extrahepatic biliary tree extends from the confluence of the hepatic ducts to the level of the cystic duct, the middle third extends from the cystic duct to the upper part of the duodenum, and the lower third extends from that level to the papilla. The reported distribution of bile duct tumors is approximately 55% in the upper third, 15% in the middle third, and 10% in the lower third. Of these tumors, 10% are diffuse. There is a slight male-to-female predominance (1.3–1) with patients presenting between 50 and 70 years of age. Risk factors include sclerosing cholangitis, choledochal cyst, Caroli disease, familial polyposis, congenital hepatic fibrosis, ulcerative colitis, parasitic infection, and biliary-enteric anastomosis.

The most common presenting symptoms in patients with hilar or extrahepatic cholangiocarcinoma are abdominal pain, jaundice, weight loss, and anorexia. There are three types of cholangiocarcinomas: mass forming, periductal infiltrating/sclerosing, and papillary intraductal. Mass-forming tumors typically involve the intrahepatic ducts, have central necrosis and fibrosis, and contain satellite nodules. In the periductal infiltrating/sclerosing type, the tumor tracks along the bile duct wall and produces mural thickening and stricturing, with a dense fibroblast reaction. Intraductal papillary cholangiocarcinomas presents as an intraluminal tumor with partial duct obstruction and upstream dilation. These may track along the mucosal surface, however, and affect several segmental ducts. One very unusual type of lesion is a papillary neoplasm that produces large amounts of mucin, which may obstruct biliary flow proximally and dilate the main duct down to the papilla (distal to the lesion).

On imaging, staging of cholangiocarcinomas is difficult and depends in part on the specific morphology or lesion type. An intrahepatic cholangiocarcinoma is a poorly marginated mass that has more prominent enhancement within viable portions of the tumor typically located in the periphery of the lesion, accompanied by central necrosis. Because of the presence of fibrous tissue, the central portions of the tumor enhance during images obtained at 10 minutes or greater delay on both CT and MRI. The dense fibrosis also causes hepatic capsular retraction, seen in up to 20% of cases. Hilar cholangiocarcinomas may present as a focal area of duct thickening, an intraductal mass, or an infiltrating mass. When they arise from the right or left intrahepatic duct, by the time of diagnosis, they tend to be large and have infiltrated the hepatic parenchyma. When located in the common hepatic or common bile duct, patients present earlier because of painless jaundice. Lobar atrophy and crowding of dilated intrahepatic ducts may be seen with cross-sectional imaging in approximately one-fourth of patients presenting with hilar lesions. Lymphatic metastases are most often to the portacaval and peripancreatic lymph nodes. The extent of tumor in the bile duct determines resectability and is categorized according to the Bismuth classification (Table 51-4).

Cholangiocarcinomas involving the distal CBD tend to have a better prognosis than more central tumors. With this type of lesion, MRC or ERC may demonstrate a short stricture and/or polypoid mass that mimics a pancreatic cancer and produces biliary obstruction.

Mimics of cholangiocarcinoma are protean, include those resembling a sclerosing cholangitis pattern such as AIDS cholangiopathy, autoimmune pancreatitis, PSC, chemotherapy-induced sclerosis, and recurrent pyogenic cholangitis and those that may present with focal disease such as xanthogranulomatous cholangitis, Mirizzi syndrome, sarcoidosis, hepatocellular carcinoma, metastases, lymphoma/leukemia, and primary carcinoid tumors. In patients with sclerosing cholangitis, accurate identification of cholangiocarcinoma is difficult. Differentiating benign from developing malignant strictures in PSC patients may be aided by the following observations that tend to occur in patients with malignant lesions: clinical deterioration, acute elevation of CA 19-9, increased bile duct dilation above a dominant stricture, or a polypoid ductal mass that measures 1 cm or greater.

TABLE 51-4 Bismuth Classification of Cholangiocarcinomas

Type I	Involvement of the common hepatic duct
Type II	Involvement of the bifurcation without involvement of the secondary intrahepatic ducts
Type IIIa	Extends into the right secondary intrahepatic duct
Type IIIb	Extends into the left secondary intrahepatic duct
Type IV	Involvement of the secondary intrahepatic ducts on both sides

OTHER NEOPLASMS

Biliary cystadenomas and cystadenocarcinomas are rare tumors of the biliary tree, which usually arise in the liver rather than the extrahepatic ducts. They are much more common in women and tend to occur in patients older than 30 years of age. Presenting symptoms are nonspecific, despite the tumors being large at presentation (most greater than 10 cm, range 3–25 cm). Like their counterpart in the pancreas, the mucinous cystic neoplasm, these lesions are most often multiloculated cystic masses containing internal septations and enhancing nodules. Unilocular lesions do occur and more frequently indicate a malignant cystadenocarcinoma rather than the benign cystadenoma. Both lesions should be resected, as cystadenocarcinomas are thought to arise from cystadenomas and the lesions cannot be reliably differentiated with imaging, biopsy, or even examination of the macroscopic specimens. Surgical resection is curative in most cases.

Periampullary tumors are described as those that arise within 2 cm of the papilla of Vater. These include ampullary, pancreatic, bile duct, and duodenal cancers; it may be difficult with imaging to determine the exact origin. Most patients with periampullary lesions present with biliary dilation extending to the ampulla, and identification of masses may be difficult to detect on CT. The most favorable resectability rates and survival occur in patients with distal cholangiocarcinomas (5-year overall survival 15%–28%) and periampullary tumors (5-year overall survival 50%–60%).

Biliary papillomatosis is a rare condition characterized by multiple papillary adenomas that may involve the intra- or extrahepatic biliary tree. These multifocal lesions are considered benign but have a high potential for malignant transformation. There are associations with Caroli's disease, choledochal cyst, familial polyposis coli, ulcerative colitis, and cirrhosis caused by hepatitis B and C. The condition is more common in men (2:1 male-to-female ratio) with clinical symptoms of jaundice, abdominal pain, and acute cholangitis. It may be difficult to distinguish biliary papillomatosis from other inflammatory conditions. On CT, dilation of both intra- and extrahepatic bile ducts may be seen along with hypoattenuating, intraductal soft-tissue masses. As opposed to cholangiocarcinomas, on MRI, the papillomas may remain hypointense relative to the adjacent parenchyma after intravenous contrast administration; however, enhancement patterns are diverse. On ERC, multiple filling defects, dilated biliary tree, and serration of the bile duct wall may be present. The disease may be confined to intra- or extrahepatic bile ducts.

Biliary intraductal papillary mucinous neoplasm (IPMN) arise from stem cells of the bile duct cells, biliary epithelium, or peribiliary gland epithelium and are characterized by papillary growth or mucosal spread along the bile duct. Hypersecretion is a frequent manifestation, and this produces marked dilation of the affected ducts. Occasionally, portions of the biliary system not affected by the neoplasm are also dilated due to mucin production. The gross and microscopic appearance of biliary IPMN depends on epithelial proliferation versus the amount of mucin secretion. When the former predominates, intraductal papillary mass formation is evident, and when the latter predominates, the ducts are grossly dilated and filled with mucin. When there is recognizable lobar or segmental bile duct dilation without a mass, accompanied by severe hepatic peripheral atrophy of the affected segment, the possibility of a biliary IPMN should be considered. Treatment is surgical, and if successful, long-term survival is good.

Gallbladder lymphoma is rare and may be secondary to systemic disease or represent a primary non-Hodgkin lymphoma arising from mucosal associated lymph tissue (MALT). In addition to lymphoma, other rare primary tumors of the biliary tree include carcinoid, extrahepatic biliary cystadenoma and cystadenocarcinoma (much more commonly seen in the liver rather than in the extrahepatic bile duct), and embryonal rhabdomyosarcoma (sarcoma botryoides). Biliary metastases are not uncommon. The bile ducts may be directly invaded by adjacent gallbladder carcinoma, hepatocellular carcinoma, and colorectal cancer metastases. The extrahepatic bile duct is affected by metastases to periportal lymph nodes, which may arise from a variety of tumors, most commonly colorectal carcinoma, but also seen in breast, lung, prostate, and other common cancers. Rare, hematogenous metastases to the biliary system may be seen in patients with melanoma; when isolated, these are surgically resected.

TRANSPLANTATION

Preoperative imaging is important in the evaluation of potential living hepatic donors. Parenchymal (focal or diffuse) disease as well as biliary or vascular abnormalities or variations that may alter the surgical methodology and/or morbidity for partial hepatectomy can be detected preoperatively with imaging. Comprehensive MRI examination includes assessment of the biliary tree, but the examination may be limited for the detection and definition of intrahepatic biliary anatomic anomalies because the donor systems are usually nondilated. Ductal anomalies such as aberrant drainage of right posterior segmental branch into the left hepatic duct or into the bifurcation (producing a biliary "trifurcation") preclude a single duct-to-duct biliary anastomosis and require additional biliary anastomosis to be performed, possibly increasing morbidity. In general, three-dimensional, heavily T2-weighted "fluid-sensitive" MRC images provide superior biliary visualization compared to 2D T2-weighted MRC images caused by increased signal to noise in these nondilated systems. Potential off-label use of gadolinium products that are excreted through the biliary pathway may aid in visualization of the bile ducts, but their role in preoperative assessment is not yet established.

After transplantation, the most common and clinically significant complications include arterial venous thromboses and stenoses, fluid collections, rejection, and biliary disorders. Biliary complications occur in an estimated 25% of liver transit recipients typically within the first 3 months following transplantation. Complications include stenosis/obstruction, bile leaks, stone formation, sphincter of Oddi dysfunction, and recurrent biliary disease. In transplant recipients, the usual biliary anastomosis is a choledochocholedochostomy, with a T tube left in place across the anastomosis for 3 to 6 months. A Roux-en-Y choledochojejunostomy may be performed when there is a discrepancy in donor and recipient duct size, or when there is an existing disease affecting the recipient duct such as biliary atresia, sclerosing cholangitis, or primary biliary cirrhosis. Evaluation of the ducts is usually carried out with ultrasound and T-tube cholangiography during the initial months after transplantation, however, after removal of the biliary catheters, MRC, ERC, or percutaneous transhepatic cholangiography may be employed.

Obstruction is the most common postliver transplant biliary complication, is usually caused by stenosis at the anastomotic site, and results from fibrotic proliferation and narrowing of the bile duct lumen. Occasionally, ischemia related to hepatic arterial thrombosis or stenosis may lead to bile duct stricturing. Strictures located elsewhere along the duct may be related to pretransplant biliary diseases such as sclerosing cholangitis. Diffuse ductal dilation may result from papillary dyskinesia brought on by devascularization or denervation of the papilla of Vater during surgery. The incidence of bile leaks in liver transplant recipients is approximately 5%. These usually present early, with 70% occurring in the first month after surgery. Leaks are generally from the T-tube site and treatment includes stent placement, plus drainage of any focal collections. Ductal ischemia results from stenosis or thrombosis of the hepatic artery, upon which the bile ducts depend entirely for the blood supply. Ductal ischemia may lead to necrosis resulting in bile leak, biloma, and duct scarring with fibrosis.

Following laparoscopic cholecystectomy, a spectrum of biliary complications may occur. Early recognition and diagnosis of these complications helps to minimize morbidity. Biliary complications include retained stones in the cystic duct or common duct, bile leak, iatrogenic bile duct obstruction or injury, and delayed biliary obstruction with stricture. MRC is an effective method for depicting remnant stones, which may produce biliary obstruction after laparoscopic cholecystectomy. Bile leakage is the most common complication, with most leaks occurring from the cystic duct stump. Other causes of bile leak in the postlaparoscopic cholecystectomy patient include unintentional laceration, duct transection, or thermal injury. Bile leaks are often diagnosed with a hepatoscintigraphy or ERC, the latter also providing a mechanism for therapy. Acute bile duct obstruction is twice as common with a laparoscopic approach compared to open cholecystectomy. Classically, the surgeon mistakes the CHD for a cystic duct and places a clip on the CHD resulting in acute biliary obstruction. Failure of recognition of anomalous bile ducts may lead to clipping of these structures as well, producing segmental biliary obstruction. In the past, percutaneous transhepatic cholangiography was used to identify the upstream-obstructed duct and ERC the location of the obstruction and "missing" upstream duct from below. Both may be visualized with MRC nowadays. Injuries to the main bile ducts are grouped according to the Bismuth classification, which designates types I through IV from the lowest part of the CHD to progressively higher levels. When a ligation or excision injury is present, the length of the intact common duct distal to the biliary confluence determines whether a choledochojejunostomy or hepaticojejunostomy is performed. Late strictures of the extrahepatic ducts are probably caused by thermal injury with mild (nontransmural) effects on the bile duct that result in stricturing from fibrosis. Abscess and retention of peritoneal gallstones that are spilled during the laparoscopic cholecystectomy may be observed readily with CT.

Other surgeries resulting in alterations of the biliary tract such as hepatic resection and biliary-enteric anastomosis may be evaluated with imaging. In particular, biliary-enteric anastomosis may preclude the option for ERC, and the use of MRC is most advantageous in these cases. Biliary-enteric anastomosis may be associated with anastomotic structuring as well as stone formation, even when the anastomosis is fully patent.

TRAUMA

Biliary tract injuries may result from blunt abdominal trauma. The most common location of biliary injury is the gallbladder, occurring in approximately 3% of blunt trauma patients undergoing laparotomy. There is a high association with additional injuries, including hepatic (up to 91%), splenic (up to 54%) and duodenal (up to 54%). Injuries to the gallbladder may be classified into three categories: contusion, laceration/perforation, or complete avulsion. Contusions, or intramural hematomas, are the mildest form of gallbladder injury and are generally treated conservatively. Lacerations and perforations are full-thickness wall injuries and require cholecystectomy. Avulsion of gallbladder may involve all or portions of the gallbladder as well as the cystic duct and cystic artery, the latter leading to major blood loss. CT signs of gallbladder injuries caused by blunt trauma include collapsed gallbladder in a fasting patient, ill-defined or thickened wall, pericholecystic fluid, and active extravasation caused by transection of the cystic artery.

Injuries to the extrahepatic bile duct are the second most common type of biliary injury and typically occur at sites of anatomic fixation after blunt trauma or deceleration mechanism. Delayed complications may result from biliary leakage; symptoms tend to be present when the leaking bile is infected and may include vague abdominal pain, nausea and vomiting, and occasionally jaundice. Intrahepatic bile duct injury occurs rarely and is seen only in patients with severe liver lacerations. While MRCP is commonly used to evaluate iatrogenic injuries, its use in the setting of acute trauma is not established. ERCP is often most helpful for identifying the level of bile extravasation, with the added potential for stenting in appropriate cases.

SUGGESTED READING

Bornman PC, van Beljon JI, Krige JEJ. Management of cholangitis. *J Hepatobiliary Pancreat Surg*. 2003;10:406-414.

Catalano OA, Sahani DV, Kalva SP, et al. MR imaging of the gallbladder: a pictorial essay. *Radiographics*. 2008;28:135-155.

Chung YE, Kim MJ, ParkYN, LeeYH, Choi JY. Staging of extrahepatic cholangiocarcinoma. *Eur Radiol*. 2008;18:2182-2195.

Gore RM, Shelhamer RP. Biliary tract neoplasms: diagnosis and staging. *Cancer Imaging*. 2007;7:S15-S23.

Gupta A, Stuhlfaut JW, Fleming KW, Lucey BC, Soto JA. Blunt trauma of the pancreas and biliary tract: a multimodality imaging approach to diagnosis. *Radiographics*. 2004;24:1381-1395.

Hoeffel C, Azizi L, Lewin M, et al. Normal and pathologic features of the postoperative biliary tract at 3D MR cholangiopancreatography and MR imaging. *Radiographics*. 2006;26:1603-1620.

Lim JH, Kim SY, Park CM. Parasitic diseases of the biliary tract. *AJR Am J Roentgenol*. 2007;188:1596-1603.

Menias CO, Surabhi VR, Prasad SR, Wang HL, Narra VR, Chintapalli KN. Mimics of cholangiocarcinoma: spectrum of disease. *Radiographics*. 2008;28:1115-1129.

Sainani NI, Catalano OA, Holalkere NS, Zhu AX, Hahn PF, Sahani DV. Cholangiocarcioma: current and novel imaging techniques. *Radiographics*. 2008;28:1263-1287.

Weismueller TJ, Wedemeyer J, Kubika S, Strassburg CP, Manns MP. The challenges in primary sclerosing cholangitis: aetiopthogenesis, autoimmunity, management and malignancy. *J Hepatol*. 2008;48:S38-S57.

Wilcox CM, Mönkemüller KE. Hepatobiliary diseases in patients with AIDS: focus on AIDS cholangiopathy and gallbladder disease. *Dig Dis*. 1998;16:205-213.

Yu J, Turner MA, Fulcher AS, Halvorsen RA. Congenital anomalies and normal variants of the pancreaticobiliary tract and the pancreas in adults: part I, biliary tract. *AJR Am J Roentgenol*. 2006;187:1536-1543.

QUESTIONS AND ANSWERS

1. What is the most common type of choledochal cyst?
   A. Type I
   B. Type II
   C. Type III
   D. Type IV

   ANSWER: A. A type I choledochal cyst involves the extrahepatic bile duct; type Ic, fusiform dilation of the extrahepatic bile duct, represents 80% to 90% of all choledochal cysts.

2. What is the most common anomalous drainage of the biliary system?
   A. Trifurcation of the confluence
   B. Right posterior duct insertion into left hepatic duct above the confluence
   C. Drainage through ducts of Luschka
   D. Cystic duct insertion into left hepatic duct

   ANSWER: B. The most common anomalous drainage of the biliary system is drainage of the right posterior duct into the left hepatic duct above the confluence. Although triple confluence is also common, it is not as common as the correct response. The other answers are much less common.

3. Which of the following conditions are represented by the "interrupted rim sign" on CT or MR imaging of the gallbladder in a patient with right upper quadrant pain?
   A. Adenomyomatosis
   B. Pericholecystic varices in portal hypertension

C. Acalculous cholecystitis
D. Gangrenous cholecystitis

ANSWER: D. Gangrenous acute cholecystitis is characterized by focal areas of necrosis in the wall, which are represented by patchy enhancement of the gallbladder mucosa on contrast-enhanced CT or MRI in patients with acute cholecystitis. Adenomyomatosis would give rise to a thickened but enhancing wall, pericholecystic varices would be brighter than the wall but the mucosal enhancement would not be patchy, and acalculous cholecystitis could be severe enough to developed gangrene, but is not as correct as the key.

4. Impaction of a stone in the gallbladder neck producing inflammation of the adjacent common hepatic duct and intrahepatic bile duct dilation describes which of the following conditions?
A. Choledocholithiasis
B. Charcot triad
C. Mirizzi syndrome
D. Carcinoid syndrome

ANSWER: C. This syndrome was described as impaction of gallstone within the gallbladder neck or cystic duct leading to extrinsic common hepatic duct compression and biliary obstruction in a patient with or without gallbladder. Choledocholithiasis refers to stones located within the biliary tree that may produce obstruction; Charcot triad is the constellation of jaundice, fever, and right upper quadrant pain that described the classic presentation of patients with cholangitis. Carcinoid syndrome describes symptomatic abnormalities present when there are carcinoid metastases in the liver.

5. What percentage of patients with acute cholecystitis have no gallstones?
A. 10%
B. 20%
C. 30%
D. 40%

ANSWER: A. Approximately 10% of all patients presenting with acute cholecystitis have no gallstones.

6. What percentage of patients with primary sclerosing cholangitis have associated inflammatory bowel disease?
A. 15%
B. 25%
C. 40%
D. 65%

ANSWER: D. Approximately 62% to 72% of patients with PSC have concomitant inflammatory bowel disease. Ulcerative colitis is much more common (80%) than Crohn disease in patients with both PSC and inflammatory bowel disease.

7. Which location in the biliary tree is most commonly affected by cholangiocarcinoma?
A. Intrahepatic ducts
B. Hilar/upper third of extrahepatic bile duct
C. Middle third of extrahepatic bile duct
D. Lower third of extrahepatic bile duct (periampullary)

ANSWER: B. The majority of cholangiocarcinomas arise from the epithelium of the bile duct in the upper third or perihilar region (Klatskin tumors). Although cholangiocarcinomas may arise within intrahepatic ducts and other locations along the course of the biliary tree, they are not as common as lesions in and around the confluence.

8. What is the most common biliary complication encountered in patients after liver transplantation?
A. Bile duct leak from the cystic duct stump
B. Obstruction/stenosis at the anastomosis
C. Recurrent stone formation
D. Sphincter of Oddi dysfunction

ANSWER: B. Obstruction is the most common postliver transplant biliary complication and is usually caused by stenosis at the anastomotic site. The other answers are all potential complications after liver transplant surgery, but are not as common.

9. What is the most common biliary complication encountered in patients after laparoscopic cholecystectomy?
A. Bile duct leak from the cystic duct stump
B. Acute bile duct obstruction
C. Retained stones
D. Delayed biliary obstruction with stricture

ANSWER: A. This typically occurs from the cystic duct stump. Acute bile duct obstruction caused by incorrect clip placement is twice as common during laparoscopic compared to open cholecystectomy, but is not the most common complication overall. Retained stones and delayed biliary obstruction are possible but less common.

10. Which location is the most common site of biliary tract injury caused by blunt abdominal trauma?
A. Intrahepatic ducts
B. Gallbladder

C. Extrahepatic bile duct
D. Intrapancreatic bile duct

ANSWER: B. The most common location of biliary injury is the gallbladder, occurring in approximately 3% to blunt trauma patients who undergo laparotomy. The extrahepatic bile duct is the second most common location. The portions of the bile duct within the liver and within the pancreas are relatively more protected and less commonly injured.

52 SPLEEN

Andrew S. Ferrell, Katherine P. Lursen, and Robert E. Koehler

THE NORMAL SPLEEN

ANATOMY

The spleen is located in the peritoneal cavity of the left upper abdomen, posterior and lateral to the stomach. By the age of 15, it normally reaches approximately 12 cm in length, 7 cm in width, and 3 cm in thickness. The splenic artery usually arises from the celiac artery, the most common alternate origins being the aorta and superior mesenteric artery. The splenic artery and vein course behind the pancreas to the splenic hilum, where each of them divides into multiple branches before entering the spleen. The splenic artery is essentially an end vessel with relatively little collateral flow, although there is some communication with small arteries in the pancreas and with short gastric arteries extending from the greater curvature of the stomach. Occlusion of the splenic artery therefore often results in splenic infarction.

The spleen is nearly entirely covered by peritoneum and is suspended by several supporting peritoneal ligaments. The gastrosplenic ligament passes from the splenic hilum to the greater curvature of the stomach and is formed by fusion of the lesser and greater peritoneal sacs. It contains the short gastric and left gastroepiploic vessels. The splenorenal ligament passes from the spleen to the left kidney and contains the splenic artery and vein and a portion of the tail of the pancreas. The phrenicocolic ligament connects the lower pole of the spleen to the splenic flexure of the colon and to the diaphragm.

HISTOLOGY AND FUNCTION

The splenic parenchyma consists of "red pulp" and "white pulp," the red pulp being the predominant tissue in the normal spleen. The white pulp is made up of lymphoid tissue arranged in sheaths around the arterioles that deliver blood to the spleen. This is where splenic T and B lymphocytes interact immunologically with the plasma.

From the white pulp, blood flows on through an array of splenic cords and venous sinuses, which together comprise the red pulp. The cords and blood-filled sinuses of the red pulp are lined with macrophages, which phagocytize abnormal erythrocytes and those at the end of their 100-to 120-day life, aging white blood cells and platelets, and circulating bacteria.

The spleen also serves as a reservoir for blood. Its capsule contains smooth muscle that enables it to function as an expandable and contractible sac, changing in size in response to variations in the body's blood volume. Although the spleen serves as a site of red blood cell production in the fetus, it does not normally exhibit hematopoietic activity after infancy.

IMAGING APPEARANCE

The spleen has a lobular contour and may have prominent clefts, which should not be mistaken for lacerations. It is normally less dense than the liver on both unenhanced and contrast-enhanced CT images. The spleen is normally at least 15 HU less dense than the liver on noncontrast CT images. If it is not, then either the liver is fatty or the spleen contains excess iron. On contrast-enhanced CT images, if the spleen is more than 25 HU denser than the liver, then hepatic steatosis is usually present. On MRI T1-weighted images, the spleen is hypointense to the liver, while it appears hyperintense to the liver on T2-weighted images.

The normal splenic parenchyma has a diffusely homogeneous appearance on CT and MR images. An exception to this is seen on images obtained by either method a few seconds after administration of intravenous contrast material. These arterial-phase images show marked heterogeneity in parenchymal enhancement because of the variable rate at which the contrast agent reaches different regions within the spleen. The resulting appearance is sometimes referred to as showing multiple "pseudomasses." On ultrasound images, the spleen has a homogeneous echotexture with midlevel echoes, slightly more echogenic than the liver, and equal to or greater than the adjacent left kidney.

Splenic clefts are commonly seen on imaging studies. They are thought to be due to the fact that the spleen forms by coalescence of multiple cellular aggregates, sometimes leaving spaces between incompletely fused embryologic tissues. Clefts are most commonly seen along the lateral or superior borders and are of no clinical significance other than occasionally being mistaken for lacerations in the setting of trauma.

CONGENITAL ABNORMALITIES

Accessory Spleens

One or more accessory spleens, also known as splenules, are present in 10% to 20% of individuals. They are derived from embryological splenic tissue that fails to fuse with the remainder of the spleen. Accessory spleens are usually spherical, smoothly marginated, and 2 cm or less in size. Most lie near the splenic hilum or in one of the suspensory peritoneal ligaments of the spleen, often the gastrosplenic ligament.

The CT attenuation value and MR signal characteristics of accessory splenic tissue mimic those of normal splenic parenchyma. This is also true of the uptake and clearance of a variety of intravenously administered CT and MRI contrast agents. Uptake and retention of Tc-99m-sulfur colloid by reticuloendothelial tissue in an accessory spleen is similar to that of normal splenic tissue, so radionuclide imaging with this agent can be used to distinguish an accessory spleen from a lymph node enlarged by lymphoma.

After splenectomy for treatment of a variety of hematologic conditions, such as autoimmune hemolytic anemia and idiopathic thrombocytopenic purpura, an accessory spleen that was not removed at the time of splenectomy may later hypertrophy and present as an abdominal mass. Hypertrophy of an accessory spleen can also lead to recurrence of the original hematologic disease.

Situs and Heterotaxia Syndromes (Polysplenia/Asplenia)

The term situs solitus is derived from the Latin words situs, meaning position, and solitus, meaning customary. Situs solitus is the normal anatomic arrangement in which the cardiac apex, stomach, spleen, and abdominal aorta lie on the left of the midsagittal plane, and the liver and inferior vena cava lie on the right.

Abdominal situs inversus is said to exist when there is a mirror image location of the abdominal viscera, opposite to that in persons with situs solitus. There are two subtypes, one associated with levocardia and the other with dextrocardia. Situs inversus with dextrocardia is more common with the cardiac apex, spleen, stomach, and aorta, all located on the right and the liver and inferior vena cava on the left. Congenital heart disease is present in only 3% to 5% of such cases. Situs inversus with levocardia is extremely rare and is characterized by mirror image location of the abdominal viscera and a left-sided cardiac apex. Nearly, all affected individuals have congenital heart disease, which usually leads to diagnosis in early infancy.

Situs ambiguous, also known as heterotaxia, is an abnormal arrangement of viscera and great vessels that is variable and does not fit the pattern of either situs solitus or situs inversus. Congenital heart disease coexists in 50% to 100% of cases according to Fulcher, and there may also be malrotation of the gut, biliary atresia, immunodeficiency, and other serious conditions. Situs ambiguous typically occurs in association with either polysplenia or asplenia and this feature can be used to classify the condition into these two subtypes.

Situs ambiguous with asplenia (Ivemark syndrome), also referred to as right isomerism or bilateral right-sidedness, is characterized by ambiguous location of the abdominal organs and congenital absence of most or all normal splenic tissue. A rudimentary amount of splenic tissue may be present. Approximately two-thirds of reported cases are in males. Congenital heart disease is present in most or all cases. Affected individuals often die within the first year of life because of the associated severe congenital heart disease and immunodeficiency related to the absence of the spleen.

Situs ambiguous with polysplenia, also referred to as left isomerism or bilateral left-sidedness, is characterized by midline or ambiguous location of multiple abdominal organs and the presence of multiple spleens. Associated congenital heart disease, when present, tends to be less severe than in persons with situs ambiguous with asplenia. Absence of the hepatic portion of the inferior vena cava is characteristic, with an enlarged azygous vein carrying venous blood from the abdomen to the right atrium (azygous continuation).

Wandering Spleen

The term wandering spleen is applied when there is a normally formed and functioning spleen that lies out of its expected left upper abdominal location. This is because of laxity of the spleen's supporting peritoneal ligaments in association with abnormalities of intestinal rotation. A wandering spleen may be found anywhere in the abdomen and may present as a palpable abdominal mass. If the lax splenic ligaments become twisted, the resulting torsion of the splenic pedicle can cause ischemia and acute or chronic abdominal pain. Chronic torsion may lead to splenomegaly or gastric varices. If this prevents arterial blood from reaching the spleen, the spleen will not enhance with intravenously administered radiologic contrast agents.

Splenomegaly

Splenomegaly is the most common radiologically demonstrable abnormality of the spleen. It has many

TABLE 52-1 Causes of Splenomegaly

Causes
Venous obstruction, e.g., cirrhosis, portal vein thrombosis, congestive heart failure
Lymphoma, leukemia
Metastasis
Primary splenic cysts and tumors
Posttraumatic pseudocyst following subcapsular hematoma
Extramedullary hematopoiesis, e.g., myelofibrosis, osteopetrosis, congenital hemolytic anemias
Splenic hyperplasia caused by infection
Chronic viral infections, e.g., Ebstein-Barr, cytomegalovirus
Bacterial, fungal, and protozoal infections, e.g., schistosomiasis
Collagen vascular diseases
Entities mainly seen in children
Acute viral infections
Juvenile rheumatoid arthritis
Histiocytic disorders, e.g., Langerhans cell histiocytosis
Storage diseases, e.g., Gaucher, Niemann-Pick (accumulation of abnormal lipids in splenic macrophages)

TABLE 52-2 AAST Grading System for Splenic Injury

Grade	Injury
Grade I	Subcapsular hematoma of less than 10% of surface area
	Capsular tear of less than 1 cm in depth
Grade II	Subcapsular hematoma of 10%–50% of surface area
	Intraparenchymal hematoma of less than 5 cm in diameter
	Laceration of 1–3 cm in depth and not involving trabecular vessels
Grade III	Subcapsular hematoma of greater than 50% of surface area or expanding and ruptured subcapsular or parenchymal hematoma
	Intraparenchymal hematoma of greater than 5 cm or expanding
	Laceration of greater than 3 cm in depth or involving trabecular vessels
Grade IV	Laceration involving segmental or hilar vessels with devascularization of more than 25% of the spleen
Grade V	Shattered spleen or hilar vascular injury

causes (Table 52-1), most related to diseases originating in other organs. There are vascular, hematologic, infectious, neoplastic, immunologic, and metabolic causes of splenomegaly. The most common cause of splenomegaly in adults is portal hypertension.

Trauma

The spleen is the most commonly injured solid thoracoabdominal organ representing approximately 25% of all significant injuries to the abdominal viscera because of blunt trauma. Combine this with the fact that the spleen contains approximately 1 unit of blood at a given time, and splenic injury poses a potentially life-threatening situation. Splenic trauma may have a surprisingly subtle clinical presentation. Abdominal tenderness and distention are seen in approximately 50% of patients, while hypotension is a presenting sign in only 25% to 30% of patients. In the modern setting, contrast-enhanced CT is the diagnostic method of choice with a sensitivity and specificity of nearly 100%. The limitations of CT in this context are related to motion artifact, misinterpretation of the normal heterogeneous perfusion seen on early arterial phase images, and mistaking a normal splenic cleft for a laceration. The use of intravenous contrast material is important because acute splenic hematomas frequently exhibit similar CT attenuation to that of normal splenic parenchyma on CT images without contrast enhancement. CT is also useful for demonstrating extravasation of intravascular contrast material in patients who are actively bleeding at the time of the scan.

Blunt splenic trauma can cause subcapsular hematoma, intraparenchymal hematoma, laceration, or massive fragmentation resulting in autosplenectomy. The Organ Injury Scaling Committee of the American Association for the Surgery of Trauma revised its splenic injury grading system in 1994. This system (Table 52-2) can be used as a guide to classifying the severity of CT findings of splenic injury; however, it has not been proven to correlate closely with clinical prognosis.

Splenosis

Splenosis refers to implants of viable splenic tissue that are disseminated at the time of splenic trauma or splenectomy. The implants are usually multiple and grow into spherical nodules varying from a few mm to 3 cm in size. They typically lie in the peritoneal cavity of the upper abdomen, but can develop in the thorax if the original splenic injury was associated with diaphragmatic rupture. Splenosis is reported to occur in 40% to 60% of splenic injuries. The splenic nature of the nodules can be confirmed with Tc-99m-sulfur colloid imaging since they retain their original reticuloendothelial activity.

SPLENIC MASSES

Cysts

Posttraumatic cysts, or pseudocysts, are the most common cystic lesions of the spleen. They occur as a result of previous splenic hemorrhage, infarction, or infection. Pseudocysts have no epithelial lining. They may have a thick wall, septations, or prominent curvilinear calcifications. They typically display sonographic findings similar to those of simple cysts in the kidneys or other organs, that is, hypoechoic contents and acoustic enhancement behind the lesion. Alternatively, the fluid within a posttraumatic splenic pseudocyst may contain echoes related to blood products, cholesterol crystals, or cellular debris.

Epidermoid cysts are congenital in origin. They result from infolding or entrapment of peritoneum within the spleen during its formation. They are therefore lined with epithelium, unlike pseudocysts, which lack an epithelial lining and cystic lymphangiomas and hemangiomas, which are lined with endothelium. Epidermoid cysts grow slowly and are usually asymptomatic. They have an average size of 10 cm at the time of discovery, typically in persons aged 10 to 30 years. Eighty percent are unilocular and solitary. Curvilinear wall calcification occurs in up to one quarter of these lesions, and they often have internal septations and a trabeculated wall. Traumatic rupture and infection are very rare but have been described. Epidermoid cysts are often difficult to distinguish from posttraumatic pseudocysts on imaging studies.

Hydatid or echinococcal cysts are caused by infection with *Echinococcus granulosus*. They usually are seen in association with similar lesions in the liver or lung. While *E. granulosus* infection is the most common cause of calcified splenic cysts worldwide, this organism is rare outside its usual geographic range and hydrated cysts are rarely seen in North America. Hydatid cysts consist of a spherical mother cyst that usually contains smaller daughter cysts that may be seen within it. There can also be internal septations and debris, referred to as hydatid sand. Thick ringlike wall calcification may be seen.

Pancreatic pseudocysts may extend from the pancreatic tail into the splenic hilum. From there, they may erode into the splenic parenchyma or subcapsular space. Associated imaging features of pancreatitis and the presence of other peripancreatic fluid collections usually make the imaging diagnosis straightforward. A variety of splenic neoplasms can also appear cystic as can resolving splenic infarction (Table 52-3).

Lymphoma

Lymphoma is the most common malignant tumor of the spleen. It is usually seen as a manifestation of systemic disease. Lymphadenopathy is usually detectable on imaging studies. The most frequent finding is splenomegaly, and this may be the only finding in patients with low-grade lymphomas. Hodgkins lymphoma and higher-grade lymphomas usually show discrete nodules of tumor.

On ultrasound images, lymphomatous deposits typically appear as focal, ill-defined, heterogeneous, and hypoechoic lesions. On contrast-enhanced CT, they are typically lower in density than the surrounding parenchyma, while on MRI they are low on T1-weighted images and varied in signal intensity on T2-weighted images. Lymphomatous nodules usually enhance with intravenous contrast agents. The reported accuracy of contrast-enhanced CT for detecting splenic involvement varies from 37% to 91%. Fortunately the foci of lymphoma within the spleen show increased radionuclide uptake on FDG PET, which has a reported sensitivity approaching 100%.

Metastasis

Splenic metastases are commonly found at autopsy but often go undetected on radiologic studies. When they are seen, they may be visible only on arterial-phase contrast-enhanced images. According to Rabushka et al., the most common primary tumor to metastasize to the spleen is carcinoma of the breast. Malignant melanoma and carcinoma of the lung, ovary, stomach, and prostate are also relatively common (Table 52-4). On CT, metastases appear as low attenuating cystic or solid lesions. Contrast enhancement can be heterogeneous or homogenous. Necrosis is common while calcification is rare. Sonographically, splenic metastases are usually hypoechoic.

Primary Malignant Tumors

Other than lymphoma, the spleen is rarely the site of primary malignant tumors. Of those that do occur, Abbott reports angiosarcoma to be the most common tumor. It is an aggressive tumor with a poor prognosis. CT shows a poorly defined area of heterogeneous or low attenuation in an enlarged spleen. These tumors may contain areas of necrosis and be associated subcapsular hematoma. The spleen can rupture spontaneously in patients with splenic hemangiosarcoma. Contrast enhancement is usually poor. On ultrasound, one sees an enlarged spleen with one or more solid heterogeneous echogenic masses. MR findings are varied and not specific.

TABLE 52-3 Cystic Lesions of the Spleen

Congenital (epidermoid) cyst
Abscess (hydatid, bacterial)
Hematoma, posttraumatic pseudocyst
Infarction
Cystic neoplasms (hemangioma, lymphangioma, lymphoma, metastasis)
Pancreatic pseudocyst

TABLE 52-4 Tumors That Metastasize to the Spleen

TUMOR TYPE	PERCENT OF SPLENIC METASTASES (%)
Breast carcinoma	21
Bronchogenic carcinoma	18
Ovarian carcinoma	8
Gastric carcinoma	7
Melanoma	6
Prostatic carcinoma	6

Benign Tumors

While a variety of benign neoplasms can affect the spleen, hemangioma is the most common. It consists of vascular channels lined by endothelium. On CT, a hemangioma may appear as a smooth, well-marginated nodule, which demonstrates marked homogenous enhancement with delayed washout. The peripheral nodular contrast enhancement and centripetal fill-in typically seen with hepatic hemangiomas is often lacking, especially if the tumor is smaller than 2 cm. Small splenic hemangiomas may show no contrast enhancement at all. There may be punctate central or peripheral curvilinear calcification. Ultrasound demonstrates a well-defined echogenic solid or complex cystic mass. On MRI, the lesion is low in intensity on T1 and high intensity on T2, with a variable contrast enhancement pattern. The imaging appearance of splenic hemangiomas is sufficiently variable that differentiation from angiosarcoma is usually not possible on radiologic grounds.

Lymphangiomas are very rare in the spleen. They are often indistinguishable from cysts on ultrasound, CT, and MR and can contain peripheral rim calcifications.

Splenic hamartomas are also rare benign neoplasms and are usually detected incidentally. They are usually less than 3 cm in diameter. Larger lesions can present with splenomegaly, palpable mass, or rupture. Sequestration of hematopoietic cells in large hamartomas can cause thrombocytopenia or anemia. Splenic hamartomas sometimes occur in association with tuberous sclerosis.

Most splenic hamartomas appear hypodense or isodense on unenhanced CT and show moderate heterogeneous enhancement when intravenous contrast material is administered. They can, however, appear hyperdense on unenhanced CT because of hemosiderin deposition. Sonographically, they appear as solid masses with mixed echogenicity, with or without small cystic and hyperechoic areas. On MR imaging, hamartomas appear isointense on T1 and hyperintense on T2.

The radiologic characterization of other splenic neoplasms of vascular origin is further complicated by the fact that some have variable biologic behavior that makes their benign or malignant nature difficult to predict. These include littoral cell angioma, hemangioendothelioma, and hemangiopericytoma.

INFECTION

Granulomatous Infection

The most common radiologically detected splenic infection is histoplasmosis Radiographs, CT, MRI, and ultrasonography all show multiple, punctate, round calcifications in the splenic parenchyma that are less than 1 cm in size. These lesions represent calcified granulomas that are no longer active. Granulomas in longstanding inactive splenic tuberculosis can have a similar radiologic appearance, but tuberculosis is a less common cause of small-calcified splenic granulomas than histoplasmosis. If more than five small-calcified splenic granulomas are seen, histoplasmosis is the likely diagnosis.

Rarely brucellosis can also cause calcified granulomas of the spleen. The granulomas are usually solitary and 2 cm or larger in size. They may have a low-density center encircled by a calcified outer layer, giving the lesion a bull's-eye appearance.

Abscess

Bacterial abscesses, although rare in the spleen, carry a high mortality rate unless diagnosed and treated early. They are typically caused by hematogenous seeding. On CT, they usually appear as well-defined, low attenuating lesions, sometimes with rim enhancement. Unfortunately, their imaging appearance is not specific, although the occasional finding of gas within the abscess is a rare but fairly specific finding.

Fungal abscesses in the spleen, usually because of *Candida albicans*, have a different appearance. They occur in immunocompromised individuals and, like bacterial abscesses, are usually a sequela of bloodborne infection. The typical CT appearance is one of multiple, round, low-density lesions that are usually 5 to 20 mm in size. On ultrasound images, they are hypo- or anechoic and ill-defined. MRI shows multiple small lesions with low signal intensity on T1-weighted images and high signal intensity on T2-weighted images.

On rare occasions, patients with severely immunocompromised function can develop disseminated infection with *Pneumocystis carinii.* In the spleen, this takes the form of multiple small abscesses. CT shows multiple, round, well-circumscribed, low attenuation lesions that may be associated with calcification.

VASCULAR ABNORMALITIES

Splenic Artery Aneurysm

Splenic artery aneurysm is the most common visceral arterial aneurysm. These can be caused by atherosclerosis, pancreatitis, or trauma. The incidence is higher in females than males and in women of childbearing age who have had two or more pregnancies. Although usually asymptomatic, left upper quadrant pain or fullness is sometimes a complaint. The aneurysm is usually saccular in the mid-to-distal artery. Calcification of the aneurysm wall is usually more irregular than that seen in splenic cysts. Diffuse calcification of the splenic artery should suggest atherosclerosis as the cause. Rupture of a splenic artery aneurysm is rare but can be fatal when it does occur and for this reason, aneurysms over 2 to 3 cm and those in younger patients are sometimes treated by transcatheter embolization or surgery.

Splenic Vein Thrombosis

Splenic vein thrombosis is a relatively common sequela of pancreatitis. It can also be related to other inflammatory conditions such as diverticulitis or Crohn enteritis. Splenic vein occlusion leads to the development of varices of the gastric cardia and proximal stomach (short gastric veins).

Infarction

Splenic infarction is a consideration in patients who present with acute left upper abdominal pain. A number of conditions predispose patients to the development of splenic infarction (Table 52-5). These include arterial embolization for various reasons, for example, embolization of left atrial thrombus in patients with atrial fibrillation. Sludging of abnormal erythrocytes in the spleen in patients with sickle cell anemia can also be a cause. Any condition that significantly enlarges the spleen can cause it to outstrip its blood supply. Splenic infarcts typically appear as peripheral, irregular, or wedge-shaped, low attenuating defects in contrast enhancement on contrast-enhanced CT or MRI after injection of gadolinium-based contrast agents. Splenic infarction may rarely lead to rupture and perisplenic hematoma.

TABLE 52-5 Conditions That Predispose to Splenic Infarction

Infiltrative diseases
Lymphoma
Myeloproliferative diseases
Storage diseases
Cardiac diseases
Arrhythmias
Valvular disease
Conditions that affect the splenic artery
Aneurysm
Vasculitis
Pancreatitis
Compression by extrinsic tumor
Wandering spleen
Splenic torsion
Portal hypertension
Hypercoagulable states
Hemoglobinopathies
Trauma

MISCELLANEOUS CONDITIONS

Sarcoidosis

Sarcoidosis is a disease of unknown etiology in which noncaseating granulomas form in various tissues and organs of the body. It has a predilection for the lymphatic system. The spleen is involved in 50% to 80% of patients with sarcoidosis but usually is asymptomatic. Severe cases can lead to hypersplenism and spontaneous rupture. The spleen is enlarged in approximately one-third of patients and frequently there is associated lymphadenopathy. Splenomegaly is usually the only radiologically detected splenic abnormality. However, aggregates of granulomatous splenic tissue in some patients may appear on CT as numerous, discrete 1 to 2 cm hypoattenuating nodules that usually have irregular borders.

Gamma Gandy Bodies

Gamma Gandy bodies represent small foci of hemorrhage in the splenic parenchyma that are usually associated with portal venous hypertension. These can be seen as low signal intensity on T2-weighted MR images.

Sickle Cell Disease

Homozygous sickle cell disease affects approximately 1 in 500 African American infants at birth, whereas heterozygous sickle cell trait is found in 8% to 10% of the African American population in the US. Splenic crisis with the resultant sickling and trapping of red blood cells within the splenic sinusoids may lead to loss of splenic function as early as 5 months of age in homozygous patients. Patients with heterozygous sickle cell trait, however, typically retain partial splenic function with splenomegaly persisting into adulthood. Ultimately, sometimes even in patients with sickle cell trait, multiple bouts of spontaneous splenic infarction caused by sickled red blood cells render patients functionally asplenic (autosplenectomy). CT typically demonstrates a shrunken and partially calcified spleen. MRI reveals a small spleen with lower than normal signal intensity on both T1- and T2-weighted images because of hemosiderin deposits.

Peliosis

Peliosis is a rare condition, characterized by multiple blood-filled cystlike spaces within a solid organ, usually the liver (peliosis hepatis). When it occurs, splenic peliosis is usually seen in conjunction with hepatic peliosis; isolated splenic peliosis is exceedingly rare. No definite etiology is known, but there are multiple associations, including anabolic steroid use, oral contraceptives, ethanol abuse, Hodgkin lymphoma and other malignant neoplasms, and chronic renal disease. Although most patients remain asymptomatic, spontaneous splenic rupture can occur.

Suggested Reading

Abbott RM, Levy AD, Aguilera NS, Gorospe L, Thompson WM. From the archives of the AFIP: primary vascular neoplasms of the spleen: radiologic-pathologic correlation. *Radiographics.* 2004;24:1137-1163.

Bhatt S, Huang J, Dogra V. Littoral cell angioma of the spleen. *Am J Roentgenol.* 2007;188:1365-1366.

Elsayes KM, Narra VR, Mukundan G, Lewis JS, Menias CO, Heiken JP. MR Imaging of the spleen: spectrum of abnormalities. *Radiographics.* 2005;25:967-982.

Freeman JL, Jafri SZ, Roberts JL, Mezwa DG, Shirkhoda A. CT of congenital and acquired abnormalities of the spleen. *Radiographics.* 1993;13:579-610.

Fulcher AS, Turner MA. Abdominal manifestations of situs anomalies in adults. *Radiographics.* 2002;22:1439-1456.

Klepac SR, Samett EJ. Spleen, trauma. http://emedicine.medscape.com/article/373694-overview. Accessed January 5, 2009.

Koyama T, Ueda H, Togashi K, Umeoka S, Kataoka M, Nagai S. Radiologic manifestations of sarcoidosis in various organs. *Radiographics.* 2004;24:87-104.

Lashbrook DJ, James RW, Phillips AJ, Holbrook AG, Agombar AC. Splenic peliosis with spontaneous splenic rupture: report of two cases. http://www.biomedcentral.com/1471-2482/6/9. Accessed January 5, 2009.

Mortele KJ, Mortele B, Silverman SG. CT features of the accessory spleen. *AJR Am J Roentgenol.* 2004;183:1653-1657.

Paterson AA, Frush DP, Donnelly LF, Foss JN, O'Hara SM, Bisset GS. A Pattern-oriented approach to splenic imaging in infants and children. *Radiographics.* 1999;19:1465-1485.

Rabushka LS, Kawashima A, Fishman EK. T1 Imaging of the spleen: CT with supplemental MR examination. *Radiographics.* 1994;14:307-332.

Rini JN, Leonidas JC, Tomas MB, Palestro CJ. 18F-FDG PET versus CT for evaluating the spleen during initial staging of lymphoma. *J Nucl Med.* 2003;44:1072-1074.

Singh-Ranger G, Rajarajan N, Aftab S, Stoker D. Splenic peliosis—a potentially fatal condition which can mimick malignancy. *Int Semin Surg Oncol.* 2007;4:27.

Urrutia M, Mergo PJ, Ros LH, Torres GM, Ros PR. Cystic masses of the spleen: radiologic-pathologic correlation. *Radiographics.* 1996;16:107-129.

QUESTIONS AND ANSWERS

1. Which one of the following primary neoplasms most commonly metastasizes to the spleen?
   A. Renal cell carcinoma
   B. Small cell lung cancer
   C. Malignant melanoma
   D. Breast carcinoma

   ANSWER: D. Breast carcinoma (see Table 53-4).

2. A contrast-enhanced abdominal CT shows focal areas of high CT attenuation within an epidermoid splenic cyst. What do the high attenuation areas most likely represent?
   A. Daughter cysts caused by infection with *Echinococcus granulosus*
   B. Proteinaceous material
   C. Internal septations
   D. Resolving areas of hemorrhage that occurred at the time of cyst formation

   ANSWER: D. Epidermoid cysts of the spleen are caused by infolding of peritoneal and mesothelial tissue trapped in splenic sulci during development. They frequently contain internal septations.

3. Regarding epidermoid cysts of the spleen, which one of the following is *true*?
   A. They are a sequela of previous traumatic hematoma.
   B. They are usually over 4 cm in size at the time of detection.
   C. Calcification of the cyst wall is useful in differentiating the lesion from hydatid cysts.
   D. Occurrence as a single splenic lesion makes this diagnosis unlikely.

   ANSWER: B. Epidermoid cysts typically grow quite large before being discovered incidentally on radiologic studies. They are congenital in origin and are usually solitary. The cyst wall commonly calcifies, but this is also true of hydatid (echinococcal) cysts and posttraumatic splenic pseudocysts.

4. Concerning splenic involvement in sarcoidosis, which one of the following is *true*?
   A. It occurs in less than 20% of patients with sarcoidosis.
   B. The spleen is rarely enlarged.
   C. Abdominal lymph node enlargement is common.
   D. Multifocal low-density splenic lesions are the most common radiologic abnormality.

   ANSWER: C. Most patients with sarcoidosis involving the spleen have splenomegaly and lymphadenopathy. Radiologically detectable, focal, low-density lesions can occur in the spleen in a minority of patients.

5. What is the most likely cause of multiple, small, round lesions in the spleen on contrast-enhanced CT in an immunocompromised patient?
   A. Lymphoma
   B. *Pneumocystis carinii* infection
   C. Fungal abscesses
   D. Multiple infarcts

ANSWER: C. Splenic microabscess caused by fungal infection are the most likely cause for this appearance in immunocompromised patients. They represent approximately 25% of splenic abscesses.

6. Which of the following conditions is most frequently associated with severe congenital heart disease?
   A. Situs inversus with dextrocardia
   B. Situs ambiguous with polysplenia
   C. Situs solitus
   D. Situs ambiguous with asplenia

   ANSWER: D. Situs ambiguous with asplenia is strongly associated with severe congenital heart disease, which is often fatal in infancy.

7. Which one of the following is the most common benign tumor of the spleen?
   A. Hamartoma
   B. Hemangioma
   C. Lymphangioma
   D. Littoral cell angioma

   ANSWER: B. While a variety of benign neoplasms can affect the spleen, hemangioma is the most common one. The CT appearance is typically that of a smooth, well-marginated nodule. Contrast enhancement is variable and not as characteristic as that of hepatic hemangiomas.

8. Isolated gastric varices are most often caused by which of the following?
   A. Splenic vein thrombosis
   B. Cirrhosis
   C. Congestive heart failure
   D. Occlusion of the inferior vena cava

   ANSWER: A. Gastric varices associated with esophageal varices are usually caused by portal hypertension. The presence of isolated gastric varices without accompanying esophageal varices should suggest splenic vein occlusion, often caused by pancreatitis or pancreatic carcinoma.

9. Concerning peliosis, which one of the following is *false*?
   A. It is more common in the spleen than in the liver.
   B. It is usually asymptomatic.
   C. Splenic rupture occurs in some cases.
   D. It is associated with the use of anabolic steroids.

   ANSWER: A. Peliosis is more common in the liver than in the spleen. Cases of splenic rupture have been reported. A number of drugs and toxins have been implicated in its causation.

10. What is the most significant complication of wandering spleen?
    A. Compression of the inferior vena cava by the spleen
    B. Splenic torsion
    C. Splenic contusion
    D. Diaphragmatic herniation

    ANSWER: B. Torsion of the spleen around its lax, elongated pedicle leading to splenic ischemia.

53 PANCREAS

Desiree E. Morgan

PANCREAS

CONGENITAL MALFORMATIONS

Pancreas divisum is the most common anatomic variant of the human pancreas, reported in 5% to 10% of autopsy series and 5% to 8% of endoscopic retrograde cholangiopancreatography (ERCP) series. This condition results from lack of fusion of the dorsal and ventral pancreatic anlagen in the developing embryo at approximately 7 weeks. The main portion of the pancreas, including the anterior part of the head, body, and tail, is drained by the dorsal pancreatic duct through the minor (accessory) duodenal papilla, and the posterior portion of the pancreatic head drains through the major papilla (ampulla of Vater). Because the ventral pancreas arises along with the bile duct from the hepatic bud on the ventral aspect of the embryonic gut, the duct of Wirsung always empties into the major papilla along with the common bile duct. The dorsal pancreas arises in the dorsal mesogastrium and when not fused with the ventral duct, the main pancreatic duct supplying this portion of the pancreas empties separately via the duct of Santorini through the minor papilla. Clinical relevance includes an increased incidence of recurrent acute pancreatitis in patients with pancreas divisum.

Other congenital anomalies of the pancreas include annular pancreas, absence of either the dorsal or ventral anlagen, or an anomalous pancreaticobiliary ductal union. Annular pancreas is a rare congenital anomaly and may be one of two types: extramural or intramural. In the extramural type, the ventral pancreatic duct encircles the duodenum to join the main pancreatic duct. In the intramural type, pancreatic tissue is located in the wall of the duodenum (intermingled with muscle fibers) and is drained via small ducts into the duodenal lumen.

In general, annular pancreas produces obstruction of the duodenum in approximately 10% of cases, and about half of symptomatic cases present in infancy. Pancreatic agenesis is extremely rare and incompatible with life. When there is absence of the dorsal or ventral anlagen, the condition is referred to as pancreatic hypoplasia or partial agenesis. Partial agenesis of the dorsal pancreas is more common than agenesis of the ventral pancreas; complete dorsal agenesis is very rare. On cross-sectional imaging, dorsal pancreatic hypoplasia is present when there is varying degree of truncation of pancreatic tissue beyond the head region. In adults, it is important to exclude a pancreatic carcinoma that has resulted in severe upstream glandular atrophy before diagnosing the defect as congenital. An anomalous pancreatobiliary duct union occurs when the fusion of the pancreatic duct and common bile duct is outside the duodenal wall, proximal (upstream) to the sphincter of Oddi. This condition is present when there is more than 1.5 cm of conjoined pancreatic and bile duct (also known as the common channel) and may allow reflux of pancreatic juice into the biliary tree. There is an association with choledochal cyst or, rarely choledochal web formation. Conversely, when bile can reflux into the pancreatic duct, pancreatitis may occur.

PANCREATIC INFLAMMATION

Acute Pancreatitis

Patients with acute pancreatitis present clinically with either mild (80%) or severe (20%) disease. In western countries, acute pancreatitis is most commonly caused by gallstones or ethanol use, with less common etiologies including tumor, trauma, hyperlipidemia, medications, and iatrogenic causes (ERCP, surgery). Symptoms of nausea, vomiting, and abdominal pain are often present, but are relatively nonspecific. More specific signs of acute pancreatitis include Cullen sign (periumbilical ecchymosis) or Gray-Turner sign (flank ecchymosis), both generally indicative of hemorrhagic pancreatitis. Typical laboratory abnormalities indicating the presence of acute pancreatitis include serum amylase and lipase elevation. According to the 2007 Acute Pancreatitis Classification Working Group revision of the Atlanta Classification, the clinical definition of acute pancreatitis now requires two of the three following features: abdominal pain suggestive of pancreatic origin, serum amylase or lipase greater than or equal to three times normal, and characteristic findings on intravenous contrast-enhanced CT (CECT). Onset of pancreatitis has now been defined by the working group as the beginning of abdominal pain.

CECT is the mainstay of imaging patients with acute pancreatitis; however, unenhanced CT may be utilized for patients with renal insufficiency, or MRI using three-dimensional T1-weighted fat-suppressed spoiled gradient-echo sequences may also be employed. The differentiation between severe and nonsevere (mild) acute pancreatitis depends on clinical findings in the first week and morphologic findings depicted on CECT or MRI thereafter. Various clinical scoring systems have been used to characterize disease severity. Marshall score is the recommended clinical tool for assessing disease severity in the first week. Radiologically, the CT severity index has been used for years as a prognosticator for morbidity and mortality in patients with acute pancreatitis, especially in research settings where comparison of disease severity among populations is important. This index is based on the grade of pancreatic inflammation plus the degree of glandular necrosis. The presence of necrosis is critical for the radiologist to recognize both in research and in everyday clinical operations, because the complications of pancreatic necrosis account for 70% to 86% of deaths caused by acute pancreatitis.

The new morphologic classification system in patients with acute pancreatitis is based on CT or MR findings after 1 week, and has been proposed to better identify patients at risk for developing complications. Acute pancreatitis is divided into either acute interstitial edematous pancreatitis or acute necrotizing pancreatitis. The necrosis may be isolated to the pancreatic gland, isolated to the peripancreatic fat, or may involve both. On CECT, pancreatic glandular necrosis is generally depicted as one or more focal or geographic areas of nonenhancing pancreatic parenchyma. Pancreatic gland necrosis is typically accompanied by varying degrees of peripancreatic fat necrosis. Isolated peripancreatic retroperitoneal fat necrosis is more difficult to identify, but may be suggested when there is incorporation of retroperitoneal fat into a complex but predominately low-attenuation (often fluid density) collection surrounding the pancreas. Potential imaging pitfalls resulting in overestimation of pancreatic glandular necrosis on CT include apparent diminished enhancement in patients with normal fatty infiltration of the pancreas, diffuse parenchymal edema in patients with severe interstitial pancreatitis, and intrapancreatic focal fluid collections. Furthermore, once a large complex collection is present, there may be compression of normal enhancing pancreatic tissue, resulting in overestimation of necrosis, especially in the central gland. Typical CT features of pancreatic necrosis may occasionally not be evident up to 48 hours after onset of symptoms hence the recommendation to characterize the morphologic changes with CT after 1 week of acute pancreatitis symptoms being present.

Infection of pancreatic necrosis is defined as culture positivity of pancreatic and/or peripancreatic necrotic tissue. This typically is polymicrobial, occurs in the second to third week following onset of symptoms, and occurs in 36% to 71% of all patients with glandular necrosis. With imaging, infected necrosis may be suggested by the presence of gas within a complex retroperitoneal collection; however, proof is achieved by fine needle aspirate and culture. Other explanations for gas being present in retroperitoneal collections associated with acute pancreatitis include spontaneous fistulization to bowel, or introduction of air through drainage catheters. Once drainage is attempted, either percutaneous, endoscopic, or surgical, there may be colonization and/or secondary infection of the residual solid necrotic debris. This debris can be successfully evacuated over time if measures to irrigate the retroperitoneal cavity and large drainage tracts are employed.

Definition of Retroperitoneal Collections Associated with Acute Pancreatitis

Recent revision of the nomenclature for imaging findings in patients with acute pancreatitis has been proposed. Figure 53-1 compares prior definitions of the 1992 Atlanta Classification to the terms recommended by the 2007 Acute Pancreatitis Working Group. *Acute peripancreatic fluid collection* refers to enzyme-rich pancreatic juice that is located predominantly adjacent to the pancreas, lacks a wall, arises early (within 48 hours) in up to 50% of patients with acute pancreatitis, typically

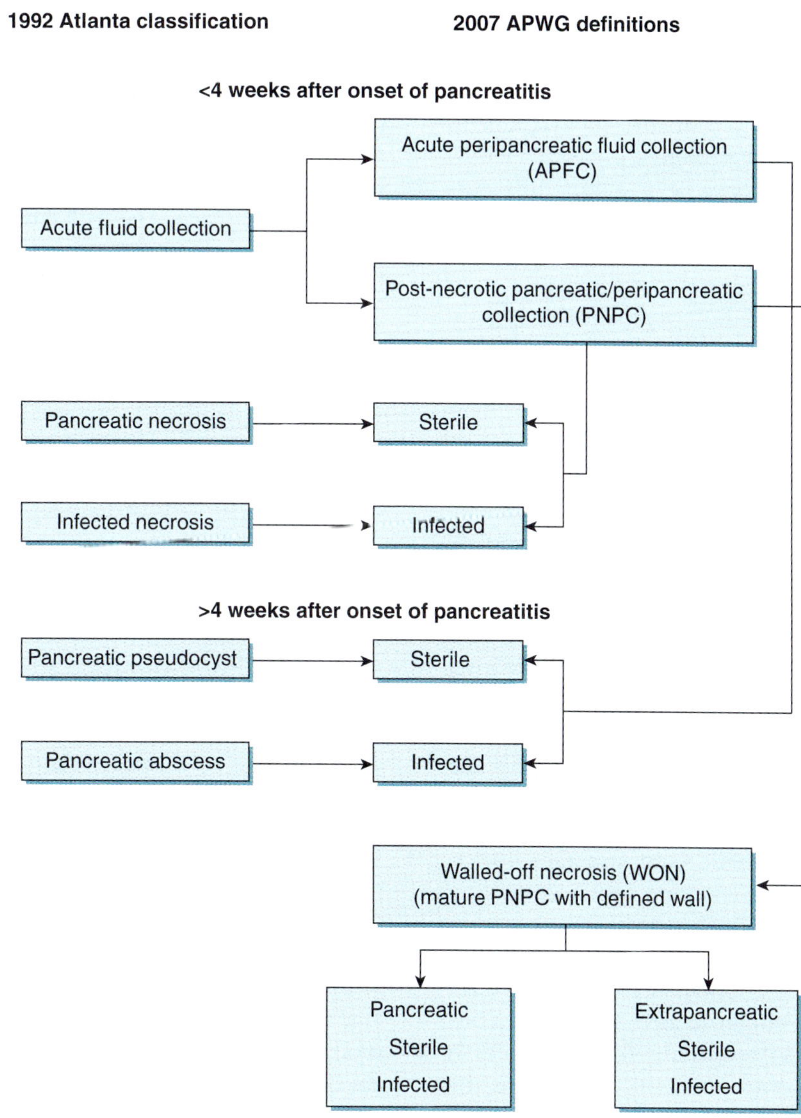

FIG. 53-1 Acute pancreatitis collection nomenclature.

remains sterile, and resolves spontaneously within 2 to 4 weeks. *Postnecrotic pancreatic collection* is the new term for enzyme-rich pancreatic fluid combined with necrotic pancreatic parenchyma and/or peripancreatic fat. These postnecrotic collections are present up to 4 weeks following onset, and may remain sterile or become infected. The intrapancreatic versus extrapancreatic nature of these collections should be distinguished, as those containing glandular necrosis are more likely to have complications related to duct disruption. If allowed to evolve, eventually postnecrotic pancreatic collections become walled-off necrosis. *Walled-off necrosis* is the new term that describes postnecrotic pancreatic collections that are present more than 4 weeks following onset of symptoms. Prior terms for this condition included organized pancreatic necrosis, pseudocyst associated with necrosis, and central cavitary necrosis, but these should now be avoided. As with postnecrotic collections, it is critical to recognize that in patients with walled-off necrosis, CECT and MRI demonstrate replacement of pancreatic tissue by the collection. This feature helps differentiate walled-off necrosis from a pseudocyst arising from acute pancreatitis on CT. Surgical, percutaneous, and endoscopic procedures have been successfully performed on patients with walled-off necrotic collections, so long as measures are undertaken to remove the necrotic debris during drainage. Both postnecrotic pancreatic collections and walled-off necrosis may remain sterile or become infected, and the presence of gas within one of these types of collection should be treated as an urgent finding by the imager, as prompt drainage is mandated. *Pancreatic pseudocyst* is defined as a collection of pancreatic juice contained by granulation tissue that requires 4 weeks or greater to form and contains little or no necrosis. These collections may resolve spontaneously when small, and are generally not intervened upon unless symptomatic. On CT, pseudocysts are well-defined, homogeneous, low-attenuation, thin-walled collections that are typically adjacent to an otherwise normal-appearing pancreas. If drainage is clinically necessary, identification of potential ductal communication is important. Patients whose upstream main pancreatic ducts fill the pseudocyst but are disconnected from the downstream duct that empties through the papilla are at risk for pancreaticocutaneous or pancreaticoenteric fistula formation. According to the new working group definition, pancreatic pseudocyst should be classified as noninfected or infected (suppurative). Infected pseudocyst is the new name to replace the term pancreatic abscess. An infected pseudocyst is a circumscribed collection of pus located near the pancreas that requires at least 4 weeks to form and has little or no necrosis. On CT or MRI, the wall of an infected pseudocyst is slightly thicker and more irregular than that of a sterile pseudocyst.

Systemic complications arising from acute pancreatitis may also be depicted on CT, and include signs of multisystem organ failure, such as pulmonary edema, pleural effusions, or infiltrates caused by adult respiratory distress syndrome, for example, in the respiratory system. Other intraabdominal findings including gastric outlet obstruction, colonic inflammation, retroperitoneal hemorrhage, pseudoaneurysm formation, ileus, pancreatic ascites, and renal obstruction may be seen in patients with acute pancreatitis; some of these abnormalities are due to mechanical compression by the retroperitoneal collections and others may arise from release of pancreatic enzymes and systemic inflammatory response syndrome.

Chronic Pancreatitis

Chronic pancreatitis is characterized by prolonged pancreatic inflammation and fibrosis with irreversible morphologic and/or functional abnormalities.

There is a strong association of alcohol abuse and chronic pancreatitis; other etiologies include familial hyperlipidemia, hyperparathyroidism, cystic fibrosis (CF), cholelithiasis, and hereditary pancreatitis that is thought to be inherited in an autosomal dominant fashion with variable penetrance. The pathognomonic features on CT in patients with chronic pancreatitis are scattered glandular and ductal calcifications, and ductal dilatation. In addition, parenchymal atrophy, fluid collections, focal pancreatic enlargement that may mimic neoplasm and biliary ductal dilatation may also be present.

As stated previously, smooth or beaded dilatation of the main pancreatic duct is most commonly associated with carcinoma, and irregular dilatation is more frequently seen in chronic pancreatitis. On CT, a ratio of duct width to total gland width less than 0.5 favors the diagnosis of chronic pancreatitis. Chronic pancreatitis severity has been traditionally characterized by the Cambridge classification (Table 53-1), originally described for ERCP. However, similar ductal abnormalities may be well seen with magnetic resonance cholangiopancreatography (MRCP). Secretin stimulation during MRCP thick-slab technique can result in better visualization of the main and side branch pancreatic duct to assess for changes of chronic pancreatitis. Also, the efflux of pancreatic juice can be observed, giving functional information about the gland. The use of diffusion-weighted MRI to help distinguish between focal, mass-like pancreatitis and pancreatic adenocarcinoma is a current area of investigation, but remains problematic. One of the strengths of endoscopic ultrasound (EUS) is to sample indeterminate focal masses in patients that have other EUS evidence of chronic pancreatitis.

Chronic pancreatitis also can be associated with obstruction of the bile duct. In most instances, the lumen of

TABLE 53-1 Cambridge Classification of Chronic Pancreatitis

GRADE	ENDOSCOPIC RETROGRADE PANCREATOGRAM FINDINGS	
	Main pancreatic duct	Side branch pancreatic ducts
Normal	Normal caliber	Normal
Equivocal ducts	Normal caliber	Three or fewer dilated
Mild	Normal caliber	> Three dilated ducts
Moderate	Abnormal dilation	> Three dilated ducts
Severe	Abnormal dilation with calculi, obstruction, extravasation, or cavity formation	> Three dilated ducts

Reproduced with permission from Akisik MF, Sandrasegaran K, Aisen AA, Maglinte DDT, et al. Dynamic secretin-enhanced MR cholangiopancreatography. *Radiographics.* 2006;26:665-677.

the obstructed bile duct tapers gradually through the inflamed region versus an abrupt transition commonly associated with neoplasm. Chronic pancreatitis may be associated with splenic and portal venous obstruction. Pseudocysts associated with chronic pancreatitis are different than those arising from acute pancreatitis. In general, there is side branch disruption, likely related to obstructive disease of the main pancreatic duct, with extravasation of pancreatic enzymes that may track throughout the abdomen or into the chest; it is not uncommon to see pseudocysts arising from chronic pancreatitis tracking into the gastric wall or along the splenic capsule.

AUTOIMMUNE PANCREATITIS

Autoimmune pancreatitis (lymphoplasmacytic sclerosing pancreatitis) is a chronic inflammatory process of the pancreas that is caused by an autoimmune mechanism, with morphologic hallmarks being periductal infiltration by lymphocytes and plasma cells together with granulocytic epithelial lesions and destruction of the duct epithelium. Serum IgG or gamma globulin elevations are associated in some patients, and there is usually a response to steroid therapy. Typical CT findings include diffuse or focal enlargement of the pancreas without dilation of the main pancreatic duct. Multiple pancreatic masses may be present. The enlarged portion/mass may be isoattenuating or hypoattenuating relative to the pancreatic parenchyma. Although not present in all patients, a rim of low-attenuation tissue surrounding the gland is characteristic and has been reported in 12% to 80% *of cases*. This is a specific sign, but the sensitivity varies widely (12%–80% of reported cases). On MRI, the affected portion is generally hypointense on T1-weighted images, and the capsule-like rim may be hypointense on T2-weighted images and show delayed enhancement (suggesting fibrosis) on postgadolinium T1-weighted sequences. Other features include mural thickening and enhancement of the bile duct (obstructive jaundice seen in 63%–75%), rare peripancreatic stranding, venous occlusion, and peripancreatic lymph node enlargement. The incidence of associated extrapancreatic manifestations of autoimmune pancreatitis is reported from 19% to 50% and consists of sclerosing changes of the intrahepatic bile ducts (appearance similar to primary sclerosing cholangitis), retroperitoneal fibrosis, renal involvement (low-attenuation parenchymal masses), mediastinal adenopathy, and lung disease. When focal, distinguishing autoimmune pancreatitis from pancreatic adenocarcinoma may be difficult. Features that might help include absence of main pancreatic duct enlargement, absence of glandular atrophy, and absence of involvement of the major peripancreatic vessels in patients with autoimmune pancreatitis. Also, notably absent are parenchymal calcifications and duct dilation, features that help distinguish autoimmune pancreatitis from other forms of chronic pancreatitis.

OTHER CHRONIC CONDITIONS

Cystic Fibrosis (CF) results from dysfunction of exocrine glands and is an inherited disease characterized by chronic bronchopulmonary infections and malabsorption secondary to pancreatic insufficiency. Pancreatic manifestations include acute pancreatitis, fatty replacement, calcifications, cysts, duct abnormalities, and carcinomas. Complete fatty replacement of the pancreatic parenchyma is the most common imaging finding in adult CF patients, with mean age of this finding being 17 years. The amount of fatty replacement correlates with the degree of pancreatic exocrine, but not endocrine dysfunction. Exocrine gland insufficiency affects 85% to 90% of patients, and endocrine gland dysfunction has been reported in 30% to 50%. CF patients with lesser exocrine dysfunction are at risk for pancreatitis. Other disease patterns include one or more macroscopic fluid-density cysts scattered through the fatty replaced gland, or rarely complete replacement of the gland by true epithelium-lined cysts, pancreatic cystosis.

Primary hemochromatosis is a hereditary disease in which iron is deposited in the parenchyma of various organs. Liver, pancreas, and heart are primarily affected. Deposition of iron in the pancreas tends to occur later in the disease course, after liver damage is irreversible, and may be best seen on T2-weighted MRI.

NEOPLASM

Pancreatic Adenocarcinoma

The clinical presentation of patients with pancreatic neoplasm varies according to the type of tumor. The most common pancreatic neoplasm is pancreatic adenocarcinoma; it is the ninth most common malignancy overall, but represents the fourth most common cause of cancer-related death. Peak incidence occurs in the seventh and eighth decade. These patients present with weight loss, abdominal pain, and jaundice if the tumor is located in the pancreatic head region and obstructs the bile duct. Imaging studies play a critical role in the diagnosis and management of patients with pancreatic neoplasms. Pancreatic adenocarcinoma is the tumor most likely to be spread beyond the organ of origin at diagnosis. At presentation, approximately 45% of patients have distant metastatic disease; 40% have locally advanced tumors that have invaded the peripancreatic vessels; and up to 15% have resectable lesions. Surgical therapy is the only option for cure at present, although patients may receive neoadjuvant or adjuvant therapy that has been shown to have a modest effect on survival. State-of-the-art multiphasic multidetector CECT consists of isometric data sets acquired through the upper abdomen/pancreas prior to contrast and during the pancreatic parenchymal phase, and throughout the abdomen and pelvis in the portal venous phase. With this technique, the overall sensitivity of CT for detection and diagnosis of pancreatic adenocarcinoma is high (89%–97%), and the positive predictive value for determining unresectability is very high (89%–100%). Accurate prediction of resectability is lower because of false-negative errors resulting from lack of detection of small hepatic and peritoneal metastases as well as underestimation of vascular invasion. At present, the criteria for diagnosing vascular invasion by tumor favor specificity over sensitivity, as it is important to avoid errors that result in denying a patient potential curative resection.

During the pancreatic parenchymal phase, typically hypovascular pancreatic adenocarcinoma appears as a low-attenuation, poorly demarcated mass within the more brightly enhancing pancreatic parenchyma. The sensitivity of CT for detection of pancreatic adenocarcinoma is high (89%–97% for larger lesions); however, identification of smaller tumors remains problematic. One recent study reported only 67% detection sensitivity for tumors that were less than or equal to 15 mm diameter, and another study reported 77% sensitivity for detection of pancreatic tumors less than or equal to 2 cm in size. It is this lesion size for which accurate detection with imaging may have the largest impact on patient survival. In addition, approximately 11% of pancreatic adenocarcinomas are isoattentuating to the remainder of the pancreas on multiphasic CECT. Dilation of the bile duct and pancreatic duct may be present because of obstruction by tumor. Pancreatic adenocarcinomas are most commonly located in the pancreatic head region (approximately 60%). If located elsewhere in the pancreas, upstream main pancreatic duct dilation and glandular atrophy may be present. The duct interruption sign, where there is abrupt termination rather than tapering through a focal low-attenuation mass in the pancreatic parenchyma, favors pancreatic adenocarcinoma over focal mass-like chronic pancreatitis. Local pancreatitis induced by obstruction of the main pancreatic duct may obscure tumor boundaries. On portal venous phase images, the pancreatic primary tumor may be less distinct; however this phase is important for assessment of the peripancreatic veins (superior mesenteric vein and portal vein) as well as for the detection of hepatic metastases. With the volumetric data acquired on multidetector CT, postprocessing may aid in assessing vascular involvement and local extension. Curved multiplanar reformations along the main pancreatic duct or vessels have also been explored and may be helpful in the case of an isoattenuating pancreatic mass.

The American Joint Commission on Cancer recently revised the TNM staging for pancreatic adenocarcinoma (Table 53-2). Tumor staging, or T staging, is as follows: TX, tumor cannot be assessed; T0, no evidence of primary tumor; Tis, carcinoma in situ; T1, tumor confined to pancreas and smaller than 2 cm; T2, tumor confined to pancreas and larger than 2 cm; T3, tumor extension beyond the pancreas but no invasion of major peripancreatic vessels or nerves; T4, tumor invasion of major peripancreatic vessels or nerves. Criteria for resectability of pancreatic lesions currently includes absence of distant metastatic disease, no evidence of tumor involvement of major peripancreatic arteries (superior mesenteric artery, hepatic artery, or celiac axis), and either uninvolved major peripancreatic vein (superior mesenteric vein and portal vein) or suitable limited venous involvement to allow for venous reconstruction. When assessing vascular invasion, degree of contact between the vessel and tumor estimated at greater than 50% represents an "optimal" threshold for predicting vascular invasion, with sensitivity of 84% and specificity of 98%. To avoid denying surgery to patients with potentially resectable disease, it may be preferable to increase the threshold to 75% contact with the circumference of an affected vessel. The shape of the vessel should be commented on as well, as narrowing or teardrop configuration of the superior mesenteric vein for example may indicate tethering caused by tumor infiltration. In addition, it has been proposed that criteria for diagnosing vascular invasion by tumor should differ between arteries and veins—areas of continued investigation. While peripancreatic lymph nodes may be detected on CT, the finding of an enlarged lymph node should not preclude

TABLE 53-2 TNM Staging of Pancreatic Adenocarcinoma

STAGE	TNM	DESCRIPTION	5-YEAR RELATIVE SURVIVAL
0	Tis, N0, M0	Tumor confined to superficial pancreatic duct epithelium (pancreatic carcinoma in situ or pancreatic intraepithelial neoplasia III (PanIn III)	
IA	T1, N0, M0	Tumor confined to pancreas, less than 2 cm; no LN or distant metastases	37
IB	T2, N0, M0	Tumor confined to pancreas, larger than 2 cm; no LN or distant metastases	21
IIA	T3, N0, M0	Tumor extends beyond pancreas but no vascular, LN, or distant metastases	12
IIB	T1-3, N1, M0	Tumor confined to pancreas or peripancreatic extension; no vascular involvement regional LN metastases, but no distant metastases	6
III	T4; any N, M0	Tumor invasion of vessels or major nerves ± lymph nodes, no distant metastases	2
IV	Any T; any N, M1	Distant metastases	1

attempted resection, as the lymph nodes are resected en bloc with the primary lesion.

Other imaging studies utilized in the evaluation of pancreatic adenocarcinoma include MRI and EUS. On MRI, pancreatic adenocarcinomas are typically hypointense on precontrast T1-weighted fat-suppressed three-dimensional spoiled gradient-echo images, and are relatively hypovascular on pancreatic parenchymal and portal venous phase. The sensitivity of MRI for detection of pancreatic adenocarcinoma is slightly less than helical CT; however, the two modalities are equivalent for determining resectability. Positron emission tomography may be used in patients with pancreatic cancer, with the largest impact being on detection of distant metastases. However, sensitivity for accurate depiction of small hepatic metastases is lower. Combining positron emission tomography and CT as an adjunct to multiphasic pancreatic contrast-enhanced multidetector CT resulted in 88% sensitivity for staging.

Cystic Pancreatic Neoplasms

When a cystic lesion is present in the pancreas, the diagnosis of an inflammatory pseudocyst arising from acute pancreatitis, an acute pancreatitis episode superimposed on chronic pancreatitis, or from chronic pancreatitis should first be excluded. Occasionally, history is unrevealing. Aspiration of cysts contents (Table 53-3), typically via EUS fine needle aspirate, may be performed to differentiate between potential etiologies of pancreatic cystic lesions, especially when the imaging appearance is not definitive. However, sampling errors are not uncommon, and interpretation of cyst aspirate results must be performed in conjunction with careful patient history and interpretation of radiologic findings; if the nature of the cystic lesion cannot be definitively established by these combined measures, surgical resection may be warranted.

Simple Cysts

Epithelial line cysts of the pancreas are rare. They occur in patients with von Hippel-Lindau (VHL) disease, polycystic kidney disease with hepatic and pancreatic involvement, and CF.

Serous Cystadenoma

Serous cystadenoma (former names, microcystic adenoma and glycogen rich adenoma) is a benign cystic neoplasm of the pancreas, more common in females (2:1 ratio) than males, occurs in the seventh decade, and often is not associated with symptoms unless large. On CT, serous cystadenomas have classically been described as heterogeneous mixed-density lesions made up of multiple small cysts (0.2–2.0 cm) that resemble the cut surface of a natural sponge. A minority of patients will have lesions that demonstrate a characteristic central stellate scar with calcification. Individual cysts may be larger than 2 cm, and rarely serous cystadenomas may be unilocular. When the individual cysts are large, this lesion may be mistaken for mucinous cystic neoplasm. In general, combined features of location in the pancreatic head (rather than tail), lobular contour, and the presence of a thin capsule without enhancement or projections/nodules may help to distinguish a serous

TABLE 53-3 Cyst Aspirate Assessment

	AMYLASE	CEA CA19–91	MUCIN	GLYCOGEN-RICH CELLS
Serous cystadenoma	+			+++
Mucinous cystic neoplasm	+	+++	+++	
IPMN	++++		+++	
Inflammatory pseudocyst	+++++			

cystadenoma from a mucinous cystic neoplasm. At ultrasound, these lesions may appear as a solid echogenic mass because of the many interfaces produced by the numerous cysts. Occasionally smaller lesions may appear solid on CT and MRI, depending on the size of individual cysts and amount of fibrous tissue. Aspiration of cyst contents (obtained during EUS with fine needle aspirate) may be helpful in differentiating between the two, as the serous cystadenomas contain epithelial cells that are rich in cytoplasmic glycogen.

Mucinous Cystic Neoplasm

Mucinous cystic neoplasms (MCN; older terms, macrocystic adenoma and macrocystic adenocarcinoma) are more common in females than males (9:1 ratio), occur in the fifth to sixth decade of life, and are usually located in the body or tail of pancreas. At diagnosis, the tumor histology may be benign, atypical, or frankly malignant. All are considered premalignant and require surgical resection. The mucinous cystic neoplasm cavity is lined by tall mucin-producing columnar cells. The cavity is filled with low-attenuation mucinous material and may have papillary projections and nodules that demonstrate progressive enhancement on CT. On MRI, high T2-weighted signal fills the cystic spaces, and enhancement of the wall, septations, and excrescences is apparent after gadolinium administration on TI fat-suppressed spoiled gradient–recalled echo imaging. While the presence of enhancing nodules and septations correlates with malignancy, absence of these findings does not preclude malignancy. There is generally no communication of MCN with the pancreatic ductal system. Curvilinear calcifications may be noted in the tumor periphery/capsule in 10% to 25% of cases. When multilocular, individual cystic spaces in MCN tend to have diameter greater than 2 cm. In general, the greater the degree of complexity, the more likely the tumor will be malignant at time of diagnosis.

Intraductal Papillary Mucinous Neoplasm

Intraductal papillary mucinous neoplasm (IPMN; older term, duct/ectatic mucinous tumor) is a mucin-producing tumor that arises from the pancreatic duct epithelium. As with MCN, at diagnosis these lesions may be benign, atypical, or frankly malignant. Unlike MCN, IPMNs lack an associated ovarian-type stroma. There is a 2:1 male-to-female predominance, with patients typically presenting in the seventh to ninth decade. Symptoms, malignant potential, prognosis, and imaging features vary according to whether the lesion arises from a side branch duct or from the main pancreatic duct, or both (mixed or combined type). On CT, a side branch–type IPMN typically appears as a small cystic mass, often within the uncinate portion of head of pancreas. The mass is unilocular or may resemble a group of small clustered cysts. Lesions less than 3 cm are usually, but not always, benign. Communication of this cystic lesion with the main pancreatic duct may be identified on thin-section CT and even more readily on MRCP. If copious amounts of mucin are produced in the side branch IPMN, this may result in main pancreatic duct enlargement downstream from the site of ductal communication. Main duct-type IPMN produces diffuse dilation of the main pancreatic duct. Atrophy of the gland and dysmorphic calcifications may be present, mimicking findings of chronic pancreatitis. However, patients with main duct-type IPMN present at a later age than patients with chronic pancreatitis and may have a bulging papilla because of mucin production. Main duct-type tumors are more likely than side branch IPMNs to be malignant. Approximately 7% to 34% of IPMNs treated with surgical resection will contain carcinoma in situ; more importantly 25% to 44% of IPMNs will contain invasive carcinoma. Imaging features associated with malignancy or invasive carcinoma include main duct diameter greater than 1.5 cm, diffuse or multifocal involvement, enhancing nodules or excrescences within the duct, or the presence of a focal hypovascular soft tissue mass, and bile duct obstruction. If the lesion is a side branch– or combined-type IPMN, large size of the mass suggests malignancy. MR imaging with MRCP demonstrates in the full extent of ductal involvement, and when combined with standard T2- and contrast-enhanced T1-weighted images can be utilized for determination of resectability. The presence of a communication between the cystic lesion and the main pancreatic duct is one of the most reliable findings for the diagnosis of IPMN. The communicating track of malignant IPMNs is typically larger than in benign lesions. All main duct lesions are considered to be malignant, if not frankly malignant at the time of diagnosis, and should be considered for surgical resection. The surgical method may be altered (more radical resection or lymph node dissection) if invasive carcinoma is predicted with imaging.

Follow-up of suspected IPMNs in patients with asymptomatic side branch IPMNs is controversial; in general, if there is no evidence of malignancy these maybe closely followed with imaging. Although there is no consensus, one strategy is to follow patients with small (less than 3 cm), unilocular, asymptomatic cystic lesions at 6-month intervals for the first year, at yearly intervals for 3 years, and if stable, consider discontinuing surveillance at that time.

Solid Pseudopapillary Tumor of the Pancreas

Solid pseudopapillary tumor (SPT; former terms, solid and papillary epithelial neoplasm, papillary and cystic tumor) is an uncommon, low-grade malignant tumor that occurs in young women (third decade), is generally large at presentation, and is typically located in the pancreatic tail region. With CECT and MR imaging, SPTs may demonstrate progressive fill-in of the solid portions of the mass over time, and may contain hemorrhage or fluid/debris levels of blood products in areas of cystic degeneration or necrosis. The absence of high T1 (hemorrhagic) signal within the lesion does not exclude the diagnosis however. When the lesions are small, distinguishing them from other solid pancreatic neoplasms is more problematic.

Pancreatic Neuroendocrine Tumors

Pancreatic neuroendocrine tumors (NETs) are uncommon neoplasms that arise from neural crest cells or well-differentiated neuroendocrine cells of the pancreas, and are classified as functioning (syndromic) or nonhyperfunctioning (nonsyndromic); all produce and secrete hormones to varying degrees. Although most NETs occur sporadically, an increased prevalence of these tumors is seen in patients with VHL syndrome, multiple endocrine neoplasia type I (MEN I), neurofibromatosis type 1, and tuberous sclerosis. Despite their rarity, these tumors are important because they have a high rate of malignancy, ranging from 60% to 92%. Functioning NETs are generally named for the predominant hormone produced and are associated with specific clinical symptoms related to the hormone production (Table 53-4). Hormonally active tumors are typically diagnosed when small. The most common functioning NETs are insulinomas and gastrinomas, with glucagonomas, VIPomas, and somatostatinomas much less common. NETs may also be multiple, especially gastrinomas. Risk of malignancy varies with histology. In general, 5% to 10% of insulinomas are malignant, but 50% to 90% of the other NETs are malignant. Insulinomas are the most common syndromic NET and produce the classic Whipple triad: fasting serum glucose less than 50 mg/dL, hypoglycemia symptoms, and response to glucose administration. Gastrinomas are the second most common syndromic NET and produce symptoms related to excessive gastrin production, Zollinger-Ellison syndrome: epigastric pain related to intractable peptic ulcer disease, diarrhea related to excess acid delivery to the small bowel. These tumors are often multiple and extrapancreatic, located in either the pancreatic wall or an area termed the "gastrinoma triangle," an area bounded by the junction of the cystic and common hepatic duct superiorly, the second and third portions of the duodenum inferiorly, and the junction of the neck and body of the pancreas medially. Glucagonomas are rare syndromic NETs and are associated with a characteristic rash—necrolytic migratory erythema. In addition to the dermatosis, these patients may also have diarrhea, depression, and deep vein thrombosis, hence the term 4D syndrome. VIPomas secrete a variety of hormones, most notably vasoactive intestinal peptide that is responsible for fluid and electrolyte secretion into the small bowel and the characteristic watery diarrhea suffered by these patients. Gastrin production is also inhibited; therefore the syndrome is referred to as watery diarrhea, hypokalemia, achlorhydria (WDHA), or sometimes Verner-Morrison syndrome after the men who first described it in 1958. Somatostatinomas are exceedingly rare lesions; the excess somatostatin results in a syndrome of diarrhea, cholelithiasis, indigestion, and hypochlorhydria.

Nonhyperfunctioning tumors represent approximately 20% to 50% of lesions reported in case series of NETs. In general, they are clinically silent unless they produce symptoms caused by metastatic disease or size. These tend to be larger than the syndromic variety; 30% of these lesions are greater than 10 cm at presentation. In addition, when NETs are cystic or necrotic, they are usually nonhyperfunctioning. These lesions are malignant in up to 80% of cases.

On CECT, functioning NETs are generally hypervasular lesions compared to normal pancreatic parenchyma. Because of the brisk enhancement during the arterial or pancreatic parenchymal phase, in the past these lesions were sometimes mistaken for vessels on thicker section axial images alone, but with state-of-the-art multiphasic CT, especially with coronal reformatted

TABLE 53-4 Syndromic Pancreatic Neuroendocrine Tumors

	HORMONE	SYNDROME	LOCATION	CELL ORIGIN	MALIGNANT
Insulinoma	Insulin	Whipple triad	Pancreas	Beta	10%
Gastrinoma	Gastrin	Zollinger-Ellison	Gastrinoma triangle		30%
Glucagonoma	Glucagon	"4D" (dermatosis, diarrhea, depression, deep vein thrombosis)	Body or tail	Alpha	60%
VIPoma	Vasoactive intestinal peptide	WDHA (watery diarrhea, hypokalemia, achlorhydria)	Tail	D1	75%
Somatostatinoma	Somatostatin	Diarrhea, cholelithiasis, indigestion, hypochlorhydria	Pancreas or duodenal wall	Delta	50%

images, this is now not as common. Some lesions, despite the propensity for being hypervascular, are hypoattenuating on early phases and are best seen on portal venous phase. Location of the lesion depicted on CT may alter surgical approaches for smaller lesions; if near the surface, enucleation is often employed. CT features that aid in distinguishing between nonfunctioning NET and other solid lesions such as adenocarcinoma include the presence of coarse calcifications, lack of vascular encasement or invasion despite large size, and cystic degeneration when large. Rarely, nonfunctioning and functioning NETs may appear completely cystic on CT. MR imaging using T1-weighted fat-suppressed three-dimensional spoiled gradient-echo images readily identify pancreatic NETs and have been shown to be at least as effective as CT. Other MR imaging features that help distinguish NETs from ductal adenocarcinomas include higher signal intensity on T2 fat-suppressed images and homogeneous enhancement on immediate post-gadolinium T1-weighted images. In addition, liver metastases are typically hypervascular and well depicted with MR.

Other Neoplasms

Pancreatic lymphoma may be caused by primary (intrapancreatic) lymphoma or by invasion of the pancreas from peripancreatic nodal involvement. In general, when the pancreas is involved by lymphoma, the lesion is larger than that typically seen with adenocarcinoma, and there is no pancreatic duct dilation despite the large size of the tumor.

Pancreatic metastases most commonly arise from breast, lung, kidney, prostate primaries, or melanoma. In general, there is imaging evidence of other metastatic disease except in the case of renal carcinoma metastases, which may occur many years after the primary tumor is diagnosed and may be an isolated pancreatic finding. The enhancement pattern of pancreatic metastases varies depending on the primary tumor, with renal and melanoma metastases being hypervascular on pancreatic parenchymal phase.

Other rare pancreatic lesions include pleomorphic carcinoma, acinar cell carcinoma, giant cell tumor, sarcoma, and small cell carcinoma. Pancreatic tumors are rare in infants and children, the commonest being pancreatoblastoma, a rare tumor of acinar cell origin in children between ages of 1 and 8.

Periampullary tumors are defined as those arising within 2 cm of the major papilla. These may be difficult to differentiate from pancreatic adenocarcinomas as they commonly obstruct the bile duct and produce a focal mass in the head of pancreas. They are often treated with Whipple procedure, and in general have a better prognosis than pancreatic adenocarcinoma. Lesions include ampullary villous adenoma, ampullary adenocarcinoma, distal cholangiocarcinoma, and duodenal adenocarcinoma.

Other focal masses that may mimic pancreatic pathology include intrapancreatic accessory spleen and duodenal diverticulum. Intrapancreatic accessory spleen follows the enhancement of the spleen on all phases of contrast on all modalities; heterogeneous enhancement during arterial or pancreatic parenchymal phases may be a diagnostic clue on CT or MRI. In addition, on MRI with super-paramagnetic iron oxide enhancement, the "mass" will demonstrate signal drop on T2- or T2*-weighted images similar to the spleen. A second portion medial duodenal diverticulum may mimic a cystic neoplasm when fluid filled and a negative oral contrast agent has been used; careful review of prior CTs may demonstrate air in the lesion or obtaining follow-up CT using a positive oral contrast medium may be of help.

SYNDROMES

VHL disease is an autosomal dominant multisystem disorder characterized by development of a variety of benign and malignant tumors. Pancreatic lesions are important to recognize because they may precede other abdominal manifestation by years. Pancreatic involvement includes simple pancreatic cysts in 50% to 91%, serous cystadenomas in 12%, pancreatic NETs in 5% to 17%, and rarely adenocarcinomas. It is uncommon for neuroendocrine lesions and cystic lesions to be present together. NETs occur more frequently in VHL patients who have pheochromocytomas; both lesions are derived from neural crest cells. The frequency of malignancy and metastatic disease in NET associated with VHL is low (less than 10%), whereas sporadic pancreatic NET metastasize in 60% to 92% of cases. Owing to the low malignant potential, these lesions may be followed in VHL patients, and when surgery is indicated pancreas-sparing procedures are employed.

Patients with MEN I have an increased prevalence of pancreatic NETs, usually of the syndromic (functioning) variety. Approximately 10% of patients with insulinomas have MEN I; however, the most common NET in patients with MEN I is gastrinoma.

TRAUMA

Pancreatic injuries occur in 2% to 12% of patients with blunt abdominal trauma. Either blunt or penetrating abdominal trauma may cause pancreatic ductal disruption, with development of the entire spectrum of acute pancreatitis. Most commonly, pancreatic injuries are caused by crushing injury due to impact against the vertebral column; two-thirds of pancreatic injuries occur in the pancreatic body. Associated injuries to the liver, stomach, duodenum, and spleen occur in more than 90% of cases; isolated pancreatic injury is extremely uncommon. Early recognition of disruption of the main pancreatic duct is important because disruption is the principal cause of delayed complications such as pseudocyst, abscess, or fistula. CT can readily demonstrate pancreatic parenchymal injuries such as lacerations and contusion in the acute setting, and although duct disruption cannot be directly imaged with CT, the extent of parenchymal laceration can help suggest its presence. Direct CT findings of pancreatic injury include pancreatic enlargement, focal laceration with linear nonenhancement coursing a variable distance through the parenchyma, or heterogeneous enhancement. Secondary findings of pancreatic injury are peripancreatic stranding, peripancreatic fluid collections that may communicate with a laceration, fluid between the splenic vein and pancreas, hemorrhage, or fluid tracking/thickening along the left anterior pararenal fascial planes. The most accepted scoring system for pancreatic injury is the American Association for the Surgery of Trauma (AAST) system, which assesses variable of location (proximal vs. distal), type of injury (hematoma, laceration, or transection) and main pancreatic duct integrity (Table 53-5).

Although CT is the standard for evaluation of post-traumatic abnormalities, ductal integrity can be evaluated with MRI and specifically MR pancreatography. Fluid-sensitive MRCP images focused on the main pancreatic duct may help delineate ductal integrity and demonstrate fluid collections upstream to the site of duct transaction. ERCP remains important in the assessment of ductal disruption in traumatic pancreatitis as it can be used for primary therapy with stent placement or serve as a guide for surgical repair. When CT or MRI are suggestive of main pancreatic duct disruption, it is imperative that the imager notify the primary service; delay in therapy longer than 72 hours after the initial trauma may result in a higher complication rate and prolonged hospitalization in patients with traumatic pancreatitis.

TABLE 53-5 AAST Scoring System for Pancreatic Trauma

GRADE	INJURY	DESCRIPTION
I	Hematoma	Minor contusion without duct injury
	Laceration	Superficial laceration without duct injury
II	Hematoma	Major contusion without duct injury
	Laceration	Major laceration without duct injury
III	Laceration	Distal transaction or parenchymal injury with duct injury
IV	Laceration	Proximal transaction or parenchymal injury involving the ampulla or bile duct
V	Disruption	Massive disruption of the pancreatic head

Reproduced with permission from Jurkovich GJ. Duodenum and pancreas. In: Mattox KL, Feliciano DV, Moore EE, eds. *Trauma.* 4th ed. New York, NY: McGraw-Hill; 2000; 735-762.

TRANSPLANTATION

The majority of pancreatic transplants are combined with renal transplants in patients with end-stage renal disease because of severe type 1 diabetes mellitus. Two methods of pancreatic transplantation may be utilized. The traditional procedure places the graft in an intraperitoneal location of the iliac fossa opposite the renal transplant, with the vascular pedicle (donor splenic artery and superior mesenteric artery) anastomosed to the common or external iliac arteries by way of a vascular Y graft, and the pancreatic venous outflow emptying into the common or external iliac vein; the accompanying cuff of duodenum may be anastomosed to the bladder or small bowel. Alternatively, for portoenteric venous drainage, the graft may be placed in an intraperitoneal location within the upper abdomen, with the vascular pedicle anastomosed to the common or external iliac arteries by way of a longer vascular Y graft, and the pancreatic venous outflow emptying into the superior mesenteric or splenic vein; the accompanying cuff of duodenum is anastomosed to small bowel. The graft may be lost in the immediate perioperative period, most commonly because of vascular thrombosis (arterial or venous), reported from 2% to 19%, and less commonly because of infection, pancreatitis, bleeding, and anastomotic leaks. CT is helpful in evaluating postoperative complications such as anastomotic leaks, hemorrhage or other peripancreatic fluid collections, or graft pancreatitis, and with CTA techniques has the potential to identify vascular thrombosis. In particular, CT may aid in differentiating between acute rejection and pancreatitis, which may appear similar on ultrasound and can readily identify gas in patients with emphysematous pancreatitis of the graft, because of either infection or major vascular thrombosis. Vascular thrombosis is detectable with Doppler ultrasound and MRI. MRI is particularly useful when there is renal allograft dysfunction precluding administration of iodinated contrast medium, and with high-resolution three-dimensional or four-dimensional time of flight MRA and three-dimensional T1-weighted fast-spoiled gradient-echo sequences, investigation of vascular anatomy and abnormalities in addition to evaluation of the graft for reject and infarction.

Suggested Reading

Akisik MF, Sandrasegaran K, Aisen AA, et al. Dynamic secretin-enhanced MR cholangiopancreatography. *Radiographics*. 2006;26:665-677.

Hagspiel KD, Nandalur K, Pruett TL, et al. Evaluation of vascular complications of pancreas transplantation with high spatial-resolution contrast enhanced MR angiography. *Radiology*. 2007;242:590-599.

Horton KA, Hruban RH, Yeo C, Fishman EK. Multi-detector row CT of pancreatic islet cell tumors. *Radiographics*. 2006;26:453-464.

Kawamoto S, Horton KA, Lawler LP, Hruban RH, Fishman EK. Intraductal papillary mucinous neoplasm of the pancreas: can benign lesions be differentiated from malignant lesions with multidetector CT? *Radiographics*. 2005;25:1451-1470.

Leung RS, Biswas SV, Duncan M, et al. Imaging features of von Hippel Lindau disease. *Radiographics*. 2008;28:65-79.

Linsenmaier U, Wirth S, Reiser M, Körner M. Diagnosis and classification of pancreatic and duodenal injuries in emergency radiology. *Radiographics*. 2008;28:1591-1601.

Manfredi R, Graziani R, Cicero C, Frulloni L, et al. Autoimmune pancreatitis: CT patterns and their changes after steroid treatment. *Radiology*. 2008;247:435-443.

Morgan DE. Imaging of acute pancreatitis and its complications. *Clin Gastroenterol Hepatol*. 2008;10:1077-1085.

Mortelé KF, Rocha TC, Streeter JL, Taylor AF. Multimodality imaging of pancreatic and biliary congenital anomalies. *Radiographics*. 2006;26:715-731.

Robertson MB, Choe KA, Joseph PM. Review of the abdominal manifestations of cystic fibrosis in the adult patient. *Radiographics*. 2006;26:679-690.

Sahani DV, Kadavigere R, Saokar A, et al. Cystic pancreatic lesions: a simple imaging-based classification system for guiding management. *Radiographics*. 2005;25:1471-1484.

Siddiqi AJ, Miller F. Chronic pancreatitis: ultrasound, computed tomography, and magnetic resonance imaging features. *Semin Ultrasound CT MR*. 2007;28:384-394.

To'o KF, Raman SS, Yu NC, et al. Pancreatic and peripancreatic diseases mimicking primary pancreatic neoplasia. *Radiographics*. 2005;25:949-965.

Wong JC, Lu DSK. Staging of pancreatic adenocarcinoma by imaging studies. *Clin Gastroenterol Hepatol*. September 27, 2008. (Epub ahead of print).

QUESTIONS AND ANSWERS

1. Concerning blunt pancreatic trauma, which of the following is the most important determinant of pancreas-related complications?
   A. Pancreatic hematoma
   B. Pancreatitis
   C. Main pancreatic duct disruption
   D. Pancreatic necrosis

   ANSWER: C. Pancreatic hematoma is possible but generally would be more self-limited than duct disruption. Pancreatitis may develop after trauma, but does not lead to the severe and prolonged complications that disruption of the main pancreatic duct would produce. Pancreatic necrosis could conceivably occur as a complication of posttraumatic pancreatitis and may lead to severe complications, but in the setting of acute trauma main pancreatic duct disruption is the determining factor for disease severity.

2. Which of the following is the most common pancreatic abnormality in adult patients with CF?
   A. Pancreatic cystosis
   B. Complete fatty replacement
   C. Partial agenesis of the dorsal duct
   D. Pancreatic adenocarcinoma

   ANSWER: B. Pancreatic cystosis is a rare manifestation of CF, while partial agenesis of the dorsal duct is not associated with CF. Pancreatic adenocarcinoma may occur in patients with CF, but is not nearly as common as fatty replacement.

3. What is the most appropriate term for an enzyme-rich collection of peripancreatic fluid accompanied by focal (<30%) gland necrosis in a patient hospitalized for 10 days with acute pancreatitis?
   A. Pancreatic necrosis
   B. Postnecrotic pancreatic collection
   C. Pancreatic pseudocyst
   D. Acute fluid collection

   ANSWER: B. Pancreatic necrosis describes diminished perfusion of the pancreatic parenchyma. Pancreatic pseudocyst requires 4 weeks to form and by definition has no necrosis. Acute fluid collection is the older term for enzyme-rich pancreatic juice that is not contained and is released acutely into the retroperitoneum in acute pancreatitis.

4. Which of the following is the correct T stage for a pancreatic adenocarcinoma that measures 3.5 cm longest diameter, extends beyond the margins of the pancreas, but does not clearly encase the peripancreatic vessels?
   A. T1
   B. T2
   C. T3
   D. T4

   ANSWER: C. T1 stage refers to smaller lesions confined to the pancreas (less than 2 cm). T2 stage refers to larger lesions confined to the pancreas (greater than 2 cm). T4 stage refers to locally advanced tumors that involve the adjacent peripancreatic vessels or nerves.

5. An EUS with fine needle aspirate of primary pancreatic lesion in addition to a nearby lymph node confirms moderately differentiated pancreatic adenocarcinoma. There are no distant metastases detected on contrast-enhanced multiphasic MDCT. Which of the following is the correct TNM stage?
   A. IIa
   B. IIb
   C. III
   D. IV

   ANSWER: B. Stage IIa is node negative. Stage III is incorrect, as T4 lesion (local invasion of vessels) is part of this definition. Stage IV disease refers to pancreatic adenocarcinoma with distant metastatic disease, absent in the above-described case.

6. Which of the following is the most common anatomical variant of the pancreas?
   A. Pancreas divisum
   B. Partial dorsal agenesis
   C. Anomalous pancreatobiliary duct union
   D. Annular pancreas

   ANSWER: A. Pancreas divisum is found in 5% to 10% of the population in autopsy series. Others are much less common anatomic variants.

7. What percentage of non-hyperfunctioning (nonsyndromic) pancreatic NETs are malignant?
   A. 10%
   B. 30%
   C. 50%
   D. 80%

   ANSWER: D. The majority of non-hyperfunctioning or endocrine tumors are malignant.

8. In a patient with a hyperfunctioning pancreatic neuroendocrine tumor, which of the following syndromes corresponds to the symptom complex of fasting serum glucose < 50 mg/dL, hypoglycemia symptoms, and response to glucose administration?
   A. Verner-Morrison syndrome
   B. Zollinger-Ellison syndrome
   C. Whipple triad
   D. WDHA syndrome

   ANSWER: C. The symptom complex (fasting serum glucose < 50 mg/dL, hypoglycemia symptoms, and response to glucose administration) describes the classic Whipple triad. Verner-Morrison syndrome describes clinical findings associated with VIPoma. Zollinger-Ellison syndrome describes clinical symptoms associated with a gastrinoma. WDHA syndrome is another term to describe the syndrome associated with VIPoma.

9. Which of the following tumors does the patient described in question 8 have?
   A. Glucagonoma
   B. VIPoma
   C. Gastrinoma
   D. Insulinoma

   ANSWER: D. Whipple triad describes the syndrome seen in patients with insulinomas.

10. A 72-year-old woman had an abdominopelvic CT scan to evaluate left lower quadrant pain, suspected diverticulitis. A 4-cm unilocular cystic pancreatic head mass was incidentally discovered. EUS confirmed the unilocular nature, and fine needle aspirate revealed mucin, elevated CEA, and no amylase. Which of the following is the most likely diagnosis?
    A. Oligocystic serous cystadenoma
    B. Side branch-type IPMN
    C. Inflammatory pseudocyst
    D. Mucinous cystic neoplasm

    ANSWER: D. Elevated mucin within a cystic pancreatic mass that appears unilocular is classic for mucinous cystic neoplasm. Oligocystic serous cystadenoma is possible given the imaging findings, but less likely as an oligocystic serous cystadenomas would contain glycogen-rich cells rather than mucin in the aspirate. Although side branch IPMN may appear cystic and reach a size of 4 cm, elevated CEA level is not characteristic. Inflammatory pseudocysts typically demonstrate elevated amylase levels.

54 PERITONEAL CAVITY AND ABDOMINAL WALL

Bhavik N. Patel, Sanjiv K. Bajaj, and Cheri L. Canon

NORMAL ANATOMY

PERITONEUM

The peritoneum forms the lining of the abdominal cavity. It consists of two layers of pleura, the parietal pleura (lining the abdominal wall) and visceral pleura (lining the organs), which appose to form a double layer that transmits vessels, nerves, and lymphatics. This double layer forms infoldings that divide the abdomen into compartments and support the abdominal organs. The intraperitoneal organs include the liver, spleen, gallbladder, stomach, first portion of the duodenum, small bowel, and transverse and sigmoid colons. The retroperitoneal organs include the adrenal glands, kidneys, ureters, urinary bladder, inferior vena cava, aorta, pancreas, esophagus, second and third portions of the duodenum, ascending and descending colons, and rectum. The dome of the liver ("bare area") is not covered by peritoneum. It is surrounded by peritoneal reflections in a rounded configuration ("coronary ligament").

The two major divisions of the abdominal cavity are the greater and lesser sacs. The lesser sac is a normally collapsed space posterior to the stomach that communicates with the greater sac, the remainder of the abdominal cavity, via the foramen of Winslow (epiploic foramen). Its anterior boundaries include the stomach and lesser omentum, a layer of peritoneum hanging from the stomach, and its posterior boundary is the retroperitoneum, including the pancreas. Its inferior margin is formed by the transverse colon and greater omentum and its superior margin by the liver and diaphragm (Fig. 54-1). The spleen bounds it on the left, and the epiploic foramen allows inflow and outflow from the right.

Within the greater sac, peritoneal reflections separate the cavity into distinct zones. The falciform ligament separates the right and left subphrenic spaces. The right subphrenic space communicates easily with Morison pouch, the hepatorenal space, the most dependant portion of the abdomen in supine individuals. The pouch of Douglas, the rectouterine pouch, is the most dependent portion of the abdomen and pelvis in upright women. The left subhepatic and left subphrenic spaces communicate with each other, but they do not communicate with the left paracolic gutter because of the phrenicocolic ligament.

MESENTERY AND OMENTUM

Developing from the mesenchyme, the mesentery attaches the foregut, midgut, and hindgut to the posterior abdominal wall and later gives rise to the dorsal mesentery during embryonic development. The dorsal mesentery then becomes the respective structures based on its location. For example, the dorsal mesentery near the stomach becomes the greater omentum (Table 54-1). During embryonic development, the mesentery segments of the duodenum, ascending colon, and descending colon becomes fixed to the retroperitoneum. The jejunum, ileum, transverse colon, and sigmoid mesenteries remain mobile. The mesentery serves as an avenue for the vascular, lymphatic, and neural channels to and from the bowel.

The greater omentum is an apronlike double sheet of peritoneum that hangs inferiorly from the stomach and proximal duodenum and drapes over the small bowel. On CT, it appears as a simple fatty layer between the abdominal wall and is anterior to the stomach, small bowel, and transverse colon. The descending portions of the greater omentum fuse to form the gastrocolic ligament that connects to the transverse colon. Similarly, the gastrosplenic and gastrophrenic ligaments attach to the spleen and thoracic diaphragm, respectively. The greater omentum serves as a visceral fixation and a shield limiting pathologic spread. However, because it is bathed in peritoneal fluid, it is a common site of neoplastic and infectious seeding. The hepatoduodenal and gastrohepatic ligaments, collectively known as the lesser omentum, connect the lesser curvature of the stomach and proximal duodenum with the liver. The gastrohepatic ligament contains the left gastric vessels and lymph nodes and can be identified on CT as a triangular fat-containing region between the stomach and the liver. The hepatoduodenal ligament contains the common bile duct, portal vein, and hepatic artery, and its inferolateral margin forms the anterior margin of the epiploic foramen or the foramen of Winslow. It is through the epiploic foramen that the lesser sac, a peritoneal space between the stomach and the pancreas, communicates with the peritoneal cavity.

ABDOMINAL WALL

The abdominal wall is defined superiorly by the xiphoid process, inferiorly by the pubic symphysis, and posteriorly by the vertebral column and is composed of multiple layers (Table 54-2). The subcutaneous tissue consists of a fatty, superficial layer of fascia known as Camper fascia and a deeper, fibrous connective tissue layer known as Scarpa fascia. The external oblique, internal oblique, and transversus abdominis are the three muscles making up the anterolateral wall and enclose a large portion of the torso. Their fibers run oblique to one another and their aponeuroses fuse anteriorly to form the rectus sheath that encases the rectus abdominis muscles. The external oblique arises from the lower seven to eight ribs and courses inferomedially with its inferior portion of the aponeurosis rolled up on itself posteriorly and superiorly forming the Poupart or inguinal ligament. This portion of the external oblique extends from the anterior iliac spine to the pubic tubercle and forms a groove in which the spermatic cord lies. The iliacus, psoas, and pectineus muscles, and the femoral artery, nerve, and vein run underneath the inguinal ligament. A femoral hernia traverses posterior to the inguinal

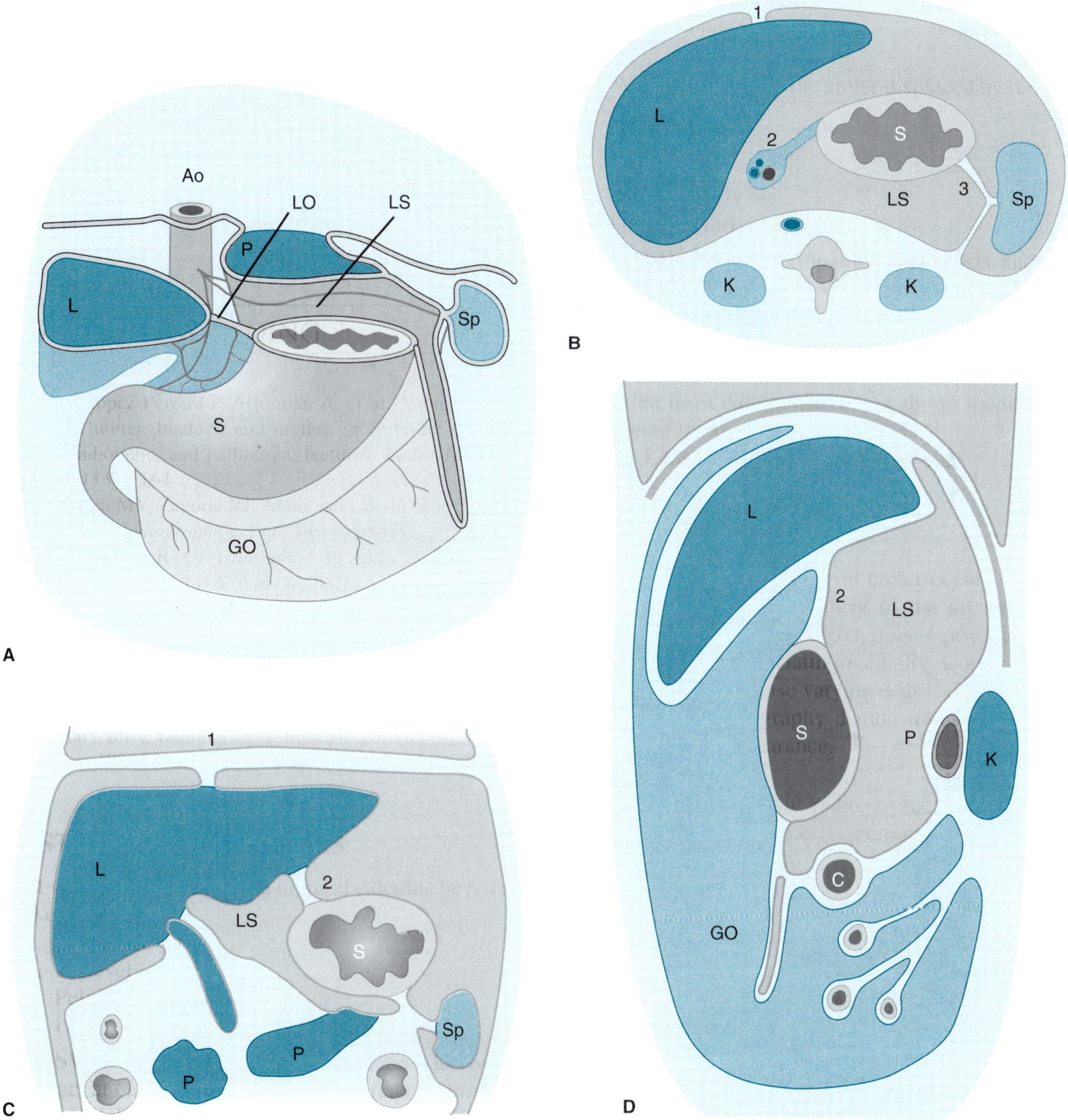

FIG. 54-1 Drawing of the anatomy of the greater and lesser omenta (A) and axial (B), coronal (C), and sagittal (D) diagrams of the upper abdomen. The greater omentum (GO) is composed of a double layer of peritoneum that extends from the greater curvature of the stomach (S) inferiorly. Its descending and ascending portions usually fuse to form a four-layer vascular fatty apron; the resulting space is contiguous with the lesser sac (LS). The lesser omentum (LO) connects the lesser curvature of the stomach and proximal duodenum with the liver (L) and contains blood vessels, nerves, and lymph nodes. The lesser sac is empty and collapsed so that only parts of its boundaries, such as the posterior gastric wall and pancreatic body, are observed on axial CT scans. Ao, aorta; C, colon; K, kidney; P, pancreas; Sp, spleen; 1, = falciform ligament; 2, = gastrohepatic ligament; 3, = gastrosplenic ligament.

SOURCE: Reprinted with permission from Yoo E, Kim JH, Kim MJ, et al. Greater and lesser omenta: normal anatomy and pathologic processes. *Radiographics*. 2007;27:707-720.

ligament, while an inguinal hernia passes anterior and superior to it. The internal oblique muscle fibers run in the opposite direction of and lie immediately below the external oblique muscle. Its inferior most fibers run along the spermatic cord and form the cremasteric muscle in the inguinal canal. The transversus abdominis muscle is the deepest of the three muscles and courses transversely from the lower six costal cartilages, lumbar vertebral spinous processes, and the iliac crest to the rectus abdominis muscle.

TABLE 54-1 Dorsal Mesentery Derivatives Based on Location

REGION	STRUCTURE
Stomach	Greater omentum
Colon	Mesocolon
Jejunum and ileum	Mesentery proper

TABLE 54-3 Borders of the Hesselbach Triangle

MARGIN	STRUCTURE
Floor	Transversalis fascia
Inferior	Inguinal ligament
Lateral	Inferior epigastric artery/vein
Medial	Lateral border of rectus sheath

Lying between the transversus abdominis and the extraperitoneal fat, the thin aponeurotic membrane of the transversalis fascia forms the fascial layer that lines the abdominal cavity giving it its structural integrity. A hernia results when there is a defect in this layer. The transversalis fascia forms the floor of Hesselbach triangle (Table 54-3) through which a direct inguinal hernia passes. The preperitoneal space contains adipose tissue through which the inferior epigastric artery and vein course before their entry into the rectus sheath. In addition, three fetal structures also lie within this space: the median umbilical ligament representing the remnant urachus, the medial umbilical ligament representing the vestigial umbilical artery, and the ligamentum teres representing the obliterated umbilical vein. The rectus abdominis muscles are paired midline muscles that are encased within the rectus sheath and extend from the xiphoid to the pubic symphysis. Along the paired muscles, there are approximately three to five tendinous interruptions of the muscle providing a site of attachment for the anterior rectus sheath. The anteroposterior layers of the rectus sheath come together at the midline to form the linea alba. Thinning of the linea alba, or diastasis recti, can lead to protrusion of the anterior abdominal wall. However, as long as the transversalis fascia is intact, there is no true hernia.

PATHOLOGY

PERITONEUM

Carcinomatosis/Metastatic Deposits

Metastatic cancers frequently involve the peritoneum. Intraperitoneal tumors commonly spread by direct implantation, when their cells become mobile in ascitic fluid. Gastric, colonic, and ovarian cancers frequently spread by this route, often to dependant areas, such as Morison pouch, ileocecal region, and the pouch of Douglas. These metastases distort the architecture of the surrounding abdominal organs, leading to fixed, retracted segments of bowel on barium examinations. Nodular, enhancing implants are seen on CT, often with associated ascites. Ultrasound demonstrates frequently hypoechoic nodules or masses, often with internal Color Doppler flow, in the setting of ascites. Treatment targets the primary neoplasm.

TABLE 54-2 Layers of the Anterolateral Abdominal Wall

Skin
Subcutaneous tissue
Superficial fascia
External oblique muscle
Internal oblique muscle
Transversus abdominis muscle
Transversalis fascia
Preperitoneal fat
Peritoneum

Peritoneal Lymphoma

Peritoneal involvement by lymphoma is rare and is nearly always of the Non-Hodgkin type. It classically occurs in patients with HIV. The disease presents similarly to peritoneal carcinomatosis, with peritoneal soft-tissue density nodularity and ascites. Treatment is with chemotherapy.

Pseudomyxoma Peritonei

Pseudomyxoma peritonei most commonly arises when appendical adenocarcinoma gives rise to a thick, mucinous material that spreads throughout the abdomen on appendiceal rupture. Other mucinous cancers, especially ovarian, more rarely give rise to this entity. Patients present with abdominal fullness, pain, and weight loss and many progress to bowel obstruction as the bowel becomes compressed by mucinous masses. Pseudomyxoma peritonei appears on CT as low attenuation ascites that causes nodular impressions upon the visceral organs. The liver surface characteristically has a "scalloped" appearance. The fluid may contain calcifications and appear complex. Ultrasound demonstrates echogenic ascites without mobile reflectors with fixed, displaced bowel loops and scalloping of the liver surface. The prognosis from this entity is extremely poor. Surgical therapy aims to ameliorate symptoms rather than provide a cure.

Malignant Mesothelioma

Primary peritoneal mesothelioma arises from neoplasia of peritoneal mesothelial cells in patients with asbestos exposure. It carries a similarly dismal prognosis to its thoracic counterpart, but is rare, occurring in approximately one-third of thoracic cases. CT detects enhancing nodular masses on the peritoneum and mesentery that spread by direct extension and can invade abdominal organs. Ultrasound demonstrates nodules that aggregate in layers or plaques with a small amount of associated ascites.

PERITONITIS

Peritonitis represents inflammation of the peritoneum and may arise from many different etiologies. Patients commonly present with signs of an acute abdomen, abdominal pain, guarding, and rebound tenderness. Many acute causes of peritonitis require emergent surgery.

Localized peritonitis can develop from inflammatory processes in adjacent organs, such as appendicitis and diverticulitis. The findings and treatment are of the primary process.

Intraperitoneal abscesses can arise from multiple etiologies, including perforated appendicitis or diverticulitis. Patients typically present with abdominal pain and fever in the relevant setting. Radiographs can demonstrate ileus and displacement of bowel loops when abscesses are large. CT demonstrates loculated fluid collections, classically with enhancing walls after the administration of intravenous contrast. Their density may be higher than simple fluid, and they may contain septations or gas. Ultrasound can show loculated fluid collections with internal reflectors and gas, sometimes with a thickened wall. Treatment involves antibiotics and drainage.

Spontaneous Bacterial Peritonitis

Spontaneous bacterial peritonitis presents with ascites, fevers, rigors, and abdominal pain and occurs when intraperitoneal fluid becomes infected after translocation of bacteria from the gut. Radiographs reveal ascites and sometimes ileus. CT can demonstrate enhancement and thickening of the peritoneum in the setting of ascites. Ultrasound can show the complicated, loculated ascites with floating debris and often thickened peritoneum. However, the diagnosis requires aspiration of fluid and culture. Untreated spontaneous bacterial peritonitis can lead to intraperitoneal abscess and carries high morbidity and mortality, although timely treatment with antibiotics provides effective cure.

Tuberculous Peritonitis

Tuberculous peritonitis likely develops after hematogenous seeding of acid-fast bacilli, most commonly in the HIV-afflicted population in the United States. Three patterns are described: wet, fibrotic, and dry. The wet type of tuberculous peritonitis presents as loculated or free high attenuation ascites. The fibrotic type can appear like peritoneal carcinomatosis, with soft-tissue density enhancing nodules and sometimes omental caking. The dry type presents with mesenteric soft-tissue replacement, nodules, and adhesions. All patterns are associated with lymphadenopathy, sometimes low in attenuation. Treatment targets the primary tuberculous infection. Peritoneal sarcoid involvement can mimic tuberculous infection.

Chemical Peritonitis

Chemical peritonitis arises from noninfectious causes, most typically gastric, biliary, or pancreatic rupture with inflammation caused by the relevant fluid. Barium sulfate contrast spillage into the peritoneum, ruptured teratoma, and meconium peritonitis in children are other etiologies. Patients are typically postoperative from biliary or pancreatic procedures or have risk factors for bowel perforation, such as nonsteroidal anti-inflammatory drug use, ulcer disease, or history of trauma. They present with sudden onset of severe abdominal pain, hypotension, and sometimes shock. Imaging studies can show ascites, peritoneal enhancement, and free gas or fluid/fluid levels in certain etiologies. Treatment is aimed at the inciting pathology and at stabilization and support.

Sclerosing Peritonitis

Sclerosing peritonitis arises in the setting of peritoneal dialysis and exposure to certain drugs. Patients present with failure of effective dialysis; they later develop abdominal pain and bowel obstructions. Pathology shows fibrotic soft-tissue thickening of the peritoneum, progressing to encasement of bowel loops. The precise etiology is unclear. Imaging studies demonstrate increased peristalsis, dilated bowel loops, calcifications, and septated, loculated ascites with fibrous soft-tissue thickening that eventually encases bowel loops. Prognosis remains poor despite surgical treatment for the amelioration of symptoms.

MESENTERY

SCLEROSING MESENTERITIS (PANNICULITIS)

Sclerosing mesenteritis is an idiopathic, inflammatory disease of the mesentery adipose tissue. Also known as mesenteric panniculitis, mesenteric lipodystrophy, retroperitoneal xanthogranuloma, sclerosing lipogranulomatosis, lipogranuloma of the mesentery, retractile mesenteritis, and primary mesenteric liposclerosis, sclerosing mesenteritis most commonly involves the small bowel mesentery and to a lesser degree the mesocolon. The disease is characterized by thickened, nodular, and fibrotic mesentery with fat necrosis and nonneoplastic mass like lesions. Ultimately, this leads to a short, thickened, and scarred mesentery that may distort the bowel. Sclerosing mesenteritis commonly presents in males in their fifth to sixth decade of life with abdominal pain and, on occasion, a palpable abdominal mass. Often, distortion of the bowel may lead to signs and symptoms of small bowel obstruction. Sclerosing mesenteritis does not display the typical infiltrative histological appearance that is commonly seen in mesenteric desmoid. On CT, sclerosing mesenteritis may appear as a spiculated, soft-tissue mass with calcification that may surround the mesenteric vessels without involving the perivascular fat, giving an appearance that has been termed the "fat ring sign." MRI will reveal low T1 and T2 signal images. Although metastatic carcinoid may appear radiologically similar to mesenteric panniculitis, a somatostatin receptor scintigraphy scan will allow distinction. Prognosis is usually favorable with treatment ranging from observation to surgical intervention. Surgery is usually performed to establish the diagnosis by biopsy or in cases of small bowel obstruction.

Mesenteric Cysts

Mesenteric cysts are benign lesions that commonly occur in the small bowel mesentery or the mesocolon. The cause is unknown and typically occurs more commonly in middle-aged women. They may be completely asymptomatic or present with symptoms of mass effect. The cysts usually contain a clear serous fluid and can be diagnosed on ultrasonography or CT. Symptomatic treatment includes surgical excision rather than aspiration, which carries a high risk of recurrence.

Mesenteric Adenitis

Mesenteric adenitis is a self-limited disorder characterized by inflammation of the mesenteric lymph nodes usually presenting in the pediatric patient population. Because the nodes in right lower quadrant are most commonly involved, the presentation and diagnosis is often confused for acute appendicitis. Etiology is most commonly viral; however, bacterial pathogens, most commonly *Yersinia enterocolitica,* parasites, and fungi have also been implicated. Often times, patients undergo surgery for presumed appendicitis only to find a normal-appearing appendix. In addition, a number of cases may involve the adjacent small bowel mucosa, giving rise to cecitis and ileocolitis. Ultrasonography is the preferred diagnostic modality and reveals enlarged lymph nodes with increased blood flow. CT may be employed and used to exclude mesenteric adenitis in the case of acute appendicitis. In addition, CT findings of clustered, large lymph nodes in the right lower quadrant with a normal appearing appendix further support the diagnosis.

Mesenteric Carcinoid

Carcinoid tumors are a type of neuroendocrine tumors that arise from the enterochromaffin cells and produce vasoactive substances such as serotonin. The gastrointestinal and bronchopulmonary tracts are the most common sites for these tumors. They are slow growing and many patients present with metastatic disease. They are the most common small bowel tumors and can involve the mesentery via direct extension or lymphatogenous spread. Serotonin produced by these tumors elicits a desmoplastic reaction in the mesentery, leading to fibrosis and ischemia. CT may reveal mesenteric fibrosis, mesenteric lymphadenopathy, and nodular deposits that may contain calcifications. In addition, octreotide scintigraphy scan demonstrates positive uptake of the radiotracer by the mesenteric nodules.

Mesenteric Desmoid

Mesenteric desmoid, also known as intra-abdominal or mesenteric fibromatosis, is part of a group of diseases known benign fibroproliferative processes. It occurs in a wide patient age range and has no race predilection. It is particularly common in patients with familial adenomatous polyposis and has even as stronger association with the subset of patients with Gardner syndrome. Prior abdominal surgery, most commonly a total colectomy, has been associated with an increased risk of developing mesenteric desmoid in patients with familial adenomatous polyposis. This correlation is significantly weaker in sporadic cases. Patients with mesenteric desmoid present with small bowel signs and symptoms, such as abdominal pain, obstruction, perforation, and fistula formation. A hallmark histological finding of these tumors is infiltration into the muscularis propria of the bowel wall that some authors have termed "tentacular or melting insinuation." Mesenteric desmoid can be often be radiologically and histologically mistaken for gastrointestinal stromal tumor (GIST). However, special immunohistochemical staining allows for differentiation between these two entities.

Radiological features of mesenteric desmoid includes mass effect with displaced bowel segments, partial or complete small bowel obstruction, perforation, or fistula formation. Ultimately, the histological characteristics (especially the degree of infiltration) determine radiological appearance. CT and MRI are the preferred imaging modalities. The degree of collagenous and myxoid stroma components of mesenteric desmoid determines its CT and MRI characteristics. It has minimal contrast enhancement on CT and typically has low to intermediate signal intensity on T1-weighted images and intermediate to high signal on T2-weighted images. Treatment of mesenteric fibromatosis varies. Although complete resection with free margins is commonly preferred, there is a high recurrence rate. In addition, many cases may be complicated by sequelae of the infiltrative nature of the tumor, such as obstruction and fistula formation. Because of a high recurrence rate, some authors recommend medical management in advanced cases. Sporadic cases typically carry lower disease morbidity and mortality associated compared to those patients with familial adenomatous polyposis.

ABDOMINAL WALL

HERNIAS

An abdominal hernia occurs when there is a protrusion of abdominal contents through a defect in the abdominal wall. Hernias are electively repaired surgically to prevent complications that arise when a hernia becomes irreducible or incarcerated and strangulated. A hernia is incarcerated when it cannot be reduced and can lead to bowel obstruction. A strangulated hernia is one in which there is compromise of the vascular supply (arterial or venous) leading to bowel ischemia and necrosis. CT is the preferred diagnostic imaging modality as it will detect the location and contents of the hernia sac as well as early signs of the aforementioned hernia complications. However, hernias may also be detected on other imaging modalities such as conventional radiographs, contrast fluoroscopy studies, and ultrasonography.

Ventral Hernias

Ventral or anterior abdominal wall hernias occur as a result of a congenital or an acquired defect through the abdominal wall musculature and fascia. The protruding peritoneal sac may contain fat, omentum, and/or bowel loops. Patients can present with abdominal pain, signs and symptoms of bowel obstruction in complicated hernias, and an anterior abdominal bulge that increases with Valsava. However, some patients may be asymptomatic or difficult to examine because of body habitus thus making imaging of greater utility in diagnosis and early detection of complications. CT imaging may detect ventral hernias either by direct visualization of the hernia sac content or through identification of the fascial defect (Table 54-4).

Groin and Pelvic Hernias

Groin and pelvic hernias typically present with vague groin pain and, like ventral hernias, carry an associated risk of strangulation and incarceration. Thus, surgical repair is indicated. CT and contrast fluoroscopy are commonly used to identify these hernias. While inguinal hernias are more common in men, femoral and obturator hernias are more prevalent in women (Table 54-5).

Internal Hernias

Internal hernias are rare and occur when the small bowel protrudes through the mesentery into another cavity. These hernias occur as a result of congenital developmental defects, such as abnormal mesentery fixation and enlarged foramen, and iatrogenic mesenteric defects (i.e., surgically created). With the increase in laparoscopic (minimally invasive) surgical procedures, postsurgical internal hernias are now the most common etiologic type. The most common clinical manifestation is that of small bowel obstruction. CT is the preferred imaging modalities (Table 54-6).

OTHER ABDOMINAL WALL ABNORMALITIES

Abdominal Wall Desmoid Tumor

Unlike mesenteric desmoids, which commonly occur in patients with familial adenomatous polyposis, abdominal wall desmoid tumors occur sporadically. Abdominal wall desmoids are common in young women and have

TABLE 54-4 Ventral Hernias

TYPE	LOCATION	FEATURES
Umbilical/paraumbilical	Midline, at the umbilical ring	Most common ventral hernia
		Congenital in infants, usually close spontaneously by 4 y of age
		In adults, it is a result of chronic increased intra-abdominal pressure. Common in obese and multiparous women
		Repair indicated in large and symptomatic hernias and in children older than 5 y with persistent congenital hernia caused by risk of incarceration
Epigastric & hypogastric	Midline, through linea alba above and below the umbilicus, respectively	Same acquired risk factors as in umbilical hernia
Richter	Midline	Only one side of bowel wall within hernia sac
		Bowel wall remains patent and thus there is no risk of obstruction. Risk of incarceration still present
Spigelian	Lateral, at the junction of the semicircular and semilunar lines	Occurs below the arcuate line where there is an absence of posterior rectus sheath
		Results in an interparietal hernia making detection difficult
Incisional	Prior surgical incision site	Increased risk factors include obesity, immunosuppression, postoperative wound infection, and malnutrition

TABLE 54-5 Groin and Pelvic Hernias

TYPE	LOCATION	FEATURES
Direct inguinal	Medial to the epigastric vessels and through Hesselbach triangle	Because of an acquired defect of the transversalis fascia
Indirect inguinal	Lateral to the epigastric vessels	Most common abdominal hernia Occurs because of patent processus vaginalus leading to entry of the hernia contents through the internal ring, into the inguinal canal, and exiting the external ring May extend into the scrotum or labia
Pantaloon	Hernia on both sides of the epigastric vessels	Combined direct and indirect inguinal hernia
Femoral	Femoral canal, below the inguinal ligament and medial to the femoral vein	Occurs because of a defect in the transversalis fascia attachment at the pubis Carries a high risk of incarceration
Obturator	Obturator canal	Occurs because of a defect in the obturator membrane Hernia contents frequently involve bowel accounting for high incidence of obstruction and incarceration Howship-Romberg sign: impingement of the obturator nerve causing medial thigh pain

been associated with increased estrogen states. Just as in mesenteric desmoid, there is some association between prior abdominal surgery and the development of abdominal wall desmoid tumors. They arise either from the abdominal musculature fascia or their aponeurosis. The tumors arising from the superficial fascia are slow growing as oppose to those arising from the aponeurosis. Patients typically present with a painless abdominal wall mass. The histological, CT, and MRI findings are similar to those of mesenteric desmoid tumors and biopsy will provide definitive diagnosis and exclude other neoplasms such as lipomas or sarcomas. Treatment includes complete resection; however, high recurrence rates are common.

Abdominal Wall Hematomas

The rectus sheath contains a collateral network of vessels including the penetrating epigastric vessels. Damage to these vessels can lead to formation of a rectus sheath hematoma. The extent of the hematoma depends on whether the bleeding occurs below or above the semicircular line. Above this line, the hematomas are

TABLE 54-6 Internal Hernias

TYPE	CHARACTERISTICS	RADIOLOGICAL FEATURES (CT)
Paraduodenal (mesocolic)	Most common type of nonsurgical internal hernia, left more common than right Left—small bowel herniates behind the mesocolon into the fossa of Landzert Right—small bowel herniates into the fossa of Waldeyer	Left paraduodenal hernia will demonstrate crowded loops of dilates small bowel within in a sac located between the pancreas and stomach. The mesenteric vessels supplying the herniated loops will be engorged and part of the hernia sac
Pericecal	Occurs as a result of absent or enlarged ileocecal recesses allowing small bowel to herniation	Cluster of dilated loops of small bowel in the right lower abdomen, lateral to the ascending colon
Transmesenteric/Transomental	Small bowel herniates through defects in the mesentery or omentum resulting in small bowel segments lying anterior to and displacing large bowel	Signs of volvulus and clustered loops of small bowel overlying large bowel and without omental fat. Involved mesenteric vessels may be crowded and engorged
Foramen of Winslow	Small bowel herniates through an enlarged foramen of Winslow	Mesentery will be present between the inferior vena cava and portal vein, dilated loops of small bowel in the foramen of Winslow, and absence of the right colon in the right lower quadrant
Intersigmoid	Small bowel herniation into the intersigmoid fossa	Dilated loops of small bowel will be seen in the intersigmoid fossa, left of the sigmoid mesocolon
Supra-/perivesical and pelvic	Herniation into the supravesical fossa, perirectal fossa, or through a defect in the broad ligament	Dilated loops of small bowel within the respective cavities

Reprinted with permission from Takeyama N, Gokan T, Ohgiya Y, et al. CT of Internal hernias. *Radiographics.* 2005;25:997-1015 and Blachar A, Federle M, Dodson SF. Internal hernia: clinical and imaging findings in 17 patients with emphasis on CT criteria. *Radiology.* 2001;218:68-74.

well confined and can be controlled by tamponade from the rectus sheath. However, below this line, there is no such confinement and the hematoma can rapidly expand. Bleeding into the rectus sheath can occur as a result of trauma, iatrogenic causes (injections), sudden contraction or stretching of the rectus muscles, or spontaneously in patients on anticoagulation therapy. Patients typically present with abdominal pain and an abdominal wall mass or bulge. CT and ultrasonography can be used to confirm the diagnosis. Treatment depends on the extent of the hematoma and may range from observation to resuscitation to surgical evacuation and vessel ligation.

MISCELLANEOUS DISORDERS

WHIPPLE DISEASE

Whipple disease arises after infection with *Tropheryma whipplei*, which leads to infiltration of lymph nodes by "foamy" macrophages on pathology. Patients present with protean symptoms from multiple body systems, including abdominal pain, diarrhea, arthritis, and ocular and neurologic symptoms. CT demonstrates small bowel wall thickening and intestinal lipodystrophy and low attenuation lymphadenopathy secondary to fatty accumulation in the lymph nodes of the small bowel mesentery. Treatment aims at curing the underlying infection.

CASTLEMAN DISEASE

Castleman disease, or angiofollicular lymph node hyperplasia, presents similarly to lymphoma, with fevers of unknown origin, weight loss, and abdominal masses, often in the setting of HIV infection. CT demonstrates brightly enhancing lymph node masses. The plasma cell type presents more commonly in the abdomen, while the hyaline type is more common in the mediastinum. Both variants carry an increased risk of lymphomatous transformation, although the primary process is nonneoplastic. The prognosis is poor.

SUGGESTED READING

Aguirre D, Santosa A, et al. Abdominal wall hernias: imaging features, complications, and diagnostic pitfalls at multi–detector row CT. *Radiographics.* 2005;25:1501-1520.

Blachar A, Federle M, Dodson SF. Internal hernia: clinical and imaging findings in 17 patients with emphasis on CT criteria. *Radiology.* 2001;218:68-74.

Hamrick-Turner JE, Chiechi MV, et al. PL abbitt, neoplastic and inflammatory processes of the peritoneum, omentum, and mesentery: diagnosis with CT. *Radiographics.* 1992;12:1051-1068.

Harrison LA, Keesling CA, et al. Abdominal wall hernias: review of herniography and correlation with cross-sectional imaging. *Radiographics.* 1995;15:315-332.

Levy A, Arnáiz J. From the Archives of the AFIP: primary peritoneal tumors: imaging features with pathologic correlation. *Radiographics.* 2008;28:583-607.

Levy A, Rimola J, et al. From the archives of the AFIP: benign fibrous tumors and tumorlike lesions of the mesentery: radiologic-pathologic correlation. *Radiographics.* 2006;26:245-264.

Miller PA, Mezwa DG, et al. Imaging of abdominal hernias. *Radiographics.* 1995;15:333-347.

Sheth S, Horton KM, Garland MR, et al. Mesenteric neoplasms: CT appearances of primary and secondary tumors and differential diagnosis. *Radiographics.* 2003;23:457-473.

Takeyama N, Gokan T, Ohgiya Y, et al. CT of internal hernias. *Radiographics.* 2005;25:997-1015.

Yoo E, Kim JH, Kim M, et al. Greater and lesser omenta: normal anatomy and pathologic processes. *Radioraphics.* 2007;27:707-720.

QUESTIONS AND ANSWERS

1. What is the most dependent space of the abdomen in the supine patient?
   A. Morison pouch
   B. Pouch of Douglas
   C. Left paracolic gutter
   D. Right paracolic gutter
   E. Lesser sac

   ANSWER: A. Morison pouch, the hepatorenal fossa, is the most dependant portion of the abdomen in supine patients. The pouch of Douglas is the most dependent portion of the abdomen in upright women. The right and left paracolic gutters are dependent areas in supine patients, but Morison pouch is more dependent. The lesser sac is an enclosed intraperitoneal space separated from the remainder of the abdominal cavity.

2. Hyperenhancing retroperitoneal lymph nodes are identified on CT. What is the most likely diagnosis?
   A. Tuberculous peritonitis
   B. Peritoneal lymphoma
   C. Whipple disease
   D. Castleman disease
   E. Pseudomyxoma peritonei

   ANSWER: D. Castleman disease (angiofollicular lymph node hyperplasia) gives enhancing lymph nodes. The lymph nodes in tuberculous peritonitis and Whipple disease are low attenuation. Peritoneal lymphoma gives soft-tissue density lymphadenopathy. Pseudomyxoma peritonei is characterized by low attenuation mucinous material that exerts mass effect upon the adjacent organs.

3. Which of the following is *true* of pseudomyxoma peritonei?
   A. Excellent prognosis
   B. Fluid is typically high in attenuation.
   C. Fluid exerts mass effect on adjacent organs.
   D. Primary process is usually infectious.
   E. Ovarian carcinoma is the most common etiology.

   ANSWER: C. The mucinous fluid from pseudomyxoma peritonei classically exerts mass effect upon the abdominal organs, causing a scalloped appearance. The prognosis is dismal, and the fluid is classically low in attenuation. The primary process is neoplastic, usually secondary to appendiceal or ovarian mucinous adenocarcinoma. Appendiceal carcinoma is a more common cause than ovarian.

4. Which of the following is *true* regarding tuberculous peritonitis?
   A. Typically results from primary peritoneal infection
   B. Only occurs in the third world
   C. Can mimic peritoneal carcinomatosis on CT
   D. Lymph nodes are usually normal in size.
   E. No ascites is seen.

   ANSWER: C. Tuberculous peritonitis can mimic peritoneal carcinomatosis, with nodular, enhancing soft-tissue thickening and adhesions. The infection is usually secondary to hematogenous spread and can occur in any location. In the US, it most commonly occurs in patients with HIV. There is usually lymphadenopathy, often low in attenuation. There is typically ascites, sometimes loculated.

5. Where is the anatomic defect in a Spigelian hernia?
   A. Diastasis recti
   B. Semicircular and semilunar lines
   C. Linea alba
   D. Umbilical ring

   ANSWER: B. Spigelian hernias are lateral, occurring at the junction of the semicircular and semiluna lines. Diastasis recti is a ventral eventration (not a true hernia) typically seen in patients with increased abdominal pressure (multiparous women, obesity). Epigastric and hypogastric hernias occur in the midline through the linea alba. Umbilical hernias are defects in the umbilical ring.

6. What is the most common etiology of mesenteric adenitis?
   A. Yersinia enterocolitica
   B. Viral
   C. Parasitic
   D. Fungal
   E. Bacterial

   ANSWER: B. Mesenteric adenitis is a self-limited inflammatory condition most commonly caused by a viral pathogen. *Yersinia enterocolitica* has been implicated the most common bacterial cause. Bacterial, parasitic, and fungal can all cause mesenteric adenitis but are not as common as viral.

7. What is the anatomic opening between the greater and lesser sacs?
   A. Epiploic foramen
   B. Gastrohepatic ligament
   C. Coronary ligament
   D. Fossa of Waldeyer

   ANSWER: A. The epiploic foramen (Foramen of Winslow) connects the greater and lesser sacs. The coronary ligament defines the bare area at the dome of the liver. The fossa of Waldeyer is the location of small bowel herniation in a right paraduodenal hernia.

8. Which of the following is the most common type of nonidiopathic internal hernia?
   A. Left paraduodenal hernia
   B. Right paraduodenal hernia
   C. Foramen of Winslow hernia
   D. Intersigmoid hernia

   ANSWER: A. Overall, most internal hernias are postsurgical, usually transmesenteric Paraduodenal hernias are the most common type of congenital internal hernia. The left paraduodenal hernias are more common than the right with the small bowel herniating behind the mesocolon into the fossa of Landzert.

9. Concerning umbilical hernias, which of the following is *true*?
   A. Most common type of abdominal hernias
   B. Low risk of incarceration and rarely require repair
   C. Common in patients with chronically increased intra-abdominal pressure
   D. Children in which the hernia has not closed by 2 years of age require repair.

   ANSWER: C. Umbilical hernias are the most common ventral hernia and occur in patients with increased intra-abdominal pressure, particularly obese patients. They carry a high risk of incarceration and are repaired. Children with umbilical hernias should have spontaneous closure by the age of 4.

10. In distinguishing mesenteric desmoid and abdominal wall desmoid tumors, which of the following is *true*?
    A. Abdominal wall desmoid tumors are more commonly associated with FAP as opposed to mesenteric desmoid.
    B. They have different histological findings.
    C. Abdominal wall desmoids have no association with prior abdominal surgery as do mesenteric desmoids.
    D. Most cases of abdominal wall desmoid are sporadic as oppose to mesenteric desmoid.

ANSWER: D. Abdominal wall and mesenteric desmoid are both fibroproliferative diseases that have similar histological findings and an association with prior abdominal surgery or trauma. Abdominal wall desmoid cases are usually sporadic, whereas mesenteric desmoid commonly occur in patients with FAP.

Section 5
GENITOURINARY TRACT

55 INTRAVENOUS CONTRAST AGENTS AND REACTIONS

Philip J. Kenney

INTRODUCTION: UTILITY OF CONTRAST

Shortly after the discovery of x-rays and their potential for diagnostic imaging, researchers began looking for materials that would enhance the detection of disease by introducing differential radiographic density of anatomic structures. In the 1920s, Moses Swick had the first reasonable success in developing an intravenously administered agent that aided visualization of the urinary tract, Uroselectan. For many years, the intravenous urogram was a standard method for initial evaluation of urologic disorders. By injecting an agent that could not cross cell membranes, was excreted by glomerular filtration and incorporated the k-edge properties of iodine, the kidneys, ureters, and bladder could be reasonably well visualized using conventional radiography. The quality was eventually improved by addition of x-ray tomography. With the development of CT, the uses of iodinated intravenous contrast agents exponentially increased and the detection of enhancing lesions in the brain, liver, and extremities became possible. This led to much broader use of these agents. Iodinated contrast also was a necessary factor in development of angiography, initially performed with direct catheter injection into arteries with radiographic imaging, now largely replaced by CT angiography.

Iodinated contrast is successfully used in many nonintravascular procedures. Contrast is necessary and useful for visualization of the bladder, urethra, ureters, uterus, and fallopian tubes by direct installation. These procedures include cystography, voiding cystourethrography, retrograde urethrography, antegrade and retrograde direct pyelo/ureterography, and hysterosalpingography (HSG). Iodinated contrast has also been useful in various gastrointestinal and other nonvascular routes of administration.

The advantage and utility of iodinated contrast is in its ability to aid accurate diagnosis by introducing a differential in radiographic density (whether on radiographic images or CT) between anatomic structures or pathology and background, thus the term contrast. The term "dye" should not be used, as these agents are all colorless. Except for differences in concentration of different formulations, and major differences in osmolality, strikingly little difference in performance has been noted between different specific agents in the same class.

However, despite the great utility, iodinated contrast agents have always had risks of adverse events. Over time, agents with less toxicity have been developed, but adverse events still occur and knowledge of the risk factors, methods for avoidance, and treatments of such events are critical parts of the skill set for the practitioners of radiology.

MRI was a great advance, initially thought to provide inherent contrast such that no injected agents would be necessary. However with further experience, limitations in the inherent tissue contrast and diagnostic capabilities of differences from T1, T2, and proton density factors became recognized. The introduction of gadolinium-based intravenous contrast agents was rapidly adopted. Gadolinium diethylenetriamine penta-acetic acid (DTPA) was the initial agent, still used. Limited to extracellular space and excreted solely by glomerular filtration, this agent mimicked the physiology of iodinated contrast, although the mechanism of action (increasing T1 relaxation time) was very different. Initial research revealed this agent to be remarkably well tolerated, with much lower rates of adverse events compared to iodinated contrast. Additional agents using gadolinium as the active heavy metal with different chelating agents were soon introduced, also well tolerated in studies, with similar low incidence of adverse events.

Only relatively recently has a previously unrecognized serious adverse outcome from exposure to gadolinium contrast agents come to light. Some 10 years after initial release of gadolinium contrast agents, reports of a new potentially fatal systemic illness, now defined as nephrogenic systemic fibrosis (NSF) appeared in the literature, stimulating the U.S. Food and Drug Administration (FDA) to place a "black-box" warning on all such agents approved for use. It is now also critical for radiologists to understand current recommendations for screening for risk factors and avoidance of this iatrogenic illness.

GENERAL PRINCIPLES

Current iodinated contrast agents are designed to increase differences in attenuation utilizing the properties of iodine for absorption of x-rays. All are based on a tri-iodinated benzoic acid ring. All are stable, not metabolized, with 99% excretion by glomerular filtration from the kidney, and with no significant tubular secretion or reabsorption. Approximately 1% is excreted in bile, tears, sweat, saliva, or breast milk if renal function is normal. The agents all have low lipid solubility, poor protein or membrane binding and are hydrophilic. Upon injection, they initially mix in the vascular pool, then spread through the extracellular space, but do not cross cell walls. With normal renal function, more than 90% is excreted within 24 hours. Thus the mechanism of action of various agents is quite similar. Some agents have higher concentration, which can affect selection of volume of administration. Some have greater or lesser viscosity, which is a consideration when injecting through small catheters.

There are three general classes of iodinated contrast agents. The older class are ratio 1.5 agents, ionic monomers with two soluble particles for every three iodine atoms, since the agents dissociate into the iodinated benzoic acid anion and the cation such as sodium or methylglucamine. These have the highest osmolality, up to five times that of plasma. Newer ratio 3 agents, three iodine atoms for every soluble particle, may be nonionic monomers such as iopamidol or ionic dimmers such as ioxaglate. The newest and lowest osmolality ratio 6 agents, six iodine atoms for each soluble particle, are nonionic dimers, such as iodixanol. Because of the large molecular size, these agents also have the highest viscosity.

Utility of iodinated contrast agents is very similar in studies comparing image quality or diagnosis. One major difference affecting the incidence of adverse events is osmolality; however, comparative studies have usually shown equivalence in diagnostic capability of the high osmolar ionic agents when compared to lower osmolar nonionic agents.

A number of physiologic effects have been reported from intravascular administration of iodinated contrast agents. These physiologic effects are seen to a significantly lesser degree with low osmolar iodinated agents. Such effects include inotropic depression.

ADVERSE EVENTS

Certain physiologic effects of the injection of iodinated contrast may cause patient discomfort. These are accentuated with high osmolar contrast. Such effects include pain at the injection site, flushing sensation, warmth, altered taste, nausea, and vomiting (much more likely with a full stomach and high osmolar contrast media [HOCM]). These are not true "reactions" or toxicity, and therefore, do not require therapy.

Cardiovascular events can be stimulated by iodinated contrast injection: inotropic depression, stimulation of arrhythmias, and decreased perfusion. These effects are greater with higher osmolar contrast, intra-arterial injection, and affect the organ closest to injection site. For example, injection of contrast, especially high osmolar, directly into a coronary vessel causes significant inotropic depression; injection directly into a renal artery causes decrease in renal perfusion; injection into aorta or intravenous administration causes much less effect.

Of most concern are allergic-like reactions. Research has shown such adverse events are not true allergies, although the term is often incorrectly used. This is because many of the symptoms and physiologic actions are similar to true allergic reactions, but the exact mechanism of contrast reactions remains unclear. Antibodies to contrast have not been demonstrated and cell-mediated immunity does not play a role.

Because of the potential for harm, whenever a patient is evaluated for a contrast-enhanced examination, three goals must be met: administer appropriate contrast given the indication, minimize the chance for a reaction, and treat a reaction should it occur.

AVOIDANCE OF ADVERSE EVENTS

The most important factor in avoidance of significant adverse events is accurate and consistent screening for risk factors. The most significant factor is history of a prior allergic-like reaction to iodinated contrast. If the patient gives such a history, investigating the details of that reaction and what treatment if any was needed is important. Any history of allergy, especially if severe, increases the risk of contrast reaction. Shellfish allergies are now *not* considered of greater significance than allergies to other substances. Patients with asthma, especially if requiring treatment, have elevated risk as do patients with cardiovascular disease, congestive heart failure, and recent myocardial infarction.

If a patient has moderate risk factors, in particular a prior but not life-threatening reaction, pretreatment may be used if there is a strong indication for a contrast study. HOCM should not be used in such instances. No data indicate a significant difference in reaction rates of low osmolar contrast media (LOCM) versus isosmolar contrast media (IOCM). There is some published data and much experience suggesting pretreatment reduces the likelihood of a repeat reaction, although the likelihood is not completely eliminated. Pretreatment regimens usually combine a histamine (H1 or H2) antagonist with steroids. Steroids must be administered for at least 12 hours prior to exposure to contrast in order to adequately reduce contrast reaction. One regimen that has been shown to reduce reactions combines oral methylprednisolone 32 mg, 12 and 2 hours prior to contrast. Another recommended regimen includes three doses of 50 mg oral prednisone every 6 hours prior to contrast with 50 mg oral or intramuscular injection diphenhydramine 1 hour before contrast administration. However, there are few if any publications comparing different regimens.

If a patient has had a prior life-threatening reaction, it may be best to avoid iodinated contrast altogether and alternates such as MRI may be used. There does not appear to be strong correlation of reactions to iodinated contrast with reactions to gadolinium, so that this alternative can be used without premedication.

COMMON REACTIONS AND TREATMENTS (Table 55-1)

A variety of distinct types of reactions have been described, all of which vary in severity. Most reactions are mild, self-limited, and resolve without treatment. Moderate reactions are defined as those somewhat more severe but not life threatening; these usually require some treatment. Severe reactions are uncommon, may be life threatening, and require treatment, sometimes vigorous. It has been shown that all reactions occur less commonly with LOCM than HOCM; however, reactions do occur with LOCM. There has not been convincing evidence that fatal reactions are significantly less common with LOCM, but are quite rare. With LOCM, overall incidence of reactions has been reported as 0.2% with severe reactions 0.05%. Luckily, the vast majority of contrast reactions (98%) occur within a short time after contrast injection while the patient is still in the radiology department. Fatal reactions almost always begin immediately or within the first 20 minutes after injection.

Some general principles must be recognized. Since reactions occur and are unpredictable, appropriate items including drugs useful for treating reactions must be kept stocked wherever contrast is administered. Personnel should be trained as to the location and use of these items, and a physician should be in attendance whenever and wherever contrast is administered. There also must be access to a rapid response code team. Oxygen should

TABLE 55-1 Management of Acute Reactions in Adults

Hives (urticaria)
a. Stop injection
b. Most cases require no treatment, careful monitoring until resolved
c. H1 antihistamine: diphenhydramine (Benadryl) po or IM, 25–50 mg
d. If severe, widespread, and nonresponding: epinephrine SC (1:1000), 0.1–0.3 mL (.01–03 mg)

Laryngeal edema
a. Oxygen 6–10 L/min via mask
b. Epinephrine SC or IM (1:1000) 0.1–0.3 mL (0.1–0.3 mg)
c. If hypotensive, epinephrine IV (1:10 000) 1–3 mL (0.1–0.3 mg); repeat as needed to maximum 1 mg

Bronchospasm
a. Oxygen 6–10 L/min via mask, monitor: ECG, pulse oximeter, blood pressure
b. Beta-agonist inhaler 2–3 puffs repeat as needed
 Metaproterenol (Alupent), terbutaline (Brethaire) albuterol (Proventil or Ventolin)
c. If not responding, epinephrine SC or IM (1:1000) 0.1–0.3 mL (0.1–0.3 mg)
d. If hypotension developing, epinephrine IV (1:10 000) 1–3 mL (0.1–0.3 mg), repeat as needed to maximum 1 mg.

Pulmonary edema
a. Oxygen 6–10 L/min via mask
b. Elevate torso
c. Furosemide (Lasix) 20–40 mg slow IV push
d. Consider morphine 1–3 mg IV
e. Transfer to ED or ICU if needed

Hypotension with bradycardia (vasovagal reaction)
a. Monitor vital signs
b. Elevate legs 60 degrees or Trendelenburg
c. Assure airway open, oxygen 6–10 L/min via mask
d. Secure intravenous access administer normal saline or Ringer's lactate 500–700 mL in 20–30 min, continue as needed
e. Atropine 0.6–1 mg slow IV
f. If not responding repeat atropine to total dose 0.04 mg/kg (2–3 mg adults)
g. Do not discharge until hypotension and bradycardia completely resolved

Hypotension with tachycardia
a. Elevate legs 60 degrees or Trendelenburg
b. Monitor ECG, pulse oximeter, blood pressure
c. Oxygen 6–10 L/min via mask
d. Intravenous normal saline or Ringer's lactate, 500–700 mL/20 min, continue as needed
e. If not responding, epinephrine IV (1:10 000) 1–3 mL (0.1–0.3 mg), repeat as needed to maximum 1 mg.

Severe hypertension
a. Oxygen 6–10 L/min via mask
b. Monitor ECG, pulse oximeter, blood pressure
c. Nitroglycerine 0.4 mg SL may repeat × 3
d. If no response, consider labetalol 20 mg intravenous, 20–80 mg intravenous every 10 min to maximum 300 mg.
e. If patient with pheochromocytoma, phentolamine 5 mg IV, may use labetalol

Seizures
a. Oxygen 6–10 L/min via mask
b. Monitor vital signs including pulse oximeter, due to concern of respiratory depression from benzodiazepine
c. Consider diazepam (Valium) 5 mg IV, repeat if needed (alternate midazolam (Versed) 0.501 mg IV)
d. If longer treatment needed, obtain consultation, consider phenytoin (dilantin) IV 15–18 mg/kg at 50 mg/min

be available. Knowledge of the drugs and dosages is important: particularly regarding epinephrine. This is supplied in two concentrations: 1:1000 (1 mg epinephrine in 1 mL) for subcutaneous or intramuscular administration; 1:10 000 (1 mg in 10 mL) for intravenous administration. Physicians must recognize the difference in these by sight and know appropriate use. Epinephrine can cause serious adverse effects itself even in young and healthy individuals, for example, hypertensive crisis and myocardial ischemia. In general, practitioners must know specific treatments for particular reactions, but must also avoid overtreatment particularly of mild reactions. In addition to the side effects of the treatment, this can cause confusion at times of future evaluation for contrast administration.

Should a reaction occur, a physician must assess the patient, including state of consciousness, vital signs, symptoms, and objective findings. Examination of the skin and respiratory system as well as pulse and blood pressure are key. Careful monitoring for any improvement or progression whether treated or not is important. Some reactions affect a single system, such as respiratory, but some can cascade with increasing severity. Although radiologists should be trained to recognize and treat reactions, especially with very severe reactions such as an unresponsive pulseless patient, there should be no hesitation to "call a code."

CUTANEOUS REACTIONS

Cutaneous reactions are fairly common. Most often urticaria (hives) occur, more often in upper body, face, neck chest, and arms. They may be single or multiple. Although usually associated with pruritis, if they are few in number and symptoms not disturbing, treatment is not necessary. If more severe, treatment with H1 antihistamine diphenhydramine (Benadryl), 50 mg oral or intramuscular, is recommended. Benadryl causes drowsiness, so care must be taken if the patient is alone so that they do not leave while still obtunded. In severe cases, H1 blockers (cimetidine or ranitidine, 50 mg in 20 mL fluid slow intravenous push) may also be needed.

Erythema or edema can occur either localized (usually around the face) or generalized. Often this does not need treatment, but if severe, can be treated with H2 antihistamines, H1 blockers, and if very severe, epinephrine.

RESPIRATORY REACTIONS

Upper airway and laryngeal edema is characterized by a feeling of throat tightness, difficulty breathing, alteration of voice due to vocal cord edema, and inspiratory stridor. This can be a very serious event and is best treated with oxygen and epinephrine and aggressively retreated if not initially responding. H2 receptor blockers are second-line drugs. If laryngeal edema persists, early intubation may be performed, as it may become impossible later if swelling becomes severe enough, necessitating tracheotomy.

Bronchospasm may be more likely in patients with history of asthma, and these patients may be refractory to lower doses of beta-agonist inhalers. Patients with bronchospasm usually have normal speaking voice but have difficulty breathing and audible wheezing. They may complain of chest tightness. If mild, two or three treatments with beta-agonist inhaler may be sufficient. This can be repeated. Oxygen should be administered. If not responding treatment, epinephrine should be given.

While patients having severe anxiety may complain of chest tightness and feeling of difficulty breathing, this is a diagnosis of exclusion. Overtreatment should be avoided. Decision should be based not only on described symptoms but also objective finding such as vital signs and breath sounds.

Contrast can uncommonly stimulate pulmonary edema. This is more common with history of heart disease and congestive heart failure. Treatment includes elevation of upper body, oxygen, diuretics (20–40 mg furosemide), and intravenous morphine (1–3 mg, repeat every 5–10 minutes if needed). Pulmonary edema management will likely require the code team or transfer to emergency department or intensive care unit.

HYPOTENSIVE AND HYPERTENSIVE REACTIONS

Hypotensive reactions may occur as isolated events or in association with (sometimes following) cutaneous or other types of reactions. Systolic blood pressure less than 90 mm Hg, diminished tissue perfusion, and altered mental status are defining features. If responsive, patients sense light headedness and weakness but may become unresponsive. Oxygen should be administered even while obtaining blood pressure. Large volumes of intravenous fluid can be administered (normal saline or lactated Ringer's solution, 500–700 mL in 20 minutes).

Vasovagal reactions are typified by hypotension in association with bradycardia (pulse rate less than 60 beats per minute). If the patient does not quickly respond to leg elevation, oxygen, and fluid, administration of atropine 0.6 to 1 mg slow intravenous push can be given and repeated every 3 to 5 minutes if needed to total dose of 0.04 mg/kg (2–3 mg in adults).

Patients who are tachycardic and hypotensive have a form of anaphylactoid reaction. In addition to the general measures of leg elevation, oxygen, and intravenous fluids, administration of intravenous epinephrine (1:10 000) slowly repeatable up to total dose of 1 mg.

Hypertensive reactions are less common than hypotensive ones. These can be difficult to treat and may require transfer to the emergency department or intensive care unit. In addition to oxygen and close monitoring, administration of sublingual nitroglycerine, which can be repeated up to three times, may be advanced to labetalol 20 mg, intravenous if needed. In patients who have a known pheochromocytoma and develop a hypertensive reaction, administration of phentolamine 5 mg intravenous (or labetalol) is recommended. However, LOCM, IOCM, and gadolinium contrast are not known to stimulate a hypertensive crisis in these patients.

CENTRAL NERVOUS SYSTEM REACTIONS

Seizures may occur following contrast administration. Although this can occur in subjects with no predisposition, it is of greater likelihood in patients with brain metastases because they have an altered blood–brain barrier. Treatment includes turning the patient's head to the side to protect the airway, monitoring of vital signs, oxygen, and consideration of administration of diazepam 5 mg intravenous (repeated if needed) or midazolam 0.5 to 1 mg intravenous.

DELAYED REACTIONS

Delayed reactions are defined as adverse events following intravenous contrast injection with onset more than 1 hour but less than 1 week after exposure; in most instances, symptoms appear within 3 days. The incidence of delayed reactions is greater than commonly recognized, since they are often not brought to the attention of the radiologist because of the late onset (and may not be considered associated with contrast administration by the patient). Investigations have reported the incidence between 1% and 9%. These do not have association with anaphylactoid reactions and in general are not life threatening. They have been reported following both high and low osmolar iodinated contrast administration, but not following gadolinium contrast agents.

Cutaneous reactions are most common, with an exanthem variable in size and distribution, macular or maculopapular, sometimes similar to angioneurotic edema. Patients usually have pruritis, but hives are uncommon. If a limited cutaneous reaction is observed, treatment with topical steroids may be effective.

Other common symptoms reported include fever, chills, dizziness, arthralgias and musculoskeletal pain, diarrhea, vomiting, headache, and rarely hypotension. Most cases are mild to moderate and many are self-limited.

The only significant association is that delayed reactions are clearly more common in patients treated with interleukin II for malignancy; these cases have similar symptoms but may be more severe.

The etiology of delayed reactions remains unclear. Treatment is largely supportive. Antipyretics, anti-inflammatory agents and antihistamines for pruritus may be used as needed. For more severe cases, systemic steroids have been recommended. There is a relatively high rate of recurrence, as much as 25%. Pretreatment may be used, although there is no published literature documenting effectiveness or comparing different regimens. Recommendations are to follow the same protocol for patients with prior moderate acute reaction, using steroids and antihistamines.

Additional types of adverse events after contrast administration may be called "very late reactions," defined as those occurring more than 1 week after exposure. NSF following intravenous gadolinium contrast would fall in this category. Others are thyrotoxicosis and acute parotitis following intravenous iodinated contrast administration. Risk factors for thyrotoxicosis include untreated Grave disease and multinodular goiter with thyroid autonomy especially if in an iodine deficient area. Patients with normal thyroid function are *not* at risk. Prophylaxis is not recommended, rather iodinated contrast should be. If iodinated contrast absolutely must be given to a patient at risk, they should be monitored by an endocrinologist.

Following intravenous iodinated contrast administration, radioiodine diagnostic tests or therapy should be avoided for 2 months owing to decreased uptake by the gland. Thus patients with thyroid cancer should be screened with this specific concern.

CONTRAST-INDUCED NEPHROTOXICITY

INCIDENCE

Despite advances, especially lower osmolality iodinated contrast, impairment of renal function due to exposure to contrast remains a serious issue. Radiologists must be knowledgeable about methods to minimize this potential serious adverse event (Table 55-2). Although there is a considerable body of literature, much remains unclear and much of the literature is conflicting. Uncertainty about contrast-induced nephrotoxicity (CIN) arises from the variability in its definition. Most until recently defined CIN based on a rise in serum creatinine, but some used an absolute rise (e.g., 0.5 or 1, or even 2 mg/dL), others a percentage (25% or 50%); some specified the time of serum creatinine determination, others did not, and the timing of the testing could affect results. More recently, alterations

TABLE 55-2 Screening for and Avoidance of Nephrotoxicity

Screen for risk factors including
Preexisting renal dysfunction (eGFR < 60 mL/min/1.73 m^2)
Diabetes mellitus
Volume depleted state
Congestive heart failure, heart disease
Concomitant use nephrotoxic drugs
Aminoglycosides, NSAIDs, amphotericin, chemotherapeutic agents, ACE inhibitors, prostaglandins, diuretics
Multiple myeloma
Nephrotic syndrome, other proteinemic states
Kidney transplant, prior nephrectomy
Liver cirrhosis
Age older than 70 y
Hyperuricemia
If risk factors present
Establish absolute necessity of contrast procedure no equivalent alternate
Determine eGFR
Consider delaying procedure
If procedure necessary and patient high risk (eGFR < 60 mL/min/1.73 m^2 with additional risk factors)
Administer intravenous 0.9% NaCl or Na HCO_3
Use low osmolar or isosmolar contrast
Limit dose of contrast
Consider administration N-acetylcysteine 600 mg po bid
Monitor serum creatinine

in estimated glomerular filtration rate (eGFR) have been used. Normal serum creatinine level may be maintained until GFR is reduced to half of normal. However, formulas for calculating eGFR are known to have varying accuracy with differing levels of renal function, tending to be less accurate with either normal or very reduced GFR. Very few studies have had true control groups, such as a matched group of hospitalized patients who did not get iodinated contrast. Some studies report on intravenous administration, others intra-arterial, often coronary angiography, and whether results from one route can be applied to another remains controversial. Thus, even the exact incidence of CIN remains surprisingly unclear. Most episodes are self-limited, with serum creatinine beginning to rise within 24 hours of exposure to contrast, peaking at approximately 96 hours (4 days), and returning to baseline within 7 to 10 days. The course may be more severe, especially with greater degrees of preexisting renal disease, or concurrent insults whether cardiovascular or other nephrotoxic drugs. Some patients may require short-term dialysis, and a small number require chronic dialysis.

PATHOGENESIS

Prevention and intervention are also limited by a lack of full understanding of the pathogenic mechanism. Most current theories are based on some evidence of renal hemodynamic changes due to vasoconstriction resulting from contrast and due to direct toxicity to tubule cells. There may be agent-specific chemotoxicity, and osmotic mechanisms may play a role. Oxygen free radicles may also have some role. Cofactors such as state of hydration can potentiate this scenario, for example, by increasing the time contrast resides in the tubules or by enhancing perfusion changes. The role of contrast viscosity is unclear but may be significant.

Because many of the demonstrated physiologic effects of contrast are to some degree proportional to the osmolality, it was expected these effects would be reduced with development of LOCM, and this to some degree has been proven correct. There may be some differences between agents with similar osmolality (although this is not proven). The osmolality of LOCM, which is typically 600 to 700 mOsm/kg, is much less than that of HOCM (greater than 1500 mOsm/kg) but still higher than that of blood (280 mOsm/kg). Whether the near isosmolar agents result in significantly lower rate of permanent renal impairment than low osmolar agents for all routes of administration remains unclear. The lowest osmolality agents, nonionic dimmers, also have the highest viscosity.

PREVENTION

Renal insufficiency is variably defined but may be considered present when eGFR is less than 60 mL/min/1.73 m^2, serum creatinine greater than 1.5 mg/dL or 133 mmol/L. Renal failure may be defined as eGFR less than 30 mL/min/1.73 m^2. Studies have revealed fairly consistent risk factors for CIN. The patients at greatest risk have diabetes and preexisting renal insufficiency. Renal insufficiency without diabetes is an independent risk factor, as is diabetes alone but somewhat less. Dehydration, cardiovascular disease especially recent myocardial infarction or shock, use of nephrotoxic drugs, especially aminoglycosides, diuretics, NSAIDs, ACE inhibitors, prostaglandins; myeloma (or other proteinemic states), hyperuricemia, hypertension, prior nephrectomy, and advanced age are additional risk factors.

Other factors that increase likelihood and severity of CIN include dose of contrast (both for single study and cumulative dose for multiple examinations over 24 hours), osmolality, and potentially, route of administration (intra-arterial especially directly into renal artery, versus intravenous, with virtually no nephrotoxicity expected from nonvascular administration such as HSG). A large meta-analysis provided strong evidence that LOCM (ratio 3 agents) are less nephrotoxic than HOCM (ratio 1.5 agents), and subsequent studies have confirmed this finding. It holds true for patients with preexisting renal disease and diabetes. Evidence is much more mixed whether ratio 6 agents, near isosmolar, produce significantly less renal impairment than LOCM.

A reasonable practice is to screen all patients for risk factors for CIN before administering contrast (Table 55-2). Although blood testing is not mandated by any society, it may be justified as interviewing patients has limits; many are poorly informed about their own condition. Point-of-service blood test devices are also available. If serum creatinine is measured, it is recommended to calculate eGFR, which provides more reliable information about degrees of renal insufficiency. For any patient with a risk factor, LOCM should be used, and dose should be limited to that necessary for diagnostic quality images. A consensus on strict cutoff values does not exist. For patients with GFR greater than 60 mL/min/1.73 m^2, there is essentially no risk of CIN; with GFR less than 30 mL/min/1.73 m^2, risk is quite high; with GFR between 30 and 60 mL/min/1.73m^2, the risk is moderate.

INTERVENTION

When giving contrast to a patient with high risk of CIN, preventative intervention is advisable (Table 55-2). However, the only intervention well supported by extensive studies to be effective is hydration. Diuretics including furosemide and mannitol have been shown to be harmful. Normal saline has been shown to be more effective than one-half normal saline and intravenous hydration superior to oral. Limited, unconfirmed studies, suggest hydration with sodium bicarbonate may be more effective than normal saline, but either can be justified. The most effective hydration protocols, however, require intravenous administration for several hours preceding and following the procedure, limiting its implementation in an outpatient setting. Administration of 1 mL/kg/h of normal saline for 4 hours before and 6 hours following contrast has been recommended; alternatively, Merten et al. used infusion of isotonic sodium bicarbonate 3 mL/kg/h for 1 hour prior and 6 hours postprocedure.

Many other interventions have been tried, but none has been consistently shown to be useful. These include atrial natriuretic peptide, prostaglandin E, fenoldopam, dopamine, adenosine inhibitors, endothelin, and calcium channel blockers. Acetylcysteine has yielded conflicting results, although not shown in any study to be harmful, and is relatively inexpensive, so is recommended by some (600 mg orally twice daily the day before and day of the examination).

Patients already on chronic dialysis for end-stage renal disease may safely be given intravascular iodinated contrast. However, LOCM or IOCM should be used. Contrast is poorly protein bound that is cleared readily by dialysis, which does not have to be scheduled to immediately follow contrast administration, unless very high doses are used. Although dialysis clears contrast, evidence that it prevents CIN is not solid. Patients on intermittent or occasional dialysis should have an alternate study.

TABLE 55-3 Medications Containing Metformin

GENERIC SUBSTANCES	TRADE NAME
Metformin	Glucophage
	Glucophage XR
	Fortamet
	Glumetza
Glyburide/metformin	Glucovance
Glipizide/metformin	Metaglip
Pioglitazone/metformin	ActoPlus Met
Rosiglitazone/metformin	Avandamet

METFORMIN

Patients given intravenous contrast are at potential risk for a serious adverse event if they are taking an oral antihyperglycemic agent containing metformin. This is a biguanide oral medication for non–insulin-dependent diabetes. It decreases hepatic glucose production and enhances peripheral glucose uptake. It has the advantage of rarely causing hypoglycemia. The active drug, metformin, is included in several medications with different trade names (Table 55-3).

Metformin accumulates unmetabolized in the urine by glomerular filtration with 90% excreted within 24 hours after administration, if renal function is normal. However, in the setting of renal dysfunction, there is potential for accumulation of metformin at levels that can lead to lactic acidosis. This could occur if the patient has preexisting renal failure. Of most concern is a patient who may suffer acute renal dysfunction because of contrast-associated nephropathy. Thus, the greatest concern is a patient with risk factors for CIN (mainly diabetes and preexisting mild-to-moderate renal insufficiency). Metformin itself is not nephrotoxic. There is no direct drug interaction between iodinated contrast and metformin.

The symptoms of lactic acidosis (blood pH less than 7.25) are vomiting, somnolence, nausea, epigastric pain, anorexia, hyperpnea, lethargy, diarrhea, and thirst. Morbidity rate is as high as 50% (usually with comorbidities such as cardiac disease). Although it is life threatening, its actual incidence is low.

The key factor in management is avoidance. Patients must be consistently screened for metformin. Patients with normal renal function and no comorbidities are not at risk (with no cases of lactic acidosis reported). Patients with significant renal failure should not be given contrast and are not good candidates for metformin, which is excreted by the kidney. Patients with normal renal function but other comorbidities including diabetes, liver dysfunction, and cardiac disease should have metformin discontinued at the time (just prior to) of the contrast administration and resumed after a delay of 48 hours. Patients with mild renal insufficiency, especially if diabetic, should have metformin administration stopped at the time of or before the administration of contrast and held for 48 hours. Ensuring good hydration and limiting the dose of contrast may be helpful. It is judicious to remeasure the serum creatinine to assure it has not changed before resuming metformin in these cases.

Gadolinium Contrast

In general, gadolinium-based contrast agents are very well tolerated. This may in part be due to the lower overall volumes usually used compared with dosing for CT. Some of the gadolinium agents are hyperosmolar, some less osmolar. Idiosyncratic reactions similar to those occurring with iodinated contrast have been reported, but at much lower rates, overall approximately 2.4% and with severe reactions much less than 1%. Mechanism has not been determined; however, it is not likely to be due to the gadolinium itself. Since reactions are uncommon, little literature exists. Most treatments respond to similar treatment for the same symptoms occurring after an iodinated contrast reaction. If a repeat study is needed, and a patient has had a prior moderate reaction to a gadolinium-based agent, pretreatment with a similar regimen as for iodinated contrast can be used. It would also be wise to use a different agent. There has not been a significant increase in reaction rates to gadolinium contrast in patients with prior reaction to iodinated contrast. However, patients with prior reaction to gadolinium are believed to be at significant risk of repeat reactions.

Nephrogenic Systemic Fibrosis

Contrast agents for use in MRI were developed and released in the 1980s, with gadopentetate dimeglumine (Gd-DTPA) being the first and it was found useful for improving diagnostic capability. It was early recognized that gadolinium agents were well tolerated and not nephrotoxic. Although excretion was prolonged in patients with renal insufficiency, they did not seem to impair renal function even in those with preexisting renal disease. Thus, gadolinium agents became used as an alternate for iodinated contrast in patients with increased CIN risk.

Despite many years of use, it was not until 2000 and thereafter that a previously unrecognized illness was reported. Because of the predominance of cutaneous manifestations, this was initially labeled nephrogenic fibrosing dermopathy (NFD), but was renamed nephrogenic systemic fibrosis (NSF) when the multisystem aspect of the disease was recognized. The earliest recognized case was identified in 1997.

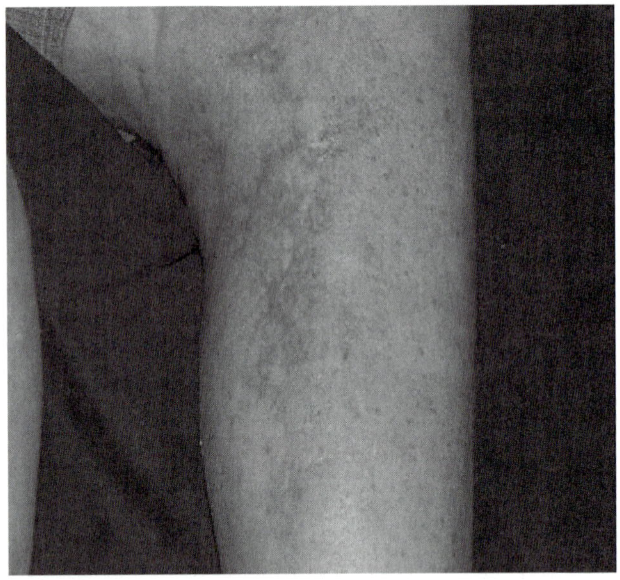

FIG. 55-1 Typical woody plaque-like lesions along anterior surface of lower extremity in patient with NSF. Extremities are most commonly affected, trunk less so with sparing of the face and upper chest.
Source: Courtesy of Sundararman Swaminathan, MD, Division of Nephrology and Philip J. Kenney, MD, Department of Radiology, University of Arkansas for Medical Sciences, Little Rock, Arkansas.

NSF is a fibrosing illness involving predominantly skin and subcutaneous tissues but also lungs, esophagus, heart, and skeletal muscles (Fig. 55-1). The typical patient is middle aged with renal failure, most on either peritoneal or hemodialysis. Cases have been reported about equally in men and women, and no racial or ethnic predilection is known. No case has been reported under age 7 years. A few years after the initial identification of this disease, it was recognized that nearly all patients had prior exposure to an intravenous gadolinium contrast agent.

Numerous investigations have been published and several registries organized to develop information. Although criteria for diagnosis has varied (not all pathologically proven), incidence is reported between 1% and 7% in patients with renal disease. No case has to date been reported in a patient exposed to any of the gadolinium contrast agents with normal renal function.

The typical course includes onset of symptoms within a few days and up to 3 months from time of exposure; swelling of distal parts of extremities with skin induration, sometimes extension to thighs, antebrachium, and lower abdomen, with pain, muscle restlessness, and loss of skin flexibility. The disease may progress to development of contractures and cachexia and may involve internal organs including heart, liver,

TABLE 55-4 Gadolinium-Based Contrast Agents

AGENT	TRADE NAME	LIGAND	NSF INCIDENCE
Gadobenate dimeglumine	Multihance	Ionic linear	No unconfounded case
Gadobutrol	Adovist*	Nonionic linear	No unconfounded case
Gadodiamide	Omniscan	Nonionic linear	3%–7% if at risk
Gadofosveset trisodium	Vasovist*	Ionic linear	Limited experience
Gadopentetate dimeglumine	Magnevist	Ionic linear	0.1%–1% if at risk
Gadoterate meglumine	Dotarem*	Ionic cyclic	No unconfounded case
Gadoteridol	Prohance	Nonionic cyclic	No unconfounded case
Gadoversetamide	Optimark†	Nonionic linear	Unconfounded cases

*Not approved by FDA for use in USA.

†Not approved for use in Europe.

Confounded case means this agent used but also another agent at different examination.

Data from Thomsen H. ESUR Guideline: gadolinium-based contrast media and nephrogenic systemic fibrosis. *Eur Radiol.* 2007;17:2692-2696.

lungs, and diaphragm, possibly resulting in death. No curative treatments have yet been reported.

Initially it was recognized that NSF patients invariably had renal disease. It eventually became clear that there was a strong association with exposure to intravenous gadolinium contrast. Almost all cases have had exposure to gadolinium, although some have not. In some cases, this may be due to inaccurate records. In some cases, patients did not have MRI but were exposed to gadolinium when used as an alternate intravascular contrast agent for radiographic studies such as angiography in patients with renal failure (a practice no longer acceptable). The great majority (at least 90%) have been exposed to the linear chelate agent gadodiamide (Table 55-4). Other agents have also been associated although some only in patients who also received gadodiamide.

Most NSF patients have had severe renal disease, many requiring dialysis. This seems to be the highest risk group and may be even more so if gadolinium is given some time before dialysis commences. Cases have been reported with lower levels of renal disease but the risk seems considerably higher with GFR less than 15 mL/min/1.73 m^2, less so with GFR between 15 and 30 mL/min/1.73 m^2 and rather low, probably less than 1% between 30 and 60 mL/min/1.73 m^2. No documented cases have been reported with GFR greater than 60 mL/min/1.73 m^2 even with gadodiamide. Since many, in fact the majority, of renal failure patients exposed to gadolinium do not contract NSF, other factors must be involved. However, none of the cofactors have been proven consistently. Although many studies seem to show greater risk from higher doses (and a stronger correlation with MRA often done with double or triple dosing) or high cumulative dose, numerous cases have been reported after a single routine dose. Additional proposed factors include liver failure especially acute; metabolic acidosis; increased iron, calcium, or phosphate levels; abnormal iron metabolism; high-dose erythropoietin therapy; immunosuppression; vasculopathy, acute proinflammatory event; and infection. It is difficult to discern which associated factors derive merely from the accepted indications for MRI/MRA at the time versus true etiologic factors, and none are established as independent risk factors.

The exact pathologic mechanism of the disease is unclear, although there are prevailing theories with some supportive evidence. Partly based on demonstration of deposition of gadolinium ion in skin in NSF patients, a prevailing theory rests on dissociation of the gadolinium ion from the chelate. This is called transmetallation, wherein another heavy metal ion replaces the gadolinium allowing it to associate with other anions such as phosphate. Because of the known heavy metal toxicity of gadolinium, all contrast agents use a chelate to reduce the toxicity. Some are linear, some macrocyclic, some ionic, some nonionic (Table 55-4). One factor of concern is the stability of the binding of the gadolinium ion by the chelate; it has been shown that gadodiamide has greater likelihood for transmetallation than some other agents (although at very low levels, and transmetallation occurs to some degree with all agents). Some theories report altered iron metabolism and metabolic acidosis may enhance transmetallation. Free gadolinium can bind with anions and become deposited. Stimulated by some mechanism, an inflammatory process with activated fibroblasts develops and produces progressive fibrosis.

Because no effective treatment has been reported, the necessary approach is to avoid this potentially devastating illness by avoiding unnecessary exposure to patients at risk. This primarily consists of screening patients for renal disease, with concern also for liver failure, especially acute. This may be done by history, but laboratory testing with serum creatinine determination and calculation of eGFR is best particularly for high-risk groups, or in a practice where the linear agent gadodiamide may be used. American College of Radiology recommends eGFR should be performed within 6 weeks of exposure. In general, using the lowest reasonable contrast dose, having an accepted indication for the study, and confirming no equivalent alternative examinations exist are recommended especially with risk groups.

In patients with end-stage renal disease on dialysis, primary consideration should be for CT with iodinated contrast as CIN is not an issue. If for some reason MRI with gadolinium must be given, the lowest possible dose and immediate dialysis may be done, but there is no good evidence that dialysis prevents NSF in this circumstance, and several cases have been reported of NSF developing despite immediate dialysis. Investigation has shown that 9 total hours of dialysis in three separate sessions is needed to effectively remove all gadolinium.

If eGFR is less than 15 mL/min/1.73 m^2, contrast of any type probably should be avoided if at all possible. With eGFR 15 to 30 mL/min/1.73 m^2 gadolinium contrast of type not commonly associated with NSF (gadobenate dimeglumine, gadobutrol, gadoterate meglumine, gadoteridol) may be safer than iodinated contrast although risk may not be zero. With eGFR over 30 mL/min/1.73 m^2, risk is very low, and no cases have been reported with eGFR over 60 mL/min/1.73 m^2 with any agent. Patients in acute severe renal failure, especially if associated with acute hepatic failure, probably should receive no contrast.

EXTRAVASATION OF CONTRAST

Extravasation of contrast into soft tissues adjacent to the injection site can result in significant adverse outcome. Although some facts are clear, much remains controversial, particularly regarding treatment. The incidence of extravasation has been varyingly reported between 1/100 and 1/1000 patients. It can occur with either hand or power injection, although it is more likely with the latter. It does not appear to be clearly related to injection flow rate (perhaps because most injectors will monitor pressure and alter flow rate). Defined risk factors include use of power injector, poor injection sites (poor venous access, small veins such as in hand, wrist, foot, and ankle), large volume of injection, obesity, and inability of the patient to communicate. Lines in place for more than 24 hours and veins subject to multiple venipunctures may also be at risk. Factors such as arterial insufficiency, poor lymphatic or venous drainage, and higher osmolality contrast agent may increase the degree of injury, although they probably do not increase risk of the event.

Symptoms and signs include swelling, tightness, stinging, or burning pain although some patients express little discomfort. Edema, erythema, and tenderness are common. The extravasated contrast stimulates a local inflammatory response, worse with higher osmolality contrast and larger amounts. While most extravasations produce a limited effect with no permanent injury, skin ulceration and tissue necrosis can occur. A compartment syndrome may be produced, independent of extravasation volume. Because the clinical course is uncertain, close follow-up for several hours is recommended.

There is no clear consensus on treatment, largely because attempts at investigation and comparison of different treatments have produced variable and conflicting results. Conservative management is adequate in most instances. Elevation of the affected limb is recommended (although there is no study proving this). Both warm and cold compresses have been advocated, with cold having improved pain relief, but warm compresses would be expected to speed resorption of contrast. Most now recommend ice packs, as symptomatic relief seems more effective. Aspiration of the contrast and local injection of steroids or hyaluronidase are not supported. Outpatients may be sent home with instructions but should be advised to self-monitor and return for medical attention if symptoms worsen or if skin ulceration or paresthesias develop. Surgical consultation is recommended if the patient develops increasing swelling or pain for more than 2 hours after the event, and if there is poor capillary refill, change in sensation, or skin ulceration.

In the event of an extravasation, documentation in the medical record (either in the radiology report or incident report) should include site of extravasation, type of contrast agent and estimated volume extravasated, physical findings, treatment, and advice to the patient.

CONTRAST IN PREGNANCY AND LACTATION

Studies have shown both intravenous iodinated and gadolinium contrast agents administered to the mother will cross the placenta and are excreted in fetal urine, subsequently swallowed by the fetus. It is possible that a small amount is absorbed across the fetal GI tract. While there has been no documented evidence of harm to the fetus from either agent, convincing evidence of safety has also not been established. Thus for administration of contrast to a pregnant woman, special consideration should be given to the clinical indication for the study, whether exposure to contrast is justified, that the information derived will affect care during the period of the pregnancy and thus cannot be delayed until after delivery, and that there are no reasonable alternatives. Documented informed consent by the patient is recommended.

Investigation has shown that both intravenous iodinated contrast and gadolinium contrast agents are secreted in small quantities in breast milk. Less than 1% of iodinated contrast appears in milk; since the infant will absorb less than 1% of this from the GI tract, the baby is exposed to less than 0.01% of the dose to the mother and less than 1% the recommended dose for a newborn examination. The risks are considered to be minimal. Less than 0.04% of gadolinium contrast administered to the mother is secreted in breast milk; again since only 1% is absorbed, the baby is exposed to 0.0004% of the dose given to the mother. There is no evidence this miniscule oral ingestion is harmful to the baby.

Thus, if contrast must be administered to a breast-feeding woman, she should be reassured there is no evidence of risk to the baby from the tiny amounts of contrast in the milk. If the mother is apprehensive about this, she may abstain from breast-feeding for 24 hours, discarding expressed milk during that period, and then resume as by 24 hours all the contrast will have been cleared assuming if she has normal renal function.

CONTRAST FOR HYSTEROSALPINGOGRAPHY

For many years HSG has been a valuable test primarily for investigating infertile women. Although indications are fewer with advances in sonography, hysterosonography, MRI, and laparoscopy, HSG is still performed. A variety of contrast agents have been used. An oil-based agent, Lipiodol, was developed in the 1920s. Another oil-based agent Ethiodol (an ethyl alcohol ester of poppy seed oil with 37% iodine) was introduced in the 1950s. While the oil-based agents were quite effective and relatively well tolerated, there were two major concerns: absorption from the peritoneal cavity was very slow (although, because of this, delayed images could be done to assess performed for adhesions); and intravasation could lead to oil embolism to the lungs (Table 55-5). However, in a study of 593 patients having oil contrast HSG, 6.9% of all patients had intravasation, most with tubal blockage, but only 1% had oil emboli and none developed significant symptoms.

Water-soluble agents, initially ionic, were developed. Methylglucamine iothalamate and methylglucamine diatrizoate were both used. Sinografin a combination of diatrizoate meglumine and iodipamide meglumine was preferred by some due to higher viscosity. The water-soluble agents have improved mucosal detail of the tubes. However, although well tolerated at the time of the examination, investigations have shown patients have greater delayed pain (perhaps due to peritoneal irritation) with water-soluble HOCM than with oil-based agents. At present, because of availability and cost factors, LOCM is commonly used. While the viscosity and density may not be optimal, they are effective for determination of tubal patency and uterine morphology, which are the two items of greatest interest.

TABLE 55-5 Adverse Events with Hysterosalpingography

Contrast-related	Idiosyncratic contrast reaction
	Intravasation (with potential pulmonary oil embolism)
	Abdominal pain (peritoneal irritation)
	Granuloma formation (peritoneal irritation)
Procedure-related	Pain from uterine distension
	Infection
	Hemorrhage
	Uterine perforation

Although HSG is not intravascular procedure, because of possibility of intravasation, there is concern if a patient has had prior contrast reactions. As in all such situations, one must consider the risk benefit ratio. Using LOCM and premedication are recommended. In circumstances of extremely severe prior reaction, use of gadolinium may be considered (Table 55-5).

Controversy existed for years regarding fertility rate following HSG. Some argued the procedure itself improved fertility. A number of practitioners believed oil-based agents would have greater effect on enhancing fertility (due to higher viscosity). Conflicting results were reported in the literature, although some showed advantage for oil-based agents, methodology was criticized. The most recent research, which included low osmolar contrast compared with oil-based, demonstrates no significant difference in conception or live birth rates.

CONTRAST ISSUES FOR THE FUTURE

While much progress has been made in reducing the negative impact of diagnostic contrast agents, issues remain for the future. The use of LOCM and screening has reduced the incidence of serious contrast reactions to the point where they are unexpected and personnel may not be emotionally prepared to deal with them. Maintaining infrastructure and training are necessary. Careful applications of policies described above should limit the incidence and severity of nephrotoxicity. Proper screening and procedures has virtually eliminated lactic acidosis associated with metformin. With proper screening and policies, incidence of NSF has dropped dramatically.

Further research is needed to determine for certain whether isoosmolar contrast or some new agent may truly reduce nephrotoxicity. Additional study may prove usefulness of some other intervention besides hydration. If an agent or treatment could be developed to prevent NSF, perhaps from better understanding of etiologic processes, patients with severe renal failure might be able to benefit from gadolinium-enhance MR procedures.

It will behoove practicing radiologists to continue with life-long learning to keep aware of new developments that may lead to safer use of contrast.

Suggested Reading

ACR Contrast Media Manual. Version 6.0 p.23, May 2008.

Aspelin P, Aubry P, Fransson S, et al. Nephrotoxic effects in high risk patients undergoing angiography. *N Engl J Med.* 2003; 348:491-499.

Barrett BJ, Carlisle EJ. Meta-analysis of the relative toxicity of high and low osmolality contrast media. *Radiology.* 1993; 188:171-178.

Choyke PL, Miller DL, Lotze MT, et al. Delayed reactions to contrast media after interleukin 2 immunotherapy. *Radiology.* 1992;183:111-114.

Cochran ST, Bomyea K, Sayre JW. Trends in adverse events after IV administration of contrast media. *AJR Am J Roentgenol.* 2001;176:1385-1388.

Cowper SE, Robin HS, Steinberg SM, et al. Scleromyxoedema-like cutaneous disease in renal dialysis patients. *Lancet.* 2000;356:1000-1001.

Greenberger PA, Patterson R, Tapiro R. Prophylaxis against repeated radiocontrast media reactions in 857 patients. *Arch Intern Med.* 1985;145:2197-2200.

Lasser EC. Pretreatment with corticosteroids to prevent reactions to IV contrast material. *AJR Am J Roentgenol.* 1994;162:523-526.

Lindquist S, Rasmussen F, Larsen C. Use of iotrolan vs ethiodized poppy seed oil in hysterosalpingography. *Radiology.* 1994;191:513-517.

Merten GJ, Burgess WP, Gray LV, et al. Prevention of contrast induced nephropathy with sodium bicarbonate. *JAMS.* 2004; 291:3328-3334.

Mueller L, Buerkle HJ, Buether HJ, et al. Prevention of contrast media-associated nephropathy: randomized comparison of two hydration regimens. *Arch Intern Med.* 2002;162:329-336.

Nelson KL, Gifford LM, Lauber-Huber C, et al. Clinical safety of gadopentetate Dimeglumine. *Radiology.* 1995;196:439-443.

Nikolsky E, Mahren R. Understanding the consequences of contrast induced nephropathy. *Rev Cardiovasc Med.* 2003;4:S10-S18.

Solomon R, Biguiri C, Bettmam M. Selection of contrast media. *Kidney Int.* 2006;69:S39-S45.

Spring DB, Barkan HE, Pruyn SC, et al. Potential therapeutic effects of contrast materials in hysterosalpingography: a prospective randomized clinical trial. Kaiser Permanente Infertility Work Group. *Radiology.* 2000;214:53-57.

Thomsen H. ESUR Guideline: gadolinium-based contrast media and nephrogenic systemic fibrosis. *Eur Radiol.* 2007;17:2692-2696.

Thurmond A. Hysterosalpingography. In: Katzberg RW, ed. *The Contrast Media Manual.* Philadelphia, PA: Lippincott Williams & Wilkins; 1992:131-142.

Trimedi HS, Moore H, Nasr S. Randomized prospective trial to assess role of saline hydration in development of contrast induced nephropathy. *Nephron Clin Pract.* 2003;93:C29-C34.

QUESTIONS AND ANSWERS

1. Which of the following is the most significant risk for iodinated contrast reaction?
   A. History of prior iodinated contrast reaction
   B. History of shellfish allergy
   C. History of asthma
   D. History of cardiovascular event

   ANSWER: A. Although all are considered risk factors, prior adverse event carries the greatest risk for another such event.

2. A patient is undergoing a contrast-enhanced CT and becomes agitated. Upon questioning, you notice a distinct change in his/her voice. After administration of oxygen, what is the next best step?
   A. Diphenhydramine IM, 50 mg
   B. Diphenhydramine IV, 50 mg
   C. Epinephrine (1:1000), 0.1 to 0.3 mL SC
   D. Metaproterenol inhaler, 2 to 3 puffs

   ANSWER: C. Voice changes suggest laryngeal edema, and after administration of oxygen by mask, subcutaneous or intramuscular epinephrine (1:100) is indicated.

3. What is the most appropriate next step in a patient (in need of a contrast-enhanced, cross-sectional imagining examination) with a prior history of a significant life-threatening contrast reaction requiring intravenous epinephrine and intubation?
   A. Any type of contrast-enhanced examination is contraindicated in this patient.
   B. Gadolinium-enhanced MRI
   C. Gadolinium-enhanced MRI after premedication
   D. Noncontrast CT

   ANSWER: B. A patient with a history of a severe reaction should probably not undergo another study with iodinated contrast. Instead, MRI can be considered and is likely more informational than noncontrast study. There are no studies to support premedication before gadolinium administration in a patient with iodinated contrast allergy.

4. What is the minimum time needed after pretreatment with steroids in a patient with history of moderate contrast reaction before intravenous contrast can be safely administered?
   A. 2 hours
   B. 8 hours
   C. 10 hours
   D. 12 hours

   ANSWER: D. At least 12 hours are needed to prevent reaction.

5. What is the concentration of epinephrine that is administered intravenously?
   A. 1 mg/1 mL
   B. 1:1000
   C. 1:10 000
   D. 1:100 000

ANSWER: C. 1:10 000 is concentration used for intravenous administration. 1 mg/10 mL = 1:10 000 concentration, which is the dose for intravenous administration. Concentration of 1:1000 is used subcutaneously.

6. What is the time frame of occurrence for a contrast reaction to be considered delayed?
   A. 1 day to 1 week
   B. 1 hour to 1 week
   C. 1 day to 2 weeks
   D. 1 hour to 2 weeks

   ANSWER: B. Delayed reactions occur after 1 hour and within 1 week, most within 3 days of administration.

7. What is the only proven intervention for contrast-induced nephrotoxicity?
   A. Intravenous hydration
   B. Intravenous hydration with diuretic
   C. Oral hydration
   D. Intravenous hydration with acetylcysteine

   ANSWER: A. Hydration is the only proven preventative measure for CIN, and intravenous hydration is a more effective route than oral.

8. A patient is undergoing contrast-enhanced CT and is currently taking metformin. What is the recommendation for discontinuing the drug?
   A. 48 hours before and after the examination
   B. 48 hours before the examination
   C. 48 hours after the examination
   D. No action needs to be taken since the patient has no other comorbidities.

   ANSWER: C. There is no need to discontinue metformin before contrast, only for 48 hours after contrast in patients with comorbidities. Presumably most (not all) patients taking metformin are diabetic, although it has other limited applications.

9. What is the eGFR below which a Gadolinium-enhanced MRI should not be performed?
   A. 20 mL/min/1.73 m^2
   B. 30 mL/min/1.73 m^2
   C. 40 mL/min/1.73 m^2
   D. 50 mL/min/1.73 m^2

   ANSWER: B. Unless the benefits significantly outweigh the risks of NSF, gadolinium should not be administered in the setting of acute of significant chronic renal disease (eGFR less than 30 mL/min/1.73 m^2).

10. What is the recommendation for a breast-feeding mother who is to undergo contrast-enhanced CT?
    A. There is no evidence of risk to the baby, so no measures need to be employed.
    B. Because of a small risk to the baby from contrast excreted in breast milk, breast milk should be discarded for 24 hours after the examination.
    C. A non-contrast examination should be performed.
    D. A contrast MRI should be performed.

    ANSWER: A. There is no study demonstrating a risk to the baby from contrast secreted in breast milk. Therefore, there are no additional actions to be taken, assuming that the study is truly indicated. If she chooses (because of anxiety), a mother can discard her milk for 24 hours, at which time all contrast should be cleared.

56 KIDNEYS

Michelle M. McNamara and Mark E. Lockhart

ANATOMY

NORMAL ANATOMY

The kidneys and renal pedicle are located in the perirenal space which is bounded by the anterior and posterior renal (Gerota) fascia. The renal pedicle consists of the renal artery, renal vein, collecting system, and lymphatics. The kidneys are approximately 10 to 12 cm long (spanning three to four lumbar vertebral bodies), and approximately 5 to 7 cm wide. Left and right kidney length should not vary more than 2 cm. The right kidney is 1 to 2 cm lower than the left kidney and slightly more lateral. The collecting system consists of minor (usually 10–14 in number) and major calyces and the renal pelvis. Intravenous pyelograms overestimate true renal length secondary to magnification and renal engorgement from osmotic diuresis. Ultrasound may underestimate true renal length because of technical difficulties in imaging the entire kidney.

VARIANT ANATOMY

Persistent fetal lobulation can be identified in approximately 5% of adult patients. The kidneys have a scalloped appearance. The number of lobes depends on the overall calyceal number and represents a vestige of lobar development of the kidney, which is visible at birth. With cellular multiplication, lobar anatomy is usually obscured by age 4 to 5 years. Persistent lobulation is of no clinical significance but may be mistaken for another entity such as tumor. With persistent fetal lobulation, renal parenchymal thickness should be normal (approximately 10 mm), and the renal indentations should be smooth and regular. An important finding in identifying persistent fetal lobulation is that the calyces are centered between indentations. This differs from indentations caused by reflux nephropathy in which indentations in the renal parenchyma overlie the calyces. The indentations, which may result from papillary necrosis, also overlie the necrotic renal papilla and its subtending calyx. Lobulation can also be mimicked by multiple renal infarcts when interlobar vessels are involved, most commonly seen in patients with small vessel disease such as chronic diabetes. In this circumstance, indentations in the renal parenchyma occur between calyces, but overall renal parenchyma thickness is diminished by atrophy.

ABNORMAL NUMBER OF KIDNEYS

Renal agenesis results from failure of the ureteric bud to reach the metanephric blastema secondary to either failure of formation or premature degeneration of the ureteric bud. Induction of the functional nephron does not occur. The resulting Mullerian duct anomalies are considered part of the Mayer-Rokitansky-Kuster-Hauser syndrome in females. In 70% of women with unilateral renal agenesis, associated genital anomalies are present; these include absence or atresia of the uterus or vagina, a unicornuate uterus with absence or atresia of the vagina and ovary, or duplication anomalies of the genital tract. In 20% of male individuals with renal agenesis, there is absence of the ipsilateral epididymis and vas deferens, or presence of an ipsilateral seminal vesicle cyst. Absence of the ipsilateral adrenal gland is associated with renal agenesis in 10% of patients. Compensatory hypertrophy of the contralateral kidney is usually evident. Renal agenesis can be diagnosed by ultrasound, CT, or radionuclide renography. Findings may be seen on conventional radiographs of the abdomen. With absence of one kidney, bowel (usually colon) will occupy the empty renal fossa. The colonic flexure on the affected side will be displaced medially. This is better appreciated in the case of left renal agenesis.

SUPERNUMERARY KIDNEYS

In this rare anomaly, more than two discrete kidneys are present on one side. It is likely a result of formation of two ureteral buds on one side. A supernumerary kidney is more often seen on the left side, caudal to the normal kidney, and is often hypoplastic. The supernumerary kidney may be drained by a bifid ureter, which also drains the second kidney on the ipsilateral side. Alternatively, a separate ureter may drain the supernumerary kidney.

ABNORMAL POSITION

Malrotation and nonrotation of the kidneys is commonly seen. This is a result of failure to rotate about the vertical renal axis. Nonrotation results in an anterior position of the ureteropelvic junction, with some calyces located medial to the renal pelvis. Overrotation of the kidney is rare and results in the ureteropelvic junction oriented posteriorly. Pelvic kidney is a common renal ectopia without fusion.

ABNORMAL FUSION

Horseshoe kidney is a common renal anomaly and occurs more frequently in males. An isthmus forms between the two developing masses of renal tissue. This connection may consist of a fibrotic band or a functioning renal parenchyma. Normal renal ascent is arrested when the horseshoe kidney becomes caught under the origin of the inferior mesenteric artery. There is an increased incidence of renal vascular and urinary tract anomalies associated with horseshoe kidney. Complications of horseshoe kidney include obstruction, stone formation, urinary tract infections, and increased risk for certain malignancies, include transitional cell carcinoma (TCC), Wilms tumor, and rarely renal carcinoid. The horseshoe kidney is susceptible to injury during blunt abdominal trauma.

Crossed fused ectopia is a rare congenital renal anomaly in which one kidney crosses the midline and fuses to the opposite kidney. The ureters insert in their normal positions, with the ureter from the crossed kidney crossing the midline. The left kidney more commonly crosses the midline to lie on the right retroperitoneum.

ABNORMAL VESSELS

Vascular anomalies of the kidney most often include duplicate renal arteries and supernumerary renal veins. Anomalies of renal vasculature are much more common with ectopic kidneys. A crossing vessel near the ureter is commonly seen in patients with ureteropelvic junction obstruction. However, most anomalous renal vessels are of no clinical significance, although recognition, of these vessels may be important for surgical planning in certain cases.

TABLE 56-1 Renal Cell Cancer Staging, TNM

TX	Primary tumor cannot be assessed
T0	No evidence of primary tumor
T1	Tumor 7 cm or less in diameter and limited to the kidney
T2	Tumor more than 7 cm in greatest dimension limited to the kidney
T3	Tumor extends into major veins or invades the adrenal gland or perinephric tissues, but not beyond Gerota's fascia
T4	Tumor invades beyond Gerota's fascia
NX	Regional lymph nodes cannot be assessed
N0	No regional lymph node metastases
N1	Metastasis in a single regional lymph node
N2	Metastasis in more than one regional lymph node
MX	Distant metastasis cannot be assessed
M0	No distant metastasis
M1	Distant metastasis

RENAL MASSES

Renal cell carcinoma (RCC) is the most common primary renal malignancy. It arises from renal tubular epithelium and usually develops in renal cortex. It is bilateral in 2% of cases. RCC is usually solid, although a small percentage is predominately cystic. Calcification occurs in approximately 25% to 30% of tumors overall, and intratumoral fat is very rarely seen. Direct tumor invasion into the renal vein or IVC may affect tumor staging (Table 56-1). Risk factors include family history, male gender, tobacco use, chronic dialysis, and advancing age. There is an increased incidence of bilateral renal tumors in Von Hippel-Lindau disease.

Lymphoma rarely primarily involves the kidneys. The kidney is commonly involved by hematogenous lymphoma metastases or by direct invasion of retroperitoneal adenopathy, usually non-Hodgkin lymphoma. Patterns of renal involvement include diffuse enlargement of the kidney, multiple bilateral solid renal masses, solitary bulky tumor, tumor invasion into the renal sinus, and perirenal tumor surrounding the kidneys. On CT, lymphoma is seen as a homogeneous poorly enhancing mass; extensive adenopathy supports the diagnosis.

Metastatic disease involving the kidneys often appears as multiple bilateral small irregular renal masses. Solitary hypervascular masses may be indistinguishable from RCC. Most renal metastases are detected late in the course of malignancy, and common primary tumors include lung, breast, and colon cancer as well as melanoma. Unlike RCC, which is typically exophytic, most metastases do not disrupt the cortical margins, but those from colon cancer may.

TCC is a uroepithelial tumor, which may arise anywhere within the collecting system. Tumors are often multifocal. TCC often has an infiltrative appearance and may diffusely invade along the collecting system urothelium. Calcifications in upper tract TCC are rare, less than 5%, and vascular invasion is not generally present.

Oncocytoma is a rare benign solid tumor, which rarely demonstrates hemorrhage or necrosis. The mass may disrupt the cortical margins, similar to RCC. Large tumors may demonstrate a stellate central star that is suggestive of the diagnosis but can be seen in malignant renal tumors. Therefore, oncocytomas are not distinguishable from RCC by standard imaging methods.

Angiomyolipoma (AML) is a rare benign tumor composed of variable amounts of fat, smooth muscle, and abnormal vessels. Tumors larger than 4 cm are susceptible to spontaneous hemorrhage. Most are solitary unilateral tumors incidentally discovered. Approximately 10% of AMLs are seen in patients with tuberous sclerosis; 80% of patients with tuberous sclerosis have AMLs, typically multiple bilateral lesions. However, less than half of patients with AML have tuberous sclerosis. CT demonstration of gross fat density within a solid renal tumor without calcification is considered diagnostic of AML.

Multilocular cystic nephroma is a rare benign thick-walled neoplasm comprising a cluster of noncommunicating cysts of varying size separated by thin connective tissue septations. It is seen most commonly in male children younger than 4 years and middle-aged women in the fourth to sixth and decade of life.

CYSTIC DISEASE

Autosomal recessive polycystic kidney disease is detectable in utero and usually presents in the neonate. The condition is characterized by involvement of the kidneys and occasionally the liver. There is a spectrum of disease from infantile polycystic disease with severe renal disease at birth to juvenile polycystic disease with relatively mild renal disease and development of hepatic fibrosis and liver failure in childhood.

Autosomal dominant polycystic kidney disease can be detected in neonates and children, but usually becomes clinically apparent between the third and fifth decades of life, with hypertension and renal failure. The renal parenchyma is progressively replaced by multiple noncommunicating cysts of varying size and complexity. The renal volume increases with the number and size of the cysts. Cysts may be seen in other organs, often the liver (60%), pancreas (10%), and rarely spleen. Extrarenal cysts are seldom clinically significant. There is an association with intracranial aneurysms (3%–20%) as well as mitral valve prolapse, bicuspid aortic valve, and aortic aneurysms/dissections.

Medullary sponge kidney is dysplastic dilatation of the collecting tubules in the papilla. This results in urinary stasis causing stone formation and sometimes infection. There is no genetic predisposition. The kidneys remain of normal size. The condition may be bilateral and symmetric or may be focal and asymmetric. Excretory urography demonstrates striations or saccular contrast collections in the papilla. Stones in the papilla result in increased density seen on CT and increased medullary echogenicity seen on ultrasound.

Multicystic dysplastic kidney is usually diagnosed in utero or at birth. It appears as a mass of noncommunicating cysts of varying sizes. The kidney progressively atrophies; by adulthood there is only a small focus of often calcified tissue remaining.

ACQUIRED CYSTIC DISEASE

Hemodialysis and end-stage renal disease may result in the development of multiple cysts in the native kidneys, also called acquired cystic kidney disease. The atrophic kidneys demonstrate predominately cortical cysts generally no greater than 2 cm in size. There is significantly increased risk of RCC in these patients.

SIMPLE CYST

The most common renal mass in the adult is the cyst. They may be solitary or multiple and arise anywhere within the kidney. Cysts tend to increase in size and number over years. They are usually asymptomatic but if large can cause mass effect leading to hypertension or obstruction of the collecting system. If imaging criteria for simple cyst are met on CT or ultrasound, no further evaluation is needed. Bosniak classification of cystic renal lesions is used to assess risk of neoplasm in renal lesions and to address risk of neoplasm in a complex-appearing renal cyst (Table 56-2).

TABLE 56-2 Bosniak Classification

Bosniak I	Simple renal cyst, uniformly water density, no enhancement, imperceptible or barely perceptible margin	Benign No intervention
Bosniak II	Thin septations, nonenhancing high density or thin peripheral calcification and smaller than 3 cm	Benign No intervention
Bosniak IIF	Lesions which would otherwise be considered Bosniak II but are larger than 3 cm, including high attenuation lesions. Lesions with multiple thin septae, mildy thick or nodular septae or wall, or perceived enhancing thin septa. No measureable enhancement.	Probably benign Follow-up to prove stability
Bosniak III	Thick irregular calcifications, thick or enhancing septations, areas of nodularity, thick wall or multilocular appearance	Indeterminate. Biopsy, ablation/excision, or follow-up
Bosniak IV	Irregular solid nodules, irregular shaggy walls and solid enhancing areas	Malignant Ablation or excision

INFECTION/INFLAMMATION

Pyelonephritis usually results from an ascending urinary tract infection caused by gram-negative organisms. Often, there are no imaging abnormalities. Edema and swelling associated with acute infection may cause wedge-shaped defects in the enhancing parenchyma, referred to as a striated nephrogram (Table 56-3). Abscess may form as a complication of acute pyelonephritis.

Emphysematous pyelonephritis is a rapidly progressing and life-threatening form of acute pyelonephritis with gas in the renal parenchyma. Risk factors include diabetes, obstruction, or immune system compromise. Mixed flora infection with gram-negative organisms is most common.

Chronic pyelonephritis is a chronic interstitial nephritis caused by infection. When associated with vesicoureteral reflux it is referred to as reflux nephropathy. In adults, chronic pyelonephritis is most commonly associated with conditions resulting in urinary stasis, such as stones with chronic obstruction, neurogenic bladder, and ileal conduit. Imaging demonstrates focal scarring overlying dilated calyces, often with normal calyces intervening.

Xanthogranulomatous pyelonephritis is more frequently seen middle-aged females in the setting of recurrent urinary tract infections. Infection-based stones are common, and the stones may be fragmented during the swelling of the kidney. Imaging demonstrates renal enlargement with a hypo- or nonfunctioning inflammatory mass, which may mimic malignancy, often with perinephric inflammatory change. These lesions are irreversible and surgical intervention may be required.

Renal tuberculosis may occur as a late complication of primary pulmonary tuberculosis, up to 10 to 15 years later. In cases of renal tuberculosis, 30% show chest radiograph evidence of prior tuberculosis, and 10% show findings of active tuberculosis. Patients may present with asymptomatic hematuria or sterile pyuria. Imaging suggests the diagnosis with findings of parenchymal

TABLE 56-3 Etiologies of Striated Nephrogram

COMMON	UNCOMMON	RARE
Pyelonephritis	ADPKD	Radiation nephritis
Acute ureteral obstruction	Acute renal vein thrombosis	
	Renal contusion	

destruction and cavity formation with eventual fibrosis causing strictures of the collecting system and ureter. Granuloma formation may result in parenchymal masses, and calcification is frequent.

Nephrolithiasis refers to the presence of calculi in the intrarenal collecting system. Nearly all stones appear high attenuation on noncontrast CT, with attenuations ranging from approximately 150 to 1000 HU, depending on composition. The uncommon exception is crystalline stones previously associated with the use of protease inhibitors in the treatment of HIV infection. High attenuation of stones on CT facilitates differentiation of calculi from other collecting system lesions such as tumors, hematoma, fungus balls, or sloughed papilla, which generally are less than 50 HU.

Types of stones:

Calcium. Approximately 80% of renal calculi contain sufficient calcium oxalate or calcium phosphate to be apparent on radiographs.

Struvite (magnesium ammonium phosphate) stones are formed in the presence of alkaline urine and infection. They make up approximately 15% of renal calculi and are also somewhat radiopaque on radiographs.

Urate/xanthine stones account for approximately the remaining 3% to 4% of renal stones. These are typically radiolucent on radiographs.

Nephrocalcinosis (Table 56-4) is the pathologic deposition of calcium in the renal parenchyma. It is usually bilateral and secondary to systemic disorders. Medullary nephrocalcinosis is the more common form and is usually related to hypocalcemia or hypercalciuria. Imaging demonstrates dense or echogenic renal pyramids. Cortical nephrocalcinosis is rare (less than 5%).

Delayed/persistent nephrogram has a broad differential diagnosis (Table 56-5). Contrast enhanced imaging shows retention of contrast in the kidneys. If the finding is bilateral and symmetric this reflects medical disease. Asymmetric or unilateral involvement is usually secondary to an underlying disorder requiring surgical intervention.

TABLE 56-4 Differential Diagnosis for Nephrocalcinosis

MEDULLARY	CORTICAL
Hyperparathyroidism	Acute cortical necrosis (severe ischemia)
Medullary sponge kidney	Chronic glomerulonephritis
Renal tubular acidosis Type 1	Primary hyperoxaluria
Milk alkali syndrome	
Hypervitaminosis D	
Hypocalcemia/ hypercalciuric states	
Primary hyperoxaluria	

TABLE 56-5 Etiologies for Delayed Nephrogram

Intrarenal (70%)
Acute tubular necrosis: drugs, including IV contrast, ischemia
Acute glomerulonephritis
Interstitial nephritis: drug reaction, especially antibiotics
Papillary necrosis: sickle cell, DM, analgesics
Prerenal (15%)
Hypovolemia/hypotension
Low cardiac output
Renal artery stenosis
Renal vein thrombosis
Postrenal (15%)
Obstructive uropathy

PARENCHYMAL DISEASE

Bilateral small kidneys (less than 9 cm) imply renal injury secondary to a systemic disease process (Table 56-6).

Unilateral small kidney implies global injury to the renal parenchyma (Table 56-7). The contralateral kidney can sometimes show compensatory hypertrophy.

Bilateral large kidneys (greater than 13 cm) imply systemic disease that adds to the renal size by deposition of protein, cells, or fluid (Table 56-8).

Unilateral large kidney may result from infiltrating neoplasm, duplicated collecting system and compensatory hypertrophy as well as a number of acute processes. A small contralateral kidney suggests compensatory hypertrophy as the etiology. Acute processes include acute renal vein thrombosis, acute arterial infarction, obstructive uropathy, and acute pyelonephritis.

RENAL VASCULAR DISEASE

The two most common causes of renal artery stenotic disease are atherosclerosis and fibromuscular disease (FMD). Patients with atherosclerotic renal disease are usually older than 60 years and may clinically present with hypertension, renal failure or both. FMD is the most common cause of renovascular hypertension in patients younger than 40 years. Atherosclerotic disease typically affects the renal artery ostia, and often requires stenting with dilatation. With FMD, the mid and distal portions of the vessel are most frequently affected and FMD typically responds well to dilatation alone. There are three

TABLE 56-6 Differential Diagnosis for Bilateral Small Kidneys

Uremic medullary disease
Chronic glomerulonephritis
Arterial hypotension (acute contrast reaction)
Generalized arterial atherosclerosis
Nephrosclerosis secondary to systemic hypertension

TABLE 56-7 Differential Diagnosis for Unilateral Small Kidney

Renal artery stenosis
Postobstructive uropathy
Postinflammatory atrophy
Global renal infarction
Radiation nephritis
Congenital hypoplasia (less than 5 lobes)

types of FMD, intimal (7%–8%), medial (85%), and periarterial (7%–8%). Medial fibroplasia demonstrates the classic "string of beads" appearance.

RENAL TRANSPLANT

A normal transplant kidney appears well defined and elliptical with preserved corticomedullary differentiation. Ultrasound echogenicity should be similar to liver echogenicity.

Renal transplant complications: peritransplant collections include hematoma, abscess, urinoma, and lymphocele. Hematoma may be seen in the immediate postoperative period. Acute hematoma is hyperechoic by ultrasound, and there may be an associated decrease in hematocrit. Abscess, appearing as a complex fluid collection and associated with fever, may develop within weeks. Urinoma tends to occur within the first month and appears as a bland collection on ultrasound. In the absence of active leak, it will not demonstrate activity on a nuclear medicine study. Lymphocele is seen in up to 20% of transplants and tends to occur at 1 to 4 months after transplantation surgery. These collections often contain thin septations and are of no consequence unless they result in obstruction or pain.

Reversal of diastolic flow in the renal vein implies compromise of drainage by the transplant renal vein or high resistance in intrarenal vessels. Differential considerations include severe rejection (most common), acute tubular necrosis, renal vein thrombosis, intimal flap, and extrinsic compromise secondary to peritransplant collection. Although only 10% of cases, renal vein thrombosis must be considered due to poor outcomes if left untreated.

TABLE 56-8 Differential Diagnosis for Bilateral Large Kidneys

Proliferative disorders	Parenchymal edema
Acute glomerulonephritis	Acute tubular necrosis
Lupus nephritis	Acute cortical necrosis
Diabetic glomerulosclerosis	Acute bilateral Pyelonephritis
Cell infiltration	Protein deposition
Lymphoma	Multiple myeloma
Leukemia	Amyloidosis
	Urate deposition
	Urate nephropathy

Arterial stenosis is suggested by an elevated peak systolic velocity and elevated renal artery to iliac artery ratio with tardus parvus waveforms in segmental renal arteries. This is the most common vascular complication of renal transplant.

Rejection is characterized by elevated resistive indices greater than 0.7–0.8 by Doppler ultrasound and demonstrates decreased perfusion on nuclear medicine study. Hyperacute rejection occurs within the first 24 hours. Accelerated acute rejection occurs between 1 and 5 days and acute rejection between 1 and 5 weeks (usually within 3 months) after transplant placement. Chronic rejection is seen months to years posttransplant. Chronic rejection diagnosed by scintigraphy can often not be differentiated from cyclosporin toxicity, renal artery stenosis, or ureteral stenosis.

Acute tubular necrosis is the most common form of acute reversible renal failure in transplant patients. It is usually seen within 24 hours of transplant and rarely occurs beyond 1 month posttransplant. Nuclear medicine study will demonstrate normal flow with reduced excretion. Causes include renal ischemia and nephrotoxicity.

Cyclosporin toxicity is uncommon within the first month after transplant. Renal scintigraphy shows decreased perfusion and function with decreased excretion, but biopsy is often required for definitive diagnosis.

Hydronephrosis may be associated with urinoma or other peritransplant collection, stone formation, or stricture.

SUGGESTED READING

Brandt WE, Helms CA. *Fundamentals of Diagnostic Radiology*. Vol 3. 3rd ed. Philadelphia, PA: Lippincott, Williams & Wilkens; 2006:chap 25 and 33.

Brown ED, Chen MYM, Wolfman NT, et al. Complications of renal transplantation: evaluation with US and radionuclide imaging. *Radiographics*. 2000;20:607.

Israel GM, Bosniak MA. How I do it: evaluating renal masses. *Radiology*. 2005;236:441-450.

Lee JKY, Sagel SS, Stanley RJ, et al. *Computed Body Tomography with MRI Correlation*. Vol 2. 4th ed. Philadelphia, PA: Lippincott, Williams & Wilkens; 2006; chap 18.

Zagoria RJ. The kidney and retroperitoneum: anatomy and congenital abnormalities; Renal masses; The kidney: diffuse parenchymal abnormalities. In: Thrall JH, ed. *The Requisites Genitourinary Radiology*. Philadelphia, PA: Mosby; 2004:chap 2–4.

QUESTIONS AND ANSWERS

1. What is the most common primary renal malignancy?
   A. Transitional cell carcinoma
   B. Renal cell carcinoma

C. Metastasis
D. Lymphoma

ANSWER: B. Renal cell carcinoma accounts for approximately 3% of adult malignancies and 90% to 95% of neoplasms arising from the kidney. It arises from the proximal renal tubular epithelium and is most often cortical location.

Transitional cell carcinoma accounts for approximately 90% of renal pelvic tumors and is the second most common primary malignancy of the kidney. The vast majority of urothelial tumors arise in the bladder. Urothelial tumors of the renal pelvis and ureter are rare, comprising approximately 5% to 6% of all urothelial tumors and 5% to 9% of renal cancers.

Primary lymphoma of the kidneys is rare. The incidence of renal lymphoma in patients with known lymphoma may be as high as 50%. Renal involvement is more often seen with non-Hodgkin than Hodgkin lymphoma.

Renal metastases are most often found in patients with known malignancies, usually in association with metastatic disease.

2. Which of the following has an increased incidence of bilateral renal cell carcinoma?
   A. Von Hippel-Lindau disease
   B. Tuberous sclerosis
   C. Klippel-Trenaunay Syndrome
   D. Sturge-Weber Syndrome

   ANSWER: A. Von Hippel-Lindau syndrome is an autosomal dominant, inherited, phakomatosis, characterized by a predisposition to bilateral and multicentric retinal angiomas, central nervous system hemangioblastoma; renal cell carcinoma; pheochromocytoma; islet cell tumor of the pancreas; endolymphatic sac tumor; and renal, pancreatic, and epididymal cysts. Tuberous sclerosis is an autosomal dominant disorder characterized by hamartoma/benign tumor formation in the skin, brain/nervous system, and kidneys, including angiomyolipoma. Clinical triad of epilepsy, low intelligence, and adenoma sebaceum is seen. Klippel-Trenaunay syndrome is a congenital vascular disorder of unknown cause, characterized by a triad of symptoms: port-wine stain covering one or more limbs, congenital vascular anomalies, and hypertrophy or atrophy of the limb.

   Sturge-Weber syndrome is a congenital, nonfamilial disorder of unknown incidence and cause. It is characterized by a congenital facial birthmark and neurologic abnormalities.

3. Which of the following is commonly associated with renal angiomyolipoma?
   A. Von Hippel-Lindau disease
   B. Tuberous sclerosis
   C. Klippel-Trenaunay Syndrome
   D. Sturge-Weber Syndrome

   ANSWER: B. See explanation for question 2.

4. Most patients with renal angiomyolipoma have tuberous sclerosis.
   A. True
   B. False

   ANSWER: B. Eighty percent of patients with tuberous sclerosis have angiomyolipomas, typically multiple bilateral lesions. Less than half of patients with AML have tuberous sclerosis.

5. A 2.5-cm renal cyst with thin peripheral calcification and no solid enhancing component is seen. What is its Bosniak Classification?
   A. I
   B. II
   C. IIF
   D. III

   ANSWER: B. A Bosniak II lesion demonstrates thin septations and/or thin peripheral calcification and are smaller than 3 cm. Hyperdense cysts are included in this category.

   Bosniak IIF are lesions that would otherwise be considered Bosniak II but are larger than 3 cm, including high attenuation lesions. Also included in this category are lesions that are slightly more complex, demonstrating multiple septations, and/or mild septal or wall thickening/nodularity without measurable contrast enhancement.

6. What is the most common type of renal calculus?
   A. Calcium
   B. Struvite
   C. Xanthine
   D. Crystalline

   ANSWER: A. Calcium rich calculi constitute approximately 80% of urinary tract stones. Struvite stones make up approximately 15%, and xanthine approximately 3% to 4%. Crystalline stones are rare.

7. What type of renal calculus may not be visualized on CT?
   A. Calcium
   B. Struvite
   C. Xanthine
   D. Crystalline

   ANSWER: D. Crystalline stones are a result of treatment with a protease inhibitor. They are nonopaque on CT imaging. They are suspected in the appropriate clinical setting with imaging findings of obstructive uropathy without stone or other obstructing lesion visualized.

8. Renal scintigraphy demonstrates normal flow with reduced excretion in a transplanted kidney on post-transplant day 1. What is the most likely diagnosis?
   A. Arterial stenosis
   B. Rejection
   C. Acute tubular necrosis
   D. Cyclosporin toxicity

   ANSWER: C. Acute tubular necrosis and cyclosporine toxicity typically demonstrate normal flow with reduced excretion. Decreased perfusion may be seen with cyclosporine toxicity. ATN typically develops within 24 to 48 hours posttransplant and is rare after 1 month. Cyclosporine toxicity is not typically seen within the first month following transplant and is associated with elevated cyclosporine levels. Rejection typically demonstrates decreased flow and reduced excretion. A major point of distinction between acute tubular necrosis and rejection is that perfusion is preserved in ATN. Transplant renal artery stenosis is best assessed sonographically and may appear similar to chronic rejection on radionuclide imaging.

9. A peritransplant collection is identified 6 months after renal transplant. What is the most likely diagnosis?
   A. Lymphocele
   B. Hematoma
   C. Urinoma
   D. Abscess

   ANSWER: A. Lymphoceles are the most common peritransplant fluid collection. They develop as a result of leakage from disrupted lymphatic channels. They generally require approximately 1 to 2 months before they become large enough to produce symptoms. They are usually asymptomatic but may cause obstruction secondary to mass effect.

   Hematoma is typically seen as a small peritransplant collection immediately after surgery. Differential diagnosis is seroma. These often appear mildly complex and maybe echogenic if they are acute.

   Urinoma is a relatively rare complication following transplant. Urine leaks generally occur within the first 2 weeks postoperative. On ultrasound, a urinoma appears as a well-defined anechoic fluid collection that rapidly increases in size. Septations are uncommon.

10. A patient has developed an intimal flap in the transplant vein in the immediate postoperative period. What is the expected sonographic finding?
   A. Tardus parvus wavefrom
   B. Reversal of diastolic flow
   C. Triphasic waveform
   D. Square wave

   ANSWER: B. Reversal of diastolic flow may be caused by a variety of factors. Less than 24 hours from transplant, renal vein thrombosis, vascular kinking, and perigraft hematomas are more common. In the longer term, reversal of diastolic flow is associated with chronic rejection. Tardus parvus waveform is variably seen with arterial stenosis. A triphasic waveform is a normal high resistance arterial waveform. A square wave is a kind of waveform commonly used to represent digital information.

57 URETERS

Heather L. Haddad and Mark E. Lockhart

NORMAL ANATOMY

The ureters range in length 25 to 30 cm and are retroperitoneal in location. They course from the renal pelvis caudally, anterior to the psoas muscle. Ureters cross over the distal common iliac or proximal external iliac vessels and continue caudally along the lateral pelvic walls. At the level of the inferior greater sciatic foramen, they course medially and run obliquely through the bladder wall to empty at the lateral angles of the bladder trigone.

The ureters consist of three layers:

1. The outer fibrous layer, the adventitia, is continuous with the renal capsule and adventitia of the urinary bladder.
2. The muscularis consists of outer circular and inner longitudinal muscular layers.
3. Transitional epithelium forms the mucosal layer beneath which lies the submucosal connective tissue of the lamina propria.

DEVELOPMENTAL ABNORMALITIES

Vesicoureteral reflux is retrograde flow of urine from the bladder into the ureters. It results due to a primary maturation abnormality of the ureterovesicular junction (UVJ) or due to submucosal segment of the ureter that is too short as it travels through the bladder wall; disrupting the ureteral valve mechanism. Reflux is categorized by a grading system of the International Reflux Committee (Table 57-1).

TABLE 57-1 Grades of Vesicoureteral Reflux

Grade I	Reflux into the distal ureter
Grade II	Reflux reaches the level of the kidney without dilation of the collecting system
Grade III	Reflux to the kidney with mild dilation of the collecting system
Grade IV	Moderate dilation of the ureter, pelvis, and calyces. Obliteration of sharp forniceal angles
Grade V	Marked tortuosity of the ureter with massive dilation of the ureters, pelvis, and calyces loss of papillary impressions on calyces

TABLE 57-2 Medial Deviation of the Ureter

Retroperitoneal fibrosis
Retrocaval ureter
Iliopsoas hypertrophy (distal ureter)
Iliac lymphadenopathy
Iliac artery aneurysm
Pelvic lipomatosis
Lateral retroperitoneal mass

Megaureter is a ureteral diameter greater than or equal to 7 mm in a child or 10 mm in an adult. Primary megaureter develops when there is a short, aperistaltic segment of ureter near the UVJ, with the most severe dilatation just proximal to this segment. The ureter is usually most dilated just above the more normal caliber aperistaltic segment. Primary megaureter can be distinguished from ureteral obstruction as the intraparenchymal collecting system typically remains normal in caliber with primary megaureter and dilates with ureteral obstruction. Reflux is uncommonly (20%) associated with primary megaureter. The condition is more prevalent in males with a left-sided predominance.

An ectopic ureter, secondary to an abnormal ureteral bud migration, usually inserts caudal to the normal ureteral insertion at the trigone. Approximately 70% to 80% are associated with complete ureteral duplication, each ipsilateral ureter inserting separately into the bladder.

WEIGERT-MEYER RULE

In a duplicated renal collecting system, the upper pole moiety ureter inserts inferior and medial to the ureter draining the lower pole moiety. The upper pole is associated with an ureterocele and obstruction. The lower pole ureter inserts at or near the normal location and is associated with reflux secondary to a short intravesicular ureteral segment.

Ectopic ureter is more common in females and can result in incontinence when the ureter inserts distal to the external sphincter in the vestibule, uterus, or vagina. Ectopic ureter is not associated with incontinence in males as the ureter inserts proximal to the external sphincter.

An ureterocele is cystic dilation of the intravesicular ureteral segment secondary to obstruction at the ureteral orifice. The outer wall consists of bladder epithelium and the inner wall consists of ureteral epithelium. Intravenous urography demonstrates the "cobra head" sign: contrasted urine within the ureterocele surrounded by the thin, radiolucent wall of the epithelium, protruding into the contrast-filled bladder. Approximately 75% of ureteroceles are associated with the upper pole moiety of a duplicated collecting system.

Retrocaval ureter occurs secondary to anomalous development of the infrarenal inferior vena cava (IVC), when the IVC forms from a persistent right posterior cardinal vein instead of the right supracardinal vein. The proximal right ureter passes posterior to the IVC, abruptly deviating medially (Table 57-2). Compression of the ureter can cause varying degrees of obstruction. Intravenous urography demonstrates a reverse "J" or fishhook appearance of the ureter.

Congenital narrowing at the ureteropelvic junction (UPJ) causes varying degrees of hydronephrosis depending on the severity of the narrowing. Approximately 20% to 30% of UPJ obstructions are bilateral. The majority are intrinsic to the ureter, while some are associated with extrinsic compression by a crossing vessel. Imaging reveals hydronephrosis without accompanying ureterectasis. UPJ obstruction is the most common cause of antenatal hydronephrosis.

NONNEOPLASTIC CONDITIONS

The vast majority of ureteral calculi result from the migration of renal calculi into the ureter (Table 57-2). The calculi are prone to lodge within the ureter at locations of anatomic narrowing including the UPJ, the UVJ, and the pelvic brim. Ureteral calculi can be confused with phleboliths. Ureteral calculi generally demonstrate uniform opacity and a soft tissue rim of the surrounding ureter on CT where as phleboliths are often multiple, do not exhibit a soft tissue rim sign, and have central lucency because of recanalization of the thrombosed vein. Calcification within the ureteral wall can occur secondary to infection with tuberculosis or schistosomiasis but is uncommonly seen in the United States.

Ureteritis cystica reveals multiple tiny (2–3 mm) subepithelial fluid-filled cysts in the wall of the ureter (Table 57-3). Development of the condition can be associated with urinary calculi, chronic inflammation, or urinary tract infection (UTI). Intravenous urography demonstrates multiple tiny smooth ureteral filling defects.

TABLE 57-3 Ureteral Filling Defects

Ureteral Filling Defects
Calculus
Transitional cell carcinoma
Blood clot
Fungus ball
Polyp
Sloughed papilla
Squamous cell carcinoma
Metastasis
Pyeloureteritis cystica
Malakoplakia
Leukoplakia

Ureteral pseudodiverticulosis consists of multiple, tiny pseudodiverticula. This is typically bilateral, more common in the proximal and mid ureter. Development of pseudodiverticuli can be associated with urinary calculi, obstruction, and infection. There is a possible association with transitional cell carcinoma (TCC).

Malacoplakia is an inflammatory condition that occurs in the setting of chronic UTIs. Plaque-like or nodular intramural lesions develop as a result of defective macrophage digestion of bacteria, which are incompletely phagocytized and form intracellular inclusion bodies termed Michaelis-Gutmann bodies. These are identifiable with histologic evaluation. The bladder is more commonly affected than the ureters. This condition is not considered premalignant and usually regresses with antibiotic treatment.

Leukoplakia is squamous metaplasia of the urothelium secondary to of chronic irritation from chronic UTI or urolithiasis. The bladder is affected more commonly than the ureters. Imaging findings in the ureter include mural filling defects. Leukoplakia is considered premalignant; there is an association with the development of squamous cell carcinoma.

URETERAL NEOPLASMS

TCC accounts for approximately 90% of renal collecting system neoplasms. Approximately 75% of ureteral TCC occur in the distal one-third of the ureter. Risk factors include tobacco, dyes used in manufacturing such as aniline, chemicals used in rubber, gas, printing and plastic industries, and drugs including chronic phenacetin abuse and cyclophosphamide. It has been theorized that bathing of the collecting system with a renally excreted carcinogen leads to the development of synchronous and metachronous lesions. The majority of metachronous bladder lesions develop within 18 to 24 months. The most common clinical symptoms include hematuria, urinary frequency, dysuria, and pain. Diagnosis can be made with retrograde pyelography, CT urography, and intravenous urography. Retrograde pyeloureterography demonstrates the "goblet or champagne glass sign." Slow growth of the TCC leads to expansion of the ureter above and below the tumor giving the dilated ureter the appearance of cupping the tumor. TCC metastasizes via lymphatics to regional lymph nodes. Hematogenous metastasis occurs to the liver, lungs, and bones.

Squamous cell carcinoma occurs much less frequently than TCC, and predisposing factors include calculi, chronic infection, and schistosomiasis infection. It infiltrates and spreads superficially.

A fibroepithelial polyp is a benign tumor of the ureter, which consists of a stalk of loose fibrous and vascular tissue covered by urothelium. These polyps are usually located in the proximal ureter and produce a smooth, oblong, mobile filling defect on urography.

SECONDARY INVOLVEMENT OF THE URETER

Retroperitoneal fibrosis is a process of progressive fibrosis, often idiopathic in etiology. Known causes include inflammatory aortic aneurysm, retroperitoneal metastasis, hematoma, abscess, and medications such as hydralazine and ergot alkaloids. Encasement of the ureters can lead to urinary obstruction. On CT, retroperitoneal fibrosis appears as a confluent mass centered at the L4 level. Classically, the ureters are medially deviated centered at the L3-L5 level (Table 57-2).

Retroperitoneal adenopathy can displace or encase the ureters. The upper ureters are displaced laterally and anteriorly by retroperitoneal adenopathy and the distal ureters are displaced medially by iliac adenopathy (Tables 57-2 and 57-4). Direct extension of metastatic disease can cause irregular strictures of the ureter. Primary sites of malignancy include cervix, prostate, bladder, uterus, and sarcomas.

Hematogenous metastasis to the ureters occurs most commonly from breast, gastrointestinal, prostate, cervix, and renal primaries. Metastasis may infiltrate the periureteral soft tissues, demonstrate transmural involvement

TABLE 57-4 Lateral Deviation of Ureter

Lateral Deviation of Ureter
Retroperitoneal adenopathy
Aortic aneurysm
Retroperitoneal mass/hematoma
Central pelvic mass
Psoas hypertrophy (proximal ureter)

of the ureteral wall, or may manifest as submucosal nodules. The majority of patients are asymptomatic; however, presenting symptoms may include hematuria or urinary obstruction.

Genitourinary tuberculosis occurs as a result of hematogenous seeding. Ureteral involvement includes wall thickening, abnormal peristalsis, and strictures resulting in proximal dilation. Urothelial calcifications may occur.

SUGGESTED READING

Berrocal T, Lopez-Pereira P, Arjonilla, A, et al. Anomalies of the distal ureter, bladder, and urethra in children: embryologic, radiologic, and pathologic features. *Radiographics.* 2002;22:1139-1164.

Dyer DB, Chen MY, Zagoria RJ. Abnormal calcifications in the urinary tract. *Radiographics.* 1998;18:1405-1424.

Silverman S, Cohan R. *CT Urography: An Atlas.* Philadelphia, PA: Lippincott, Williams & Wilkins; 2007.

Wasserman NF, La Pointe S, Posalaky IP. Ureteral pseudodiverticulosis. *Radiology.* 1985;155:561-566.

Winalski CS, Lipman JC, Tumeh SS. Ureteral neoplasms. *Radiographics.* 1990;10:271-283.

Wong-You-Cheong JJ, Wagner BJ. Transitional cell carcinoma of the urinary tract: radiologic—pathologic correlation. *Radiographics.* 1998;18:123-142.

QUESTIONS AND ANSWERS

1. At which location would a ureteral calculus be *least* likely to impact?
   A. UPJ
   B. L4 level
   C. Pelvic brim
   D. UVJ

   ANSWER: B. A ureteral calculus is most likely to impact at one of the three points of ureteral narrowing, the UPJ, the pelvic brim, and the UVJ.

2. The Weigert-Meyer rule states that in a duplicated collecting system:
   A. Lower pole moiety ureter inserts inferior and medial.
   B. Lower pole moiety ureter inserts inferior and lateral.
   C. Upper pole moiety ureter inserts inferior and medial.
   D. Upper pole moiety ureter inserts inferior and lateral.

   ANSWER: C. The upper pole moiety inserts inferior and medial to the lower pole moiety. The upper pole moiety tends to obstruct, and the lower pole moiety tends to reflux.

3. Which direction is the ureter displaced by retroperitoneal fibrosis?
   A. Medially
   B. Laterally
   C. Anteriorly
   D. Posteriorly

   ANSWER: A. Retroperitoneal fibrosis and retrocaval ureter typically displace the ureter medially, while adenopathy and aortic aneurysm displace laterally.

4. What most commonly causes abrupt medial deviation of the proximal right ureter?
   A. Lymphoma
   B. Retroperitoneal hematoma
   C. Retrocaval ureter
   D. Retroperitoneal fibrosis

   ANSWER: C. Retrocaval ureter occurs secondary to anomalous development of the infrarenal IVC. The proximal right ureter passes posterior to the IVC, abruptly deviating medially. Compression of the ureter can cause varying degrees of obstruction. Intravenous urography demonstrates a reverse "J" or fishhook appearance.

5. What is the classic radiographic sign describing ureteral transitional cell carcinoma?
   A. Cobra head sign
   B. Soft tissue rim sign
   C. Fishhook sign
   D. Goblet sign

   ANSWER: D. Slow growth of the TCC leads to expansion of the ureter above and below the tumor giving the dilated ureter the appearance of cupping the tumor. Cobra head sign describes the appearance of an ureterocele. The soft tissue rim sign helps distinguish a ureteral calculus from a phlebolith as a ureteral calculus will have a rim of ureteral tissue surrounding it.

6. What is the most likely diagnosis with radiographic findings of multiple tiny smooth filling defects in the ureter of a patient with chronic UTI?
   A. Ureteritis cystica
   B. Malacoplakia
   C. Leukoplakia
   D. Ureteral pseudodiverticulosis

   ANSWER: A. Ureteritis cystica reveals multiple tiny (2–3 mm) subepithelial fluid-filled cysts in the wall of the ureter. Development of the condition can be associated with stone disease, chronic inflammation, or UTI. Malacoplakia is also associated with chronic UTI, but the findings include plaque-like or nodular lesions in the bladder more commonly than ureter.

7. A smooth, mobile filling defect in the proximal ureter is most likely
   A. Transitional cell carcinoma
   B. Squamous cell carcinoma
   C. Fibroepithelial polyp
   D. Calculus

   ANSWER: C. Benign fibroepithelial polyp is usually located in the proximal ureter and produces a smooth, oblong, mobile filling defect on urography.

8. Concerning malacoplakia, which of the following is true?
   A. More common in ureters than the bladder
   B. Histology reveals gamma-Gandy bodies.
   C. Premalignant
   D. Regresses with antibiotic treatment

   ANSWER: D. Malacoplakia is not considered premalignant and usually regresses with antibiotic treatment. It occurs more commonly in the bladder. Bacteria are incompletely phagocytized and form intracellular inclusion bodies termed Michaelis-Gutmann bodies, which are visible upon histologic evaluation.

9. Which of the following concerning ectopic ureter is true?
   A. Upper pole moiety ureter obstructs.
   B. More common in males
   C. Leads to incontinence in males
   D. Lower pole moiety ureter typically has a ureterocele.

   ANSWER: A. In a duplicated collecting system, the upper pole is associated with an ureterocele and obstruction. The lower pole ureter inserts at or near the normal location and is associated reflux.

10. Where does transitional cell carcinoma of the ureter most commonly occur?
    A. Ureteropelvic junction
    B. Proximal third
    C. Middle third
    D. Distal third

    ANSWER: D. Transitional cell carcinoma accounts for approximately 90% of renal collecting system neoplasms. Approximately 75% of ureteral TCCs occur in the distal third of the ureter.

58 URINARY BLADDER

Heather L. Haddad and Mark E. Lockhart

NORMAL ANATOMY

The urinary bladder is located in the extraperitoneal space and is composed of four layers. The inner, luminal layer is lined by transitional urothelium. The majority of bladder neoplasms arise from this urothelial layer. The lamina propria lies deep to the epithelium. The third layer is the muscularis propria, which consists of bundles of smooth detrusor muscle. The outer adventitial layer is formed by connective tissues. The dome of the bladder is covered by peritoneum.

DEVELOPMENTAL ANOMALIES OF THE URINARY BLADDER

Bladder diverticula usually occur in males and are caused by congenital muscular anomalies of the bladder wall. A periureteric diverticulum, also known as a Hutch diverticulum, is often associated with vesicoureteral reflux. Diverticula can also be seen in patients with Ehlers-Danlos syndrome or secondary to chronic bladder obstruction, such as prostatic hypertrophy.

Bladder duplication results from a rare disturbance in the embryogenesis of the hindgut. The most common form is sagittal duplication in which two bladders lay side-by-side and are separated by a fold of peritoneum. Each bladder is drained by its own urethra.

Prune belly syndrome consists of a triad of three major findings including undescended testes, abnormal urinary tract, and renal dysmorphism. These individuals have a wrinkled and lax abdominal wall due to absence of the rectus muscles. The urinary bladder is enlarged and elongated without trabeculation and is seen in association with tortuous dilated ureters and a dilated prostatic urethra.

With cloacal malformation, the urinary, genital, and gastrointestinal tracts drain through a common perineal opening due to persistence of an early embryologic state. This condition occurs only in females.

BLADDER NEOPLASMS

Rhabdomyosarcoma is the most common bladder neoplasm in children younger than 10 years (Table 58-1). It arises from primitive fetal muscle cells demonstrating various stages of maturation. Genitourinary sites include

TABLE 58-1 Bladder Neoplasms

MALIGNANT		BENIGN	
Rhabdomyosarcoma	Most common bladder neoplasm in children	Leiomyoma	Most common mesenchymal tumor
Transitional cell carcinoma	Most common overall Risk factors: environmental agents, drugs, and tobacco	Neurofibroma	NF I or isolated
Squamous cell carcinoma	Risk factors: chronic inflammation, schistosomiasis, and tobacco	Paraganglioma	Extra-adrenal pheochromocytoma (NF, VHL, Sturge-Weber, TS, MEN)
Adenocarcinoma	Risk factors: chronic inflammation, urachal, remnant, exstrophy	Hemangioma	
Small cell	Neuroendocrine (can have carcinoid variant)	Inflammatory pseudotumor (pseudosarcomatous fibromyxoid tumor)	Non-neoplastic
Leiomyosarcoma		Nephrogenic adenoma	Metaplastic

bladder, prostate, testes, paratesticular tissues, penis, perineum, vagina, and uterus. These tumors often have an infiltrative growth pattern and the exact site of origin can be difficult to determine. In males, tumors are grouped into paratesticular rhabdomyosarcomas and bladder-prostate rhabdomyosarcomas. Symptoms include hematuria, bladder outlet obstruction, abdominal distention, dysuria, and urinary tract infections. Metastases are most commonly to lungs, cortical bone, and lymph nodes. Ultrasound, CT, and MRI show a heterogeneous mass, which may invade adjacent structures. On MRI, rhabdomyosarcoma demonstrates low T1 signal and high T2 signal with heterogeneous enhancement. Botryoid variant produces a polypoid mass, which resembles a cluster of grapes.

Greater than 90% of bladder carcinomas are transitional cell carcinoma (TCC). Risks factors include tobacco, manufacturing dyes such as aniline, cyclophosphamide, and long-term phenacetin use. Synchronous and metachronous upper urinary tract and bladder TCCs are common. Development of TCC occurs as a result of renally excreted carcinogenic substances bathing the urothelial surfaces. Approximately 90% to 95% of the TCCs occur in the urinary bladder. A propensity for bladder TCC development is hypothesized to result secondary to the longer exposure time of the bladder mucosa to urine and the larger surface area of the bladder as compared with the upper tracts.

TCC, now termed urothelial carcinoma, can be papillary, sessile, or nodular and occurs most frequently in the bladder base. Superficial papillary neoplasms are most common. Approximately 20% of tumors are invasive at presentation, extending into the detrusor muscle layer. There is a male predilection, and patients often present with gross hematuria. On imaging, TCC can appear as focal wall thickening or a papillary/nodular mass. At the time of diagnosis, up to one-third of bladder TCCs are multifocal. On ultrasound, lesions appear hypoechoic. On MRI, lesions are isointense to bladder muscle on T1-weighted images and mildly hyperintense to muscle on T2-weighted images. On both CT and MRI, tumors demonstrate early enhancement following intravenous contrast administration. MRI is the best modality for determining extent of invasion into the bladder wall and perivesicular fat. Tumors metastasize to pelvic lymph nodes, lung, liver, and abdomen.

Development of squamous cell carcinoma (SCC) in the bladder is associated with chronic inflammation from etiologies such as chronic UTI, bladder calculi, and chronic indwelling catheters. Tobacco use is also a risk factor. In countries with schistosomiasis, the majority of SCCs result from chronic bilharzial infection. Most patients present with gross hematuria. SCC can vary in appearance occurring as wall thickening or a mass. There is a predilection for the bladder trigone and the lateral walls. Often, the disease is advanced at presentation, and muscle wall invasion is common. On CT and MRI, SCC enhances following contrast administration. On delayed CT images, the tumor can be seen as a low attenuation filling defect against the contrasted urine. On T2-weighted images, the lesion is slightly higher in signal than the bladder wall. SCC invades locally and metastasizes to regional lymph nodes, bone, lung, and bowel.

Adenocarcinoma accounts for less than 2% of bladder neoplasms and may be primary or metastatic. Risk factors include persistent urachus, bladder exstrophy, and intestinal metaplasia from chronic mucosal irritation in cystitis glandularis. Of primary adenocarcinomas, only one-third are urachal in origin. Nonurachal primary adenocarcinomas are most common in the bladder base. Ninety percent of urachal carcinomas are located at the dome of the bladder in the midline. Both urachal and nonurachal adenocarcinomas are generally mixed solid and cystic with the cystic component composed of mucin. Calcifications are common, as is bladder wall invasion and extravesical spread.

Small cell/neuroendocrine tumors are rare bladder neoplasms believed to originate from dedifferentiated neuroendocrine cells. Patients often present with hematuria.

Tumors most commonly involve the lateral bladder walls and are usually large with a nodular or polypoid configuration. Tumors exhibit local invasion, peritoneal metastasis, and lymph node metastasis. The carcinoid variant of neuroendocrine tumors is rare. These tumors are small and round, located at the bladder neck or trigone.

Leiomyoma is a mass that originates in the submucosa and is the most common mesenchymal bladder tumor. Tumors may be small and incidentally discovered, or may grow large causing symptoms of obstruction, urinary frequency, hematuria, and pressure. The most common location of these lesions is the trigone. On MR imaging, leiomyomas have intermediate T1 signal and low signal on T2-weighted images. Tumors can be solid and homogeneous, or demonstrate degenerative changes with cystic components and heterogeneous signal. Leiomyoma and leiomyosarcomas can be difficult to distinguish radiographically. Leiomyosarcomas are generally poorly circumscribed with regions of necrosis.

Neurofibroma is a rare bladder neoplasm, which can occur in association with neurofibromatosis type 1 or as an isolated lesion. Neurofibroma arises from the nerve plexus of the bladder. They can be localized, diffuse, or plexiform in configuration. These tumors can grow to involve surrounding pelvic structures. On MRI, neurofibromas are low in signal on T1; they demonstrate a characteristic target appearance on T2 with a low signal center surrounded by high signal myxoid stroma.

A paraganglioma is an extra-adrenal pheochromocytoma. Bladder paragangliomas account for 0.1% of bladder tumors. Most tumors occur sporadically but can be seen in association with neurofibromatosis, Von Hippel-Lindau, Sturge-Weber, tuberous sclerosis, and MEN. Catecholamines can be released during micturition causing symptoms including headache, sweating, anxiety, hypertension, and syncope. Lesions are submucosal in location and demonstrate marked enhancement on contrasted CT and MRI. When present, peripheral ring calcification suggests the diagnosis.

Hemangiomas are detected in both childhood and adulthood. Patients usually present with gross hematuria. CT and MRI reveal a hypervascular mass.

INFLAMMATORY AND NON-NEOPLASTIC CONDITIONS

Inflammatory pseudotumor, also termed pseudosarcomatous fibromyxoid tumor, is a non-neoplastic lesion composed of myofibroblastic spindle cells and inflammatory cells with myxoid components. The lesion may develop in response to infection, inflammation, or malignancy; however, the pathogenesis not fully delineated. Patients often present with hematuria. At imaging, the tumors appear as an exophytic or polypoid mass, sometimes demonstrating ulceration. These lesions can act aggressively, invading through the bladder to involve adjacent structures. Inflammatory pseudotumors are often heterogeneous on T2-weighted MRI with central hyperintense necrosis surrounded by a hypointense periphery. Contrast-enhanced CT and MRI images reveal enhancement of the non-necrotic periphery.

Nephrogenic adenoma is a reactive, metaplastic process in the urothelium, which results from chronic irritation by calculi, infection, or surgery. Patients present with hematuria or irritative voiding symptoms. Imaging findings are nonspecific, demonstrating a polypoid mass, sessile mass, or wall thickening.

Malacoplakia is a rare, chronic granulomatous condition predominantly found in women. The pathogenesis is thought to involve impaired host defenses and defective phagocytosis. Macrophages ingest but do not completely destroy bacteria, which become mineralized and result in calcified intracellular inclusions—Michaelis-Gutmann bodies. Malacoplakia is highly associated with *Escherichia coli* infection and is commonly seen in diabetic patients and immunocompromised individuals. Patients present with hematuria and urinary tract infection symptoms. Malacoplakia varies in appearance from plaque-like wall thickening to a polypoid vascular mass.

Cystitis cystica and cystitis glandularis are rare chronic reactive inflammatory disorders. Chronic irritation caused by infection, calculi, or outlet obstruction induces metaplasia of the urothelium. The abnormal urothelium grows into the lamina propria and differentiates into cystic deposits (cystitis cystica) or glandular deposits (cystitis glandularis). Usually there is a combination of the two elements that causes a nodular mass in the lamina propria. CT and MR imaging reveal a hypervascular, polypoid mass. Imaging characteristics can overlap with urothelial carcinoma; however unlike carcinoma, cystitis should not involve the muscular layer of the bladder. Cystitis glandularis can occur in association with pelvic lipomatosis.

Emphysematous cystitis can occur secondary to infection with *E. coli*, *Aerobacter aeogenes*, and *Candida*. Imaging demonstrates foci of gas within the bladder wall. It is generally a non–life-threatening condition treated by antibiotics.

Eosinophilic cystitis, where eosinophils infiltrate into the bladder wall, is a rare chronic inflammatory condition of the bladder. Inflammation can eventually lead to fibrosis and muscle necrosis resulting in a small, contracted bladder. Patients most commonly present with hematuria and frequency. At imaging, a single mass is seen more often than multiple masses. On MR, the mass is hyperintense to muscle on T1-weighted images, isointense on T2-weighted images, and enhances following contrast administration.

Tuberculosis of the bladder is rare in the United States. The upper urinary tracts are usually primarily involved with secondary involvement of the bladder. In the acute phase, the mucosa is irregular with thickening and trabeculation of the bladder wall. There can be ureteral thickening with stricture or a patulous ureterovesical junction with reflux. In the chronic phase, the bladder is thick walled and contracted with small volume because of fibrosis. Bladder wall or upper tract urothelial calcifications can be seen with healing.

Schistosomiasis, infection with *Schistosoma haematobium*, is rare in the United States but is more commonly seen in North Africa. Eggs are deposited in the vessels supplying the bladder wall. The presence of the eggs incites a chronic inflammatory response, predisposing to the development of SCC. The granulomatous reaction initially causes nodular wall thickening and eventually leads to a contracted, fibrotic bladder containing curvilinear calcifications representing calcified eggs. Associated ureteral findings include calcification, stricture, dilation, and vesicoureteral reflux.

Chemotherapy and radiotherapy can cause hemorrhagic cystitis by denuding the urothelium. The bladder wall appears irregularly thickened, and intraluminal blood clot may be present. Chronic radiation changes are a result of ischemic changes from obliterative endarteritis and interstitial fibrosis. Patients experience frequency and urgency because of the contracted bladder.

Fistulous connections between the bladder and bowel can result as complications from Crohn disease, diverticulitis, colon carcinoma, and pelvic radiation. Patients present with complaints of UTI symptoms, fecaluria, and pneumaturia. On imaging, thickening of the bladder wall with intraluminal gas or orally administered contrast in the bladder are indicative of a fistulous communication. Vesicovaginal fistulas can result from gynecologic malignancy, gynecologic surgery, and pelvic radiation. Delayed contrast CT or cystogram may demonstrate contrast in the vagina.

Neurogenic bladder can result from spinal trauma, meningomyelocele, central nervous system tumor, diabetes, polio, and multiple sclerosis. Neurogenic bladder has two forms, spastic with a small contracted bladder and atonic with a large dilated bladder. Neurogenic bladder leads to urinary stasis, chronic infection, stone formation and vesicoureteral reflux.

Acquired bladder diverticula are usually associated with bladder outlet obstruction such as neurogenic bladder and prostatic hypertrophy. They are most commonly located near the UVJ. Diverticula can lead to stasis with development of TCC or SCC, calculi, and infection.

TABLE 58-2 Conditions Associated with Development of Bladder Calculi

Chronic outlet obstruction
Neurogenic bladder
Bladder diverticula
Bladder infection (*Proteus mirabilis*)
Migration of upper tract calculus
Foreign body nidus

Bladder calculi can develop secondary to stasis associated with chronic outlet obstruction, neurogenic bladder, and bladder diverticula or secondary to infection with organisms such as *Proteus mirabilis* (Table 58-2). A renal calculus, which has migrated into the urinary bladder or a foreign body within the bladder, can act as a nidus for calculus growth. Patients can present with microhematuria and suprapubic pain. Chronic bladder irritation caused by the presence of the calculus may predispose to the development of TCC or SCC. Calculi will appear echogenic on ultrasound with posterior acoustic shadowing, radiopaque on CT, and as an intraluminal signal abnormality with variable signal intensity on MRI.

Bladder rupture is classified as intraperitoneal or extraperitoneal in location. Extraperitoneal bladder rupture occurs due to puncture of the bladder by a bone fragment from a pelvic fracture. On conventional or CT cystogram, contrast extravasates into the extraperitoneal space including the perivesical space, the anterior abdominal wall, the groin/thigh, and retroperitoneum. The extravasated contrast is amorphous in shape or occasionally flame shaped and does not outline bowel loops. Intraperitoneal bladder rupture occurs when blunt force causes a rise in intravesicle pressure with rupture of the bladder dome. In contradistinction to intraperitoneal rupture, conventional or CT cystogram findings of intraperitoneal bladder rupture demonstrate extravasated contrast surrounding intraperitoneal bowel loops and layering in the paracolic gutters. A combined injury demonstrates features of both intraperitoneal and extraperitoneal rupture. Pelvic hematoma can cause extrinsic compression of the bladder (Table 58-3).

TABLE 58-3 Extrinsic Bladder Compression

Pelvic hematoma
Urinoma
Lymphadenopathy
Pelvic lipomatosis
Psoas muscle hypertrophy
Unopacified bladder diverticulum
Iliac artery aneurysms

Suggested Reading

Agrons GA, Wagner BJ, Lonergan GJ, et al. Genitourinary rhabdomyosarcoma in children: radiologic-pathologic correlation. *Radiographics*. 1997;17:919-937.

Berrocal T, Lopez-Pereira P, Ajronilla A, et al. Anomalies of the distal ureter, bladder, and urethra in children: embryologic, radiologic, and pathologic features. *Radiographics*. 2002;22:1139-1164.

Dyer DB, Chen MY, Zagoria RJ. Abnormal calcifications in the urinary tract. *Radiographics*. 1998;18:1405-1424.

Silverman S, Cohan R. *CT Urography: An Atlas*. Philadelphia, PA: Lippincott, Williams & Wilkins; 2007.

Wong JT, Wasserman NF, Padurean AM. Bladder squamous cell carcinoma. *Radiographics*. 2004;24:855-860.

Wong-You-Cheong JJ, Wagner BJ. Transitional cell carcinoma of the urinary tract: radiologic – pathologic correlation. *Radiographics*. 1998;18:123-142.

Wong-You-Cheong JJ, Woodward PJ, Manning MA, et al. Neoplasms of the urinary bladder: radiologic – pathologic correlation. *Radiographics*. 2006;26:553-580.

Wong-You-Cheong JJ, Woodward PJ, et al. Inflammatory and nonneoplastic bladder masses: radiologic—pathologic correlation. *Radiographics*. 2006;26:1847-1868.

QUESTIONS AND ANSWERS

1. A patient with history of multiple subcutaneous nodules presents with a bladder mass. This mass demonstrates low signal central core surrounded by high signal rim. What is the most likely diagnosis?
   A. Paraganglioma
   B. Neurofibroma
   C. Leiomyoma
   D. Adenocarcinoma

   ANSWER: B. Bladder neurofibromas can be a manifestation of neurofibromatosis type 1 and may demonstrate a characteristic target sign on T2 with a low signal center surrounded by high signal myxoid stroma.

2. Where is contrast leakage identified on CT cystogram in a patient with intraperitoneal bladder rupture?
   A. Retroperitoneum
   B. Suprapubic space
   C. Perivesical fat
   D. Surrounding small bowel loops

   ANSWER: D. Small bowel loops are intraperitoneal in location; therefore, contrast outlining small bowel indicates in intraperitoneal bladder rupture.

3. What histologic type of mass develops in an urachal remnant?
   A. Squamous cell carcinoma
   B. Adenocarcinoma
   C. Transitional cell carcinoma
   D. Small cell carcinoma

   ANSWER: B. A persistent urachus is a risk factor for developing adenocarcinoma. Most urachal carcinomas are located at the dome of the bladder in the midline.

4. What is the most common type of bladder carcinoma?
   A. Squamous cell carcinoma
   B. Adenocarcinoma
   C. Urothelial carcinoma
   D. Small cell carcinoma

   ANSWER: C. The urinary bladder is lined by transitional epithelium. Greater than 90% of bladder carcinomas are transitional cell (urothelial) carcinoma.

5. Where is a Hutch diverticulum located?
   A. Bladder neck
   B. Bladder dome
   C. Anterolateral bladder wall
   D. Near ureterovesical junction

   ANSWER: D. A periureteric diverticulum is also known as a Hutch diverticulum and is often associated with vesicoureteral reflux.

6. A patient experiences syncope during micturition and is found to have an enhancing bladder mass. What is the most likely diagnosis?
   A. Paraganglioma
   B. Neurofibroma
   C. Neuroendocrine tumor
   D. Nephrogenic adenoma

   ANSWER: A. A paraganglioma is an extra-adrenal pheochromocytoma. Catecholamines can be released during micturition causing symptoms including headache, sweating, anxiety, hypertension, and syncope.

7. A diabetic patient with chronic *E. coli* infection demonstrates multiple nodular bladder masses. Pathology reveals Michaelis-Gutmann bodies. What is the most likely diagnosis?
   A. Nephrogenic adenoma
   B. Malakoplakia
   C. Pseudotumor
   D. Cystitis cystica

   ANSWER: B. Malacoplakia is a rare, chronic granulomatous condition predominantly found in women. Macrophages ingest but do not completely destroy bacteria, which become mineralized and result in calcified intracellular inclusions, Michaelis-Gutmann bodies. Malacoplakia is highly associated with *E. coli* infection and is commonly seen in diabetic patients and immunocompromised individuals.

8. A paraplegic patient with a long-term suprapubic catheter presents with a bladder mass. What is the most likely diagnosis?
   A. Adenocarcinoma
   B. Rhabdomyosarcoma
   C. Transitional cell carcinoma
   D. Squamous cell carcinoma

   ANSWER: D. Chronic irritation such as that due to an indwelling catheter is a risk factor for developing squamous cell carcinoma.

9. Concerning rhabdomyosarcoma, which of the following is true?
   A. Most common bladder neoplasm in young adults
   B. Noninfiltrative growth pattern
   C. Botryoid variant produces a grape-like mass.
   D. Occurs only in females

   ANSWER: C. Rhabdomyosarcoma is the most common bladder neoplasm in children younger than 10 years. These tumors often have an infiltrative growth pattern, and the exact site of origin can be difficult to determine. Botryoid variant produces a polypoid mass that resembles a cluster of grapes.

10. What is the best modality for determining depth of urothelial carcinoma invasion into the bladder musculature?
    A. MRI
    B. CT
    C. Ultrasound
    D. Cystogram

    ANSWER: A. The ability of MRI to display soft tissue differentiation allows for visualization of the bladder wall layers and determination of tumor depth.

59 ADRENAL GLANDS

Mark E. Lockhart and Mark D. Little

NORMAL ANATOMY

The adrenal glands play an important role in endocrine function and are a frequent site of disease. The paired glands in the retroperitoneum are located along the superior-medial aspect of both kidneys, invested in perinephric fat and bound by Gerota fascia. Positioned adjacent to the diaphragmatic crus, the glands normally have a "V" or "Y" shape configuration composed of two limbs, medial and lateral, which communicate through the apex or body. Each limb is approximately 3 to 6 mm thick, and the entire width of the gland should not be greater than 1 cm.

The adrenal glands have a complicated vascular supply. Each gland is supplied by superior, middle, and inferior adrenal arteries. The superior adrenal artery originates from the inferior phenic, the middle from the aorta, and the inferior from a branch of the ipsilateral renal artery. Each gland is drained by a single vein. Because of the position of the inferior vena cava on the right, the right adrenal vein drains directly into the cava, while the left vein drains into the left renal vein.

Each adrenal gland has a cortex and medulla. The cortex is derived from the mesoderm and has three distinct layers, organized superficial to deep: zona glomerulosa, zona fasciculata, and zona reticularis. Each cortical zone has a distinct endocrine function, which becomes important when evaluating hyperfunctioning adrenal lesions. The zona glomerulosa produces aldosterone. The zona fasciculata produces cortisol. Androgens are derived from the zona reticularis. Production of each of these hormones is regulated by adrenocorticotropic hormone (ACTH), produced by the anterior pituitary gland. The medulla originates from neural crest cell migration and produces catecholamines such as epinephrine and norepinephrine.

PATHOLOGY

The central imaging question to be answered when confronted with an incidental adrenal mass is whether or not this represents a benign or malignant lesion. In addition, adrenal masses can be divided into functioning or nonfunctioning lesions (Table 59-1), based on whether or not the lesion hypersecretes hormones. The majority of adrenal tumors encountered in clinical practice will be adenomas, usually incidental, nonfunctional, and benign. Unilateral versus bilateral adrenal lesion(s) determines differential diagnosis (Table 59-2). CT is usually the initial imaging modality of choice when evaluating the adrenal glands owing to its superior spatial resolution and defined diagnostic criteria. In such instances when CT is equivocal, MRI with opposed phase imaging may be used.

CONN SYNDROME (PRIMARY ALDOSTERONISM)

Hypersecretion of aldosterone is characterized clinically by mild hypertension and hypokalemia. Approximately 80% of patients demonstrate a functioning adrenal

TABLE 59-1 Functional Adrenal Lesions

Cushing disease	Increased cortisol, glucocorticoids	Ectopic ACTH production from pituitary adenoma
Cushing syndrome	Increased cortisol, glucocorticoids	Adenoma, hyperplasia, carcinoma, paraneoplastic
Conn syndrome (adenoma)	Increased aldosterone	Adenoma, hyperplasia
Adrenogenital syndrome (adenoma)	Increased sex hormones	Hyperplasia (enzymatic deficiency), adenoma, carcinoma
Pheochromocytoma	Increased catecholamines	Unilateral, bilateral, syndromic (MEN IIa, MEN IIb, familial)
Cortical carcinoma	50% functional	

adenoma on thin slice CT. These lesions are usually small (less than 2 cm in diameter), eccentrically located within the adrenal gland and appear uniformly low in attenuation, secondary to lipid laden cells of the zona fasciculata. When an adenoma is demonstrated in these patients, they are often treated with unilateral adrenalectomy.

The other 20% of patients demonstrate adrenal gland hyperplasia, usually bilateral. On imaging, the adrenal glands may appear enlarged, thickened (greater than 1 cm), and mildly nodular. However, up to one-third of patients with adrenal hyperplasia have normal-appearing glands. In such instances, adrenal vein sampling for elevated levels of aldosterone may be performed. Patients with primary aldosteronism from hyperplasia are often treated pharmacologically. In rare cases, primary aldosteronism can be caused by adrenal carcinoma.

CUSHING SYNDROME

Cushing syndrome is characterized by increased serum glucocorticoids, particularly cortisol. Clinically, patients present with obesity, hypertension, muscle wasting, bruising, and abdominal striae. In addition, abnormal glucose metabolism results in diabetes mellitus in a minority of patients.

Hypersecretion of glucocorticoids can be divided as either ACTH-dependent or independent forms. When the increase in secretion is dependent on ACTH (approximately 80% of patients), the condition is termed Cushing disease and is usually secondary to a hyperfunctioning ACTH-producing pituitary adenoma. Consequently, initial workup for patients with hypercortisolism usually involves pituitary brain MRI, plasma or urinary cortisol levels, and a dexamethasone suppression test. In Cushing disease, dexamethasone should suppress glucocorticoid production by negative feedback inhibition of pituitary gland ACTH production. Adrenal morphology in Cushing disease is variable. The adrenals may appear normal, diffusely enlarged, micronodular, or macronodular.

TABLE 59-2 Adrenal Masses

UNILATERAL	BILATERAL
Adenoma	Hyperplasia
Hemorrhage	Adenoma
Cyst	Hemorrhage
Myelolipoma	Infection (granulomatous, histoplasmosis, TB)
Metastasis	Metastasis
Pheochromocytoma	Pheochromocytoma (rare)
Cortical carcinoma	

Cushing syndrome is distinguished by increased cortisol production secondary to an adrenal adenoma. These adenomas are similarly low in attenuation, but are usually larger than the adenomas seen in Conn syndrome, measuring approximately 2 to 4 cm in size. Interestingly, when a functional cortisol producing adenoma is present, the remaining adrenal tissue should appear hypoplastic/atrophic owing to inhibition of ACTH production.

In rare instances (less than 5%), increased cortisol production may be secondary to ectopic ACTH production, primarily from lung, ovary, or pancreatic islet cell neoplasms. In addition, approximately 50% of adrenal cortical carcinomas, a rare tumor, secrete cortisol as well.

ADRENOGENITAL SYNDROME

Adrenogenital syndrome is rare and presents clinically as the excess secretion of sex hormones resulting in precocious puberty, feminization, or virilization. The syndrome can either be congenital or acquired. Congenital adrenal hyperplasia is usually secondary to an enzymatic deficiency in steroid synthesis. Less commonly, an acquired adrenal adenoma or carcinoma may be the cause.

PHEOCHROMOCYTOMA

Pheochromocytomas are paraganglionic neuroendocrine tumors usually arising from the adrenal medulla. These tumors are typically unilateral and may secrete catecholamines, such as epinephrine, dopamine, and norepinephrine. Patients present clinically with episodic palpitations, tachycardia, flushing, and severe hypertension. Pheochromocytomas are extremely rare, responsible for less than 1% of hypertensive patients. Approximately, 10% of pheochromocytomas are nonfunctional and are therefore usually larger in size when discovered incidentally.

In suspected patients, initial evaluation includes measurements for elevated serum catecholamines and increased 24 hours urine metanephrines and vanillylmandelic acid. The majority of pheochromocytomas originate in the adrenal gland. However, as paragangliomas these tumors can arise anywhere along the sympathetic chain. The most common extra-adrenal location being the organ of Zuckerkandl, located between the origin of the inferior mesenteric artery and the aortic bifurcation. As a general rule, approximately 10% of pheochromocytomas are extra-adrenal, 10% are malignant, and 10% are bilateral. When bilateral, consideration should be made of a syndrome. Specifically, pheochromocytomas are associated with MEN IIA (pheochromocytoma, medullary thyroid carcinoma, parathyroid adenoma) and MEN IIB (pheochromocytoma, medullary thyroid carcinoma, mucosal ganglioneuromas). Additionally, these tumors may be associated with neurofibromatosis type I, von Hippel-Lindau, and familial pheochromocytomas.

Pheochromocytomas are vascular tumors and therefore demonstrate significant heterogenous enhancement. These lesions may also demonstrate a characteristic "lightbulb bright" T2 hyperintense signal on MRI imaging, due to internal necrosis or cystic change. If no tumor is localized in suspected patients by cross-sectional imaging, further radiopharmaceutical evaluation with I-131 or I-123 MIBG or, less commonly, In-111 octreotide may be performed. Surveillance for recurrence and metastases may also be similarly performed with MIBG avid tumors. If biopsy or surgery is contemplated, alpha-adrenergic blockade is usually required to prevent inciting a hypertensive crisis. Surgery is usually curative for solitary pheochromocytomas.

ADENOMA

As discussed earlier, the majority of incidental adrenal masses are benign nonfunctioning adenomas. In fact, adenomas are very common, seen in approximately 2% to 8% of the population, and increase in frequency with age, hypertension, or diabetes mellitus. However, in certain clinical settings, the importance of differentiating benign and malignant adrenal masses is important for patient management. Specifically, when an incidental adrenal mass is discovered during imaging workup for an unrelated condition, or when the adrenal mass is the only possible evidence of metastasis in a patient with a known primary neoplasm, accurate characterization of the adrenal mass may have profound impact on patient outcome. Typically, the CT imaging characteristics of an adenoma are a small, well-circumscribed homogeneous low density adrenal mass. These lesions are often round or oval, bilateral or multifocal, and may be central or eccentrically located within the gland. Accurate CT characterization of these lesions takes advantage of the increased lipid content of these lesions. On nonenhanced CT, a lipid rich adrenal adenoma will demonstrate an attenuation of less than 10 HU with 98% specificity. Adenomas enhance homogeneously, similar to some metastases, but also demonstrate increased washout. Therefore, 15 minutes delayed CT images may be performed to help characterize indeterminate adrenal lesions. Two strategies are employed to help diagnose indeterminate adrenal lesions as lipid poor adenomas.

Relative washout criterion for adenoma

$$(\text{enhanced} - \text{delayed})/\text{enhanced} \times 100 = \text{greater than } 40\%$$

Absolute washout criterion for adenoma

$$(\text{enhanced} - \text{delayed})/(\text{enhanced} - \text{unenhanced}) = \text{greater than } 60\%$$

If CT evaluation is still equivocal, the lipid content of adenomas can be exploited for MRI evaluation as well. Using opposed phase MRI compared to in-phase sequence, intravoxel lipid signal will be suppressed compared to nonlipid tissue, resulting in near 90% specificity for the diagnosis of adenomas. Finally, if an indeterminate adrenal mass cannot be confidently characterized as an adenoma by imaging, percutaneous retroperitoneal biopsy or PET-CT may be indicated.

MYELOLIPOMA

Myelolipomas are unique but rare, benign tumors most commonly involving the adrenal gland. They are made up of fat and bone marrow elements and usually present incidentally. Typically, these tumors can be confidently diagnosed by CT or MRI characteristics without the need for biopsy. On CT, myeloliopomas characteristically demonstrate macroscopic fat with associated small soft tissue components. Calcification is unusual. Similarly, the macroscopic fat on MRI demonstrates high T1 and T2 signal that is suppressed by fat saturation. Large lesions can occasionally present with flank pain from mass effect or internal hemorrhage or necrosis. As a result, differentiation from a liposarcoma may be difficult and biopsy is indicated. Myelolipomas are often treated conservatively unless symptoms develop.

ADRENAL CYSTS

Cysts of the adrenal gland are rare and can be characterized as epithelial, endothelial, parasitic, or posttraumatic.

True epithelial cysts are uncommon and most cystic lesions of the adrenal gland are endothelial or posttraumatic pseudocysts. These lesions can appear simple or complex, demonstrating thick walls, multiple septations, or increased attenuation due to internal hemorrhage or protein, making differentiation from malignancy difficult. These lesions occasionally calcify; however, they should not enhance. On unenhanced CT, simple cysts can occasionally be confused with adenomas due to there similar attenuation characteristics.

HEMORRHAGE (Table 59-3)

The most common cause of adrenal hemorrhage is blunt trauma, occurring more commonly on the right side. Occasionally, unilateral hemorrhage can result from adrenal vein thrombosis following catheterization or as the presentation of a hemorrhagic metastasis. When bilateral, hemorrhage is usually the result of anticoagulation, blood dyscrasia, or sepsis. An important cause of childhood bilateral adrenal hemorrhage is meningococcal sepsis resulting in Waterhouse-Friderichsen syndrome and associated adrenal insufficiency. However, adrenal insufficiency from hemorrhage is rare, necessitating destruction of approximately 90% to 98% of adrenal tissue.

On unenhanced CT, adrenal hemorrhage is usually characterized by an adrenal mass with adjacent periadrenal fat stranding and increased attenuation between 50 and 90 HU. However, on enhanced CT, it may be difficult to differentiate hemorrhage from neoplasm. In contrast to tumor, hemorrhage decreases in size and attenuation on follow-up imaging. Additionally, MRI may be useful in certain instances when CT is equivocal. Subacute adrenal hemorrhage typically demonstrates areas of increased T1/T2 signal consistent with methemoglobin. In cases of chronic hemorrhage, the adrenal mass may demonstrate a T1/T2 hypointense ring consistent with hemosiderin deposition. Late sequelae of adrenal hemorrhage can result in calcification or cyst formation.

TABLE 59-3 Adrenal Hemorrhage

UNILATERAL	BILATERAL
Trauma/Surgery	Anticoagulation
Adrenal vein thrombosis	Sepsis
Metastasis	Blood dyscrasia
	Hypotension
	Hypoxemia
	Birth trauma

INFECTION

Adrenal infection is most often caused by histoplasmosis, tuberculosis, or other granulomatous infections. Involvement of the adrenal glands is usually bilateral and asymmetric with imaging characteristics that are nonspecific. Typically, the adrenal glands are acutely enlarged, but they may also demonstrate hemorrhage, cystic change, or calcification. Rarely, infection, such as tuberculosis or meningococcemia, can result in chronic adrenal insufficiency—Addison disease. Clinically, these patients present with fatigue, hypoglycemia, orthostatic hypotension, nausea, and emesis. Interestingly, these patients also demonstrate hyperpigmentation. When the adrenal glands are destroyed, decreased cortisol results in unregulated increased ACTH production. Melanocyte stimulating hormone shares the same precursor molecule as ACTH and therefore is also increased, resulting in the characteristic "bronzed appearance" of the skin. Addison disease can also be caused by autoimmune destruction, bilateral metastases, or hemorrhage.

MALIGNANT NEOPLASMS

METASTASES

The adrenal glands are a common location for metastasis, occurring in approximately 27% of patients with a known malignancy. The most common responsible tumors are melanoma, breast, and lung, particularly small cell carcinoma. Adrenal metastases are typically large, (greater than 3 cm), more ill defined, and may be solitary or bilateral at presentation. Calcification is rare. With increased size, metastases usually demonstrate more heterogeneous enhancement due to the areas of hemorrhage or necrosis, therefore making imaging characterization easier. However, when small, these lesions can often be difficult to differentiate from benign tumors. Small metastases often appear homogeneous on enhanced CT, but demonstrate decreased relative or absolute washout characteristics on delayed images. Similarly, an adrenal metastasis will not demonstrate loss of signal on opposed phase MRI images due to lack of intracellular lipid seen in adenomas. Finally, for indeterminate adrenal masses in cancer patients where there is no other evidence of metastatic disease, percutaneous CT-guided biopsy may be indicated. Collision tumors occur when an adrenal metastasis occurs with a preexisting adenoma.

Metastatic involvement of the adrenal glands can also be a manifestation of lymphoma. Primary adrenal lymphoma is rare, with secondary involvement of retroperitoneal lymphoma, usually non-Hodgkin type, being more common. The imaging characteristics are often nonspecific. However, the diagnosis can usually be inferred due to the presence of coexistent retroperitoneal adenopathy. Involvement of the adrenal glands is usually bilateral and may be masslike or present as diffuse adeniform enlargement. Typically, lymphoma enhances relatively poorly. On MRI, lymphoma demonstrates hypointense T1 and hyperintense T2 signal.

ADRENOCORTICAL CARCINOMA

Carcinoma of the adrenal glands is extremely rare and occurs in 2/1 000 000 patients. Approximately 50% of these tumors are functional, most often producing cortisol, and may present with Cushing type symptoms. As a result, functional adrenocortical carcinomas usually present earlier and are smaller in size. In general, however these tumors are large when discovered, often greater than 10 cm, and have a dismal prognosis because of the high rate of liver, lung, and lymph node metastases seen at the time of presentation. On CT, these lesions are well defined but heterogeneously enhancing, large adrenal masses with central areas of necrosis. Approximately 30% of these tumors calcify. If surgical excision is considered, attention should be given to possible vascular invasion of the renal vein or cava.

OTHER RARE LESIONS

HEMANGIOMA

Adrenal hemangioma is a benign tumor, which is usually discovered incidentally. It commonly presents as large, unilateral, hypervascular lesion with persistent peripheral nodular enhancement on delayed CT images. It is often calcified, either from prior hemorrhage or phleboliths, and may have a central fibrous scar. On MRI, this lesion typically shows low T1 and high T2 signal. Occasionally, internal high T1 signal may be seen due to the presence of methemoglobin from prior hemorrhage. Hemangiomas, and especially malignant hemangiosarcomas, are rare.

GANGLIONEUROMA

Similarly, ganglioneuromas is a rare, benign tumor that occasionally originates from the adrenal medulla. However, this lesion may arise anywhere along the sympathetic chain and are most often extra-adrenal. It is nonfunctional, presents incidentally, and therefore typically large (greater than 20 cm) at presentation. Their imaging characteristics are nonspecific.

NEUROBLASTOMA

Neuroblastomas are primary tumors of neural crest cell origin and rarely seen in adults. These tumors may originate anywhere along the sympathetic chain and may have imaging characteristics similar to pediatric cases. Typically, neuroblastomas appear as large, ill defined, inhomogeneous, soft tissue masses with stippled calcification and necrosis. However, adult neuroblastoma is less often calcified and is usually widely metastatic at presentation. As a result, it can be confused with other malignancies and biopsy is usually required.

SUGGESTED READING

Boland GL, Blake MA, Hahn PF, et al. Incidental adrenal lesions: principles, techniques, and algorithms for imaging characterization. *Radiology.* 2008;249:756-775.

Caoili EM, Korobkin M, Francis IR, et al. Adrenal masses: characterization with combined unenhanced and delayed enhanced CT. *Radiology*. 2002;222:629-633.

Dunnick NR, Korobkin M. Imaging of adrenal incidentalomas: current status. *AJR Am J Roentgenol*. 2002;179:559-568.

Dunnick NR, Korobkin M, Francis I. Adrenal radiology: distinguishing benign from malignant adrenal masses. *Am J Roentgenol*. 1996;167:861-867.

Haider MA, Ghai S, Jhaveri K, et al. Chemical shift MR imaging of hyperattenuating (>10 HU) adrenal masses: does it still have a role? *Radiology.* 2004;231:711-716.

Korobkin M, Lombardi TJ, Aisen AM, et al. Characterization of adrenal masses with chemical shift and gadolinium- enhanced MR imaging. *Radiology.* 1995;197:411-418.

Lockhart ME, Smith JK, Kenney PJ. Imaging of adrenal masses. *Eur J Radiol*. 2002;41(2):95-112.

Mayo-Smith WW, Boland GW, Noto RB, et al. State-of-the-art adrenal imaging. *Radiographics*. 2001;21:995-1012.

Song JH, Chaudhry FS, Mayo-Smith WW. The incidental adrenal mass on CT: prevalence of adrenal disease in 1049 consecutive adrenal masses in patients with no known malignancy. *AJR Am J Roentgenol*. 2008;190:1163-1168.

QUESTIONS AND ANSWERS

1. A 40-year-old man presents with obesity, mild hypertension, and abdominal striae. What is the most likely diagnosis?
   A. Pheochromocytoma
   B. Adrenal carcinoma
   C. Adrenal adenoma
   D. Pituitary adenoma

   ANSWER: D. The case describes Cushing type symptoms secondary to increased glucocorticoid secretion. The more common ACTH-dependent form, Cushing disease, is secondary to a pituitary adenoma.

2. A 62-year-old man with a history of lung cancer and a homogeneous left adrenal mass with attenuation of −40 HU on CT. What is the most likely diagnosis?
   A. Pheochromocytoma
   B. Myelolipoma
   C. Metastasis
   D. Adenoma

   ANSWER: B. Negative attenuation suggests macroscopic fat, consistent with a myelolipoma.

3. A 70-year-old woman with history of metastatic breast cancer and a homogenous left adrenal mass with attenuation of 8 HU on CT. What is the most likely diagnosis?
   A. Metastasis
   B. Adenoma
   C. Myelolipoma
   D. Angiomyolipoma

   ANSWER: B. Lipid rich lesions with attenuation less than 10 HU are 98% specific for adenomas.

4. A 35-year-old man presents with mild hypertension, metabolic alkalosis, and hypokalemia. What is the most likely cause?
   A. Adrenal adenoma
   B. Adrenal hyperplasia
   C. Pheochromocytoma
   D. Pituitary adenoma

   ANSWER: A. The case describes the typical symptoms of Conn syndrome, which is secondary to an adrenal adenoma in 80% of patients.

5. A 41-year-old man with Conn disease has a small adrenal lesion on MRI. When compared with in-phase images, what will out-of-phase images of the lesion most likely demonstrate?
   A. Increase in signal
   B. No change in signal
   C. Decrease in signal
   D. Enhancement

   ANSWER: C. Eighty percent of patients with Conn syndrome present with an adrenal adenoma. Typically, adrenal adenomas drop signal on out of phase MRI imaging.

6. A 64-year-old man has lung cancer. A right adrenal lesion has pre- and postcontrast attenuation of 20 and 60 HU, respectively. Delayed images at 15 minutes demonstrated an attenuation of 40 HU. What is the most likely diagnosis?
   A. Metastasis
   B. Adenoma
   C. Pheochromocytoma
   D. Myelolipoma

   ANSWER: A. The calculated absolute washout of 50% ((enhanced − delayed)/(enhanced − unenhanced)) is less than the expected 60% seen in adenomas. Therefore, metastasis should be suspected.

7. A 32-year-old woman is in a motor vehicle collision and presents with a right adrenal lesion with unenhanced attenuation of 17 HU. What is the most likely diagnosis?
   A. Metastasis
   B. Hematoma
   C. Lipid poor adenoma
   D. Myelolipoma

   ANSWER: C. Incidental adrenal lesion detected in a patient without a history of cancer is most likely adenomas. The attenuation is less than the 50 to 90 HU expected of hemorrhage.

8. A 49-year-old woman with breast cancer demonstrates increased 24 hours urine metanephrines and vanillylmandelic acid. On MRI, a T2 hyperintense lesion will most likely discovered within:
   A. Organ of Zuckerkandl
   B. Pararenal space
   C. Morison pouch
   D. Gerota fascia

   ANSWER: D. The case describes the typical findings of a pheochromocytoma, which are most likely found in the adrenal gland. The adrenal gland is contained by Gerota fascia.

9. A 35-year-old man with a history of left renal cell carcinoma, severe hypertension, and new enhancing right adrenal mass. What is the most likely diagnosis?
   A. Neurofibromatosis
   B. Multiple endocrine neoplasia (MEN)
   C. Familial pheochromocytoma
   D. Von Hippel-Lindau

   ANSWER: D. Pheochromocytoma is associated with multiple syndromes. Von Hippel-Lindau has a high incidence of renal cell carcinoma.

10. A 56-year-old woman with melanoma is involved in a motorcycle accident. Initial routine enhanced CT demonstrates a right adrenal mass with attenuation of 70 HU. Follow-up thoracic MRI 1 month later demonstrates decreased size of the lesion. What is the most likely diagnosis?
    A. Metastasis
    B. Adenoma

C. Hematoma
D. Angiomyolipoma

ANSWER: C. In the setting of trauma, adrenal lesions with attenuation between 50 and 90 HU should suggest adrenal hemorrhage/hematoma. Decreased size on follow-up imaging makes this the most likely diagnosis.

60 MALE REPRODUCTIVE SYSTEM

Therese M. Weber and
Heather L. Haddad

NORMAL MALE ANATOMY

PROSTATE

The normal prostate gland weighs up to 10 g with an upside-down pear appearance. The base is cephalad and the apex is caudal. Three separate zones within the prostate have been described. The peripheral zone contains true prostatic tissue and represents the bulk of the prostate gland. Approximately 70% of prostate cancers involve the peripheral zone. The central gland contains the central and transitional zones, which can undergo hypertrophy.

VAS DEFERENS

The vas deferens are paired structures that arise from the tail of the epididymis, course along the spermatic cord, and enter the pelvis through the internal spermatic ring. In the pelvis, the vas deferens follows the lateral pelvic wall and crosses superficial to the external iliac vessels and ureter. The vas deferens becomes convoluted and dilated as it crosses the ureter, the ampulla of the vas deferens. As the ampulla courses to the midline it joins the excretory duct of the seminal vesicle. The distal ampulla and excretory duct join to form the ejaculatory duct. The ejaculatory duct passes through the prostate posteriorly to empty into the verumontanum.

SEMINAL VESICLES

The seminal vesicle is a blind-ending tube, which is coiled and convoluted, with an appearance of multiple diverticula. The lower end of the seminal vesicle is funneled to form the excretory duct, which joins with the distal end of the ampulla of the vas deferens to form the ejaculatory duct. The distal posterior surface of the seminal vesicle is closely adjacent to the base of the prostate.

URETHRA

ANTERIOR URETHRA

The anterior urethra extends from the external meatus to the inferior edge of the urogenital diaphragm and consists of the penile and bulbous portions (Fig. 60-1). The penile urethra extends from the external meatus to the penoscrotal junction inferiorly, and to the suspensory ligament superiorly. The penile urethra has a slightly dilated segment proximal to the external meatus, which represents the fossa navicularis, approximately 1 to 1.5 cm in length. The bulbous urethra extends from the penoscrotal junction to the inferior fascia of the urogenital diaphragm. The diameter of the anterior urethra is greatest in the proximal half of the bulbous urethra, which represents the bulbous urethral sump, approximately 2 to 3 cm in length. The bulbous urethral sump is the most inferior part of the urethra.

The anterior urethra is lined by stratified columnar epithelium except at the external meatus, where it changes to stratified squamous epithelium, which covers

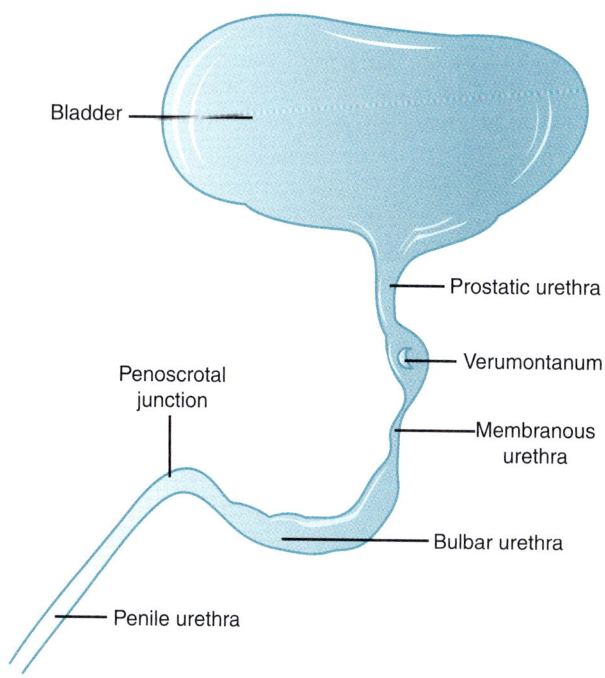

FIG. 60-1 Male urethra.
SOURCE: Courtesy of Anthony F. Zagar, UAB, Department of Radiology, Birmingham, Alabama.

the glans penis. Small, mucus-secreting submucosal glands, glands of Littre, are found along the length of the anterior urethra, and are more numerous in the bulbous sump and in the superior aspect of the penile urethra. Two ducts from the glands of Cowper, which lie on either side of the membranous urethra within the urogenital diaphragm, empty into the bulbous urethral sump. Cowper glands secrete mucus during sexual stimulation.

A small musculotendinous sling of the bulbocavernous muscle, known as the musculus compressor nuda, extends from the anterior and lateral surfaces of the proximal bulbous urethra. This structure may indent the proximal bulbous urethra on dynamic retrograde urethrography or, rarely, on voiding urethrography, and should not be mistaken for a stricture.

Posterior Urethra

The anterior and posterior urethra are separated by the urogenital diaphragm. The posterior urethra extends from the bladder neck to the inferior aspect of the urogenital diaphragm and consists of the prostatic and membranous portions. The prostatic urethra passes through the prostate gland and continues as the membranous urethra.

The prostatic urethral mucosa is continuous with the bladder mucosa and composed of transitional epithelium, but changes to stratified columnar epithelium at the membranous urethra.

The verumontanum contains three distinct orifices. The most proximal central orifice is the prostatic utricle, a vestigial remnant of the mullerian duct. Below the prostatic utricle on either side of midline, two additional openings are the ejaculatory ducts, formed at the junction of the ampulla of the vas deferens and the short duct of the seminal vesicles. The verumontanum tapers inferiorly to continue as the urethral crest, which continues to the membranous urethra. The verumontanum and urethral crest form a smooth muscle organ, which lengthens the posterior urethra during voiding, and shortens the urethra at the end of voiding. This muscular organ is likely involved in contracting the posterior urethra during emission and ejaculation, directing the emission through the membranous urethra into the bulbous urethra for ejaculation by contraction of the bulbocavernous muscle.

URETHRAL SPHINCTERS

Two separate smooth muscle sphincters in the posterior urethra function as muscles maintaining passive continence. The internal urethral sphincter lies in the trigourethral area at the bladder neck and is the primary muscle of passive continence. A second smooth muscle sphincter, the intrinsic sphincter lies below the verumontanum in the distal one-third of the prostatic urethra, surrounding the membranous urethra. If the internal sphincter at the bladder neck is ablated in prostatectomy or as a result of trigourethral injury in pelvic fracture, the intrinsic sphincter becomes the primary smooth muscle of passive continence.

The external sphincter, which surrounds the membranous urethra peripheral to the intrinsic sphincter, is a striated voluntary muscle involved in active continence or interruption of micturition.

PENIS

The penis contains two separate bodies of cavernous tissue. The urethra passes though the corpus spongiosum. The corpora cavernosa are symmetric, parallel cavernous bodies, which become separated proximally at the root of the penis, with each firmly attached to the rami of the pubic arch.

PATHOLOGY

BENIGN PROSTATIC HYPERTROPHY

Benign prostatic hypertrophy (BPH) is due to hyperplasia of the periurethral glands in the transitional zone. After 50 years of age, 50% of men have some degree of BPH. Excretory urography images may show bladder-base elevation, indenting of the bladder base, and "J-ing" or "hooking" of the distal ureters. As the prostate enlarges, evidence of bladder outlet obstruction may increase with large postvoid residual, bladder trabeculation, or bladder diverticula. On CT or ultrasound examination of the bladder, prostate enlargement indenting the bladder base should not be confused for a bladder mass. With long-standing, severe bladder outlet obstruction, the upper urinary tract will become dilated in a bilaterally symmetric fashion with ureteral dilatation to the level of the ureterovesical junction (UVJ). Asymmetric or unilateral ureteral obstruction should raise the question of prostate cancer extension into the distal ureter. Bladder stones may result from long-standing outlet obstruction by BPH.

PROSTATE CANCER

Prostate cancer is now the most common cancer in men other than skin cancer. The majority of prostate neoplasms are adenocarcinomas arising from the peripheral zone of the prostate. Other rare prostate tumors include squamous cell carcinoma (SCC), endometrioid carcinoma arising from the prostatic utricle, carcinosarcoma, melanoma, rhabdomyosarcoma, leiomyosarcoma, and fibrosarcoma. Small cell carcinoma of the prostate is extremely rare and usually occurs in association with adenocarcinoma.

PROSTATE CANCER SCREENING

Prostate-specific antigen (PSA) is a serine protease normally secreted only into the ductal system of the prostate. PSA can leak from the acini into the stroma of the gland and enter the circulation through lymphatics and capillaries if there is derangement of the prostate architecture. Elevated PSA levels can be found in association with prostatitis, prostatic infarct, acute urinary retention, BPH, and interventional procedures involving the prostate or bladder. Serum PSA level has an upper limit of normal of 4.0 ng/mL. PSA velocity (the rate of PSA increases over time) may be a more useful indicator of malignancy. An increase of 20% or more in serum PSA per year is far more suggestive of prostate cancer than of BPH.

The digital rectal examination (DRE) is another screening tool, which detects only approximately 40% of prostate cancers less than 1.5 cm in diameter. A large number of prostate cancers will be clinically advanced at the time they are detected by DRE. There is, however, a significant benefit in combining DRE with PSA. If both DRE and PSA are positive, 60% of those patients will have prostate cancer. If both DRE and PSA are normal, only 2% will have cancer.

Although prostate cancer screening remains a controversial subject, both the American Cancer Society and the American Urological Association recommend annual DRE and PSA beginning at 50 years of age. In high-risk men, such as those with a strong family history of prostate cancer or African American men, screening is recommended earlier, at 40 years of age.

HISTOLOGY

The Gleason system is commonly used for grading prostate cancer. Correlation between tumor grade and degree of spread is usually good. The tumor is studied histologically with identification of predominant and secondary tumor patterns. Each of these is assigned a score of 1 through 5. A better differentiated tumor will have a lower tumor grade. The higher the grade, the less differentiation is present. These numbers are added for the final score, between 2 and 10. Tumors with a Gleason score of 2 to 4 rarely have metastatic lymphadenopathy, while tumors with Gleason scores of 8 to 10 do.

TABLE 60-1 Comparison of Staging Systems for Prostate Cancer

WHITMORE-JEWETT	TNM	DESCRIPTION
	T0	No evidence of tumor
A	T1	Nonpalpable tumor
B	T2	Palpable tumor continued to the prostate
C	T3	Extracapsular tumor extension
	T4a	Invasion of bladder neck, external sphincter, or rectum
	T4b	Invasion of levator muscles or fixation to pelvic sidewall
D1	N	Regional (pelvic) node involvement
D2	M	Distant metastases

PROSTATE CANCER STAGING

Staging can be done with the Whitmore-Jewett staging method or the TNM staging method (Table 60-1). The Whitmore-Jewett staging method is commonly used in North America. Stage A carcinoma has no clinical manifestations and is not palpable on DRE. Stage A carcinoma is usually found incidentally in pathology specimens or autopsy specimens. Stage B carcinoma is a clinically palpable, firm nodule in the peripheral zone without evidence of capsular or distant extension. Stage C carcinoma extends beyond the capsule. Differentiation of stage B and C tumors with DRE may be difficult. At least 50% of patients with Stage C carcinoma have metastatic pelvic lymphadenopathy. Stage D carcinoma patients may present with urinary symptoms, palpable extension of tumor beyond the prostate, bone metastases, and hydronephrosis due to ureteral obstruction by carcinoma at the UVJ.

PROSTATE CANCER DISSEMINATION

Spread of prostate cancer occurs by three methods: direct extension, lymphatic spread, and hematogenous spread. Prostate cancer typically originates in the peripheral zone closer to the prostatic capsule than to the urethra. Capsular extension allows the tumor to spread to perineural lymphatics and to the periprostatic venous plexus of Santorini, allowing distant metastases to the viscera and axial skeleton. Tumor spreads locally to the seminal vesicles, urethra, bladder neck, bladder base, and interureteric ridge, which will cause asymmetric or unilateral ureteral obstruction. Less commonly tumor may spread posteriorly and superiorly to grow into the rectosigmoid colon.

Lymphatic spread starts within prostate lymphatics with spread to the pelvic lymph nodes. Nodal groups most commonly involved include the obturator, external iliac, and internal iliac nodes. The common iliac, para-aortic, mediastinal, and supraclavicular lymph nodes may be involved in advanced disease.

Hematogenous spread is to the axial skeleton or viscera. In patients dying with prostate cancer, 85% will have bony metastases in the axial skeleton, most frequently the lumbar spine, proximal femur, bony pelvis, thoracic spine, ribs, sternum, skull, and proximal humerus, in decreasing frequency. The intervertebral venous plexus of Batson, which directly communicates with the periprostatic venous plexus of Santorini, provides the route of early hematogenous spread to the spine and pelvis. The majority (greater than 90%) of prostatic metastatic lesions to bone are blastic.

In order to more accurately predict the pathologic stage of the cancer, especially whether or not tumor has extended beyond the prostatic capsule, nomograms have been developed, known as the Partin Tables. The Partin Tables combine clinical stage (determined by DRE), serum PSA levels, and the Gleason grade in the biopsy specimen.

Transrectal Ultrasound

Once prostate cancer is suspected based on DRE, PSA, or both, transrectal ultrasound (TRUS) is usually performed for further evaluation and to guide biopsy. Prostate cancer is most frequently seen on TRUS as a hypoechoic lesion; however, this is nonspecific and other entities, such as prostatitis, infarct, abscess, etc., can also appear as a focal hypoechoic lesion. Antibiotics are recommended before the biopsy to reduce the incidence of infection.

Radionuclide Bone Scintigraphy

Recent studies indicate that it is extremely rare to find bony metastases in patients with PSA of 10 ng/mL or less. Therefore, bone scans should be reserved for those patients with PSA levels greater than 10 ng/mL at the time of diagnosis, or for patients with localized bone pain suggesting osseous metastases. Most metastatic bone lesions will occur in the thoracolumbar spine, pelvis, and ribs, with the majority being blastic (90%).

Prostate cancer can be so diffusely metastatic that all bones are involved, and no focal areas of uptake are identified. The key finding will be absence of visualization of the kidneys. In patients with diffuse osseous metastases, the radionuclide is completely absorbed by the bones, leaving little for the kidneys to excrete. This pattern is known as a "super bone scan." The differential diagnosis of diffuse bone uptake includes myelosclerosis, urticaria pigmentosa, and fluorine poisoning, in addition to diffuse blastic metastases.

Magnetic Resonance Imaging

On T2-weighted images the central gland is medium to low-signal intensity and frequently heterogeneous, while the normal peripheral zone shows high signal intensity. Prostate cancer is typically seen on MRI as an area of lower signal intensity in the otherwise high-signal peripheral zone. MRI is not useful for early detection of prostate cancer but can be useful for staging prostate cancer after this diagnosis has been made. A 1.5T magnet is used with an endorectal coil in a pelvic phased-array coil or images can be obtained using a 3T magnet without or with an endorectal coil. Gross extension of tumor beyond the prostate into an adjacent structure is usually readily seen with MRI. More subtle extension of tumor beyond the prostate gland may be more difficult to determine. A smooth or irregular bulge in the contour of the gland in the region of the tumor or asymmetry of the fat plane surrounding the neurovascular bundle should increase suspicion. Smooth capsular bulge is predictive of tumor extension in approximately 25% of cases, while an irregular bulge is predictive of tumor extension in 75% of cases. The normal seminal vesicles will show high-signal intensity on T2-weighted images, while tumor involvement of the seminal vesicles appears as areas of lower signal. An exception will be patients who have received radiation or hormonal therapy, which may show lower than normal signal intensity in the seminal vesicles. Accuracy of MRI in detecting seminal vesicles involvement in patients with prostate cancer is reported as greater than 90%. The major limitation in widespread use of MRI in staging has been the lack of consistent prediction of tumor extent because of microscopic involvement. Magnetic resonance spectroscopy of the prostate is a potentially useful adjunctive study that may be helpful in evaluating patients with elevated serum PSA level with previous negative biopsy specimens.

SEMINAL VESICLE STONES

Seminal vesicle stones, which are uncommon, are related to stone disease elsewhere in the urinary tract or ectopic insertion of a ureter into the ipsilateral seminal vesicle. Stones should not be confused with seminal vesicle wall calcification, which can be seen in diabetic men. Small stones may result in pain and hematospermia if they become impacted in the duct from the seminal vesicle or the ejaculatory duct.

SEMINAL VESICLE CYSTS

Seminal vesicle cysts are also uncommon. There is an association with ipsilateral renal agenesis in at least two-thirds of patients with a congenital seminal vesicle cyst. In rare cases, cystic dilatation of a seminal vesicle may be related to a small dysplastic kidney with its ureter ectopically inserting into the ipsilateral seminal vesicle. When a seminal vesicle cyst is identified, imaging of the kidneys is usually indicated. Acquired seminal vesicle cysts may be related to obstruction or inflammation. Congenital or acquired cysts may become quite large and indent the bladder posteriorly. Hemorrhage into the lumen of a cyst may be differentiated with MRI, which will show high signal intensity on both T1- and T2-weighted images. Seminal vesiculitis in conjunction with prostatitis is common, although imaging findings are nonspecific. The most common cause of neoplastic involvement of the seminal vesicles is direct invasion by prostate cancer.

ACQUIRED URETHRAL STRICTURES IN MEN

Urethral strictures may be the result of infectious or inflammatory etiology, iatrogenic, or traumatic (Table 60-2).

Approximately 40% of all urethral strictures in the United States are caused by gonorrhea. The proximal bulbar urethra is the site of stricture in 70% of patients with gonococcal urethritis because of the high concentration of periurethral glands in this area and the dependent position of this portion of the male urethra. Infectious strictures may be multiple and of various lengths. Serial strictures are common. At urography, the Littre glands may be opacified when strictures are present because of inflammatory dilation of duct ostia. An important clue to the urodynamic significance of a stricture may be backfilling of ducts or glands that empty into the urethra proximal to a stricture. Pseudodiverticulum formation results from a gonococcal periurethral abscess that eventually ruptures into the urethra leaving a cavity. Occasionally, a large periurethral abscess will extend to and penetrate the perineum, resulting in an urethrocutaneous fistula, which may be multiple. Urine may pass through these perineal fistulae, resulting in the "watering can perineum," which is more typical of tuberculosis or schistosomiasis rather than of gonorrhea.

TABLE 60-2 Urethral Stricture

ETIOLOGY	LOCATION	APPEARANCE
Nongonococcal urethritis, gonococcus, or rarely tuberculosis	Bulbar urethra strictures	Multiple and serial
Iatrogenic (surgery, instrumentation, catheterization)	Membranous urethra or penoscrotal junction	
Traumatic; occurs after complete rupture	Goldman type II—V injuries	Solitary, short stricture

Urethral surgery, instrumentation, or catheterization may result in stricture formation. These strictures occur most often in parts of the urethra that are anatomically fixed and narrow (i.e., the membranous urethra and the penoscrotal junction of the anterior urethra). The majority of instrument-related urethral strictures occur in the bulbomembranous region, with less than 20% occurring at the penoscrotal junction. An iatrogenic stricture can be focal and short, multifocal or long.

Urethral injury is a common complication of pelvic trauma. The most common injury involves the posterior urethra. Traumatic stricture will occur more commonly after complete transection of the urethra; a partial laceration will more likely heal without significant narrowing. The majority of patients with injuries to the posterior urethra who develop strictures will require repeated dilatations or urethroplasty regardless of initial treatment. Traumatic strictures are usually solitary, less than 2 cm in length, and flanked by segments of urethra that are normal in caliber. Traumatic strictures form more rapidly than inflammatory strictures.

Straddle injury occurs most commonly when a male patient falls astride a hard object such as a bicycle crossbar, or a steel or wooden beam. Straddle injuries involve the bulbous urethra. Coexisting pelvic fractures are less common with a straddle injury. This injury results from compression of the anterior urethra against the pubis. The typical straddle injury will result in a focal stricture in the proximal third of the bulbous urethra on follow-up examination.

The two most commonly used systems of classification or urethral injuries are the American Association for the Surgery of Trauma (AAST) and the one originally proposed by Colapinto and McCollum and revised by Goldman et al. The unified classification system proposed by Goldman et al. uses the anatomic location of injury, whether is it nearer to the urogenital diaphragm or the external sphincter, and includes a category for bladder injuries that involve or simulate posterior urethral injury (Table 60-3). Accurate classification of urethral injuries plays an important role in effective treatment planning. If a complete urethral transaction is observed on initial retrograde urethrogram, the length of the defect must be accurately demonstrated for effective urethroplasty planning. The length of the defect can be effectively demonstrated by performing simultaneous antegrade and retrograde studies.

Stricture formation rarely is the sole manifestation of a urethral carcinoma; however, when stricture formation

TABLE 60-3 Goldman System for Classification of Urethral Injuries at Urethrography

INJURY TYPE	INJURY DESCRIPTION	URETHROGRAPHIC APPEARANCE
I	Stretching or elongation of the otherwise intact posterior urethra	Intact but stretched urethra
II	Urethral disruption above the urogenital diaphragm while the membranous segment remains intact	Contrast agent extravasation above the urogenital diaphragm only
III	Disruption of the membranous urethra, extending below the urogenital diaphragm and involving the anterior urethra	Contrast agent extravasation below the urogenital diaphragm, possibly extending to the pelvis or perineum; intact bladder neck
IV	Bladder neck injury extending into the proximal urethra	Extraperitoneal contrast agent extravasation; bladder neck disruption
IVa	Bladder base injury simulating a type IV injury	Periurethral contrast agent extravasation; bladder base disruption
V	Isolated anterior urethral injury	Contrast agent extravasation below the urogenital diaphragm, confined to the anterior urethra

Reprinted with permission from Goldman SM, Sandler CM, Corriere JN, Jr., et al. Blunt urethral trauma: a unified, anatomical mechanical classification. *J Urol*. 1997;157:85-89. Copyright © Elsevier.

occurs in an elderly patient with no previous medical history of urethral surgery, instrumentation, or infection, carcinoma should be suspected. Radiology evaluation should assess the location, length, severity, and multiplicity of these strictures.

Penetrating injuries to the male urethra from gunshot or knife wounds are uncommon. Penetrating injuries more commonly affect the anterior, rather than the posterior urethra. These injuries usually require immediate surgical exploration and antibiotic therapy.

URETHRAL TUMORS

BENIGN TUMORS

Benign urethral neoplasms include the fibrous polyp (also known as congenital urethral polyp or fibroepithelial polyp), transitional cell, and squamous cell papillomas.

MALIGNANT TUMORS

Carcinoma of the urethra is the only epithelial malignancy of the urinary tract that occurs more frequently in women, with the peak age range of 40 to 60 years. Carcinoma of the male urethra occurs predominantly in men older than 50 years. SCC, the most common type, occurs in 75% of these patients, followed by transitional cell carcinoma (TCC). Adenocarcinoma is the most common malignancy in a urethral diverticulum due to the origin of diverticula, as they arise secondary to infection in paraurethral Bartholin's glands. The tumor type involving the male urethra varies by location of involvement. TCC involves the prostatic urethra. Adenocarcinoma involves the glands of Littre and Cowper's glands. SCC involves the anterior urethra and is associated with prior urethral stricture in up to 75% of cases. Lymphogenous spread occurs before hematogenous dissemination.

Risk factors associated with carcinoma of the male urethra include a medical history of chronic urethral inflammation or sexually transmitted disease and urethral stricture. The majority of carcinomas of the male urethra, almost 80%, are SCCs. Two-thirds arise in the bulbar or membranous urethra. The majority of the remaining carcinomas are found in the anterior urethra, especially the fossa navicularis. Approximately 15% of male urethral carcinomas will be TCC, arising in the posterior urethra in most patients. There is an association between TCC of the prostatic urethra and previous transurethral resection of bladder carcinoma. Initial spread of tumor is again predominantly lymphogenous. Bulbar and posterior urethral carcinomas spread to the internal iliac or obturator nodes, prior to spread to more proximal nodal groups. Carcinoma of the penile urethra spreads to the deep inguinal and external iliac lymph nodes. The diagnosis of urethral carcinoma is made with urethroscopy of urethrography. The diagnosis should be suspected on urethrography when the margin of a stricture is irregular or poorly defined.

METASTASES TO THE URETHRA

Bladder and colorectal carcinomas can involve the urethra through extensive local spread. Prostate, cervical, and vaginal cancers also may invade the urethra.

PENILE CANCER

Primary penile cancer is rare, representing only 0.4% of all malignancies in the male population in the United States. The majority of penile cancers (95%) are SCCs, and usually occur in the sixth and seventh decades of life. The most predisposing factor is the presence of a foreskin, which results in the accumulation of smegma. Penile cancers, therefore, are most commonly located on the glans penis and are usually solitary, ill defined, and infiltrative in nature. The primary factors involving survival are the depth of invasion of the primary tumor and the extent of involvement of the draining inguinal lymph nodes. MRI is the most sensitive method for evaluation of these characteristics. Penile cancer is typically low signal intensity relative to the corpora on both T1- and T2-weighted images. Tumors will enhance following gadolinium administration, although with less enhancement than seen in the corpora cavernosa. T2-weighted and gadolinium enhanced T1-weighted sequences are the most useful sequences for determining the extent of tumor into the tunica albuginea, corpora, or the urethra.

Metastatic tumors to the penis will most commonly arise from a primary tumor in the genitourinary system. The typical MRI appearance will be multiple discrete masses in the corpora cavernosa and corpus spongiosum, which are low signal intensity relative to the normal corporal tissue on both T1- and T2-weighted images.

POSTOPERATIVE URETHRAL CHANGES

URETHROPLASTY

Urethroplasty performed for treatment of anterior urethral strictures, especially two-stage procedures, may result in saccular dilatation of the urethra, more frequently near the proximal and distal ends of the repair. When these sacculations become large, they may resemble urethral diverticula. Large sacculations may collect urine during voiding, resulting in postvoid dribbling. Retrograde urethrography will differentiate these urethroplasty sacculations from acquired diverticula.

PROSTATECTOMY

Possible complications from radical prostatectomy include lymphocele formation after pelvic lymph node dissection and vesicourethral anastomotic leak. During radical prostatectomy the entire prostate including the prostatic urethra and seminal vesicles are removed. The lower urinary tract continuity is reestablished by anastomosing the bladder neck to a stump of the membranous urethra extending from the urogenital diaphragm. This surgical intervention results in a funnel-shaped bladder base that extends below the top of the pubic symphysis. This finding is essentially pathognomonic of a radical prostatectomy.

SUGGESTED READING

Colapinto V, McCollum RW. Injury to the male posterior urethra in fractured pelvis: a new classification. *J Urol.* 1977;118:576-580.

Goldman SM, Sandler CM, Corriere JN, Jr., et al. Blunt urethral trauma: a unified, anatomical mechanical classification. *J Urol.* 1997;157:85-89.

Hricak H, Choyke PL, Eberhardt SC, Leibel SA, Scardino PT. Imaging prostate cancer: a multidisciplinary perspective. *Radiology.* 2007;243:28-53.

Ingram MD, Watson SG, Skippage PL, Patel U. Urethral injuries after pelvic trauma: evaluation with urethrography. *Radiographics.* 2008;28:1631-1643.

Moore EE, Cogbill TH, Malagoni MA, et al. Organ injury scaling. *Surg Clin North Am.* 1995;74:293-303.

National Cancer Institute. What You Need to Know About Prostate Cancer. www.cancer.gov/cancertopic/wyntk/prostate. Updated October 2007. Accessed January 10, 2009.

NCCN Prostate Cancer. In: Mohler J, Anglin CL, Bahnson RR, et al. *NCCN Clinical Practice Guidelines in Oncology*, Version 2. Fort Washington, PA: NCCN; 2009.

QUESTIONS AND ANSWERS

1. Concerning seminal vesicle cysts, which of the following is true?
   A. Imaging will differentiate congenital from acquired seminal vesicle cysts.
   B. Most frequently an association with trauma.
   C. Association with ipsilateral renal agenesis.
   D. Association with multicystic dysplastic kidney.

   ANSWER: C. There is an association with ipsilateral renal agenesis in at least two-thirds of patients with a congenital seminal vesicle cyst. In rare cases, cystic dilatation of a seminal vesicle may be related to a small dysplastic kidney with its ureter ectopically inserting into the ipsilateral seminal vesicle.

2. From what structure does the vas deferens arise?
   A. Verumontanum
   B. Seminal vesicles

C. Ampulla of the vas deferens
D. Tail of the epididymis

ANSWER: D. The vas deferens arises from the tail of the epididymis and after entering the pelvis, become the ampulla of the vas deferens. The ampulla courses toward the midline of the pelvis and joins the excretory duct of the seminal vesicle to form the ejaculatory duct, and eventually empties into the verumontanum.

3. A man with a straddle injury has difficulty urinating. What is the most likely location of stricture?
   A. Bulbous urethra
   B. Membranous urethra
   C. Penile urethra
   D. Posterior urethra

   ANSWER: A. Straddle injury occurs most commonly when a male patient falls astride a hard object such as a bicycle crossbar, or a steel or wooden bean. Straddle injuries involve the bulbous urethra.

4. Patient presents with PSA of 8, what do you do?
   A. Nothing
   B. Endorectal coil MRI
   C. Nuclear medicine bone scan
   D. Ultrasound guided biopsy

   ANSWER: D. Normal PSA is <4 ng/mL. Abnormal PSA, alone, does not confirm prostate cancer. TRUS of the prostate with ultrasound-guided biopsy is the most likely of the group to differentiate BPH from prostate cancer. Bone scans should be reserved for those patients with PSA levels greater than 10 ng/mL at the time of diagnosis, or for patients with localized bone pain suggesting osseous metastases. Endorectal coil MRI is most helpful for staging prostate cancer after the diagnosis has been made with biopsy.

5. What percent of prostate cancers involve the peripheral zone?
   A. 33%
   B. 62%
   C. 70%
   D. 82%

   ANSWER: C. The bulk of the prostate is the peripheral zone and is involved in 70% of prostate cancers.

6. At what age does the American Cancer Society and the American Urological Association recommend annual DRE and PSA screening in an African American man?
   A. 35 years
   B. 40 years
   C. 45 years
   D. 50 years

   ANSWER: B. In high-risk men, such as those with a strong family history of prostate cancer or African American men, screening is recommended to begin at 40 years of age.

7. Using the Gleason system of grading a prostate cancer, which of the following statements is true?
   A. Stage A carcinoma is usually found incidentally in pathology specimens or autopsy specimens.
   B. Better differentiated tumor will have a higher grade.
   C. Gleason scores of 8 to 10 frequently have metastatic pelvic lymphadenopathy.
   D. Highest Gleason score is the result of the histology of an aggressive tumor divided by the estimated volume of the prostate gland.

   ANSWER: C. The tumor is studied with identification of the predominant and secondary histological patterns of tumor, with each assigned a score of 1 through 5, for a total maximum score of 10. A better-differentiated tumor will have a lower tumor grade.

8. What venous plexus directly communicates with the plexus of Batson?
   A. Vesuvius
   B. Galen
   C. Santorini
   D. Virchow

   ANSWER: C. The vertebral plexus of Batson directly communicates with the periprostatic venous plexus of Santorini and provides the route of early hematogenous spread to the spine and pelvis.

9. The glands of Littre are found in what part of the urethra?
   A. Anterior urethra
   B. Posterior urethra
   C. Prostatic urethra
   D. Semimembranous urethra

   ANSWER: A. These are small, mucus secreting glands that are found along the length of the anterior urethra and are more numerous in the bulbous sump and in the superior aspect of the penile urethra.

10. What is the location in the urinary tract where uroepithelial malignancy is more common in women than men?
    A. Renal pelvis
    B. Proximal ureter

TABLE 61-6 Benign Versus Malignant Epithelial Tumors

	BENIGN	MALIGNANT
Wall thickness	Thin	Thick, >3 mm, irregular
Septa	None or thin septations	Thick septations, >3 mm septal nodularity
Internal structure	Lacking	Papillary projections, solid components

and malignant. Serous cystadenocarcinoma accounts for over half of all ovarian malignancies. Benign serous lesions are usually unilocular cystic lesions but can contain a small amount of tissue. Malignant lesions contain a larger component of papillary soft tissue and may be multilocular. Up to a quarter of benign lesions and up to half of malignant lesions are bilateral. Calcification of peritoneal metastasis has been reported in up to one-third of cases.

Mucinous neoplasms include benign mucinous cystadenomas and malignant cystadenocarcinomas. Mucinous cystadenomas are the second most common benign epithelial neoplasm after serous cystadenomas. These tumors are often very large and multilocular. The locules may demonstrate slightly varying densities at imaging, which is due to differences in viscosity of the protein content. This finding is in contrast to serous tumors, which are generally simple fluid attenuation. Mucinous cystadenocarcinomas are much less likely than serous carcinomas to be bilateral. Rupture of a mucinous adenocarcinoma produces pseudomyxoma peritonei.

Endometrioid cancer accounts for approximately 10% to 15% of ovarian cancers. Endometrioid carcinomas are almost always malignant. Bilateral ovarian involvement can be present in 25% to 50% of cases. These lesions are complex cystic and solid masses at imaging. Synchronous endometrial carcinoma or endometrial hyperplasia occurs in up to a third of cases.

Clear cell carcinoma represents approximately 5% of ovarian carcinomas. These lesions are always malignant. Imaging appearance is similar to serous neoplasms displaying a large cyst with solid protrusions. Both endometrioid and clear cell carcinomas can arise from endometriosis.

Brenner tumors represent approximately 2% to 3% of ovarian tumors. These lesions are rarely malignant. Histologically, the tumors are composed of transitional cells and fibrous stroma. At imaging, lesions are small predominately solid masses or multiloculated cystic and solid masses. Amorphous calcifications can be present within the solid component. The fibrous stroma is low in signal on T2-weighted MR imaging. Brenner tumors can occur in association with mucinous cystic tumors.

GERM CELL TUMORS

Germ cell tumors are the second most common group of ovarian tumors after epithelial tumors. These lesions account for 20% to 30% of all ovarian tumors. Malignant germ cell tumors can produce elevated levels of alpha-fetoprotein and human chorionic gonadotropin.

A mature teratoma is named as the most common benign ovarian tumor in some series. Approximately 15% to 20% are bilateral. It is the only benign neoplasm in the germ cell tumor group. Malignant transformation is rare. These lesions are derived from all three germ cell layers: mesoderm, endoderm, and ectoderm. The ectodermal components usually predominate. Teratomas are lined by squamous epithelium and filled with sebaceous material. Hair, muscle, bone, and teeth can also be present within teratomas. A soft-tissue protuberance called a Rokitansky nodule or a dermoid plug can be seen projecting into the cyst. If present, bone or teeth are usually located with the soft-tissue protuberance. At ultrasound imaging, the classic finding is the echogenic dermoid plug with posterior acoustic shadowing termed the "tip of the iceberg" sign. At CT, fat attenuation and teeth can be seen. On MR imaging, the fatty sebaceous material follows fat signal. Teratoma which is primarily composed of thyroid tissue is termed struma ovarii.

Less than 1% of all teratomas are immature teratomas. They contain immature tissue from all three germ cell layers. These lesions are malignant and occur in the first two decades. In contrast to mature teratomas, an immature teratoma contains small scattered foci of fat, prominent solid components, and scattered calcifications.

Dysgerminoma is a rare ovarian neoplasm occurring in children and young women. Imaging reveals a multilobulated solid mass with prominent fibrovascular septa. Speckled calcifications and areas of necrosis and hemorrhage can be present. Approximately 5% of dysgerminomas will produce human chorionic gonadotropin. Seminoma is the testicular counterpart of dysgerminoma.

Endodermal sinus tumor is a rare ovarian tumor, which usually occurs in the second decade of life. This lesion is also known as a yolk sac tumor. Imaging reveals a large complex mass with cystic and solid components. Elevated serum alpha-fetoprotein levels are detectable.

SEX CORD-STROMAL TUMORS

Sex cord-stromal tumors derive from coelomic epithelium or mesenchymal cells of the embryologic gonads. These tumors account for approximately 8% to 10% of ovarian neoplasms and occur in all age groups.

Granulosa cell tumor is the most common malignant sex cord-stromal tumor. These lesions predominately occur in perimenopausal and postmenopausal women. At imaging, the lesions vary widely in appearance from cystic to solid masses. Granulosa cell tumor is the most common ovarian neoplasm to produce estrogen. Estrogenic effects on the endometrium can result in endometrial hyperplasia and uterine hemorrhage. Endometrial carcinoma can occur in up to 25% of women with granulosa cell tumors.

Fibrothecomas contain varying quantities of thecoma and fibroma. Thecoma is lipid rich and exhibits estrogenic activity while fibroma contains fibroblasts and collagen and exhibits no hormonal activity. Ovarian fibroma is the most common sex cord tumor. These lesions occur in both premenopausal and postmenopausal women. The imaging appearance is a solid mass which may contain dense calcifications. The collagenous component appears low in signal on both T1- and T2-weighted MR imaging. Meigs syndrome is a triad of fibroma, ascites, and pleural effusions.

Rare sex cord-stromal tumors occurring in young women include sclerosing stromal tumor and Sertoli-Leydig cell tumor. Imaging of a sclerosing stromal tumor reveals a cystic and solid mass demonstrating early peripheral enhancement with centripetal progression. Sertoli-Leydig cell tumors appear as enhancing solid masses with intratumoral cysts. Approximately 30% of tumors are hormonally active producing virilizing changes.

METASTATIC OVARIAN TUMORS

Approximately 5% of all ovarian tumors are metastases. Colon and stomach carcinomas are the most common primary neoplasms to metastasize to the ovaries. Breast, lung, and contralateral ovarian neoplasms also metastasize to the ovary. Krukenberg tumors are ovarian metastases from gastrointestinal tract carcinomas, classically the stomach, which are composed of mucin-secreting signet-ring cells.

MISCELLANEOUS OVARIAN LESIONS

Endometriosis is the presence of endometrial tissue outside of the uterus. The ovary is the most commonly affected site. Chronic cyclic hemorrhage results in a cyst containing hemorrhagic material surrounded by a thick fibrous wall. These cysts are high signal intensity on T1-weighted MR images and can be either high or low in signal on T2-weighted images. The low T2 signal occurs because of T2 shortening associated with the high iron concentration related to chronic hemorrhage and is termed "shading." Fluid-fluid and fluid-debris levels may be seen. The imaging appearance of some endometriotic cysts, high T1 and T2 signal, can overlap with that of hemorrhagic functional cysts; however, hemorrhagic functional cysts are usually solitary and regress within 2 months.

Tuboovarian abscess usually manifests as a complication of pelvic inflammatory disease (PID)—infection of the upper genital tract caused by ascending infection from the lower genital tract. The most common infectious sources are chlamydia and gonorrhea. Patients present with fever and pelvic pain. The diagnosis is often made on ultrasound, which reveals a multilocular thick-walled fluid collection. Contrasted CT and MRI images demonstrate enhancement of the thickened walls.

Polycystic ovarian syndrome is an endocrine disorder. Women with the syndrome have abnormal production and metabolism of androgen, abnormal metabolism of estrogen, and peripheral insulin resistance. Obesity compounds these abnormalities. Secondary effects include hirsutism, obesity, anovulation with oligomenorrhea or amenorrhea, and reduced fertility. Ultrasound or MR imaging may reveal enlarged ovaries with numerous subcentimeter follicles located peripherally in the cortex. The ovaries may demonstrate increased echogenicity on ultrasound.

HYSTEROSALPINGOGRAMS

Hysterosalpingograms (HSG) are used primarily as a component of routine infertility evaluation. Other indications for HSG include evaluation for repeated abortions, abnormal uterine bleeding, assessing for successful tubal occlusion in tubal ligation, locating an intrauterine device, and postsurgical evaluation. HSG is performed during the follicular phase of the menstrual cycle. The cervix is cannulated with an "acorn" tip cannula or a balloon catheter. Oil- or water-soluble contrast is injected into the uterus and fallopian tubes under fluoroscopic visualization. With oil-based agents, there is increased risk of oil embolization to the lungs via venous intravasation. In animal models, slow resorption of the oil-based contrast from the peritoneal cavity may lead to inflammatory or granulomatous reactions. Water-based contrast provides better uterine and ampullary mucosal detail; however, it also has a higher incidence of pain and bleeding following the procedure (Tables 61-7 and 61-8).

TABLE 61-7 HSG Risks

Pain
Bleeding
Vascular intravasation
Contrast reaction
Uterotubal perforation
Postprocedure infection
Radiation to fetus

TABLE 61-8 HSG Contraindications

Active infection (PID)
Recent uterine or tubal surgery
Active uterine bleeding
Pregnancy

There is a purported therapeutic effect of HSG leading to increased rates of pregnancy. This therapeutic effect may be due to lavage of the fallopian tubes, stimulation of cilia, release of peritubal adhesions, alteration of cervical mucus, concomitant therapy, or bacteriostatic effect. There is debate in the literature whether the choice of contrast material leads to significant differences in live birth rates.

UTERUS

NORMAL ANATOMY

The normal uterus is triangular in shape with the fundus forming the base. The fundus is usually straight in contour but may also demonstrate a mildly concave or convex contour.

UTERINE ABNORMALITIES

Uterine filling defects and irregularities can be caused by a number of etiologies (Table 61-9). Smooth uterine filling defects include air bubbles, polyps, leiomyomas, and adenomyomas. Air bubbles are injected through the tubing and cause transient filling defects. Leiomyomas can be intramural, submucosal, or subserosal in location. The majority is intramural in location. Submucosal and large intramural tumors can distort, enlarge, and fill portions of the uterine cavity. Uterine fibroids can also obstruct the cornua or intramural portions of the fallopian tube.

Adenomyosis appears as single or multiple cavities in the uterine wall. Adenomyosis is usually seen in the upper body and fundus, while lower uterine segment cavities are often dilated glands near the cervical isthmus. Synechiae are intrauterine adhesions, which result from trauma such as dilation and curettage. They manifest as focal or diffuse filling defects, which are irregular and angulated in shape. Asherman syndrome is extensive intrauterine adhesive disease associated with infertility.

Diethylstilbestrol (DES) is synthetic estrogen, which was used in the 1940s to 1960s to prevent pregnancy. In female fetuses, exposure to DES interferes with development of mesenchymal layers of the genital tract. Associated anomalies include a hypoplastic uterus with a small, irregular cavity in a T-shape configuration, narrowed endocervical canal with irregular contour, and short irregular fallopian tubes. Females exposed to DES in utero have twofold risk of abortion and ninefold risk of ectopic pregnancy. There is also an association with the development of clear cell carcinoma of the vagina.

TABLE 61-9 Uterine Filling Defects and Irregularity

Air bubble	Synechiae
Leiomyoma	Congenital fold
Polyp	Septation
Adenomyosis/adenomyoma	IUD
Pregnancy	Blood clot
Retained products of conception	Mucus

A caesarian section performed utilizing a lower uterine segment incision can produce an irregular defect, which may reveal unilateral or bilateral outpouchings at HSG.

FALLOPIAN TUBES

NORMAL ANATOMY

The fallopian tubes arise at the uterine cornua and are 10 to 12 cm in length. They are divided into four segments—the interstitial segment which travels through the myometrium, the isthmus, the ampulla, and the fimbria. Patent fallopian tubes show free spill of contrast into the peritoneum. Cornual spasm or tubal mucoid plug can mimic tubal occlusion (Table 61-10).

PID is caused by an ascending infection from the lower genital tract and is the most common cause of tubal obstruction leading to infertility. PID causes salpingitis, inflammation of the tubes. Resolving salpingitis is associated with mucosal scarring and peritubal adhesions. The ampullary portion of the tube is the most common site of obstruction. Scarring of the fimbria can lead to ampullary dilation with serous or purulent fluid, termed hydrosalpinx and pyosalpinx respectively. On HSG, hydrosalpinx appears as contrast filling a dilated distal tube. Peritubal adhesions can lead to contrast loculations seen at HSG.

Salpingitis isthmica nodosa (SIN) is glandular mucosal proliferation with tubal irregularity and multiple

TABLE 61-10 Tubal Filling Defects and Irregularity

Air bubble
Polyp
Neoplasm
SIN
Diverticula
Tubal ligation
Tubal pregnancy
Tuberculosis
Endometriosis

diverticula. It usually occurs in the isthmic portion of the tube. SIN is suspected to be postinflammatory in etiology and is associated with PID, infertility, and ectopic pregnancy.

Tubal ligation is performed with clips, bands, rings, ligatures, division, resection, and microinserts. HSG can show bulbous termination of the isthmic portion.

CONGENITAL UTERINE MALFORMATION

The uterus and fallopian tubes develop from paired Müllerian ducts. There is a spectrum of failure of ductal elongation and fusion (Fig. 61-1). Agenesis can occur involving any segment of the duct. The most common

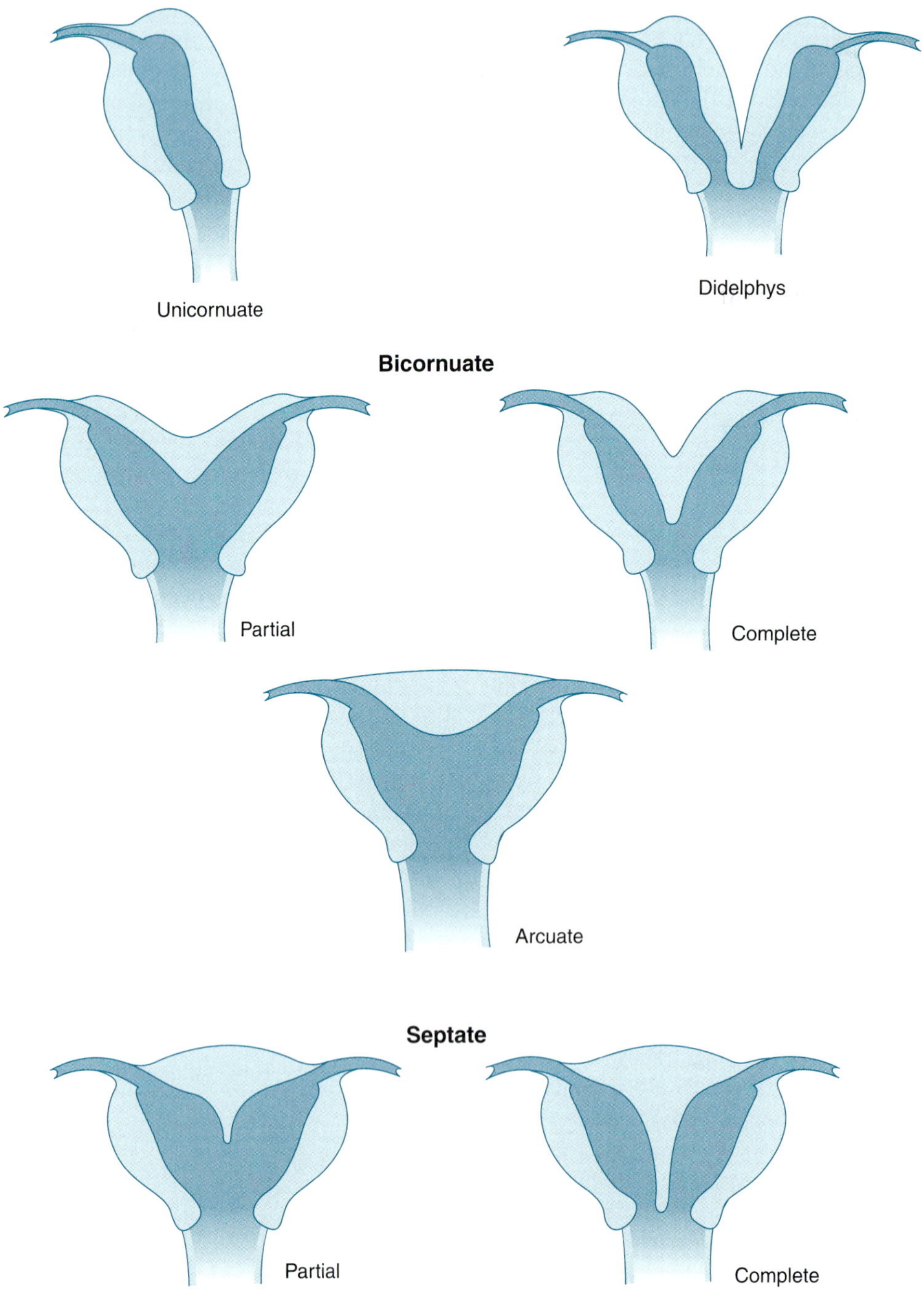

FIG. 61-1 Classification of congenital uterine abnormalities.
SOURCE: Courtesy of Anthony F. Zagar, UAB, Department of Radiology, Birmingham, Alabama.

TABLE 61-11 Bicornuate Versus Septate Uterus

	CONGENITAL MALFORMATION	INTERCORNUAL ANGLE	INTERCORNUAL DISTANCE	EXTERNAL FUNDAL CONTOUR
Bicornuate uterus	Partial nonfusion of Müllerian ducts	Obtuse >105 degrees	>4 cm	Cleft between horns
Septate uterus	Partial or complete failure of septal resorption	Acute <75 degrees	<4 cm	Normal

form of agenesis is Mayer-Rokitansky-Kuster-Hauser syndrome, which is agenesis of the uterus, cervix, and upper portion of the vagina. The development of the urinary and genital systems is related embryologically. Congenital urinary anomalies can be seen in association with uterine anomalies including unilateral renal agenesis, renal ectopia, cystic renal dysplasia, and duplicated collecting system.

A unicornuate uterus results because of the failure of one of the Müllerian ducts to elongate. The endometrial cavity of a unicornuate uterus is fusiform in shape on HSG. The incompletely developed Müllerian duct may exist as a rudimentary horn or may be absent. The rudimentary horn can have no endometrial cavity, or it can have an endometrial cavity, which may or may not communicate with the unicornuate uterine cavity. Unicornuate uterus carries an increased risk of abortion and premature labor.

Uterus didelphys occurs because of complete failure of the ducts to fuse. There are two separate uterine cavities and cervixes. HSG demonstrates two separate fusiform uterine horns flexed in opposite directions. There may be vaginal duplication or vaginal septum. Uterus didelphys carries an increased risk of spontaneous abortion.

Bicornuate uterus results because of partial nonfusion of the ducts. There is a spectrum of degree of abnormal fusion. In a partial bicornuate uterus, there are two divergent horns, which are fused caudally with communication of the two endometrial cavities. In a complete bicornuate uterus, the myometrial cleft between the horns extends to the internal cervical os, termed bicornuate unicollis. In a bicornuate bicollis uterus, the myometrial cleft extends to the external cervical os. Arcuate uterus is a mild form of bicornuate uterus in which HSG reveals mild concavity of the fundal uterine contour. Gestations are normal term with arcuate uterus.

Septate uterus results due to partial or complete failure of the septum dividing the Müllerian ducts to rcsorb. This is the most common developmental abnormality. With complete failure of septal resorption, the septum extends from the fundus to the lower uterine segment. With partial failure of septal resorption, the fundal portion of the septum remains. On HSG, contrast fills two separate uterine horns. There is a high incidence of spontaneous abortion and premature labor because of vascular deficiency of the septum.

On HSG, bicornuate uterus and septate uterus can have overlapping appearances with two separate horns (Table 61-11). The intercornual angle, the intercornual distance, and the external fundal contour can be used to distinguish between the two entities. The bicornuate uterus has an obtuse intercornual angle more than 105 degrees while the septate uterus has an acute intercornual angle less than 75 degrees. The bicornuate intercornual distance is more than 4 cm while the septate intercornual distance is less than 4 cm. The external fundal contour of a bicornuate uterus demonstrates an indentation between the horns, while the external fundal contour of a septate uterus is normal. The multiplanar capability of MRI makes it an excellent modality in assessing the external fundal contour (Table 61-1).

Suggested Reading

Fulcher AS, O'Sullivan SG, Segreti EM, Kavanagh BD. Recurrent cervical carcinoma: typical and atypical manifestations. *Radiographics*. 1999;19:S103-S116.

Jung SE, Lee JM, Rha SE, et al. CT and MR imaging of ovarian tumors with emphasis on differential diagnosis. *Radiographics*. 2002;22:1305-1325.

Krysiewicz S. Infertility in women: diagnostic evaluation with hysterosalpingography and other imaging techniques. *AJR Am J Roentgenol*. 1992;159:253-261.

Nicolet V, Carignan L, Bourdon F, Prosmanne O. MR imaging of cervical carcinoma: a practical staging approach. *Radiographics*. 2000;20:1539-1549.

Ott DJ, Fayez JA, Zagoria RJ. *Hysterosalpingography: A Text and Atlas*. 2nd ed. Baltimore, MD: Williams & Wilkins; 1998.

Prasad SR, Menias CO, Narra VR, et al. Cross-sectional imaging of the female urethra: technique and results. *Radiographics*. 2005;25:749-761.

Ryu J, Kim B. MR imagining of the male and female urethra. *Radiographics*. 2001;21:1169-1185.

Troiano RN, McCarthy SM. Mullerian duct anomalies: imaging and clinical issues. *Radiology*. 2004;233:19-34.

Viswanathan AN, Buttin BM, Kennedy AM. Oncodiagnosis Panel: 2006, ovarian, cervical, and endometrial cancer. *Radiographics*. 2008;28:289-307.

Weber TM, Sostman HD, Spritzer CE, et al. Cervical carcinoma: determination of recurrent tumor extent vs. radiation changes with MR imaging. *Radiology*. 1995;194:135-139.

Yoder IC, Hall DA. Hysterosalpingography in the 1990's. *AJR Am J Roentgenol*. 1991;157:675-683.

QUESTIONS AND ANSWERS

1. Which of the following is the most common location of a periurethral diverticulum in a female with respect to the urethra?
   A. Anterior
   B. Posterior
   C. Anterolateral
   D. Posterolateral

   ANSWER: D. Periurethral diverticula most commonly occur along the posterolateral wall of the midurethra.

2. A cyst is identified in the anterolateral wall of the vagina. Which of the following is the most likely diagnosis?
   A. Bartholin cyst
   B. Gartner cyst
   C. Periurethral cyst
   D. Skene cyst

   ANSWER: B. Gartner cyst arises from remnants of the Wolffian (mesonephric) duct and is lined by nonmucinous epithelium. Gartner cysts are located in the anterolateral wall of the vagina posterior to the urethra.

3. HSG reveals a distorted and enlarged uterine cavity with a smooth filling defect. Which of the following is the most likely diagnosis?
   A. Polyp
   B. Synechiae
   C. Leiomyomas
   D. DES exposure

   ANSWER: C. Leiomyomas can distort and enlarge the endometrial cavity. Submucosal fibroids produce smooth filling defects on HSG.

4. HSG reveals two fusiform uterine horns, which are fused caudally with communication of the endometrial cavities. The horns are flexed in opposite directions with an obtuse intercornual angle. Which of the following is the most likely diagnosis?
   A. Bicornuate uterus
   B. Septate uterus
   C. Uterus didelphys
   D. Unicornuate uterus

   ANSWER: A. Bicornuate uterus results because of a defect in Müllerian ductal fusion. Classically, the uterine cavity is fused caudally with two divergent horns, which are fusiform in shape. There is an obtuse intercornual angle and a dip in the external fundal contour.

5. Which of the following is the most common malignant ovarian neoplasm?
   A. Teratoma
   B. Mucinous cystadenocarcinoma
   C. Serous cystadenocarcinoma
   D. Dysgerminoma

   ANSWER: C. Serous cystadenocarcinoma accounts for more than one-half of all malignant ovarian neoplasms.

6. Which of the following is the most common primary female urethral malignancy?
   A. Adenocarcinoma
   B. Transitional carcinoma
   C. Squamous cell carcinoma
   D. Sarcoma

   ANSWER: C. Approximately 60% to 70% of urethral carcinomas are squamous cell carcinomas. Approximately 20% of urethral malignancies are TCC, with adenocarcinomas representing only 10% of urethral carcinomas.

7. Where do most periurethral cysts originate?
   A. Periurethral glands of Skene
   B. Cowper glands
   C. Glands of Littre
   D. Vaginal structures

   ANSWER: D. Most periurethral cysts originate from the vaginal structures and do not communicate with the urethra. These cysts have their origin from the Müllerian and Gartner ducts and the Bartholin glands.

8. The most common ovarian tumors have their origin from which of the following cell type?
   A. Epithelial tumors
   B. Germ cell tumors
   C. Sex cord-stromal tumors
   D. Metastatic tumors

   ANSWER: A. Epithelial tumors are the most common lesions, accounting for 60% to 70% of all ovarian neoplasms and more than 85% of malignant neoplasms.

9. Up to what percent of serous cystadenocarcinomas will be bilateral?
   A. 15%
   B. 22%
   C. 50%
   D. 75%

   ANSWER: C. Up to 25% of serous cystadenomas and 50% of serous cystadenocarcinomas will be bilateral.

10. Which of the following can be used to distinguish a bicornuate uterus from a septate uterus?
   A. Bicornuate uterus will have an intercornual angle of more than 105 degrees.
   B. The external fundal contour of a septate uterus demonstrates an indentation.
   C. The septate uterus intercornual distance is more than 4 cm.
   D. The external fundal contour of a septate uterus demonstrates a pleated fold.

   ANSWER: A. A bicornuate uterus will have an intercornual angle of more than 105 degrees, demonstrate a contour with an indentation, and have an intercornual distance of more than 4 cm.

Section 6
ULTRASOUND

62 ULTRASOUND PHYSICS

Kenneth Hoyt and Franklin N. Tessler

BASIC PROPERTIES OF SOUND

DEFINITION OF SOUND AND SOURCES

Sound is a form of mechanical energy that possesses the capacity to do work. In response to a transmitted pressure wave, molecules and particles within a medium (e.g., tissue) physically vibrate against each other, causing the energy to propagate. Sound is produced by a vibrating source. In medical ultrasound, the source is a piezoelectric transducer that converts high-frequency electrical energy to sound and vice versa. When placed in contact with tissue, the transducer acts like a piston, producing short bursts or pulses of mechanical energy that propagate through the tissue in a beam-like fashion.

LONGITUDINAL VERSUS TRANSVERSE WAVES

Ultrasound can be classified by the direction of wave propagation in relation to particle vibration. Longitudinal waves, which are used in medical ultrasound, propagate along the axis of particle vibration. However, wave propagation perpendicular to particle vibration can also occur in solid tissue. Termed transverse waves, they propagate over considerably shorter distances than longitudinal waves since they are not transmitted as effectively. In general, only longitudinal waves are considered important in medical ultrasound.

COMPRESSION AND RAREFACTION

A propagating ultrasound wave causes local disturbances in tissue as the particles move back-and-forth. This mechanical energy is conducted to neighboring particles and allows the wave to propagate further. Compared to unperturbed tissue, *zones of compression* describe regions of slightly higher particle density, while zones of *rarefaction* define regions of slightly lower particle density.

WAVE MOTION

A propagating ultrasound wave may be visualized as a sinusoidal signal that varies in amplitude over time. The *frequency* of the wave is the number of oscillations (cycles) that it undergoes per second (Fig. 62-1). The unit for frequency is hertz (Hz), where 1 Hz equals 1 cycle/s. In medical ultrasound, wave frequency is typically between 2 and 20 MHz, although higher frequencies are used for special applications.

The *period* of a wave is the reciprocal of its frequency, and denotes the time required for the wave to oscillate one full cycle (Fig. 62-2). The physical distance a wave travels over one full cycle is termed the *wavelength*.

Propagation speed is a measure of how quickly ultrasound travels in a given tissue and is influenced by both tissue density and stiffness. An increase in tissue stiffness or a decrease in tissue density results in a corresponding increase in the speed of sound through that tissue (Fig. 62-3). In medical ultrasound imaging, the speed of sound in the human body is assumed to be 1540 m/s.

Typically, ultrasound propagates at a given frequency that is defined as the fundamental (transmit) frequency. However, as the wave propagates, its shape gradually changes, resulting in energy redistribution and generation of waves at multiples of the fundamental frequency. Termed harmonics, these waves contain useful information that can be isolated and exploited to improve visualization of tissues or ultrasound contrast agents.

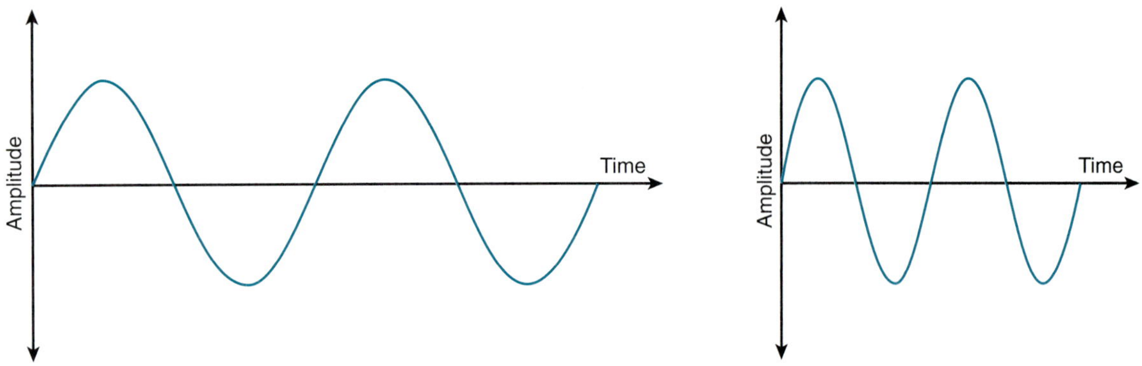

FIG. 62-1 Amplitude versus time plots describing a low- (left) and high- (right) frequency sinusoidal signal. Note the low-frequency signal has a longer period.

ACOUSTIC PRESSURE AND INTENSITY

The strength or *amplitude* of an ultrasound wave is typically measured by its pressure. Zones of *compression* have a higher pressure than undisturbed tissue, whereas zones of *rarefaction* have a lower pressure. In fact, it is this cyclic oscillation between states of high and low pressure that compel the particles to vibrate back-and-forth and allow ultrasound wave propagation. The plots illustrated in Figs. 62-1 and 62-2 describe signal amplitude, but pressure could be used interchangeably.

An alternative measure of ultrasound strength is *acoustic intensity*. At any point along the path of a propagating ultrasound wave, the intensity is proportional to the square of the pressure. Signal intensity is typically denoted in *decibel*, which denotes the logarithmic ratio of two intensities (or amplitudes). For example, a 40-dB difference between two sounds is equivalent to a 10 000-fold intensity change.

INTERACTION OF ULTRASOUND BEAMS WITH TISSUE

SOURCES OF ATTENUATION

As ultrasound propagates through tissue, there is a loss of energy termed *attenuation*. This progressive reduction in signal amplitude is attributed to two sources. The first results from reflection and scattering of ultrasound as it passes through the tissues and the second is due to absorption, the conversion of wave energy to heat energy. Absorption is the dominant source of ultrasound attenuation in soft tissues.

FREQUENCY DEPENDENCE OF ATTENUATION

Ultrasound attenuation in tissue is highly dependent on signal frequency. Specifically, higher-frequency ultrasound waves are attenuated more than lower-frequency waves in

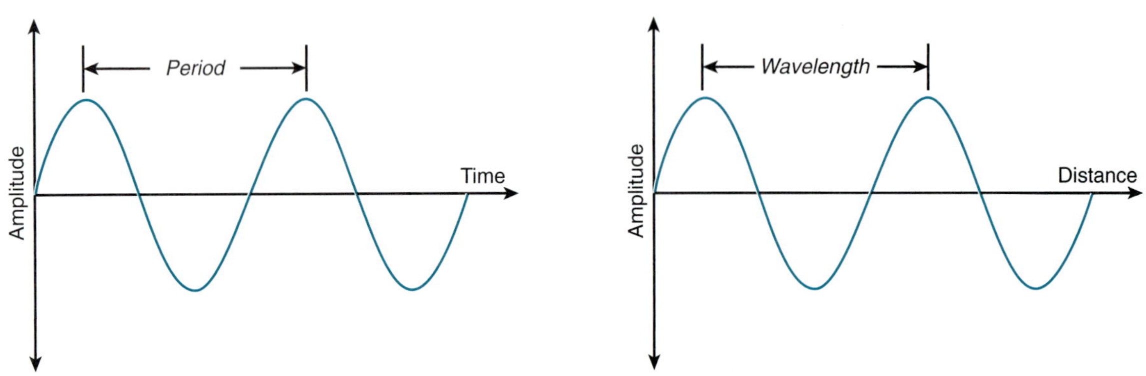

FIG. 62-2 Sinusoidal signals describing the physical concept of period (left) and wavelength (right).

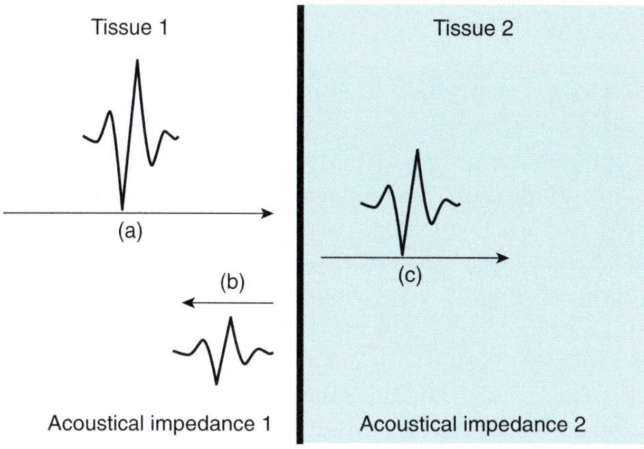

FIG. 62-3 An ultrasound wave orthogonally incident on a boundary between two tissues characterized by different acoustical impedances. As shown, ultrasound incident at the interface (a) is separated into lower amplitude reflected (b) and transmitted (c) waves.

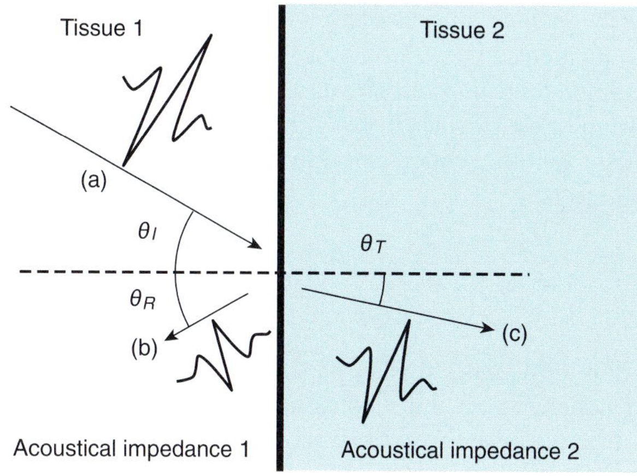

FIG. 62-4 An ultrasound wave obliquely incident on a boundary between two tissues characterized by different acoustical impedances (or ultrasound propagation speeds). As shown, ultrasound incident on the interface at an angle θ_I (a) is separated into lower amplitude reflected (b) and transmitted (c) waves with angles to the normal θ_R and θ_T, respectively. The transmission angle is governed by the difference in propagation speeds between tissues 1 and 2.

any given tissue. This means that tissue penetration is compromised at higher frequencies, limiting the amount of useful information that can be extracted at depth. However, since spatial resolution improves with ultrasound frequency, there is a fundamental trade-off between tissue penetration and spatial resolution that must be taken into account during every ultrasound examination.

ACOUSTICAL IMPEDANCE

Ultrasound imaging is based on the detection and display of reflected ultrasound waves called echoes, which are produced at tissue interfaces. In ultrasound imaging, these interfaces represent boundaries between tissue that differs in a property called *acoustical impedance*, which is defined as the product of a tissue's density and the speed of sound within that tissue. Spatial variations in acoustical impedance proportionally influence the amplitude of echoes that are detected to generate the ultrasound image.

If an area of tissue produces echoes of greater amplitude than the surrounding tissue, then this region is referred to as *hyperechoic* or *echogenic*. Alternatively, a tissue region that generates echoes lower in amplitude than the surrounding tissue is termed *hypoechoic*. Lastly, a region of tissue is referred to as *anechoic* if ultrasound passes through with no discernible backscatter. All three terms are used to characterize ultrasound findings.

REFLECTION AND TRANSMISSION

Ultrasound striking a smooth tissue boundary produces a *reflection*. The amount of reflection at an interface is dependent on the acoustical impedance of the two tissues on either side of the boundary, as well as on the angle of incidence of the ultrasound wave. Specifically, ultrasound that strikes a boundary at 90 degrees results in a fraction of the wave being reflected back toward the source, termed specular reflection. The reflected wave (called backscatter) has a lower amplitude. The remainder of the wave is transmitted across the interface (Fig. 62-3).

Ultrasound striking a boundary obliquely also results in wave reflection and transmission. However, the lower-amplitude reflected wave is redirected back away from the source at an angle equal to the incident angle (Fig. 62-4). If the tissue interface is not orthogonal to the ultrasound beam, the reflected wave will not reach the imaging transducer and the echoes will go undetected. Most soft-tissue interfaces encountered in the human body possess relatively small differences in acoustical impedance, which leads to a majority of the incident waves being transmitted into the deeper tissues.

SCATTERING

Scattering is the weak reflection of ultrasound by structures with dimensions smaller than the wavelength of the incident wave (i.e., micrometer scale), and is encountered at rough surfaces or in heterogeneous organs such as the liver. Such reflectors produce reflections in multiple directions, with intensity directly proportional to the frequency and scatterer size. Since specular reflection is highly angle-dependent, images of tissue interfaces or organ boundaries are generally attributed to the mechanism of scattering, which is less dependent on the incident angle. Furthermore, it is the simultaneous detection and interference of echoes from many neighboring scattering sites that produces the characteristic image texture, called speckle that is associated with solid organs.

REFRACTION

When ultrasound traverses a tissue boundary, the wave may change direction, indicating that the incident angle is different than the transmission angle (Fig. 62-4). This change in direction is termed *refraction* and is attributed to the difference in the speed of sound in the two tissues and on the obliqueness of the incident wave.

ULTRASOUND IMAGING PRINCIPLES

PULSED ULTRASOUND

In medical ultrasound, short bursts of acoustical energy are produced by a transducer and pass through the tissues in a beam-like pattern. As the ultrasound pulses propagate, echoes are generated that travel back to the tissue surface. This backscatter is continuously detected by the transducer and is recorded as a function of time. Assuming an average speed of sound in tissue of 1540 m/s, the time elapsed between transmission and echo detection is used to calculate the depth of the structure that produced the echo. This pulse-echo principle is the foundation for the vast majority of ultrasound imaging.

AMPLITUDE MODE

Mapping the reflected echo amplitude along the beam path as a function of depth is termed amplitude-modulated (or A-mode) imaging. This produces a single scan line or line of sight for a given imaging angle. Beyond some ophthalmic applications, this modality is now rarely used clinically.

MOTION MODE

Motion-modulated (or M-mode) imaging is similar to A-mode ultrasound described in the previous paragraph. An M-mode display maps echo amplitudes to a color scale over time. Today, the M-mode display is most often used in cardiac applications and to document cardiac motion in small embryos.

BRIGHTNESS MODE AND REAL-TIME IMAGING

Sequential acquisition of multiple scan lines produces a two-dimensional cross-sectional image. This is termed brightness-modulated (or B-mode) imaging, since the echo amplitude is mapped to a brightness scale (Fig. 62-5). Typically, the background (absence of echoes) is black and successively lighter shades of gray represent higher echo amplitudes (originating from stronger ultrasound reflectors). Hence, these images are commonly referred to as grayscale images. Transmission of a single pulse and detection of echoes is sufficient to produce a scan line. However, several transmissions may be required if multiple focal points are used, since each focus requires a separate pulse-echo sequence.

Generation of multiple images in rapid succession results in an illusion of motion that is referred to as real-time ultrasound. The time required to collect echoes from the deepest lying reflectors at a given imaging depth determines the delay before the next scan line can be acquired. Because image acquisition depends on the depth and number of scan lines, a deep or wide imaging field of view limits the achievable frame rate. Typical frame rates for pulsed ultrasound imaging are in the order of tens of frames per second and are suitable for real-time visualization of tissue structures and organs. High frame rates are needed to image fast-moving structures such as the fetal heart.

THREE-DIMENSIONAL IMAGING

In three-dimensional ultrasound imaging, the ultrasound system collects echoes from a volume of tissue. The resultant data may be analyzed to produce two-dimensional images in any arbitrary plane or shaded, volumetric images.

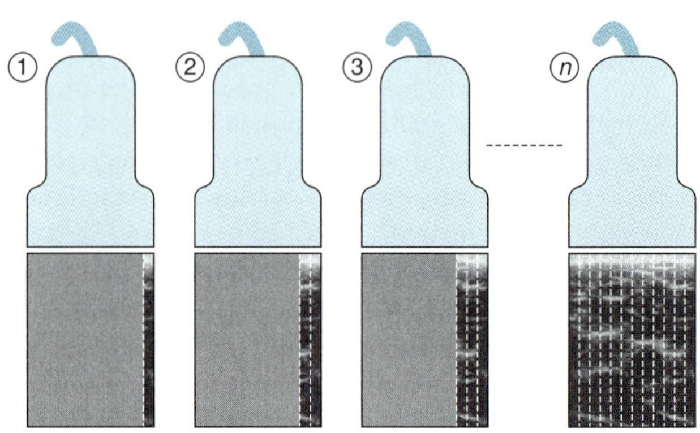

FIG. 62-5 A pulse-echo sequence allows acquisition of one scan line of ultrasound data. The subsequent acquisition of scan lines produces a two-dimensional cross-sectional B-mode (grayscale) ultrasound image for a fixed tissue depth. The number of scan lines used in image formation determines the image width.

RESOLUTION

One measure of ultrasound image quality is the spatial resolution, which is defined as the ability to resolve closely spaced objects as distinct structures. *Axial resolution* describes the ability to distinguish objects along the ultrasound beam path and is determined by the transmit pulse length. In ultrasound, the pulse length is a product of the wavelength and number of transmit cycles (typically two or three). Since wavelength is the inverse of frequency, shorter pulses improve axial resolution through increases in ultrasound frequency. But, as noted, increasing the ultrasound frequency also increases attenuation, minimizing penetration depth. Therefore, the selection of ultrasound frequency for any application is always a compromise between spatial resolution and depth.

Lateral resolution is defined as the ability to distinguish objects located at right angles to the ultrasound beam, parallel to the transducer surface. Lateral resolution is primarily influenced by the ultrasound beam width. For unfocused transducers, the lateral resolution is highest in the Fresnel zone closest to the transducer, and decreases as the beam diverges in the far field, or Fraunhofer zone. However, most modern transducers are focused either mechanically or electronically to produce beams that are optimized for a specific depth.

Finally, *elevational resolution* refers to the spatial resolution perpendicular to the imaging plane. Decreasing the elevational resolution results in a greater effective slice thickness, which produces echoes from structures adjacent to the imaging plane. It is especially important in three-dimensional imaging applications.

PULSED DOPPLER

In medical ultrasound imaging, the Doppler effect refers to the change in frequency of a sound beam as it interacts with moving structures, typically red blood cells. The Doppler frequency (f_D) and the received ultrasound frequency (f_0) are related to the velocity (v) of the moving scatterers by the following equation:

$$v = \frac{f_D c}{2 f_0 \cos\theta}$$

where c and θ denote the speed of sound and angle between the ultrasound beam and moving scatterers, respectively. A positive Doppler shift indicates that scatterers are moving toward the ultrasound beam while a negative Doppler shift denotes motion away. Note that there is no Doppler shift at an angle of 90 degrees. Doppler imaging is typically performed at an angle of 60 degrees or less to minimize the effects of errors in setting the Doppler angle.

Blood velocity measurements using ultrasound are made using the pulsed Doppler technique, which detects Doppler shifts within a small area of interest called the sample volume. The operator adjusts the sample volume to match the size and depth of the vessel being examined. In pulsed Doppler, a series of ultrasound pulses are transmitted at a given rate (termed pulse repetition frequency, PRF) and echoes are acquired periodically. (An older Doppler technique uses continuous insonation along a line of sight, but it is rarely used in radiology.)

The sample volume typically encompasses a range of blood flow velocities at any given instant; therefore, the pulsed Doppler signal encodes a corresponding range of Doppler shift frequencies. Contributions from much slower-moving tissue structures such as blood vessel walls are removed from the Doppler signal using wall filters, which allow higher-frequency signals to pass.

The Doppler spectrum is computed using a mathematical technique known as the fast Fourier transform. The resultant Doppler spectral tracing is presented as a moving graph, where the vertical axis represents the magnitude of the Doppler shift frequency (or velocity), corrected for the Doppler angle, and the horizontal axis denotes time. The Doppler spectrum is usually displayed along with a grayscale or color Doppler ultrasound image, which lets the operator adjust the Doppler angle to match the flow axis. Since the Doppler shift frequency is within the human audible frequency range, it is also typically played through speakers on the ultrasound system.

COLOR DOPPLER

Color Doppler imaging uses color coding to denote flow velocity and direction within a region of interest. Similar to B-mode ultrasound, a sequence of pulsed beams generates signals from a given region. Velocity information is derived in the same manner as in pulsed Doppler, but a large number of volumes are sampled along each beam. Depending on the size of the imaging field of view, the number of sample volumes can easily reach thousands. Therefore, pulse-echo acquisitions from a given location are limited to 4 to 24 echo sequences (termed the ensemble length or packet size). The rate at which this occurs is determined by the PRF. Since echoes from deeper-lying structures must be received before another pulse-echo sequence can be initiated, color flow imaging at depth requires a longer delay between pulses, which means a lower PRF.

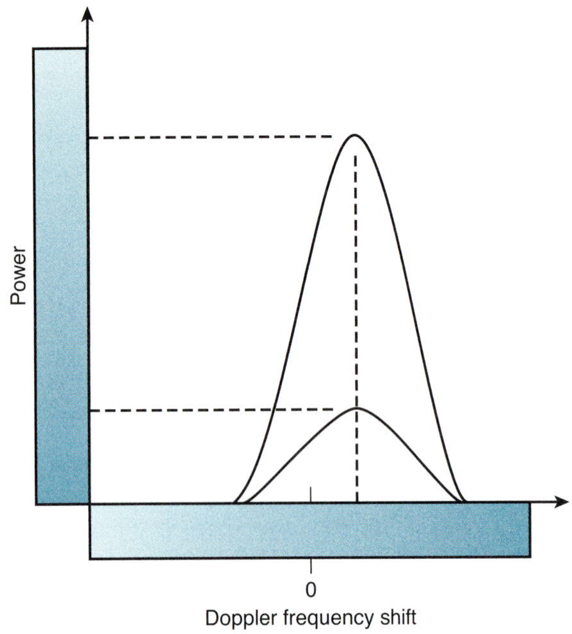

FIG. 62-6 Illustration of color flow and power Doppler signal mapping. The spectra of two different Doppler signals are depicted. For a given Doppler signal and sample volume, color flow Doppler estimates and maps the mean Doppler frequency shift and power Doppler measures and maps the signal amplitude.

Because the ensemble length used for color flow Doppler is considerably shorter than that used for pulsed Doppler, an alternative mathematical technique called autocorrelation is employed to give an estimate of the Doppler shift frequency after wall filtering. The blood velocity estimates derived using this technique are cruder than those used in pulsed Doppler imaging. However, color Doppler is still very helpful to depict flow within a relatively large area, as opposed to the small sample volume used in pulsed Doppler.

In color flow imaging, the sign and mean value of velocity estimates are mapped to a color scale at each location within the region of interest. Typically, red and blue denote flow toward or away from the transducer, respectively (Fig. 62-6). The color flow image is overlaid on a B-mode image for anatomical mapping. Owing to the amount of processing needed, the frame rate is usually less than that for grayscale imaging alone. However, the frame rate can be improved by reducing the size of the color region of interest.

POWER DOPPLER

As mentioned in the previous section, color flow Doppler estimates the mean Doppler frequency shift using a sequence of pulse-echo acquisitions and maps these measurements to an image. An alternative but similar imaging technique, known as power Doppler, estimates and maps the total strength (power) of the Doppler signal within each sample volume (Fig. 62-6). For blood flow applications, the power Doppler value corresponds to the number of red blood cells in a given sample volume. Power Doppler imaging offers more sensitive detection of blood flow, allowing improved depiction of slow flow and small vessels, but at the expense of eliminating directional information.

CONTRAST IMAGING

Ultrasound contrast agents are composed of gas-filled micrometer-sized spheres, typically known as microbubbles. The use of low-diffusivity gas and thin stabilizing shell permits a circulatory lifetime in the order of tens of minutes. Because of a large acoustical impedance difference between the microbubbles and the surrounding blood, they are excellent ultrasound scatterers and improve the sensitivity to blood flow.

Ultrasound contrast agents undergo an oscillatory movement, or resonate, in response to an ultrasound field, a process called stable cavitation. Under sufficiently high ultrasound pressures, this can lead to nonlinear scattering and generation of echoes with frequency components at harmonic multiples of the transmit frequency. These harmonic signals can be selectively isolated from the backscatter signals using various signal processing and pulsing techniques to improve image contrast. At present, contrast agents are only approved for echocardiographic applications in the United States, although they are widely employed elsewhere.

ULTRASOUND INSTRUMENTATION

TRANSDUCER ARRAYS

An ultrasound transducer converts electrical signals to acoustical energy and vice versa. In any medical ultrasound system, the transducer transmits the acoustic pulses that propagate through tissue and receives the echoes that are generated. The received echoes are then converted to electrical signals for processing. To allow the sound pulses to pass from the transducer into the patient, a coupling gel is placed between the transducer and the skin.

The active elements in a typical ultrasound transducer are small piezoelectric elements. When excited with a very short high-frequency electrical signal, a piezoelectric element mechanically vibrates and generates an ultrasound pulse. The dominant frequency of this ultrasound pulse is the same as the electrical signal used for excitation. However, there are also additional frequencies that are above and below this nominal frequency. This spread or range of frequencies is termed the bandwidth of the ultrasound pulse. The transducer bandwidth defines the range of frequencies that can be transmitted and received. Higher-bandwidth transducers (often called broadband) are suitable for a wider range of clinical settings.

The piezoelectric elements that make up a transducer can be arranged in a variety of configurations to suit various applications. The most common types are linear, curved, and phased arrays. Linear and curved arrays are composed of 120 to 250 elements. Small subgroups of elements are activated sequentially to produce pulses and receive echoes along a series of scan lines to make up the image. The number of transducer elements activated and the timing sequence determines the transmit focal depth. Linear arrays produce a series of beams that are parallel to each other, resulting in a rectangular image. Curved arrays have a convex shape, so the beams diverge at depth, producing a sector format image that is wider at the bottom. Phased arrays are typically made of 120 or more elements and are much smaller than linear and curved arrays. They function by firing all the elements to form an ultrasound beam. Through proper timing of individual element excitation, the ultrasound beam can be steered through a field of view to produce a sector image.

As noted above, modern ultrasound transducers are also designed to focus at particular depths. Electronic focusing, which is achieved by applying electronic delays when the ultrasound pulses are transmitted and received, is the most flexible. This allows the operator to adjust the focal zone to match the depth of the area of interest.

BASIC FUNCTIONAL LAYOUT OF AN ULTRASOUND SYSTEM

Modern ultrasound systems are highly complex. However, their basic functional layout includes transducer probes, a central processing unit (CPU), system controls, display, keyboard, print network, and storage (Fig. 62-7).

The CPU directs the overall operation of the ultrasound system and is usually a collection of microprocessors. Under direction from the CPU, the transducer receives a high-voltage signal and acquires echoes that are amplified and transferred back to the CPU for processing and display. External controls allow the operator to optimize the image for a particular examination. The operator typically adjusts the system using a

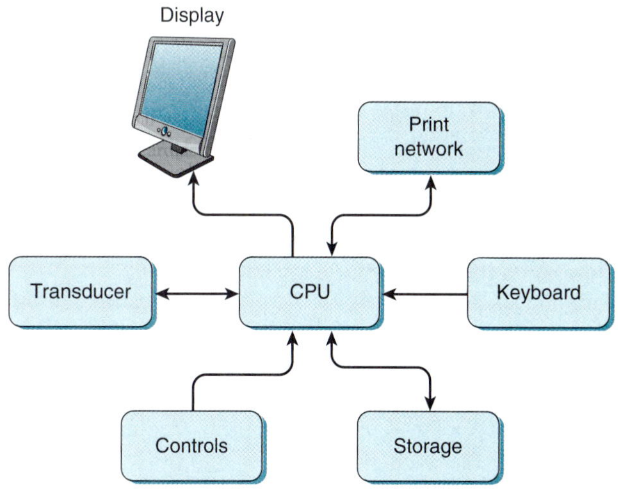

FIG. 62-7 Block diagram illustrating the basic functional layout of a typical ultrasound imaging system.

keyboard and a series of switches and dials. The resultant images are viewed on a monitor and printed or saved digitally for subsequent review.

IMAGING PARAMETERS AND CONTROLS

In ultrasound imaging, the received echoes are typically very weak and must be amplified. An adjustable master gain control allows amplification of all the echoes. However, since the ultrasound beam is attenuated as it passes through tissue, echoes from deeper structures are weaker. To compensate for this, depth-dependent amplification, known as time gain compensation, is used. In older equipment, the time gain compensation controls were set by the operator. However, many newer machines set the time gain compensation automatically.

The received echoes span a very wide range of values (up to 120 dB), which is called the dynamic range. However, since ultrasound system can only display a much smaller range (usually approximately 40 dB), the echo data are compressed logarithmically before it is displayed. In most ultrasound systems, dynamic range mapping is under the operator's control. Lower values are typically used to improve grayscale contrast between vessels and adjacent structures, while higher settings are used for soft-tissue imaging.

Other common user-adjustable parameters include pre- and postprocessing, grayscale mapping, smoothing, and frame averaging. The last control, which averages successive frames to produce a more pleasing image, also has the effect of blurring small moving structures such as the embryonic heart. This emphasizes the importance of optimizing the machine controls for each clinical application.

Various controls also exist for Doppler imaging. In pulsed Doppler, the sample volume size and position are defined by the user. The sample volume size determines the transmitted pulse length and its depth along the beam axis establishes the PRF. Although the sample volumes are fixed in color flow and power Doppler imaging, the depth is adjustable and establishes an upper limit on the achievable frame rate. The frame rate is also limited by the Doppler packet size (ensemble length). A larger packet size improves flow velocity estimates but lowers the frame rate.

In all Doppler imaging modes, wall filters remove low-frequency clutter below a certain cutoff frequency from the Doppler signal. This cutoff frequency is adjustable by the user. In color flow and pulsed Doppler, the zero point of the Doppler display, called the baseline, is also adjustable. When the baseline is centered, there is equal room above and below it to display flow toward or away from the transducer. However, if flow in a vessel is unidirectional, the baseline may be adjusted accordingly.

ULTRASOUND ARTIFACTS

PROPAGATION

Ultrasound reverberations occur when echoes shuttle back-and-forth between two highly reflective structures. For example, strong echoes (such as those originating at the wall of a cyst) may reflect off the transducer surface and be redirected into the body, only to return to the transducer after an additional delay. This produces spurious echoes deep to the interface. In some situations, multiple reflections occur within or adjacent to small structures such as gas bubbles. This produces a train of equally spaced echoes that are called ringdown or comet-tail artifacts. Multiple reflections also may occur if a structure lies between the transducer and a highly reflective interface such as the diaphragm, producing a mirror image artifact.

Refraction occurs when an ultrasound beam strikes a tissue boundary obliquely, changing the beam's direction. This is attributed to a difference in the speed of sound in the two tissues. Echoes produced from a refracted ultrasound beam are misregistered by the ultrasound system, resulting in image distortion and a loss of resolution. As noted previously, ultrasound systems assume that the speed of sound in tissue is a constant 1540 m/s. However, the actual speed varies from tissue to tissue (Table 62-1), and even within a particular type of tissue. Any deviation from the assumed speed of sound leads to misregistration, as well.

TABLE 62-1 Propagation Speed of Ultrasound in Various Biological Tissues

TISSUE TYPE	SPEED OF SOUND (m/s)
Air	330
Fat	1450
Water	1480
Soft tissue (average)	1540
Liver	1550
Kidney	1560
Blood	1570
Muscle	1580
Tendon	1750
Bone	4080

Side lobe artifacts result from the interactions of off-axis components of the sound beam with tissues. Although these components are weak, they produce low-level echoes that may simulate debris in cystic structures. Similarly, slice thickness or beam width artifacts occur when the ultrasound beam interacts with structures just outside the desired imaging plane. This can produce spurious echoes at the margins of vessels and other fluid-containing structures.

ATTENUATION

When an ultrasound beam encounters structures that absorb or reflect it strongly, the pulses that are transmitted to the deeper tissues are weakened. In some cases, deeper echoes are minimal or absent, leading to artifacts known as *acoustic shadows*, which are analogous to shadows in beams of light. Acoustic shadowing is most often associated with interfaces where there is a large difference in acoustical impedance, such as bone, calcium, metal, or gas. Conversely, when the beam passes through a structure that transmits sound more readily than the tissues on either side of it, deeper structures appear more echogenic. This artifact, termed *acoustic enhancement* or increased-through transmission, is helpful to distinguish fluid from solid structures.

PULSED DOPPLER

Sampling theory requires that PRF for a pulsed Doppler system be at least twice the Doppler shift frequency to be detected. This limit is known as the Nyquist sampling rate. Because the PRF is restricted by the time required to collect echoes from each pulse before the next one is sent, this limits the maximum Doppler frequency shift (velocity) that can be accurately detected. When the PRF is not high enough, the system cannot determine the true Doppler shift. Known as aliasing, this artifact is easily recognized by appearance of the spectral tracing "wrapping around" from the top to bottom of the pulsed Doppler display window, suggesting a reversal of blood flow. This artifact may be eliminated by increasing the system PRF, adjusting the baseline, reducing the Doppler frequency, or increasing the Doppler angle.

COLOR DOPPLER

The Nyquist limit also applies to color Doppler imaging. If the color Doppler PRF is not sufficiently high, aliasing occurs, and high-frequency signals appear incorrectly as reversed flow. Aliasing artifacts can generally be removed in color Doppler by increasing the PRF.

Color Doppler not only detects motion from blood flow but also from slow-moving adjacent structures such as vessel walls. These signals, called clutter, are removed by wall filters, which suppress low-frequency signals below a cutoff frequency. Although wall filters are effective in removing low-frequency noise, care must be taken so that signals from slowly moving blood are not eliminated.

Twinkling artifact is unique to color flow imaging. It results from interaction of the sound beam with the irregular surface of stones and other calcifications, and appears as alternating bands of color deep to the stone. In some cases, it is helpful to distinguish stones from other small reflective structures.

BIOLOGICAL EFFECTS OF ULTRASOUND

THERMAL

Ultrasound is a form of mechanical energy that is absorbed by tissue and converted to heat as it propagates. The temperature rise is tissue-dependent and is more pronounced in highly attenuating tissues such as bone. Heat is also produced at the transducer surface. Factors that determine the amount of heating include the tissue's ability to conduct heat, tissue perfusion, and the ultrasound intensity and exposure time. The thermal index has been adopted as a standard to minimize any thermal bioeffects associated with ultrasound exposure. Displayed on the scanner monitor for reference, the thermal index value represents the ratio between the current ultrasound power and the intensity that will result in a maximum temperature rise of 1°C.

MECHANICAL

The propagation of ultrasound through tissue imparts a low-level radiation force that perturbs the tissue along the beam path. This absorption-based mechanical effect can induce fluid movements termed streaming and may also stress cells and tissue interfaces. However, radiation forces associated with diagnostic ultrasound exposures are generally considered unlikely to promote any adverse bioeffects.

CAVITATIONAL

Cavitation describes the ultrasound-induced formation and behavior of gas bubbles at high negative peak pressures. Stable cavitation denotes an oscillatory movement of gas bubbles in response to ultrasound and its cyclic pressure variations. If the oscillations become too large, gas bubbles may implode. Termed inertial cavitation, this can lead to extremely high localized temperatures and significant tissue destruction. Therefore, the mechanical index was adopted as a standard to quantify the likelihood of cavitation-related bioeffects. Commercially available ultrasound scanners are limited to a maximum mechanical index value of 1.9 for most diagnostic purposes.

ALARA PRINCIPLE

An acronym for "as low as reasonably achievable," ALARA is an important concept in ultrasound imaging, as well as in other medical imaging modalities. The ALARA principle is based on the assumption that any amount of exposure to ultrasound energy can increase (even minutely) the risk of adverse bioeffects. The guiding principle of ALARA is to keep the patient exposed to ultrasound energy as low as possible for a given diagnostic result. In general, Doppler ultrasound deposits more energy in the tissues than grayscale imaging—therefore, its use in very early pregnancy should be restricted. However, it is generally agreed that ultrasound exposure in typical clinical applications, including early obstetric imaging, is very safe.

SUGGESTED READING

Cosgrove D. Ultrasound contrast agents: an overview. *Eur J Radiol*. 2006;60:324-330.

Fenster A, Downey DB, Cardinal HN. Three-dimensional ultrasound imaging. *Phys Med Biol*. 2001;46:67-99.

Jensen JA. Medical ultrasound imaging. *Prog Biophys Mol Biol.* 2007;93:153-165.

Merritt CRB. Update on ultrasonography. *Radiol Clin North Am.* 2001;39:385-397.

Miller DL, Averkiou MA, Brayman AA, et al. Bioeffects considerations for diagnostic ultrasound contrast agents. *J Ultrasound Med.* 2008;27:611-632.

Robbin ML. Ultrasound contrast agents: a promising future. *Radiol Clin North Am* 2001;39:399-414.

Wells PNT. Ultrasound imaging. *Phys Med Biol.* 2006;51:83-98.

York G, Kim Y. Ultrasound processing and computing: review and future directions. *Annu Rev Biomed Eng.* 1999;1:559-588.

QUESTIONS AND ANSWERS

1. Concerning ultrasound, which of the following is *true*?
   A. Transverse waves propagate over longer distances.
   B. Bone conducts sound more slowly than soft tissue.
   C. It is a form of mechanical energy.
   D. Period is the distance a wave travels during one full cycle.

   ANSWER: C. Like all sound, ultrasound is a form of mechanical energy that is transmitted through a solid, liquid, or gaseous medium.

2. Concerning the frequency of ultrasound, which of the following is *true*?
   A. Higher-frequency ultrasound penetrates more readily than lower-frequency sound.
   B. Frequency is directly related to spatial resolution.
   C. Modern transducers produce a narrower range of frequencies.
   D. Most ultrasound transducers operate at 15–20 MHz.

   ANSWER: B. As the frequency goes up, the spatial resolution increases at the expense of penetration.

3. Concerning ultrasound imaging modes, which of the following is *true*?
   A. A-mode produces images along a single line of sight.
   B. M-mode produces images along multiple lines of sight.
   C. Increasing the image depth results in a higher frame rate.
   D. In B-mode scanning, the returning echo frequency is mapped to a gray scale.

   ANSWER: A. A-mode ultrasound detects echoes from structures along a single line of sight.

4. Which of the following statements about spectral Doppler ultrasound is *true*?
   A. Doppler angle should not be less than 60 degrees.
   B. Lower the PRF, the higher the Nyquist limit.
   C. Wall filters remove high-frequency components from the Doppler signal.
   D. In medical applications, frequency shifts are usually in the audible range.

   ANSWER: D. Doppler shifts are typically in kilohertz, and so fall well within the range of human hearing. Experienced ultrasound operators can grossly estimate a stenosis based on the pitch of the audible shift.

5. Which of the following statements about color Doppler imaging is *true*?
   A. Less accurate than spectral Doppler
   B. Depicts flow over a smaller region of interest than spectral Doppler
   C. Frame rates are higher than for grayscale imaging.
   D. No directional information

   ANSWER: A. Color Doppler imaging provides a less accurate measure of flow velocity than spectral Doppler, but depicts blood flow over a much larger area.

6. Concerning ultrasound transducers, which of the following is *true*?
   A. Phased arrays are larger than linear arrays.
   B. Convert one form of energy to another
   C. Coupling agent is used for patient comfort.
   D. Most transducers have a single element.

   ANSWER: B. Ultrasound transducers convert electrical signals to sound at transmit and do the opposite at receive.

7. Which of the following statements about ultrasound artifacts is *true*?
   A. Aliasing occurs with spectral Doppler, but not color Doppler imaging.
   B. Twinkling artifact is only seen with grayscale imaging.
   C. The assumption of a constant ultrasound transmission speed in tissues is responsible for some artifacts.
   D. Comet-tail artifacts appear between the transducer and the interface that produced them.

   ANSWER: C. Pulse-echo imaging is based on the assumption that the speed of ultrasound in tissue is a constant 1540 m/s. However, this assumption is incorrect for some types of tissue, resulting in misregistration artifacts.

8. Which of the following will reduce aliasing when flow is toward the transducer?
   A. Increasing the PRF
   B. Increasing the Doppler frequency
   C. Reducing the Doppler angle
   D. Moving the baseline up

   ANSWER: A. Increasing the PRF raises the Nyquist limit, and hence makes it possible to detect higher-velocity flow without aliasing. All the other choices have the opposite effect.

9. Concerning bioeffects, which of the following is *true*?
   A. Gas bubble implosion is a thermal effect.
   B. Thermal index uses the intensity needed to cause a temperature rise of 0.5°C as a reference point.
   C. Stable cavitation is related to cyclic pressure variation in the ultrasound beam.
   D. Doppler imaging results in less energy deposition than grayscale imaging.

   ANSWER: C. Stable cavitation refers to oscillation of tiny gas bubbles in tissue in response to pressure variations in the ultrasound beam.

10. Concerning the interaction of ultrasound with solid organs, which of the following is *true*?
   A. Interfaces with large differences in acoustical impedance cause weak reflections.
   B. Specular reflections predominate.
   C. Speckle in solid organs results from scattering and interference.
   D. Low-frequency sound is absorbed at a higher rate than high-frequency ultrasound.

   ANSWER: C. In solid organs like the liver, scattering and interference predominate to produce a typical echotexture that is called speckle.

63 ABDOMINAL ULTRASOUND

Franklin N. Tessler

LIVER

NORMAL ANATOMY AND ULTRASOUND APPEARANCE

The liver is the largest organ in the abdomen and is usually the anchor point for any nonfocused abdominal sonogram. It is divided into right and left lobes, which are separated by an oblique plane that intersects the middle hepatic vein and the gallbladder fossa. The right lobe, in turn, is divided into anterior and posterior segments, which are demarcated by a roughly horizontal plane that follows the course of the right hepatic vein. The intersegmental fissure divides the medial and lateral segments of the left lobe. Finally, the fissure for the ligamentum venosum bounds the caudate lobe anteriorly. All of the structures that demarcate the hepatic lobes and segments are usually well visualized on ultrasound, and knowledge of typical anatomy and common variations is essential for localization of focal liver lesions.

Sonographically, the hepatic parenchyma is of medium-level echogenicity that is slightly higher than that of the adjacent right renal cortex. Superiorly, the liver is bounded by the diaphragm, which appears as a curvilinear bright reflector. Liver size varies greatly, but the craniocaudal span of the right lobe is typically less than 15 to 16 cm in adults. The liver is traversed by portal and hepatic veins, which are usually readily visible as anechoic structures. The hepatic arteries are generally not as prominent on grayscale ultrasound, although they are easily depicted on color Doppler imaging. The inferior vena cava (IVC) is also easily seen as it courses craniocaudally along the posterior aspect of the liver.

CIRRHOSIS AND STEATOSIS

The liver usually appears normal in early cirrhosis. As cirrhosis advances, the liver becomes increasingly coarse and nodular, although these changes may be subtle. The gross morphologic changes in cirrhotic livers that are manifest on CT and MRI, including contour nodularity and enlargement of the caudate lobe, are also visible sonographically. Surface nodularity is most easily appreciated by scanning the anterior liver margin with a high-frequency linear array transducer. Visualization of the hepatic contour is also facilitated in the presence of ascites.

Deposition of fat in the liver produces an appearance that often results in a coarse echotexture. This is usually accompanied by an increase in backscatter, which causes the liver to appear much more echogenic than the cortex of the right kidney. Fatty deposition also attenuates the sound beam, so specular reflectors such as the diaphragm and the walls of the portal veins appear less prominent. Unfortunately, these are subjective findings, and it is easy to over- or undercall steatosis sonographically. As well, because echogenicity is a relative term, it is important to be aware that steatosis may significantly alter the appearance of focal liver lesions.

INFECTION

Acute viral hepatitis may cause the portal triads to appear more echogenic than their surroundings, resulting in the so-called starry sky pattern, but the liver is often normal appearing. *Bacterial infection* may cause one or more abscesses, which often appear solid early in their course, progressing to a cystic appearance as they liquefy. *Amebic abscesses* have a similar appearance, and may be differentiated on the basis of serologic testing and the patient's clinical history. *Hepatic candidiasis*, which is most commonly encountered in immunocompromised patients, typically appears as multiple, hypoechoic foci. However, in some cases, the sonographic finding of hypoechoic lesions with a central echogenic focus may be a helpful clue to the diagnosis. Finally, *echinococcal infection* may affect the liver, resulting in cysts that vary from simple to complex.

FOCAL FATTY CHANGE AND SPARING

In addition to the diffuse pattern noted earlier in this chapter, fat may be deposited in a focal or multifocal pattern that simulates solitary or multiple echogenic masses. Unlike true space-occupying lesions, however, focal fat tends not to distort normal structures such as vessels. In problematic cases, CT or MRI can be helpful to confirm the diagnosis. Conversely, fatty livers may harbor spared areas that contain less fat than the adjacent liver parenchyma and hence appear less echogenic. Often, these appear in characteristic locations, notably in the medial segment adjacent to the portal vein and adjacent to the gallbladder. While focal sparing may simulate neoplasm, it generally has an elongated or geographic appearance. And, like focal fatty change, focal sparing tends not to distort vessels.

CYSTS

Hepatic cysts are common incidental findings on liver sonograms. Most are benign epithelial cysts that have little or no clinical significance unless they become large or infected, a rare occurrence. Although benign cysts may appear complex, the greater the number of septations or mural nodules, the higher the suspicion for biliary cystadenoma or cystadenocarcinoma, which may be further assessed with multiphasic CT or MRI. Multiple cysts are also commonly seen in patients with the adult form of polycystic kidney disease.

BENIGN HEPATIC NEOPLASMS

Cavernous hemangiomas are the most common benign liver neoplasms. They are encountered frequently as incidental findings in clinical practice. The typical lesion is small, well defined, and uniformly echogenic, without a hypoechoic halo. Often, they exhibit slightly increased through transmission because they contain multiple vascular spaces. In the setting of steatosis, however, they may appear less echogenic than the adjacent reflective liver parenchyma. In young asymptomatic patients without known or suspected malignancy, they may be safely ignored. If there is any doubt as to the diagnosis, further imaging with multiphasic CT or MRI may be warranted for confirmation. (In some centers, contrast-enhanced ultrasound is a viable alternative for sonographic evaluation of hemangiomas and other focal liver lesions).

Focal nodular hyperplasia is a benign tumor that is most often encountered in young women. The ultrasound appearance is usually nonspecific, although at times ultrasound may demonstrate a characteristic central scar. Similarly, the sonographic findings in *hepatic adenoma*, a benign neoplasm that is associated with oral contraceptive use in women, are not specific. In both instances, other imaging modalities or percutaneous biopsy are often needed to make the diagnosis.

MALIGNANT HEPATIC NEOPLASMS

Hepatocellular carcinoma (HCC) is the most common form of primary liver malignancy. It is most commonly encountered in patients with cirrhosis, particularly the alcoholic variety. The ultrasound findings range from solitary, fairly well-defined masses to subtle, diffuse infiltration, which may be echogenic, hypoechoic, or mixed. Invasion of the portal and hepatic veins is an important distinguishing feature, especially if arterial flow is demonstrated within malignant tumor thrombus using color and spectral Doppler ultrasound.

A variety of other primary malignant tumors may arise in the liver; however, their ultrasound appearance is nonspecific. Much more common are *metastatic liver lesions*, which have extremely variable ultrasound appearances that range from focal masses to subtle, diffuse alterations of liver architecture. Colorectal and other gastrointestinal cancer metastases tend to be echogenic, as do metastases from carcinoid tumors and renal cell cancers. Calcifications may be seen in tumors with a mucinous component. Lymphomatous liver involvement tends to be hypoechoic, but there is considerable overlap, and percutaneous biopsy under ultrasound or CT guidance may be required to establish a diagnosis before initiating therapy.

PORTAL HYPERTENSION

Increased portal venous pressure may be caused by intrahepatic pathology (typically cirrhosis) or extrahepatic conditions, such as portal vein or splenic vein thrombosis. As the portal venous pressure rises, flow in the main portal vein as depicted by color or spectral Doppler sonography slows and eventually reverses. There is an intermediate stage in which the portal vein is patent, but the flow rate is below the Doppler detection threshold. In these instances, grayscale sonography may demonstrate to-and-fro motion within the portal vein, avoiding the misdiagnosis of portal vein thrombosis. This pitfall highlights the role of grayscale imaging in diagnosing nonocclusive thrombosis anywhere in the portal or hepatic venous system, as small thrombi may be obscured on color flow, particularly if the gain and scale settings are incorrect.

Over time, thrombosis of the portal vein may lead to *cavernous transformation*, which refers to the development of periportal collateral vessels. These collaterals may become quite large, mimicking the portal vein itself. In some patients, collaterals that develop around the gallbladder may be a clue to the diagnosis.

With increasing portal venous pressure, flow is preferentially directed through portosystemic collaterals, which may be seen sonographically. These include the coronary vein, perigastric and perisplenic varices, and the paraumbilical veins, which course from the left portal vein to run along the falciform ligament toward the umbilicus. Indirect signs of portal hypertension include ascites and splenomegaly, which are easily depicted sonographically.

Therapy of Portal Hypertension

Historically, surgical shunts played an important part in the treatment of portal hypertension. Their role has diminished over time, but operative shunts are still sometimes performed or otherwise encountered in clinical practice. These shunts, which are surgically created anastomoses between the portal and systemic circulations, include mesocaval (portal vein to superior mesenteric vein), portocaval (portal vein to inferior vena cava), and splenorenal (splenic vein to left renal vein) shunts. With meticulous technique, it is often possible to demonstrate shunt patency.

In recent years, transjugular intrahepatic portosystemic shunts (TIPS) have assumed a greater role in the treatment of patients with portal hypertension. These shunts are placed via the transjugular route, and consist of one or more metallic stents that course from the portal vein to the right or middle hepatic vein. Because TIPS are prone to complications that lead to shunt failure, ultrasound surveillance is vital for management of these patients.

Doppler assessment of TIPS includes color flow and spectral Doppler interrogation of the shunt itself, as well as the entire portal venous system and the hepatic veins. Peak flow velocities should be measured in the main portal vein beyond the shunt orifice, at the portal vein terminus, at midshunt, and in the hepatic vein terminus of the shunt. Flow velocities typically rise toward the outflow end of the shunt. Flow in the main portal vein should be antegrade (into the liver), while flow within intrahepatic portal vein branches usually is retrograde.

Shunt thrombosis is usually easily demonstrated, but criteria for the diagnosis of stenosis remain controversial. Because stenosis decreases flow, shunt velocity has received the widest attention. A flow rate of 90 cm/s has been recommended as a normal lower limit, but this is not universally accepted. Changes from baseline also may be a clue to developing stenosis. It is therefore helpful to obtain baseline flow measurements within 1 week after shunt placement, although acoustic shadowing may impair visibility in the first few days.

BUDD-CHIARI SYNDROME

Budd-Chiari syndrome refers to the effects of obstruction to hepatic venous outflow at any level, whether caused by intrinsic (e.g., thrombi, webs) or extrinsic causes (e.g., masses obstructing the cavoatrial junction). Sonographically, flow in the hepatic veins may be dampened, reversed, or absent. As well, grayscale ultrasound may demonstrate enlargement of the caudate lobe and signs of associated portal venous hypertension, such as ascites and splenomegaly. Similarly, bone marrow transplant and other patients with *hepatic venoocclusive disease* may show diminished portal venous flow, although sonography is insensitive for detection of this condition.

Patients with right heart dysfunction may have large hepatic veins with increased pulsatility. Increased pulsatility is also sometimes demonstrated in the portal vein in these patients, although this is often a normal finding in young individuals. Conversely, hepatic vein flow may be dampened or monophasic in patients with cirrhosis.

Portal Venous Gas

Gas in the portal venous system almost always results from extrahepatic pathology. Gas in the portal vein was formerly thought to be a premorbid condition associated with gastrointestinal tract necrosis, but it also may occur in patients with benign intestinal pneumatosis. On ultrasound, portal vein gas appears as bright echoes that move in the direction of blood flow. They may be distinguished from red cell clumps, which are a clinically insignificant finding, by the presence of sharp spikes in the portal vein spectral Doppler tracing.

HEPATIC TRANSPLANTATION

Ultrasound plays a central role in the evaluation of patients after whole and partial liver transplants. Because the hepatic artery assumes the primary role in supplying blood to the liver following transplantation, verification of arterial patency is the most important part of the sonogram. Hepatic arterial thrombosis is an early complication that has a high mortality rate. Signs of hepatic arterial thrombosis include absent flow in the hepatic artery and its intrahepatic branches, although intrahepatic flow may be demonstrated in the presence of collaterals, especially in children.

Hepatic arterial stenosis may be an early or late complication. An attempt should be made to image the anastomosis between the donor and recipient hepatic arteries directly. A perianastomotic velocity rise (more than 200 cm/s) and turbulence are considered suspicious, especially in the setting of declining hepatic function. Often, however, the anastomosis cannot be visualized because of overlying bowel gas and dressings. Indirect signs of stenosis include a decrease in the resistive index within intrahepatic arterial branches to less than 0.5. Decreased echogenicity within the liver parenchyma and along the bile ducts is worrisome for necrosis.

In addition to the hepatic arterial system, the postoperative scan should evaluate the portal vein and IVC to look for velocity gradients or luminal narrowing at their respective anastomoses. Surveillance for hematomas, bilomas, seromas, and abscesses is also essential. Finally, although rejection is an important clinical concern, ultrasound plays little role in its diagnosis.

GALLBLADDER

NORMAL, CHOLELITHIASIS, AND SLUDGE

The gallbladder typically lies in the right upper quadrant, extending obliquely from the interlobar fissure, although its position varies considerably. Anatomic variants include prehepatic and intrahepatic locations; occasionally, the gallbladder may extend through the foramen of Winslow into the lesser sac. Variations in size and configuration are even more frequent, and folds or kinks are seen commonly. The normal gallbladder usually measures no more than 4 to 5 cm in transverse diameter. Bile is anechoic or nearly so, accounting for the echolucent appearance of the normal gallbladder on grayscale ultrasound. An echogenic wall that measures up to 3 mm in thickness bounds the gallbladder. Because the gallbladder contracts after a meal, biliary sonography is best performed after a fast. Contraction makes it more difficult to visualize calculi and other pathology, and may lead to artifactual wall thickening.

Sonography is a mainstay in the noninvasive diagnosis of *cholelithiasis*. Gallstones typically appear as dependent echogenic structures that exhibit acoustic shadowing, although the latter sign may not be present if the scanning frequency is too low or the focal zone is not set correctly. Most gallstones consist primarily of cholesterol, with a minority consisting of calcium bilirubinate. Minute calculi, also called "biliary sand," may not exhibit shadowing unless they are clumped. Turning the patient to move the stones toward the fundus facilitates this. Even if the gallbladder appears normal with the patient in the supine position, rotating the patient into the left lateral decubitus or prone-oblique position may cause stones hidden in the neck to move into the body or fundus, where they are more readily identified.

As the number of calculi increases, the residual lumen becomes less apparent, and it may be very difficult to distinguish the stone-filled gallbladder from adjacent structures. The so-called wall-echo-shadow sign is often helpful to distinguish a contracted gallbladder filled with stones from bowel. This sign comprises two echogenic lines (the gallbladder wall and the anterior margin of the calculi) separated by a thin hypoechoic layer. Care must be taken not to confuse this sign with mural calcification (porcelain gallbladder) or gallbladder wall air (emphysematous cholecystitis), neither of which possesses the trilayered appearance.

The term *gallbladder sludge* refers to viscous material that consists of minute bile crystals. Sludge is a common incidental finding in hospitalized patients and usually is not clinically significant. Sonographically, sludge appears as a dependent layer of medium-level echogenicity that slowly changes position as the patient moves. Occasionally, however, sludge may form aggregates (so-called tumefactive sludge or sludge balls) that have a mass-like appearance. As with layering sludge, these aggregates move or alter their configuration as the patient's position changes.

CHOLECYSTITIS

Acute cholecystitis is usually caused by obstruction of the gallbladder neck by stones, which leads to progressive inflammation of the gallbladder wall. If left untreated, the changes may progress to frank gangrene. Patients with acute cholecystitis typically present with right upper quadrant pain, fever, nausea, and vomiting, but these symptoms may be encountered in various

TABLE 63-1 Etiology of Sonographic Gallbladder Wall Thickening

Acute cholecystitis
Chronic cholecystitis
Gallbladder carcinoma
Adenomyomatosis
Hepatic, cardiac, or renal dysfunction
Hypoproteinemia
Sepsis
Portal hypertension

other conditions, including acute pyelonephritis and pancreatitis.

The most sensitive sonographic findings in patients with acute cholecystitis are gallstones and tenderness over the gallbladder, the sonographic Murphy sign. In eliciting this sign, it is important to have the patient indicate if they experience pain as the transducer is moved over the right upper quadrant, rather than simply asking if pressing on their abdomen causes discomfort. As well, the sonographic Murphy sign may be diminished or absent if the patient has received analgesic medication shortly before the sonogram. Other less specific signs of acute cholecystitis include pericholecystic fluid and gallbladder wall thickening. The latter is particularly nonspecific, as it is associated with a broad range of conditions (Table 63-1).

Gangrenous cholecystitis, which may lead to gallbladder perforation and sepsis, is a particularly dire complication of acute inflammation. As inflammation and necrosis progress, the gallbladder mucosa detaches and is visualized as linear intraluminal echoes that parallel the wall. Microperforations are usually not perceptible, but frank perforation may be seen as a discontinuity of the gallbladder wall, with or without a focal fluid collection. Interestingly, patients with perforation may report a sudden improvement in their pain as the increased luminal pressure is relieved.

Emphysematous cholecystitis is another form of acute inflammation that is associated with high morbidity and mortality. It is often associated with diabetes, and its hallmark is the presence of infection with gas-forming organisms in the gallbladder wall. Gas may be visible sonographically as high-level echoes associated with ringdown artifacts, which appear as diminishing echo trains deep to the gas.

As its name implies, *acalculous cholecystitis* is characterized by inflammation in the absence of gallbladder calculi. It is most often encountered in hospitalized patients with serious illnesses that may limit evaluation for the sonographic Murphy sign, which is the most specific finding in the intensive care unit patient population. Other signs, including gallbladder distension and wall thickening, are nonspecific. Therefore, percutaneous cholecystostomy is sometimes recommended in septic patients with at least one of these sonographic signs and no other evident etiology.

ADENOMYOMATOSIS AND CHOLESTEROLOSIS

Adenomyomatosis and cholesterolosis comprise the so-called hyperplastic cholecystoses. *Adenomyomatosis* is a benign condition of uncertain etiology that is characterized by focal or diffuse mural hyperplasia and the formation of intramural diverticula that are termed Rokitansky-Aschoff sinuses. The sinuses often contain minute calculi that produce comet-tail artifacts which are V-shaped echoes that are similar to the ringdown artifacts associated with gas bubbles. The segmental form of adenomyomatosis causes constriction of the gallbladder contour. The focal form of adenomyomatosis, which results in a mass-like appearance at the gallbladder fundus, may be difficult to distinguish sonographically from gallbladder carcinoma.

Cholesterolosis is characterized by multiple fatty deposits within the lamina propria of the gallbladder wall that result in a gross appearance termed strawberry gallbladder. Sonographically, cholesterolosis appears as multiple echogenic foci with comet-tail artifacts within the gallbladder wall. Unlike adenomyomatosis, however, there is no wall thickening.

POLYPS AND GALLBLADDER CARCINOMA

Polyps are frequently discovered incidentally at gallbladder sonography. They usually can be readily distinguished from stones by their nondependent, fixed position and lack of acoustic shadowing, although some calculi that are adherent to the gallbladder wall may have a similar appearance. Approximately 90% of gallbladder polyps are cholesterol polyps that are of no clinical significance. The remaining 10% are adenomas, which may have some malignant potential. Although it is difficult to distinguish small cholesterol polyps from adenomatous polyps, lesions that measure less than 10 mm do not require follow-up or surgery unless they enlarge over time.

Gallbladder carcinoma is most often seen in elderly women. It is associated with cholelithiasis, chronic gallbladder infection, and porcelain gallbladder. Signs and symptoms are nonspecific. At ultrasound, gallbladder cancer presents as a hypoechoic mass that occupies part or all of the lumen, or as focal or diffuse wall thickening that mimics chronic cholecystitis. Invasion of the contiguous liver is a frequent associated finding. The focal form of gallbladder carcinoma may be impossible to distinguish sonographically from metastases to the gallbladder.

BILE DUCTS

NORMAL APPEARANCE

Normal intrahepatic bile ducts appear as tubular structures that measure 1 to 2 mm in diameter and accompany portal vein branches. Ducts from the right and left lobes converge at the porta hepatis to form the right and left hepatic ducts, which unite to form the common hepatic duct. It joins the cystic duct at a variable distance from its origin to form the common bile duct, which courses caudally and obliquely through or behind the pancreatic head to enter the duodenum. The cystic duct is not usually visualized as a separate structure, but the common hepatic and common bile ducts are readily identified in almost every patient owing to their fixed relationship to the portal vein and the hepatic artery.

Much has been written about the diameter of the common duct. However, as a rule of thumb, it should not measure more than 6 mm in patients younger than 60 years. There is some evidence to suggest that the duct dilates with advancing age, and an upper limit of 8 to 9 mm may be appropriate for patients older than 80 years. Whether the common duct enlarges following cholecystectomy is more controversial, although some studies suggest that this does occur.

BILIARY DILATION AND OBSTRUCTION

The hallmark of biliary obstruction from any cause is dilation of the segments that lie proximal to the obstructing process. For example, a mass that fortuitously obstructs the right hepatic duct will only result in right-sided dilation, but a stone in the distal common duct will cause intrahepatic and extrahepatic enlargement. Early intrahepatic dilation may be difficult to distinguish from normal, and dilated intrahepatic arterial branches may mimic dilated bile ducts if color Doppler sonography is not used. With progressive dilation, intrahepatic bile ducts become increasingly conspicuous as tortuous tubular structures that follow the portal veins, an appearance that has been termed the "too many tubes" sign. The dilated ducts also frequently exhibit posterior acoustic enhancement.

Dilation of the extrahepatic duct is more sensitive for obstruction below the hepatic duct confluence. As already noted, the diagnosis depends on distinguishing a normal from a dilated common duct, which can be challenging in elderly patients or in individuals who are post cholecystectomy. In equivocal cases, correlation with laboratory indices of biliary obstruction may be helpful.

If the common duct is dilated, an effort should be made to identify the obstructing process. Choledocholithiasis may be diagnosed sonographically in as many as 80% to 90% of patients with common duct stones. The appearance of common duct calculi is similar to that of stones in the gallbladder. Placing the patient in the Trendelenburg position, which causes distal stones to move proximally, may enhance visualization.

Neoplastic causes of biliary obstruction, including distal cholangiocarcinomas and pancreatic carcinomas, appear as hypoechoic masses, although conventional ultrasound usually does not play a major role in establishing the diagnosis. (On the other hand, endoscopic sonography is often extremely helpful in this regard.) Common duct strictures and ampullary carcinomas are usually not visible sonographically.

OTHER BILE DUCT CONDITIONS

Caroli disease is a rare condition that has an autosomal recessive inheritance and is associated with infantile polycystic kidney disease and congenital hepatic fibrosis. Patients are prone to developing recurrent bacterial infections, abscesses, and intrahepatic biliary stones, and also have an increased risk of cholangiocarcinomas. Ultrasound usually reveals multiple fusiform or saccular dilations of intrahepatic bile ducts that are bridged by fibrovascular bundles.

Pneumobilia, which refers to the presence of gas within the bile ducts, is most often encountered in patients with biliary stents, following sphincterotomy, or after surgical biliary-enteric anastomoses. Regardless of the etiology, pneumobilia appears as linear bands of high echogenicity that follow the ductal system and are associated with acoustic shadowing and ringdown artifacts. In patients with biliary stents, the stent may be appreciated as a tubular echogenic structure within the duct lumen.

AIDS cholangiopathy refers to the syndrome of biliary infection and obstruction in patients with AIDS, usually secondary to cryptosporidium, cytomegalovirus, or mycobacterium avium-intracellulare. Ultrasound findings include wall thickening that involves the gallbladder and bile ducts as well as ductal dilation. In some patients, the edematous papilla of Vater appears as an echogenic focus at the distal common bile duct.

SPLEEN

NORMAL APPEARANCE

The spleen is visualized in the left upper quadrant using a coronal approach. It is slightly more echogenic than the liver, although direct comparison of the echogenicity of the two organs is generally not possible unless the left lobe extends far to the left, as occasionally occurs as a normal variant or in the setting of hepatomegaly. In such cases, the relatively hypoechoic liver may simulate a left subphrenic collection. The spleen has a fairly fine-grained echotexture. Unlike the liver, vessels of the spleen are usually not prominent features. In adults, the spleen usually measures no more than 13 cm in length.

SPLENOMEGALY

The spleen may become enlarged in a wide variety of disorders, hence the ultrasound finding of an enlarged spleen is generally nonspecific. However, massive splenomegaly is most often associated with myelofibrosis, a condition in which the bone marrow is replaced by fibrous tissue, resulting in extramedullary hematopoiesis within the spleen. Splenic enlargement is also seen in hematologic conditions such as lymphoma and leukemia, as well as in infectious mononucleosis.

FOCAL SPLENIC LESIONS

Focal lesions are classified as cystic or solid. Cystic splenic lesions include congenital cysts, which are lined by epithelium, and pseudocysts that develop because of infection, trauma, or acute pancreatitis. Whatever their etiology, splenic cysts appear as anechoic or hypoechoic masses with increased through transmission and variable internal echoes. Splenic abscesses have a similar appearance, although they are usually less well defined than other cysts. Lymphangiomas, which are more often seen in children than adults, are rare tumors that are usually cystic, with or without internal septations or debris.

Splenic hemangiomas are said to be relatively common at autopsy, but are rarely encountered sonographically. They may occur in isolation or as part of the Klippel-Trénaunay syndrome. Hemangiomas have sonographic appearances that range from echogenic, similar to hemangiomas in the liver, to hypoechoic or mixed. Metastases to the spleen, which occur most often in patients with malignant melanoma or lymphoma, are typically hypoechoic, and are seen more commonly.

PANCREAS

NORMAL ANATOMY AND APPEARANCE

The pancreas lies obliquely in the retroperitoneum, extending from the duodenal sweep to the splenic hilum. It is divided into four portions—head and uncinate process, neck, body, and tail—that blend imperceptibly with each other and are demarcated chiefly by their relationship to adjacent structures. The splenic vein, which lies deep to the body and tail, is the easiest landmark to identify sonographically, and is often a good starting point for pancreatic sonography. However, it is vital to remember that an axial sonogram that encompasses the splenic vein only includes a portion of the pancreas and that complete visualization requires considerable angulation and movement of the transducer.

The pancreatic duct is most readily identified in the pancreatic body, where its walls lie at right angles to the insonating beam. With high-frequency transducers, the duct appears as thin parallel echogenic lines that course through the pancreatic parenchyma. Its normal diameter is 3 mm or less in the head; the duct tapers toward the body and tail. Pancreas divisum, a congenital abnormality in which the dorsal and ventral pancreatic buds fail to fuse during development, results in separate dorsal and ventral ducts, which may be seen sonographically with meticulous technique.

The echogenicity of the normal pancreas is usually greater than or equal to that of the overlying left hepatic lobe. With advancing age, fatty infiltration of the pancreas may increase its echogenicity considerably, making it very difficult to distinguish from peripancreatic fat. Complete fatty replacement is also seen in patients with cystic fibrosis. Published values for the AP dimension of the normal pancreas vary, but the head usually measures no more than approximately 2.5 cm.

ACUTE PANCREATITIS

Sonography is rarely the primary imaging modality used in patients with acute pancreatitis because of its insensitivity to early changes and complications such as pancreatic necrosis and distant pseudocysts. However, ultrasound is often performed to evaluate patients who present with nonspecific upper abdominal pain or to diagnose associated conditions such as gallstones. In the acute phase, the pancreas becomes edematous and its echogenicity diminishes. Over time, intrapancreatic and peripancreatic fluid collections develop; these are usually complex in appearance, and may contain shadowing gas if they become infected. Pancreatic pseudocysts, which are postinflammatory collections that are bounded by a fibrous, nonepithelialized wall, are usually discovered at CT, but may be monitored sonographically. As well, ultrasound is often helpful to guide percutaneous placement of drainage catheters. Other complications that may be seen sonographically include pseudoaneurysms affecting the hepatic artery and other regional vessels and splenic vein thrombosis.

CHRONIC PANCREATITIS

Repeated bouts of pancreatitis may result in progressive, irreversible replacement of the pancreas by fibrous tissue, with an associated decline in pancreatic function. The gland may decrease in size, although this change is often difficult to detect sonographically. Pancreatic echogenicity increases as the parenchyma is replaced by fat and fibrosis, but this may also be seen with fatty replacement that occurs with advancing age. Pancreatic echotexture becomes increasingly heterogeneous and ductal dilation is often observed.

Intraductal or parenchymal pancreatic calcifications are the most important distinguishing ultrasound feature. Like calcifications elsewhere, they appear as small, echogenic foci that are accompanied by acoustic shadowing. However, the latter finding may be subtle, and high-frequency imaging with close attention to focal zone placement and other settings is critical.

CYSTIC PANCREATIC MASSES

True pancreatic cysts are uncommon, but may be seen in patients with adult polycystic kidney disease. Most cysts are acquired, and include serous cystadenomas, mucinous cystadenomas, and intraductal papillary mucinous neoplasms. Serous cystadenomas, which are benign tumors that are most common in women in the sixth or seventh decade of life, are often composed of multiple minute cysts that have a solid aggregate appearance. A central scar containing calcifications may be present.

In contrast, mucinous tumors have a malignant potential. Sonographically, they appear as cystic masses of varying complexity that do not communicate with the ductal system. They are also more common in women. The term intraductal papillary mucinous neoplasm is reserved for mucin-producing tumors that involve the main pancreatic duct, its side branches, or both. Conventional ultrasound usually plays little role in the workup of cystic tumors. However, endoscopic sonography is valuable to characterize their internal architecture, gauge their relationship to adjacent vessels and organs, and guide placement of sampling needles.

SOLID PANCREATIC MASSES

As with cystic masses, conventional ultrasound is much less important than endoscopic sonography for the detection and staging of solid pancreatic tumors. Approximately 90% are adenocarcinomas, with endocrine and other primary and secondary tumors comprising the remainder. The most common sonographic appearance is a hypoechoic mass, which may obstruct the pancreatic duct and/or the common bile duct, depending on its location. If ultrasound is the initial imaging modality, it is important to search for signs of unresectability, such as invasion and encasement of major regional vessels and liver metastases.

PANCREATIC TRANSPLANTS

Pancreatic transplantation is most often performed in diabetic patients, often in conjunction with a simultaneous or prior renal transplant. The right lower quadrant is the most frequent site of placement. Initially, bladder drainage via a surgical anastomosis between the pancreaticoduodenal graft and the bladder was the predominant technique. In recent years, enteric drainage, in which the donor duodenal segment is attached to a recipient small bowel loop, has become more popular.

The goal of pancreatic transplant sonography is to look for peripancreatic fluid collections, evaluate the allograft parenchyma, and exclude thrombosis in the transplant vasculature. Although imaging may be compromised by overlying bowel, an attempt should be made to demonstrate intrapancreatic venous and arterial flow, as well as assess the supplying arteries and draining veins. In the bladder drainage technique, both the donor arteries and veins are anastomosed to the recipient iliac vessels; in the enteric drainage procedure, venous drainage is usually to the recipient superior mesenteric vein.

Ultrasound has a limited role in the diagnosis of rejection, as transplant pancreatitis and vascular compromise may have a similar appearance. In patients with transplant dysfunction in whom the diagnosis is in doubt, ultrasound-guided percutaneous biopsy may be performed.

ADRENAL GLANDS

In adults, CT and MRI are usually preferred to evaluate patients with known or suspected adrenal pathology. It is often challenging to visualize the adrenal glands sonographically, particularly on the left side. The normal adrenal glands, which lie superomedial to the upper renal poles, typically appear hypoechoic, with an echogenic core that represents the medulla.

Adrenal masses often have a nonspecific ultrasound appearance, although it should be possible to diagnose cysts with a high degree of confidence. Similarly, the finding of a highly echogenic mass suggests fat content in a myelolipoma, but confirmation with CT or MRI is recommended. Other masses, including adenomas, pheochromocytomas, and metastases, have a variable ultrasound presentation, ranging from hypoechoic to mixed. In general, however, the concern for malignancy is higher in large heterogeneous masses.

KIDNEYS, URETERS, AND BLADDER

NORMAL ANATOMY AND APPEARANCE

The kidneys are easily visualized sonographically using a coronal or an anterior approach, although a posterior vantage point may be advantageous in patients with copious bowel gas. In adults, they measure approximately 9 to 13 cm in length, have a typical bean-like shape, and are well defined, usually with little or no lobulation. Normal variants include the "dromedary hump," an apparent bulge in the left kidney caused by impression from the adjacent spleen, the hypertrophied column of Bertin, invagination of cortical tissue between renal pyramids, and persistent fetal lobation, fine indentations along the surface demarcating renal lobes. Other more striking congenital anomalies that may be visible with ultrasound are agenesis, ectopia, and horseshoe kidney.

On ultrasound, normal kidneys have three components: the echogenic central sinus, which includes the collecting systems, vessels, and other supporting tissues, hypoechoic pyramids, and the intermediate echogenicity cortex. The echogenicity of the normal cortex is less than or equal to that of the adjacent right hepatic lobe, an appearance that is accentuated in the presence of hepatic steatosis.

The collecting systems may be mildly distended in the absence of obstruction, particularly if the bladder is distended or if the patient has been hydrated. The normal ureters are rarely visualized. The urine-filled bladder is readily identified as an anechoic structure in the pelvic midline. Wall thickness is usually no more than approximately 5 mm, but varies with the degree of distension. Flow of urine from the ureters into the bladder is often visible as ureteral jets, which may be seen on grayscale or color Doppler imaging. They are thought to result from differences in specific gravity, and are helpful to verify gross ureteral patency.

DIFFUSE RENAL CONDITIONS

Many conditions that affect the kidneys reverse the normal relationship between the renal cortex and the adjacent right hepatic lobe, causing the kidneys to appear echogenic. Cortical echogenicity is particularly increased in certain conditions, including AIDS nephropathy, amyloidosis, and lupus nephritis. However, this appearance, which some term *medical renal disease,* is therefore nonspecific, and biopsy is often required for a definitive diagnosis.

Ultrasound and other imaging modalities usually play little role in patients with uncomplicated *bacterial pyelonephritis*, as management may be guided clinically. The kidneys are usually normal in appearance sonographically, although they may be edematous, and power Doppler interrogation may demonstrate areas of hypoperfusion. In refractory cases, ultrasound is sometimes helpful to detect renal abscesses and guide percutaneous sampling. As well, sonography may suggest the diagnosis of *emphysematous pyelonephritis* in diabetic patients by demonstrating gas within the renal parenchyma or collecting system.

Nephrocalcinosis, which encompasses conditions that result in calcium deposition within the kidneys, is classified as medullary, cortical, or mixed, and has a variety of causes (Table 63-2). The ultrasound appearance of these deposits ranges from faint areas of slightly increased echogenicity to highly reflective aggregates with strong acoustic shadowing. *Medullary sponge kidney*, a developmental condition that is characterized by cystic dilatation of the collecting ducts within one or more medullary pyramids, may have a similar appearance, even in the absence of calculi.

UROLITHIASIS

The sensitivity of ultrasound for detecting stones in the urinary tract depends on a number of factors, including

TABLE 63-2 Causes of Nephrocalcinosis

Medullary	Hypervitaminosis D
	Medullary sponge kidney
	Metastatic carcinoma to bone
	Milk alkali syndrome
	Multiple myeloma
	Primary hyperparathyroidism
	Renal tubular acidosis
	Sarcoidosis
Cortical	Acute cortical necrosis
	Alport syndrome
	Chronic membranous glomerulonephritis
	Congenital oxalosis

the size, location, and composition of the calculus; the patient's body habitus; and the equipment used. The diagnosis rests on the demonstration of an echogenic focus with posterior acoustic shadowing. Unfortunately, the latter may be absent if the stone does not block the ultrasound beam sufficiently because it is too small, the frequency is too low, or the focal zone is set incorrectly. Conversely, other structures in the kidneys, such as calcified vessels, may mimic calculi. In recent years, a color Doppler finding called the twinkling artifact has been applied successfully. This artifact, which appears as a band of alternating color deep to a stone, is related to its surface roughness. Because it improves sensitivity, color Doppler interrogation should be performed routinely when urinary calculi are suspected.

In women with suspected distal ureteral calculi, sensitivity and specificity may be enhanced by endovaginal sonography, which readily visualizes the uretrovesical junctions. In addition, if a bladder calculus is demonstrated via the transabdominal or endovaginal route, turning the patient to one side will cause the stone to move if it is lying freely within the bladder lumen.

OBSTRUCTIVE UROPATHY

Ultrasound is often performed to exclude obstruction in the setting of acute renal dysfunction. While most such examinations are noncontributory (most patients with acute renal failure do not have obstructed ureters), grayscale sonography is certainly capable of demonstrating hydronephrosis when obstruction is present. (The value of the arterial resistive index in determining the presence and severity of ureteral obstruction remains controversial.)

Dilation may be classified as mild, moderate, or severe, depending on the degree of distension of the collecting system and pelvis. As the obstructed collecting system expands, the overlying parenchyma thins, although this is usually a chronic finding. As noted earlier in the chapter, mild dilation may be seen in normal patients with a distended bladder or following aggressive hydration; however, this is usually readily apparent. In any patient with unilateral or bilateral hydronephrosis, an attempt should be made to identify the level and cause of obstruction. Clearly, the likelihood of success depends on the clinical setting, but it should be possible to at least determine if the proximal ureter is dilated in most patients.

Because hydronephrosis predisposes the patient to infection, the sonologist should search for debris within the dilated collecting system. This typically appears as layering material of medium echogenicity that is similar to gallbladder sludge. This finding is highly suspicious for pyonephrosis, although hemorrhagic debris may have a similar appearance. In addition, immunocompromised patients may develop intraluminal mycetomas that appear as echogenic, nonshadowing filling defects.

CYSTIC RENAL MASSES

Renal cysts are exceedingly common incidental findings in adults with no history of renal disease, and it is vital to distinguish those that do not need follow-up from those that require further imaging with CT or MRI. This determination rests on ultrasound's ability to demonstrate solid elements (septations, mural nodules, or calcifications) within cysts. To a large extent, this mirrors categorization of cysts using the Bosniak classification, which is widely used to guide clinical management of patients with complex renal cysts. However, some features in this classification system, notably septal and mural enhancement, cannot be reliably assessed with grayscale and color/power Doppler sonography, and care should be taken when assigning Bosniak category based solely on these techniques. (The availability of contrast-enhanced ultrasound will likely change this.)

Masses that meet all the sonographic criteria for simple cysts (Table 63-3) need no follow-up or intervention, unless they are symptomatic because of their size or location. Complex cysts present a range of appearances, which include septations, calcifications, mural nodules, and amorphous echoes. Cysts with hairline septations or slight calcification also need no follow-up. With increasing complexity, further evaluation with CT or MRI is usually warranted.

Because of their central location within the kidney, multiple *parapelvic cysts* may be mistaken for a dilated collecting system. Differentiation depends on demonstrating interconnection between the fluid-filled components in the latter condition. *Calyceal diverticula*, which are lined by transitional epithelium and communicate with a calyx or the renal pelvis, also present a diagnostic challenge. The finding of mobile, dependent echoes representing milk of calcium strongly suggests the diagnosis.

Multilocular cystic nephroma is an uncommon cystic mass that occurs in very young children and in adults between 40 and 60 years. The ultrasound appearance is that of a highly complex cystic mass that

TABLE 63-3 Sonographic Signs of a Simple Cyst

Anechoic
Good through transmission
Very thin, sharply defined wall
Round shape

cannot be reliably distinguished from other complex cysts, and excision is often required for a definitive diagnosis.

SOLID RENAL MASSES

Renal cell carcinoma is the most common solid renal tumor in adults. It most frequently presents in the fifth to seventh decade of life, and has an overall 5-year survival of approximately 60%. Clear cell adenocarcinomas predominate, with papillary, chromophobe, and other subtypes occurring less frequently. Predisposing conditions include von Hippel-Lindau disease and hereditary papillary renal cancer, as well as acquired renal cystic disease in dialysis patients.

At ultrasound, renal cell carcinomas usually appear iso- or hypoechoic to the renal cortex. Small lesions tend to be higher in echogenicity. When encountered incidentally, it is important to search for local extension into the perinephric fat, regional adenopathy, or thrombus within the ipsilateral vein or IVC. Doppler sonography may be helpful to distinguish bland from tumor thrombus by demonstrating arterial flow within it.

Angiomyolipomas are composed of blood vessels, smooth muscle, and fat in variable proportion. Lesions with high fat content tend to appear echogenic on ultrasound, particularly when they are small, but reliable differentiation from renal cell carcinoma is often problematic without CT or MRI. The presence of acoustic shadowing suggests fat in an angiomyolipoma, however.

Other primary and metastatic renal neoplasms, including *transitional cell carcinomas*, have a nonspecific ultrasound appearance, and further imaging or biopsy may be required to establish the diagnosis. *Renal lymphoma* is usually secondary, and may cause hypoechoic masses that mimic cysts. However, the degree of through transmission tends to be less than would be expected for a cyst of equivalent size.

POLYCYSTIC AND END-STAGE KIDNEYS

Adult polycystic kidney disease is an autosomal dominant condition that is characterized by replacement of the kidneys by innumerable cysts of varying size. The kidneys are frequently too large to encompass on a single sonographic image unless extended field-of-view techniques are employed, measuring 20 cm or more craniocaudally. The primary role of sonography is to detect complications such as cyst infection or hemorrhage and renal cell carcinomas. Unfortunately, this can be exceedingly difficult owing to the size of the kidneys and the multiplicity of cysts. As in other cysts, mural nodules and thick septations are worrisome. Contrast-enhanced sonography may be helpful in this regard.

No matter what the etiology, chronic renal failure tends to produce a common sonographic appearance in which the kidneys become small and echogenic. Often termed *end-stage kidneys*, they may be difficult or impossible to detect, and exclusion of solid masses within them may not be feasible sonographically.

RENAL VASCULAR CONDITIONS

Verification of gross renal vein patency is usually easily accomplished with color and spectral Doppler ultrasound, although demonstration of nonocclusive thrombi may be challenging, particularly in the longer left renal vein. Ultrasound is also able to detect postbiopsy arteriovenous fistulas and pseudoaneurysms in selected patients.

The role of sonography in the workup of patients with suspected renovascular hypertension is controversial. Some centers tend to reserve ultrasound for patients who cannot undergo contrast-enhanced CT or MRI because of renal failure, on the premise that stenotic accessory renal arteries may be missed sonographically. In other labs, ultrasound is a first-line investigation in hypertensive patients.

Two classes of signs of hemodynamically significant renal artery stenosis have been described. The first group comprises findings within the intrarenal arteries, which can be visualized and interrogated in most patients. These findings include alterations of the normal waveform to produce a so-called tardus-parvus pattern, which refers to a decreased amplitude and rounded configuration of the waveforms.

The second group of signs requires direct visualization of the stenosis, which is more challenging technically, but these signs are more widely accepted. A peak systolic velocity of 200 cm/s is often used as the cutoff for diagnosing significant stenosis. This is combined with calculation of the ratio of the peak systolic velocity in the renal artery to the peak systolic velocity in the proximal abdominal aorta, with 3.5 or more indicating significant stenosis.

RENAL TRANSPLANTATION

The transplanted kidney is essentially identical in appearance to the normal native kidney on ultrasound, although it is usually better seen because of its superficial location. Grayscale imaging is done initially to detect complications that may compromise renal function or transplant survival, including hydronephrosis and adjacent fluid collections. The latter, which include urinomas, hematomas, seromas, and abscesses, have a nonspecific appearance, although complexity suggests hemorrhage or infection. Sterile collections may be significant if they are large and compress the transplant ureter sufficiently to cause obstruction.

Doppler ultrasound is an important part of the post-transplant examination. Power and color Doppler imaging show an arborized flow pattern that extends to the renal capsule. Spectral interrogation of the interlobar and segmental arteries shows a low medium-resistance pattern with a resistive index of 0.8 or lower.

Timely detection of renal arterial or venous thrombosis is mandatory to avoid graft loss. The main renal artery and vein should be followed to their anastomoses with the iliac vessels, and care should be taken to image accessory arteries. Arterial thrombosis is usually readily apparent, but the diagnosis of renal vein thrombosis may be more challenging. The finding of a very high resistive index (1.0) or reversed diastolic flow is a clue to its presence, although this finding is also seen in patients with acute tubular necrosis, severe rejection, or allograft compression.

The diagnosis of renal artery stenosis is based on the demonstration of high-velocity turbulent flow just beyond the anastomosis, which is the most frequent site of involvement. A peak systolic velocity of 300 cm/s has been recommended as a threshold. The ratio of the velocity in the main renal artery to the velocity in the iliac artery proximal to the anastomosis is also used in some centers, with 2.0 as a suggested cutoff.

Ultrasound is invaluable to guide needle placement for renal transplant biopsy, and it is also helpful to demonstrate biopsy-related complications, including extrarenal flow along the needle track and arteriovenous fistula. The latter often appears as a focal zone of random color assignment within the kidney; spectral Doppler interrogation shows high-velocity turbulent flow.

URINARY BLADDER

OBSTRUCTION, MASSES, AND MISCELLANEOUS CONDITIONS

Because of its fluid content, the urinary bladder is ideally suited to ultrasound evaluation. Despite this, sonography is not often used to detect bladder masses. Nevertheless, bladder tumors, including benign papillomas, transitional cell carcinomas, and squamous cell carcinomas, may be visualized sonographically as masses that project into the bladder lumen. The finding of flow within the lesion with color and spectral Doppler imaging increases the level of suspicion, although cystoscopy is required for a definitive diagnosis. In patients with hematuria, blood clots within the bladder lumen may mimic masses—turning the patient to elicit movement usually differentiates them.

In patients with suspected outlet obstruction, ultrasound is helpful to estimate the volume of the bladder prior to and after voiding. Many ultrasound scanners include software that computes the bladder volume based on linear measurements obtained in three orthogonal planes. Sonography is also helpful to verify the position of transurethral and suprapubic catheters. *Diverticula*, outpouchings of the bladder wall, are often encountered incidentally. Most are acquired in patients with bladder outlet obstruction.

Cystitis has a nonspecific ultrasound appearance that is characterized by focal or diffuse mural thickening. As in the gallbladder, the presence of shadowing echogenic foci within the wall of the bladder suggests emphysematous cystitis, which is often associated with diabetes. *Fungus balls* may also be seen in patients with diabetes or compromised immune systems.

AORTA, IVC, AND RETROPERITONEUM

The abdominal aorta can be visualized in most patients using an anterior or a coronal approach. Normally, it is smooth in contour and tapers craniocaudally. Spectral Doppler interrogation usually demonstrates a high-resistance waveform.

The primary role of ultrasound is to detect and measure abdominal aortic aneurysms (AAA), which are defined as an outer aortic AP diameter of 3 cm or more. Most are atherosclerotic, with inflammatory and mycotic aneurysms comprising a small minority. Risk factors for atherosclerotic AAA include gender (male > female), smoking, and age. When measuring AAA, care must be taken not to image the aorta obliquely. The ideal plane for measurement of the AP diameter of an aneurysm lies perpendicular to its long axis, which may not parallel the sagittal plane of the patient if the aorta is tortuous.

The relationship of the aneurysm to the renal arteries should be determined, and the presence of any mural thrombus noted. The proximal iliac arteries should be imaged for extension below the bifurcation. Although CT is usually preferred over ultrasound in patients with suspected AAA rupture, sonography may demonstrate retroperitoneal or intraperitoneal fluid. The role of sonography in evaluating patients following endostent placement has yet to be defined, but early studies suggest that contrast-enhanced ultrasound may be helpful.

Abdominal aortic dissections are more often evaluated with CT than ultrasound, in part because identification of the origin of the dissection, which usually is in the chest, is mandatory to guide management. Hypertension is an important risk factor. On ultrasound, dissection appears as curvilinear structure representing the intimal flap within the aortic lumen. Color flow imaging is helpful to demonstrate flow in the false and true lumens and to determine their relationship to the splanchnic and renal vessels.

The proximal (hepatic) segment of the IVC should be included in every complete abdominal sonogram. Extension of thrombi from the renal veins may be evident in patients with renal cell carcinoma, and IVC filters should be assessed for clot cephalad to them. Visibility of the IVC below the renal veins is variable, depending on the patient's body habitus and the amount of overlying bowel gas.

Most retroperitoneal masses and collections are best imaged with CT or MRI. However, retroperitoneal adenopathy, whether due to lymphoma, metastatic disease, or any other cause, may be visible sonographically, particularly in the upper abdomen. The enlarged lymph nodes are typically hypoechoic, and they may be so confluent that measurement of individual nodes cannot be performed.

GI TRACT AND APPENDIX

Although a detailed description of anatomy is beyond the scope of this chapter, in general, the GI tract has a multilayered "signature" of alternating echogenic and echopenic bands that is common to all segments. Mural thickness and configuration vary depending on the segment that is being examined, as well as on the degree of distension. Peristalsis is usually readily apparent at real-time imaging. The content of the GI tract also varies widely, ranging from almost hypoechoic to highly reflective.

Many types of bowel pathology may be visualized sonographically. These range from infectious and inflammatory conditions, which tend to cause segmental or extensive mural thickening, to neoplasms, which result in focal masses. Overlap is considerable, however. Sonography occasionally may be helpful to suggest the diagnosis of obstruction in patients who present with nonspecific abdominal pain.

The appendix deserves special mention, as it is often studied with ultrasound. The normal appendix is a blind-ending tubular structure that is typically located in the right lower quadrant. Because loops of bowel often lie between the appendix and the anterior abdominal wall, so-called graded compression sonography, in which gradually increasing pressure is applied to the abdomen, is used. Acute appendicitis should be suspected when the diameter is more than 6 mm, particularly if there is focal tenderness or an appendicolith is visible. The presence of a focal fluid collection or infiltration of periappendiceal fat suggests perforation.

MESENTERIC VESSELS

While technically challenging, Doppler ultrasound is valuable for assessing patients with suspected mesenteric insufficiency. Imaging is performed after a fast to minimize interfering bowel gas. The examination includes visualization and velocity measurements within the abdominal aorta, the celiac axis, the superior mesenteric artery, and the inferior mesenteric artery. As in other vessels, the diagnosis of stenosis is based on the presence of focal high-velocity flow and turbulence; however, there is disagreement concerning appropriate thresholds for peak-systolic or end-diastolic velocities. As a rule of thumb, however, flow rates more than 200 cm/s in the celiac axis or inferior mesenteric artery and 275 cm/s in the superior mesenteric artery are associated with significant stenosis.

PERITONEAL CAVITY AND ABDOMINAL WALL

Ultrasound is quite sensitive for the detection of peritoneal fluid, which is the basis of its role in assessing patients with abdominal trauma. Sonography is also helpful to guide needle or catheter placement in patients who require diagnostic or therapeutic paracentesis. Peritoneal carcinomatosis, in which there are disseminated peritoneal tumor deposits from ovarian or other malignancies, also may be characterized sonographically, although CT is usually more effective in this regard.

The abdominal wall may be assessed for masses, collections, or hernias using a high-frequency linear array transducer. Herniated bowel or omentum is easily recognized if a hernia is large, although small defects may be challenging to demonstrate.

SUGGESTED READING

Ackerman S, Irshad A. The role of sonography in liver transplantation. *Ultrasound Clin*. 2007;2(3):377-390.

Bhatt S, Ghazale J, Dogra VS. Sonographic evaluation of the abdominal aorta. *Ultrasound Clin*. 2007;2(3):437-453.

Brancatelli G, Vilgrain V, Federle MP, et al. Budd-Chiari syndrome: spectrum of imaging findings. *AJR Am J Roentgenol*. 2007;188(2):W168-76.

Hosseinzadeh K, Wong-You-Cheong J. Ultrasound imaging of pancreatic transplantation. *Ultrasound Clin*. 2007;2(3):423-435.

Israel GM, Bosniak MA. How I do it: evaluating renal masses. *Radiology*. 2005;236(2):441-450.

Martinez-Noguera A, D'Onofrio M. Ultrasonography of the pancreas. 1. Conventional imaging. *Abdom Imaging*. 2007;32(2): 136-149.

Middleton WD, Teefey SA, Darcy MD. Doppler evaluation of transjugular intrahepatic portosystemic shunts. *Ultrasound Q.* 2003;19(2):56-70.

Ng CS, Wood CG, Silverman PM, et al. Renal cell carcinoma: diagnosis, staging, and surveillance. *AJR Am J Roentgenol.* 2008;191(4):1220-1232.

Prasad SR, Surabhi VR, Menias CO, et al. Benign renal neoplasms in adults: cross-sectional imaging findings. *AJR Am J Roentgenol.* 2008;190(1):158-164.

Rubens DJ. Ultrasound imaging of the biliary tract. *Ultrasound Clin.* 2007;2(3):391-413.

QUESTIONS AND ANSWERS

1. Concerning hepatic hemangiomas, which of the following is *true*?
   A. They often possess a hypoechoic halo.
   B. Echogenicity varies with the degree of steatosis.
   C. Through transmission is not seen.
   D. Biopsy is recommended for definitive diagnosis.

   ANSWER: B. In the presence of steatosis, hemangiomas, which are usually echogenic, may appear hypoechoic compared to the adjacent echogenic parenchyma.

2. Concerning focal fatty sparing, which of the following is *true*?
   A. Pericholecystic location is rare.
   B. Typically echogenic.
   C. May simulate neoplasm
   D. Vessels are usually displaced.

   ANSWER: C. Although the location and configuration of focal fatty sparing usually make the diagnosis straightforward, it may occasionally have a mass-like appearance that simulates neoplasm.

3. Concerning hepatic tumors, which of the following is *true*?
   A. Cholangiocarcinoma is the most common primary malignancy.
   B. Metastases are less common than HCC.
   C. Lymphoma is usually echogenic.
   D. The presence of flow within thrombus suggests HCC.

   ANSWER: D. The finding of flow within tumor thrombus on Doppler ultrasound distinguishes it from bland thrombus, and is highly suggestive of HCC.

4. Concerning portosystemic shunts, which of the following is *true*?
   A. Color Doppler ultrasound alone is adequate to assess TIPS.
   B. TIPS stents usually extend from the portal vein to the left hepatic vein.
   C. Goal of shunting is to improve hepatic blood flow.
   D. Absent flow on color Doppler ultrasound does not always indicate thrombosis.

   ANSWER: D. Very slow flow in an otherwise patent TIPS may not be detectable sonographically, although it is highly worrisome for impending shunt failure. As well, some types of shunts may be obscured by acoustic shadowing soon after placement.

5. Which of the following statements about gallstones is *true*?
   A. Most are cholesterol stones.
   B. Decreasing the ultrasound frequency improves demonstration of acoustic shadowing from small calculi.
   C. Stones are a frequent cause of acute cholecystitis when they become impacted at the gallbladder fundus.
   D. Wall-echo-shadow sign consists of two parallel lines.

   ANSWER: A. The majority of gallstones are cholesterol stones.

6. Concerning the spleen, which of the following is *true*?
   A. Spleen is larger in myelofibrosis than lymphoma.
   B. Normal adult spleen measures up to 15 cm in length.
   C. Lymphangiomas do not contain internal septations.
   D. Normally the spleen is less echogenic than the liver.

   ANSWER: A. Although splenomegaly is encountered in both disorders, it is usually more pronounced in patients with myelofibrosis.

7. Which of the following is the most frequent subtype of renal cell carcinoma?
   A. Chromophobe
   B. Papillary
   C. Clear cell
   D. Other

   ANSWER: C. Clear cell adenocarcinomas account for 80% of renal cell carcinomas.

8. Concerning GU tract stones, which of the following is *true*?
   A. Color Doppler sonography improves sensitivity.
   B. Lowering the ultrasound frequency improves stone detection.
   C. Acoustic shadowing is not related to the beam width.
   D. Most midureteral calculi are easily detectable with ultrasound.

ANSWER: A. The presence of the twinkling artifact on color Doppler imaging helps distinguish stones from other normal echogenic foci, although calcified vessels may still be problematic.

9. Concerning cystic renal masses, which of the following is *true*?
   A. Multilocular cystic nephromas are readily distinguished from other cystic masses.
   B. Assignment of some Bosniak categories may be done with ultrasound alone.
   C. Calyceal diverticula do not contain calcium.
   D. Cysts and lymphomatous masses exhibit similar through transmission.

   ANSWER: B. Grade I and II cysts often may be confidently diagnosed with sonography alone.

10. Concerning aortic aneurysms, which of the following is *true*?
    A. AP measurements are best done in the sagittal plane.
    B. Ultrasound is sensitive for the detection of rupture.
    C. AP diameter more than 2.5 cm is considered aneurysmal.
    D. More common in women.

    ANSWER: A. Measurements performed in the axial plane may overestimate the AP diameter of the aorta if the plane of section is oblique. Therefore, the AP dimension should be measured in a plane that is perpendicular to the long axis of the aneurysm, which is usually sagittal.

64 FEMALE PELVIC ULTRASOUND

Arthur C. Fleischer and Robert S. Morrison III

INTRODUCTION

The role of pelvic sonography in the evaluation of gynecologic disorders is universal and well accepted by patients and practitioners. It provides clinically important information in a variety of gynecologic disorders such as evaluation of patients for pelvic masses, endometrial or uterine disorders, pelvic pain, and inflammatory disorders.

Pelvic sonography requires that the operator has extensive scanning skills and have interpretation expertise in addressing common and less common clinical questions.

TABLE 64-1 Normal Uterus

Prepubertal	Mostly cervix
Postpubertal	Cervix and corpus/fundus about equal in size
Nulliparous	6–8 cm in length, 3–5 cm in anterior-posterior and transverse axes
Parous	1–2 cm larger than nulliparous
Postmenopause	3–4 cm smaller, thin endometrium

It behooves medical professionals to be up-to-date with current scanning technology and clinical application.

SCANNING TECHNIQUES AND INSTRUMENTATION

When imaging the pelvic structures, two techniques are commonly used. Transvaginal sonography (TVS) provides detailed depiction of the uterus, endometrium, myometrium, ovaries, and cul-de-sac (Tables 64-1 to 64-3). Transabdominal sonography (TAS) provides an overview of these pelvic structures but it has limitations because of the fact that it is degraded by gas-filled bowel and requires that the urinary bladder be distended.

TVS requires an empiric approach to providing optimal images. The first images of the pelvis include long and short axes of the uterus. This requires some anterior angulations of the probe for anteflexed uteri. Retroflexed uteri are imaged without much manipulation of the probe once it is introduced. The endometrial bilayer thickness should be measured in the greatest anteroposterior plane. The ovaries are best delineated in an oblique semicoronal plane. It is important to assess the relative mobility of the ovaries as they are displaced from the uterus with minimal pressure using the probe. Finally, the cul-de-sac and cervix need to be evaluated.

Transabdominal sonography is helpful in the delineation of masses larger than 5 cm, particularly those that are displaced anteriorly or superior to the urinary bladder.

Both TVS and TAS have color Doppler capabilities. The major feeding vessels to the ovaries and some of the larger arcuate and radial vessels can be interrogated with pulse Doppler sonography. The relative impedance (high, intermediate, or low) can be calculated.

Three-dimensional pelvic sonography can be obtained with transabdominal or transvaginal probes that contain a curved array of transducer elements that are automatically swept through a region of interest.

TABLE 64-2 Normal Endometrium

Menstrual phase	Irregular interface representing sloughed endometrium and blood clots, 3–5 mm bilayer
Follicular phase	Isoechoic, 5–6 mm
Periovulatory	Multilayered, 5–8 mm
Luteal phase	Echogenic, 5–12 mm

TABLE 64-3 Normal Ovaries

Premenarche	2 × 2 × 1 cm
Postmenarche	3 × 2 × 1 cm with antral follicles of various sizes
Childbearing	3 × 2 × 2 cm with multiple follicles of various sizes of development
Postmenopause	2 × 2 × 1 cm without follicles

Three-dimensional pelvic sonography provides images in any selectable scan plane and is particularly useful in assessment of endometrial/myometrial disorders.

PATHOLOGY

PELVIC MASSES

Pelvic sonography is the diagnostic modality of choice for evaluation of most pelvic masses. It provides information as to the mass' organ of origin, internal consistency, and vascularity. Each of these parameters is clinically important in determining the most likely diagnosis, whether the mass is most likely benign or malignant and optimal management. (Table 64-4). In most patients, the differential diagnosis can be narrowed to one or two entities based upon the clinical features and laboratory values. There are some relatively specific TVS findings (Table 64-5). Selective use of MR, CT, or PET/CT can further clarify the nature of some masses. These modalities may also be needed when sonography is equivocal or limited.

TABLE 64-4 Sonographic Differential Diagnoses of Pelvic Masses*

CYSTIC	COMPLEX	SOLID
Completely cystic	**Predominantly cystic**	**Uterine**
Physiologic ovarian cysts	Cystadenomas	Leiomyoma (sarcoma)
Cystadenomas	Tubo-ovarian abscess	Endometrial carcinoma, sarcoma
Hydrosalpinx	Ectopic pregnancy	
Endometrioma	Cystic teratoma	
Paraovarian cyst	**Predominantly solid**	**Extrauterine**
Hydatid cyst of Morgagni	Cystadenoma/ cystadenocarcinoma	Solid ovarian tumor
	Germ cell tumor	
Multiple		
Endometriomas		
Multiple follicular cysts		
Septated		
Cystadenoma (carcinoma)		
Mucinous		
Serous		
Papillary		

*Based on most common appearance.

TABLE 64-5 Sonographic Findings of Pelvic Masses

Ovarian Epithelial Tumors	Septated or Nonloculated
Hydrosalpinx	Endosalpingeal folds as echogenic intraluminal projections
Endometriomas	Ground glass internal texture, echogenic foci
Dermoid cysts	Variable appearance can contain echogenic sebum, mural calcifications
Hemorrhagic corpus luteum	Peripheral vascular rim, echogenic interfaces

OVARIAN MASSES

The ovary is the site of a variety of adnexal masses that range histologically from benign to malignant. It is important to correlate the clinical features of each patient to the sonographic findings to provide the most likely diagnosis. For example, physiologic cysts are common in women of childbearing age and uncommon after menopause. Similarly, there are two major peak years for torsion: in the postmenarche girl who begins to ovulate and in the postmenopause woman, secondary to an ovarian epithelial neoplasm acting as a leading mass.

The ovaries are characteristically ovoid structures residing lateral to the body of the uterus. The size of the ovaries changes throughout a woman's life, increasing in size until menarche and then atrophying once menopausal. During the menstruating years, they may vary in size from 1 to 3 cm depending on if they contain mature follicles or corpora lutea. With each menstrual cycle, several follicles begin to develop during the follicular phase. Of these, a dominant follicle (more than 10 mm) forms and contains inside it an oocyte. The cumulus oophorus, which surrounds the maturing oocyte, can occasionally be seen sonographically as a small (1–2 mm) hyperechoic structure along the inner wall of the dominant follicle. At the midpoint of the menstrual cycle, luteinizing hormone surges and the dominant follicle (ranging from 18–25 mm) ruptures, releasing its oocyte and a small amount (3–5 cm^3) of free fluid into the cul-de-sac. This dominant follicle subsequently involutes with thickening and serration of the wall and becomes the progesterone-secreting corpus luteum. Occasionally, the dominant follicle will bleed internally and increase in size. This can be seen as a complex intraovarian area termed as hemorrhagic cyst. This hemorrhagic cyst characteristically resolves within one to two menstrual cycles. The remaining nondominant follicles also shrink following dominant follicle rupture. The uterus is primed for implantation; however, if this does not occur, then the follicles will involute and the cycle will begin again.

Cysts within the ovary can range from 3 to more than 20 cm. Most are smooth walled and demonstrate no internal echogenicity. They can be identified as arising from the ovary by recognizing the compressed remaining ovarian tissue surrounding the cystic component. Cystic ovarian masses may contain multiple septations or irregular solid components. Papillary excrescences that arise from the wall usually indicate either a borderline or malignant pathology. Cysts may contain echogenic material, such as sebum, within dermoid cysts or inflammatory debris within a tuboovarian abscess. Mucin within a cyst can be seen in mucinous tumors whereas serous tumors usually have anechoic fluid.

Follicles (functioning cysts) are under the influence of the female sex hormones and thus vary with size depending on the stage of menstruation. A simple cyst that does not change or increase in size between menstrual cycles is considered to be independent from hormonal influence and is termed nonfunctional. If this cyst measures less than 5 cm, then simple observation will suffice as these are almost always benign. However, if a nonfunctional cyst measures more than 5 cm, then the differential for that cyst includes nonphysiologic causes. In these patients, color Doppler sonography (CDS) and three-dimensional sonography can provide useful information as to which patients may be followed is those that may require surgery. Those features which suggest malignancy include papillary excrescences, focal wall irregularity, low-impedance flow within centrally located cluster vessels.

Complex or semisolid ovarian masses are usually dermoid cysts, endometriosis, or in the patient who is febrile, a tuboovarian complex. The greater the degree of variability within a cyst, and in particular the more solid components present, the higher the likelihood for malignancy. For instance, those with increased wall thickness, papillary excrescences, thick septations, and increased echogenicity are significantly more concerning for malignancy. Dermoids are benign neoplasms that are present from birth. These structures contain a myriad of mature epithelial structures, including skin, hair, and teeth. Hydrosalpinges are typically fusiform but can mimic a cystic ovarian mass. However, the endosalpingal folds within a hydrosalpinx can help identify the cystic mass as arising from the tube and not the ovary. Endometrioma typically contain echogenic internal content termed as ground glass appearance. Occasionally, echogenic foci associated with fibrinolyzed blood products can be seen within the endometrioma. This finding may also be observed in dermoid cysts.

Ovarian tumors typically contain focally thickened walls and papillary excrescences. If the tumor has spread through the capsule of the ovary, intraperitoneal fluid is usually present. On color Doppler sonography, most ovarian neoplasms contain central vessels with low-impedance flow in the morphologically abnormal area, as well as clusters of abnormal vessels (Table 64-6). Three-dimensional sonography can be used to depict papillary excrescence. Additionally, the use of color Doppler sonography may show abnormally branching vessels with an irregular caliper exhibiting focal areas of stenosis and microaneurysm.

PELVIC PAIN

TVS has a vital role in the evaluation of patients presenting with pelvic pain. The main clinical concern is evaluation for adnexal (ovarian and tubal) torsion.

Ovarian torsion is an infrequent but significant cause of lower abdominal pain and accounts for some 3% of operative emergencies in gynecology—the fifth most common cause of gynecologic emergencies. It typically occurs unilaterally in an enlarged ovary and commonly involves torsion of both the ovary and the fallopian tube. Although torsion may occur in a normal ovary (as is common in pediatric patients), it typically involves an adnexa abnormality with an ovarian mass being implicated in almost 60% of all cases. Torsion typically occurs during the early reproductive years; however, it may occur at any stage in a woman's life. The median age for torsion to occur is 28 years.

TABLE 64-6 Sonographic Features of Benign and Malignant Pelvic Masses

	BENIGN		MALIGNANT	
	TVS	CDS	TVS	CDS
Morphology	Smooth-walled, anechoic		Papillary excrescences, mural nodules, irregular solid areas	
Vessels		Regularly spaced		Irregularly spaced, clustered
Impedance		High		Low
Velocity		Low		High
Change in size	Regression or no change		Increase or no change	
Other findings	No ascites; no liver masses or lymphadenopathy		Ascites; liver masses, lymphadenopathy	

TVS: transvaginal sonography; CDS: color Doppler sonography.

In its most common presentation, ovarian torsion presents as the sudden onset of severe unilateral lower abdominal pain that may be intermittent. This sharp stabbing pain often radiates to the back, pelvis, or thigh. Physical examination is relatively nonspecific, but may reveal a tender adnexa or adnexal mass. Given the ovaries intraperitoneal location, examination findings of peritonitis may be present and signify advanced disease. Laboratory studies are of limited value in ovarian torsion; however, a pregnancy test is certainly necessary. TVS is best at helping to identify ovarian torsion but it has limitations in distinguishing torsion from other adnexal masses.

Most frequently, the affected ovary is enlarged and relatively irregular in texture, probably related to intravenous hemorrhage and edema. The increased weight and reduced venous return of the affected ovary precipitates torsion. On color Doppler sonography, the affected ovary and tube typically have reduced to absent venous flow. Arterial flow may be present in less affected portions of the ovary, probably a reflection of the dual arterial supply. Waveforms that demonstrate reversed diastolic flow indicate severe ischemia. The affected adnexa may be surrounded by intraperitoneal fluid.

Another sonographic finding associated with pelvic pain includes pelvic inflammatory disease. In this condition, corps luteum can become a locus for infection appearing as a hypoechoic mass adjacent to a hydrosalpinx. Guided TVS can provide a means to aspirate the contents of a tuboovarian abscess.

Ectopic pregnancy is an important consideration when considering pelvic pain. By definition, an ectopic pregnancy is one in which the fertilized egg is implanted outside of the endometrial cavity. More than 95% of the time, the improperly implanted embryo can be found within the fallopian tubes; rarely these ova can implant within the adnexa or intraperitoneal surfaces. Clearly, serum beta-hCG testing is necessary to evaluate for ectopic pregnancy in any female with pelvic pain and clinical suspicion. In early healthy intrauterine pregnancies, the serum beta-hCG value should double approximately every 2 days. In the case of an ectopic pregnancy, this doubling rule is not met or may show a beta-hCG value that is slightly decreasing. In practicality, the difficulty with relying on serial laboratory values lies in the delay in establishing a diagnosis. Therefore, ultrasound (US) is often an effective means of helping to identify ectopic pregnancies.

TVS is able to detect an intrauterine gestational sac in cases in which the serum beta-hCG is 1500 to 1800 mIU/mL (approximately 6000 mIU/mL on transabdominal US). If the serum value is at this threshold level and a gestational sac is not visualized within the endometrial cavity, then the pregnancy can typically be considered to be extrauterine.

ENDOMETRIAL DISORDERS

TVS has a vital role in the evaluation of women with suspected endometrial disorders. It provides a means to determine which patients need to be sampled or undergo hysteroscopy versus those who are best managed medically.

It is important to realize that of all postmenopause women who experience bleeding, only 10% to 15% will have hyperplasia, polyps, or carcinoma. The majority will have endometrial atrophy as the cause of their bleeding.

When assessing a patient's endometrium, it is important to consider their menarchal/menstrual state. For example, a collection of fluid within the endometrial cavity of a fertile woman can be completely normal with menstruation, but in a postmenopause woman this same finding may be the result of cervical stenosis or an obstructing endometrial or cervical tumor.

In general, an endometrial bilayer less than 6 mm in postmenopause women who experience bleeding is typically associated with atrophy; those women with a thicker endometrial bilayer are best served by biopsy with management based upon the results. TVS has an important role in recognizing polyps as focal echogenic thickening that with CDS have a feeding vessel. Endometrial cancer can appear as a polypoid lesion, occasionally disrupting the endometrial myometrial junction due to invasion. If there is a question regarding the presence of a polyp, a saline infusion sonohysterogram can be performed to determine the presence of polyps, submucous fibroids, or synechae.

Another finding to consider when a mass is identified within the endometrial cavity is retained products of conception. These can have various appearances, but should particularly be considered when the patient is known to have recently been pregnant or undergone an elective or nonelective abortion. It is important to identify these products as they may result in uterine infection, synechiae, and metaplasia. One way to help distinguish retained products of conception is through the use of color Doppler sonography, which should show vascular flow to the retained products that have not sloughed. Clots and sloughed tissue typically do not demonstrate flow, however.

UTERINE DISORDERS

By far the most common uterine masses that are seen on sonography are uterine fibroids. They may be submucosal, intramural, or subserosal, and vary from hypoechoic to moderately hyperechoic with echogenic foci consistent with calcification. Additionally, fibroids will show some degree of shadowing particularly arising from their pseudocapsate. Fibroids are benign soft-tissue masses that have increased frequency in women of African descent and those of middle age. When clinically symptomatic, fibroids often cause pain and vaginal bleeding, which is often disassociated with menstruation. Occasionally, these fibroids will outgrow their blood supply and necrose resulting in an area of hypoechoic or anechoic echotexture present within the solid areas. It is important to document the location of a fibroid relative to the endometrium so that those amenable to intraluminal extraction are distinguished from those that require an open approach.

Adenomyosis is a common cause of excessive bleeding and pain. Sonographically, it appears as an ill-defined disruption of thickened myometrium/endometrium with streaking. This has been described as a moth-eaten appearance that is due to the multiple, small hypoechoic masses seen within the myometrium. As opposed to fibroids that typically exhibit peripheral vascularity, the vascularity associated with adenomyosis is diffuse.

Three-dimensional pelvic sonography provides an accurate means to characterize uterine malformations. Septated uteri can be seen as having a smooth fundal contour and bicornate uteri are noted to have a fundal cleft. Three-dimensional sonography is also useful in assessing the location of an intrauterine contraception device.

MISCELLANEOUS CONDITIONS

TVS has a vital role in the management of gynecologic infertility from follicular monitoring to guided follicular aspiration. Similarity, it is helpful in guided aspiration of tuboovarian abscess and other pelvic fluid collections.

SUGGESTED READING

Callen P. *Ultrasonography in Obstetrics and Gynecology*. 5th ed. New York, NY: Elsevier; 2007.

Chang HC, Bhatt S, Dogra VS. Pearls and pitfalls in diagnosis of ovarian torsion. *Radiographics.* Sep–Oct 2008;28(5):1355-1368.

Fleischer AC. *Sonography in Gynecology and Obstetrics: Just the Facts*. New York, NY: McGraw Hill Publishers; 2004.

Fleischer A, Manning F, Jeanty P, Romero R. *Sonography in Obstetrics and Gynecology: Principles and Practice*. 6th ed. New York, NY: McGraw-Hill Publishers; 2001.

Kuligowska E, Deeds L III, Lu K III. Pelvic pain: overlooked and underdiagnosed gynecologic conditions. *Radiographics.* 2005; 25(1):3-20.

Potter AW, Chandrasekhar CA. US and CT evaluation of acute pelvic pain of gynecologic origin in nonpregnant premenopausal patients. *Radiographics.* 2008;28(6):1645-1659.

Williams PL, Laifer-Narin SL, Ragavendra N. US of abnormal uterine bleeding. *Radiographics.* 2003;23(3):703-718.

QUESTIONS AND ANSWERS

1. You perform a transvaginal US and identify a pelvic mass with ground glass internal texture. Which of the following is the most likely diagnosis?
   A. Epithelial ovarian tumor
   B. Endometrioma
   C. Dermoid cyst
   D. Corpus luteum cyst

   ANSWER: B. Ground glass appearance is classic for an endometrioma.

2. Which of the following is the most likely etiology for the enlarged ovary seen in torsion?
   A. Hemorrhagic cyst
   B. Dermoid
   C. Hydrosalpinx
   D. Hemorrhage and edema

   ANSWER: D. Although torsion is usually associated with an ovarian mass, ovarian enlargement is thought to be due to hemorrhage and edema, likely from venous outflow obstruction.

3. What does reversed diastolic flow indicate in the setting of torsion?
   A. Severe ischemia
   B. Infarction
   C. Reversibility
   D. Has no clinical/prognostic significance

   ANSWER: A. Reversed diastolic flow suggests severe ischemia.

4. Which of the following is the most common cause of postmenopause bleeding?
   A. Endometrial carcinoma
   B. Polyp
   C. Atrophy
   D. Cervical carcinoma

   ANSWER: C. Atrophy of the endometrium is the most common cause of postmenopause bleeding.

5. How is the vascularity of adenomyosis different from fibroids?
   A. Fibroids—peripheral; adenomyosis—diffuse
   B. Fibroids—diffuse; adenomyosis—peripheral
   C. Their vascularity is identical.
   D. There is no typical vascular signature of either entity.

   ANSWER: A. The vascularity of fibroids is typically peripheral, while that of adenomyosis is more diffuse.

65 OBSTETRICAL ULTRASOUND

Rochelle F. Andreotti, Reagan R. Leverett, and Libby L. Shadinger

FIRST TRIMESTER OBSTETRIC ULTRASOUND

ANATOMY

The blastocyst adheres to the endometrial epithelium on day 6 and is completely surrounded by endometrial epithelium by day 10 of gestation (Fig. 65-1). A normal intrauterine pregnancy will demonstrate the following structures (Fig. 65-2):

- Yolk sac
- Amnion
- Chorion
- Embryo

Note that the chorionic sac may be considered the same as the gestational sac and a portion of it will eventually form the placenta. The yolk sac provides nutrients for the embryo until the establishment of placental circulation and is the first structure identified by sonogram within the gestational sac. A portion of the yolk sac will remain connected to the embryo by the omphalomesenteric duct (secondary yolk sac) and become part of the primitive gut. The amnionic and chorionic membranes fuse at approximately 14 to 16 weeks gestation.

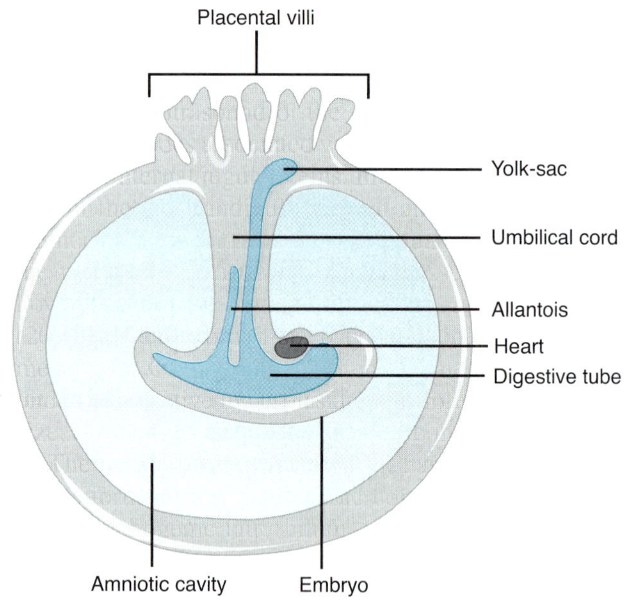

FIG. 65-2 Early intrauterine pregnancy.
SOURCE: Reprinted with permission for use granted by Bartleby.com, Inc.

FIRST TRIMESTER SONOGRAPHIC EVALUATION MAY INCLUDE

- Cervix
- Uterus
- Adnexa
- Number and location of gestational sacs
- Number of embryos
- Crown-rump length

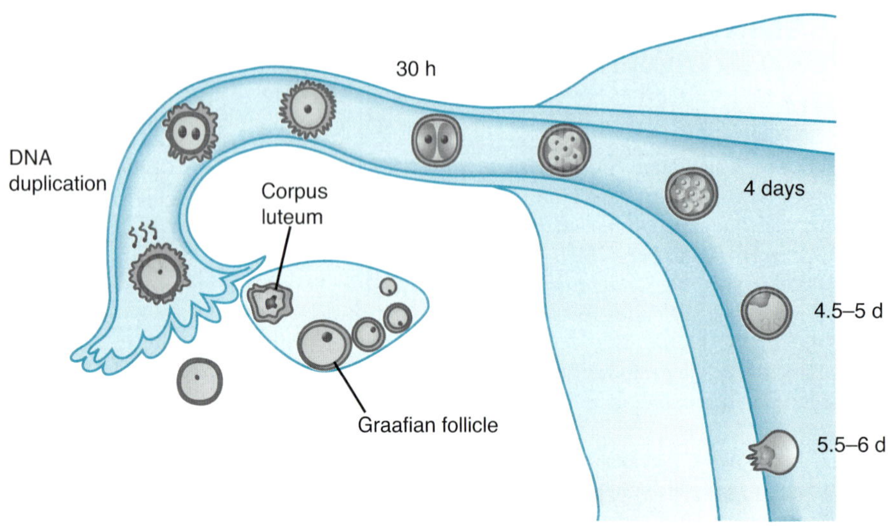

FIG. 65-1 Diagram of ovulation/fertilization sequence.
SOURCE: Courtesy of Anthony F. Zagar, UAB, Department of Radiology, Birmingham, Alabama.

- Cardiac activity
- Membranes
- Placenta
- Nuchal translucency

INDICATIONS FOR FIRST TRIMESTER ULTRASOUND

Dating by Sonography

Sonography, if performed early during pregnancy, can greatly enhance the obstetrician's ability to determine the gestational age. The most accurate measurement is the crown-rump length (CRL) when performed between 6 and 12 weeks gestation, confidence level of 95% with a range of 4 to 5 days. The mean sac diameter (MSD) may be used to date the pregnancy if the embryo is not visualized and is equal to the sum of the length, width, and diameter of the gestational sac divided by three.

Clinical dates are calculated from the first day of the last menstrual period with the assumption that ovulation and conception take place on approximately day 14 after the last menstrual period (LMP). It is not uncommon for a patient to be unsure of her dates, have irregular menstrual periods with occasional prolonged cycles, or have some bleeding at the time of implantation of the blastocyst, which is mistaken for a normal menstrual period. The most accurate estimate of gestational age can be made only in patients followed by various clinical methods such as basal body temperatures, luteinizing hormone (LH) surge assays, and ultrasound assessment of follicular growth, while undergoing infertility evaluation.

Determination of a Live Embryo Using Transvaginal Sonography

Using transvaginal sonography (TVS), a gestational sac should be seen by 4.5 weeks, a yolk sac by 5.5 weeks, and an embryo by 6.5 weeks. A yolk sac should be identified by TVS, with a MSD of 8 mm, and an embryo should be seen within a gestational sac of with a MSD of 16 mm or more. The double bleb sign is a transvaginal sonographic sign of a normal intrauterine pregnancy at approximately 5 to 6 weeks, where two cystic structures (the primary yolk sac and amniotic sac) are identified with the developing embryo in between. An embryo with a CRL of 5 mm without cardiac motion is consistent with a failed intrauterine pregnancy (IUP). Note that some radiologists use slightly less strict criteria, typically 8 to 10 mm. A follow-up sonogram may be warranted to ensure that a live pregnancy is not mistaken for a failed pregnancy. A normal early heart rate is greater than 100 bpm. A heart rate of less than 90 bpm has an associated 79% risk of demise.

A saclike structure without a yolk sac or embryo, which appears separate from the endometrial cavity probably represents a true gestational sac. This may be represented by two important sonographic signs.

- The double decidual sign with the inner decidua being the gestational sac and the outer sac being the endometrial cavity.
- The intradecidual sign is when the sac is eccentrically located with respect to the endometrial cavity within the endometrium.

If no gestational sac is seen within the uterus, the following should be considered:

- Complete or incomplete abortion
- Early IUP (normal or abnormal)
- Ectopic pregnancy

Serial serum beta-human chorionic gonadotropin (hCG) levels are usually obtained to differentiate among these possibilities: a gestational sac should be visualized by 1000 to 2000 mIU/mL (IRP), a yolk sac should be visualized by 7000 mIU/mL, and cardiac activity by 11000 mIU/mL.

Vaginal Bleeding

In the first trimester, the earliest bleeding may be secondary to implantation from the blastocyst burrowing into the endometrium, approximate day 20 to 23. Between 5 and 8 weeks gestation, there is sloughing of the decidua capsularis, which covers the chorion levae, also sometimes referred to as a type of implantation bleeding. Blood may be visualized within the endometrial cavity surrounding the gestational sac giving a "Y" shaped configuration. Retrochorionic hemorrhage occurs following fusion of the chorion with the uterine wall when fluid is demonstrated elevating the chorion from the endometrium and may dissect between chorion and endometrium posterior to the placenta. Prominent vascularity in the region of the cervix may be demonstrated in some patients with vaginal bleeding in the early second trimester in whom no other reason for bleeding has been demonstrated. Other causes of first trimester bleeding include spontaneous abortion, ectopic pregnancy, and gestational trophoblastic disease.

Suspected Ectopic Pregnancy

If the serum hCG is positive, the next step in evaluation of suspected ectopic pregnancy is pelvic sonography. Sonographic confirmation of an IUP effectively excludes ectopic pregnancy because of the extremely low incidence of concomitant ectopic and intrauterine gestations (historically 1/27 000 although the incidence may now be as high as 1/6000 in patients being treated for infertility). An

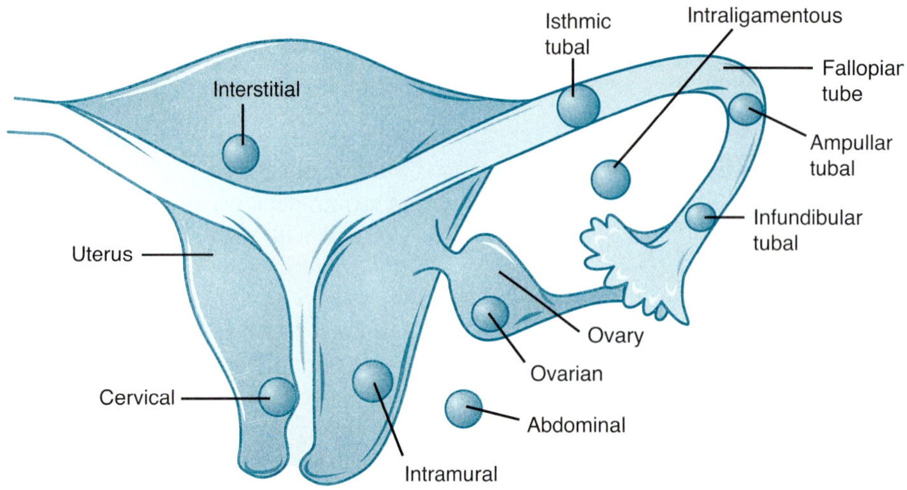

FIG. 65-3 Diagram of ectopic pregnancy.
SOURCE: Courtesy of Anthony F. Zagar, UAB, Department of Radiology, Birmingham, Alabama.

ectopic pregnancy may be suggested by a hCG of 1000 to 2000 mIU/mL (IRP) and an empty uterus by TVS. In order to confirm an IUP, a sac should be demonstrated within the uterus separate from the endometrial cavity. Although this is a fairly reliable finding, there may still be some confusion between a true sac and fluid within the endometrial cavity (pseudosac), which may be associated with an ectopic pregnancy. A pseudosac of an ectopic pregnancy may be suggested by the presence of an abnormal appearing sac. This would include a sac with angles or a collapsed sac. The absence of the intradecidual and double decidual signs would also warrant a search for an ectopic pregnancy. Adnexal signs vary and may include a living extrauterine pregnancy, a tubal ring, which may contain a yolk sac and/or embryo, a complex cystic or solid adnexal mass, or free fluid, often hemorrhagic in appearance. A tubal ring must be separate from the ovary in order to differentiate it from the corpus luteum.

Doppler imaging may also be of use in identifying an ectopic pregnancy. A tubal ring will appear as a "ring of fire" with color Doppler. Again the "ring of fire" of an ectopic should be determined to be separate from the ovary in order to differentiate it from color Doppler signal that may surround a corpus luteum. Pulsed Doppler may be used to evaluate the tissue surrounding a sac within the uterus. A true gestational sac will have low resistance or high diastolic arterial waveforms, whereas a pseudosac will not. Pulsed Doppler of a tubal ring will demonstrate low resistance/high diastolic arterial waveforms as well, although this is nonspecific because of the presence of the same low resistance waveforms seen in such things as a corpus luteum cyst or ovarian tumors.

The majority (95%–97%) of ectopic pregnancies are tubal, which include both the ampullary and isthmic portions of the fallopian tube. Other types of ectopic pregnancies are rarely seen although interstitial ectopic pregnancies are the most common of these infrequent locations (Fig. 65-3).

MULTIPLE GESTATIONS

Dizygotic twins (two eggs) are always dichorionic (two placentas) and diamniotic (two amniotic sacs).

Monozygotic twins (one egg) may be

- dichorionic/diamniotic if division is prior to day 3
- monochorionic/diamniotic if division is between days 4 to 8.
- monochorionic/monoamniotic if division is between days 4 to 14.
- conjoined twins if division is after day 14.

DETERMINATION OF AMNIONICITY AND CHORIONICITY

Determining the amnionicity and chorionicity is an important objective for the first trimester sonogram. Important distinguishing signs include the twin peak sign or lambda sign and the T sign. The twin peak sign or lambda sign is a thick intervening membrane and is consistent with dichorionic/diamniotic pregnancy. The T sign is a thin intervening membrane and is consistent with monochorionic/diamniotic twins. No intervening membrane is seen with monochorionic/monoamniotic twins.

NUCHAL TRANSLUCENCY

The nuchal translucency measurement is performed between 11 and 14 weeks gestation and refers to the hypoechoic region along the posterior aspect of the fetal neck. This measurement is part of screening process for chromosomal abnormalities including trisomies 21, 13, and 18. The pathophysiology of abnormally thickened nuchal translucency is mulitfactorial, including cardiac dysfunction, venous congestion in the head and neck, altered composition of the extracellular matrix, failure of lymphatic drainage, fetal anemia (because of genetic causes), fetal hypoproteinemia, and fetal infection. Venous congestion in the head and neck may be seen with amniotic rupture, diaphragmatic hernia, and skeletal dysplasias because of obstruction of return of blood to the heart. In trisomies 21, 13, and 18, the etiology is because of altered composition of the extracellular matrix. Fetal infection is more likely if the increased nuchal translucency evolves into hydrops by the second or third trimester. Problematic lymphatic drainage is usually a consequence of hypoplastic lymphatics such as in Turner syndrome.

Measurements vary with gestational age but greater than 3 mm is always considered abnormal. Technique is very important and the unfused amnion should not be mistaken for the fetal skin line. Adding serum two serum markers, pregnancy-associated plasma protein (PAPP-A) and the free beta-subunit of human chorionic gonadotropin (hCG) markers, have also been found to increase sensitivity. According to Malone et al., at 11 weeks of gestation, adding PAPP-A and hCG determinations to measurement of nuchal translucency increases the detection rate of Down syndrome from 70% to 87%, with a 5% false positive rate.

SECOND AND THIRD TRIMESTER OBSTETRIC ULTRASOUND

In the US most women who seek prenatal care receive sonographic evaluation of their pregnancies in the second trimester, usually at around 20 weeks gestational age. While the vast majority of fetuses are structurally normal, sonographic evaluation at this stage enables the patient to make informed choices about the pregnancy and allows for adequate antenatal preparation for delivery and care of infants with a wide variety of anomalies. As fetal surgical interventions continue to advance, early and accurate detection of potentially correctable abnormalities becomes ever more crucial.

In addition to its role in anatomic survey, second and third trimester sonography is a valuable tool in the evaluation of fetal well-being, position, growth, and can help answer clinically relevant questions regarding placentation, umbilical cord configuration and insertion, etiology of vaginal bleeding, status of the cervix particularly as it pertains to preterm labor, and multiple gestations. While first trimester crown-rump length is more precise in pregnancy dating, parameters within the second and third trimesters allow dating with reasonable accuracy.

FETAL ANATOMY

A complete fetal anatomic survey should include examination of the cerebral ventricles, posterior fossa, full length of the spine, stomach, urinary bladder, kidneys, extremities, anterior abdominal wall umbilical cord insertion site, and four chamber views of the fetal heart. If possible, the cardiac outflow tracts should be evaluated.

FETAL NERVOUS SYSTEM

The normal size and configuration of three key intracranial structures can exclude a majority of CNS anomalies: the ventricular atria, cisterna magna, and cavum septum pellucidum. The average measurement of the ventricular atrium is 7 mm; atria over 10 mm are considered abnormal. The choroid plexus may appear to "dangle" in the lateral ventricle. Ventricular enlargement is occasionally seen in normal pregnancies as an isolated finding, but its presence should prompt careful evaluation for underlying hydrocephalus or CNS abnormalities. The presence of a cavum septum pellucidum excludes midline developmental anomalies such as holoprosencephaly and septo-optic dysplasia, and also rules out complete corpus callosal dysgenesis, which is also commonly associated with CNS malformations. Cisterna magna measurements greater than 10 mm may be normal, but should trigger careful analysis for posterior fossa abnormalities.

Hydrocephalus is a common CNS abnormality with a myriad of origins, categorized as obstructive or nonobstructive. Usual underlying etiology is obstructive and causes include spina bifida, aqueductal stenosis, encephalocele, Chiari malformation, and Dandy-Walker syndrome. Nonobstructive causes include intracranial hemorrhage and infection.

Neural tube defects are the most common CNS malformation and have been associated with maternal folic acid deficiency. Maternal serum alpha-fetoprotein level can be elevated in these disorders, which may be the impetus for the sonographic examination. Like many CNS disorders, neural tube defects may be associated with polyhydramnios because of neurologic impairment of swallowing. Neural tube defects include anencephaly, encephaloceles, and Chiari II and III malformations.

Anencephaly is one of the most common fetal CNS anomalies, with a frequency of 1:1000. This lethal anomaly may be detected during first trimester evaluations, but is reliably demonstrated during the second trimester. Ultrasound reveals calvarial absence above the orbits.

Chiari II malformations are complex anomalies affecting the brain, skull, and spinal cord. The most serious neurologic effects are due to the almost invariable present myelomeningocele as well as the obstructive hydrocephalus caused by anatomic abnormalities of the brain. Radiographic features include a small posterior fossa, herniation of the cerebellar vermis through the foramen magnum, upward herniation of the cerebellum through the incisura ("towering cerebellum"), wrapping of the cerebellum around the pons ("banana" configuration), effacement of the cisterna magna, diminution of the fourth ventricle, beaking of the tectum, corpus callosal dysgenesis, and narrowing of the frontal bone angles which confers a "lemon" shape to the skull. The associated myelomeningocele may be visualized at any level along the spinal cord. Chiari III is defined as the typical findings of Chiari II with an associated encephalocele.

While strongly associated with Chairi malformations, meningomyeloceles and myeloceles may be found as isolated defects. They occur most commonly in the sacral region and are sonographically identified by splaying of the vertebral body lateral masses with posterior protrusion of a cystic mass of neural elements through the osseous defect. These diagnoses cannot be made with confidence prior to 20 weeks gestation as sacral ossification centers may not be completely ossified earlier in the pregnancy.

Cephaloceles are skull defects that contain herniated neural tissues. They are generally midline and associated with other entities such as Meckel-Gruber syndrome and Chiari III malformations. While 80% are occipital, other locations include parietal, frontal, nasoethmoidal, sphenoidal, and lateral defects.

Posterior fossa malformations include the spectrum of Dandy-Walker malformation, Dandy-Walker variant, and megacisterna magna. The pathophysiology of Dandy-Walker malformation is thought to be at least partially due to atresia of the foramina of Luschka and Magendie. Radiographically, the entity is characterized by agenesis or hypoplasia of the cerebellar vermis, dilatation of the fourth ventricle, and cystic enlargement of the posterior fossa. Typically, progressive hydrocephalus develops after birth. Dandy-Walker variant, which is more common, has similar findings. However, the posterior fossa is not dilated because of patency of the foramen of Magendie. Megacisterna magna, defined as cisterna magna measurement of greater than 1 cm, consists of an enlarged posterior fossa with normal cerebellar vermis and fourth ventricle. As an isolated finding, it is usually clinically inconsequential. Its importance therefore lies in differentiating it from the more clinically significant Dandy-Walker malformation.

Aqueductal stenosis is the most common cause of congenital hydrocephalus. It may be congenital, secondary to chromosomal abnormalities, or acquired through in utero infection. Much more rarely, it may be caused by an underlying congenital mass such as germinoma or teratoma. Prognosis depends upon the degree of ventriculomegaly and response to postnatal shunting.

Holoprosencephaly is failure of the embryonic forebrain to divide into right and left cerebral hemispheres. The manifestations of this disorder range from the most severe, alobar form, to the moderate semilobar form, to the milder lobar form. Midline facial anomalies ranging from cyclopia to mild facial dysplasia are common. The severity of these defects correlates with the severity of the holoprosencephaly. Similarly, the clinical expressions of holoprosencephaly, which include developmental delay, seizures, hydrocephalus, and pituitary dysfunction, correspond to the degree of the anomaly. While the radiographic features vary between the alobar, semilobar, and lobar forms, the unifying finding is absence of the septum pellucidum.

Hydrencephaly is characterized by near complete absence of supratentorial structures, particularly the cerebral cortex. The thalami, midbrain, pons, and cerebellum develop normally. While the exact etiology is unknown, an in utero event leading to ischemia or infarction of the anterior circulation bilaterally is suspected. Ultrasound reveals a cystic appearance of the cranial cavity with near absence or total absence of the cortex. Prognosis is uniformly poor, and most infants die within the first year. While the children may appear physically normal at birth, developmental delays quickly become apparent (Table 65-1).

While they are not abnormalities of the CNS, cleft palate, cleft lip, and cystic hygroma should be considered when examining the fetal head and neck. Cystic hygromas are fluid-filled structures caused by lymphatic malformation or obstruction. Their prognosis depends upon size and associated anomalies. Large cervical hygromas are associated with fetal hydrops and intrauterine

TABLE 65-1 Comparisons Between Major Cystic Supratentorial Central Nervous System Abnormalities

HOLOPROSENCEPHALY	HYDRANCEPHALY	SEVERE HYDROCEPHALUS
Cerebral cortex fused across midline	Cerebral cortical tissue absent	Cortical tissue present (thin rim)
Falx absent	Falx present	Falx present
Thalami partially or totally fused	Normal thalami	Normal thalami
Abn karyotypes common (especially trisomy 13)	No association with karyotype abnormalities	± Karyotype abnormalities
Midline facial defects	Normal face and midline structures	Normal face and midline structures

demise. The association with chromosomal abnormalities, especially Turner syndrome, is strong. Cystic hygromas outside the head and neck do not have the same risks of chromosomal abnormalities and adverse outcome. Cleft lip is a superficial soft-tissue abnormality, which is caused by failure of fusion of the maxillary and medial nasal processes during formation of the primary palate. Cleft palate is caused by failure of fusion of the formation of the secondary palate, which is formed by the lateral palatine processes, the nasal septum, and medial palatine processes. Cleft palate is usually accompanied by cleft lip. The two processes may be isolated or may be seen in chromosomal abnormalities or midline neurologic abnormalities such as holoprosencephaly.

FETAL THORAX

Cardiac Abnormalities

Structural cardiac defects are present in as many as 8/1000 live births. These defects may be difficult to detect because of the small fetal heart size, often confusing fetal orientation with respect to ultrasound scan planes, and rapid fetal heart rates. However, the four-chamber and outflow tract views can allow detection of many abnormalities. M-mode scanning also allows discovery of fetal arrhythmias. Key to interpretation of fetal cardiac images, especially when fetal lie is variable, is understanding that the left atrium should be the chamber nearest the spine. Additionally, the right ventricle must be differentiated from the left. The right ventricle is retrosternal and contains the moderator band. Normally, both ventricles are approximately the same size. The left ventricle is posterior and to the left of the right ventricle, and the mitral valve insertion is just slightly cephalad to that of the tricuspid valve.

Ventricular septal defect (VSD) is common among the cardiac abnormalities, comprising up to 40% of congenital heart defects. It results from abnormal development of or improper resorption of portions of the muscular septum and endocardial cushions. The presence of a VSD allows left-to-right ventricular shunting of blood. While it may be found in isolation, VSD has an association with trisomy 21. It is best detected on the four-chamber view, and Doppler analysis may be helpful in confirming smaller defects.

Endocardial cushion defect, also readily diagnosed on the four-chamber view, is much less common and is caused by failure of the endocardial cushions to fuse. Regurgitation at the atrioventricular valve level is always present. A common atrioventricular valve exists rather than seperating tricuspid and mitral valves. The association with trisomy 21 is somewhat higher than that of VSD.

Hypoplastic left heart represents up to 4% of congenital heart defects, and its pathophysiology is largely unknown. A leading theory is that cardiac chamber development is dependent upon chamber blood flow and that some impedance to left chamber blood flow results in a disproportionately small left heart and aorta. The abnormality is best detected on the four-chamber view. The left ventricle appears small, and the mitral valve and aorta appear small. Sustainment of the life of the newborn infant outside of the uterus depends upon the maintenance of a patent ductus arteriosus and shunting through a large atrial septal defect to supply the necessary blood flow to the body beyond the aorta.

Tetralogy of Fallot has four classic features: VSD, overriding aorta, right ventricular outflow tract stenosis, and right ventricular hypertrophy. It is caused by unequal division of the conus resulting from anterior displacement of the truncoconal system. The conus then divides into a smaller anterior right ventricular segment and a larger posterior left ventricular segment, which subsequently gives rise to an overriding aorta and stenosis of the right ventricular outflow tract. This disorder is best visualized on the heart base and outflow tract images, which may demonstrate failure of normal crossing of the great vessels at the base of the heart. The relatively large aorta will override the comparatively small pulmonary artery.

Complete transposition of the great arteries occurs in 0.2 to 0.4/1000 live births. In normal development, the truncus arteriosus divides into a pulmonary artery arising from the right ventricle and an aorta arising from the left ventricle. This division is a result of spiraling of the conal truncal ridge. Caudal growth of the septum without spiraling of the conal truncal ridge results in abnormal relationship between the ventricles and great vessels. The great vessels assume a parallel rather than crossing orientation, apparent on the outflow tract images.

Truncus arteriosus is a less common abnormality, which results when the conal-truncal ridges fail to fuse and descend toward the aortic sac. The truncus arteriosus is formed by the fusion of two opposing ridges in the cephalic portion of the truncus, which grow caudally toward the aortic sac. Normally, these ridges spiral and divide the truncus into the more anteriorly located pulmonary artery and the more posterior aorta. When conal-truncal ridge fusion and spiral fail, a single truncal vessel overrides the ventricular septum. A ventricular septal defect is usually associated. The diagnosis may be made on outflow tract views or on a base view of the heart, which depicts a single vessel originating from the ventricles.

M-mode or Doppler interrogation can be useful for the assessment of fetal arrhythmias. Premature atrial contractions are the most common fetal arrhythmia. Both premature atrial and ventricular contractions are generally benign and often resolve before birth. Supraventricular tachycardia (heart rate greater than 180 beats per minute) is the most common tachyarrhythmia. A minority of these cases is associated with a congenital heart defect. The clinical importance lies in the possible development of fetal hydrops, and these arrhythmias are often treated medically during the pregnancy. Bradycardia is defined as heart rate less than 100 beats per minute sustained for longer than 10 seconds and is indicative of hypoxic distress. Fetal heart block is highly associated with congenital heart disease as well as maternal systemic lupus erythematosus.

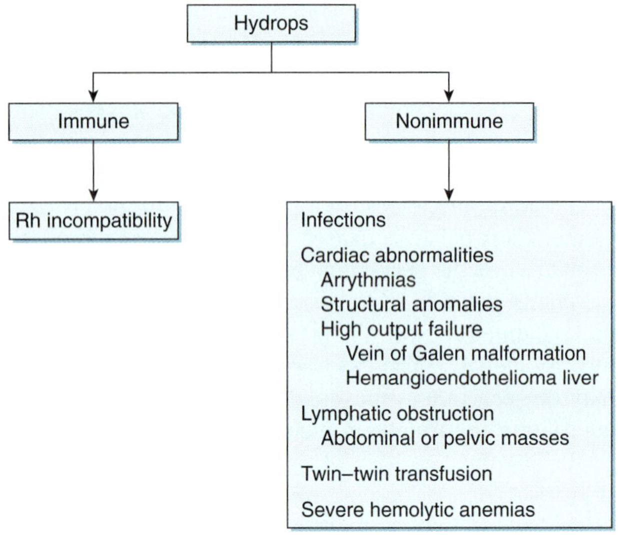

FIG. 65-4 Causes of fetal hydrops.

FETAL HYDROPS

Fetal hydrops is defined as the accumulation of fluid within at least two separate fetal body compartments. Suggestive sonographic features include the presence of ascites, pleural effusions, pericardial effusion, subcutaneous edema, placental enlargement, and polyhydramnios. The presence of oligohydramnios in combination with other findings suggestive of hydrops is a very poor prognostic indicator.

Hydrops is categorized into immune and nonimmune causes, which comprise approximately 10% and 90% of cases, respectively. Immune hydrops is usually because of maternal–fetal rhesus (Rh) blood antigen-antibody incompatibility. An Rh− mother develops immunoglobulins during her first pregnancy with an Rh+ fetus. In a subsequent pregnancy with an Rh+ fetus, and antigen-antibody reaction causes hemolysis of fetal red blood cells. This anemia triggers a chain of events, which culminate in fetal hydrops. This immune reaction is largely preventable by the administration of anti-Rh antigen immunoglobulin to Rh− mothers at 28 weeks. In cases in which immune hydrops develops, effective therapeutic intervention is possible by fetal blood transfusion via the umbilical cord.

The more common nonimmune fetal hydrops has a multitude of possible causes and has a relatively poor prognosis as the etiologies are generally not correctable in utero. The majority are cardiac-related. Other causes include chromosomal abnormalities, infection, twin–twin transfusion, and nonimmune types of fetal anemia (Fig. 65-4).

NONCARDIAC THORACIC ABNORMALITIES

Pulmonary hypoplasia may be idiopathic, but is more often a sequela of other malformations. Oligohydramnios, particularly secondary to renal agenesis, may severely impede lung growth by preventing proper lung distention. Skeletal abnormalities, such as many forms of dwarfism, which result in decreased thoracic cavity size, may prevent adequate lung expansion. Structural abnormalities such as diaphragmatic hernias and pulmonary adenomatoid malformations can prevent adequate development and maturity of one or both lungs. Congenital diaphragmatic hernia is the herniation of abdominal contents into the thoracic cavity resulting from a failure of closure of the pleuroperitoneal canals. Ninety percent of these hernias are left sided, with most of the remainder on the right. Rarely the entity may be bilateral. While it may be seen in association with abnormal karyotypes, many are isolated anomalies. The outcome of this condition depends upon the severity of consequential events including polyhydramnios caused by bowel obstruction and impairment of swallowing, pulmonary hypoplasia, ascites caused by impeded venous return to the heart, and mass effect upon the heart itself. Herniation of the liver through a right-sided defect also portends a poor prognosis.

Sonographic evaluation demonstrates contralateral displacement of the heart within the thoracic cavity in relation to the diaphragmatic defect. Often the abdominal circumference is decreased as the abdominal contents lie within the thorax. If the stomach and bowel are involved in the hernia, real-time sonography may reveal peristaltic motion of these structures within the chest. The position of the liver may be ascertained by the use of Doppler interrogation of the portal vein to determine its relationship with the diaphragm.

Cystic masses within the chest include bronchogenic cyst, esophageal duplication cyst, congenital teratoma, and congenital pulmonary adenomatoid malformation (CPAM). While the former three entities tend to favor the mediastinum, CPAM is a hamartomatous anomaly found in the lung parenchyma. It is generally subdivided into three types. Type I CPAMs, which generally have a favorable a prognosis, are composed of one or more cysts which are each 2 to 10 cm in size. Type II includes cysts less than 2 cm. Prognosis is fairly poor as this type has an association with renal and gastrointestinal abnormalities. Type III may appear as a sonographically solid mass which is actually a conglomeration of macroscopic cysts; prognosis tends to be poor.

Bronchopulmonary sequestration is a nonfunctioning nest of pulmonary tissue, which does not communicate with the tracheobronchial tree. It is thought to arise from an accessory lung bud, which migrates caudally from the developing normal lung. Sequestrations are categorized as intralobar or extralobar types, and 80% occur on the left side of the body. Intralobar sequestrations are usually an isolated abnormality. Extralobar types are often associated with other structural abnormalities, particularly congenital diaphragmatic hernias. While both types tend to have a systemic arterial supply, extralobar types typically have systemic venous drainage, while intralobar sequestrations usually drain via pulmonary veins. Extralobar sequestrations are enveloped by a separate pleura, while intralobar are enclosed within the pleura of the adjacent normal lung. Generally, only the extralobar type is prenatally detected. In these cases, ultrasound may demonstrate an echogenic mass at the lung base with systemic vascular supply.

FETAL GASTROINTESTINAL TRACT

Evaluation of the stomach is helpful in detection of upper gastrointestinal tract abnormalities. The stomach should be reliably visualized beyond 20 weeks gestation. Lack of visualization of the stomach beyond this point may imply several abnormalities, including neurologic impairment of swallowing, physical obstruction by an oral, cervical, or thoracic mass, esophageal atresia, or more rarely gastric atresia. Esophageal atresia is often associated with other anomalies, one of which is the VACTERL complex. VACTERL is an acronym that encompasses a constellation of *v*ertebral body anomalies, *a*nal atresia, *c*ardiac defects, *t*racheoesophageal fistula, *e*sophageal atresia, renal anomalies, and *l*imb malformations.

When the stomach and duodenum appear dilated, duodenal obstruction is suspected, often attributable to atresia, stenosis, annular pancreas, or peritoneal bands. The exact etiology may be difficult to elucidate during fetal life. Duodenal atresia has a relatively high association with chromosomal abnormalities, particularly trisomy 21. Muliple dilated loops of small bowel may herald ostructive processes such as volvulus, malrotation, and peritoneal bands.

Echogenic bowel is seen in approximately 1% of second-trimester fetuses. The ultrasound appearance is that of a hyperechoic (isoechoic to bone), nonshadowing mass in the lower abdomen and pelvis. In about 50% of cases, the appearance is an isolated finding that resolves upon subsequent imaging. Differential considerations include cystic fibrosis, intraamniotic bleeding with fetal swallowing of the blood, congenital infections, and chromosomal abnormalities.

The significance of peritoneal calcifications depends upon their location and associated findings. Meconium peritonitis is manifested as scattered peritoneal calcifications which often stud the surface of the liver, and represents the sequela of in utero bowel perforation. Causes of meconium peritonitis include ileal atresia, jejunal atresia, volvulus, microcolon, and cystic fibrosis. A meconium pseudocyst, indicative of contained perforation, is a hypoechoic mass with a calcified wall. Isolated calcifications within the hepatic parenchyma rather than on the peritoneal surface are often of no consequence. However, they may be associated with congenital infections such as toxoplasmosis or cytomegalovirus (CMV) and may rarely be found in conjunction with fetal tumors such as hemangioendothelioma.

Anterior abdominal wall defects are subcategorized into midline and lateral defects (Table 65-2). Midline defects include omphaloceles and Pentalogy of Cantrel, the latter of which is very rare and associated with ectopia cordis. Lateral defects include gastroschisis, limb body wall complex, and amniotic band syndrome. Of these entities, gastroschisis and omphalocele are the most common and the most similar in appearance.

Gastroschisis is generally an isolated defect. Recent research has indicated a slightly increased risk in primparous teenage mothers. The associated morbidity and mortality are chiefly the result of complications related to bowel obstruction, bowel infarction, or sepsis.

TABLE 65-2 Distinguishing Features of Gastroschisis and Omphalocele

	GASTROSCHISIS	OMPHALOCELE
Location	Right paraumbilical	Midline
Umbilical cord insertion	Lateral to defect	Apex of defect
Size of defect	Small (2–4 cm)	Large (2–10 cm)
Covering membrane	No	Yes
Liver involvement	No	Common
Ascites	No	Common
Bowel thickening	Common at term	Rarely
Bowel atresia	Common	Rare
Bowel ischemia	Common	Rare
Cardiac anomalies	Rare (ASD, PDA)	Common
Associated karyotype abnormalities	No	Often

Ultrasound in the second trimester reveals bowel floating within the amniotic fluid outside the confines of the fetal abdomen, with insertion of the umbilical cord to the right of the defect. An omphalocele is a central abdominal wall fusion defect with a high association with chromosomal abnormalities. The midgut and occasionally the liver, spleen, or gonads are herniated into a translucent sac composed of amnion, peritoneum, and Wharton's jelly. The umbilical cord inserts centrally. The associated morbidity and mortality of omphalocele is chiefly determined by the underlying chromosomal defects.

Amniotic band syndrome is the result of amputations and defects of the abdominal wall and extremities resulting from ruptured bands of amnion within the amniotic fluid. The head may be spared, but occasionally unusually located encephaloceles are seen. The abdominal wall defects are asymmetric, eccentric, and may bear a resemblance to gastroschisis. Limb-body wall complex is a severe form of amniotic band syndrome, which is incompatible with life. The presence of both an omphalocele and severe scoliotic curvature of the fetal spine are suggestive of the diagnosis.

FETAL GENITOURINARY TRACT

The fetal kidneys can be routinely visualized beyond gestation week 16, at which point the bladder begins to fill with urine and empty every 30 to 45 minutes. A potential pitfall in the assessment of the fetal kidneys is that the presence of reniform structures in the flanks may not necessarily signify kidneys as the adrenal glands may enlarge and appear reniform shape in renal agenesis. Thus, lack of visualization of the bladder and oligohydramnios is a more reliable indicator of nonfunctioning or absent kidneys. Fetal urinary tract anomalies may include obstructive processes as well as functional impairment. The consequences of obstructive processes exist on a continuum from mild hydronephrosis to the nonfunctional multicystic dysplastic kidney.

Renal agenesis results from failure of differentiation of the metanephric blastema during the first month of embryogenesis. The affected kidney, renal artery, and ureter are absent. Unilateral agenesis, which is compatible with normal life, is at least twice as common as the lethal bilateral agenesis. This entity is heritable in approximately 15% of cases. The diagnosis of bilateral agenesis is suggested sonographically by oligohydramnios and lack of bladder filling. Potter's sequence is the clinical syndrome associated with bilateral renal agenesis and the resulting oligohydramnios. Affected infants have a typical facial appearance with a flattened nose, low-set ears, and prominent epicanthal folds. Various skeletal and cardiovascular malformations may be present. The severe pulmonary hypoplasia is incompatible with life. Bilateral agenesis may be seen in conjunction with chromosomal abnormalities, multicystic dysplastic kidney, or as part of a constellation of complex anomalies such as VACTERL.

Cystic renal diseases include multicystic dysplastic kidney disease (MCDK) and polycystic kidney disease. Polycystic kidney disease exists in two forms: the autosomal recessive (ARPKD) infantile type and the autosomal dominant (ADPKD) later (adult) onset type. The kidneys are enlarged and hypoechoic, and individual cysts cannot be identified sonographically. ARPKD is a spectrum of liver and renal disease; the severity of the hepatic and renal manifestations vary inversely. Renal disease dominates in the severe perinatal form and can result in the Potter sequence.

MCDK, which is the most common neonatal renal mass, is the end result of severe in utero obstruction. The upper third of the ureter is atretic, which prevents the metanephric blastema from producing nephrons. The collecting tubules become dilated. Ultrasound features include a paraspinal mass with numerous cysts of varying sizes. These cysts do not communicate, which allows discrimination from hydronephrosis. Contralateral renal anomalies, most commonly ureteropelvic junction (UPJ) obstruction, are present in 40% of cases. The condition is lethal if associated with contralateral MCDK or renal agenesis. Meckel-Gruber, an autosomal recessive syndrome, requires two of the three characteristic features of bilateral multicystic dysplastic kidney, occipital encephalocele, and polydactyly for the diagnosis. As 95% of the affected fetuses have bilateral MCDK, the condition is generally lethal at birth.

Common obstructive processes include UPJ obstruction, ureterovesicle junction (UVJ) obstruction, and bladder outlet obstruction. UPJ obstruction is the most common antenatal cause of hydronephrosis. Abnormal ureteral recanalization, which normally begins in the midureter and continues proximally and distally, is a leading theory in the pathogenesis of intrinsic UPJ obstruction. Extrinsic causes of UPJ obstruction are most commonly associated with compression of the ureter by aberrant or supernumerary renal vessels, usually by low insertion of a renal artery. Contralateral renal anomalies are not uncommon. Severe obstruction can cause significant mass effect within the thorax and abdomen. Congenital UPJ obstruction may lead to progressive ipsilateral renal impairment.

UVJ obstruction is less common than UPJ obstruction. As with UPJ obstruction, when the process is unilateral, amniotic fluid volume remains unaffected. Underlying etiologies include a duplicated system with obstruction of the ectopic upper pole moiety, primary megaureter, which is a functional obstruction, and distal ureteral atresia or stricture. If severe, renal function can be affected by urinary stasis and reflux.

Posterior urethral valves (PUV) in a male infant are by far the most common cause of fetal bladder outlet obstruction. A posterior urethral valve is an abnormal membrane which arises during abnormal embryological development of the Wolffian duct. Key sonographic findings include a thickened bladder wall with bladder and posterior urethral dilatation, the appearance of which has been likened to a keyhole. Urinary ascites may develop as a consequence of calyceal rupture caused by extremely high pressures generated by constant urinary reflux and stasis. Outcome depends upon the severity of the resulting renal dysfunction and oligohydramnios.

FETAL MUSCULOSKELETAL SYSTEM

Second and third trimester sonographic evaluation of the osseous structures, particularly the extremities, can be helpful in detection of a host of skeletal dysplasias. Long bone lengths greater than two standard deviations below the mean are highly suggestive of dwarfisms. A small thoracic circumference with associated pulmonary hypoplasia is ominous for lethal skeletal abnormality such as thanatophoric dwarfism, which is the most common lethal dysplasia. The most common nonlethal skeletal dysplasia is heterozygous achondroplasia. Fetuses with the lethal autosomal recessive form of osteogenesis imperfecta, OI type II, lack skull ossification and demonstrate multiple angulated long bone fractures.

Caudal regression is caused by abnormal caudal mesoderm development. While the pathogenesis is largely unknown, up to 20% of cases affect fetuses of diabetic mothers. The entity encompasses a spectrum from complete sacral absence with associated lumbar spine, lower extremity, GI, and GU abnormalities to milder sacral abnormalities without associated defects. Typically, sonographic findings will include absence of one or more vertebrae with fused appearance of the ilia and decreased distance between the femoral heads. The most severe manifestation of caudal regression syndrome is sirenomelia, in which the lower extremities are fused and bilateral renal agenesis or MCKD leads to marked oligohydramnios.

Sonographic evaluation of the hands and feet can provide valuable information about anatomic defects of these extremities, some of which are highly associated with underlying chromosomal abnormalities. The presence of a rocker bottom foot is strongly associated with trisomy 18. Equinovarus talipes, or congenital clubfoot, may be seen in isolation or in combination with other chromosomal abnormalities, neuromuscular disorders, oligohydramnios, amniotic band syndrome, or connective tissue disorders. The foot remains fixed at a right angle to the tibia, and the metatarsal bones are seen in the same imaging plane as the tibia and fibula. Fixed overlapping of the index over the other closed digits is known as clenched fist. The thumb is adducted, and the proximal interphalangeal joint of the index finger flexed. The position is constant during sonographic evaluation and is strongly associated with trisomy 18. Clinodactyly is fixed deviation of the fifth finger in the radioulnar plane. This abnormality is caused by a short middle phalanx, which causes radial angulation of the distal interphalangeal joint. Clinodactyly is associated with trisomy 21 and should prompt a search for other findings suggestive of the diagnosis.

TABLE 65-3 Sonographic Markers of Chromosomal Abnormalities

TRISOMY 21	TRISOMY 18
Thickened nuchal fold (>5 mm)	Choroid plexus cysts
Echogenic intracardiac focus	
Short femur	
Short humerus	
Pyelectasis (>4 mm)	
Absent nasal bone	

CHROMOSOMAL ABNORMALITIES AND SYNDROMES

A search for sonographic findings supportive of the diagnosis of chromosomal abnormalities may be undertaken in cases of abnormal triple or quadruple screen results, or when a sonographic finding with high association with such anomalies is discovered. Choroid plexus cysts are identified in approximately 1% of pregnancies scanned during the second trimester. The majority will resolve by the third trimester with no implications upon fetal outcome. However, the presence of choroid plexus cysts is a marker for possible increased risk of trisomy 18. Similarly, a single echogenic intracardiac focus is a marker which has been associated with trisomy 21. This echogenic focus correlates with papillary muscle mineralization. With either finding, the fetus should be carefully evaluated as additional abnormalities confer marked increased risk for aneuploidy (Tables 65-3 to 65-6).

TABLE 65-4 Additional Sonographic Findings of Chromosomal Abnormalities

TRISOMY 21	TRISOMY 18
Major cardiac abnormalities (endocardial cushion defect most common)	Persistent clenched hand
	Holoprosencephaly
	Omphalocele
	Rocker bottom feet

TABLE 65-5 Triple/Quadruple Screen Markers in Chromosomal or Structural Abnormalities Compared to Maternal Blood Serum Concentrations in Normal Subjects

MARKER	TRISOMY 21	TRISOMY 18
Alpha-fetoprotein (AFP)	Low	Low
Unconjugated estriol (uE3)	Low	Low
Human chorionic gonadotropin (hCG)	High	Low
Inhibin A (quadruple screen only)	High	Not used

DATING AND FETAL GROWTH

While crown-rump measurement in the first trimester is fairly precise for dating of pregnancy, sonographic gestational age assessment becomes increasingly less accurate as pregnancy progresses. Biparietal diameter, head circumference, and femur length are measurements used for dating which, when used in the second trimester, obtain a 95% confidence level of ±10 to 12 days with the greatest accuracy before 20 weeks gestation. The abdominal circumference measurement has been found to reflect size more so than gestational age, especially in the third trimester. Beyond 26 weeks, ultrasound is much less reliable with a 95% confidence level of ± 3 weeks. Some data suggest that femur length may be the most accurate measurement in the third trimester. The transverse cerebellar diameter has also been reported to be a fairly reliable predictor in the second and third trimester.

Third trimester pregnancy dating can become important in cases in which patients received no previous prenatal care or in cases in which fetal growth disturbances are suspected. Because of difficulty in accurately dating a pregnancy in the third trimester through measurements, investigators have tried to determine fetal age and more importantly, fetal lung maturity, by the appearance of different organ systems, including bowel, lungs, bones, and placenta. These correlations have met with a limited success. For example, a mature appearance of the placenta is usually associated with fetal lung maturity in most low-risk patients, but multiple case reports describe hyaline membrane disease in patients with a sonographically mature placenta. More recently, appearance of long bone ossification centers has been studied as a predictor of gestational age. The distal femoral epiphysis is seen by approximately 33 weeks, while the proximal humeral epiphysis is not present before 37 weeks.

TABLE 65-6 Causes of Elevated Maternal Serum Alpha-Fetoprotein Level

Fetal causes
Open neural tube defects
Fetal demise
Multiple gestation
Omphalocele, gastroschisis
Sacrococcygeal teratoma
Cystic hygroma
Maternal causes
Subchorionic or retroplacental hemorrhage
Inaccurate dating of pregnancy

SMALL FOR DATES

Patients may be referred for ultrasound examination because of small uterine size for stated menstrual age or because of known fetal or maternal abnormalities which increase risk for intrauterine growth restriction (IUGR). While a fetus below the 10th percentile for weight is at risk for growth restriction, many of these infants are normal. However, true growth restricted fetuses are at high risk for significant morbidity and mortality. Ultrasound is a helpful tool for identifying fetuses at risk with the use of fetal parameters such as abdominal circumference, weight, and body proportionality. In most cases of IUGR, the abdomen is small whereas head circumference is spared. Therefore, abdominal circumference and head circumference ratios are commonly used in the evaluation. These pregnancies are generally followed closely with ultrasound for interval growth assessment, particularly if the gestational age is uncertain.

In some cases, a small uterine size for menstrual dates is due to oligohydramnios. Decreased amniotic fluid volume can be quantitatively diagnosed if the largest vertical pocket of fluid is less than 2 cm or the amniotic fluid index, which adds the largest vertical pocket in each of the four abdominal quadrants, is less than 5 cm. Oligohydramnios may be due to intrauterine fetal demise, bilateral renal anomalies, in utero infection, premature rupture of membranes, postdates pregnancy, and chromosomal abnormalities (Tables 65-7 and 65-8).

LARGE FOR DATES

Sonographic evaluation may also be helpful in cases in which the uterus is clinically large for the patient's gestational age. Fetuses with estimated fetal weight above the 90th percentile or above 4000 or 4500 g, depending on the selected diagnostic threshold, are large for gestational age (LGA). Risk factors include maternal diabetes, maternal obesity, and a previous LGA infant. Most LGA fetuses are symmetrically large. Macrosomic infants are a subset of LGA fetuses in whom the shoulder and body are disproportionately large; these fetuses are at significantly increased risk for shoulder dystocia during delivery. Macrosomia is associated with maternal gestational diabetes (for which it may be the only diagnostic indicator) as well as preexisting insulin-dependent maternal diabetes. Other reported complications of

TABLE 65-7 Causes of Intrauterine Growth Restriction

PLACENTAL CAUSES	MATERNAL CAUSES	FETAL CAUSES
Twin–twin transfusion	Hypertension	Chromosomal abnormalities
Placental abnormalities	Chronic renal disease	Congenital infections
Chronic abruption	Severe diabetes	Multiple gestations
Placenta previa	Hemoglobinopathies	
	Autoimmune disease	
	Smoking	
	Substance abuse	
	Uterine malformations	

LGA fetuses include birth asphyxia, meconium aspiration, neonatal hypoglycemia, and birth trauma.

Other entities which may cause a larger than expected uterus include polyhydramnios, multiple gestations, and uterine leiomyomas. Uterine leiomyomas may significantly enlarge under hormone influences in the second and third trimester, causing marked uterine distortion. Multiple gestations may significantly enlarge the uterus even while the fetuses are individually small.

While many experienced practitioners accurately diagnose polyhydramnios by gestalt, it can be quantitatively defined as a single vertical pocket greater than 8 cm or an amniotic fluid index of greater than 20 cm. In many cases, increased amniotic fluid volume is idiopathic. However, the majority of pregnancies with markedly increased amniotic fluid are associated with underlying congenital abnormalities including fetal hydrops, CNS lesions, thoracic mass, GI obstruction, and twin–twin transfusion. Other causes include maternal diabetes mellitus, congenital infection, and multiple gestations (Table 65-9).

FETAL WELL-BEING

The biophysical profile (BPP) is a powerful predictor of fetal risk hypoxia, distress, and perinatal death. The results may be used to determine the timing of delivery in high-risk pregnancies. The BPP grading system is a binomial system to which scores of 0, 1, or 2 are assigned to the four variables of fetal tone, breathing movements, gross body movements, and amniotic fluid volume. These four variables are combined with the results of nonstress testing for a maximum score of 10. A BPP score of eight or higher portends a negative predictive value of approximately 99% for normal live outcome within 1 week of the test; a score of two or less is highly predictive of impending fetal demise. The intermediate scores of 4 to 7 have variable outcomes.

Umbilical artery Doppler velocity waveform analysis can further elucidate the risk of fetal morbidity and mortality in cases of suspected IUGR with hypoxemia. An abnormal Doppler ratio indicates compromise of fetal circulation, although the degree of ratio increase generally does not correlate with the severity of the distress. The ratio is obtained by comparing peak umbilical artery systole (A) to end-diastole (B). Normally, A/B ratios progressively decrease throughout the second and third trimesters from mean values of 4.25 at 16 weeks to 2.5 at term. Decreased fetal blood flow may be secondary to increased vascular resistance within the placenta, abnormalities of the fetus itself, or maternal cardiovascular problems. Analysis of the middle cerebral artery Doppler waveform may further characterize the degree of hypoxemia in the fetus with asymmetric IUGR and abnormal umbilical artery Doppler ratios. Initially, the MCA end diastolic velocity will increase, while the pulsatility index (peak systole minus end-diastole divided by the area under the curve of one waveform) will decline as autoregulation preserves brain flow at the expense of blood flow to the remainder of the body. As

TABLE 65-8 Causes of Oligohydramnios

Intrauterine fetal demise
Renal anomalies
Intrauterine growth restriction
Postmaturity syndrome
Premature rupture of membranes
Maternal use of prostaglandin synthase inhibitors of ACE inhibitors
Chromosomal abnormalities
Placental insufficiency

TABLE 65-9 Causes of Polyhydramnios

Fetal causes
CNS abnormalities
Neural tube defects
Hydrocephalous
GI abnormalities
Upper GI obstruction
Abdominal wall defects
Twin–twin transfusion syndrome
Congenital infections
Chromosomal abnormalities
Maternal causes
Maternal diabetes
Erythroblastosis fetalis

the fetal distress worsens and end-diastolic velocity decreases, autoregulation is lost and the pulsatility index rises. The loss of autoregulation is likely due to brain edema.

FETAL PRESENTATION

Sonographic evaluation of fetal lie or presentation is both time-efficient and radiation-free, which are significant advantages over the older radiographic method. At term, the fetal lie may have implications in the management of delivery.

PLACENTATION ABNORMALITIES

In most cases, placental implantation occurs well away from the internal cervical os. In a small minority of cases during the second trimester, the placenta extends to or partially or totally covers the os. Partial and complete previas partially and completely cover the os, respectively. Marginal placentas extend within 2 cm of the os. After the initial detection of these placental abnormalities, the patient is followed with repeat ultrasound early in the third trimester. Placenta previas can regress, so that at term only 0.5% of these abnormalities persist. The apparent regression of the previa has been attributed to more rapid growth of the more cranial uterus as compared to the lower uterine segment and cervical regions during pregnancy. A newer, more widely accepted theory involves involution of the placenta previa owing to lack of vascular support from the cervix (trophotropism). Should the previa or marginal placenta continue, cesarean delivery is planned before the onset of labor to prevent major hemorrhage. Potential pitfalls in the diagnosis of placenta previa include overdistention of the bladder and focal myometrial contractions at the time of the ultrasound evaluation. The patient should be reimaged after bladder emptying if placenta previa or a low-lying placenta is suspected.

In normal placentation, the endometrium prevents placental invasion into the uterine myometrium. Placenta invasion refers to the abnormal penetration of chorionic villi into or even through the uterus. Placenta accreta, which constitutes 80% of such cases, is the adherence of chorionic villi to the superficial myometrium. Approximately 15% involve deep invasion into the myometrium, termed placenta increta. In less than 5% of cases, the villi completely penetrate through the uterus and may invade adjacent organs such as the bladder. Detection of placental invasion is critical as it may result in catastrophic maternal hemorrhage at delivery or infection caused by retained placenta. Prior cesarean section or other surgical intervention of the uterus with subsequent scar formation is a known risk factor. Sonographic diagnosis is based upon demonstration of retroplacental vascularity within or projecting through the myometrium. MRI may be helpful if the diagnosis is equivocal.

UMBILICAL CORD

The normal umbilical cord contains two arteries and one vein. A two-vessel cord with a single artery and vein is associated with karyotype or structural abnormalities in singleton pregnancies; two-vessel cord in multiple pregnancy is less likely to have associated abnormalities. The cord may have only two vessels for portions of its length, but color Doppler imaging of the iliac arteries on both sides of the urinary bladder confirms the presence of two arteries at the fetal level. Evaluation of fetal growth in the third trimester is recommended given the association of two vessel cords and intrauterine growth restriction.

Anomalous umbilical cord insertion into the placenta has potentially critical ramifications. Cord insertion is normal if it occurs anywhere in the placental substance, including its margin. A velamentous cord insertion is insertion beyond the margin of the placenta. The umbilical cord arteries and vein are connected to the placenta by a pedicle and covered only by the amnion and chorion. If undetected sonographically, the vessels can rupture during labor and delivery and cause life-threatening fetal hemorrhage. If these anomalous vessels cross the internal os, the condition is termed vasa previa. Again, catastrophic fetal blood loss can occur at the time of membrane rupture or delivery.

VAGINAL BLEEDING

As previously discussed, the entities of placenta previa, placental invasion, velamentous cord insertion, and vasa previa may lead to major fetal and/or maternal peripartal hemorrhage. Another important cause of vaginal bleeding during the second and third trimester is placental abruption, which is the premature separation of the implanted placenta from the uterus. As 50% of abruptions are sonographically occult, the diagnosis is primarily clinical. Nonetheless, retroplacental hemorrhage on ultrasound is diagnostic.

CERVIX

The average length of the normal cervix at 20 weeks is 3.5 to 4.0 cm as measured along the endocervical canal. Transvaginal, rather than transabdominal, cervical length evaluation is more reliable and more reproducible. The shortest length observed during sonographic evaluation should be reported. Before 32 weeks, measurements below the 10th percentile, which is 2.5 cm, are generally considered to suggest a risk for preterm labor. Beyond 32 weeks, cervical length becomes less reliable as a predictor of achievement of term pregnancy as cervical effacement generally begins 4 to 8 weeks before delivery.

Incompetent cervix refers to the painless, premature dilatation of the cervical canal. This term is generally applied to cervical dilatation during the first or early second trimesters. Women who have a cerclage placed for incompetent cervix should be followed with serial ultrasound examinations.

MULTIPLE GESTATIONS

Multiple gestations have profound implications upon prenatal, perinatal, and postnatal clinical management. The worldwide incidence of twins is slightly less than one in every 100 births. However, twins and even higher-order multiples are occurring at increased frequency as infertility treatments are introduced and improved. The inherent risks of pregnancy, such as preeclampsia, preterm delivery, growth restriction, and umbilical cord accidents, are significantly increased in multiple gestations.

Differentiation of the different categories of twins is important as the risks for adverse outcome is significantly increased in twinning other than the dichorionic-diamniotic type. One of the feared complications of monochorionic twinning is twin–twin transfusion syndrome (TTS), in which the blood of one twin flows preferentially to the other through a shared placenta. The donor twin becomes hypovolemic and oliguric, and oligohydramnios develops in its amniotic cavity if the twins are diamnionic. Severe oligohydramnios may lead to stuck twin syndrome in which the donor twin may appear fused to the uterine wall. The recipient twin is significantly larger and may develop cardiac failure as a result of volume overload. Polyhydramnios within its amniotic cavity may cause rapid maternal abdomen enlargement. Both twins are at risk for hydrops fetalis. In utero treatments for TTS include reduction amniocentesis of the fluid surrounding the recipient twin. A few medical centers offer laser photocoagulation of chorionic plate vessels to destroy the anastomoses within the placenta allowing the abnormal circulation.

Embolization is a complication of monochorionic twinning in which the death of one twin results in a sudden hemodynamic shift of blood to the remaining twin that ultimately leads to the demise of the latter. Rarer is the acardiac twin, in which a twin with a nonfunctioning heart receives blood supply from a donor twin via arteriovenous anastomoses; the cardiac demand upon the normal twin may lead to heart failure and death. Monochorionic/monoamniotic twins carry not only the risks inherent to monochorionic pregnancies, but have an extraordinarily high risk of cord entanglement as they are not physically separated by a dividing membrane. The risk of minor and major anomalies involving one or both twins approaches 90%. The risk of intrauterine demise of one or both twins is approximately 50%. Cesarean delivery upon relative lung maturity, usually around 32 weeks gestation, is typical.

SUGGESTED READING

Barboza JM, Dajani NK, Glenn LG, et al. Prenatal diagnosis of congenital cardiac anomalies: a practical approach using two basic views. *Radiographics*. 2002;22:1125.

Bree, R et al. Transvaginal sonography in the evaluation of normal early pregnancy: correlation with HCG. *AJR Am J Roentgenol*. 1989;153:75.

Dulay A, Copel J. First-trimester ultrasound: current uses and applications. *Semin Ultrasound CT MR*. 2008;29:121-131.

Emanuel PG, Garcia GI, Angtuaco TL. Prenatal detection of anterior abdominal wall defects with US. *Radiographics*. 1995;15:517.

Epelman M, Daneman A, Blaser S, et al. Differential diagnosis of intracranial cystic lesions at head US: correlation with CT and MRI. *Radiographics*. 2006;26:173.

Frates M, Laing F. Sonographic evaluation of ectopic pregnancy: an update. *AJR Am J Roentgenol*. 1995;165:251-259.

Malone F et al. First-trimester or second-trimester screening, or both, for down's syndrome. *N Engl J Med*. 2005;353:2001-2011.

Manjiri D et al. Sonography in first trimester bleeding. *J Clin Ultrasound*. 2008;36(6):352-366.

McNamara A, Levine D. Intraadbdominal fetal echogenic masses: a practical guide to diagnosis and management. *Radiographics*. 2005;25:633.

Moore K, Persaud T. Placenta and fetal membranes. In: *The Developing Human: Clinically Oriented Embryology*. 6th ed. Philadelphia, PA: W.B. Saunders Company; 1998:129.

Nicolaides K. *The 11-13 Weeks Scan*. London, UK: Fetal Medicine Foundation; 2004:85-88.

Rypens F et al. Obstetric US: watch the fetal hands. *Radiographics*. 2006;26:811.

Thieme G, Manco-Johnson M. A pictorial review of normal obstetric ultrasound. *Ultrasound Q*. 1999;15(3):106-134.

QUESTIONS AND ANSWERS

1. Prenatal sonography demonstrates widening of the lateral masses of the lumbo-sacral spine. Which of the following is an associated intracranial finding?
   A. Effacement of the cisterna magna
   B. Monoventricle
   C. Megacisterna magna
   D. Absence of the cavum septum pellucidum
   E. Strawberry skull

ANSWER: A. Widening of the lateral masses of the lumbo-sacral spine suggests spina bifida aperta, most likely a meningomyelocele. This type of defect is consistently associated with a Chiari type II malformation of the intracranial posterior fossa, which consists of inferior displacement of posterior fossa structures through the foramen magna resulting in obliteration of the cisterna magna and a small, abnormal-shaped cerebellum (banana sign). A variable degree of ventricular enlargement as well as frontal bossing of the cranial vault (lemon sign) are frequently present. Absence of the cavum septum pellucidum is not a finding associated with spina bifida but would suggest the presence of a midline defect such as agenesis of the corpus callosum or holoprosencephaly, as would monoventricle. Strawberry-shaped skull is associated with trisomy 18.

2. Hydrops is associated with fetal ascites in which of the following?
   A. Posterior urethral valves
   B. Cardiac abnormalities
   C. Duodenal atresia
   D. Echogenic bowel
   E. Renal dysplasia

   ANSWER: B. Fetal hydrops is defined as the abnormal accumulation of fluid in at least two fetal sites, which include body cavities and soft tissues. The development of hydrops can be explained by an imbalance of intravascular and interstitial fluid compartments. Cardiac failure caused by cardiac anomalies as well as obstruction of venous and lymphatic flow by a mass are two possible mechanisms. Fetal ascites seen without other associated findings of hydrops is usually because of a GI or GU obstruction causing viscous rupture and leakage of urine or bowel contents. Etiologies would include posterior urethral valves and duodenal atresia. Echogenic bowel is considered a soft maker for trisomy 21.

3. Which of the following is used to evaluate fetuses with suspected IUGR?
   A. Quadruple screen
   B. Amniocentesis
   C. Doppler of the middle cerebral artery
   D. Chorionic villus sampling
   E. Nuchal translucency

   ANSWER: C. When IUGR is diagnosed or suspected, fetal growth and well-being should be monitored for the remainder of the pregnancy since these fetuses are at high risk for mortality and morbidity. Weekly or semiweekly studies are recommended in the third trimester. The biophysical profile score, amniotic fluid volume, and spectral Doppler waveforms of the umbilical artery and middle cerebral artery are criteria used to evaluate fetal well-being. A worsening trend of these parameters may prompt early delivery. Amniocentesis may be used to evaluate fetal lung maturity but would give no information regarding the status of a fetus with possible IUGR. The quadruple screen, chorionic villus sampling, and nuchal translucency are all used in the detection of probability of chromosomal abnormalities.

4. Which of the following is a sonographic finding associated with renal dysplasia?
   A. Polyhydramnios
   B. Cysts
   C. Mesoblastic nephroma
   D. Hydronephrosis
   E. Most often bilateral

   ANSWER: B. Renal dysplasia includes a spectrum abnormality, secondary to early renal obstruction. Multicystic dysplastic kidney is the most severe form and is secondary to atresia of the upper one-third of the ureter. Fewer cortical cysts with an echogenic parenchymal pattern is usually the manifestation of renal dysplasia secondary to severe urethral or UPJ obstruction in the first half of pregnancy. Without the presence of large cysts, these kidneys may be abnormally small. Dysplastic kidneys may be mistaken for hydronephrotic kidneys because of their cystic appearance; however, hydronephrosis is not an associated finding. Renal dysplasia is usually associated with oligohydramnios. Mesoblastic nephroma is the most common renal tumor in the fetus and can appear partially cystic, although usually appears as a solid tumor.

5. Which of the following is the most accurate sonographic measurement used for dating pregnancy in the first trimester?
   A. Biparietal diameter
   B. Crown rump length
   C. Humerus length
   D. Head circumference
   E. Abdominal circumference

   ANSWER: B. Crown-rump length is the most accurate for dating in the first trimester. Biparietal diameter, head circumference, femur length, and humerus length are measurements used for dating which, when used in the second trimester, obtain a 95% confidence level of ± 10 to 12 days with the greatest accuracy below 20 weeks. The transverse cerebellar diameter is reported to be a fairly reliable method in the second and possibly third trimester if well visualized. The abdominal circumference measurement has been found to reflect size more so than gestational age, especially in the third trimester.

6. Which of the following cardiac anomalies is best detected on outflow tract images of the fetal heart?
   A. Endocardial cushion defect
   B. Ventricular septal defect
   C. Hypoplastic left heart
   D. Tetralogy of Fallot
   E. Fetal tachyarrhythmia

   ANSWER: D. Both Tetralogy of Fallot and transposition of the great arteries are more readily apparent on outflow tract views of the fetal heart, as both the pulmonary artery and aorta should be visualized for confirming these diagnoses. The four chamber view is valuable for evaluation of chamber size (i.e., hypoplastic left heart) and atrioventricular connections so that endocardial cushion defects and ventricular septal defects may be detected. Fetal arrhythmias are detected with M-mode Doppler imaging

7. Which of the following is the most likely etiology of a dilated fetal stomach and duodenum detected upon a 20-week fetal anatomic survey?
   A. Esophageal atresia
   B. Anterior abdominal wall defect
   C. Cystic fibrosis
   D. Duodenal atresia
   E. Severe hydrocephalus

   ANSWER: D. The classic "double-bubble" sign caused by dilation of the fetal stomach and duodenum is highly suspicious for duodenal atresia, which has a relatively strong association with underlying chromosomal abnormalities. Other entities, which may cause a similar appearance indicative of some degree of duodenal obstruction include annular pancreas, high-grade duodenal stenosis, and peritoneal bands. Esophageal atresia is in the differential diagnosis for lack of fluid distention of the fetal stomach after 20 weeks and is associated with the VACTERL syndrome. Severe hydrocephalus and other neurologic defects, which may impair swallowing, may similarly be accompanied by lack of stomach distention. Cystic fibrosis may be associated with echogenic bowel or peritoneal calcifications. Anterior abdominal wall defects are a broad category of herniations of bowel outside the abdominal wall.

8. Dizygotic twinning is most readily confirmed by
   A. Presence of a thick dividing membrane
   B. Detection of twins of different gender
   C. Presence of two placentas
   D. Diagnosis of twin–twin transfusion syndrome
   E. Presence of two amniotic sacs

   ANSWER: B. Twins of different gender confirms that the twinning is dizygotic, or fraternal, rather than monozygotic, or identical. A thick dividing membrane and two placentas are seen in dichorionic–diamniotic twins. While dizygotic twins are always dichorionic–diamniotic, monozygotic twins may be dichorionic–diamniotic, monochorionic–diamniotic, monochorionic–monoamniotic, or conjoined. Their chorionicity and amnionicity is thought to depend upon the timing of the cleavage of the blastocyst into two separate developing embryos. Two separate amnions will be seen in all twins other than monochorionic–monoamniotic and conjoined twins. Twin–twin transfusion syndrome is a complication unique to monozygotic twins.

9. Which of the following is associated with decreased maternal alpha-fetoprotein levels?
   A. Down syndrome
   B. Neural tube defect
   C. Intrauterine fetal demise
   D. Multiple gestations
   E. Gastroschisis

   ANSWER: A. Alpha-fetoprotein is the major circulatory protein of the early fetus. It is formed initially by the yolk sac and the fetal intestine and later by the fetal liver. Screening with maternal serum AFP is performed at 16 to 18 weeks gestation, and values must be corrected for dates, maternal weight, and race. Elevated maternal serum AFP levels are associated with congenital defects including gastroschisis, anencephaly, open spinal defects, omphalocele, renal agenesis, and occasionally proximal fetal bowel obstruction. It may be falsely elevated by incorrect dates, multiple gestations, and intrauterine fetal demise. Low maternal serum AFP levels are seen in incorrect pregnancy dating and trisomy 21.

10. Which of the following is most strongly associated with choroid plexus cysts?
    A. Turner syndrome
    B. Trisomy 21
    C. Trisomy 18
    D. Trisomy 13
    E. Chiari malformation

    ANSWER: C. Choroid plexus cysts will be visible in approximately one-third of patients with trisomy 18 during the second trimester. However, they can be present in up to 5% of normal second trimester fetuses. Visualization of choroid plexus cysts should prompt careful anatomic evaluation for other anomalies. These cysts often resolve in the late second or early third trimester.

66 VASCULAR ULTRASOUND

Mark E. Lockhart and Heather L. Haddad

AORTA

The aorta and inferior vena cava (IVC) are the largest arterial and venous structures in the body. They are retroperitoneal structures that course through the diaphragmatic hiatus near the midline abdomen. The aorta is typically located to the left of the IVC. The wall of the abdominal aorta is composed of three layers: intima, media, and adventitia. When abdominal aortic aneurysm (AAA) develops, there is expansion of all three layers. This differs from pseudoaneurysm (PSA), which expands the aorta but no longer is contained by all three layers. The first major branch of the abdominal aorta is usually the celiac axis, but paired inferior phrenic arteries may originate cranial to the celiac artery. Both renal arteries originate from the lateral aspects of the aorta and lumbar arteries originate at each vertebral level, L1-4. The celiac artery and superior mesenteric artery supply abdominal organs. At approximately the L4 level, the aorta divides into two common iliac arteries.

In recent years, endostent placement has replaced open repair for AAA. Endoleak into the aneurysm sac around the stent after stent repair of AAA is a common complication.

The most common type of endoleak results from retrograde filling of a branch vessel such as the inferior mesenteric artery, classified as type II endoleak. Ultrasound can detect abnormal flow in the aneurysm sac around the stent and may be used to guide therapy (Table 66-1).

RENAL

RENAL ARTERY STENOSIS

The clinical presentation of renal artery stenosis (RAS) includes refractory hypertension resistant to simultaneous treatment with three or more antihypertensive medications, impaired renal function (azotemia), or acute renal failure after antihypertensive therapy with ACE inhibitors or angiotensin receptor blockers. Hypertension occurs because of effects on the renin angiotensin system. Diagnosis can be made by ultrasound, but invasive techniques like angioplasty are required for treatment. Ultrasound criteria for RAS include peak systolic velocity (PSV) greater than 200 cm/s, ratio of renal artery PSV to aortic PSV greater than 3.5, asymmetry of intrarenal resistive indices compared with contralateral kidney, segmental artery delayed acceleration, and parvus-tardus waveforms.

Beyond the diagnosis of RAS, ultrasound may also suggest which patients will benefit from angioplasty. If the resistive index (PSV-EDV/PSV) is elevated (greater than 0.80), these patients do not benefit from interventional therapy (Rademacher). However, these results have been challenged in subsequent studies.

TABLE 66-1 Aortic Stent Endoleak Classification

Type I	Attachment site leak at the proximal or distal end of the endostent
Type II	Reversed flow in branch artery
Type III	Modular failure
Type IV	Porosity of the graft
Type V	Expansion of the aneurysm with no endoleak "endotension"

RENAL VEIN THROMBOSIS

The etiologies of renal vein thrombosis (RVT) are numerous and include nephrotic syndrome, hypercoagulable states, birth control pills, antiphospholipid antibody syndrome/systemic lupus erythematosus, Behcet syndrome, renal neoplasms, trauma, and renal transplant. In infants, dehydration is the most common etiology. In adults, nephrotic syndrome, specifically membranous glomerulonephropathy, is the most common cause. On ultrasound, the kidney can acutely swell and increase in echogenicity. There may be absence of renal venous flow on color Doppler. Arterial waveforms will show high resistance flow. Rapid diagnosis is important if there is to be salvage of renal function.

HEPATIC

PORTAL HYPERTENSION

The etiology of portal hypertension may be prehepatic, intrahepatic, or posthepatic. Cirrhosis is the most common etiology and represents intrahepatic disease. There is normally no significant pressure gradient between the portal venous and hepatic venous systems. In a variety of clinical settings, the gradient may reach 13 mm Hg and lead to variceal formation or ascites. Signs of portal hypertension include dilatation of the main portal vein, monophasic hepatic venous flow, main portal vein or branch reversal, ascites, and varices.

Cavernous transformation occurs when there is collateral vessel formation in the setting of chronic portal vein thrombosis. This has clinical importance since it may prevent transplantation. On ultrasound, there will be a tangle of vessels visible in the hepatic hilum, and no normal portal vein is identified. Etiologies of portal vein thrombosis include abdominal malignancies such as hepatocellular and pancreatic carcinoma, hepatic dysfunction because of hepatitis or portal venous hypertension, abdominal infections or sepsis, pancreatitis, severe dehydration, hypercoagulable syndromes, and estrogen therapy.

TRANSJUGULAR INTRAHEPATIC PORTOSYSTEMIC SHUNT

The first-line treatment for variceal bleeding is medical management or endoscopic sclerotherapy. In patients who fail, transjugular intrahepatic portosystemic shunt (TIPS) placement is the suggested treatment. A shunt using open mesh or more recently polytetrafluorethylene graft material communicates between the right portal vein and either the right or middle hepatic vein. TIPS can also be used to treat intractable ascites. Although technical success rates are high, TIPS dysfunction is common within the first 2 years and requires surveillance.

Ultrasound is the primary method of monitoring for TIPS dysfunction. TIPS dysfunction may include stenosis, occlusion, infection, hemorrhage, or biliary leakage. On ultrasound, a variety of criteria may suggest stenosis such as low main portal vein velocity less than 30 cm/s, elevated intrashunt gradient greater than 50 to 100 cm/s, intrashunt peak velocity less than 90 cm/s or greater than 190 cm/s, reversal of portal vein branch flow from retrograde to antegrade flow. Interval change (increase greater than 60 cm/s or decrease greater than 40 cm/s) in peak intrashunt velocities compared with baseline may also herald TIPS failure.

ABDOMINAL VISCERAL

Mesenteric ischemia affects patients when there is involvement of at least two of the three major visceral vessels (celiac, superior mesenteric artery, or inferior mesenteric artery). Mesenteric ischemia can be classified as chronic or acute. Chronic mesenteric ischemia usually occurs secondary to long-standing atherosclerotic disease and less commonly caused by vasculitis. Patients typically present with postprandial abdominal pain, termed intestinal angina, and weight loss. Acute mesenteric ischemia is divided into embolic, thrombotic, and nonocclusive (vasoconstrictive and vasospastic) causes, each accounting for approximately a third of acute mesenteric ischemia cases. Patients may present with poorly localized severe abdominal pain, nausea, vomiting, and possibly prior episodes of intestinal angina. Mesenteric ischemia generally occurs in older individuals secondary to the increased prevalence of atherosclerotic disease, the most common etiology. Unlike atherosclerotic disease, vasculitis affects younger individuals, more commonly women. Sonographic findings include smooth hypoechoic thickening of the vessel wall with a halo appearance. The stenosis may occur at points other that the artery origin from the aorta.

RENAL TRANSPLANT

Transplant renal artery abnormalities are the most common vascular complications associated with renal transplant. Renal artery occlusion is devastating and typically results in allograft failure. Sonographic diagnosis relies on absence of flow in the renal artery and abnormal intrarenal perfusion. There may be persistent venous flow because of capsular arteries or an accessory renal artery supplying a portion of the kidney. RAS most commonly affects the surgical anastomosis. The artery is usually anastomosed to the external iliac artery in an end-to-side fashion, but end-to-end anastomosis to the internal iliac artery is also performed, especially in patients who undergo vascular revision.

Sonographic criteria for transplant RAS include PSV greater than 250 to 300 cm/s, renal artery to iliac artery ratio greater than 1.8, and parvus-tardus waveforms in the segmental renal arteries. Turbulence and mildly elevated velocities may occur in the absence of stenosis because of the angle at which the renal artery takes off from the external iliac artery. In chronic transplant RAS, formation of collateral vessels has been described and may hinder the diagnosis.

TRANSPLANT RENAL VEIN THROMBOSIS

Renal vein thrombosis (RTV) is more common in transplanted kidneys than in native kidneys. It is highly associated with renal allograft failure. RVT is most common in the first month after transplantation and presents with acute renal failure or pain. The kidney will appear swollen and high resistance flow is present on spectral Doppler. Although reversal of arterial diastolic flow is commonly described in RVT, this finding is more commonly because of acute rejection or ATN. Therefore, further evaluation is necessary unless thrombus is identified in the vein. Venous occlusion of the iliac vein will similarly limit outflow and have a similar presentation.

PSEUDOANEURYSM-ARTERIOVENOUS FISTULA

Development of arteriovenous fistula (AVF) occurs in as many as 10% to 15% of transplants after biopsy. Other than biopsy, rare etiologies include infection or trauma. PSA formation can also be related to needle procedure and may be mistaken for renal cyst if Doppler technique is not applied. Extrarenal AVF or PSA are rare and most commonly associated with surgical technical complication or infection. Extrarenal PSA most commonly occur at the anastomotic site.

HEPATIC TRANSPLANT

Hepatic artery thrombosis is a devastating complication that occurs when the artery acutely occludes. Doppler will not identify flow within the hepatic artery in its expected position alongside the portal vein. There may be elevated flow in the portal vein in an effort to compensate. In the setting of progressive development rather than acute occlusion, collaterals may form. The bile ducts are solely supplied by the hepatic artery and are most susceptible to ischemia. In hepatic artery thrombosis, the bile ducts necrose and fill with fluid and gas. Biliary necrosis is severe and may lead to death if transplantation is not again available.

Hepatic artery stenosis is often a precursor to thrombosis, and noninvasive diagnosis by ultrasound is important. Doppler will show focal turbulence and aliasing at the site of stenosis with a 3:1 velocity ratio relative to the upstream artery. Parvus-tardus waveforms beyond the stenosis can confirm the diagnosis but have low sensitivity. Absence of diastolic flow within the hepatic artery is an ominous finding that may predict future thrombosis. The most common location of hepatic artery stenosis is the anastomotic site. Studies have shown that Doppler velocity criteria obtained from the hepatic artery are not useful in the first 48 hours to predict thrombosis as long as diastolic flow is present.

IVC stenosis is difficult to diagnose as the etiology of transplant dysfunction. A 3:1 or 4:1 ratio of stenotic flow versus vena cava inflow suggests abnormality. Absence of transmitted cardiac pulsatility below the narrowing is another indicator of significant abnormality. In many cases, there may be only a kink in the venous structures because of positioning of the liver, but fibrotic strictures can occur.

SCROTAL

Testicular torsion affects young males and usually presents with symptoms of acute testicular pain. The testis is supplied primarily by the testicular arteries, which arise directly off the anterolateral aspect of the aorta just below the renal artery origins. Testicular torsion can be incomplete or complete, ranging between 90 and 1080 degrees. In partial or incomplete torsion, the degree of spermatic cord rotation is less than 360 degrees. Color Doppler imaging may demonstrate decreased flow and asymmetric arterial waveform as compared with the contralateral testicle. In complete torsion, the rotation is greater than 360 degrees. In 720-degree torsion, the testicle can become nonviable in as early as 6 hours. Rapid diagnosis is important since nearly 100% can be salvaged within 4 to 6 hours but only 70% can be salvaged after 6 to 12 hours, and 20% at 12 to 24 hours. Sonographic findings include absence of flow in the arteries within the testicular parenchyma, absent venous flow, and testicular enlargement. Later findings of hypoechoic echotexture of the testis occur after salvage is no longer possible (see Chapter 67, "The Scrotum").

VARICOCELE

Enlargement of the intrascrotal venous plexus can be symptomatic and palpable. It may be confused for testicular mass, but ultrasound can differentiate the two diagnoses. Intratesticular varicocele (rare) will be a linear anechoic structure with vascular flow on Doppler. However, most are extratesticular. There are two mechanisms of varicocele formation. Type I includes valvular insufficiency and type II is associated with outflow obstruction. Varicocele is more common on the left, and isolated right-sided varicocele should prompt further evaluation for outflow obstruction because of renal mass or adenopathy. Diagnosis of varicocele by ultrasound is based upon identification of dilated veins (greater than 2–3 mm) and engorgement of the veins during Valsalva. There may be persistent reversal of venous flow or reversal only during Valsalva. If there is clinical suspicion, it is important to scan the patient in standing position to increase diagnostic sensitivity for varicocele.

PERIPHERAL VENOUS

Deep venous thrombosis evaluation of the lower extremity is one of the most common Doppler studies performed. Ultrasound is critical since the clinical examination is nonspecific to differentiate cellulitis, thrombophlebitis, and DVT. The exclusion of DVT is necessary since untreated DVT may lead to pulmonary embolism or death. Pulmonary emboli may arise from a variety of sources. Clot in the atrium may dislodge in the setting of atrial fibrillation. However, dislodged clots from the deep venous system of the leg or arm are more common. Upper extremity

DVT is usually associated with venous catheter placement. Chronic occlusion and stricturing are more commonly associated with subclavian catheter placement rather than internal jugular line placement. Unilateral central occlusion will cause arm swelling. Bilateral occlusion results in arm, neck, and facial swelling, referred to as the SVC syndrome. Central venous clot or stricture can be suggested by Doppler, when there is lack of normal phasicity to baseline in the medial subclavian veins.

Lower extremity DVT is most commonly associated with surgery, trauma, and prolonged immobility. Hypercoagulable states increase the risk of thrombosis. Although the deep system above the calf has been most commonly evaluated because of higher embolic risk, intersociety guidelines now recommend calf evaluation. Approximately 50% of DVT occur in the calf veins. Extension into the deep system is the greatest embolic risk of calf clots.

Chronic thrombosis of calf veins can have a less heralded, yet serious, effect on the valves. Fibrosis and tethering of the venous valves can lead to valvular insufficiency and chronic complications characterized by pain and swelling. On ultrasound, reversal of flow greater than 1 second during Valsalva is indicative of venous insufficiency. Since superficial venous insufficiency can have a complex pattern of varices, mapping of the pattern is useful for sclerotherapy planning. The most important venous pathway involves the great saphenous vein. Other named pathways include the vein of Giacomini, which is the intersaphenous vein linking the cephalad extension of the small saphenous vein to the great saphenous veins and perforating veins, which connect the superficial to the deep system. Hunterian perforators are located at the cranial extent of the adductor canal, Dodd perforators at the lower, medial thigh, Boyd perforators at the midcalf, and Cockett perforators at the lower posteromedial calf near the ankle.

Suggested Reading

Lockhart ME, Robbin ML. Renal vascular imaging: ultrasound and other modalities. *Ultrasound Q*. 2007;23(4):279-292.

McNamara MM, Lockhart ME, Robbin ML. Emergency Doppler evaluation of the liver and kidneys. *Radiol Clin North Am*. 2004;42(2):397-415.

Middleton WD, Teefey SA, Darcy MD. Doppler evaluation of transjugular intrahepatic portosystemic shunts. *Ultrasound Q*. 2003;19(2):56-70.

Thorisson HM, Pollak JS, Scoutt L.The role of ultrasound in the diagnosis and treatment of chronic venous insufficiency. *Ultrasound Q*. 2007;23(2):137-150.

Umphrey H, Lockhart ME, Robbin M. Transplant ultrasound of the kidney, pancreas, and spleen. *US Clin*. 2008;3(1):49-65.

Weber TM, Lockhart ME, Robbin ML. Upper extremity venous Doppler ultrasound. *Radiol Clin North Am*. 2007; 45(3):513-524, viii-ix.

QUESTIONS AND ANSWERS

1. What is the most common type of abdominal aortic endoleak?
   A. Type I
   B. Type II
   C. Type III
   D. Type IV
   E. Type V

   ANSWER: B. Type II endoleak is because of retrograde filling by reversed flow in branch artery is by far the most common endoleak.

2. What is the most common cause of renal vein thrombosis in adults?
   A. Nephrotic syndrome
   B. Trauma
   C. Systemic lupus erythematosus
   D. Dehydration
   E. Neoplasm

   ANSWER: A. The most common cause of renal vein thrombosis in adults is membranous glomerulonephropathy causing nephrotic syndrome. In infants, dehydration is the most common cause.

3. Which is a criterion for diagnosis of TIPS dysfunction?
   A. Intrashunt peak velocity >100 cm/s
   B. Main portal vein velocity >30 cm/s
   C. Reversal of portal vein branch flow
   D. Interval decrease in intrashunt peak velocity >40 cm/s
   E. Hepatic artery reversal

   ANSWER: D. All of the following can indicate TIPS dysfunction: portal vein velocity <30 cm/s, intrashunt gradient >50 to 100 cm/s, intrashunt peak velocity >190 cm/s, reversal of portal vein branch flow, and finally, increase >60 cm/s or decrease >40 cm/s in peak intrashunt velocities.

4. What is the most common etiology of mesenteric ischemia?
   A. Intestinal angina
   B. Emboli
   C. Atherosclerosis
   D. Vasculitis
   E. Trauma

   ANSWER: C. Atherosclerosis is the most common cause of mesenteric ischemia.

5. What is a diagnostic criterion for transplant renal artery stenosis?
   A. Renal artery-to-iliac ratio <1.8
   B. Peak systolic velocity <250 cm/s
   C. Resistive index >0.8
   D. Tardus-parvus waveforms in segmental artery
   E. Resistive index <0.8

   ANSWER: D. Resistive index is not a criterion. The "a" and "b" are incorrect (>1.8 and >250 cm/s would be correct).

6. Concerning transplant renal vein thrombosis, which of the following statement is *true*?
   A. Most common cause of reversal of diastolic flow
   B. More common in transplant kidneys than native kidneys
   C. Transplant may be acutely shrunken and hypoechoic.
   D. Segmental artery waveforms will have low resistive index.
   E. Segmental artery parvus-tardus waveforms will be present.

   ANSWER: B. Transplant renal vein thrombosis is more common than native vein thrombosis. Parvus-tardus and low resistive indices are findings of renal artery stenosis. Rejection is most common cause of reversal of diastolic flow.

7. Concerning hepatic artery stenosis/hepatic artery thrombosis, which of the following statements is *true*?
   A. Hepatic artery thrombosis is diagnosed by a 3:1 velocity gradient.
   B. Collateral vessels may hinder diagnosis of acute occlusion.
   C. Lack of diastolic flow in the first 48 hours is normal.
   D. Elevated peak velocity of flow in the first 48 hours is normal.
   E. Bile duct necrosis occurs when portal venous flow is also impaired.

   ANSWER: D. Elevated peak velocity of flow in the first 48 hours is normal. Bile duct necrosis does not rely on portal venous abnormality since bile ducts are solely supplied by hepatic artery. Hepatic artery stenosis uses a 3:1 ratio. Lack of diastolic flow is always abnormal but peak flow varies in the first 48 hours.

8. After how many hours of torsion does the testicular salvage rate drop to less than 20%?
   A. 1 hour
   B. 2 hours
   C. 4 hours
   D. 6 hours
   E. 24 hours

   ANSWER: E. The salvage rate is 20% after 12–24 hours.

9. Concerning varicocele, which of the following statement is *true*?
   A. Isolated left varicocele necessitates exclusion of renal hilar mass.
   B. Most are intratesticular.
   C. Diagnosis is made if vein measures >4 mm diameter.
   D. Type II is because of valvular dysfunction.
   E. Reversal of venous flow is diagnostic.

   ANSWER: E. Reversal of venous flow is diagnostic of varicocele. Isolated right varicocele necessitates renal mass workup. Intratesticular varicocele is rare. Diagnosis relies on 2 to 3 mm threshold. Type I is valvular in etiology. Reversal of venous flow is diagnostic.

10. Which lower extremity venous collateral represents the cephalad extension of the small saphenous vein?
    A. Hunterian
    B. Boyd
    C. Giacomini
    D. Dodd
    E. Cockett

    ANSWER: C. Anatomic locations of venous pathways of calf:

    Hunterian–cranial adductor canal
    Boyd–midcalf
    Giacomini–intersaphenous vein
    Dodd–lower medial thigh
    Crockett–lower posteromedial calf (ankle)

67 SCROTUM

Michelle L. Robbin and Victoria E. Kraft

INTRODUCTION

Although many processes affect the testes and scrotum, in general, the four major areas of clinical concern are infection, tumors, torsion, and trauma. The scrotum is easily assessed with physical examination, but often needs further characterization of the abnormality with ultrasound. Gray scale and color Doppler ultrasound findings are extremely useful in noninvasively determining the etiology of palpable masses or scrotal enlargement and can sort between the diagnostic possibilities causing scrotal pain, without using radiation. It is highly accurate in differentiating between intra- and extratesticular pathology.

A complete scrotal ultrasound will record the upper, mid, and lower transverse planes and mid, medial, and lateral longitudinal planes of the testis. The testes need to be compared together in a single transverse image to assess for individual differences in echotexture and size. Color Doppler evaluation of testicular arterial flow should be performed in every examination. Assessment of the epididymis and spermatic cords bilaterally, and scrotal contents for abnormalities such as hydrocele and skin thickening complete the examination. If the patient has a palpable focal mass, it is best for the patient to grasp it between his fingers so a transducer can be placed directly over the lesion for further evaluation, as a nondirected examination may miss the questioned abnormality. Because of ultrasound's high spatial resolution, the only other further scrotal evaluation after the physical evaluation is surgical (if necessary).

NORMAL ANATOMY

TESTIS

Testicles are simultaneously gonads that produce spermatozoa and endocrine glands that produce male sex hormones and may thus be categorized under both the reproductive and endocrine systems. The two testicles descend from the abdomen into the scrotum in the fetus, beginning about 36 weeks in utero with the vast majority descended at birth. The testis is a cylindrical, homogenously medium-level echogenic gland measuring approximately 3 to 5 cm in length, and 2 to 3 cm in both the transverse and anteroposterior planes. A small fingerlike projection called the appendix testis (a mullerian duct remnant) is frequently present off of the cranial portion of the testis, more easily seen with a hydrocele. A tough white fibrous shell, the tunica albuginea, tightly covers the testis. The testis is lined by the visceral layer of the tunica vaginalis everywhere except where the epididymis, spermatic cord, and testis are attached to the posterior scrotal wall. The parietal layer of the tunica vaginalis lines the inside of the scrotum and forms a potential space where fluid can collect, a hydrocele.

The innermost aspect of the tunica albuginea extends as septae into the testicular parenchyma, converging posteriorly to divide the testes into lobules. A lobule comprises multiple seminiferous tubules, which open into dilated spaces within the mediastinum of the testis, termed the rete testes. The rete testis can be identified by a characteristic extension across the testicle in a craniocaudal direction toward the mediastinum testis. They can appear more echogenic than the adjacent testicular parenchyma and can be especially prominent when dilated.

The seminiferous tubules are lined with a layer of cells that begin to produce sperm cells at puberty and continue into old age. The sperm travel from the seminiferous tubules to the rete testis located in the mediastinum testis, to the efferent ducts, and then to the epididymis where newly created sperm cells mature. The sperm move into the vas deferens and are eventually expelled through the urethra and out of the urethral orifice through muscular contractions. Between the seminiferous tubules are interstitial cells, where androgens such as testosterone are formed.

The deferential, cremasteric, and testicular arteries make up the three arterial sources of testicular blood flow. The testicular artery originates just below the origin of the renal artery anteriorly off of the aorta, and then progresses through the inguinal canal to the posterosuperior testis, where it arborizes to supply the testis peripherally, perforating into the parenchyma. The deferential artery arises from the inferior vesical artery and progresses to the caudal region of the epididymis, where it forms a capillary network. The cremasteric artery originates from the inferior epigastric artery, then progresses to the tunica vaginalis, where it forms anastomoses with capillaries of other two arteries. The deferential and cremasteric arteries primarily supply the epididymis and scrotal tissues, and anastomose with the testicular artery to provide a small amount of testicular flow. Low resistance velocity waveforms are found in normal intratesticular and capsular arteries. Flow in the epididymis normally has a high vascular resistance. With current ultrasound transducers, flow is always seen in the normal adult testis and can usually be demonstrated even in the pediatric testis using a high frequency (at least a 9–12 MHz) linear array transducer with low flow settings.

EPIDIDYMIS

The epididymis is a narrow, curved, tightly coiled tube that connects the efferent ducts from the rear of each testicle to its vas deferens. The epididymis can be divided into three main regions: the head, the body, and the tail. Spermatozoa formed in the testis enter the head of the epididymis, and then progress to the body and tail of the epididymis, where they are stored. The epididymis is normally iso to slightly hyperechoic to the testis on ultrasound, with a slightly more granular echotexture. The head normally measures approximately 1.0 cm in diameter, and the body and tail usually measure less than 0.4 cm in diameter. An appendix epididymis may also be seen, typically off of the head of the epididymis, again more easily seen in the presence of a hydrocele.

SPERMATIC CORD AND SCROTUM

The spermatic cord is formed by the cremasteric, deferential, and testicular arteries, lymphatics, nerves, a pampiniform plexus of veins, and the vas deferens. The spermatic cord is enveloped in three layers of tissue: the external spermatic fascia, the cremasteric muscle and fascia, and the internal spermatic fascia and extends down from the abdomen through the inguinal canal. The scrotum develops from a fetal protuberance of abdominal skin and muscle containing the testicles, with fetal peritoneum (processus vaginalis) extending from the abdomen. The function of the scrotum appears to be to keep the testis at a temperature slightly lower than that of the rest of the body. The temperature is controlled by the contracting and relaxing of the dartos fascia in the scrotum and the cremasteric muscle in the abdomen, which moves the testicles closer to the abdomen when it is cold, and away when hot. Skin thickness greater than approximately 0.3 cm is abnormal.

TESTICULAR PATHOLOGY

MASS

The majority of intratesticular masses are malignant, whereas the majority of extratesticular lesions are benign. Risk factors for testicular neoplasm include undescended testicles (cryptorchidism), mumps orchitis, carcinoma in situ, and family history of testicular cancer. Symptoms include a lump in one testis or a hardening of one of the testicles, abnormal scrotal sensitivity (pain or numbness), increasing hydrocele, an increase or significant decrease in size of one testis, blood in the semen, or a dull ache in the lower abdomen or groin.

The goal of scrotal ultrasound in the evaluation of a mass should be to determine intra- versus extratesticular location, size, cyst versus solid, uniform versus heterogeneous, sharply circumscribed or poorly defined borders, and the presence and character of calcifications, as well as determining bilateral versus unilateral location. It is important to compare the testes directly to each other in the same transverse image on ultrasound, so mild changes in testicular echotexture and size because of diffuse tumor infiltration can be appreciated as compared to the normal contralateral testis. Concurrent physical examination can add to the differentiation between benign and malignant, as a focal tumor mass is likely to be firm and not painful, whereas focal orchitis will be soft and painful to palpation. It is extremely important to recognize that testicular masses should not be biopsied percutaneously through the scrotum. The testicle needs to be approached surgically through the inguinal canal, and the testis brought up through the level of the internal inguinal ring to be resected, or less commonly, biopsied if there is a question of a benign tumor or infection.

MALIGNANT NEOPLASMS

The majority of primary malignant testis tumors occurs in men in their forties and can be divided into seminomatous (50%) and nonseminomatous germ cell tumors (45%). Seminoma is the most common kind of single-cell testicular tumor in adults and in the cryptorchid testes. Seminoma is comparatively less aggressive than the other malignant testicular tumors, and therefore has the most favorable prognosis. Sonographically, it is typically homogenous and hypoechoic and can range from a small (usually well defined) hypoechoic nodule to virtually replacing and enlarging the testis. Rarely, portions of the seminoma can appear cystic because of necrosis.

The more aggressive nonseminomatous germ cell tumors (NSGCT) occur between puberty and age 50, but tend to occur in a younger age group than seminomas. They often invade the tunica albuginea and frequently cause visceral metastases. NSGCT may present with various combinations of teratomas, endodermal sinus or yolk sac tumors, embryonal cell carcinoma, and choriocarcinoma cell types in 40% to 60% of patients. Choriocarcinoma is the rarest form of NSGCT but is highly malignant. Although seminoma may be present in the NSGCT, it does not mean a more favorable prognosis. Sixty percent of endodermal sinus or yolk sac tumors are found in infants younger than 2 years of age and have abnormal alpha-fetoprotein in 95% of cases. Sonographically, NSGCT tumors are heterogenous, and both cystic areas and large or coarse calcifications are common. They do not have sonographic characteristics that allow further classification other than likely nonseminomatous tumor. Although most testicular tumors are hypervascular, color Doppler by itself is not useful in differentiating tumor types, nor can it definitively distinguish neoplasm from infection.

Some patients have supraclavicular, lung, mediastinal, or retroperitoneal testicular metastases despite a normal testicular physical examination. These primary testicular tumors may be too small to feel, but may still be seen sonographically. Sometimes only a small calcification with or without a soft-tissue mass or just a small soft-tissue mass may represent the primary tumor, the so-called "burnt out" testicular tumor. It is important to remove this residual tumor, as it can be a source of continued metastasis, although no tumor may be found histologically.

The gonadal stromal tumor generally is made up of Leydig or Sertoli cells and is usually benign. Gonadal stromal tumors may be composed of a single cell type or multiple cell types and account for 3% to 6% of testicular masses, 20% in children. Most stromal tumors are of Leydig cell origin, with some patients presenting with gynecomastia or impotence, while Sertoli cell tumors occur rarely.

METASTASES

Metastatic testicular tumors include lymphoma, leukemia, myeloma, and a small percentage of other metastasis to the testes. The most common bilaterally occurring testicular tumor is lymphoma, nearly always non-Hodgkin type. Lymphoma may not be clinically evident, or disseminated disease may be present. It is the most frequent testicular tumor in men older than 60 years. Patients with lymphoma generally have painless testicular enlargement. Sonographically, the tumor resembles seminoma, with increased color Doppler flow. The tumor is usually large and often replaces the normal testicular parenchyma, but smaller lesions can occur.

Second highest in occurrence in the testes, leukemia metastases are often found (particularly in children) despite bone marrow remission. The blood–testis barrier is thought to decrease the concentration of chemotherapy within the testis, increasing the chance that residual or recurrent cells will be found there. Leukemia metastasis in the testis are hypoechoic and tend to largely replace normal parenchyma. Testicular myeloma can be seen in patients with diffuse myeloma. Other metastases are infrequent and include lung, melanoma, stomach, prostate, pancreas, kidney, and colon. These are usually not clinically symptomatic and occur in patients with diffuse metastatic disease.

BENIGN MASSES

The most common benign mass in the testis is the simple cyst (no perceptible wall, no internal echoes or septations, increased through sound transmission). These are of no clinical significance and do not need to be followed for interval change. More complex cysts require follow-up or may need to be surgically evaluated, as malignant tumors can have cystic areas because of necrosis or hemorrhage. Rarely, a firm palpable nodule may be an epidermoid cyst. These have variable sonographic appearances, including a swirled onion-skin appearance, or a decreased echogenicity mass with a partially or completely calcified periphery, or central calcification. They may have a nonspecific pattern, however, and need to be surgically evaluated if newly discovered. These tumors are not vascular, in contradistinction to most malignant testis tumors. Care must be taken to avoid misdiagnosing the twinkle artifact from calcifications in an epidermoid cyst for vascular flow, when the lesions are actually avascular.

Cysts in the tunica albuginea are generally single, small and unilocular, and benign. No color Doppler flow is seen in these cysts. Prominent or dilated rete testis can simulate a tumor; the fact that there is a pattern of linearly branching structures converging into the mediastinum of the testis helps to differentiate this normal finding from a tumor. The dilatation may be bilateral and is thought to result from trauma or inflammation. Cystic dysplasia is a rare congenital condition and appears as multiple different interconnecting cysts.

Rarely, sarcoid may cause hypoechoic intratesticular masses. These can be bilateral and may need to go to surgical biopsy for differentiation from tumor. Adrenal rests are another rare cause of testicular mass and usually can be diagnosed correctly with the history of congenital adrenal hyperplasia or Cushing syndrome.

MICROLITHIASIS

Testicular microlithiasis (TM) is relatively uncommon, and the significance of the finding is debated. These findings have been increasingly detected with the current increased resolution of high frequency linear transducers. Small (1–3 mm) echogenic foci, some of which may demonstrate ring down at ultrasound, are seen in testes either unilaterally or bilaterally. In 80% of cases, both testicles are affected. The calcifications are though to be related to degeneration of seminiferous tubules. It is an asymptomatic, nonprogressive disease that has been classified as limited (less than 5 microliths in a single ultrasound image of the testis) and diffuse (greater than or equal to 5 microliths in a single image). No definite difference between the categories of limited and diffuse microlithiasis and the incidence of malignancy has been noted. An association with TM and testicular malignancy has been suggested, but the validity of the association has been questioned. Most urologists now recommend regular testicular patient self-examination and examination by a urologist, with follow-up ultrasound as needed. This recommendation is altered depending on the patient's risk profile for testicular cancer, with increased surveillance in cryptorchidism, infertility, and history of testicular cancer, among others.

TORSION

Testicular torsion occurs when the spermatic cord is twisted, thereby cutting off the blood supply to the testis. Patients typically present with acute onset of severe scrotal pain; if surgically treated within 5 to 6 hours, greater than 80% of testes can be preserved. If surgery is not instituted within 12 hours, only 20% of testes are salvaged. Intravaginal torsion is the most frequent cause of torsion and occurs when the tunica vaginalis (arising from the processus vaginalis in utero) covers the entire testis and epididymis and a portion of the spermatic cord, the so-called "bell-clapper deformity." This condition is bilateral in greater than 50% of patients. Extravaginal torsion is uncommon and typically seen in neonates. This occurs when an abnormally mobile testis (with normal tunica attachments) rotates together with the epididymis and spermatic cord, twisting at the inguinal ring.

Color Doppler ultrasound of the scrotum can make the diagnosis of torsion with a very high degree of accuracy and sensitivity. Flow is always seen in the normal postpubertal testis (and nearly always in the prepubertal testis), and the absence of flow is diagnostic for torsion given the correct clinical history. The spermatic cord twist may be seen, termed the "whirlpool sign." The testis may have a normal echotexture initially and is usually enlarged. It later becomes hypoechoic and often is heterogenous.

When evaluating for torsion, it is important to sample central intratesticular arteries for typical low resistance flow. It should be noted that some peripheral high resistance capsular artery flow can be seen from anastomoses with the deferential and cremasteric arteries in testicular artery occlusion. If only high resistance peripheral arterial flow without central arterial flow is seen, torsion is present. Careful attention to technique using low flow settings with high gain and low pulse repetition frequency along with comparison to the contralateral normal testis is very important. Surgical exploration in the neonate may be necessary if no definite flow can be seen, although further evaluation with testicular scintigraphy could be performed. Scrotal skin thickening and a reactive hydrocele with low-level echoes within may be seen.

Partial torsion (less than approximately two full cord twists) is problematic to diagnose, with arterial flow decreased but not absent; low or no venous outflow may be useful in suggesting this diagnosis. In the unusual setting of detorsion, the testis may be hyperemic, and the sonographic appearance will be similar to epididymo-orchitis. The appendix testis or epididymis may torse, causing pain and symptoms similar to testicular torsion. The appendix may be seen as an enlarged, hypoechoic mass without flow adjacent to a testis with normal flow. Central lack of arterial flow in the testis can also be seen in infarction from severe epididymo-orchitis, but these two entities are usually distinguishable clinically.

TRAUMA

Testicular trauma is an injury to one or both testicles, and generally occurs in men between 15 and 40 years of age. Types of injuries include blunt and penetrating, usually from sports injuries, assault and motor vehicle collisions. If an adequate physical examination of the testes cannot be performed because of testicular pain and swelling, and evidence of testicular rupture is compelling or there is a penetrating injury, the patient may be taken to surgery. In less obvious cases of testicular trauma, ultrasound is performed to assess for testicular rupture. If testicular rupture is present, the testicle can be salvaged if repaired within approximately 72 hours. Findings of testicular rupture include protrusion of the seminiferous tubules outside of the testicular contour, an irregular periphery of the testis, and loss of continuity of the tunica albuginea. Color Doppler can be used to assess intratesticular heterogenous areas for infarction or intratesticular hematoma and assess the overall vascularity of the testicle. The presence of clot overlying the testis in a hematocele should not be mistaken for testicular rupture.

CRYPTORCHIDISM

If the testis fails to descend into the scrotum, it can usually be felt in the inguinal canal. If it cannot be felt, ultrasound is usually the first examination of choice to determine its location and size. MRI is then used if the testis cannot be found. The testis needs to be surgically placed in the scrotum before 1 to 2 years of age to decrease the incidence of both infertility and tumor. There is a large lifetime risk of testicular tumor in the undescended testis, with an increased incidence of tumor in the normally descended testis as well.

EPIDIDYMIS—PATHOLOGY

NEOPLASMS

Most epididymal tumors are benign. The most common type is the adenomatoid tumor, usually located in the tail of the epididymis. Adenomatoid tumors generally occur singly, in well-defined round or oval shapes, and are variable in echogenicity. Leiomyomas of the epididymis are uncommon; papillary cystadenoma is rare but is frequent in men with von Hippel-Lindau disease. Lymphoma is the most common malignancy that involves the epididymis; metastases are rare.

BENIGN LESIONS

Epididymal cysts and spermatoceles are commonly seen, and are usually of no clinical significance unless they cause discomfort because of size. Epididymal cysts are lined with epithelium, are generally small, and can occur throughout the epididymis. Spermatoceles are seen most commonly in men after vasectomy and contain low-level echoes made up debris and sperm. These cysts usually occur in the epididymal head and can be quite large. Since both of these cysts are rarely evaluated operatively and appear virtually identical sonographically, common parlance terms them epididymal cysts when the epididymis is seen and they are relatively small, and spermatoceles when little if any normal epididymal head can be detected.

Sperm granulomas can be seen in men postvasectomy and represent a focal, sharply defined lesion that has decreased echogenicity with respect to the adjacent epididymis. These are usually found at the vasectomy site and only rarely cause pain.

INFECTION

Epididymitis is the most common cause for acute scrotal pain in males after puberty. Under 35 years of age, it is usually from sexually transmitted urethritis from *Chlamydia trachomatis* or *Neisseria gonorrhea*. *Escherichia coli* and *Proteus mirabilis* are usually the cause in boys younger and men older than this age range, usually from urinary tract infections (and prostatitis in the older age group). Unusual causes of epididymitis include mumps, tuberculosis, and syphilis. Discomfort while voiding or urethral discharge may develop, along with fever. Scrotal pain is usually present, sometimes radiating to the groin or flank. Epididymitis usually starts in the epididymis tail. Ultrasound findings include an enlarged epididymis with increased epididymal blood flow with respect to the contralateral side. Extension of the infection into the testis, termed epididymo-orchitis, may occur in up to 20%. Patchy (focal orchitis) or diffuse areas of decreased echogenicity along with increased testicular blood flow is diagnostic in the correct clinical setting.

When severe orchitis is present, it may progress to abscess formation and or infarction. Typically, these patients are diabetic and have a spinal cord injury or some other reason for lack of sensation and early detection of the infection. Patients with epididymitis may develop an associated hydrocele, often with low-level echoes or septations within. The infection may be unilateral or bilateral. It is important to note that if a focal testicular mass or masslike area is present in the clinical context of epididymitis or epididymo-orchitis, the patient needs to be reexamined with ultrasound after the epididymitis has resolved to exclude a coexistent tumor.

SCROTUM—PATHOLOGY

VARICOCELE

A varicocele is an abnormal engorgement of the veins that drain the testicle, the pampiniform plexus. The network of veins coalesces into the testicular vein or gonadal vein. Small one-way valves prevent backflow to ensure upward flow of blood in the veins. Defective valves can cause dilation of the veins near the testis, leading to the formation of a primary varicocele. Secondary varicoceles are usually caused by compression of the gonadal vein by extrinsic masses such as from a renal mass or renal hilar adenopathy. Varicoceles are multiple tubular veins greater than 0.2 to 0.3 cm in diameter and usually increase in size with the Valsalva maneuver. They are nearly always found on the left and are usually found near the testis-epididymal head region, extending up into the spermatic cord. They can be bilateral in up to 70% of patients. However, an isolated right-sided varicocele or a new varicocele should raise suspicions for a compressive mass in the course of the gonadal vein and should prompt a renal ultrasound to search for the cause. Color Doppler can definitively characterize the multiple vessels seen on gray scale ultrasound imaging as dilated veins. Rarely, the varicocele can extend into the testis; a dilated tubular structure with venous flow in the testis is diagnostic. Varicoceles that are not palpable still may cause infertility, and thus ultrasound can be important in the evaluation of infertile men.

HYDROCELE

A hydrocele forms in the potential space between the parietal and visceral tunica vaginalis and may result in scrotal swelling. A small amount of fluid is likely physiologic. However, hydroceles may also result from repeated chronic infection, trauma, or tumor. Low-level echoes, septations, and loculated fluid usually indicate prior trauma or infection and can be seen with torsion.

SCROTAL PEARL

Inflammation or infection in the tunica vaginalis, or torsed appendices of the epididymis or testis may slough off to lie between the parietal and visceral tunica vaginalis. Instead of involuting, this inflammatory tissue may remain, with tissue deposition around a central calcification, termed a scrotal pearl. These are usually mobile and may be palpable and are of no clinical significance.

INGUINAL HERNIAS/OTHER MASSES

Patients occasionally present with groin masses that extend into the scrotum. Ultrasound can be diagnostic, assessing for herniation of bowel, mesentery, or ascites into the scrotal sac. Compression of the inguinal canal may prompt peristalsis. Bowel peristalsis or typical bowel wall contents is diagnostic. Real time evaluation with the Valsalva maneuver is also helpful. If only mesenteric fat is present, only an echogenic mass will be seen. Rarely, a lipoma of the spermatic cord can cause this echogenic appearance; even more rarely, a liposarcoma can be present. CT can be useful for further evaluation of those inguinal and scrotal masses that are not typical bowel containing hernias.

Suggested Reading

Akin EA, Khati NJ, Hill MC. Ultrasound of the scrotum. *Ultrasound Q*. 2004;20:181-200.

Bhatt S, Dogra VS. Role of US in testicular and scrotal trauma. *Radiographics*. 2008;28:1617-1629.

Bhatt S, Rubens DJ, Dogra VS. Sonography of benign intrascrotal lesions. *Ultrasound Q*. 2006;22:121-136.

Buckley JC, McAninch JW. Diagnosis and management of testicular ruptures. *Urol Clin North Am*. 2006;33:111-116, vii.

Coley BD. Sonography of pediatric scrotal swelling. *Semin Ultrasound CT MR*. 2007;28:297-306.

Coley BD. The acute pediatric scrotum. *Ultrasound Clin*. 2006;1(3):485-496.

Dagash H, Mackinnon EA. Testicular microlithiasis: what does it mean clinically? *BJU Int*. 2007;99:157-160.

Deurdulian C, Mittelstaedt CA, Chong WK, et al. US of acute scrotal trauma: optimal technique, imaging findings, and management. *Radiographics*. 2007;27:357-369.

Dogra VS, Bhatt S, Rubens DJ. Sonographic evaluation of testicular torsion. *Ultrasound Clin*. 2006;1(1):55-66.

Dogra VS, Gottlieb RH, Oka M, et al. Sonography of the scrotum. *Radiology*. 2003;227:18-36.

Futterer JJ, Heijmink SW, Spermon JR. Imaging the male reproductive tract: current trends and future directions. *Radiol Clin North Am*. 2008;46:133-147, vii.

Hormann M, Balassy C, Philipp MO, et al. Imaging of the scrotum in children. *Eur Radiol*. 2004;14:974-983.

Khan O, Protheroe A. Testis cancer. *Postgrad Med J*. 2007;83:624-632.

Kim W, Rosen MA, Langer JE, et al. US MR imaging correlation in pathologic conditions of the scrotum. *Radiographics*. 2007;27:1239-1253.

Krege S, Beyer J, Souchon R, et al. European consensus conference on diagnosis and treatment of germ cell cancer: a report of the second meeting of the European Germ Cell Cancer Consensus Group (EGCCCG): part I. *Eur Urol*. 2008;53:478-496.

Lee JC, Bhatt S, Dogra VS. Imaging of the epididymis. *Ultrasound Q*. 2008;24:3-16.

Stewart VR, Sidhu PS. The testis: the unusual, the rare and the bizarre. *Clin Radiol*. 2007;62:289-302.

Tetreau R, Julian P, Lyonnet D, et al. Intratesticular varicocele: an easy diagnosis but unclear physiopathologic characteristics. *J Ultrasound Med*. 2007;26:1767-1773.

Turgut AT, Bhatt S, Dogra VS. Acute painful scrotum. *Ultrasound Clin*. 2008;3(1):93-107.

QUESTIONS AND ANSWERS

1. Which anatomic structure extends into the testis parenchyma as septae, forming lobules?
   A. Epididymis
   B. Visceral layer of the tunica vaginalis
   C. Parietal layer of the tunica vaginalis
   D. Tunica albuginea

   ANSWER: D. The tunica albuginea extends into the testis parenchyma to form septae, dividing the testis into lobules. The visceral layer of the tunica vaginalis surrounds the tunica, epididymis, and spermatic cord except where the epididymis and testis is fused to the scrotal wall. The parietal layer of the tunica vaginalis lines the inside of the scrotum. The epididymis is connected to the testis via the rete testis.

2. When do most testis descend into the scrotum?
   A. 28–32 weeks gestational age
   B. 32–36 weeks gestational age
   C. 36–40 weeks gestational age
   D. First month after birth

   ANSWER: C. The testis normally begin their descent from the abdomen into the scrotum at approximately 36 weeks. Nearly all testes have descended into the scrotum by 40 weeks gestation.

3. Concerning testicular neoplasms, what is the most common malignancy?
   A. Leydig cell
   B. Nonseminatous germ cell

C. Seminomatous germ cell
D. Sertoli cell

ANSWER: B. Nonseminomatous germ cell tumors are the most common malignant testis tumors, usually with multiple tumor types in the same mass. Seminomatous tumors are the next most common. Leydig and Sertoli cell tumors are both gonadal stromal tumors, uncommon, and usually benign.

4. Concerning testicular masses, what is the most common benign mass?
   A. Simple cyst
   B. Tunica albuginea cyst
   C. Sarcoid nodules
   D. Epidermoid cyst

   ANSWER: A. Simple cysts are the most common benign testicular mass, and of no clinical significance (in contradistinction to complex cysts, which require further investigation). Tunica albuginea cysts are benign and less common. Sarcoid nodules and epidermoid cysts are rare.

5. What is the most common epididymal neoplasm?
   A. Adenomatoid tumor
   B. Leiomyoma
   C. Papillary cystadenoma
   D. Sperm granuloma

   ANSWER: A. The most common neoplasm in the epididymis is benign, the epidermoid tumor. Leiomyomas and papillary cystadenomas are rare. Sperm granulomas are not neoplasms and are usually a focal epididymal lesion seen after vasectomy.

6. Concerning color Doppler of the testes to rule out torsion, which of the following findings is diagnostic for torsion?
   A. Capsular low resistance arterial flow
   B. Absence of central arterial flow
   C. Hypervascular "lesion"
   D. Absent venous flow

   ANSWER: B. Absence of central arterial flow is diagnostic of torsion, in the correct clinical setting, but can also be seen in infarction from severe epididymo-orchitis and trauma. When the testicular artery is torsed, high resistance arterial flow may sometimes be seen in capsular arteries because of collateral flow from the cremasteric and deferential arteries. A hypervascular mass is not diagnostic for torsion, although a testicular tumor can hemorrhage and cause acute testicular pain. If flow is symmetric and normal, torsion is not present. Torsion is rarely bilateral.

7. What is the most common cause of epididymitis in males aged 15 to 35 years?
   A. Prostatitis
   B. Sexually transmitted diseases
   C. Urinary tract infection
   D. Mumps

   ANSWER: B. Sexually transmitted diseases such as *Chlamydia trachomatis* or *Neisseria gonorrhea* are the most common cause of epididymitis in postpubertal males to age 35. Prostatitis or a urinary tract infection is usually the cause of epididymitis in males older than 35. Mumps is an uncommon cause of epididymitis.

8. Concerning testicular microlithiasis, which of the following is *true*?
   A. Microlithiasis causes cancer.
   B. Risk factors for testicular cancer help determine follow-up.
   C. Percutaneous biopsy should be performed.
   D. Calcifications are usually >0.5 cm in diameter.

   ANSWER: B. Microlithiasis has an unclear association with testicular tumor, but there is no evidence that it causes testicular cancer. Urologists will typically recommend monthly testicular self-examinations; whether or not follow-up ultrasounds or urologist examinations will be scheduled depends on the patient's risk factors and urologist preference. Percutaneous biopsy through the scrotal wall should never be performed if tumor is suspected. The microcalcifations seen in microlithiasis range from 0.1 to 0.3 cm in diameter.

9. Concerning an isolated right-sided varicocele, which the following is *true*?
   A. Varicocele is easily compressible.
   B. More common than an isolated left-sided varicocele.
   C. Need to assess kidney and hilar region for mass.
   D. Unlikely to cause infertility

   ANSWER: C. Isolated right varicoceles are uncommon and are concerning for a mass obstructing the right gonadal vein or its drainage pathway to the IVC (renal vein). If an obstructing mass is present, the varicocele will not be easily compressible nor change significantly with Valsalva. A renal ultrasound to evaluate the kidney for a renal or hilar mass should be performed. Varicoceles, even ones that are not palpable, can be a correctable cause of infertility.

10. Concerning cryptorchidism, what is a common clinical finding?
    A. Normal-sized testis
    B. Increased incidence of infertility

C. Nonpalpable testis
D. Increased testicular tumor risk only in cryptorchid testis

ANSWER: B. Cryptorchid testes are usually small and located in the inguinal canal and so most are palpable. If no testis is palpable, MRI may be useful to help localize prior to surgery. There is a significantly higher tumor risk in both the cryptorchid testis and the contralateral testis normally located in the scrotum.

68 THYROID, PARATHYROID, AND NECK ULTRASOUND

Mark D. Little and Franklin N. Tessler

THYROID GLAND: NORMAL ANATOMY AND APPEARANCE

The thyroid gland is located in the anterior neck, just below the thyroid cartilage. Sonographically, the gland is homogeneous, slightly hyperechoic, and is contained by a well-defined echogenic capsule. The two lobes of the thyroid gland are positioned on either side of the trachea, bounded anteriorly by the strap musculature, laterally by the common carotid artery and the internal jugular vein, and posteriorly by the longus coli muscle. The lobes communicate across the midline by a thin isthmus of thyroid parenchyma. In addition, up to 40% of patients have a pyramidal lobe lying anterior to the thyroid cartilage, originating from the isthmus. The pyramidal lobe is more often seen in childhood, usually undergoing atrophy with age, but it can be seen in hyperplastic processes such as Graves disease. Arterial supply and venous drainage are via the superior and inferior thyroid arteries and veins, respectively. The recurrent laryngeal nerve passes posterior to the thyroid gland, an important consideration at neck surgery.

The size of the thyroid is highly variable, depending on the patient's age, sex, and physiology. The normal thyroid is larger in males and in endemic areas of iodine deficiency, with a mean longitudinal dimension of approximately 4 to 6 cm and a mean anteroposterior diameter of approximately 1.3 to 1.8 cm. The isthmus measures up to approximately 4 to 6 mm anteroposterior. The estimated mean thyroid volume can be determined clinically or calculated (height × width × depth × 0.52), averaging approximately 12 to 40 cm^3. In general, however, the normal thyroid dimensions are up to 5 × 2 × 2 cm. Specifically, the thyroid gland is considered enlarged when the anteroposterior diameter is greater than 2 cm.

CONGENITAL THYROID ABNORMALITIES

Various congenital abnormalities of the thyroid can be assessed sonographically, including complete or partial thyroid agenesis or hypoplasia. Ectopic thyroid tissue can be seen in the tongue or suprahyoid neck, arising along the course of the gland's embryonic descent from the foramen cecum. Ultrasound, however, has limited utility in screening for thyroid ectopia, which is usually evaluated with radionuclide imaging.

MICROSCOPIC ANATOMY AND FUNCTION

The thyroid gland is intimately involved in regulating the body's cellular metabolism and protein synthesis, mediated through the production of thyroid hormones, thyroxine (T4), and triiodothyronine (T3). It is composed of spherical follicles that are lined by a simple epithelium surrounding a central cavity that contains colloid. Briefly, the follicular cells accumulate dietary iodide, which is subsequently organified with the amino acid tyrosine and attached to the protein thyroglobulin to produce monoiodotyrosine and diiodotyrosine. Coupling of these precursor proteins results in T3 and T4, depending on the number of iodine atoms.

T3 and T4 are cleaved from thyroglobulin under the influence of thyroid-stimulating hormone (TSH), which is produced and released by the anterior pituitary gland. The released thyroid hormones predominantly circulate in inactive form, bound to multiple serum proteins, including thyroid binding globulin, albumin, and thyroid binding prealbumin. Only a small percentage (less than 1%) of circulating free T4 and free T3 is metabolically active. T4 is released in greater quantity by the thyroid and is subsequently converted to the more metabolically active T3 in peripheral tissues. Thyroid hormone production is controlled by a negative feedback loop along the hypothalamic-pituitary axis, mediated through thyrotropin releasing hormone (TRH), which stimulates TSH production by the pituitary.

The thyroid gland also contains parafollicular cells (C-cells), which produce calcitonin, which has opposing effects to parathyroid hormone (PTH) on calcium metabolism. Calcitonin decreases serum calcium by inhibiting osteoclastic activity and reabsorption of calcium by the kidneys and intestine.

DIFFUSE THYROID DISEASE

Thyroid disease can present as focal or diffuse involvement. Diffuse disease is most often characterized by generalized glandular enlargement or hyperplasia. Clinically, patients present as hyperthyroid, euthyroid, or hypothyroid, and the diagnosis is based on the combination of diffuse enlargement and specific laboratory findings. The sonographic appearance is often nonspecific. However, ultrasound is indicated to evaluate coexistent nodular disease or response to treatment.

Diffuse thyroid disease includes multinodular goiter, Graves disease, Hashimoto thyroiditis, subacute thyroiditis, and infectious thyroiditis. The most common worldwide cause of diffuse thyroid enlargement is endemic goiter, secondary to dietary iodine deficiency. Graves disease and thyroiditis are the most common presentations within the United States.

MULTINODULAR GOITER

Multinodular goiter is a common condition that has multiple clinical presentations but is the final expression of a hyperstimulated gland. (The term "goiter" is nonspecific, referring only to an enlarged thyroid gland.) Biochemically, these patients are either hypothyroid-euthyroid or hyperthyroid and are referred to as having nontoxic or toxic multinodular goiter, respectively. Most often, they present with hypothyroidism and palpable neck masses, which occasionally exert mass effect on the trachea.

Sonographically, the thyroid gland appears enlarged with multiple nodules of varying size and complexity with intervening areas of normal or heterogeneous thyroid tissue. These hyperplastic nodules are often nonfunctional and have areas of hemorrhage, necrosis, and colloid. Multinodular goiter is more common in women. In addition, while it was once believed that there was a lower incidence of carcinoma within multinodular goiter, current understanding suggests a similar level of risk. Therefore, suspicious thyroid nodules should be evaluated and biopsied (see below).

GRAVES DISEASE

The most common cause of hyperthyroidism in the United States is Graves disease, an autoimmune, often familial condition that is more common in females. Thyroid-stimulating immunoglobulins bind to and activate TSH receptors, leading to hypersecretion of T3 and T4. Patients present with symptoms of hyperthyroidism, including tachycardia, heat intolerance, fatigue, palpitations, and unexplained weight loss. Twenty-five to thirty percent of patients also have clinical signs and symptoms of Graves ophthalmopathy, such as proptosis, lid retraction, and visual changes. Sonographically, the thyroid gland appears enlarged and heterogeneous and is often diffusely hypoechoic caused by lymphocytic infiltration or loss of parenchymal colloid. On color Doppler sonography, the gland may be diffusely hypervascular, a condition that has been termed "thyroid inferno."

HASHIMOTO THYROIDITIS

The most common cause of thyroiditis and hypothyroidism within the United States is Hashimoto thyroiditis or chronic lymphocytic thyroiditis. The condition is a result of autoimmune destruction of thyroid cells in the presence of antithyroid peroxidase, antithyroglobulin, and other antibodies, and often presents as a painless enlarged thyroid gland with clinical symptoms of hypothyroidism, including lethargy, cold intolerance, weight gain, dry skin, and fatigue. The condition is more common in young to middle-aged women. Sonographically, the gland may appear enlarged, with numerous 1 to 6 mm hypoechoic nodules with intervening areas of coarsened echogenic fibrous stroma. This appearance is termed micronodulation and is fairly specific for Hashimoto. As the condition progresses, there is increased fibrosis and atrophy of the gland. Because there is an increased risk of carcinoma, enlarging lesions should be evaluated and biopsied. In addition, similar to other autoimmune diseases, patients with Hashimoto thyroiditis are at increased risk for thyroid B-cell lymphoma.

SUBACUTE GRANULOMATOUS THYROIDITIS

The most common cause of a painful thyroid gland is subacute granulomatous thyroiditis, also known as De Quervain thyroiditis. The condition often presents as painful enlargement of the thyroid gland and is thought to be related to viral infection. The clinical course is usually benign and self-limited, but recurrence is possible. Sonographically, subacute thyroiditis is nonspecific and may appear as an enlarged diffusely hypoechoic gland or as focal areas of inhomogeneity.

INFECTIOUS THYROIDITIS

Infectious thyroiditis may be caused by viral, bacterial, or granulomatous etiologies. The involved thyroid gland may be enlarged, hypervascular, and heterogeneous. Ultrasound has limited utility in the diagnosis of infectious thyroiditis and is used primarily to evaluate for frank abscesses. Sonographically, an abscess appears as an ill-defined, complex, hypoechoic fluid collection with internal echoes, and debris. At times, gas is also present.

TABLE 68-1 Signs of Malignant Thyroid Nodules on Ultrasound

Microcalcifications
Markedly low echogenicity
Irregular margin
Irregular halo
Central flow

NODULAR THYROID DISEASE: GENERAL PRINCIPLES

Nodular thyroid disease has an estimated 50% prevalence within the United States. However, thyroid carcinoma is rare, constituting approximately 1% of all malignancies. Therefore, the vast majority of all incidentally discovered thyroid nodules will be benign. Although clinical features such as rapid growth, hoarseness, and a history of neck irradiation are suspicious for thyroid cancer, ultrasound is the modality of choice to identify nodules that require biopsy. (Nuclear scintigraphy is limited to confirming the presence of hyperfunctioning nodules in selected patients.)

The majority of nodular thyroid disease is secondary to hyperplasia. When individual thyroid acini become hyperplastic, they may undergo micro- or macronodular formation. Hyperplastic nodules have variable sonographic appearances, adding to the diagnostic challenge. Hyperplastic nodules are initially isoechoic to the adjacent parenchyma. As they accumulate colloid, however, their appearance changes. Many undergo cystic or liquefactive degeneration, typified by internal areas of necrosis, hemorrhage, and colloid. They may calcify with eggshell or coarse dystrophic calcification. Most thyroid cysts are usually degenerated hyperplastic nodules, as true epithelial thyroid cysts are rare.

ULTRASOUND ASSESSMENT OF THYROID NODULES

As the use of noninvasive neck imaging has increased, more and more incidental nonpalpable thyroid nodules, termed "incidentalomas," are being detected. In general, morphologic characteristics are more important than size for determining whether or not a nodule needs to be biopsied. If only the largest thyroid nodule is biopsied, some thyroid cancers will be missed. Similarly, because thyroid cancer appears just as commonly in patients with multiple nodules as in those with solitary lesions, careful sonographic interrogation of all nodules is mandatory.

A significant percentage of nodules contain cystic components. When a thyroid nodule is almost purely cystic, it most likely represents a degenerated benign adenoma or hyperplastic nodule. On high resolution sonography, however, these hyperplastic lesions often show areas of mural irregularity and layering debris, with or without septations. Since papillary thyroid carcinoma may have cystic components, careful examination with grayscale and color Doppler sonography is recommended to exclude other suspicious characteristics (Table 68-1). Conversely, V-shaped ("comet tail") artifacts that are associated with colloid microcrystals are found in benign nodules.

The echogenicity of nodules is compared to that of the surrounding thyroid parenchyma. Generally, thyroid carcinomas are hypoechoic. Since most thyroid nodules are benign, the likelihood that an individual hypoechoic lesion represents cancer is unlikely. However, hypoechoic nodules should be interrogated with greater suspicion. Hyperechoic and isoechoic nodules have a lower suspicion for cancer.

Taken in isolation, the marginal characteristics of individual nodules are also nonspecific. While the margins of thyroid carcinomas tend to be irregular and ill defined, this feature has significant overlap with benign nodules. Nevertheless, irregular thyroid lesions that appear to invade surrounding soft tissues or are associated with significant cervical adenopathy should be considered suspicious.

Another helpful feature is the presence or absence of a sonolucent halo. A large percentage of benign hyperplastic thyroid nodules have a peripheral hypoechoic ring that likely represents compressed normal thyroid parenchyma. This sign is present in a minority of thyroid carcinomas. In such instances, the halo may appear irregular or discontinuous.

The presence and, specifically, the pattern of calcification are useful in evaluating thyroid nodules. Approximately 10% to 15% of all thyroid nodules contain calcification. Common patterns include coarse dystrophic, eggshell, and punctate calcifications. While dystrophic calcifications are associated with a somewhat higher risk of malignancy, eggshell calcification is often predictive of a benign lesion. On the other hand, punctate microcalcifications are considered one of the most specific findings for malignant thyroid lesions. Additionally, medullary thyroid cancer may also contain small intralesional echogenic foci, which can also be seen in adjacent metastatic lymph nodes.

Color Doppler sonography has limited utility in differentiating hyperplastic from malignant nodules. However, hyperplastic nodules tend to show increased peripheral vascularity. In contrast, thyroid carcinoma and adenomas often demonstrate central vascularity. When used in combination with other sonographic findings, color Doppler imaging may be helpful in distinguishing suspicious nodules in need of biopsy.

THYROID NODULE BIOPSY

Fine needle aspiration (FNA) biopsy is a safe, effective technique for evaluating nodules that are felt to be suspicious based on the patient's clinical history or sonographic findings. Most centers perform FNA using 22 to 25 gauge needles, either using the so-called capillary technique, in which no syringe is employed, or the more traditional syringe suction technique. (Neither technique has been shown to be superior.) Core biopsy is performed rarely.

Although many clinicians perform FNA based solely on palpation, ultrasound guidance increases diagnostic confidence and accuracy. Color Doppler imaging may be helpful to avoid blood vessels, decreasing the likelihood of obtaining a nondiagnostic, bloody specimen. In general, aspirates may be classified as *inadequate* (insufficient cellular material for diagnosis), *benign*, *malignant*, or *suspicious* (follicular or Hürthle cell neoplasm). When the aspirate is insufficient, repeat FNA is recommended, although excisional biopsy may eventually be needed, particularly if the nodule has worrisome sonographic characteristics.

NEOPLASTIC THYROID NODULES

THYROID ADENOMA

Adenomas are infrequent, representing less than 10% of all thyroid nodules. They are approximately seven times more common in females and are usually solitary and nonfunctional. Rare autonomous hyperfunctional adenomas can lead to thyrotoxicosis (Plummer disease). Histologically, these lesions are difficult to distinguish from follicular carcinomas and therefore are usually surgically removed. Sonographically, thyroid adenomas are often hyperechoic, although they can be iso- or hypoechoic, as well. Additionally, they may have a thick peripheral sonolucent halo and demonstrate internal vascularity in a characteristic spoke wheel distribution.

TABLE 68-2 Classification of Primary Thyroid Cancer

Well-differentiated	Papillary carcinoma
	Follicular carcinoma (includes Hürthle cell neoplasm)
	Mixed
Poorly differentiated	Medullary carcinoma
	Anaplastic carcinoma
	Other (lymphoma, sarcoma, carcinosarcoma)

THYROID CANCER

Thyroid cancer is generally classified as well-differentiated or poorly differentiated (Table 68-2). The former group, which includes papillary and follicular carcinomas, has an overall better prognosis than the latter group.

PAPILLARY CARCINOMA

Papillary thyroid carcinoma is the most common form of thyroid cancer, accounting for approximately 75% of cases. This form of cancer most often presents as a solid, hypoechoic thyroid nodule that contains internal vascularity. These tumors may contain microcalcifications, which represent psammoma bodies. Papillary carcinoma spreads via lymphatics, and metastatic lymph nodes may contain microcalcifications, as well. Early identification and diagnosis of these tumors improves their generally good prognosis. Distant metastases are rare, but when present they are usually to lung or mediastinum.

FOLLICULAR NEOPLASIA

Follicular carcinoma is the second most common type of thyroid cancer. The term "follicular neoplasia," which includes both benign follicular adenomas and carcinomas, is used because of their nonspecific sonographic and cytological appearances. Both benign and malignant lesions often appear as well capsulated, hyperechoic masses with intrinsic vascularity and a prominent, often incomplete, sonolucent halo. Since FNA cytological analysis cannot reliably differentiate these lesions, the entire nodule must be examined for evidence of capsular invasion and atypia. Therefore, follicular lesions are surgically resected. Overall, prognosis for follicular carcinoma is good. Metastases occur hematogenously and are rare.

MEDULLARY CARCINOMA

Medullary thyroid carcinoma is the next most common subtype. These lesions are distinguished by their inclusion in the multiple endocrine neoplasia (MEN) and familial medullary carcinoma syndromes. They are neuroendocrine tumors and are derived from the parafollicular C-cells. Medullary thyroid cancer is seen in MEN types 2a and 2b. Sonographically, these lesions present as hypoechoic, solid masses, often with internal echogenic foci, typically a coarser appearing calcification than present in papillary cancers. They have a worse prognosis, and distant lymphatic metastases are common at presentation.

ANAPLASTIC CARCINOMA

Anaplastic thyroid carcinoma represents less than 5% of thyroid cancer and is more common in elderly patients. The prognosis is dismal, with local and distant metastases very common at presentation. These tumors are locally aggressive and sonographically appear as large, hypoechoic thyroid masses that commonly demonstrate internal necrosis, calcification, and direct invasion of surrounding neck structures, including the trachea.

LYMPHOMA

Primary thyroid lymphoma is rare and is usually associated with Hashimoto thyroiditis. Typically of the B-cell variety, primary lymphoma has a variable presentation. Sonographically, it may appear as a diffuse or focal hypoechoic mass involving all or part of the gland. More commonly, it appears locally invasive with involvement of adjacent neck structures.

METASTATIC DISEASE

Metastases to the thyroid gland are uncommon, usually from melanoma, breast, or renal cancers. They rarely calcify and may mimic primary thyroid tumors. Sonographically, they are typically hypoechoic and may show internal cavitation or necrosis.

CERVICAL LYMPH NODES

The primary goal of lymph node sonography is to distinguish benign from metastatic adenopathy. Early detection of nodal disease optimizes staging and may direct treatment for many cancers. Ultrasound has emerged as a sensitive modality for detection of abnormal cervical lymph nodes in need of further evaluation and biopsy.

Targeted ultrasound of the neck usually begins with the lymph nodes associated with the common carotid artery and internal jugular veins. In addition, lymph nodes within the submandibular region and posterior to the sternocleidomastoid should be evaluated. Node size is the only characteristic that can be assessed clinically, however studies have shown that a fair number (20%–40%) of normal-sized lymph nodes may harbor metastases. Conversely, nodal enlargement may be secondary to reactive hyperplasia. Therefore, in addition to size, attention should also be given to morphology.

The normal lymph node usually has a smooth, ovoid, or fusiform shaped hypoechoic cortex with a centrally located echogenic fatty hilum. Often, small blood vessels are seen entering the hilum with color or power Doppler imaging. Metastatic lymph nodes exhibit disruption of the normal architecture, along with development of a more globular shape. Heterogeneity, increased echogenicity, cystic areas, and microcalcifications are all findings that are suspicious for lymph node metastases from thyroid cancers.

POSTTHYROID SURGERY SURVEILLANCE

In recent years, ultrasound has assumed a greater role in the surveillance of patients following thyroidectomy for thyroid cancer. The examination involves evaluation of the thyroid bed for recurrent tumor as well as assessment of the regional lymph nodes for metastases, using the criteria discussed above. Any suspicious findings should be subject to ultrasound-guided FNA biopsy.

PARATHYROID GLANDS

The four parathyroid glands are typically located deep to the upper and lower poles of the thyroid gland and are supplied by branches of the thyroidal arteries. However, ectopic locations, including the substance of the thyroid gland, the retropharyngeal or retroesophageal space, or the mediastinum are not uncommon and supernumerary or absent glands are seen as well.

The parathyroid glands produce PTH, which influences the serum calcium level via several mechanisms. Primary hyperparathyroidism is diagnosed when the serum calcium level is high in the presence of an inappropriately normal or elevated PTH. Symptoms include fatigue, bone pain, and muscle weakness. Most cases are caused by an isolated parathyroid adenoma, although multiple adenomas, hyperplasia, or carcinoma may also be present. Parathyroid adenomas are also seen in MEN 1 and 2a, with the former predominating. (Primary hyperparathyroidism must be distinguished from the secondary form, which is seen in renal failure patients who develop diffuse or nodular parathyroid hyperplasia.)

Normal parathyroid glands are rarely visible sonographically because of their propensity to blend imperceptibly with adjacent tissues. Parathyroid gland enlargement may be secondary to hyperplasia, adenoma, or carcinoma. In general, it is not possible to distinguish these entities based on their sonographic appearance, as all appear hypoechoic. However, large masses that compress or invade adjacent structures are suspicious for carcinoma, as hyperplastic or adenomatous glands typically conform to their surroundings. Color or power Doppler imaging often demonstrates a vascular arc that partially encircles the gland before penetrating it.

SALIVARY GLANDS: NORMAL ANATOMY AND APPEARANCE

The *parotid gland* is located in the retromandibular fossa, anterior to the ear. It is divided into superficial and deep lobes, of which only the former is well visualized with ultrasound. The *submandibular gland* lies anterior and caudal to the parotid gland in the submandibular triangle, and the *sublingual glands* are located in the floor of the oral cavity. All the salivary glands tend to be homogeneous and at least moderately echogenic.

NONNEOPLASTIC CONDITIONS

Acute infection is most common in children and is usually viral. Ultrasound reveals an enlarged gland with decreased echogenicity. Bacterial infection is more common in elderly and diabetic patients and may proceed to abscess formation. In these cases, ultrasound may be helpful to guide aspiration to determine the causative organism.

Sjögren syndrome, an autoimmune condition that is characterized by chronic inflammation of the salivary glands, results in glands that are very heterogeneous, often showing hypervascularity on color Doppler imaging. These patients have an increased risk of lymphoma, therefore biopsy is recommended for lesions that are larger than 2 cm or that grow rapidly.

Most salivary stones are located in the submandibular gland or Wharton duct, which opens in the floor of the mouth. Sialitis appear as small echogenic foci that exhibit acoustic shadowing, although this feature may be absent with very small calculi. Dilation of the duct proximal to the stone or glandular swelling may be present if the duct is obstructed.

SALIVARY GLAND NEOPLASMS

Pleomorphic adenomas and Warthin tumors are the most common benign neoplasms, which comprise the majority of salivary gland tumors. Both tend to be hypoechoic. Of the malignant neoplasms, mucoepidermoid carcinomas and adenoid cystic carcinomas are the most frequent. They tend to be less well defined than the benign tumors, but there is considerable overlap. Examination of the cervical lymph nodes is essential in these patients.

MISCELLANEOUS NECK MASSES

A variety of cystic and cystlike masses that arise in the neck may be imaged with ultrasound. *Thyroglossal duct cysts* result from persistence of a portion of the thyroglossal duct, which runs from the base of the tongue to the anterior neck. Thyroglossal duct cysts have a sonographic appearance that ranges from simple to complex, and most are infrahyoid. Because thyroid cancer can develop within them, FNA biopsy is recommended if mural nodules are demonstrated and excision is not planned.

Branchial cleft cysts are usually located at the mandibular angle. Most are simple, but proteinaceous or other content may result in an appearance that mimics a solid mass. *Venous malformations* have a complex, multiseptated configuration. Slow flow may be evident on power Doppler imaging or grayscale sonography. Phleboliths, which are echogenic and cast acoustic shadows, are a clue to the diagnosis, but are seen in a minority of cases. Finally, *cervical abscesses* have a sonographic appearance that is similar to abscesses elsewhere, with varying internal debris and gas. Ultrasound is useful to guide percutaneous sampling or drainage.

SUGGESTED READING

Bialek EJ, Jakubowski W, Zajkowski P, et al. US of the major salivary glands: anatomy and spatial relationships, pathologic conditions, and pitfalls. *Radiographics*. 2006;26(3):745-763.

Cappelli C, Pirola I, De Martino E, et al. The role of imaging in Graves' disease: a cost-effectiveness analysis. *Eur J Radiol*. 2008;65(1):99-103.

Frates MC, Benson CB, Charboneau JW, et al. Management of thyroid nodules detected at US: society of radiologists in ultrasound consensus conference statement. *Radiology*. 2005; 237(3):794-800.

Johnson NA, Tublin ME. Postoperative surveillance of differentiated thyroid carcinoma: rationale, techniques, and controversies. *Radiology*. 2008;249(2):429-444.

Johnson NA, Tublin ME, Ogilvie JB. Parathyroid imaging: technique and role in the preoperative evaluation of primary hyperparathyroidism. *AJR Am J Roentgenol.* 2007;188(6):1706-1715.

Kim MJ, Kim EK, Park SI, et al. US-guided fine-needle aspiration of thyroid nodules: indications, techniques, results. *Radiographics.* 2008; 28(7):1869-1886, discussion 1887.

Park JS, Son KR, Na DG, et al. Performance of preoperative sonographic staging of papillary thyroid carcinoma based on the sixth edition of the AJCC/UICC TNM classification system. *AJR Am J Roentgenol.* 2009;192(1):66-72.

Reading CC, Charboneau JW, Hay ID, et al. Sonography of thyroid nodules: a "classic pattern" diagnostic approach. *Ultrasound Q.* 2005;21(3):157-165.

Reeder SB, Desser TS, Weigel RJ, et al. Sonography in primary hyperparathyroidism: review with emphasis on scanning technique. *J Ultrasound Med.* 2002;21(5):539-552.

Tublin ME, Martin JA, Rollin LJ, et al. Ultrasound-guided fine-needle aspiration versus fine-needle capillary sampling biopsy of thyroid nodules: does technique matter? *J Ultrasound Med.* 2007;26(12):1697-1701.

QUESTIONS AND ANSWERS

1. Concerning thyroid physiology, which of the following is *true*?
   A. Most thyroid hormone circulates in active form.
   B. Production of thyroid hormone is controlled by a positive feedback loop.
   C. TRH is secreted by the anterior pituitary gland.
   D. T4 is converted to T3 peripherally.

   ANSWER: D. T4 is released in greater quantity and is then converted to T3.

2. Concerning Hashimoto thyroiditis, which of the following is *true*?
   A. Micronodularity is the predominant sonographic feature.
   B. Lymphoma is not a recognized complication.
   C. Most patients present with hyperthyroidism.
   D. It has a male predominance.

   ANSWER: A. The thyroid gland in Hashimoto thyroiditis has a micronodular appearance, with multiple, small hypoechoic foci scattered throughout the gland.

3. Concerning acute Graves disease, which of the following is *true*?
   A. Males are affected more often than females.
   B. It is an autoimmune condition.
   C. The thyroid gland is small.
   D. "Thyroid storm" refers to thyroid hypervascularity on ultrasound.

   ANSWER: B. Like Hashimoto thyroiditis, Graves disease is an autoimmune condition that is caused by circulating autoantibodies.

4. Which of the following statements regarding thyroid nodules is *true*?
   A. They are malignant approximately 20% of the time.
   B. Most are hyperplastic.
   C. Epithelial cysts are more common than cystic degeneration.
   D. Calcifications are rare.

   ANSWER: B. Most thyroid nodules are hyperplastic and not neoplastic.

5. Which of the following statements about thyroid nodule calcification is *true*?
   A. Coarse calcifications are more worrisome than punctate calcifications.
   B. If coarse calcifications are present, biopsy is not warranted.
   C. Microcalcifications correspond to psammoma bodies in papillary cancers.
   D. Colloid crystals cannot be distinguished from microcalcifications by their ultrasound appearance.

   ANSWER: C. The microcalcifications in papillary cancers correspond to psammoma bodies seen microscopically. When demonstrated sonographically, they are highly suspicious for papillary thyroid cancer.

6. Concerning thyroid cancer, which of the following is *true*?
   A. Papillary cancer has a better prognosis than medullary cancer.
   B. Papillary cancer is less common than follicular cancer.
   C. FNA is sufficient to distinguish follicular adenoma from follicular carcinoma.
   D. Thyroid cancer is a common malignancy.

   ANSWER: A. Medullary cancer has a worse prognosis than papillary cancer, and nodal metastases are common at presentation.

7. Which of the following is a sign of benign thyroid nodules?
   A. Central flow on color Doppler
   B. Ill-defined halo
   C. Microcalcifications
   D. Echogenic foci with comet tail artifacts

   ANSWER: D. Echogenic foci with comet tail artifacts are representative of colloid, which is often found in benign nodules.

8. Concerning cervical lymph nodes, which of the following is suggestive of malignancy?
   A. Elongated shape
   B. Fatty hilum

C. Homogeneity
D. Cystic areas

ANSWER: D. Lymph nodes with cystic areas are suspicious for regional metastases.

9. Concerning thyroid biopsy, which of the following is *true*?
   A. Indeterminate aspirates always require surgical excision for diagnosis.
   B. Capillary technique is superior to the aspiration technique.
   C. Core biopsy is required for diagnosis approximately 25% of the time.
   D. Color Doppler ultrasound is a useful adjunct.

ANSWER: D. Color Doppler sonography may help the radiologist avoid vessels and lessen the likelihood of obtaining a bloody specimen.

10. Concerning parathyroid gland ultrasound, which of the following is *true*?
   A. Normal parathyroid glands are usually visible sonographically.
   B. Adenomas can be reliably distinguished from hyperplastic glands.
   C. Parathyroid adenomas typically have a vessel along their margin.
   D. Parathyroid adenomas are typically more echogenic than the thyroid gland.

ANSWER: C. Parathyroid adenomas usually have a prominent supplying vessel that partially encircles them.

Section 7
MUSCULOSKELETAL SYSTEM

69 MUSCULOSKELETAL ANATOMY AND BASIC PHYSIOLOGY

Andrew S. Ferrell and Matthew C. Larrison

SUBSTRUCTURE OF BONE

Compact (cortical) bone is the hard outer layer of bone containing very little intervening spaces. This accounts for approximately 80% of total bone weight and provides a significant amount of the strength of bone.

Trabecular bone consists of a porous network found in the center of bones; it contains hematopoetic elements, fat, and vascular structures. Its spongy configuration makes the overall bone lighter.

CELLULAR ELEMENTS OF BONE

Osteoblasts are mononuclear bone-forming cells derived from osteoprogenitor cells. These cells cover the surface of developing osteoid and secrete a protein-rich mixture, predominantly made of type I collagen. They also secrete other matrix proteins, hormones, and prostaglandins, which regulate bone formation. Osteoblasts are stimulated by calcitonin.

Osteoclasts are multinucleated cells responsible for bone resorption and are located in resorption pits called Howship's lacuna. These cells are derived from monocyte precursors and have phagocyte-like activity. They secrete enzymes involved in bone breakdown and turnover. Osteoclasts are stimulated by parathyroid hormone.

Osteocytes originate from osteoblasts trapped within the bone matrix in spaces known as lacunae. These cells are involved in the formation and maintenance of bone, as well as regulating bones response to stress and mechanical load.

TYPES OF BONES

- Long bones develop by endochondral ossification, and consist of a shaft (diaphysis) with two expanded articular ends (epiphysis). The metaphysis is part of the diaphysis and is the growth zone between the epiphysis and diaphysis during development. The marrow cavity of long bones is within the diaphysis. Long bones include the humerus, radius, ulna, and femur.
- Short bones are composed of an outer layer of compact bone surrounding inner spongy bone and include the carpal and tarsal bones.
- Flat bones consist of two layers of compact bone enclosing spongy bone and marrow (diploic) space. The articular surface of flat bones is lined with fibrocartilage. Ribs, sternum, scapulae, and bones of the skull vault are flat bones.
- Irregular bones include bones of mixed shape, such as those of the skull base and vertebrae.
- Sesamoid bones develop in tendons that cross the surface of long bones such as in the wrist and knee (patella), and they reduce friction.

BONE FORMATION

Endochondral ossification occurs on the foundation of a cartilaginous model and is the type of bone growth that occurs in long and short bones as well as portions of irregular bones. This type of ossification accounts for the majority of growth in childhood as well as some repair following fractures. In fetal life, a primary ossification center develops in the future diaphysis of the cartilaginous model. The perichondrium becomes vascularized and subsequently becomes the periosteum from which undifferentiated cells migrate and become osteoblasts at the primary ossification center. The osteoblasts secrete osteoid on top of cartilage secreted by chondrocytes and this ultimately calcifies. Osteoblasts secrete additional osteoid that will ultimately lead to trabecular formation. The secondary ossification center occurs in the epiphysis after birth. The epiphysis and diaphysis are separated by a growing transverse band of cartilage known as the physis.

Intramembranous ossification is the formation of bone on or in fibrous connective tissue formed from condensed mesenchymal cells. Unlike endochondral ossification, a cartilage model is not present in intramembranous ossification. Primitive mesenchymal cells proliferate and differentiate into osteogenic precursor cells, which develop into osteoblasts. Osteoblasts begin to lay down osteoid, the inorganic precursor of bone formed of collagen fibrils. The osteoid calcifies to form bone spicules, which unite to form trabeculae. This process creates flat bones such as the mandible and flat bones of the skull, and it is the primary process involved with healing of fractures.

MARROW CONVERSION

In the neonatal period, red or hematopoeitc marrow is present throughout the skeletal system. Normal physiologic conversion of red to yellow marrow occurs in a predictable pattern through childhood into adolescence. Conversion begins in the terminal phalanges and progresses proximally. There is a distal to proximal trend within individual bones as well, starting in the diaphysis followed by the distal and ultimately proximal metaphysis. Conversion is completed by age 25, with red marrow remaining primarily within the axial skeleton. Red marrow can be found in the humeral and femoral heads as a normal variant in adults.

FRACTURE HEALING

Fracture healing occurs in three phases. The first is the inflammatory or reactive phase that begins immediately following the fracture with vasoconstriction and formation of localized hematoma and lasts approximately 2 weeks. This hematoma provides limited initial stability of the fracture fragments. The cells in this area will subsequently die allowing fibroblasts to migrate into the area along with small proliferative vessels collectively forming granulation tissue. The second phase is the reparative phase. Periosoteal progenitor cells migrate into the fracture gap and form both chondroblasts and osteoblasts that produce hyaline cartilage and woven bone, respectively. Fibroblasts within the granulation tissue itself will also differentiate into hyaline-producing chondroblasts. This collection of cartilage and woven bone, known as soft callus, serves as the initial connection of the fracture gap and occurs at approximately 2 to 3 weeks. After the immature callus is formed, both endochondral and intramembranous ossification processes convert the hyaline cartilage and woven bone to more organized lamellar bone or hard callus. This occurs at approximately 4 to 8 weeks and is the point at which time the callus becomes radiographically evident. New vessels permeate the lamellar bone and recruit additional osteoblasts, which eventually serve to convert the lamellar bone into trabecular bone. In the final remodeling phase, osteoclasts migrate to create pits known as Howship's lacuna. Osteoblasts will then deposit compact bone within this pit. A balance of osteoblastic and osteoclastic activity will continue until the form of the fracture site is functionally similar to the original bone. This final phase can last for several years.

MUSCLES, TENDONS, AND LIGAMENTS—MACROSTRUCTURE

Skeletal muscles have sites of origin and insertion. Each individual muscle fiber is surrounded by endomysium. Bundles of muscles fibers are surrounded by perimysium and the entire muscle is enclosed by epimysium. Tendons are fibrous bands of connective tissue that connect muscles to bones or cartilage. Ligaments are also fibrous bands of connective tissue; however, they connect bony structures to each other rather than to muscles. Ligaments should be described by their proximal and distal attachments.

TYPES OF JOINTS

Fibrous (synarthroses) joints are held together by fibrous tissue, have no joint cavity, and are immovable. Examples include the sutures of the skull, teeth, and synchondroses. A synchondrosis is a joint of two bones united by cartilage and is seen in the epiphyseal plates in growing children.

Cartilagenous (amphiarthrosis) joints occur where two bones are held together by cartilaginous structures and like fibrous joints have no joint cavity but are slightly moveable. Symphyses are joints joined by fibrocartilage and provide slight mobility and include the symphisis pubis, intervertebral discs, and sacroiliac joints. A syndesmosis is another type of amphiarthrosis where the bony surfaces are united by an interosseous ligament, as in the inferior tibiofibular articulation.

Synovial (diarthrodial) joints are freely moveable joints with thick fibrous capsules containing synovial fluid produced by a synovial membrane. Articular cartilage (hyaline cartilage) at the ends of the adjoining bones provide for smooth motion and cushioning. The bones are also typically held together by thick ligaments. There are many types of synovial joints based on the shape of their articular surfaces and mechanics:

- Hinge (knee and elbow)
- Ball and socket (hip)
- Pivot (proximal radioulnar and atlantoaxial)
- Condyloid or ellipsoid (wrist)
- Gliding (intercarpal and intertarsal)
- Saddle (thumb carpometacarpal)

SPECIFIC JOINTS

Shoulder

The shoulder is composed of three separate joints: the glenohumeral, acromioclavicular, and sternoclavicular. The glenohumeral joint is the major one and is a ball-and-socket–type synovial joint. It is formed by the articulation of the humerus and lateral aspect of the scapula (glenoid fossa). The shallowness of the glenoid and relative loose connections of the joint capsule and surrounding muscles allow for tremendous mobility; however, this makes this joint prone to dislocation. The capsule is attached superiorly to the glenoid and inferiorly to the anatomic neck of the humerus. The capsule is reinforced by the four muscles and associated tendons of the rotator cuff and five scapulohumeral ligaments (Table 69-1). The rotator cuff circumferentially covers the humeral head and stabilizes, abducts, adducts, and rotates the shoulder. The supraspinatus lies directly over the humeral head attaching to the greater tuberosity and serves to abduct the shoulder through the first 15 degrees of motion. The infraspinatus and teres minor muscles cover the back of the humeral head, both inserting on the greater tuberosity and serving primarily as external rotators. The subscapularis attaches to the lesser tuberosity and stabilizes the glenohumeral joint as well as functioning as adductor and internal rotator.

TABLE 69-1 Rotator Cuff

Muscles
Subscapularis
Supraspinatus
Infraspinatus
Teres minor
Ligaments
Coracohumeral
Superior glenohumeral
Middle glenohumeral
Anteroinferior glenohumeral
Posteroinferior glenohumeral

Three bursa serve to lubricate the rotator cuff as it moves through the coracoacromial arch (space between the acromion and coracoacromial ligament). The subacromial bursa lies superior to the rotator cuff and facilitates supraspinatus movement beneath the coracoacromial arch. This bursa communicates freely with the subdeltoid bursa, which lies between the deltoid and joint capsule facilitating smooth movement between these structures. A third bursa, the subscapular bursa or recess, lies between the subscapularis tendon and the neck of the scapula. This bursa communicates freely with the synovial joint space, and is therefore normally opacified on arthrograms unlike the subacromial and subdeltoid bursa.

The glenoid labrum is a fibrocartilaginous rim attached around the margin of the glenoid fossa; it protects the edges of bone during motion and deepens the articular fossa. Superiorly, in most individuals, it is continuous with the long head of the biceps (biceps anchor complex). The anterosuperior portions of the labrum are loosely attached to the glenoid while the inferior portion is firmly attached, functioning as an immobile extension of the articular cartilage.

A common normal shoulder variant is a Buford complex, which consists of an absent anterior/superior labrum along with a cord-like thickened middle glenohumeral ligament.

Elbow

The elbow is a synovial hinge joint formed by three separate articulations. The first two are the humeroradial between the capitellum of the humerus and the radial head and the humeroulnar between the trochlea of the humerus and the trochlear notch of the ulna. These allow for flexion and extension. The third articulation, which allows for supination and pronation of the forearm, is the proximal radiolulnar joint between the radial head and radial notch of the ulna. Collectively these three articulations are within a common capsule.

The distal humerus has important medial and lateral epicondyles, the former being larger and the site of origin of the common flexor tendon of the forearm as well as the pronator teres. The lateral epicondyle is the site of origin of the common extensor tendon of the forearm as well as the supinator. The olecranon fossa allows for accommodation of the olecranon along the posterior aspect of the humerus during full extension while the coronoid fossa has a similar role anteriorly during flexion.

Three separate ligaments act to reinforce the elbow, the radial and ulnar collateral ligaments, as well as the annular ligament. The annular ligament is a fibrous band that encircles four-fifths of the radial head, forming a collar securing the radial head to the radial notch of the ulna at the proximal radioulnar joint. The annular ligament blends with both the radial collateral ligament and joint capsule. The radial collateral ligament is merely a thickening of the joint capsule, which extends from the lateral epicondyle of the humerus to the anterior and posterior margins of the radial notch of the ulna as well as the annular ligament. The ulnar collateral ligament is triangular in its configuration consisting of anterior, posterior, and oblique bands, and extends from the medial epicondyle of the humerus to the coronoid process and olecranon. Additionally, the lateral ulnar collateral ligament is located posterolaterally and prevents posterolateral subluxation of the radial head.

Wrist

The carpal bones are best arranged functionally into proximal and distal rows. The proximal row consists of the scaphoid, lunate, triquetrum, and pisiform, and the distal row consists of the trapezium, trapezoid, capitate, and hamate. The wrist is an ellipsoid joint formed between the radius and the proximal carpal row excluding the pisiform. The triangular fibrocartilage complex attaches the distal radius to the ulna as well as separating the lunate from the distal ulna. Dorsal and palmar radiocarpal ligaments connect the radius and ulna to the proximal carpal row. Radial and ulnar collateral ligaments connect the radial styloid to the scaphoid and the ulnar styloid to the triquetrum and pisiform respectively.

The carpal tunnel is bounded anteriorly by the flexor retinaculum and posteriorly by the carpal bones. The flexor retinaculum extends from the hook of the hamate to the tubercle of the trapezium. The carpal tunnel transmits the median nerve and tendons of the flexor pollicus longus, flexor digitorum profundus, and flexor digitorum superficialis muscles. The extensor retinaculum on the dorsum of the wrist is thinner than the flexor retinaculum and allows passages for the extensor tendons.

Hip

The femoral head articulates with the acetabular cavity, which is an elevated bony rim, incomplete inferiorly at the acetabular notch. The transverse acetabular ligament covers this deficient portion of the acetabulum. The articular surface of the acetabulum is covered by hyaline cartilage and fibocartilage (acetabular labrum) except centrally at the acetabular fossa that contains fibrofatty tissue and synovium. The femoral head is covered by articular cartilage except centrally at the fovea capitis, a central depression containing the ligamentum teres, which attaches the femoral head to the central aspect of the acetabular cavity at the transverse acetabular ligament.

A strong joint capsule attaches anteriorly and posteriorly to the acetabular rim, creating small paralabral recesses. Superiorly, it also attaches to the labrum creating a larger paralabral recess. Inferiorly, the capsule attaches to the femoral neck. Anteriorly, the capsule extends to the intertrochanteric line; however, it covers only approximately half of the femoral neck posteriorly. There is a normal communication of the joint cavity with the iliopsoas bursa in approximately 15% of individuals.

Knee

Three main joints of the knee are the femorotibial, patellofemoral, and proximal tibiofibular joints. The femorotibial articulation is a condylar-type synovial hinge joint between the condyles of the femur and tibia. The patellofemoral joint is a saddle-type joint. The proximal tibiofibular joint is a glide-type joint.

The lateral collateral ligament (LCL) extends from the proximal aspect of the lateral femoral condyle to the lateral aspect of the fibular head. The distal aspect of the ligament merges with tendon of the long head of the biceps femoris as a common attachment. The LCL serves as a stabilizer to varus forces during movement. The iliotibial band is a thickening of the fascia lata, which originates from the iliac crest and attaches to the lateral femoral condyle of the tibia at Gerdy's tubercle. Segond fracture is an avulsion fracture of the lateral tibial metaphysis, and is thought to relate to the insertion of the central portion of the lateral capsular ligament, which attaches to the proximal lateral aspect of the tibia.

The medial (tibial) collateral ligament (MCL) can be divided into both superficial and deep components. Anatomically the superficial component has a proximal attachment from the medial femoral condyle just below the adductor tubercle and extends distally to the metaphyseal region of the tibia just beneath the pes anserinus (common tendinous insertion of the sartorius, gracillis, and semitendinosus). The MCL is the primary structure responsible for resistance to valgus stress within the knee. The deep MCL anatomically consists of the meniscofemoral and meniscotibial ligaments. These structures are firmly attached to the meniscus but do not provide significant resistance to valgus force.

The anterior cruciate ligament (ACL) arises from the posteromedial aspect of the lateral femoral condyle and has a broad attachment to the tibia in front of and lateral to the anterior tibial eminence. The ACL is composed of two principle bundles, the anteromedial and posterolateral bands. The anteromedial band is tight in flexion and the posterolateral is tight in extension. The ACL serves to prevent anterior translation of the tibia with respect to the femur. It also serves as a stabilizer during rotational movement.

The posterior cruiciate ligament (PCL) originates from the anterolateral aspect of the medial femoral condyle in the intercondylar notch and extends to attach to a recessed shelf posterior and inferior to the articular surface of the tibial plateau. The PCL is approximately twice as strong and thick as the ACL, therefore it is injured much less frequently than the ACL. It serves as a stabilizer of the knee providing significant resistance to posterior tibial displacement with respect to the femur. The PCL can be divided into anterolateral and posteromedial bundles. The anterolateral bundle prevents hyperflexion while the posterolateral bundle prevents hyperextension.

Medial and lateral menisci are attached to the condylar surface of the tibia. They are separated into body, anterior, and posterior horns. Their superior surfaces are concave and the inferior surfaces are flat. The periphery of the menisci are convex and thick and attached to the joint capsule while the central portion is thinner and only loosely attached to the tibial surface. The peripheral surface is considered nonarticular and usually not involved in tears. Several ligaments also attach to the menisci including the meniscofemoral, meniscotibial, coronary, and transverse intermeniscal ligaments.

These are mostly avascular structures, except for the peripheral 10% to 25%, supplied by perimeniscal capillary plexus from the lateral and medial geniculate arteries. For this reason, peripheral tears will heal better than central ones.

The medial meniscus has an open C shape and is larger than the lateral meniscus. There is a firm attachment to the deep MCL and joint capsule at the periphery and is therefore more prone to injury. The posterior horn is roughly twice the size of the anterior horn.

The lateral meniscus has a more tight C shape and appears more circular on axial slices. The anterior and posterior horns are roughly equal in size. Unlike the medial meniscus, there is only a loose attachment to the capsule peripherally and there is no direct attachment to the LCL. This makes the lateral meniscus overall more mobile and less prone to injury. Of particular note, the posterior horn is attached to the medial femoral condyle through the ligament of Wrisberg (posterior to PCL) or ligament of Humphrey (anterior to PCL) in one-third of patients. Approximately 3% of people have both.

A common variant of the meniscus is the discoid configuration. This occurs when there is thickening of the central portion of the meniscus extending toward the intracondylar notch. On MRI, this is demonstrated as more than two consecutive sagittal images without a bowtie configuration. This is more commonly seen in the lateral meniscus. Another common variant is meniscal flounce, which is seen as a wavy appearance of the free edge of the meniscus when the knee is in approximately 10 degrees of flexion. This commonly resolves when the knee is fully extended.

Ankle

While the tibiotalar joint is the true ankle joint, functionally the ankle is composed of four joints: tibiotalar, subtalar, and the proximal and distal tibiofibular. Interaction of all of these joints is required for proper motion at the ankle.

The tibiotalar joint is a hinge joint with medial and lateral malleoli projecting inferiorly from the tibia and fibula respectively forming the medial and lateral walls. Strong ligaments reinforce the medial (deltoid) and lateral aspects of the joint while the capsule is significantly weaker both posteriorly and anteriorly.

The medial collateral ligamentous complex (deltoid ligament) has several components: tibiotalar, tibiocalcaneal, talonavicular, and the spring ligaments (between the sustentaculum tali and navicular). Functionally, and as seen on imaging studies, the deltoid ligament is best divided into superficial and deep components. The superficial portion arises from the medial malleolus and extends into three separate ligaments. The superficial part of the deltoid primarily resists eversion of the hindfoot. The deep portion arises from the medial malleolus and inserts on the nonarticular surface of the medial talus. The main function of the deep deltoid is to prevent lateral displacement and external rotation of the talus.

The lateral collateral ligamentous complex can be divided into superior and inferior groups. The superior group is composed of anterior and posterior tibiofibular ligaments. The inferior group is composed of anterior and posterior talofibular as well as calcaneofibular ligaments. The anterior talofibular ligament is the most commonly torn ligament of the ankle.

Many important tendons surround the ankle joint. Posteriorly, the Achilles tendon attaches to the posterior aspect of the calacaneus. Of note, the Achilles tendon does not have a tendon sheath but rather a paratenon. Immediately adjacent to the Achilles tendon, along its medial aspect, is the small plantaris tendon. The flexor tendons are located on the medial aspect of the ankle. In successive fashion from medial to lateral and anterior to posterior are the posterior tibial, flexor digitorum longus, posterior tibial neurovascular bundle, and flexor hallucis longus tendon (mnemonic for remembering this is Tom, Dick, and Harry). Laterally there are the primary everters of the foot, the peroneus longus and brevis, which both pass behind the lateral malleolus using this structure as a pulley. Anteriorly from medial to lateral, the main tendons seen are the anterior tibial, extensor hallucis longus, extensor digitorum longus, and peroneus terius.

Suggested Reading

Chhabra, A. Anatomic, radiographic, biomechanical, and kinematic evaluation of the anterior cruciate ligament and its two functional bundles. *J Bone Joint Surg*. 2006;88:2-10.

Massengill AD. Labrocapsular ligamentous complex of the shoulder: normal anatomy, anatomic variation, and pitfalls of MR imaging and MR arthrography. *Radiographics.* 1994;14: 1211-1223.

Recondo JA. Lateral stabilizing structures of the knee: functional anatomy and injuries assessed with MR imaging. *Radiographics.* 2000;20:S91-S102.

QUESTIONS AND ANSWERS

1. Where is normal red marrow located in the adult skeleton?
   A. Distal femur
   B. Skull
   C. Vertebral bodies
   D. Humeral diaphysis

   ANSWER: C. Vertebral bodies. In the neonatal period, red or hematopoietic marrow is present throughout the skeletal system. Normal physiologic conversion of red to yellow marrow occurs in a predictable pattern through childhood and adolescence. Conversion begins in the terminal phalanges and progresses proximally. There is a distal to proximal trend within individual bones as well, starting in the diaphysis followed by the distal and ultimately proximal metaphysis. Conversion is completed by age 25, with red marrow remaining primarily within the axial skeleton. Red marrow can be found in the humeral and femoral heads as a normal variant in adults.

2. Which of the following is the most commonly injured ankle ligament?
   A. Anterior talofibular
   B. Anterior tibiofibular
   C. Deltoid
   D. Posterior talofibular

   ANSWER: A. The anterior talofibular ligament is the most commonly torn ligament followed by the posterior talofibular and calcaneofibular ligaments. These are commonly torn with inversion injuries. In contrast, the medial deltoid ligamentous complex is significantly stronger and seldom tears.

3. Which of the following is a component of the Buford complex?
   A. Thickened common superior glenohumeral ligament
   B. Common superior glenohumeral ligament
   C. Thickened superior glenohumeral ligament
   D. Common middle glenohumeral ligament

   ANSWER: B. A common normal variant seen within the shoulder is a Buford complex, which consists of an absent anterior/superior labrum along with a cord-like thickened middle glenohumeral ligament.

4. Between which two muscle tendons is a Baker cyst located?
   A. Medial head gastrocnemius and semimembranosus
   B. Medial head gastrocnemius and semitendinosus
   C. Medial and lateral heads of the gastrocnemius
   D. Semitendinosus and semimembranosus

   ANSWER: A. A true Baker cyst as originally described lies between the tendons of the medial head of the gastrocnemius and the semimembranosus.

5. Segond fracture is an avulsion fracture of which of the following structures?
   A. Medial capsular ligament
   B. Iliotibial band
   C. LCLs
   D. ACL

   ANSWER: C. Segond fracture is an avulsion fracture of the lateral tibial metaphysis, and is thought to relate to the insertion of the central portion of the lateral capsular ligament, which attaches to the proximal lateral aspect of the tibia.

6. Which of the following is *not* found within the carpal tunnel?
   A. Median nerve
   B. Flexor pollicus longus
   C. Extensor carpi radialis brevis
   D. Flexor digitorum superficialis

   ANSWER: C. The carpal tunnel is bounded anteriorly by the flexor retinaculum and posteriorly by the carpal bones. The flexor retinaculum extends from the hook of the hamate to the tubercle of the trapezium. The carpal tunnel transmits the median nerve and tendons of the flexor pollicus longus, flexor digitorum profundus, and flexor digitorum superficialis muscles.

7. Which of the following is *not* normally opacified on shoulder arthrography?
   A. Subscapularis recess
   B. Glenohumeral joint space
   C. Biceps tendon sheath
   D. Subacromial bursa

   ANSWER: D. The subacromial and subdeltoid bursas do not normally communicate with the glenohumeral joint space, and opacification of this bursa on routine shoulder arthrography is indicative of a full-thickness rotator cuff tear. The subscapularis recess is a normal inferior extension of the joint space, which can be seen "saddle bagging" over the subscapularis on sagittal images. The long head of the biceps has an intraarticular course, and fluid or gadolinium is often seen around the tendon within the tendon sheath. Fluid or gadolinium within the tendon itself is indicative of tear.

8. Which of the following structures is found within the tarsal tunnel?
   A. Anterior tibial nerve
   B. Extensor hallucis longus tendon
   C. Sural nerve
   D. Flexor digitorum longus

   ANSWER: D. The tarsal tunnel is on the medial aspect of the ankle and is bordered medially by the bony medial aspects of the distal tibia, calcaneus, and talus and laterally by the flexor retinaculum. Through this tunnel pass the posterior tibial artery and vein; posterior tibial nerve; and tendons of the tibialis posterior, flexor hallucis longus, and flexor digitorum longus muscles.

9. The flexor retinaculum of the wrist extends from which of the following two structures?
   A. Pisiform to triquetrum
   B. Hamate to trapezium
   C. Scaphoid to hamate
   D. Trapezium to trapezoid

   ANSWER: B. The flexor retinaculum extends from the hook of the hamate to the tubercle of the trapezium.

10. Which of the following structure serves to keep the radial head in appropriate location at the proximal radioulnar joint?
    A. Annular ligament
    B. Radial collateral ligament
    C. Ulnar collateral ligament
    D. Bicipital aponeurosis

    ANSWER: A. Three separate ligaments act to reinforce the elbow, the radial and ulnar collateral, as well as the annular ligament. The annular ligament is a fibrous band, which encircles four-fifths of the radial head, forming a collar, which secures the radial head to the radial notch of the ulna at the proximal radioulnar joint. The annular ligament blends with both the radial collateral ligament and joint capsule. The radial collateral ligament is merely a thickening of the joint capsule, which extends from the lateral epicondyle of the humerus to the anterior and posterior margins of the radial notch of the ulna as well as the annular ligament. The ulnar collateral ligament is triangular in its configuration consisting of anterior, posterior, and oblique bands, and extends from the medial epicondyle of the humerus to the coronoid process and olecranon.

70 MUSCULOSKELETAL TRAUMA

Roderick F. Biosca Jr. and Matthew Larrison

CERVICAL SPINE FRACTURES

The cervical spine remains one of the most clinically significant areas of evaluation because of the dire consequences of injury. Injuries of the cervical spine predominantly occur at differing levels based on age. In the pediatric population, cervical injuries tend to involve the proximal cervical spine (C1-2), while in adults, injuries tend to involve the lower cervical spine, specifically C5-6 and C6-7. These differences are believed to be related to the relative size and mass of the child's head with respect to the cervical muscle mass.

The most devastating cervical spinal injury is a flexion teardrop fracture; it is the most common cervical spine fracture with dire consequences. The flexion teardrop fracture results from severe flexion compression that often results in a comminuted fracture of the affected vertebral body, typically C5 or C6 and spinal column. There is posterior dissociation of the upper involved vertebral body. Typically a fragment from the anterior inferior margin of the more cranial affected vertebral body is detached as is the anterior spinal ligament, which remains attached to the fragment. The anterior spinal ligament is disrupted at the level of injury, but also remains attached to the remainder of the spine. The ring of the affected vertebral level is intact and displaces posteriorly, causing marked narrowing of the spinal canal, often with cord impingement, entrapment, and injury. The cord is often struck on the ventral (anterior) surface where the greatest trauma is induced, creating an anterior cord syndrome: diminished motor function with loss of pain and temperature sensation. Proprioception and vibratory sense are intact.

Hyperextension injuries are much more subtle. The uppermost vertebral body is dislocated posteriorly for an instant, but usually self-reduces, limiting findings seen on CT and radiographs. Imaging typically reveals subtle findings, such as prevertebral soft-tissue thickening, mild posterior vertebral body displacement, and widening of the intervertebral disk space.

The most commonly missed significant cervical spine fractures involve the odontoid. Dens fractures are classified by where the fracture plane dissects the dens. Type I is often an avulsion-type injury and only involves the tip and is considered stable. Types II and III are considered unstable and involve the body of the dens or fracture into the vertebral body of C2, respectively. Findings are often subtle on radiographs, and disruption of the spinolaminar line is classic as a result of the loss of the normal posterior tilt of the dens body with respect to the anterior spinal line.

Axial loading can cause lateral displacement of the lateral masses of C1. Since the atlas is essentially a ring, for the lateral masses to move laterally, the ring has to break in two places. The weakest portion of the atlas is the anterior and posterior arches, where fractures typically occur. Once fractured through both arches, the lateral masses are free to displace laterally, resulting in an unstable injury.

Traumatic spondylolysis, commonly called Hangman fracture, typically results from a hyperextension injury with fractures through neural arches (pedicles or lamina). This injury decompresses itself as the involved vertebral body moves anterior, but the posterior neural arch remains approximately unchanged, thereby actually widening the spinal canal rather than narrowing it. These injuries typically affect C1-2 or C2-3. Disruption of the spinal laminar line is diagnostic.

Jumped, perched, and locked facets occur by a similar mechanism, and are more of a spectrum of the same injury resulting from flexion, distraction, and rotation within the spine. The most common level involved is C4-5 or C5-6.

Three types of occipital condylar fractures are seen. The first type results from axial loading and is a compression-type fracture of the condyle. The second type is unique because it is an extension into or from the occipital bone. The third type of occipital condyle fracture is the most unstable and severe. It involves a simple avulsion of the alar ligament from the occipital condyle. This increases laxity at the skull base and can result in spinal cord compression slightly below the brainstem junction.

THORACIC AND LUMBAR SPINAL INJURY

Thoracic and lumbar spine injuries are unique from cervical spinal injuries because the lower spine has greater structural stability secondary to larger support muscles, thicker ligaments, and larger overall intervertebral disks. Compression and flexion injuries account for 75% of all thoracic and lumbar spinal injuries. The most common thoracic and lumbar fracture in normal bone is an anterior wedging fracture, which usually results in depression and wedging of the superior endplate. If the force load is asymmetric, the injury can simply be a lateral compression fracture.

TABLE 70-1 Grading of Spondylolisthesis

GRADE	DEGREE OF SUBLUXATION OF VERTEBRAL BODY
1	Less than 25%
2	25%–50%
3	50%–75%
4	75% to complete subluxation

Another common thoracic/lumbar fracture is a transverse fracture through the vertebral body with extension through the posterior processes or the intervertebral disk. This injury used to be seen most commonly with a lap belt restraint (Chance fracture). Shoulder belts have decreased these types of injuries significantly to the point that falls from heights are now the most common type of insighting event.

Spondylolysis and spondylolisthesis are considered as a spectrum of injuries that are actually graded based on severity of subluxation. Spondylolysis is actually disruption of one or both pars interarticularis without dissociation or subluxation. This is usually noted by a defect and/or sclerosis of the pars on one or both sides. Spondylolisthesis is the resulting anterior subluxation of the upper vertebral body with respect to underlying level secondary to pars defect(s) disassociation(s). These abnormalities typically occur at the L4-5 or L5-S1 level (Table 70-1).

Within the cervical spine, involvement of the transverse process usually involves the transverse foramina and is associated with injury to the transiting vertebral artery. These injures commonly occur at C7, and studies have shown that less than 5% of vertebral arteries have entered the transverse foramina at C7, but rather the most common entry level is C6.

PELVIC TRAUMA

Traumatic pelvic fractures usually demonstrate a vertical pattern through the sacrum. Insufficiency sacral fractures are typically horizontal, accounting for the traditional Honda sign on bone scans. As for the most sensitive test for sacral fractures, most references state MRI is slightly more sensitive than conventional bone scan.

Approximately two-thirds of pelvic fractures are stable, that is they are single-break or avulsion-type fractures. One-third is complex and considered unstable.

Hip fractures are one of the most clinically common injuries encountered by radiologists, as they occur in both the young with severe trauma and the elderly with less severe injuries, such as ground-level falls. Hip fractures can be divided into three components based on anatomy: fractures of the acetabula, the femoral neck, and the femoral shaft. The majority of acetabular fractures can be divided based on which surface is involved—the column, the wall, or a transverse fracture involving both column and wall.

Briefly, the posterior column extends from the obturator foramen through the posterior aspect of the weight-bearing acetabular dome and then obliquely through the greater sciatic notch. Posterior column fractures account for 50% of acetabular fractures and usually occur with a force directed parallel to a flexed femoral shaft. The force is transmitted from the femur onto the posterior acetabular wall, which typically results in either a fracture through the posterior acetabular wall with subluxation or dislocation of the femoral head. If more than 40% of the posterior acetabular wall is involved, the injury is considered unstable and will require surgical fixation. A third injury with more devastating consequences is a posterior acetabular wall fracture with femoral dislocation accompanied by a femoral neck fracture (aka the Bo Jackson). On an AP pelvic radiograph, the ilioischial line is used to evaluate the posterior column for injury. Other associated injuries include sciatic nerve trauma, bladder injury, internal iliac artery injury, and posterior collateral ligament (PCL) tears. Posterior hip dislocations account for 85% to 90% of hip dislocations and patients typically present with the affected lower extremity in internal rotation. Approximately 15% of these injuries result in avascular necrosis.

Anatomically, the anterior column extends from the symphysis pubis and obturator foramen through the iliac crest. The iliopectineal line on an AP pelvic radiograph provides the best evaluation of the anterior column and many fractures involving only the anterior column are associated with anterior hip dislocations. Anterior hip dislocations account for 10% to 15% of traumatic hip dislocations and typically present with an externally rotated lower extremity and only approximately 4% develop avascular necrosis.

The remaining acetabular fractures result from a common mechanism: lateral impaction of the femoral head into the acetabulum. This force results in either a two-column (involving both the anterior and posterior columns) or a T-type fracture. The T-type fracture is a transverse two-column fracture with a third fracture line extending inferiorly into the obturator foramen (and often through the inferior pubic rami). Generally speaking, the T-type injury has a higher prevalence of poor clinical results including nerve injury, osteoarthrosis development, and avascular necrosis.

FEMUR FRACTURES

Femoral fractures can be divided into those involving the femoral head, femoral neck, intertrochanteric region, the femoral shaft, and the femoral condyles. Simple fractures of the femoral head are extremely rare and usually only result from direct-impact trauma like a gunshot wound or some other type of penetrating injury. The other option for a femoral head fracture is slipped capital femoral epiphysis, which is simply an atraumatic fracture through the hypertrophic zone of the physeal plate. These fractures are classic Salter Harris type I injuries and are seen bilaterally in 20% of those affected. This injury is associated with rickets, renal osteodystrophy, growth hormone therapy, and obesity. Absence of the line of Klein to intersect the femoral head is diagnostic. Avascular necrosis increases with severity of displacement and attempted reduction.

Femoral neck fractures are a common injury among the elderly and often occur as a result of a fall or less likely as a pathologic fracture. A general trend in femoral neck fractures is the more proximal the occurrence and the more severe the displacement, the higher the chance of developing avascular necrosis. Subcapital, transcervical, and basicervical fractures are similar in mechanism. They all are intracapsular and despite the capsule being sometimes disrupted with more severe fractures, the joint compartment actually can contribute to the increased prevalence of avascular necrosis. Fracture-associated hemorrhage often fills the capsule resulting in increased intracapsular pressure and collapse of the draining venous channels, which in effect can lead to a venous infarct and the development of avascular necrosis. Femoral neck fractures are graded based on the Gardner classification, which has four stages ranging from stage I, incomplete fracture, to stage IV, grossly displaced fracture.

Fractures involving the trochanters are not common, to the point that fractures of the lesser trochanter in an adult is considered pathologic (secondary to a metastasis or primary bone tumor) until proven otherwise. In children, however, a simple avulsion of the lesser trochanter is more common than a pathologic fracture at this same location.

Intertrochanteric fractures typical occur in older individuals and are classified based on the number of fracture fragments. The main fracture line typical runs from the greater to the lesser trochanter, and avascular necrosis and nonunion are uncommon complications.

KNEE INJURIES

Femoral condyle fractures are rare, typically occurring as either direct trauma or as a result of repetitive microtrauma, which causes a subchondral insufficiency fracture. This subchondral insufficiency fracture is usually located in the medial femoral condyle and classically seen in older women with new onset of knee pain. These injuries often progress to spontaneous osteonecrosis of the knee (SONK) and are associated with a medial meniscus tear approximately 75% of the time. Rapid subcondylar collapse of the medial anterior weight-bearing femoral condyle is diagnostic.

Patellar fractures are often comminuted and the result of direct impaction. Transverse fractures through the patella are the most common (60%) and often result in distraction of the two fragments by the contracting quadriceps muscle group. The distraction distance varies based on the degree to which the medial and lateral patellar retinacula are disrupted. A single oblique lucency through the upper lateral patella is commonly mistaken for a fracture, but is almost exclusively a bipartite patella. Patellar dislocations are almost exclusively in the lateral direction and associated with tears of the weaker medial retinaculum. A bone bruise within the lateral femoral condyle and a patellar fracture are often seen from impaction of the dislocating patella.

Actual femoral-tibial knee dislocations are rare and can occur in any direction. Because of the immediate proximity of the popliteal artery and tibial nerve, these injuries often have devastating vascular and neurologic consequences, and if not treated promptly can result in limb loss or death because of hemorrhage. The popliteal artery is injured in approximately 30% of cases.

An avulsion fracture involving the anterior lateral proximal tibia slightly below the articular surface is called a Segond fracture. The significance of this injury is its association with tears of the anterior cruciate ligament (ACL, 75%–100%) and either or both menisci (66%–75%).

MENISCUS ABNORMALITIES

The four types of meniscal tears commonly described include vertical, horizontal, radial, and bucket handle tear. The bucket handle tear is more of an extensive/severe configuration of a typical vertical tear. Tears typically appear as linear-increased signal within the meniscus. Degenerative changes within the meniscus cannot be seen on arthroscopy and are not thought to be symptomatic.

LIGAMENT INJURIES

The ACL along with the medial and fibular collateral ligaments are the dominant stabilizers of the knee. The fourth major ligament of the knee, the PCL, was typically not repaired in the past if torn; however, recent data suggest that repair/reconstruction may be preferential. The PCL prevents posterior subluxation/dislocation.

The ACL is the most commonly injured knee ligament often occurring with valgus and anterolateral rotary subluxation. The ACL is the primary stabilizer opposite the PCL, preventing anterior subluxation of the tibia on the femoral condyles. On physical examination, an ACL tear is diagnosed by the "anterior drawer sign,"–induced tibial anterior subluxation. MRI findings of an ACL tear include swelling/effusion, increased signal within the ACL on sagittal imaging, fiber disruption, and a change in ACL course. These findings have 90% specificity for ACL tear. Other ACL injury–associated findings include hemarthrosis, "kissing contusions" on the anterior lateral aspect of the lateral femoral condyle, and the posterior lateral tibial plateau.

The medial collateral ligament (MCL) is a common accompanier of ACL and medial meniscal injuries (the terrible triad seen commonly in football players). More specifically, an injury to the MCL occurs from a valgus stress often initiated from a lateral blow to the knee. Proximal disruption can result in avulsion of the MCL origin from the medial femoral condyle. Often following a remote MCL injury, posttraumatic ossification develops surrounding the ligament and is known as Pellegrini-Stieda disease.

FORELEG AND ANKLE INJURIES

Blunt trauma to the proximal lateral foreleg, over the fibular head, has the ability to result in traumatic injury to the common fibular (peroneal) nerve, which innervates the extensor muscles of the foreleg, potentially resulting in "foot drop." Fractures through the proximal fibula can result from two sources: direct blunt trauma and extension of a syndesmotic injury within the distal foreleg exiting through the proximal fibula called a Maisonneuve fracture. Distally this injury can be extremely subtle, most commonly appearing as minimal widening of the ankle mortise. Fractures of the proximal tibia include those from direct blunt trauma and injuries, such as the Segond fracture and avulsion fractures/injuries.

Tendon ruptures and muscle tears most commonly involve the gastrocnemius within either the medial head or the calcaneal (Achilles) tendon. Both injuries are commonly seen in weekend warriors who feel something pop in the back of the foreleg during activity. Achilles tendon injuries typically occur 2 to 6 cm proximal to the calcaneal insertion and result in an inability to plantar flex the foot. The injury to the medial gastrocnemius is often called tennis leg and results in a sharp burning pain in the posterior foreleg. This injury was originally believed to be due to a tear of the plantaris tendon, but has now been correctly identified as an injury to the medial head of the gastrocnemius.

A severe ankle fracture, the plafond fracture consists of a comminuted combined fracture of the ankle and distal tibial metaphysis. It usually has intraarticular extension and is complex approximately 25% of the time. Fractures

TABLE 70-2 Weber Classification of Ankle Fractures

A	Most stable supination, horizontal avulsion fracture below ankle mortise; associated medial malleolar fracture
B	Spiral/oblique fracture at mortise; associated medial malleolar fracture
C	Pronation with extrenal rotation; fibula above mortise; disrupts tibiafibular syndesmosis

of the medial malleolus and the distal anterior and posterior articulating tibial margins are often seen. The fibula can remain intact as much as 25% of the time. The mechanism is one of axial loading, and this injury is often associated with a compression fracture of the lumbar spine (most commonly L1).

Ankle fractures typically involve the medial (tibial) or lateral (fibular) malleolus. Injuries involving the fibular malleolus are graded based on their level and stability (Table 70-2).

Ankle sprains are overwhelmingly inversion injuries that put three ligaments at risk. The first ligament to tear is the anterior talofibular ligament. The second ligament to tear is the calcaneofibular ligament, and rarely the posterior talofibular ligament will be torn.

FOOT INJURIES

Seventy-five percent of talus fractures occur through the neck or body, and because of the tenuous blood supply there is an increased risk of avascular necrosis following fracture.

Fractures of the calcaneus are classified based on the Rowe classification system with type V (a comminuted intraarticular fracture) being the most common. These fractures usually occur from a fall from height (lover's leap fracture) and result in a decreased Boehler angle (normally between 28 and 48 degrees.) Seventy-five percent of calcaneal fractures are intraarticular.

Fractures of the navicular usually occur in the sagittal plane at the junction of the middle and lateral thirds, and an increased risk of avascular necrosis is seen in the lateral fragment of such fractures. Other injuries include stress fractures in runners.

Lisfranc fracture/dislocation results from a rupture of the tarsal-metatarsal ligament complex resulting in lateral subluxation of all the metatarsals (homolateral subluxation) or of the second through fifth metatarsals (divergent subluxation). The mechanism is a result of axial loading on a plantar-flexed foot or the result of a neuropathic (Charcot) joint associated with diabetes.

Jones fracture is a transverse fracture through the base of the fifth metatarsal 1.5 to 2.0 cm distal to the tuberosity. The distance is significant in differentiating this injury from a similar-appearing injury involving an avulsion of the proximal pole of the fifth metatarsal insertion of the peroneus brevis.

Stress fractures are most commonly seen in the foot, more specifically within the second or third metatarsals, often seen in marching military recruits. Turf toe is an injury resulting in a tear of the first metatarsal phalangeal joint capsule (plantar plate) allowing subluxation and possible dislocation of the joint.

The tibialis posterior muscle function is to maintain inversion of the subtalar joint. When there is paralysis or disruption of the posterior tibialis, the arch flattens and the foot moves into a valgus position as a result of the unopposed peroneus brevis action. Disruption of the posterior tibialis tendon most commonly occurs as the tendon traverses behind the medial malleolus and navicular tuberosity (hypovascular zone of the tendon). Rupture is classically described as acute discomfort and swelling overlying the posteromedial ankle in a middle-aged woman who develops a fallen arch.

UPPER EXTREMITY

SHOULDER

The shoulder is the most dynamic and unstable joint in the body, which also places this joint at risk of several injuries. The most dramatic injury is dislocation, of which 95% are in the anterior direction (the humeral head moves anterior and slightly inferior to the glenoid). Associated injuries include an impaction fracture on the posterior lateral aspect of the humeral head from contact with the inferior glenoid. This injury is called a Hill-Sachs lesion and it typically appears as a wedge-shaped defect. The counterpart to this lesion is a fracture from the anterior inferior rim of the glenoid. This lesion is called the Bankart deformity. Posterior dislocations make up the remaining significant dislocation injuries and are often associated with shock therapy or seizure episodes. The posterior rim of the glenoid is often fractured and displaced with posterior dislocations. Once posteriorly dislocated, the humerus is locked in internal rotation as the subscapularis turns the humeral shaft, unless the lesser tubercle is avulsed by the subscapularis that can occur. The subscapularis inserts on the lesser tubercle, but continues to the greater tubercle as the transverse ligament whose purpose is to contain the long head of the biceps tendon within the intertubercle groove. If the long tendon of the biceps is displaced from this location, the transverse ligament is disrupted and the subscapularis tendon is often torn. Posterior dislocations also put the innervating axillary nerve of the deltoid muscle at risk of injury as it traverses the quadrangular space.

Fractures of the clavicle typically occur through the middle third of the shaft. Fragments are typically displaced by contraction of the sternocleidomastoid, which elevates the proximal clavicular fragment. The distal fragment is typically depressed by the weight of the arm and shoulder. Clavicular articulations are at risk of dislocation with the acromioclavicular joint dislocation occurring more commonly, as this is a focus to release stress with shoulder injuries. The acromioclavicular (AC) joint is a synovial joint tightly vested with connective tissue including the AC ligament and coracoclavicular ligament complex. The weaker AC joint complex is typically disrupted first followed by the coracoclavicular complex with more severe injury. Injuries to the AC joint are graded based on the degree of disruption of the AC joint. Trauma to the distal clavicle has a propensity to develop osteolysis of the distal clavicle.

Labral tears typical occur along the superior margin and track from anterior to posterior, hence the mnemonic SLAP (superior labral tear from anterior to posterior). These lesions typically occur from overhand throwing, such as in baseball pitchers, and are seen in the majority of the elderly population. These lesions often have associated injuries to the biceps tendon as well.

Injuries to the scapula usually indicate direct high-impact blunt trauma with fractures occurring most commonly in the body, neck, glenoid, and acromion. Scapular fractures are often associated with pulmonary contusion, pneumothorax, clavicular fracture (which results in a free-floating shoulder), shoulder dislocation, and because of the proximity to the axillary artery and brachial plexus, arterial and nerve injuries.

Os acromiale is failure of complete ossification of the scapular acromion and is considered a normal variant. This is important as it can be confused with a fracture through the acromion.

HUMERUS

Fractures of the proximal humerus are injuries typically seen in elderly individuals and in those with high-impact trauma. The Neer system is used to grade these injuries based on the number of fracture fragments displaced or angulated from normal anatomic position. Fragments of significance include greater tuberosity, lesser tuberosity, anatomic neck, and surgical neck. Simple surgical neck fractures are the most common proximal humeral fracture in adults and are often associated with osteoporosis. The prognosis is good as the blood supply to the humeral head is usually intact. Anatomic humeral neck fractures are rare and often associated with a poorer outcome as the blood supply to the humeral head is often disrupted. The radial nerve is commonly injured with humeral fractures and shoulder dislocations.

Fractures through the distal half of the humerus are rare, excluding direct blunt trauma. In children, supracondylar fractures of the humerus are the most common cause of a posterior fat pad sign; in adults, it is a fracture of the radial head.

ELBOW

Radial head fractures are the most common elbow fracture in adults. These fractures are often subtle, but rarely comminuted, and require dedicated imaging to adequately define them. Subtle associated signs include a displaced anterior fat pad and more specifically, a displaced posterior fat pad. The mechanism of injury in most radial head and neck fractures is a fall on an outstretched hand, which drives the radial head into the capitellum resulting in fracture. Injuries associated with a radial head fracture include capitellum fracture, distal radial fracture, triceps tendon rupture, and radial head dislocation. Radial neck fractures are more common in children, and are usually Salter Harris type II fractures in approximately 90% of cases. Radial head and neck fractures have a propensity to develop nonunion and/or avascular necrosis because of a very mobile joint. Operative intervention occurs in more severe fractures and often results on a higher incidence of nonunion or avascular necrosis. In adults with closed physes, a radial head osteotomy is commonly performed. However, in children, this type of procedure can have disastrous consequences.

Supracondylar fractures are the most common pediatric elbow injury. Medial and lateral epicondylar fractures are also seen in pediatric populations. Lateral epicondylar fractures are the second most common elbow fracture in children (20% of pediatric elbow fractures) and result from a fall on an outstretched hand with the forearm abducted and the elbow extended. This injury is unstable and prone to nonunion as the fracture is intraarticular. Medial epicondylar fractures are the third most common pediatric elbow fracture. These injuries are usually extraarticular and usually associated with elbow dislocation. Commonly associated complications include ulnar nerve palsy, avascular necrosis, and nonunion—although this is less common in medial epicondylar fractures than in lateral epicondylar fractures.

RADIUS AND ULNA

As mentioned earlier in the chapter, radial head fractures are the most common adult elbow fracture accounting for one-half of all elbow fractures in adults. What is less common is a combined fracture of the radius with a dislocation of the adjacent ulna (Galeazzi fracture). Classically this is a radial shaft fracture near the junction between the proximal and middle third along with dislocation of the distal radioulnar joint. The fracture almost invariably occurs slightly above the pronator quadratus. A fracture of the ulnar styloid can be associated. The mechanism is a direct blow or fall on an outstretched hand. The most common distal radial fracture is the result of forced dorsiflexion of wrist, classically seen in a woman older than 50 years falling on an outstretched hand, where the dorsal surface undergoes compression and the volar surface undergoes tension, which results in a fracture with dorsal angulation of the distal radius (Colles fracture). These injuries can have intraarticular extension, scapholunate dissociation, and a triangular fibrocartilage tear resulting in increased carpal osteoarthrosis. Smith's fracture is the reverse of Colles fracture, in that the distal radial articulation is angled volar as apposed to dorsal.

A fracture of the radial styloid is known as Chauffeur fracture. It is usually an avulsion fracture and is frequently accompanied by scapholunate dissociation or perilunate dislocation.

There are four main types of ulnar fractures: those involving the coronoid, those involving the midshaft of the ulna, those involving the ulnar styloid, and those associated with radial dislocation (Monteggia fractures). The coronoid is the curved portion of the ulna that articulates with the trochlea of the humerus and it helps to resist posterior subluxation at the elbow joint. Coronoid fractures can vary from a small impaction fracture of the coronoid tip occurring with elbow dislocation, which is usually stable, to a comminuted fracture through the base of the coronoid, which is unstable. The majority is associated with elbow subluxation or dislocation and possible injuries to the anterior band of the ulnar collateral ligament and anterior joint capsule.

Nightstick fractures are blunt-trauma injuries occurring within the ulnar shaft. If they are displaced by greater than 50%, by more than 10 to 15 degrees of angulation, or associated with disruption of the interosseous membrane, they are considered unstable.

The third type of ulnar fracture is the ulnar styloid fracture. This fracture is often associated with other wrist fractures such as Colles, Smith, or Barton or can occur alone. The mechanism is either avulsion or compression.

The last ulnar fracture type is a combined ulnar fracture with radial head dislocation. The mechanism can be similar to that of a nightstick fracture or may result from a hyperpronation or hyperextension injury. The injury was originally described as a fracture through the proximal third of the ulna associated with anterior radial head dislocation. Associated comorbidities include posterior interosseous nerve or radial nerve injury, nonunion, radial-humeral ankylosis, and recurrent radial head dislocation.

WRIST AND HAND

Carpal bone fractures are uncommon, but can have devastating consequences if untreated, including avascular necrosis and extensive osteoarthrosis. The most common carpal bone fractured is the scaphoid, representing approximately 60% to 70% of all carpal bone fractures. Seventy percent of scaphoid fractures occur at the waist and are nondisplaced. Because the scaphoid receives its blood supply in a distal-to-proximal fashion, a fracture involving the proximal pole or waist has an increased risk of vascular disruption resulting in delayed union/nonunion and avascular necrosis. The actual statistics are fairly good in that 90% of scaphoid fractures unite, but some may take up to 2 years to do so. Scaphoid fractures occur by a common mechanism of falling on an outstretched hand.

The second most common carpal bone fracture involves a dorsal avulsion fracture from the triquetrum and usually only seen on lateral views. Lunate fractures are rare, but devastating because of the propensity to develop Kienbock disease, which is lunatomalacia secondary to vascular compromise and avascular necrosis. There is an association between Kienbock and repetitive lunate trauma, which is most commonly seen with negative ulnar variance, which results in increased stress on the lunate. Disruption of the scapholunate ligament complex can result in scapholunate dissociation. The normal distance between the scaphoid and lunate is 2 mm or less. If this distance is widened to 4 mm or more, the diagnosis of scapholunate dissociation can be made. This disruption and displacement can be accentuated by clenching the fist, which will cause the capitate to migrate proximally into the scapholunate interval. This instability results in arthrosis of the lunate capitate space along with narrowing and arthrosis of the radioscaphoid space known as scapholunate advanced collapse wrist. Its appearance is identical to changes seen with pseudogout (CPPD).

A lunate dislocation is more severe than a perilunate dislocation, which is more severe than scapholunate dislocation. Fracture dislocations are more common than simple dislocations and are often less stable.

The most common fracture of the hand is a fracture through the distal little or (less commonly) ring finger metacarpal from an axial load along the metacarpal shaft. The common name for this injury is a boxer fracture because a close-fisted blow is the usual mechanism of injury. The distal fracture fragment is often angulated in a palmar. If left untreated, this may result in limited range of motion.

A mallet fracture is a fracture through the dorsal base of the distal phalanx caused by an avulsion of the common extensor tendon, which occurs from flexion on a forcibly extended finger—often seen in young baseball pitchers. Open surgical repair is required if the fracture displaces more than 40% of the articular surface.

A Boutonniere deformity (buttonhole deformity) occurs when the middle slip of the extensor tendon is disrupted at the proximal interphalangeal joint, which causes flexion of the proximal interphalangeal joint and hyperextension of the distal interphalangeal joint. Surgical correction is required.

There are three main types of thumb injuries. The best-known thumb injury is the gamekeeper's thumb (aka skier's thumb) and it represents an avulsion of the thumb metacarpal phalangeal joint ulnar collateral ligament. This ligament almost always pulls away from the proximal thumb phalanx and results from valgus stress across the thumb.

Bennett fracture is the most common type of thumb fracture. The mechanism is axial loading on a partially flexed first metacarpal, often associated with a fistfight. This results in a fracture dislocation often with an oblique intraarticular fracture of the base of the thumb metacarpal and is unstable. If the intraarticular fracture through the thumb metacarpal is comminuted with dorsal subluxation, this fracture is known as Rolando fracture.

Suggested Reading

Bencardino JT, et al. Traumatic musculotendinous injuries of the knee: diagnosis with MR imaging. *Radiographics.* 2002;20:S103-S120.

el-Khoury GY, et al. Imaging of acute injuries of the cervical spine: value of plain radiography, CT, and MR imaging. *Am J Roentgenol.* 1995;164:43-50.

Hall FM. Radiographs in cervical spine trauma. *Am J Roentgenol.* 1978;131:555-556.

Lee P, et al. Musculoskeletal colloquialisms: how did we come up with these names? *Radiographics.* 2004;24:1009-1027.

Potok PS, et al. Fractures of the acetabulum: imaging, classification, and understanding. *Radiographics.* 1995;15:7-23.

QUESTIONS AND ANSWERS

1. On shoulder arthrography, contrast in which of the following locations is considered diagnostic of a complete rotator cuff tear?
   A. Along the biceps tendon within the tendon sheath
   B. Within the subacromion bursa
   C. Within the subdeltoid bursa
   D. Overlying the subscapularis
   E. Both B and C

   ANSWER: E. The subacromial and subdeltoid bursae are thought to usually communicate, and hence contrast is often seen occupying both spaces. Contrast in this space is never normal and usually represents a complete (full-thickness) tear of the rotator cuff. Contrast surrounding the biceps tendon is considered a normal variant as long as it is confined to the tendon sheath.

2. Which of the following types of acetabular fracture affects both the ilioischial and iliopectaneal lines?
   A. Transverse
   B. Posterior column
   C. Anterior column
   D. Posterior wall
   E. Anterior wall

   ANSWER: A. The iliopectaneal line on an AP pelvis is considered representative of the anterior column. The ilioischial line is considered representative of the posterior column. A transverse fracture involves both the posterior and anterior columns and hence results in disruption of both the ilioischial and iliopectaneal lines.

3. Which of the following is *not* associated with Segond fracture?
   A. ACL injury
   B. Lateral capsular ligament injury
   C. Meniscal tear
   D. Lateral collateral ligament tear

   ANSWER: D. Segond fracture is an avulsion fracture of the lateral tibial plateau below the articular surface. The mechanism of injury is internal rotation and varus stress, which causes abnormal tension on the central portion of the lateral capsular ligament resulting in avulsion of this attachement. Segond fractures are accompanied by other injuries including: ACL tears (75%–100%), medial or lateral menisci injuries (66%–75%), avulsion fracture of the fibular head, and avulsion fracture of Gerdy tubercle.

4. In an inversion ankle sprain, which of the following ligaments is most likely injured?
   A. Calcaneofibular ligament
   B. Anterior talofibular ligament
   C. Posterior talofibular ligament
   D. Deltoid ligament

   ANSWER: B. With inversion ankle sprains, the lateral ankle ligaments tear in a sequencial order from front to back depending on the severity of the inversion. The first and most commonly torn ligament is the anterior talofibular ligament followed next by the calcaneofibular ligament and finally (rarely) by the posterior talofibular ligament.

5. Which of the following shoulder tendons is disrupted with a dislocation of the long head of the biceps tendon?
   A. Subscapularis
   B. Infraspinatus
   C. Teres minor
   D. Deltoid
   E. Supraspinatus

   ANSWER: A. The tendon of the long head of the biceps runs within the intertubercular groove between the greater and lesser tubercles. The greater tubercle is the insertion of three of the four muscles of the rotator cuff, including the teres minor, supraspinatus, and infraspinatus. The lesser tubercle is the insertion of the fourth rotator cuff muscle, the supscapularis. Fibers of this insertion continue across the intertubercular groove as the transverse ligament whose fuction is to contain the long head of the biceps within the intertubercular groove. Hence if the long head of the biceps is dislocated (almost always anterior), the transverse ligament is disrupted.

6. Which of the following MR findings is *not* associated with a tear of the meniscus?
   A. Linear high signal extending to the articular surface
   B. Posterior horn appearing smaller than the anterior horn
   C. Appearance of a single "bowtie" on sagittal sequences
   D. Globular high signal within the meniscal body without extention to the articular surface

   ANSWER: D. Globular high signal within the meniscal body without extention to the articular surface can represent one of two normal variants. In the young, this can represent increased vascularity, which is often present into the early twenties, or in older individuals may represent myxoid degeneration, which some believe may put individuals at an increased risk for future tears, but does not currently represent a meniscal tear. The other descriptors listed including a linear focus of high signal extending to the articular surface, blunting of the posterior horn of the meniscus with respect to the anterior horn, and seeing less than two sequential "bowties" on sagittal sequences are all indicative of meniscal tears.

7. A patient has a bone bruise on the anterior aspect of the lateral femoral condyle acompanied by a fracture of the medial patella. This constellation of findings is most consistent with which of the following tears:
   A. Medial patellofemoral ligament
   B. MCL
   C. ACL
   D. PCL

   ANSWER: A. With a dislocation of the patella (usually laterally), associated injuries include a disruption of the medial patellar retinaculum, disruption of the medial patellofemoral ligament, and often a bone contusion on the lateral femoral condyle from the displaced patella striking the adjacent surface. A osteochondral fracture of the medial facet is also often seen.

8. A middle-aged man felt a pop followed by acute sharp pain behind his knee while playing basketball. Which of the following structures is injured?
   A. Medial head of the gastrocnemius
   B. PCL
   C. MCL
   D. Semimembranosis

   ANSWER: A. Tennis leg is characterized by the sudden onset of calf pain, often related to an injury incurred because of extension of the knee and forced dorsiflexion of the ankle, as the case would be with an acute change in direction on a tennis or basketball court. Tennis leg is characterized by an injury to one of two structures, the medial head of the gastrocnemius and the plantaris tendon. Rupture of the plantaris tendon at the medial aspect of the calf and rupture of the medial head of gastrocnemius muscle at the musculotendinous junction without concomitant injury to the plantaris tendon have been implicated in the pathogenesis of this condition and are difficult to differentiate on physical examination. MR will show a fluid collection between the aponeuroses of the medial head of the gastrocnemius and the soleus with or without rupture of the medial gastrocnemius muscle.

9. Following reduction of a posterior elbow dislocation in an adult, which of the following is the most common origin of a trapped intraarticular fracture fragment?
   A. Radial head
   B. Medial epicondyle
   C. Lateral epicondyle
   D. Olecranon
   E. Coronoid process

   ANSWER: E. Eighty to ninety percent of elbow dislocations are posterior. In adults, intraarticular fracture fragments most often originate from the coronoid process, which is often avulsed off the proximal ulna as the humerus moves anterior with respect to the ulna and radius. In children, the medial epicondylar ossifcation center can avulse and displace into the joint space.

10. What repetitive motion is most often associated with SLAP (superior labrum anterior to posterior) tears?
    A. Rowing
    B. Bench press
    C. Swinging a bat or golf club
    D. Overhead throwing

    ANSWER: D. SLAP tears involve the superior aspect of the glenoid labrum near the origin of the long head of the biceps tendon. These injuries are very common in "throwing atheletes," but are most common in individuals who have fallen or received a blow to the shoulder.

71 INFECTION

James S. Spann Jr. and Robert Lopez-Ben

INTRODUCTION

Infectious processes occurring in the musculoskeletal system can be medical emergencies and important causes of morbidity, and less commonly mortality in the postantibiotic era. Infection can involve bones, soft tissues, and joints. There are often several etiologies and pathogens. Some findings associated with infection can be protean and others more specific. The following discussion highlights the more common infectious processes of the musculoskeletal system and examines the more rare types of infectious processes with brevity.

Musculoskeletal infection occurs by three different routes of inoculation: hematogenous, contiguous spread, and direct implantation. It is important to consider these broad-category etiologies when discussing the various forms of infection involving the musculoskeletal system.

OSTEOMYELITIS

Osteomyelitis simply means inflammation of bone marrow. Although not commonly used, osteitis is a term indicating inflammatory involvement of cortical bone. The term osteomyelitis is essentially synonymous with an infectious process as the etiology.

A brief glossary of several terms regarding osteomyelitis is necessary.

- *Sequestrum* is a necrotic bone fragment separated from living bone by granulation tissue.
- *Involucrum* represents the thick periosteal reaction formed around the cortex of an infected tubular bone.
- *Cloaca* is an opening through the periosteum allowing pus from infected bone to communicate with the soft tissues.
- *Sinus tract* is a channel between infected bone and skin lined by granulation tissue. Sinus tract is different from a *fistula*, which represents a channel between two organs lined by granulation tissue.
- *Phlegmon* is a solid mass of inflammatory tissue, while *abscess* is a cavity lined by granulation tissue and filled with pus. An abscess can be drained if large enough but a phlegmon cannot be drained.

Osteomyelitis caused by hematogenous seeding leads to an immunological response. An organism hematogenously disseminated will initially seed the bone marrow with secondary extension into the cortex and soft tissues. In bone, the host response to the foreign organism leads initially to marrow edema and can progress onward if not treated to involve cortical bone destruction, cloaca formation, periosteal expansion, contiguous spread of infection into the soft tissues, abscess formation, sinus tract formation, bone infarction, and periosteal new bone formation. Abscess formation can be intraosseous within the marrow cavity, periosteal in location, or in the adjacent soft tissues.

Osteomyelitis is commonly divided into three categories: acute, subacute, and chronic. There are characteristic presentations in the infant, child, and the skeletally mature individual.

INFANT (AGE 0–1 YEARS)

In infants, osteomyelitis may be difficult to diagnose and remain clinically silent. Soft-tissue swelling may be the only initial sign. While infections caused by group B *Streptococcus* are more common in the neonate than at other ages, the most common infectious organisms for infants are *Staphylococcus aureus* and group A *Streptococcus*.

The pattern of infection in osteomyelitis can appear different because of variability in the vascular supply to long bones. In the infant, metaphyseal and diaphyseal vessels penetrate the physis, and hematogenously disseminated organisms will often deposit in the epiphyses and/or physis (growth plate). Periosteal elevation because of extracortical spread of infection followed by thick periosteal reaction (involucrum) is common. Periarticular spread is common and occurs with relative ease.

If infection continues to fester, subperiosteal abscess formation can readily occur because of the loose periosteum and subsequent elevation. In the long bones, the subperiosteal abscess can track along the shaft of the bone. Chronic osteomyelitis manifests often as bony sclerosis. In active chronic infection, there will be findings of bone loss, sequestra, and periosteal reaction. Sinus tracts and pathologic fracture are uncommon in the infant.

CHILD (1 YEAR CLOSURE OF PHYSIS)

In the child, vessels typically do not penetrate the physis, and infection will often deposit in the metaphysis because of slow flow in sinusoidal lakes in the metaphysis. Infection does not typically cross the growth plate to involve the joint until later in the course because of contiguous infection. Joint involvement can occur as well as sequestrum and involucrum formation. As in infants, subperiosteal abscess formation is common. A difference in this age group is that sinus tracts can occur.

Subacute osteomyelitis is exemplified by the Brodie abscess, which represents a walled-off fluid collection often with a sequestrum. The fluid in the Brodie abscess can be sterile. It is more common in male children and the metaphysis of the tibia and femur. The physis may be involved by progression of disease and if the lesion is intramedullary, channel-like lucencies may be encountered.

The chronic appearance of osteomyelitis may result in osteosclerosis or a mixed sclerotic and osteolytic appearance. Chronic active infection may manifest as areas of new bone destruction, sequestra, and involucrum. Pathologic fracture is uncommon in this age group. *Staphylococcus aureus* is by far the most common pathogen accounting for approximately 80% of infections. Group A *Streptococcus* is another common source of infection.

ADULT

After physeal closure in the skeletally mature individual, vessels from the diaphysis and metaphysis readily cross the physis, and hematogenous inoculation often results in localization of infection to the subchondral bone plate of the epiphysis. Joint involvement (septic arthritis) can subsequently occur because of contiguous spread. The most common source of infection in the adult is *S. aureus*.

Hematogenously disseminated osteomyelitis is less common in the adult than direct inoculation. When hematogenous dissemination occurs in the adult, it more commonly involves the small bones (hands and feet), pelvis, and spine, rather than the long tubular bones. Joint involvement and sinus tract formation are common. As opposed to children and infants, formation of involucrum, sequestra, and abscesses are less common. Pathologic fracture, although not common with adult osteomyelitis, can certainly occur in cases of neglect or chronic infection.

ACUTE OSTEOMYELITIS

Initially, bone radiographs are normal in the first week of osteomyelitis of hematogenous origin. The earliest radiographic manifestation of acute osteomyelitis may be deep soft-tissue swelling. This is followed by bone resorption after 1 to 2 weeks (osteoporosis/osteolysis), followed by periosteal reaction. A permeative or moth-eaten appearance because of bone destruction would be a later manifestation of acute osteomyelitis.

MR is excellent for the detection of osteomyelitis because of its high sensitivity but is relatively nonspecific with reported specificities ranging from 53% to 94%. MR has a very useful negative predictive value near 100%. This makes MR an excellent imaging modality, if there is clinical concern for osteomyelitis. Healed osteomyelitis in the adult can be diagnosed after return of normal high T1- and low T2-signal intensity in the marrow representing fatty marrow.

A three-phase bone scan is another excellent tool to evaluate for osteomyelitis if there is clinical suspicion for infection, and as in the case of MR, although sensitive, it lacks specificity. Bone scan imaging findings include increased radiotracer uptake on flow, blood pool, and delayed-phase imaging with technetium-labeled MDP. These findings are specific for osteomyelitis in the absence of recent fracture or surgical hardware/manipulation. The more chronic the infection, flow abnormality is less likely to be seen; however, blood pool and delayed-phase imaging would still probably be positive. More specific nuclear imaging examinations for infection like labeled WBC scans sometimes have decreased sensitivity, especially when infection is chronic.

SUBACUTE OSTEOMYELITIS (BRODIE ABSCESS)

A geographic osteolytic lesion with or without sclerosis and either intramedullary or intracortical in location is the hallmark of subacute osteomyelitis. If intramedullary, channel-like or serpiginous lucencies may be seen. The growth plate can be involved. Periosteal reaction and sequestra may be found. If epiphyses or epiphyseal equivalents are involved by a Brodie abscess, there can be confusion with chondroblastoma. Contrast-enhanced MRI can be useful in distinguishing between the two as the periphery of the lesion enhances in a

Brodie abscess, whereas there is heterogeneous enhancement of chondroblastoma.

CHRONIC OSTEOMYELITIS

Infections of more than 6 weeks duration can be labeled as chronic. Osteosclerosis caused by endosteal thickening, periosteal thickening, thickened intramedullary trabeculae, and cystic changes are common radiographic findings in chronic osteomyelitis. A sequestrum may be present. The most specific sign of active chronic osteomyelitis is a sequestrum, which is best imaged by CT. Other signs of active chronic infection at radiography would include ill-defined and new areas of osteolysis in addition to new areas of periosteal reaction. With CT and MR, findings of active chronic infection would include the presence of sequestrum, intramedullary abscess, cloaca formation, subperiosteal fluid collection, and sinus tract.

CONTIGUOUS SPREAD

When the soft tissues are the site for initial infection (cellulitis), infection that extends into bone is considered to be due to contiguous spread. This type of infection is more commonly seen in the debilitated and immunosuppressed patients, such as diabetic patients and those treated with steroids. The course of disease involves cellulitis followed by periostitis, then osteitis, and finally marrow extension indicating osteomyelitis. This "out to in" pattern of disease progression is opposite that of osteomyelitis because of hematogenous origin where the infection begins in the marrow and spreads in to out.

DIRECT IMPLANTATION

Direct implantation of infectious microorganisms can occur via multiple methods, such as iatrogenic during surgical procedures, open fractures, foreign bodies, or as the result of puncture wounds (dog/cat bites). Rose gardeners can inoculate *Sporothrix schenckii* with thorn punctures (much more prevalent in USMLE Step 1 examination questions than in reality). Human bites are polymicrobial sources of infectious organisms, while animal bites are commonly associated with *Pasteurella multocida*. Interestingly, approximately 5% of dog bites result in infection, whereas slightly less than half of cat bites may result in infection (another reason not to own a cat). Staphylococcal and streptococcal species are other common sources of infection because of animal bites, as many of these species are native skin flora.

The vast majority of cases of osteomyelitis are due to *S. aureus*. *Streptococcus*, *Haemophilus influenzae*, and gram-negative rods are other common pathogens. Several pathogens have increased prevalence in certain patient populations. For example, osteomyelitis secondary to salmonella is more common in patients with sickle cell compared with the background population. However, the overall incidence of *S. aureus* still accounts for the majority of osteomyelitis cases in patients with sickle cell. Pseudomonas is commonly associated with penetrating trauma and intravenous drug abuse. Fracture of the great toe distal phalanx with involvement of the physis is commonly associated with subsequent development of osteomyelitis.

SEPTIC ARTHRITIS

Etiologies for septic arthritis (joint infection) are hematogenous seeding, contiguous spread, or direct implantation of infectious organisms. Osteomyelitis with secondary involvement of the joint and iatrogenic implantation at the time of surgery represents examples of contiguous spread and direct implantation, respectively.

Monoarticular joint involvement represents the overwhelming majority of cases of septic arthritis (~80%). Monoarticular joint inflammation is infection until otherwise excluded. The organism responsible for septic arthritis beyond age 2 years is usually hematogenously seeded staphylococcal or streptococcal species. In the past, *H. influenzae* was one of the leading causes in children younger than 3 years; although it has become rarer in the United States after the implementation of vaccination in 1985. Septic arthritis is polyarticular in 20% of cases. The acromioclavicular, sternoclavicular, and sacroiliac (SI) joints and spine are common sites of infection in intravenous drug users. Atypical infectious etiologies such as tuberculosis and fungi may present more indolent with chronic joint space widening, although other inflammatory-related changes may be seen. The Phemister triad in TB arthritis includes juxtaarticular osteopenia, peripheral bone erosions, and gradual joint space narrowing.

Pathologically, there is a synovial inflammatory response to the hematogenously seeded organism as evidenced by hyperemia and joint fluid production. Inflammatory-related deposition of fibrin is thought to prohibit cartilage nutrition and WBC release–damaging enzymes such as collagenase. There is pannus formation causing further distention of the joint. Untreated, cartilage and bone destruction ensues.

Radiographically, a septic joint manifests as any inflammatory arthritis may appear: soft-tissue swelling, periarticular osteopenia, uniform joint space narrowing, and bone erosions. Joint space widening may be the initial finding that is due to joint effusion. In the infant or child hip, septic arthritis is a surgical emergency and the only sign may be a widened hip joint at radiography. An effusion may be seen with ultrasound. The complications of septic arthritis are related to the extent of involvement of the initial infection. Osteonecrosis, slipped epiphysis, growth disturbance, osteomyelitis, and secondary osteoarthritis may result from septic arthritis. Tendon and capsule injury in addition to synovial cyst formation may be found.

CELLULITIS AND OTHER SOFT-TISSUE INFECTIONS

CELLULITIS

Infections involving the soft tissues include cellulitis, septic bursitis, septic tenosynovitis, infectious myositis, and necrotizing fasciitis.

Cellulitis represents acute infection of the subcutaneous fat and dermis associated with pain, erythema, and edema. Cellulitis typically occurs after skin breakdown or a focus of injury allows skin flora or exogenous bacteria to infiltrate into the subcutaneous tissues. Those with peripheral vascular disease, diabetes mellitus, and immunosuppression are at particularly increased risk. Streptococcal and staphylococcal species are common organisms as is *H. influenzae*. The majority of cases of cellulitis are clinical diagnoses, with few cases requiring imaging limited to those who are at high risk of developing more complicated cellulitis, such as those who are immunosuppressed, diabetic and alcoholic patients. Imaging is utilized to assess for inflammatory changes and abscess formation. Uncomplicated cellulitis may mimic anasarca as in heart failure.

SEPTIC BURSITIS/TENOSYNOVITIS

Septic bursitis and septic tenosynovitis are usually the result of direct implantation of infectious organisms as can be seen in penetrating trauma. TB is an alternative consideration. The presence of infectious bursitis or tenosynovitis cannot be distinguished by imaging features from other inflammatory conditions.

PYOMYOSITIS

Infectious myositis (pyomyositis) is infection of muscle and is fortunately very rare, but is now more common in North America because of HIV. Penetrating trauma and hematogenous seeding in intravenous drug users and the immunocompromised patients account for the majority of cases. Although viruses, fungi, and parasites are sources of infection, bacteria represent the overwhelming majority of cases and most are due to *Staphylococcus* (~75%). Risk factors for development of pyomyositis include HIV/AIDS, strenuous activity, muscle trauma, and rhabdomyolysis. Other risk factors include contiguous spread of skin infections, direct implantation as in intravenous drug use and insect bites, and immunocompromised states like diabetes mellitus. Pyomyositis is more common in the quadriceps muscle, followed by gluteal and iliopsoas muscles, and less common in the upper extremities. Findings can be subtle, and a high degree of suspicion is required, especially in the immunocompromised.

There are three stages of pyomyositis: invasive phase, suppurative phase, and late stage. The invasive stage is characterized by muscle edema and pain while the suppurative phase represents further progression with fever and later abscess formation followed by the late stage indicating sepsis/toxicity, which is potentially life threatening. Findings may include multifocality in approximately 50% of cases, inflammatory muscle expansion, and inflammatory enlargement of intermuscular fascia. Air/gas in muscle tissue is always abnormal and can be due to gas-forming organisms.

Drainage of an abscess and appropriate antibiotic coverage usually leads to complete recovery, although scarring and dysfunction can occur. Untreated cases may evolve into a compartment syndrome or progress onward to septic arthritis and/or osteomyelitis, and if ultimately untreated can lead to death.

NECROTIZING FASCIITIS

Necrotizing fasciitis represents infection and necrosis involving the fascia. Typically, cellulitis (infection of subcutaneous tissues) can progress to involve the fascia where the infectious process can then become rapidly progressive and is associated with a high mortality rate (less than 70%). The incidence of necrotizing fasciitis, although rare, is increasing because of the increase in the numbers of immunocompromised patients, such as those with HIV, diabetes mellitus, cancer, transplants, and alcoholism. Necrotizing fasciitis is a surgical emergency as infection can rapidly spread along fascial planes. Surgical treatment of the necrotizing variety includes fasciotomy and debridement in addition to antibiotics.

Common locations include the perineum, extremities, neck, and face. If the scrotum or penis is involved, it is termed Fournier gangrene. Etiologies for Fournier gangrene include recent genitourinary manipulation, surgery, or trauma, and it is associated with immunocompromised states.

Imaging findings are generally more severe than cellulitis and include skin thickening, sometimes subcutaneous edema/gas, inflammatory fascial thickening, and potentially fluid collections. CT and MR can be used to distinguish cellulitis from necrotizing fasciitis. Lack of enhancement of fascia represents the necrotizing form. Nonnecrotizing fasciitis demonstrates enhancement of inflamed fascia. A sonographic hallmark of Fournier gangrene is subcutaneous gas.

INFECTION OF THE SPINE

Infection of the spine is usually because of hematogenous dissemination of infectious organisms, and the sequence of spine infection is different in adults and children. The adult pattern is characterized by hematogenous seeding of the marrow adjacent to the endplate of the vertebral body (osteomyelitis) followed by rapid spread to the adjacent vertebral disc. Infection spreads sequentially to the next vertebral body. Infection of disc is termed discitis, and when both the bone and the disc are infected it is termed spondylodiscitis. The childhood pattern is characterized by initial seeding of the disc because of the relatively high vascularity of the disc with spread into bone secondarily.

Given the importance of making a diagnosis quickly, MR is the modality of choice for imaging spine infection. At radiography, endplate destruction and loss of disc height may be seen. MR is aptly suited to demonstrate the bone marrow and disc involvement as well as complications related to paraspinal abscess formation and epidural abscess formation. At MR, acute osteomyelitis appears as bone marrow edema, so it is low on T1-weighted images, usually high on T2-weighted images, and will enhance on postcontrast T1 images. Involvement of the disc is usually characterized by high signal on T2-weighted images, and contrast enhancement is variable on postcontrast T1 images.

Paraspinal abscess formation appears as fluid collections typically do—low T1, high T2, and rim-enhancing mass/fluid collection on postcontrast T1 images. The majority of cases of epidural abscess are due to spondylodiscitis and contiguous spread of infection rather than seeding from another site. The earliest stage of contiguous spread may appear as a phlegmon that can progress to abscess.

MISCELLANEOUS AND RARE INFECTIONS

Foot infection is a common source of morbidity in those with diabetes and is usually the result of infection secondary to soft-tissue injury, followed by cellulitis, and can progress via contiguous spread to osteomyelitis. The presence of microvascular disease and neuropathy create the favorable environment for the development of diabetic foot infection. Pressure points, particularly the plantar surface of the first and fifth metatarsal heads, calcaneal tuberosity, distal toe phalanges, and medial and lateral malleoli, are common sites of infection. Joint effusion, soft-tissue edema, bone marrow edema, and periosteal reaction can be seen in both the neuropathic joint and the diabetic foot infection with osteomyelitis. Therefore, it is helpful to look for other features suggestive of infection such as cortical destruction, sequestrum, and intraosseous abscess in addition to the location to guide the diagnosis of diabetic foot infections. Neuroarthropathy/neuropathy always occurs at the joint, and discriminating features include destruction or fragmentation of bone, joint debris, and dislocation.

Patients with HIV/AIDS are immunosuppressed and are susceptible to common infectious organisms as well as atypical bacterial and fungal infections. As has been previously noted, immunosuppressed patients are at risk for osteomyelitis, septic arthritis, and infectious myositis. Patients with AIDS are susceptible to a rare systemic disease termed bacillary angiomatosis, which can result in osteomyelitis. The causative organisms have been isolated to two gram-negative bacteria, either *Bartonella henselae* or *Bartonella quintana*. This systemic disease results in disseminated nodules including subcutaneous nodules, and multiple osteolytic bone lesions can be seen involving the intramedullary cavity and/or cortex and possibly associated with a soft-tissue mass. Common sites of involvement are the long bones.

Chronic recurrent multifocal osteomyelitis is a form of chronic osteomyelitis, which usually affects children and adolescents, and is associated with SAPHO syndrome because of the common presentation with palmoplantar pustulosis (~40%), but is not necessary for the diagnosis. SAPHO syndrome is characterized by synovitis, acne, pustulosis, hyperostosis, and osteitis. Typical presentations of chronic recurrent multifocal osteomyelitis include symmetric involvement, mixed lytic and sclerotic appearance, and involvement of the metaphyses of the lower extremity and medial clavicle. Bone cultures are often sterile in this disease process, as no definite infectious organism can confidently be attributed to this process. Bone samples often demonstrate plasma cell predominance, and this entity has become known as a "plasma cell osteomyelitis." Chronic recurrent multifocal osteomyelitis is usually a diagnosis of exclusion.

Chronic granulomatous disease of childhood is another disease characterized by chronic osteomyelitis. Chronic granulomatous disease is a rare X-linked recessive disorder affecting neutrophils leading to susceptibility to catalase-positive organisms (*Staphylococcus*, Nocardia, TB).

TB of the musculoskeletal system is increasing in incidence because of the increasing immunocompromised patient population. One to three percent of patients with TB will have musculoskeletal system involvement. If the musculoskeletal system is involved, the majority of cases involve the spine with infection of the digits, joints, bursae, and tendon sheaths, all less common sites of involvement. TB spondylodiscitis is hematogenous in origin via Batson plexus, with L1 being the most frequent site of occurrence usually with more than one vertebral body level affected in a contiguous manner. The infection seeds the subchondral bone plate and is characterized by a slow process resulting in vertebral body destruction and later disc destruction. Paraspinal abscess is commonly associated with this process and the degree of abscess formation with relative sparing of the vertebral body and disc space in comparison with typical bacterial spondylodiscitis makes one think of TB as the etiology. Anterior endplate destruction, especially in the thoracic spine, results in the gibbus deformity.

TB osteomyelitis is rare but can affect any bone, usually at the epiphysis. TB is a less common cause of dactylitis and has a spike-like and puffed full-of-air appearance termed spina ventosa. If TB infects a joint, a monoarticular infection involving a large joint may be seen; it is a slow process/infection because of the lack of proteases. The cartilage is usually spared in TB arthritis, although over time granulation tissue leads to cartilaginous erosion. The Phemister triad appears as juxtaarticular osteopenia, slow joint space loss, and peripheral erosions. A nodular synovial thickening can be seen with joint effusion at MRI.

Leprosy represents the manifestation of infection because of *Mycobacterium leprae* and occurs in the United States (rarely), Africa, South America, and Asia. Infection occurs through the skin and mucous membranes, and there is a long incubation period between 3 and 6 years. Lepromatous leprosy is the more severe and generalized infection due in large part to higher quantities of bacilli, while tuberculoid leprosy has less bacilli, more reaction, and skin and nerve involvement. The dimorphous form features characteristics of both lepromatous and tuberculoid types. Indeterminate leprosy is another form of the disease. A specific sign related to leprosy is a lacelike osseous destructive process involving the phalanges (hands/feet) and nasal bone. Periosteal reaction and bone fragmentation as well as arthritis may be seen. An appearance termed "licked candy stick" has been associated with this disease process because of fracture, bone erosion, and bone remodeling.

Brucellosis is a rare infection that occurs in the United States caused by *Brucella* species, and can involve the spine and joints. Infection with *Brucella* species is rare in the United States because of pasteurization of milk products as most infections caused by this species occur between livestock/animals, such as cows, goats, and sheep. Infection occurs principally by ingesting contaminated milk or meat sources without adequate preparation. The musculoskeletal system is often the target because of the predilection for marrow involvement (reticuloendothelial system). A septic arthritis can occur with predilection for the knee and shoulder as well as SI joints. Most focal spinal infections that are due to brucellosis occur in the lumbar spine, particularly the L4 vertebral body. The focal form of infection results in a parrot beak osteophyte of the superior anterior endplate and also sclerotic endplate and disc gas. The diffuse form represents severe infection that can mimic osteoarthritis. It is a slow process that is usually characterized by vertebral body height preservation and less tendency to form a paravertebral abscess or epidural abscess. Disc gas can occur and is thought to represent the smoldering progression of the osteomyelitis.

Actinomycosis israelii is normal flora in the oral cavity and can also be introduced into other sites of the body because of trauma. Actinomyces infection is known to form sinus tracts and abscesses with common sites of involvement including the mandible, ribs, spine, and pelvis.

Fungal infections involving the musculoskeletal system can be seen in the immunocompromised host. Aspergillosis, blastomycosis, candidiasis, cryptococcosis, histoplasmosis, mucormycosis, and sporotrichosis represent the majority of the fungal infections affecting the musculoskeletal system. Fungal infection is characterized by large lytic and punched-out lesions, often multifocal, and with or without surrounding sclerosis. Blastomycosis is endemic in the Ohio River basin and infection can occur because of inhalation or skin entry from the soil. Coccidioidomycosis is infectious via inhalation, and the organism is endemic in the soil of southwestern parts of the United States and Mexico and can cause bone and joint involvement including a migratory arthritis. Cryptococcosis is another inhaled organism with rare features of musculoskeletal involvement.

Histoplasmosis is the most common fungal organism infection in the United States, is endemic throughout the soil, and infection is spread via inhalation. If musculoskeletal changes are seen, more common sites of involvement include the pelvis, skull, ribs, and small bones. Arthritis can occur with histoplasmosis infection.

Zygomycosis (mucormycosis) infections are encountered mainly in the immunocompromised, burn and uremic patients, and especially those with diabetes, potentially resulting in the feared complication of rhino-orbital-cerebral infection. Mucormycosis is probably the most familiar term but deadly human infection is not limited simply to the *Mucor* family. Other genera include

Rhizopus and *Cunninghamella*. Zygomycetes are a group of fungi that are spore forming and infection typically begins via inhalation with contamination of the nares and sinuses with subsequent tissue invasion. Hyperglycemia and ketoacidosis create the favorable environment for infection. A state of iron overload also fosters growth. Rhino-orbital-cerebral infection results when there is contiguous spread of infection from the sinuses to the soft tissues of the orbit and potentially the brain. It is an angioinvasive fungal infection that can rapidly spread leaving infarcted tissue behind characterized as black eschar. High morbidity/mortality is associated with the disease process.

Sporotrichosis is due to the saprophyte *S. schenckii* and inoculation can occur because of a skin wound (e.g., a rose's thorn) or via inhalation. Disseminated sporotrichosis is highly associated with musculoskeletal changes (~80%) including arthritis and osteomyelitis. The arthritis is typically monoarticular involving the knee or wrist, and osteomyelitis is usually secondary to the arthritis.

Parasitic infections are usually characterized by soft-tissue calcification or other soft-tissue involvement. For example, filariasis results in lymphatic obstruction and elephantiasis. Cysticercosis appears as a linear or oval rice grain of calcification parallel to the long axis of the muscle. Loa loa affects the soft tissues with lacelike subcutaneous soft-tissue calcifications. Echinococcal infection usually spares bone but a multiloculated cystic soft-tissue mass may be encountered.

Congenital infections, as in TORCH infections, typically result in metaphyseal lucent bands. Congenital syphilis manifests initially as osteochondritis (metaphyseal lucent bands) and/or osteomyelitis. Proliferative periosteal reaction is most common finding and at the tibia is known as "saber shin." Osteomyelitis is not common with congenital infection. If osteomyelitis occurs, nasal bone involvement can lead to a saddle nose deformity. The majority of cases are not discovered until beyond 10 years. The Hutchinson triad may be encountered characterized by Hutchinson teeth, interstitial keratitis, and sensorineural deafness. Later changes include osteomyelitis and osteitis as well as gumma formation because of caseous bone necrosis.

Lyme disease is the result of infection with *Borrelia burgdorferi* via a tick-borne vector (*Ixodes dammini*) and occurs in endemic areas in the United States (northeast). Skin lesions and joint symptoms are common sequelae. Joint involvement typically involves the knee, though no joint may necessarily be spared. Mono/oligo/polyarticular forms can occur. Soft-tissue swelling and effusion may be seen in MRI with a relative lack of subcutaneous edema. Chronic changes include erosions, joint space loss, and osteopenia.

SUGGESTED READING

Arkun R. Parasitic and fungal disease of bones and joints. *Semin Musculoskelet Radiol*. 2004;8(3):231-242.

Christian S, Kraas J, Conway WF. Musculoskeletal infections. *Semin Roentgenol*. 2007;42(2):92-101.

Frank G, Mahoney HM, Eppes SC. Musculoskeletal infections in children. *Pediatr Clin North Am*. 2005;52(4):1083-1106.

Offiah AC. Acute osteomyelitis, septic arthritis and discitis: differences between neonates and older children. *Eur J Radiol*. 2006;60(2):221-232.

Saigal G, Azouz EM, Abdenour G. Imaging of osteomyelitis with special reference to children. *Semin Musculoskelet Radiol*. 2004;8(3):255-265.

Struk DW, Munk PL, Lee MJ, Ho SG, Worsley DF. Imaging of soft tissue infections. *Radiol Clin North Am*. 2001;39(2):277-303.

QUESTIONS AND ANSWERS

1. Which of the following is the most common association with fracture of the great toe distal phalanx with physeal involvement?
   A. Septic arthritis
   B. Early degenerative change
   C. Growth arrest
   D. Osteomyelitis

   ANSWER: D. Occult open fractures can occur after stubbing the great toe because of the proximity of the nail to bone at this location. Although disruption of the growth plate from a fracture can lead to secondary growth arrest and articular incongruity, the best answer is direct implantation of infectious microorganisms leading to osteomyelitis in this location.

2. Which of the following is the most likely pathogen in a patient with sickle cell disease and osteomyelitis?
   A. *Salmonella* species
   B. *Streptococcus* species
   C. *Actinomyces* species
   D. *Staphylococcus aureus*

   ANSWER: D. Although infection with encapsulated organisms like salmonella is indeed much more common in patients with sickle cell disease when compared to other patients, the most common microbial etiology for osteomyelitis in this patient population remains *S. aureus*.

3. The presence of gas in which of the following spaces in the absence of trauma implies infection?
   A. Disc
   B. Intramuscular

C. SI joint space
D. Symphysis pubis

ANSWER: B. The vacuum phenomenon appears as a radiolucent area visible in synovial joints, intervertebral discs, and vertebrae. This phenomenon is explained by temporary gas accumulation, mostly nitrogen, related to the negative pressures that can be generated by distraction of the articular surfaces. So the remaining choices are incorrect. Intramuscular gas is not generated by vacuum and is usually due to percutaneous introduction (trauma) or gas-producing organisms.

4. Infection of which anatomic location is more prevalent in intravenous drug users when compared to the general population?
   A. Acromioclavicular, sternoclavicular, and SI joints, and spine
   B. Symphysis pubis, facet joints, and short bones of the hand and feet
   C. Sternomanubrial, humeroulnar, capitellotriquetral, and humeroglenoid joints
   D. Hip, knee, and shoulders

ANSWER: A. Although the knee is the most common joint involved by infection (greater than 50% in many series), intravenous drug users patients have a predilection for axial joint infection.

5. Which of the following is the hallmark sonographic feature of Fournier gangrene?
   A. Soft-tissue swelling
   B. Posterior acoustic enhancement
   C. Subcutaneous emphysema
   D. Engorgement of vessels of the pampiniform plexus

ANSWER: C. Ultrasound can help in the early diagnosis of Fournier gangrene by differentiating it from scrotal cellulitis. Soft-tissue swelling would not be specific as it is also identified in cellulitis. Identification of subcutaneous gas with discrete foci of posterior acoustic shadowing is diagnostic of Fournier gangrene.

6. All of the below are associated with an increased incidence of cellulitis, pyomyositis, and necrotizing fasciitis *except*
   A. HIV
   B. Diabetes mellitus
   C. Alcoholism
   D. Recent organ transplant
   E. Tobacco abuse

ANSWER: E. All other choices are all examples of immunocompromised hosts who are at higher risk for soft-tissue infections of the musculoskeleton. Although tobacco abuse can lead to COPD which when treated with chronic corticosteroid use may increase infection susceptibility, it has not been associated with soft-tissue infections in the nonimmunocompromised host.

7. Spondylodiscitis appears different in the child compared to the adult because
   A. Infection in the child usually begins at the vertebral endplate with direct extension into the disc space via contiguous spread of infection.
   B. Infection in the child usually begins at the disc space because of hematogenous seeding of the well-vascularized disc with subsequent contiguous spread to adjacent vertebral bodies.
   C. Paraspinal abscess formation is a prerequisite to vertebral body and disc infection in the child as opposed to the adult.
   D. Different pathogens are responsible for the infectious process in the child and the adult.

ANSWER: B. Infection of the spine is usually because of hematogenous dissemination of infectious organisms, with *S. aureus* being the most common pathogen for both child and adult. So, choice D is incorrect. The adult pattern is characterized by hematogenous seeding of the marrow adjacent to the endplate of the vertebral body followed by rapid spread to the adjacent vertebral disc. Choice A is thus incorrect for the child. The childhood pattern is characterized by initial seeding of the disc because of the relatively high vascularity of the disc with spread into bone secondarily. So, choice B is the best choice. Paraspinal abscesses are usually secondary to vertebral injection. So choice C is incorrect.

8. Chronic recurrent multifocal osteomyelitis is characterized by all of the following *except*
   A. Bone specimen demonstrates the majority of cells as plasma cells.
   B. More common in adolescents and children and is a diagnosis of exclusion.
   C. Almost always associated with SAPHO syndrome, a prerequisite for the diagnosis.
   D. Typical presentations include symmetric involvement, a mixed lytic and sclerotic appearance, and involvement of the metaphyses of the lower extremity and medial clavicle.

ANSWER: C. Chronic recurrent multifocal osteomyelitis usually affects children and adolescents. Bone samples often demonstrate a plasma cell predominance. Typical presentations include symmetric involvement, mixed lytic and sclerotic appearance, and involvement of the metaphyses of the lower extremity and medial clavicle. Although it can be associated with SAPHO syndrome due to the common presentation with palmoplantar pustulosis (~40%), this is not necessary for the diagnosis.

9. Why is septic arthritis/osteomyelitis in the hip of an infant or child a radiological emergency?
   A. Joint destruction rapidly occurs because of the presence of proteases including collagenase, which leads to cartilage loss and joint space destruction.
   B. Pyomyositis and/or cellulitis may occur if untreated.
   C. It is highly associated with left ventricular–infected thrombus and signals the possibility of septic emboli.
   D. Femoral head is likely to fracture in the first 24–48 hours of infection if the patient is not made non–weight bearing.

   ANSWER: A. Joint destruction can occur rapidly due to the release of proteases during the inflammatory response. Pyomyositis is typically not seen after septic arthritis. Although microbial hematogenous dissemination is a common pathway for septic arthritis, it is not highly associated with left ventricular thrombi. Pathologic fracture is a rare complication of bone infection in children.

10. The Phemister triad, which includes juxtaarticular osteopenia, slow joint space loss, and peripheral erosions, is seen with which of the following etiologies?
    A. TORCH infection
    B. Loa loa
    C. Tuberculosis
    D. *Staphylococcus aureus*

    ANSWER: C. The Phemister triad has been classically associated with mycobacterial infection. TORCH infections typically result in metaphyseal lucent bands. Loa loa is a parasitic infection usually of soft tissues and does not involve intraarticular structures. *Staphylococcus aureus* is a virulent organism associated with more rapid joint destruction.

11. Infection by a fungus from the *Zygomycetes* family, associated with the dreaded rhino-orbital-cerebral infection, occurs with which of the following:
    A. Ketoacidosis and/or hyperglycemia, and iron overload
    B. Hypoglycemia and copper deficiency
    C. Hemodynamically significant bilateral common carotid stenoses
    D. Hospital-acquired pneumonia

    ANSWER: A. Zygomycetes are a group of fungi that are spore forming, and infection typically begins via inhalation with contamination of the nares and sinuses with subsequent tissue invasion. Rhino-orbital-cerebral infection results when there is contiguous spread of infection from the sinuses to the soft tissues of the orbit and potentially the brain. Hyperglycemia and ketoacidosis create the favorable environment for infection. A state of iron overload also fosters growth.

72 BONE TUMORS AND TUMORLIKE CONDITIONS

Matthew C. Larrison and Gregory S. Elliott

INTRODUCTION

Differential diagnosis of bone tumors is best determined by conventional radiographs. MRI occasionally will aid in specificity but most often is useful for evaluating extent of disease, staging prior to treatment, and follow-up. The approach to bone tumors is based on evaluating several key factors which will help one to decide if a lesion is aggressive or nonaggressive in appearance and to help narrow the differential diagnosis. These key factors include type of matrix (cartilage, osteoid), zone of transition, presence or absence of soft-tissue mass, location in bone (cortical, medullary, juxtacortical; epiphyseal, metaphyseal, diaphyseal), and the bone involved. The age of the patient is also very important in narrowing the list of diagnostic possibilities.

OSTEOID LESIONS (Table 72-1)

GENERAL

Osteoid lesions demonstrate osseous internal content of varying degrees of maturity. The benign lesions usually contain mature bone elements while the more aggressive lesions contain less mature elements. The radiographic appearance of osteoid matrix is described as fluffy or cloudlike. As with all aggressive or malignant bone lesions, the well-defined lesion will typically have a more favorable biological behavior.

BONE ISLAND (ENOSTOSIS)

Bone islands are a typically incidental finding and are asymptomatic. They are intramedullary in location. The clinical importance of these lesions is the potential to be confused with sclerotic metastasis or low-grade intramedullary osteosarcoma. Radiographic findings include a densely sclerotic intramedullary lesion, round in shape often with spiculated margins with no or minimally increased activity on bone scan. A giant bone island is defined as greater than 2 to 3 cm in size and is most often found in the pelvis.

OSTEOMA

An osteoma is a benign tumor most often found in the cranium and sinuses. The presence of symptoms depends on size and location but can potentially cause headache or sinus disease. Exophytic lesions arise from the surface of bone/cortex. Osteomas can be associated with Gardner syndrome (Familial polyposis syndrome, also associated with desmoid tumors, and skin lesions). Radiographic findings include a well-defined sclerotic lesion arising from the surface of bone.

OSTEOID OSTEOMA

These lesions typically occur in young male patients (10–25 years of age). The classic history is that of night pain relieved with aspirin. Ten percent occur in the spine and present with "painful scoliosis." The vast majority of spine osteoid osteomas are in the posterior elements. The most common location is in the diaphyses of long bones with over 50% found in the femur or tibia. Seventy-five percent are cortical and remainder are cancellous in location. The radiographic findings include a cortical lesion with central radiolucent "nidus" surrounded by dense, solid periosteal bone formation. The intra-articular or cancellous lesions often do not have same degree of surrounding sclerosis. MR appearance may be misleading because of degree of bone marrow edema

OSTEOBLASTOMA

This rare tumor occurs in the posterior elements of the spine in 40% of the cases. It occurs in a similar age group as osteoid osteoma (10–30 years of age). Pain is the most common presentation but not as common or severe as with osteoid osteoma. Osteoblastoma can occur in association with aneurysmal bone cyst (ABC) (chondroblastoma are also associated with ABC). Radiographic findings include a lytic lesion with expansion, cortical thinning, or mild destruction. In the posterior elements of the spine, it appears as an expansile mass greater than in diameter 1.5 cm with associated soft-tissue mass. Osteoblastoma should be included in the differential diagnosis of expansile mass in the spine with any type of matrix.

OSTEOSARCOMA

This lesion is very common, second only to multiple myeloma as the most common primary bone tumor. It can occur as a primary lesion (75%) or secondary to a know precursor, most commonly is Paget disease followed by radiation and osteonecrosis. Primary osteosarcoma is classified as intramedullary (75%) and juxtacortical (approximately 10%) of cases. Rarer classifications include low-grade sclerosing, multifocal, and intracortical. Primary osteosarcoma occurs in younger patients, most commonly in the metaphyses of long bones. The majority produce extensive bony matrix as most are of the osteoblastic type and less than 10% exhibit the fibroblastic histologic pattern. Less common histologic patterns include chondroblastic and telangiectatic.

The radiographic findings depend on the histologic pattern, classification, and whether the lesion is primary or secondary. The classic, primary intramedullary osteosarcoma in children exhibits a dense osteoid matrix (also described as cloudlike) and aggressive periosteal reaction (described as "sunburst," "hair-on-end," "Codman triangle"). The majority of these lesions cross the epiphyseal plate. Juxtacortical osteosarcomas have a distinctive appearance and are divided into categories. The two most common in order are:

a. Parosteal osteosarcoma: low-grade tumor arising from outer periosteum. Classic location is posterior distal femoral metaphysis.
b. Periosteal osteosarcoma: origin is inner layer of periosteum. Broad-based diaphyseal lesion with 85% in femur or tibia. Usually, chondroblastic histology and appear as cortical thickening with erosions and aggressive periosteal reaction that rarely extends into the medullary cavity.

Telangiectatic osteosarcoma is a rare subtype but exhibits a unique appearance when compared with other osteosarcomas. These are expansile lesions, which contain cavities with blood products and necrosis. They can be confused with ABC on radiographs. Similarly, telangiectatic osteosarcomas and ABC both exhibit fluid/fluid levels on MRI. When evaluating osteosarcoma, be sure to evaluate the entire bone, for "skip metastases" or lesions in the same bone separated by normal intervening marrow.

TABLE 72-1 Osteoid Tumors

BENIGN	MALIGNANT
Enostosis: Bone island	Osteosarcoma: Young patients
Osteoma: Cranium, sinuses; Gardner syndrome	Parosteal osteosarcoma: Arises from outer layer of periosteum; posterior femoral metaphysis
Osteoid: Young males; night pain; relieved by aspirin	Periosteal osteosarcoma: Arises from inner layer of periosteum; femur and tibia diaphysis
Osteoblastoma: Young patients; spine; associated with ABC	Telangiectatic osteosarcoma: Multiple cavities; skip metastases

CHONDROID LESIONS (Table 72-2)

GENERAL

Chondroid lesions contain cartilaginous internal elements. The matrix may or may not be calcified. Those lesions that become calcified are described as having a punctuate, flocculent, or arclike pattern of mineralization.

OSTEOCHONDROMA

Osteochondroma occurs in young patients and symptoms are typically related to mass effect, bursa formation, or potential cosmetic effect. They are the only benign skeletal tumor associated with radiation. Osteochondromas have a rare potential of malignant transformation (less than 1% for solitary lesions). The width of the cartilage cap can be measured on MR and is a predictor of malignant transformation to chondrosarcoma. A cap greater than 1.5 cm in a skeletally mature individual is concerning for a malignant lesion. Pain within a previously painless osteochondroma is also ominous.

Hereditary multiple exostosis is an autosomal dominant condition in which patients have multiple osteochondromas (exostosis). This polyostotic variant presents earlier and lesions are said to exhibit a greater incidence of malignant transformation than do solitary osteochondromas. Lesions have a propensity for one side of the body. The femora and tibia are often involved in a characteristic pattern.

Trevor disease is a condition in which osteochondromas develop in an epiphyses causing significant joint deformity. For this reason, these are often treated more aggressively (this is most common in the ankle and knee). Radiographic findings include cortical and medullary continuity. The bone marrow flows freely into the lesion. In long bones, the lesion is metaphyseal and points away from the closest joint. They can be sessile or pedunculated. Look for the cartilage cap with calcification.

ENCHONDROMA

An enchondroma is a rest of hyaline cartilage within cancellous bone. They exhibit lobular growth, producing remodeling and cortical thinning. Common locations include the hands, in particular, the metacarpals. Multiple enchondromatosis is a nonhereditary condition in which polyostotic disease is present. These exhibit increased risk of malignant transformation to chondrosarcomas. Ollier disease is the more common form and presents with varying degrees of severity in childhood. Maffucci syndrome is very rare and is best differentiated from Ollier disease by the presence of multiple soft-tissue cavernous hemangiomas (look for phleboliths on radiographs.) Maffucci syndrome has the added risk of development of other malignancies such as ovarian cancer and glioma.

Imaging findings include incidentally noted, well-marginated, central metaphyseal lesion with chondroid matrix (rings and arcs). Cortical scalloping can suggest a more aggressive process such as developing chondrosarcoma. Typical metaphyseal lesion can mimic bone infarct on radiographs. In the hands, an enchondroma is often expansile and calcified chondroid matrix may be absent or difficult to appreciate. Look for T2 hyperintense lesion with a stippled pattern on MR because of the presence of hyaline cartilage.

JUXTACORTICAL CHONDROMA

This tumor arises just beneath the periosteum in the metaphyses. At least half are found in the humerus, usually in a patient younger than 30 years of age. It can be difficult to differentiate by imaging from juxtacortical chondrosarcoma. Radiographic findings include juxtacortical chondroid mass with cortical erosions, giving a characteristic "saucerization" pattern or long, smooth arc within the metaphysic, occasionally with adjacent sclerosis or periosteal reaction. The soft-tissue mass does not reliably contain chondroid calcification.

CHONDROBLASTOMA

Chondroblastoma is an epiphyseal lesion of children or young adults. At least half will extend into the metaphyses. It is considered an epiphyseal lesion, but do not forget the apophyses (epiphyseal equivalents) such as the greater trochanter can be involved. A small portion (approximately 10%) will be associated with ABC (similar to osteoblastoma). Most common differential diagnosis in a child is infection and Brodie abscess. Radiographic findings include a well-marginated epiphyseal

TABLE 72-2 Chondroid Lesions

BENIGN	MALIGNANT
Osteochondroma: Young patients; hereditary multiple exostosis; Trevor disease	Chondrosarcoma: Primary or secondary (Paget disease, radiation, malignant degerative of enchondroma or osteochondroma)
Enchondroma: Metacarpals	
Ollier syndrome: Polyostotic: increases risk for chondrosarcoma	
Muffucci syndrome: Polyostotic with hemangioma; risk of other cancers (ovarian, glioma)	
Juxtacortial chondroma	
Chondroblastoma: Children; young adults; epiphyseal	

lesion, often centrally located. Presence of chondroid matrix is not reliable. This is the only cartilage lesion that is not primarily hyaline cartilage and therefore can be intermediate or even dark in signal intensity on T2-weighted images. MR also reveals abundant surrounding edema such as that seen with osteoid osteoma. Fluid/fluid levels on MR suggest an association with ABC.

CHONDROSARCOMA

Chondrosarcoma is a malignant cartilaginous tumor occurring in patients aged 40 to 45 years. Over 50% occur in the femur or pelvis. As seen with osteosarcoma and can be primary or secondary. In addition to Paget disease and radiation, malignant degeneration of enchondroma or osteochondroma can produce a chondrosarcoma. Low-grade chondrosarcoma can be pathologically and radiographically difficult if not impossible to differentiate from enchondroma. Pain suggests chondrosarcoma rather than a benign lesion.

Radiographic findings dependant a great deal on whether the tumor is primary or secondary, the location, and the type (Table 72-3).

1. Intramedullary chondrosarcoma (the most common type) is mixed lytic and sclerotic tumor with chondroid matrix (rings and arcs). Attempts to differentiate from enchondroma are made by assessing the presence of aggressive features such as cortical scalloping (greater than two-thirds of the normal cortical thickness), expansion, and degree of permeative change.
2. Juxtacortical chondrosarcoma exhibits similar appearance to juxtacortical chondroma but is typically larger (greater than 3–4 cm).
3. Clear cell chondrosarcoma makes up only 2% of chondrosarcomas. These unique lesions are usually epiphyseal and can mimic benign lesions. They contain enough cartilage to remain very bright on T2-weighted imaging (as opposed to other common epiphyseal lesions, such as giant cell tumor and chondroblastoma)

TABLE 72-3 Classification of Primary Chondrosarcomas

Intramedullary (most common)
Juxtacortical
Clear cell
Mesenchymal

FIBROUS LESIONS (Table 72-4)

FIBROUS CORTICAL DEFECT/ NONOSSIFYING FIBROMA

This is a benign, self-limited, very common pediatric lesion. Over 80% are within the tibia or femur. The term fibrous cortical defect is used when the lesion is small (1–2 cm) and confined to the cortex. Nonossifying fibroma (NOF) extend into the medullary canal. They are clinically silent with the exception of large lesions, which have the potential to pathologically fracture. They can "heal" with sclerosis and then disappear. A healed or sclerotic NOF is termed an ossified NOF. Radiographic findings include a lucent lesion within the cortex of the metaphysis, often with a rim of sclerosis. It can be mildly expansile, but there is no associated soft-tissue mass or aggressive periosteal reaction.

FIBROUS DYSPASIA

Fibrous dysplasia is a benign developmental anomaly where fibrous tissue and spindle cells replace normal medullary bone. It occurs in children and young adults and can be monostotic or polyostotic. The polyostotic form can be associated with McCune-Albright syndrome (precocious puberty in girls, café au lait skin spots) and endocrine abnormalities (diabetes, hyperthyroidism, and hyperparathyroidism). Polyostotic disease usually presents prior to age 10. Cherubism describes an inherited variant with symmetric involvement of the mandible and maxilla. Monostotic lesions are smaller and usually asymptomatic. Common locations include femur, tibia, calvarium/facial bones, and ribs. A very small fraction are said to undergo malignant degeneration, most commonly to osteosarcoma. The radiographic appearance is varied. "Long lesion in a long bone," an often-stated quote, explains the most common location and propensity to extend a long segment of the diaphyses. "Ground glass," is a buzzword to describe the matrix of fibrous dysplasia. Ground glass appearance describes etched glass. Monostotic lesions are typically well marginated with sclerotic borders, often with mild expansion and cortical remodeling. Polyostotic disease yields more significant deformity causing leg-length discrepancies and fractures. "Shepard crook" deformity describes the angled deformity of the proximal femur. In the facial bones, they appear as smooth osseous expansion with typical ground-glass appearance. Frequency of sinus involvement is sphenoid, frontal, maxillary, and ethmoid sinuses in decreasing order. Leontiasis ossea describes "lionlike" faces in patients with extensive facial/cranial bone involvement.

OSTEOFIBROUS DYSPLASIA

This rare pediatric lesion typically occurs in the tibia and/or the fibula. Progression to bowing and fracture is not uncommon. Radiographic appearance includes an elongated, mixed lytic and sclerotic lesion, most commonly in the anterior cortex of the midtibial diaphyses. If large enough, intramedullary extension and cortical remodeling can occur.

ADAMANTINOMA

It is a rare tumor, which is similar in appearance and location to osteofibrous dysplasia. The best discriminator between the two is perhaps age, as adamantinoma occurs in those older than 25 years and osteofibrous dysplasia is rare after the teenage years. This lesion presents with pain and is considered a low-grade malignancy. Radiographic appearance is that of a mixed lytic and sclerotic lesion in the anterior tibial cortex often with expansion and cortical thickening. Often associated with soft-tissue mass.

FIBROMATOSIS: EXTRAABDOMINAL DESMOID

This asymptomatic soft-tissue mass in third to fourth decade, most commonly occurs around the shoulders. It often begins in intermuscular fascia. Treatment is difficult as recurrence is common. Radiographic appearance includes an infiltrative soft-tissue mass that is locally aggressive. MR appearance demonstrates a low T1/T2 signal mass, which enhances homogeneously. There is typically no calcification or bone involvement. The extent of tumor infiltration and neurovascular involvement is best evaluated with MRI.

TABLE 72-4 Fibrous Lesions

BENIGN	MALIGNANT
Fibrous cortical defect: Limited to cortex; common; small; tibia, femur	Malignant fibrous histiocytoma: Older patient; most common soft-tissue sarcoma in adults; primary or secondary (Paget disease, infarct, radiation therapy)
Nonossifying fibroma: Extend to medullary canal; common; tibia, femur	Adamantinoma: Rare; older than 25 years; low grade
Fibrous dysplasia	
McCune-Albright syndrome: Precocious puberty, café au lait skin pigmentation; endocrine abnormalities	
Cherubism: Inherited; mandible and maxilla	
Leontiasis ossea: Facial and cranial bones	
Osteofibrous dysplasia: Rare; young; tibia, fibula	

MALIGNANT FIBROUS HISTIOCYTOMA

This is a common primary bone or soft-tissue tumor occurring in older patients (40–60 years), which can be secondary (just like osteosarcoma and chondrosarcoma) to Paget disease, bone infarct, or radiation therapy. It cannot be distinguished from fibrosarcoma using imaging; however, fibrosarcomas often occur in younger patients (30–50 years). Soft-tissue malignant fibrous histiocytoma (MFH) is the most common soft-tissue sarcoma in adults (Table 72-5). It carries a poor prognosis, as there is a high rate of recurrence and frequency of distant metastases at time of diagnosis. Radiographic appearance of osseous MFH within the diaphyses is an aggressive, permeative lesion with cortical disruption and soft-tissue mass. If it occurs in the diametaphyses, the appearance may be less aggressive and does not extend to subchondral bone. The mass is infiltrative and the presence of extension to adjacent bone and cortical disruption is suggestive of MFH.

TABLE 72-5 Soft-Tissue Sarcomas

MFH (most common)
Liposarcoma
Rhabdomyosarcoma
Spindle cell sarcoma
Leiomyosarcoma
Synovial sarcoma (least common)

BONE MARROW TUMORS (Table 72-6)

MYELOMA

Myeloma is the most common primary bone tumor. Its distribution is that of red marrow with axial skeletal involvement being most common. Types include multiple (60%), solitary (25%), generalized (15%), plasma cell leukemia (1%), and extraskeletal (0.5%). The most common complication is pathologic fracture. Radiographic findings of multiple myeloma include numerous "punched-out" lytic lesions and "moth-eaten" appearance of the calvarium. These often scallop the inner cortex in the long bones. Plasmacytoma, also known as solitary myeloma, is a bubbly, lytic expansile lesion. A rare variant is the soft tissue or extramedullary plasmacytoma. Ninety percent of extramedullary plasmacytomas occur in the head and neck region. These are most often in the aerodigestive tract such as the nasopharynx or paranasal sinuses. Myeloma most commonly presents as generalized osteopenia (with or without spine compression fractures). MRI can reveal diffuse marrow replacement. Bone scintigraphy may be normal or reveal increased or decreased uptake depending on phase and extent of involvement. Therefore, extent is typically followed with skeletal survey.

PRIMARY LYMPHOMA OF BONE

Primary skeletal lymphoma is rare, making up approximately 5% of primary bone tumors. Almost all are of non-Hodgkin lymphoma. This can occur in any age group. Radiographic findings include an aggressive, permeative appearance, most commonly with associated soft-tissue mass. There is typically no lesional content.

EWING SARCOMA

This is a common malignant tumor in children, ages from 5 to 15 years. Derived from red marrow and histologically related to reticulum cell sarcoma, this tumor is in the category of round blue cell tumors. It typically presents with pain but can clinically mimic infection, presenting with fever, leukocytosis, and elevated sedimentation rate. Most common location is diaphyses or metaphyses of long bones (70% lower extremity). However, particularly in older patients, it is found in the flat bones including the ribs, pelvis, and scapula (locations of red marrow). Radiographic findings typically demonstrate a lytic, permeative lesion with aggressive periosteal reaction (onion-skinning or sunburst appearance) and associated soft-tissue mass. One-quarter is purely sclerotic.

LANGERHANS CELL HISTIOCYTOSIS (EOSINIOPHILIC GRANULOMA)

The underlying pathophysiology of this disease is abnormal histiocyte proliferation in the reticuloendothelial system (skeletal and extraskeletal). Occurs predominately in children (first through third decades) and can grow or expand rapidly. Eosinophilic granuloma is the term for localized osseous or pulmonary form of the disease. Clinical presentation, symptoms, and prognosis depend on degree of extraskeletal involvement. Laboratory studies are frequently normal. Isolated skeletal disease has an excellent prognosis. Osseous radiographic findings vary greatly causing this entity to be placed on the differential diagnosis of most pediatric bone tumors. The appearance in part depends on the bone involved. The skull is the most common site of osseous involvement. The tumor involves the inner and outer table to varying degrees giving a "beveled edge" appearance. Occasionally, a cortical lucency will be present with a central density or sequestrum (button sequestrum). "Floating teeth" describes a lytic lesion in the alveolar ridge that gives the impression that teeth are not held in place by bone or are "floating." Ribs are the second most common site of bony involvement, typically with multiple rib involvement. Ribs become expanded and often have associated soft-tissue mass. Spine lesions can have lytic destruction which when extensive causes vertebra plana (complete collapse of vertebral body). The adjacent disc space heights are typically normal. Pelvis and scapular lesions are often well defined often with sclerotic margins in the pelvis. Langerhans cell histiocytosis cannot be reliably differentiated from malignant lesions such as Ewing sarcoma or infection. Extraskeletal disease can involve the lungs (upper lobe interstitial disease), central nervous system (absent pituitary bright spot, thickened pituitary stalk), and gastrointestinal tract (fibrous polypoid lesion in stomach).

METASTATIC DISEASE

The most common bone tumor is metastatic and occurs as a result of tumor emboli or retrograde venous flow (via Batson Plexus). Breast, prostate, and lung make up the order of frequency of metastatic disease. Pain is the most common complaint but only occurs in two-thirds of patients with metastatic disease. Classically blastic lesions include prostate, carcinoid, and medulloblastoma. Classic lytic "blowout" lesions include renal and thyroid metastases. Bone mets in children are typically because of neuroblastoma, leukemia, lymphoma, or medulloblastoma. Radiographic findings can simulate primary bone tumors and appear both indolent and

TABLE 72-6 Bone Marrow Tumors

Myeloma	Most common primary bone tumor
Lymphoma	Non-Hodgkin type; rare
Ewing sarcoma	Common; children
Langerhans cell histiocytosis	Eosinophic granuloma; children; skull most common, then ribs

aggressive. Bone scintigraphy is helpful to evaluate extent of disease. PET is also helpful in FDG-avid malignancies.

OTHER BONE TUMORS AND CYSTIC BONE LESIONS

GIANT CELL TUMOR

This adult tumor formed from osteoclast-like giant cells commonly present with pain. Fifteen percent are associated with ABC and ten percent are malignant. The only way to determine if a giant cell tumor is malignant is the presence of metastatic disease. Radiographic findings typically include a lytic, sometimes expansile, epiphyseal lesion commonly extending from the epiphysis and metaphyses. It occurs almost exclusively after fusion of physeal plate, is solitary and often eccentric, and exhibits narrow zone of transition with fading sclerosis.

UNICAMERAL BONE CYST

This common pediatric tumor (85% occur in patients younger than 20 years) often presents with pathologic fracture. It is twice as common in males than females and is typically treated with bone graft or curettage. Radiographic findings include a lytic, mildly expansile lesion without periosteal reaction (unless fractured). It is most often in long bones (except in adult patient, where it can reside in the pelvis or calcaneous) and originates at metaphyses. The "fallen fragment" sign describes fragment of bone layering dependently within a fractured unicameral bone cyst.

ANEURYSMAL BONE CYST

This osseous vascular malformation is made up of multiple blood-filled, thin-walled cavities. It occurs in pediatric patients and can occur as a primarily lesion or secondarily within another bone tumor. Associate tumors include giant cell tumor, chondroblastoma, and osteoblastoma. Bone cysts can grow rapidly and cause pain, sometimes with pathologic fracture. Treatment involves grafting or curettage. Up to 20% will recur, although it has no malignant potential. Radiographic findings include an eccentric, markedly expansile lesion with remodeled but usually intact surrounding cortex (unless in most aggressive phase of growth). Majority are metaphyseal with fewer in diaphyseal location. MRI exhibits multiple cysts with varying degrees of T1 signal intensity (blood products) and fluid/fluid levels.

INTRAOSSEOUS LIPOMA

Usually, this is an incidental lesion, but pain has been reported as a presenting symptom. It is most commonly reported in adults (fourth to fifth decade). Although intraosseous lipoma can occur throughout the skeleton, most common locations include proximal femur (34%) and calcaneus. Radiographic findings include a lucent lesion sometimes with mild expansile remodeling of the medullary canal, fat density and signal characteristics of fat on CT and MR, respectively. Lesion can exhibit central or peripheral ossification. In particular, central calcification in a lucent calcaneal body lesion is essentially pathognomonic for intraosseous lipoma.

EPIDERMOID INCLUSION CYST

Epidermoid inclusion cyst is most common in the third and fourth decades. It is a benign proliferation of epidermal cells. The intraosseous form is usually diagnosed in the terminal phalanx, but can also be found in the skull. Gardner syndrome has an association with epidermoid inclusion cysts. Radiographic findings typically demonstrate a well-defined lucent lesion in the terminal phalanx with surrounding sclerosis.

VASCULAR OR LYMPHATIC TUMORS OF BONE AND SOFT TISSUE

HEMANGIOMA

Hemangioma is the most common vascular soft-tissue abnormality (represents 7% of all soft-tissue tumors). Osseous hemangiomas have a characteristic appearance and are common within the spine in adults. Soft-tissue hemangiomas can be pathologically classified as capillary, cavernous, venous, arteriovenous, and mixed (Table 72-7). An alternate classification schema categorizes high-flow (arteriovenous) or low-flow (capillary, cavernous, venous) lesions.

Maffucci syndrome describes multiple cavernous soft-tissue hemangiomas in the setting of enchondromatosis.

TABLE 72-7 Soft-Tissue Hemangioma Classification

Capillary	Infantile hemangioma; typically involute without treatment
Cavernous	"Vascular birthmark," deeper than capillary hemangiomas; older children; do not involute spontaneously; most common intraorbital tumor in adults
Venous	Deep structures; abdomen and extremities
Arteriovenous	Persistent fetal capillary bed causes shunting; can be deep or superficial

Klippel-Trenaunay-Weber is a nonhereditary condition of extensive unilateral capillary or arteriovenous hemangiomas in a lower extremity.

Osseous hemangiomas are most common in the vertebral bodies and exhibit vertical striations. In long bones, expansion and bone overgrowth are common. Soft-tissue cavernous hemangiomas are best diagnosed on conventional radiographs with phleboliths, occurring in about one-half of lesions.

GLOMUS TUMOR

This painful, often pulsating tumor commonly occurs in the hand with the majority being subungual in location. Radiographic findings include remodeling of adjacent bone, which is typically along the dorsal margin of the terminal phalanx. Soft-tissue tumor is very bright on T2-weighted images because of vascular nature.

TUMOR-LIKE CONDITIONS AND OTHER SOFT-TISSUE MASSES

SYNOVIAL METAPLASIAS

Pigmented Villonodular Synovitis (PVNS)

This idiopathic condition typically presents with pain in the young adult. Treatment is synovectomy. The localized form is also called giant cell tumor of the tendon sheath and is most common in the hand. The diffuse form is seen most commonly found in the hip, shoulder, knee, in decreasing order Radiographic findings of the diffuse form demonstrate erosions at the joint margins, often with preservation of the joint space and without other findings of arthritis. The localized form often presents as a small soft-tissue mass. Because of presence of hemosiderin (pigmented), these lesions are typically dark on MR sequences.

Synovial Chondromatosis

This idiopathic condition presents with joint pain and decreased range of motion. The most common location is the knee. Males are involved at least twice as commonly as females. Treatment includes synovectomy, but recurrence is common. This condition produces proliferation of metaplastic synovium with eventual fragmentation. These fragments grow and eventually will ossify. Radiographic findings depend on the degree of ossification of the intra-articular bodies. There are typically many more intra-articular bodies present than depicted on radiographs. Tight joints such as the hip will demonstrate earlier erosions and secondary osteoarthrosis. In contrast, capacious joints such as the knee often appear essentially normal except for the presence of multiple loose bodies. MR better depicts both the ossific and cartilaginous bodies and the synovial proliferation.

POPLITEAL CYST (BAKER CYST)

Most commonly recognized synovial cyst (herniation of synovial membrane through the joint capsule) resulting from a communication between the knee joint and a distended gastrocnemius-semimembranosus bursa. The most common complication is rupture, which can clinically mimic a deep venous thrombosis. Radiographic findings are best depicted on ultrasound or MR, with fluid signal/cyst extending between the medial head of the gastrocnemius and the semimembranosus tendons.

MYOSITIS OSSIFICANS

Myositis ossificans describes the heterotopic bone formation that occurs most commonly in young adults following trauma, although a significant percentage have no trauma history. In the early stages, this can be confused with an aggressive lesion such as a surface osteosarcoma. Myositis ossificans progressiva is an autosomal dominant condition with dysmorphic skeletal features and an average age of onset of 5 years. Radiographic findings include a focal soft-tissue calcification beginning 2 to 6 weeks following trauma. Over time, this exhibits a pattern of peripheral maturation (dense bone at the periphery of the lesion). CT best demonstrates this maturation pattern, especially early in the course.

SOFT-TISSUE LIPOMA

Lipoma is the most common soft-tissue tumor, a slow growing fatty tumor, surrounded by a thin fibrous capsule. It is usually asymptomatic and presents as a palpable mass. No intervention is required, but these often removed for cosmetic reasons and to exclude liposarcoma. Radiographic findings include a well-circumscribed

TABLE 72-8 Soft-Tissue Sarcomas

Malignant fibrous histiocytoma (MFH)	Most common
Liposarcoma	Second most common; usually painless; extremities; may not contain fat, although many do
Synovial sarcoma	Does not arise from synovium; resembles synovial tissue on microscopy; greater than 90% occur away from a joint; most common sarcoma of the foot and ankle
Rhabdomyosarcoma	Most common soft-tissue sarcoma in children; embryonal is most common type and typically involves the head/neck region or GU tract. The alveolar type is seen more commonly in older children and young adults and involves the extremities more commonly. The pleomorphic type is rare and found in adults

mass that exhibits signal characteristics of subcutaneous fat on all MR sequences but exhibits no significant enhancement. If there are septations, any degree of heterogeneity, or enhancement, then liposarcoma should be considered.

SOFT-TISSUE SARCOMAS (Table 72-8)

Radiographic findings depend on type of sarcoma, however findings relatively nonspecific and often require biopsy or resection to establish diagnosis. MR is most useful in assessing extent of the neoplasm, operative planning, and follow-up. Synovial sarcomas can appear small, cystic, and benign. Enhancement helps to differentiate this lesion from a cyst on MR. On radiographic findings, synovial sarcomas occasionally exhibits "stippled" calcifications. Liposarcomas usually appear as large, enhancing masses with components of fat and soft tissue. Low-grade liposarcomas are difficult to differentiate from atypical lipomas on MR.

SUGGESTED READING

Cerase A, Priolo F. Skeletal benign bone-forming lesions. *Eur J Radiol*. 1998;27(suppl 1):S91-S97.

Levine SM, et al. Cortical lesions of the tibia: characteristic appearances at conventional radiography. *Radiographics*. 2003; 23:157-177.

Miller TT. Bone tumors and tumorlike conditions: analysis with conventional radiography. *Radiology*. 2008;246: 662-674.

Murphy MD, et al. The many faces of osteosarcoma. *Radiographics*. 1997;17:1205-1231.

QUESTIONS AND ANSWERS

1. A popliteal cyst protrudes through which two anatomic structures?
   A. Semitendonosis and lateral head of the gastrocnemius
   B. Gracilis and medial head of the pes anserinus
   C. Semimembranosus and medial head of the gastrocnemius
   D. Popliteus and the lateral head of the gastrocnemius

   ANSWER: C. Popliteal cyst is a synovial cyst, which is a herniation of the joint capsule between the medial head of the gastrocnemius and the semimembranosus.

2. What is the most common soft-tissue sarcoma in the adult ankle/foot?
   A. Synovial sarcoma
   B. Malignant fibrous histiocytoma
   C. Liposarcoma
   D. Rhabdomyosarcoma

   ANSWER: A. Synovial sarcoma is the most common sarcoma in the foot in the adult and often exhibits stippled calcification on plain films. This lesion can appear cystic on MR and therefore enhancement can be very important to verify that a solid lesion is present. MFH is the most common overall sarcoma. Rhabdomyosarcoma is the most common in the pediatric population.

3. Which of the following typically has little or no surrounding edema on MR?
   A. Osteoid osteoma
   B. Chondroblastoma
   C. Intraosseous abscess
   D. Enchondroma

   ANSWER: D. Enchondromas are often incidental findings typically without a great deal of surrounding edema. The other lesions by comparison are known for surrounding edema. In fact, osteoid osteomas and chondroblastomas are occasionally mistaken for more aggressive lesions.

4. Which of the following does *not* help differentiate enchondroma from chondrosarcoma?
   A. Degree of enhancement
   B. Pain
   C. Degree of cortical thinning
   D. Aggressive periosteal reaction

   ANSWER: A. Both tumors can enhance, so this does not help a great deal. Aggressive features such as periosteal reaction and cortical thinning favor chondrosarcoma. Pain favors a malignant lesion as well.

5. Which of the following is *not* associated with fluid/fluid levels on MR?
   A. Aneurysmal bone cyst
   B. Eosinophilic granuloma
   C. Telangiectatic osteosarcoma
   D. Chondroblastoma

   ANSWER: B. ABC and telangiectatic osteosarcoma are known to be associated with fluid/fluid levels on MR and chondroblastoma can be associated with ABC. Eosinophilic granuloma does not have fluid/fluid levels.

6. Which of the following has no or only mild uptake on bone scintigraphy?
   A. Fibrous dysplasia
   B. Bone island
   C. Paget disease
   D. Primary osseous lymphoma

   ANSWER: B. Bone islands typically have no or mild uptake. The other lesions are known for marked uptake on bone scintigraphy.

7. Imaging reveals an aggressive bone lesion which exhibits a sequestration and an associated soft-tissue mass. What is the most likely diagnosis?
   A. Chondrosarcoma
   B. Primary lymphoma of bone
   C. Multiple myeloma
   D. Ewings Sarcoma

   ANSWER: B. Primary lymphoma of bone has a documented associated with sequestra though it is only associated 15% of the time. The other lesions are not associated with sequestration formation.

8. What is the most common risk factor leading to secondary osteosarcoma?
   A. Radiation
   B. Osteonecrosis
   C. Paget disease
   D. Fibrous dysplasia

   ANSWER: C. Over 60% of secondary osteosarcomas are diagnosed in patients with Paget disease.

9. Of the synovial metaplasias, which one typically exhibits low signal intensity on all MR pulse sequences?
   A. Lipoma arborescens
   B. Synovial chondromatosis
   C. PVNS
   D. Inflammatory arthropathy

   ANSWER: B. PVNS and giant cell tumor of the tendon sheath are pigmented lesions and exhibit hemosiderin. Therefore, they have low signal intensity on MR pulse sequences and, in particular, a gradient sequence. Inflammatory arthropathy is a synovial hyperplasia rather than a metaplasia.

10. Patient presents with an osteolytic, painful lesion at the dorsal aspect of the terminal phalanx. What is the most likely diagnosis?
    A. Enchondroma
    B. Hemangioma
    C. Aneurysmal bone cyst
    D. Glomus Tumor

    ANSWER: D. Glomus tumors are vascular lesions that are characteristically subungual in location, painful, and cause osteolysis.

73 ARTHROPATHIES

Mark Sultenfuss and Robert Lopez-Ben

OVERVIEW

Arthritis is most easily approached from an etiologic standpoint. Changes within an articulation can occur from direct injury to the joint, systemic inflammatory processes, or from metabolic abnormalities resulting in deposition of products within and surrounding the joint. The pathophysiology of the underlying disease can explain the radiographic findings. Important distinguishing characteristics include the distribution of involvement, the presence or absence of bony proliferation, and the presence or absence of erosions. Taking these factors into consideration, most forms of arthritis can be accurately characterized.

DEGENERATIVE JOINT DISEASE

Degenerative joint disease or osteoarthrosis is a noninflammatory process of synovial joints, resulting from presumably mechanical joint destruction and repair. Degenerative osteoarthrosis is considered primary when abnormal forces applied to a normal joint lead to joint disruption, and secondary when normal forces applied to an abnormal joint lead to the same disruptive changes. Degenerative osteoarthritis can affect any articulation, but most commonly affects large weight-bearing joints, such as the hips, knees, and spine. Cartilage disruption or degeneration within affected joints results in nonuniform joint space narrowing, and subchondral bone fracture and/or collapse. Loss of articular cartilage is accentuated in areas, where there is increased pressure within the joint, accounting for asymmetric joint space loss within an articulation. As the joint is disrupted, joint instability and subluxation occurs, further increasing the abnormal biomechanical forces applied to the articulation. Eventually, the subchondral bone fractures and collapses, and new bone is produced, which is characterized by subchondral eburnation (sclerosis) radiographically. In an attempt to increase the surface area of the articulation and offset the increasingly abnormal forces within the joint, marginal osteophytes are created at low-stress points. Periarticular subchondral lucencies/cysts, which are commonly seen in degenerative osteoarthrosis, are thought to occur from extruded synovial fluid into the disrupted subchondral bone and/or bony marrow contusion/involution. The overall lack of inflammation explains the normal bone mineralization and absence of erosions.

EROSIVE OSTEOARTHRITIS

Erosive osteoarthritis is an inflammatory form of degenerative osteoarthrosis, most characteristically affecting bilaterally and symmetrically the interphalangeal joints of postmenopausal females. The characteristic central erosions help distinguish this entity from other inflammatory arthritides, which have marginal erosions. Inflammation leads to enzymatic loss of articular cartilage and subsequent collapse of the subchondral bone. The repair process results in marginal osteophyte formation, as seen with degenerative osteoarthrosis, another distinguishing feature from other forms of inflammatory arthritis. These marginal osteophytes, in combination with central erosions, can lead to a gull-wing appearance of the interphalangeal joints. Occasionally, new bone formation can result in ankylosis.

RHEUMATOID ARTHRITIS

Rheumatoid arthritis is an immune-mediated inflammatory process of synovial joints, thought to occur from a type III hypersensitivity reaction to an unknown antigen. Synovial joints of both the axial and appendicular skeleton are involved. Although any synovial joint can be involved, the hands and feet are most commonly affected. Inflammatory cells target and infiltrate the synovium of these joints, forming granulation tissue known as "pannus." Immune mediators released from these inflammatory cells stimulate capillary proliferation, further increasing the inflammatory response and pannus formation. Periarticular osteopenia develops from the resultant hyperemia. Articular bone and cartilage are both directly affected by the inflammatory response. Enzymes released from inflammatory cells create symmetric uniform cartilage destruction, while direct pannus interaction with bone leads to osseous erosions. Since the margins of synovial joints are devoid of articular cartilage, these "bare" areas of bone are affected first, demonstrated radiographically as marginal erosions.

The articular surfaces become incongruous from cartilage and subchondral bone destruction, and the articular capsule and ligaments become weakened from inflammation. As these processes progress, joint laxity and subluxation develop. Subluxations characteristically occur along the ulnar side of the articulation. There is a distinct lack of new bone formation.

Synovium lining the tendon sheaths and bursae can also be affected by the inflammatory infiltration of rheumatoid arthritis, referred to as tenosynovitis and bursitis. The inflammation creates soft-tissue swelling and subjacent bone erosion. Classic examples include ulnar styloid erosion from extensor carpi ulnaris tenosynovitis and posterior calcaneal erosions from retrocalcaneal bursitis. The tendons can spontaneously rupture, contributing to articular subluxation.

JUVENILE RHEUMATIOD ARTHRITIS

Juvenile rheumatoid arthritis (JRA) combines five forms of inflammatory arthritis, which occur in children and adolescents. These forms of arthritis include Still disease, polyarticular JRA, seronegative and seropositive JRA, and juvenile ankylosing spondylitis.

Still disease is a systemic process affecting children younger than 5 years. The child presents with fever, anemia, leukocytosis, lymphadenopathy, and polyarticular arthritis. Radiographic changes of arthritis are typically mild and nonspecific.

Pauciarticular disease is the most common form of juvenile arthritis, accounting for approximately 40% of cases. The patients are typically female and are seronegative for rheumatoid factor. One to three joints are involved and usually affect larger joints, such as the knee, elbow, or ankle. Patients can also have a chronic iridocyclitis. Radiographic changes are more pronounced than Still disease, with periarticular osteoporosis, soft-tissue swelling, and a variable presence of joint space loss and erosions.

Polyarticular disease can be seen in both seronegative and seropositive patients. Seronegative polyarticular JRA accounts for about 25% of all JRA patients and is defined as a symmetric arthritis involving multiple articulations in a patient who does not produce rheumatoid factor. The arthropathy is similar to adult-type RA in distribution and radiographic changes. Some features of long-standing involvement include ankylosis of apophyseal joints in the cervical spine, creating hypoplasia of the cervical vertebrae and discs, as well as ankylosis of the carpal and tarsal bones. Seropositive polyarticular disease accounts for only about 5% of patients and is similar in appearance and distribution to adult-type RA. Symptoms typically begin during the second decade and primarily affect females. Rheumatoid factor is present on serologic examination.

Juvenile ankylosing spondylitis is essentially a young-onset form of adult-type ankylosing spondylitis. There are many similarities between juvenile and adult ankylosing spondylitis, including male predominance, and an association with HLA-B27. Radiographic changes are similar as well, with ankylosis of involved articulations, primarily the sacroiliac joints and spine.

In all forms of JRA, distinguishing features include overgrowth of epiphyses from hyperemia, leading to a ballooned appearance of the epiphysis. Advanced skeletal maturation also occurs from premature physeal closure, resulting in shortened limbs. Soft-tissue swelling and metaphyseal osteopenia are also common radiographic findings. Loss of joint space and erosions are typically late manifestations of the disease.

COLLAGEN VASCULAR DISEASES

SCLERODERMA

Scleroderma is an autoimmune collagen vascular disease, which primarily affects the dermis, although many other organ systems, including the heart, GI tract, and kidneys, can be involved. There is a low-grade inflammatory response to an unknown inciting antigen, with inflammatory cells surround the vasculature and depositing collagen. These alterations result in fibrosis of the soft tissues, atrophy of the dermal appendages, and thrombotic occlusion of arterioles. This is most pronounced radiographically within the digits, where resorption and fibrosis of soft tissues results in a sausage-shaped digit. The soft tissues of the fingertips are frequently absorbed and can be associated with osseous erosions of the distal phalangeal tufts, which is termed acro-osteolysis. The tuft can alternatively be sclerotic, which is termed acrosclerosis.

Amorphous calcification of the periarticular soft tissues is also a common feature and is most pronounced in the hands. Infrequently, erosive arthropathy can occur at the interphalangeal joints and the first carpometacarpal joint in patients with scleroderma. A common finding is thickening of the periodontal membrane on mandible radiographs in patients with scleroderma. Although the erosive changes may resemble those of rheumatoid arthritis, distal interphalangeal involvement may help distinguish scleroderma from RA.

SYSTEMIC LUPUS ERYTHEMATOSUS

Systemic lupus erythematosus (SLE) is an autoimmune collagen vascular disease of unknown etiology. Arthritis in SLE is a result of autoantibody-induced synovial inflammation and hyperemia, without pannus formation. Changes of soft-tissue swelling and periarticular osteoporosis occur in a bilateral and symmetric distribution. Since there is a lack of pannus formation, cartilage destruction is absent and joint spaces are therefore maintained. Erosive changes are distinctly absent. The inflammation weakens and disrupts tendons, resulting in flexion and extension deformities, as well as ulnar-sided articular subluxations. The metacarpal phalangeal (MCP) joints of the hand and large weight-bearing joints are the most common sites of involvement. Subchondral cysts are though to occur from the alteration of articular mechanics. Most of these patients require steroid therapy to control the systemic inflammation, which can lead to osteonecrosis.

POLYMYOSITIS/DERMATOMYOSITIS

Polymyositis and dermatomyositis are inflammatory processes involving the striated muscle and dermis respectively. The etiology is unknown, but may be a cell-mediated autoimmune process. Chronic inflammatory cell infiltration of muscle fibers and dermis lead to edema, followed by fibrosis and atrophy. Resulting necrosis leads to soft-tissue calcifications, which are the radiographic hallmark of both disease entities. Articular involvement is rare, with periarticular soft-tissue swelling and calcification seen most commonly. Rarely erosions or articular subluxations can occur.

SERONEGATIVE SPONDYLOARTHROPATHIES

ANKYLOSING SPONDYLITIS

Ankylosing spondylitis is a chronic inflammatory arthritis of unknown etiology, likely related to an autoimmune response in patients with HLA-B27 antigen. The disease affects young adults, with a strong male predominance. The low-grade inflammatory process involves both synovial and cartilaginous articulations as well as ligamentous attachment to bone. Involvement is typically bilateral and symmetric in distribution. Sacroiliitis and a lack of articular subluxations and subchondral cysts are all important features of this disease.

The synovial joints most commonly affected in ankylosing spondylitis are the sacroiliac joints, hips, and shoulders. Inflammation within the synovial joint results in loss of articular cartilage, joint space narrowing, and osseous erosions. The articular cartilage becomes hyperemic from the inflammatory response, with metaplasia of the cartilage occurring over time. The metaplastic cartilage subsequently ossifies, resulting in intra-articular ankylosis.

The cartilaginous joints most commonly affected in ankylosing spondylitis are the intervertebral disc/body junction as well as the symphysis pubis. The inflammation results in cartilage calcification, angiogenesis, and ultimately ossification. These thin bridges of ossification are known as syndesmophytes, which ultimately progresses to bony ankylosis once the bridge across the articulation is complete. The radiographic result is a "bamboo" appearance of the spine.

Inflammation of ligament/tendon attachments to bone (enthesitis) results in subligamentous bone erosion/eburnation, which are termed "shining corner" when it affects the vertebral body. As healing occurs, bony excrescences develop at these ligamentous attachments, which are termed enthesophytes. These inflammatory enthesophytes are nonspecific and can also be demonstrated with reactive arthritis and psoriasis.

REACTIVE ARTHRITIS (FORMERLY TERMED REITER SYNDROME)

This is a triad of ureteritis, conjunctivitis, and inflammatory arthritis, most commonly affecting young male patients. The arthritis associated with Reiter syndrome is thought to occur from immune-mediated inflammatory cell infiltration of the synovial membrane. The inflammatory process results in periarticular soft-tissue swelling as well as osteoporosis from associated hyperemia. Inflammatory cartilaginous and osseous changes include joint space narrowing and erosions, which begin at the joint margin and extend centrally. New bone is produced in response to the inflammatory process (periostitis), beginning as cartilaginous fibroplasias/metaplasia, which subsequently ossifies, resulting in intra-articular ankylosis. Reiter's characteristically involves the small joints of the foot as well as the hand and wrist.

PSORIATIC ARTHRITIS

Psoriasis is a skin disorder, with articular involvement in only a small percentage of patients (less than 30%). Synovial inflammation and effusions result in fusiform soft-tissue swelling. The degree of synovial inflammatory infiltrate, however, is less than with rheumatoid arthritis. The articular cartilage is destroyed by the inflammatory process, resulting in uniform loss of the joint space. Erosions also develop from direct inflammatory infiltration of bone, beginning at the articular margin and extending centrally. New bone proliferation does occur as an exaggerated healing response, creating excrescences, which accompany osseous erosions.

A characteristic finding is the "pencil-in-cup" deformity, representing telescoping of bone into the central erosion. Arthritis from psoriasis most commonly involves the interphalangeal joints of the hand and foot, MCP and metatarsal phalangeal (MTP) joints, and the calcaneus. Sacroiliac and spine involvement is also common. Psoriatic arthritis is also one of the cause of acro-osteolysis or distal tuft erosion. Additionally, the distal tuft can have increased density, termed "ivory phalanx."

ENTEROPATHIC ARTHRITIS

Articular changes similar to those of psoriasis and reactive arthritis can occur from enteropathic disease processes and infections. Enteric diseases such as ulcerative colitis, Crohn disease, and Whipple disease, as well as enteric infections, such as salmonella, shigella, and yersinia, can all have nonspecific articular changes. These findings include soft-tissue swelling, periarticular osteoporosis, joint space narrowing, and osseous erosions. There is a predilection for larger joints, as opposed to the small joint involvement seen in psoriatic and reactive arthritis.

METABOLIC/BIOCHEMICAL ARTHRITIS

GOUTY ARTHRITIS

Gouty arthritis occurs from the inflammatory response stimulated by sodium monourate crystal deposition in tissues with poor blood supply. Sodium monourate crystals develop from hyperuricemia, either in response to an inborn error of metabolism (primary gout) or from a disease state that creates hyperuricemia secondary to increased production or decreased excretion of uric acid (secondary gout). Radiographic changes are evident in only half of patients with gout, most commonly affecting the MTP of the great toe. Other common areas of involvement include the hands, wrists, elbows, and knees.

Eccentric crystal deposition in the soft tissues, along with the associated inflammatory response, leads to prominence of soft tissues as well as calcification of the soft tissues over time. These crystal deposits are referred to as tophi. Destruction of cartilage within a joint is asymmetric, usually preserving the joint space until the late stages of disease. Punched-out intra- and juxta-articular erosions, with sclerotic borders, occur at sites of tophus formation. The edges of cortex can create an elevated bony margin, as the bone covers a tophaceous nodule, with bone absorption occurring adjacent to the nodule.

CALCIUM PYROPHOSPHATE CRYSTAL DEPOSITION ARTHROPATHY

Arthropathy from calcium pyrophosphate crystal deposition (CPPD) results from deposition of calcium pyrophosphate crystals into articular tissues. The process can be hereditary, idiopathic or degenerative, or secondary to other diseases, such as hyperparathyroidism, hemochromatosis, hypothyroidism, and many others. Crystals are deposited within the articular cartilage, synovium, articular capsule, and periarticular soft tissues. Deposition of crystal within fibrocartilage accounts for chondrocalcinosis, which is characteristic radiographically. The inflammatory response to intra-articular crystals results in enzymatic destruction of cartilage and ultimately joint space narrowing. Subchondral bone becomes sclerotic and thickened, either from collapse or subchondral new bone formation. Periarticular mineralization remains normal, a finding that suggests a lower-grade inflammatory response and/or the lack of hyperemia within the articulation.

Although findings of CPPD arthropathy seem similar to osteoarthritis, there are several features, which help distinguish the two. The distribution is slightly different; although the knee is most commonly affected, other articulations affected in CPPD, such as the wrists and MCP joints, are less commonly affected by osteoarthritis. Wrist involvement is very distinctive for CPPD, with chondrocalcinosis and degenerative tearing of the triangular fibrocartilage complex. Also, degeneration of the lunate articulations and ligamentous attachments can lead to scapholunate articular collapse (SLAC).

The distribution of CPPD also includes the hands, hips, shoulder, and elbow. When compared with osteoarthritis, CPPD can atypically affect certain areas of the joint, such as selective patellofemoral involvement of the knee. Subchondral cysts that form in the bones of affected articulations are larger and more numerous than those demonstrated with simple osteoarthritis. Destructive changes are more severe and progressive, when compared with osteoarthritis. Finally, osteophyte formation in joints affected by CPPD is variable; some patients may produce exuberant osteophyte formation, while others demonstrate none.

CALCIUM HYDROXYAPATITE CRYSTAL DEPOSITION DISEASE

Calcium hydroxyapatite crystal deposition disease (HADD) is also known as calcific tendonitis/peritendinitis/bursitis. It occurs from deposition of hydroxyapatite crystals into periarticular soft tissues, with subsequent loss of normal soft-tissue structure, mild inflammatory response, and possibly necrosis. The articulations adjacent to these calcific deposits can be normal, or may have nonspecific destructive changes such as loss of joint space, subchondral eburnation, and possibly erosions with articular derangement. The etiology is unknown, but local, systemic, and metabolic factors may be contributory.

The shoulder is the most commonly affected joint in HADD, with calcific deposits in the rotator cuff tendons, and other periarticular soft tissues. These deposits stimulate an inflammatory response, leading to subsequent derangement of the joint. Intra-articular involvement of the shoulder with marked loss of articular cartilage, osseous erosions, and rotator cuff degeneration, represent an entity of pain and decreased mobility in elderly patients termed Milwaukee shoulder syndrome. This can sometimes be confused clinically with infection or neuropathic arthropathy. Other joints can also be affected by hydroxyapatite crystal deposition, including the elbow, wrists, hips, and knee. In the cervical spine, soft-tissue swelling, along with amorphous calcium deposition in the prevertebral soft tissues, representing calcific tendonitis of the longus colli muscle, can suggest hydroxyapatite deposition disease.

The periarticular calcification of hydroxyapatite deposition can be simulated by other disease entities. Altered calcium/phosphorous metabolism, such as in renal osteodystrophy, calcinosis in the presence of normal calcium metabolism (idiopathic tumoral calcinosis), and dystrophic calcification in devitalized tissue, can all lead to periarticular calcifications.

HEMOCHROMATOSIS

Hemochromatosis is an iron deposition disorder from either an autosomal recessive inborn error of increased iron absorption (primary hemochromatosis) or iron overload (secondary hemochromatosis). Many years of iron deposition are required for clinical symptoms to occur; therefore, the age of onset is typically the fifth through seventh decades of life.

Arthropathy from iron deposition is more common in patients with primary hemochromatosis, and there is an association of hemochromatosis with CPPD. Iron is deposited within the synovium and cartilage, with calcification of the articular cartilage, either isolated or in association with CPPD. Osseous changes from iron deposition are similar to those of CPPD arthropathy, including subchondral eburnation and cyst formation.

Distinguishing hemochromatosis from CPPD relies on a few subtle findings. Arthropathy of hemochromatosis primarily affects the second and third MCP joints, with less common involvement of the remaining MCP joints. Hooklike osteophytes along these MCP articulations are also subtle distinguishing radiographic characteristics. Additionally, the radiocarpal articulation is less severely affected by hemochromatosis, when compared with CPPD arthropathy. Finally, the arthropathy of hemochromatosis is less progressive than CPPD arthropathy.

Suggested Reading

Brower AC, Flemming DJ, et al. *Arthritis in Black and White*. 2nd ed. Philadelphia, PA: W.B. Saunders; 1996:195-306, 325-404.

Buchmann RF, Jaramillo D. Imaging of articular disorders in children. *Radiol Clin North Am*. 2004;42(1):151-168.

Chew FS. Radiology of the hands: review and self-assessment module. *AJR Am J Roentgenol*. 2005;184(6 suppl):S157-S168.

Hayes CW, Conway WF. Calcium hydroxyapatite deposition disease. *Radiographics*. 1990;10:1031-1048.

Monu JU, Pope TL Jr. Gout: a clinical and radiologic review. *Radiol Clin North Am*. 2004;42(1):169-184.

Resnik D, Kransdorf MJ, et al. *Bone and Joint Imaging*. 3rd ed. Philadelphia, PA: Elsevier Saunders; 2005:209-334, 445-493.

QUESTIONS AND ANSWERS

1. Which arthropathy presents with central erosions with marginal osteophyte formation, producing a gull-wing appearance to the interphalangeal joints?
   A. Psoriatic arthritis
   B. Reactive arthritis
   C. Erosive osteoarthritis
   D. Calcium pyrophosphate crystal deposition disease

   ANSWER: C. Erosive osteoarthritis characteristically has central erosions, along with marginal osteophyte formation to create a gull-wing appearance of the interphalangeal joint.

2. Enteropathic arthritis when compared to psoriasis is distinguished by which of the following?
   A. Joint space narrowing
   B. Periarticular osteopenia
   C. Large joint involvement
   D. Erosions

   ANSWER: C. Soft-tissue swelling, periarticular osteopenia, joint space narrowing, and osseous erosions are common for both psoriasis and enteropathic arthritis, but the latter has more of a predilection for involvement of larger axial joints.

3. Seronegative arthropathy is often associated with which of the following?
   A. Periostitis
   B. Thickening of the periodontal membrane
   C. Subcutaneous nodules
   D. Hooklike osteophytes

   ANSWER: A. Periostitis is another term for reactive new bone proliferation, a common finding in seronegative arthropathies, as well as enthesitis.

4. Radiographic findings of advanced scapholunate articular collapse are typically found in which crystal deposition disease?
   A. Hemochromatosis
   B. Wilson disease
   C. Gouty arthritis
   D. Pyrophosphate deposition disease

   ANSWER: D. Pyrophosphate deposition disease (also known as calcium pyrophosphate deposition disease or CPPD) commonly affects the lunate articulation, with arthropathy and ligamentous disruption, and subsequent radiographic findings of scapholunate articular collapse (SLAC). The other entities are not usually associated with this radiographic finding.

5. The most common arthropathy to present as hooklike osteophytes of the second and third MCP joints?
   A. Hemachromatosis
   B. Osteoarthritis
   C. Wilson disease
   D. Gout
   E. CPPD

   ANSWER: A. Second and third MCP joint involvement with hooklike osteophytes is a distinctive finding for hemachromatosis. The other choices do produce this distinctive presentation, although this finding can also be seen sometimes with DJD of the dominant hand in manual laborers. CPPD and hemochromatosis are commonly associated, but CPPD by itself typically does not account for the hooklike osteophytes in these joints.

6. A 4-year-old child presents with fever, anemia, lymphadenopathy, and mild polyarticular arthritis. What is the most likely diagnosis?

A. Juvenile ankylosing spondylitis
B. Pauciarticular juvenile rheumatoid arthritis
C. Polyarticular juvenile rheumatoid arthritis
D. Stills disease

ANSWER: D. Still disease is a mild polyarticular arthritis occurring in children younger than 5 years of age. Systemic symptoms include fever, leukocytosis, lymphadenopathy, and anemia. Although the remaining choices can produce arthritis in children, the presentation is typically more severe than that seen with Still disease.

7. Sclerosis of the anterior margin of the vertebral body is most commonly associated with which of the following?
A. Rheumatoid arthritis
B. Psoriatic arthritis
C. Reactive arthritis
D. SLE
E. Ankylosing spondylitis

ANSWER: E. Ankylosing spondylitis is commonly associated with enthesitis of the ligamentous attachment to the vertebral body, termed "shining corner."

8. Which of the following arthropathies is associated with calcification in the cervical spine prevertebral soft tissues?
A. SLE
B. Hydroxyapatite deposition disease
C. Gout
D. Rheumatoid arthritis

ANSWER: B. Hydroxyapatite deposition disease (HADD) is associated with calcific tendonitis of the longus colli muscles, producing calcification in the prevertebral soft tissues. Although SLE is commonly associated with soft-tissue calcifications, this specific involvement is more commonly seen with HADD. Rheumatoid arthritis can affect the cervical spine, but more commonly causes erosive arthropathy, especially at the atlantoaxial articulation.

9. Ulnar subluxation of the MCP joints without significant loss of joint space or destructive arthropathy is most commonly seen with which of the following?
A. CPPD
B. HADD
C. SLE
D. Hemochromatosis
E. Ankylosing spondylitis

ANSWER: C. Articular changes from SLE are primarily derived from soft-tissue derangement. Tendon laxity and rupture allow for subluxation in the absence of significant cartilage and bone derangement.

10. The "pencil-in-cup" deformity is most commonly associated with which of the following?
A. SLE
B. JRA
C. Gout
D. Psoriasis

ANSWER: D. Pencil in cup deformity results from telescoping of bone into a central erosion of the interphalangeal joint. This is most commonly associated with psoriatic arthritis. The other choices do not commonly demonstrate this abnormality.

74 ENDOCRINE AND METABOLIC BONE DISEASE

Michael A. Bruno and Robert Lopez-Ben

OSTEOPOROSIS

Osteoporosis is a systemic skeletal disease characterized by low bone mass and microarchitectural deterioration of bone tissue, with a consequent increase in bone fragility and susceptibility to fracture. It is the most common metabolic disease of bone and one of the most common skeletal disorders worldwide. Osteoporotic fractures are one of the leading causes of morbidity in the elderly after arthritis.

The most common cause for osteoporosis is primary osteoporosis that can be further classified into type I (postmenopausal) and type II (senile or age-related). In these categories, type I affects women after menopause and is associated with wrist fractures and vertebral crush fractures. Type II is age-related, or senile, osteoporosis, affects men and women older than age 70, and is associated with hip fractures and vertebral wedge fractures.

Involutional changes in bone density happen as both sexes age. This is caused by alterations in the normally coordinated functions of the bone remodeling units of osteoclasts and osteoblasts within the skeleton. The resulting mismatch of the rate of bone resorption to bone formation leads to a decrease in bone mass and abnormal bone morphology. Postmenopausal women will have an accelerated phase of bone loss as compared to age-matched men secondary to the absence of the anabolic effects of estrogen. Because women typically achieve a lower peak bone mass than men during bone growth and formation, they are at higher risk of osteoporosis development because of their increased rate of bone loss and lower starting point for bone mass. There is predominantly a loss of trabecular bone and not cortical bone. Although serum calcium and phosphorus levels are typically normal, these patients may have increased urine calcium excretion.

Secondary osteoporosis is because of other etiologies that are not related to menopause or aging. It is important to search for these conditions in order to tailor therapy appropriately. These include endocrine causes like hypogonadism in men (like estrogen, testosterone is also a potent anabolic hormone for bone formation and its deficiency can lead to osteoporosis). Other endocrine causes include hyperparathyroidism, hypercortisolism from functioning adrenal tumors, and hyperthyroidism. Prolonged disuse will lead to generalized bone loss. This can be encountered in space travel but closer to earth is seen when patients with chronic illness have prolonged bedrest or neurologic deficits that impede ambulation and weightbearing. Nutritional disorders (such as malnutrition, vitamin D deficiency, scurvy, and alcoholism) and certain medications (predominantly corticosteroids but also anticonvulsants and heparin) can lead to abnormal bone mass and morphology. Congenital causes include osteogenesis imperfecta, homocystinuria, Marfan syndrome, and Gaucher disease.

Osteoporosis is typically asymptomatic but these patients have increased risk of fractures that can occur without significant preceding trauma (bone fragility fractures). Patients may present with a painful fracture or a progressive kyphosis from loss of height because of multiple vertebral compression fractures. Radiographs will show only advanced disease, as greater than 30% to 50% of bone mass needs to be lost to become detected by this technique. There may be cortical thinning and prominence of weight-bearing trabecula present, especially in the hip. Typical vertebral compression fractures are classified as anterior wedging, biconcave endplates, and posterior wedging fracture patterns. MRI is helpful in distinguishing osteoporotic compression fractures from other pathologic fractures because of tumor replacement of the marrow.

Evaluation of bone densitometry is typically done with dual x-ray absorptiometry (DXA). Usually, central areas of bone mineral density (BMD) measurement including the lumbar spine and hip are performed, although peripheral areas like the wrist can also be measured. Other less commonly used methods include quantitative CT and quantitative ultrasound. These BMD measurements are compared to the sex-matched population of young adults at their estimated peak bone mass. A T-score is calculated as the number of standard deviations of the BMD measurements from that young adult mean, which is a good predictor of relative fracture risk when less than 2.5 and is used to diagnose osteoporosis. A "Z" score is also generated when BMD of the patient is compared to a reference database of BMD from sex and age-matched individuals. This "Z" score helps determine if there are secondary causes of osteoporosis present.

The WHO system is the most often used BMD criteria for the densitometric diagnosis of osteoporosis at central sites. Categories are:

Normal: BMD or bone mineral content (BMC) not more than 1 SD below the young adult mean (T-score above −1).

Osteopenia (or low bone mass): BMD or BMC between 1 and 2.5 SD below young adult mean (T-score between −1 and −2.5).

Osteoporosis: BMD or BMC 2.5 SD or more below the young adult mean (T-score at/or below −2.5).

Severe osteoporosis (or established osteoporosis): BMD or BMC 2.5 SD or more below the young adult mean in the presence of one or more insufficiency (i.e., fragility) fractures.

Assessment of fracture risk is possible with densitometry measurements as bone strength correlates with BMD. Each standard deviation decrease in BMD is associated with a 1.5 to 3.0 fold increase in risk of future fracture. Pharmacological therapy including bisphosphonates, estrogen, or selective estrogen receptor modulators has been shown to be effective in preventing future bone loss in this patient population and reducing fracture risk. Therapy can be monitored with DXA, usually performed at 2 year intervals.

DISORDERS OF CALCIUM AND PHOSPHATE METABOLISM

HYPERPARATHYROIDISM

Primary hyperparathyroidism is characterized by the excessive, unregulated excretion of parathyroid hormone and is usually secondary to a hyperfunctioning solitary parathyroid adenoma. In 10% to 20% of cases, it is secondary to a diffuse hyperplasia of the parathyroid glands and in less than 1% of cases, it is caused by a parathyroid carcinoma. It is also associated with MEN syndromes 1 and 2. Ectopic secretion of a parathyroid hormonelike protein can also rarely occur in some paraneoplastic syndromes. Transient hyperparathyroidism of the neonate can occur secondary to maternal hyperparathyroidism but will resolve spontaneously after birth. Secondary hyperparathyroidism is usually secondary to chronic renal insufficiency but can also be seen in certain malabsorption states.

Patients with hyperparathyroidism will have elevated serum calcium and decreased serum phosphorus levels.

This is secondary to parathyroid hormone's effects in increasing calcium mobilization from the skeleton via osteoclast activation, increased gastrointestinal reabsorption of calcium (by promoting conversion of vitamin D to the active metabolite, dihydroxyvitamin D), and increased phosphate excretion from the renal tubules.

Because of the increased use of laboratory blood screening, most patients today with primary hyperparathyroidism are asymptomatic. When skeletal changes are present, the most common (but least specific) finding is generalized osteopenia. These patients will have abnormally decreased BMD when measured with DXA, but as opposed to patient with primary osteoporosis, the areas of bone loss will be more substantial at anatomic sites that contain a higher proportion of cortical bone (like the midradius).

Bone resorption at sites of ongoing mechanical stresses are typically present and can be classified as subperiosteal, subligamentous, subchondral, trabecular, endosteal, and intracortical. Hand radiographs will characteristically show subperiosteal bone resorption of the radial aspects of the middle phalanges of the index and middle fingers, although loss of the distal tufts outline is felt to happen earlier in the disease. Skull radiographs will show typical "salt and pepper" patchy bone resorption and/or patchy bone sclerosis. Subchondral bone resorption can be dramatic in the distal clavicles and sacroiliac joints. Resorption of bone from the margins of joints can lead to an "erosive" appearance atypically. Brown tumors (osteoclastomas) are focal well-circumscribed lytic lesions because of accumulation of giant cells and are seen in both primary and secondary hyperparathyroidism, although they are more commonly seen with primary hyperparathyroidism. Similarly, chondrocalcinosis is predominantly seen in primary hyperparathyroidism.

RENAL OSTEODYSTROPHY

Renal osteodystrophy is a term used to describe the abnormal bone metabolism in the setting of chronic renal failure and is a combination of the above effects of parathyroid hyperplasia but with abnormal low vitamin D levels with resultant osteomalacia. These patients will have increased serum phosphate levels, increased parathormone levels (PTH), and diminished dihydroxyvitamin D levels. The spectrum of renal osteodystrophy includes patients, where the hyperparathyroidism effects are predominant (high bone turnover disease) or osteomalacia effects are more prevalent (low bone turnover disease).

Renal osteodystrophy, when compared to primary hyperparathyroidism, shares a lot of the previously described radiographic findings of parathyroid hormone mediated bone resorption. However, it may also show more soft-tissue calcification and osseous "sclerosis" secondary to the abnormal deposition of unmineralized osteoid seams in bone because of osteomalacia. In children, typical changes of rickets may be more prevalent. The "rugger jersey" radiographic appearance of the spine in adults is characteristic; there is excess mineralization of excess osteoid at the end plates and resorption of bone from the midportion of the vertebral body, resulting in a horizontal striped or bandlike appearance (hence the rugby jersey analogy) with dense endplates and a lucent central region. Patients with renal osteodystrophy can also demonstrate "Looser zones" and other manifestations of osteomalacia.

HYPOPARATHYROIDISM

Typically results from a deficiency of parathyroid hormone: usually postsurgical from resection of the parathyroid glands during thyroidectomy. These patients will typically have low serum calcium levels, increased serum phosphate levels, and normal renal function.

The imaging appearance is that of widespread osseous sclerosis. This must be distinguished from osteoblastic metastasis, Paget disease, fluorosis, and renal osteodystrophy. Manifestations in the skull include thickening of the calvarium, hypoplastic teeth with blunted roots, and intracranial calcifications, especially within the basal ganglia (these are also seen in pseudohypoparathyroidism [PHP]). Subcutaneous calcifications can be present as well. In the spine, there may be marked calcification of the longitudinal ligaments, which can mimic the appearance of diffuse idiopathic skeletal hyperostosis (DISH).

PSEUDO AND PSEUDO-PSEUDOHYPOPARATHYROIDISM

PHP is because of abnormal tissue receptors for parathyroid hormone. It is sometimes referred to as Albright's hereditary osteodystrophy. Like in patients with hypoparathyroidism, there will usually be serum hypocalcemia and hyperphosphatemia. The imaging findings in PHP are similar to hypoparathyroidism with marked osseous sclerosis and calcifications. These patients will also show other bony abnormalities like cone-shaped epiphyses, exostoses, and shortening of the metatarsal and metacarpal bones, predominantly the fourth. The latter is a nonspecific finding, which can also be encountered in patients with other disorders like Turner syndrome. Pseudo-pseudohypoparathyroidism

(PPHP) is the normocalcemic form; the two syndromes are otherwise indistinguishable.

RICKETS AND OSTEOMALACIA

Rickets and osteomalacia are encountered when there is impaired mineralization of otherwise normal osteoid matrix and a secondary excess of unmineralized osteoid develops. Rickets is basically the occurrence of osteomalacia in an immature skeleton with decreased mineralization of the growth plate. There are three main causes: nutritional, including vitamin D deficiency from any cause (lack of sunlight, drug side-effect, malabsorption, liver disease), vitamin D-resistant rickets (caused by renal tubular loss of phosphate and also seen in certain oncogenic osteomalacia syndromes), and renal osteodystrophy (secondary or "renal rickets").

The most common imaging finding in a patient with rickets and osteomalacia is generalized osteopenia. Flared metaphyses with widened physeal plates are characteristic of rickets and are most commonly encountered in knee radiographs as the distal femur and proximal tibia growth plates have some of the most rapid rates of bone growth in the child. When encountered in the infant rib costochondral junctions, it can lead to the development of *rachitic rosary.* There is secondary bowing of weakened long bones when chronically present. In older children, slipped capital femoral epiphysis can be seen. In adults with osteomalacia, Looser zones are characteristic insufficiency fractures that can occur bilaterally symmetrical in the proximal femurs concave sides, pubic rami, and scapula.

OTHER ENDOCRINE SYNDROMES

ACROMEGALY

Acromegaly is caused by excess human growth hormone (HGH) secretion, usually because of a pituitary adenoma, with secondary bone and soft-tissue growth. This leads to a direct hormonal stimulation of the growth plates and in the skeletally immature patient will present as pituitary gigantism. In the adult, this can lead to enlargement of the *acral* parts (hands, feet, mandible), which is the source of the term *acromegaly.* Fatigue/lethargy is the most common complaint. Proliferation of articular cartilage can lead to widening of joint spaces because of direct stimulation of chondrocytes by HGH and secondarily to osteoarthritis, when the thick cartilage prevents adequate chondrocyte nutrition. Imaging findings include increased thickness of the heel pad with greater than 21 mm thickness felt by some to be pathognomonic. In the hands, there is marked prominence of the tufts of the terminal phalanges of the fingers and beaklike osteophytes arising from the metacarpal heads. In the spine, there is elongation and widening of the vertebral bodies and this is one of the causes of scalloping of the posterior margins of the vertebral bodies.

THYROID DISEASE

Hyperthyroidism

Excess thyroid hormone secretion will result in both bone resorption and bone formation but bone resorption will be more evident in the patient. This may present as a secondary cause of osteoporosis with secondary insufficiency fractures. Some of the descriptions of hyperthyroid osteoporosis have specifically described cortical striations in the metacarpal bones. Thyroid acropachy in euthyroid patients has been observed after the successful treatment of hyperthyroidism but is also seen in patients with Graves disease and ophthalmopathy. It is polyostotic pattern with asymmetric periosteal new bone formation/thick, shaggy periostitis that can mimic hypertrophic osteoarthropathy. As opposed to hypertrophic osteoarthropathy, soft-tissue swelling and periostitis are mostly in the acral regions—hands and feet, and not in the long bones.

Hypothyroidism

Hypothyroidism in adults can be because of prior surgery or antithyroid medications as well as iodine deficiency. In children, it is associated with marked osseous deformities and delayed skeletal maturation. Imaging findings include epiphyseal deformities, with "fragmented" epiphyses in childhood. Absence of the epiphyses of the distal femur and proximal tibia in infant is also encountered. In the skull, wormian bones can be seen. Vertebral deformities, including bullet-shaped vertebrae and gibbus deformity, are seen in the spine. SCFE can occur, along with other hip deformities. In adults, only generalized osteopenia is seen.

CUSHING SYNDROME

Cushing syndrome results when there is excess corticosteroid. It may be endogenous from adrenal overproduction or exogenous (as in glucocorticoid therapy). Glucocorticoids can decrease calcium absorption, increase calcium secretion, and have direct effects on osteoblasts and osteoclasts. Endogenous causes include ACTH hypersecretion (Cushing disease) and adrenal hyperplasia. Ectopic ACTH secretion (small cell carcinoma of the lung, carcinoid tumors, etc.) can also be present. The principal musculoskeletal manifestation will be secondary osteoporosis and/or osteonecrosis.

PAGET DISEASE

Paget disease is a disease of unknown, presumably viral, etiology that is characterized by abnormal remodeling of bone with secondary enlargement. It affects males slightly more commonly than females and is usually seen in patients older than 40 years of age. Paget disease is usually polyostotic but may be monostotic.

Although often asymptomatic and discovered incidentally, patients with Paget disease may have bone pain at sites of involvement. Bowing deformities of the long bones are typical and pathologic fractures are a known complication, as is deafness secondary to cranial nerve compression from an enlarging skull base or direct involvement of the middle ear ossicles. Most pagetic bone fractures heal normally. Spinal canal narrowing and nerve compression similarly is seen with vertebral or skull base involvement. Premature degenerative joint disease secondary to acquired articular incongruities may develop. Secondary osteosarcomas of bone are an unusual but dreaded complication. This should be evaluated for in the patient with long-standing disease and new pain or new focal areas of bone destruction or soft-tissue mass. MRI can be helpful in this setting to evaluate for marrow signal changes and soft-tissue extensions of secondary sarcomas.

There are usually three sequential radiographic stages, although they may coexist occasionally. The lytic phase is usually seen initially, with geographic lesions with well-demarcated borders that can be "flame-shaped" in the tubular bones. The intermediate stage is a mixed pattern between lytic and sclerotic areas, and, lastly, the sclerotic phase will show progressive enlargement and density of the bone.

The most common site of involvement is the lumbar spine. The so-called ivory vertebra appearance of a single sclerotic vertebral body can also be seen in osteoblastic metastatic disease and lymphoma. One important differentiating aspect of the vertebra affected by Paget disease as compared to other etiologies for ivory vertebra is the expansion in size typically present in Paget disease and not usually seen in metastatic disease. The pelvis is another common site of involvement. When present, cortical thickening of the iliopectineal line is very suggestive. In the skull, the initial round lytic phase is termed osteoporosis circumscripta and is very suggestive of Paget. As sclerotic foci appear with disease progression, these are described as "cotton-wool" spots. Basilar invagination can occur in up to one-third of patients. In the tubular bones, the initial lytic phase begins in the subarticular bone with an advancing "blade of grass" border toward the diaphysis. The exception is the tibia, where the lytic phase may begin in the middle of the diaphysis. In more advanced stages, the bones will appear diffusely sclerotic and enlarged, with both trabecular and cortical thickening present.

SUGGESTED READING

Boutin RD, Sptiz DJ, Newman JS, et al. Complications in paget disease at MR imaging. *Radiology*. 1998;209:641-651.

Consensus Development Conference: diagnosis, prophylaxis, and treatment of osteoporosis. *Am J Med*. 1993;94:646-650.

Finberg, Laurence. Metabolic Bone Disease, e-medicine Specialties (Pediatrics) http://www.emedicine.com/ped/topic2854.htm/ Up-dated Dec. 18, 2003.

Lenchik L, Sartoris DJ. Orthopedic aspects of metabolic bone disease. *Orthop Clin North Am*. 1998;29(1):103-134.

Pitt MJ. Rickets and osteomalacia are still around. *Radiol Clin North Am*. 1991;29:97.

Tigges S, Nance EP, Carpenter WA, et al. Renal osteodystrophy: imaging findings that mimic those of other disorders. *AJR Am J Roentgenol*. 1995;165:143-148.

QUESTIONS AND ANSWERS

1. Which of the following is *not* a cause of secondary osteoporosis?
   A. Postmenopausal
   B. Hypogonadism
   C. Bedrest
   D. Malnutrition

   ANSWER: A. Secondary osteoporosis is because of etiologies that are not related to menopause or aging. Postmenopausal osteoporosis is classified as primary osteoporosis, type I.

2. How much bone loss is necessary to appreciate osteopenia on radiographs?
   A. 10%
   B. 20%–30%
   C. 30%–50%
   D. >75%

   ANSWER: C. Bones appear lucent on radiographs with loss of cortical thickness as well as trabecula. This requires 30% to 50% bone mass loss to be detectable.

3. According to the WHO classification, a person with a T-score of −2.4 is
   A. Normal
   B. Osteopenic
   C. Severe osteopenic
   D. Osteoporotic

ANSWER: B. *Osteopenic* (or low bone mass) is diagnosed on bone densitometry, when the BMD or BMC is between 1 and 2.5 SD below young adult mean (T-score between −1 and −2.5). There is no category labeled severe osteopenia.

4. What is the most common cause of primary hyperparathyroidism?
   A. Parathyroid hyperplasia
   B. MEN type 2
   C. Parathyroid carcinoma
   D. Parathyroid adenoma

   ANSWER: D. The excessive secretion of parathyroid hormone in primary hyperparathyroidism is secondary to a hyperfunctioning solitary parathyroid adenoma in approximately 80% of cases. In 10% to 20% of cases, it is secondary to a diffuse hyperplasia of the parathyroid glands and in less than 1% of cases, it is because of a parathyroid carcinoma. Although MEN syndrome type 2a is associated with parathyroid tumors and hyperparathyroidism (as well as pheochromocytoma and medullary thyroid carcinoma), it is not a common clinical occurrence.

5. Patients with primary hyperparathyroidism will typically have what findings in their blood work?
   A. Decreased parathyroid hormone levels
   B. Increased serum phosphate levels
   C. Decreased vitamin D levels
   D. Increased urine phosphate

   ANSWER: D. Hyperparathyroidism patients will have elevated parathyroid hormone levels and subsequent elevated serum calcium and decreased serum phosphorus levels. Parathyroid hormone increases the renal tubular excretion of phosphate.

6. Which findings are more commonly seen in secondary hyperparathyroidism when compared to primary hyperparathyroidism?
   A. Brown tumors
   B. Chondrocalcinosis
   C. Soft-tissue calcifications
   D. Subperiosteal bone resorption

   ANSWER: C. Brown tumors occur in both primary and secondary hyperparathyroidism but are more commonly encountered in primary hyperparathyroidism. Chondrocalcinosis is usually seen with primary hyperparathyroidism. Subperiosteal bone resorption is typically seen in both. Soft-tissue calcifications are usually seen in secondary hyperparathyroidism because of the increased calcium phosphate product leading to metastatic deposits.

7. The radiographic findings of hypoparathyroidism in the spine resemble what other disease process?
   A. DISH
   B. Renal cell carcinoma metastases
   C. Hypothyroidism
   D. Rheumatoid arthritis

   ANSWER: A. The imaging appearance of hypoparathyroidism is of widespread osseous sclerosis. This must be distinguished from osteoblastic metastasis, Paget disease, and renal osteodystrophy. Patients with renal cell carcinoma metastases typically have osteolytic lesions. Adult patients with hypothyroidism will typically show generalized osteopenia. Patients with rheumatoid arthritis will also show generalized osteopenia. In the spine there may be marked calcification of the longitudinal ligaments resembling DISH.

8. Which of the following is *not* associated with acromegaly?
   A. Fatigue
   B. Thickness of the heel pad
   C. Joint space widening
   D. Acro-osteolysis

   ANSWER: D. Acromegaly is associated with fatigue and increased joint space widening and thickness of the heel pads. In the hands, there is marked prominence of the tufts of the terminal phalanges of the fingers, which is the opposite of acro-osteolysis where there is loss of the tuft.

9. Absence of visualization of the epiphyses of the distal femur and proximal tibia in the infant is associated with which endocrine anomaly?
   A. Cushing disease
   B. Acromegaly
   C. Hyperparathyroidism
   D. Hypothyroidism

   ANSWER: D. Hypothyroidism in the infantile and childhood stages is associated with abnormal epiphyseal development, including fragmented epiphyses in the child and stippled or radiographically inapparent epiphyses in the infants.

10. The lytic phase of Paget disease can begin in the middiaphyses of which bone?
    A. Humerus
    B. Radius
    C. Tibia
    D. Metacarpals

    ANSWER: C. In the tubular bones, the initial lytic phase of Paget disease begins next to a joint in the subarticular bone with an advancing "blade of grass" border toward the diaphysis. The exception is the tibia, where the lytic phase may begin in the middle of the diaphysis.

75 HEMATOPOIETIC AND MISCELLANEOUS MUSCULOSKELETAL DISORDERS

Bhavik N. Patel, Joshua P. Smith, Matthew C. Larrison, and Gregory S. Elliott

HEMATOPOIETIC DISORDERS

Bone marrow is a key component of the hematopoietic system. Disorders of the hematopoietic system, therefore, often exhibit skeletal findings. There is considerable overlap in the appearance of these disorders in part owing to their similar compensatory mechanisms. For example, the "hair-on-end" appearance of the skull is classically discussed with relation to thalassemia and is caused by increased marrow production in the calvarium. However, this hair-on-end appearance is not specific to thalassemia and can be seen in sickle cell disease, hereditary spherocytosis, and Gaucher disease. In the following text, we discuss the most common disorders of the hematopoietic system, which exhibit radiologic findings.

SICKLE CELL DISEASE

Sickle cell trait occurs in approximately 7% of African Americans, and sickle cell anemia is estimated to occur in 0.3% to 1.3% of African Americans. Clinical presentation most commonly involves a painful "crisis" that can begin at age 2 to 3 years. One-third of patients present with dactylitis, or "hand-foot" syndrome. Dactylitis most commonly begins at ages 6 months to 2 years and is said to be a complication of small vessel occlusion. Nonmusculoskeletal imaging findings include cholelithiasis (or evidence of cholecystectomy), cardiomegaly, splenomegaly (heterozygous disease), or autosplenectomy with dense, calcified spleen (homozygous disease). Musculoskeletal imaging findings relate to complications of marrow hyperplasia, bone infarction, infection, and complications of treatment. Patients with sickle cell disease are prone to develop osteomyelitis, classically associated with *Salmonella*, but more commonly caused by staphylococci.

Radiographic findings include marrow hyperplasia in the skull that yields thickening of the diploic space with thin inner and outer tables. The "hair-on-end" periosteal new bone formation is more often seen with thalassemia. "Lincoln-log" or "H-type" vertebral bodies describe the shape of vertebral bodies as demonstrated in the lateral view. Osteonecrosis of the epiphyses is more common in adults than in children and is most commonly seen in the proximal humerus and femur. A bone-within-bone appearance of the long bone diaphyses is caused by diaphyseal infarction. Occasionally, patchy or diffuse osteosclerosis will result from advanced medullary infarction. Osteomyelitis is most common in the long bones and can yield bone abscesses, involucrum formation, and cortical sequestrations.

THALASSEMIA

This group of disorders shares an inherited globin production abnormality. Thalassemia major is the term for the homozygous form and thalassemia minor is the term for the heterozygous form. The major form is significantly more severe. It is most common (and originally described) in those of Mediterranean descent but has been reported in many different populations. Radiographic findings most commonly relate to marrow hyperplasia, but this disorder can also cause growth disturbance as well as pathologic fractures. A "hair-on-end" appearance of the skull is caused by marrow hyperplasia and osseous proliferation of the outer table. Marrow expansion creates an Erlenmeyer flask appearance of the distal femurs, most common in thalassemia. Obliteration of the paranasal sinuses and abnormal facies can result from expansion of the temporal and nasal bones in a child. Marrow hyperplasia leads to diffuse osseous expansion, cortical thinning, and osteopenia. Extramedullary hematopoiesis produces paravertebral, posterior mediastinal, retroperitoneal, and pelvic masses. Osteonecrosis is less common than in sickle cell disease.

HEREDITARY SPHEROCYSTOSIS

Hereditary spherocytosis is an autosomal dominant, inherited disease, most commonly found in those of Northern European descent. Spectrin deficiency causes spherocyte formation, which are trapped in the microcirculation of the spleen, and presents with jaundice and splenomegaly. Radiographic and MR findings are nonspecific showing only bone marrow hyperplasia. Diploic spaces are widened with thinning of the outer table of the cortex.

FANCONI ANEMIA/THROMBOCYTOPENIA ABSENT RADIUS

These two syndromes are often categorized together radiographically as both present with absence or hypoplasia of the radius. Fanconi anemia is characterized by anemia, congential anomalies, and brown pigmentation. Thrombocytopenia absent radius (TAR) consists of thrombocytopenia and often results in hemorrhage and more severe skeletal anomalies. TAR often has an earlier presentation (first few months of life) as compared with Fanconi anemia (age 5–10 years). Radiographic appearance of Fanconi anemia includes anomalies of the radius and radial side of the hand ranging from hypoplasia to absence. It is also associated with short stature, developmental hip dysplasia, and renal abnormalities. TAR exhibits bilateral absence of the radius often with hypoplastic ulnae. Absent or small thumbs in Fanconi anemia help differentiate it from TAR. Holt-Oram is a genetic disease that can also present with an absent or small radius.

MYELOFIBROSIS

Marrow replacement by fibrotic tissue is usually diagnosed in the middle-aged to elderly population. This idiopathic condition generally has a poor prognosis. Fibrosis of the bone marrow begins in the locations of active hematopoiesis in adults (spine, pelvis). Compensatory marrow hematopoiesis is then found in the long bones or extramedullary location, but long bones eventually exhibit medullary fibrosis as well. Radiographic findings include osteosclerosis in the axial skeleton and proximal long bones. Prior to osteosclerosis, osteoporosis is demonstrated. Extramedullary hematopoiesis can yield splenomegaly and paraspinal masses. On bone scintigraphy, the resulting diffuse skeletal uptake is one of the causes of a "superscan."

MISCELLANEOUS DISORDERS

PYKNODYSOSTOSIS

Pyknodysostosis is a congenital disorder of osteoclast activity which results in deficient bone resorption. Sclerosis of long bones with transverse fractures is also seen. Phenotypically, there are short statures (vertebral segmentation anomalies), shortened hands, and hypoplastic nails. Hypoplasia or aplasia of the distal tufts can also be seen.

OSTEOPOIKILOSIS

Osteopoikilosis is an autosomal dominant, asymptomatic disorder that results in multiple sclerotic foci throughout the skeleton, predominately in a periarticular distribution in long bones, but also involving the hands, feet, scapula, and pelvis. The sclerotic foci are small, typically well circumscribed, round, or ovoid lesions, somewhat symmetrically distributed. Symmetric distribution helps differentiate it from other disease processes, such as tuberous sclerosis, mastocytosis, or osteoblastic metastases. The lesions may involute or grow on serial radiographs, but do not demonstrate uptake increase on MDP bone scans. They are pathologically similar to bone islands or enostoses. Like bone islands, they can also have thorny spiculations that blend into the surrounding trabeculae. This disorder has been associated with other sclerosing diseases such as melorheostosis.

MELORHEOSTOSIS

Melorheostosis is another sclerosing disease that results in cortical thickening of the long bones, described as "wavy hyperostosis." Cortical expansion can encroach on the medullary cavity and has a characteristic description of "dripping candle wax" on radiography. This often affects only one side of the bone, involving the periosteum as well as endosteum. The disease can be painful, resulting in contracture, deformities, limb shortening, and circulatory problems. It typically affects a single limb or ray, usually in the lower extremity. This can be associated with other sclerosing diseases such as osteopoikilosis or osteopetrosis. Periarticular soft-tissue calcifications can be seen. Unlike osteopoikilosis, this entity can demonstrate increased uptake on MDP bone scintigraphy.

TARSAL COALITIONS

Tarsal coalitions are ankylosis of the tarsal bones which are most commonly congenital, but can be secondary to trauma/surgery/inflammatory arthropathy. Tarsal coalitions can be osseous, cartilaginous, or fibrous. Classically, the incidence is 1%, though may be more prevalent as many cases go undetected. Bilateral lesions are seen in about 25% to 50% of the cases. Coalitions are more common in males.

Coalition occurs most commonly at the talocalcaneal joint than at the calcaneonavicular joint. These are both greater in frequency than talonavicular, calcaneocuboid, and cubonavicular locations.

The first two entities comprise greater than 90% of all cases, with calcaneonavicular being the most likely to be bilateral. There is a familial inheritance pattern, and the disease can be associated with rare musculoskeletal conditions.

Clinically, patients in their second decade present with painful flatfoot in their second decade. Peroneal spasm may accompany the disorder. Talocalcaneal coalition is typically the most symptomatic. Radiographically, the coalitions can be bony, cartilaginous, or fibrous. Talocalcaneal coalition shows dorsal and anterior osteophyte of the talus at the talonavicular joint ("breaking") (differential diagnosis includes diffuse idiopathic skeletal hyperostosis and rheumatoid arthritis) and the "C-sign," where there is continuity between the posterior talus and the calcaneus (sustentaculum tali), forming a C-shape. Radiography is sensitive, but CT is better for talocalcaneal coalitions, especially in cartilaginous or fibrous unions. The coalition most commonly involves the middle facet of the joint. Calcaneonavicular coalitions demonstrate the "anteater sign," where the anterior process of the calcaneus is elongated and is best seen on 45-degree internal oblique radiographs. Bone scintigraphy can be positive at the joints adjacent to the coalitions, as they are subjected to abnormal forces, as well as at the site of coalition itself. MR and/or joint arthrography is used in cases of nonosseous union.

MADELUNG DEFORMITY

The Madelung deformity is a disorder of growth disturbance (though other etiologies often lead to a similar appearance) of the distal radius. The volar and ulnar tilt of the radius causes the wrist and hand translate to volarly, with a protuberant ulna dorsally at the wrist.

The etiologies are many and the resultant differential diagnoses are numerous (Tables 75-1 and 75-2). Madelung deformity is seen more often in females, in part because of the association with Turner syndrome.

PROXIMAL FEMORAL FOCAL DEFICIENCY

This deficiency is a rare, sporadic, congenital, developmental defect (also having association with toxins, particularly thalidomide), and this disease is characterized by complete or partial agenesis of the proximal femur. This results in obvious deformity, with the distal femur normally formed. There are various degrees of severity, and the most mild form is characterized by nonossified cartilage in the proximal femur persisting long past normal, but eventually self-healing through ossification. For this reason, MRI may be the best modality to evaluate this disorder. A dysplastic acetabulum suggests worsening severity, and the shortened femur may pseudoarticulate with the pelvis. The proximal musculature is often normal contributing to the mechanical problems. Despite the name, the abnormality is often associated with other defects in the same limb and can be bilateral in a minority of cases. Treatment consists of a leg-lengthening procedure for mild cases and amputation for more severe cases. A Van Ness rotationplasty can be performed, where the lower leg is rotated 180 degrees and the ankle joint acts as a functional knee. The appearance is fairly pathognomonic, though the mild form could be confused with infantile coxa vara, where the femoral neck angle is less than 120 degrees.

TABLE 75-1 Classification of Madelung Deformity

Posttraumatic
Dysplastic
Genetic (Turner syndrome)
Primary (Idiopathic)

TABLE 75-2 Differential Diagnosis of Madelung Deformity

Enchondromatosis
Multiple hereditary osteochondrous
Mucopolysaccharidoses
Achondroplasia
Dyschondrosteosis (Leri-Weill disease: autosomal dominant, varying penetrance, short-limbed mesomelic dwarf. Involves proximal radius, unlike Madelung deformity)

MUCOPOLYSACCHARIDOSES

These autosomal, recessive disorders (Hunter syndrome is the only exception and is X-linked) are a phenotypically heterogenous group that share a common biochemical abnormality: the inability to break down glycosaminoglycans, found many places throughout the body, but notably in synovial fluid, bones, connective tissue, and tendons. The incomplete breakdown products accumulate in lysosomes, resulting in cellular dysfunction; thus, these are classified as lysosomal storage disorders. Any one of eleven enzymes may be deficient, resulting in different manifestations. The most common are types I, II, II, IV, and VII or Hurler, Hunter, Sanfilippo, Morquio, and Sly syndromes, respectively.

All these diseases have similar manifestation but differ in acuity. Hydrocephalus and mental retardation are often seen, except in Morquio syndrome, where the patients are neurologically normal. Peripheral nerve root compression, corneal abnormalities, and hearing loss are common phenotypic features. Phenotypic appearance includes coarse facial features, coxa vara, hypoplastic odontoid, oar-shaped ribs, and shortened long bones.

SARCOID

Sarcoid is a systemic, immune disorder affecting various organ systems, including the musculoskeletal system. Its exact cause is unknown, and it commonly affects young and middle-aged patients with a higher predilection for African Americans. Diagnosis is made by clinical, radiologic, and histologic findings.

Musculoskeletal involvement of sarcoid is seen with generalized disease. Joint involvement is more common, and rare involvement of muscles and bones typically indicates a prolonged or chronic disease state. Involvement of joints, most commonly knees, ankles, elbows, proximal interphalangeal joints, and wrists, usually presents as inflammatory arthralgia. Articular involvement may manifest as an acute or chronic polyarthritis. Arthralgia in the acute pattern is a result of the effects of inflammatory cytokines on the joints and not as a result of granulomatous change. Tenosynovitis and joint effusion may be detected on ultrasonography. Acute polyarthritis with periarticular ankle joint involvement can be seen as a part of Löfgren syndrome, along with mediastinal lymphadenopathy and erythema nodosum. Granulomatous arthritis with synovitis leading to irreversible joint damage may be seen in the chronic pattern. Acute and chronic sarcoid arthropathy is largely a clinical diagnosis as radiologic evidence of joint involvement is rarely seen.

Skeletal muscle involvement may be of the myopathic or nodular type. Myopathic types have nonspecific findings of symmetric proximal muscle atrophy with fat replacement. They may show hyperintensity on T2-weighted MRI. Sarcoid nodules usually manifest as multiple, bilateral focal intramuscular masses commonly in the lower extremities. They have a characteristic "dark star" appearance on MRI as the central fibrosis appears hypointense on all sequences and the peripheral area of granuloma appears hyperintense on T2-weighted images.

Lesions involving the skeleton are multiple and commonly seen in the hands and feet. Nuclear scintigraphic findings are positive and often precede radiographic manifestations. A combination of cystlike radiolucencies, lacelike honeycomb appearance, bony lytic lesions, and tenosynovitis is diagnostic.

RADIATION-INDUCED INJURY

Radiation-induced injury to the bone may occur as a result of radiation therapy to a metastatic bone lesion or secondarily from inclusion in a radiation field for treatment of adjacent cancer. Radiation effects on the bone include growth arrest, scoliosis, osteonecrosis, and neoplasm formation.

Direct chondrocyte injury and injury to the physeal blood vessels from radiation can lead to growth arrest. The epiphysis is the most sensitive to radiation effects, with growth disturbances seen with a total of 20 Gy; the diaphysis, however, is more resistant. Damage to the epiphysis may increase the risk of plate trauma and slipped capital femoral epiphysis. Injury to the metaphysis may lead to bowing, fraying, and sclerosis. When an entire bone is exposed, shaft narrowing and decrease in size can be seen. In a mature skeleton, growth disturbance is seen in the form of osteonecrosis. The necrosis is dose-dependent with radiation osteitis seen at 30 Gy and necrosis at 50 Gy.

Scoliosis from radiation can be seen in the growing spine, especially in children younger than 2 years of age. More frequent and severe deformities have been associated with asymmetric radiation with changes seen with a total of 10 Gy.

Tumor formation can also manifest secondary to radiation administration. Benign tumors are usually seen if the exposure was prior to 2 years of age, whereas in adults, tumors are likely to be malignant. Osteochondromas are the most common tumors in the pediatric population, while osteosarcoma and fibrosarcoma are seen in adults from radiation exposure.

SCOLIOSIS

Scoliosis is marked by lateral curvature of the spine and vertebral rotation. There are several etiologies of scoliosis (Table 75-3). Approximately 80% of scoliosis cases are of the idiopathic type.

Anteroposterior (AP) and lateral views of the entire spine should be obtained in evaluating for scoliosis. Scoliotic curve is assessed in the anteroposterior view. The most common method of assessment is the Cobb method. First, the type of curvature (thoracic, thoracolumbar, lumbar, major double curve) should be noted followed by the presence of any anomalies and spondylolisthesis or spondylolysis.

NEUROFIBROMATOSIS

Neurofibromatosis 1 (NF1), also known as von Recklinghausen disease, is part of the phakomatosis or neurocutaneous syndromes. It is a result of a defect in

TABLE 75-3 Etiologies of Scoliosis

Nonstructural	Postural, compensatory
Transient	Sciatic, hysterical, inflammatory
Structural	Congenital, neuromuscular, neurofibromatosis, mesenchymal disorders, trauma

chromosome 17 and carries an autosomal dominant pattern of inheritance. Specific findings of NF1 involving the musculoskeletal system include sphenoid dysplasia known as the empty orbit sign, pseudarthrosis, ribbon rib deformity, and bowing of long bones. Radiologic findings of NF1 involving the spine include thoracic kyphoscoliosis, vertebral scalloping, enlarged neural foramina, and a lateral thoracic meningocele.

MARFAN SYNDROME

A connective tissue disorder affecting both sexes, Marfan syndrome is commonly seen in athletes with the classic habitus of tall stature, long extremities, and tapered phalanges. It is an autosomal dominant, inherited disorder; however, sporadic mutations have been reported. It affects many organ systems including ocular, cardiovascular, skeletal, pulmonary, central nervous, dermatologic, and musculoskeletal.

Skeletal abnormalities include tall stature, arachnodactyly, hyperextension, scoliosis, pectus deformity, and osteopenia. Hypermobility and subluxation leading to joint deformity, premature arthritis, asymmetric bone growth, arm span greater than for height, and decreased ratio of upper body segment to lower body segment size can also be seen.

Scoliosis is frequently seen in over one-half of patients, with the right thoracic or major double curve being the most common types of curvature. Unlike idiopathic scoliosis, scoliosis in Marfan syndrome can be seen in both sexes and is typically more severe and progressive, often requiring surgery. Scoliosis and straight back can contribute to cardiopulmonary compromise. Dural ectasia can lead to posterior vertebral body scalloping. Many patients have a widened lumbosacral canal with thinned lamina, pedicles, and erosion of the foramina leading to neurologic symptoms. Over two-thirds of Marfan patients have chest wall deformities with pectus excavatum or carinatum from longitudinal overgrowth of ribs. Severe pectus deformity with or without scoliosis can lead to pulmonary function compromise.

EHLERS-DANLOS SYNDROME

Ehlers-Danlos syndrome consists of a group of inherited disorders in which there is a defect in the structure, production, or processing of collagen or defect in the proteins associated with collagen. Symptoms vary from mild-to-severe and result in weakened connective tissue in the skin, bones, blood vessels, and various organs resulting in the clinical presentation of the disorder.

TABLE 75-4 Osteogenesis Imperfecta

TYPE	FEATURES
I	A mild form in which collagen is of normal quality but insufficient in quantity. Findings include blue-gray sclera, loose joints, fragile bones, and early hearing loss
II	Severe form with insufficient quality and quantity and not compatible with life
III	Quantity of collagen is sufficient but the quality is not leading to bone fractures, deformities, short stature, discolored sclera, loose joints, and hearing loss
IV	Similar to type III but without the progressive nature, discolored sclera, and is less severe
V	Similar clinical features as type IV but has a meshlike appearance of bone on histology. Classic triad consists of exuberant callus, radiopaque band adjacent to growth plates, and radioulnar interosseous membrane calcification
VI	Similar clinical features as type IV but has a fish scale appearance of bone on histology
VII	Involves cartilage associated protein
VIII	Associated with the protein leprecan

The most common type is the hypermobility type. The main clinical manifestation is joint hypermobility. Radiologic findings include soft-tissue calcification in the extremities and periarticular regions, recurrent joint or bursal effusions, knee osteoarthritis with chondrocalcinosis, kyphoscoliosis, spondylolysis, spondylolisthesis, and joint malalignment, subluxation, and dislocation.

OSTEOGENISIS IMPERFECTA

Also known as brittle bone disease, osteogenesis imperfecta (OI) is a connective tissue disorder with an autosomal dominant inheritance. The disorder is characterized by inability to produce collagen or production of improper collagen affecting the skeleton, ligaments, skin, and the sclera. There are eight types with type I being the most common (Table 75-4). Short stature may be seen as a result of defective collagen synthesis as well as a result of fractures. Osteopenia is a common radiographic finding along with fractures and deformity as a result of fractures. Multiple fractures in different stages of healing may be seen, and thus child abuse must be excluded. Classic features of OI are blue sclera, fragile bones, Wormian skull bones, and odontogenesis imperfecta.

OSTEOPETROSIS

Also known as marble bone or Albers-Schonberg disease, osteopetrosis is a rare, inherited disorder resulting from defective osteoclastic activity. Findings include dense but brittle bones, stunted growth, pancytopenia, neural foraminal stenosis, and deafness. Three clinical forms exist: benign type (autosomal dominant), malignant type (autosomal recessive), and carbonic anhydrase II deficiency (type III RTA).

Suggested Readings

Ejindu V et al. Musculoskeletal manifestations of sickle cell disease. *Radiographics*. 2007;27:1005-1021.

Koyama T et al. Radiologic manifestations of sarcoidosis in various organs. *Radiographics*. 2004;24:87-104.

Mitchell MJ, Logan PM. Radiation-induced changes in bone. *Radiographics*. 1998;18:1125-1136.

Newman J, Newberg A. Congenital tarsal coalition: multimodality evaluation with emphasis on CT and MR. *Radiographics*. 2000;20:321-332.

QUESTIONS AND ANSWERS

1. What is the most commonly symptomatic tarsal coalition?
   A. Calcaneonavicular
   B. Talocalcaneal
   C. Talonavicular
   D. Calcaneocuboid
   E. Cubonavicular

   ANSWER: B. Talocalcaneal coalitions are the most commonly painful tarsal coalition, though there is some debate as to which is the most common overall, with different sources citing calcaneonavicular versus talocalcaneal. At any rate, these two are much more common than the other rare choices.

2. Acro-osteolysis, sclerotic bone changes, and transverse fracture of long bones are identified in a patient. What is the most likely diagnosis?
   A. Thermal injury
   B. Reflex sympathetic dystrophy
   C. Pyknodysostosis
   D. Psoriasis
   E. Scleroderma

   ANSWER: C. Acro-osteolysis is seen in all of the above, but transverse fractures of the bone as well as sclerotic bone changes are seen only in pyknodysostosis, reflecting abnormality of the bone matrix itself.

3. Basilar invagination is seen in all of the following *except*:
   A. Chiari I malformation
   B. Osteogenesis imperfecta
   C. Osteopetrosis
   D. Achondroplasia
   E. Rickets

   ANSWER: C. All of the above can be associated with basilar invagination except osteopetrosis. Sclerosis of the skull base is seen osteopetrosis.

4. Posterior scalloping of a vertebral body can be seen in which of the following?
   A. Pyknodysotosis
   B. Marfan syndrome
   C. Osteopetrosis
   D. Rare association with tarsal coalition
   E. Scoliosis

   ANSWER: B. Posterior vertebral body scalloping can be seen in syndromes associated with dural ectasia such as neurofibromatosis, Marfan and Ehlers-Danlos syndromes. Other abnormalities can cause the finding, such as a syrinx or a spinal canal tumor. Congenital disorders associated with this include achondroplasia, the mucopolysaccharidoses, osteogenesis imperfecta, and acromegaly.

5. What is the etiology of osteogenesis imperfecta?
   A. Inability to properly precipitate hydroxyapatite
   B. Delayed enchondral ossification
   C. Defect in collagen synthesis
   D. Deficient cartilage production

   ANSWER: C. The root cause of OI is a defect in type I collagen formation.

6. What is the etiology of the chest wall deformity in Marfan syndrome?
   A. Rib overgrowth
   B. Defect in cartilage production
   C. Underlying pulmonary defect
   D. Hyperlaxity of joints

   ANSWER: A. The chest wall deformity, pectus excavatum, or carinatum is secondary to rib outgrowth. Although these patients have joint hypermobility, this does not contribute to the chest deformity.

7. Findings associated with NF1 include all of the following *except*:
   A. Sphenoid dysplasia
   B. Pseudarthroses
   C. Ribbon rib deformity
   D. Bowing of long bones with Looser lines

   ANSWER: D. While bowing of the long bones can be seen in NF1, Looser lines are not seen and are more commonly associated with rickets The other findings are commonly associated with NF1.

8. What organism is most commonly implicated in osteomyelitis in patients with sickle cell disease?
   A. *Staphylococcus*
   B. *Salmonella*
   C. *Enterobacter*
   D. *Streptococcus*

   ANSWER: A. Thoughs *Salmonella* osteomyelitis is more commonly seen in sickle cell disease patients than in the general population, *Staphylococcus* remains the most common etiology.

9. You are presented with a 5-year-old male child with short stature and radiographs revealing an absent radius and thumb. What is the most likely diagnosis?
   A. Thrombocytopenia absent radius (TAR)
   B. Holt-Oram
   C. Fanconi anemia
   D. Ellis-van Creveld

   ANSWER: C. TAR typically has normal thumbs. Additionally, TAR would typically present at a younger age. Ellis-van Creveld is a syndrome characterized by thoracic dysplasia and death in infancy in 50%.

10. The "hair-on-end" appearance of the calvarium has been reported to occur in all the following *except*:
    A. Sickle cell disease
    B. Thalassemia
    C. Myelofibrosis
    D. Gaucher disease

    ANSWER: C. The "hair-on-end" calvarium is not a specific sign. It is most severe and commonly reported with thalassemia. However, it is also associated with sickle cell disease and Gaucher's disease.

Section 8
BREAST RADIOLOGY

76 BREAST ANATOMY AND IMAGING MODALITIES

Heidi R. Umphrey, Cheryl R. Herman, and David E. Hogg

BREAST ANATOMY

The breasts are located within the superficial fascia of the chest wall. The deep layer of the superficial fascia lies on the posterior surface of the breast parenchyma and rests upon the pectoral fascia of the chest wall that overlies the pectoralis major muscle. There is a distinct space between the deep layer of the superficial fascia and the pectoral fascia, termed the retromammary bursa that contributes to the mobility of the breast. Cords of fibrous connective tissue (Cooper ligaments) extend between the deep layer of the superficial fascia and the dermis of the skin.

The breasts are highly modified apocrine sweat glands, derived from ectodermal elements that develop along embryological lines termed the "milk lines," which extend from the axillary region to the groin. Failure of regression can lead to the development of accessory breast tissue termed polymastia or accessory nipples known as polythelia. Absence of mammary glands is termed amastia. Each breast is composed of 15 to 25 independent secretory units, lobes, which are arranged in a radial pattern around the nipple. The lobes are embedded in adipose tissue that is incompletely subdivided by collagenous septae. A lobe is composed of a main duct system and terminal duct lobular units. Each lobe drains via a main lactiferous duct that has an opening at the nipple and measures 2.0 to 4.5 mm. Just proximal to the opening at the nipple, each main lactiferous duct contains a dilated portion in the subareolar region called a lactiferous sinus. The main lactiferous ducts branch dichotomously eventually forming terminal duct lobular units.

The normal terminal duct lobular unit (TDLU) ranges from 1 to 4 mm in diameter and is composed of an extralobular terminal duct and associated lobule (Fig. 76-1). The extralobular terminal duct is lined by low columnar epithelium with an outer layer of myoepithelial cells and a distinguishing coat of elastic fibers. A lobule is composed of an intralobular terminal duct and ductules (acini). The intralobular terminal duct is lined by a layer of cuboidal epithelium and by an outer layer of myoepithelial cells without surrounding elastic fibers. Ductules are composed of a single layer of cuboidal epithelium with discontinuously interspersed myoepithelial cells. A continuous basement membrane supports the entire glandular epithelium. The lobules are surrounded by intralobular connective tissue. There is cyclic proliferation of TDLU during reproductive age prior to ovulation and cyclic involution during menstruation. TDLU show regression with fatty replacement after menopause. The distinction between the TDLU and larger duct system is essential for understanding breast pathology. The TDLU is the site of origin for ductal carcinoma in situ (DCIS), lobular carcinoma in situ (LCIS), infiltrating ductal carcinoma (IDC), infiltrating lobular

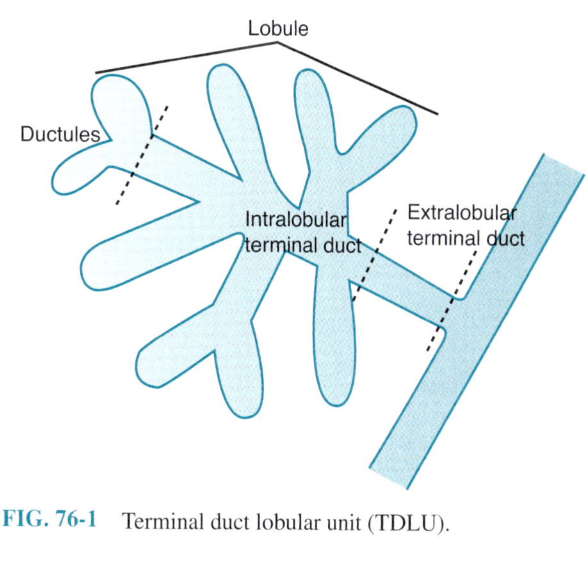

FIG. 76-1 Terminal duct lobular unit (TDLU).

carcinoma (ILC), components of fibrocystic change (microcysts, apocrine metaplasia, adenosis, and epitheliosis), and cysts. The main lactiferous duct and its branches are the origin for intraductal papillomas, papillary neoplasms, and duct ectasia.

BREAST IMAGING MODALITIES

MAMMOGRAPHY

Mammography is primarily a screening tool and will be discussed in detail in the chapter to follow; however, mammographic views in addition to the routine screening views, mediolateral oblique (MLO), and craniocaudal (CC) views have a role in diagnostic imaging. Additional views are obtained to localize a lesion, to characterize a lesion, or to confirm or exclude the presence of a lesion. The location of a lesion is described in a clock-face manner as if the observer is standing in front of the patient (Fig. 76-2).

The straight lateral view is a 90-degree lateral view that can be performed in lateromedial or mediolateral positioning. The location of the lesion is essential when determining a particular view. For example, a lateral lesion would be imaged in the mediolateral view since the lesion would be in closest proximity to the image receptor (film) on this view with compression from the medial aspect. If a lesion is seen on the MLO view only, a true lateral view may be beneficial in triangulating the lesion. A medial lesion moves superiorly on a true lateral view when compared to the MLO view. A lateral lesion moves inferiorly on a true lateral view when compared to the MLO view.

The axillary tail view also known as the Cleopatra view or XCCL view shows the axillary tail (the tail of Spence) of the breast. A cleavage view is a modified CC view that improves visualization of medial and posterior breast tissue.

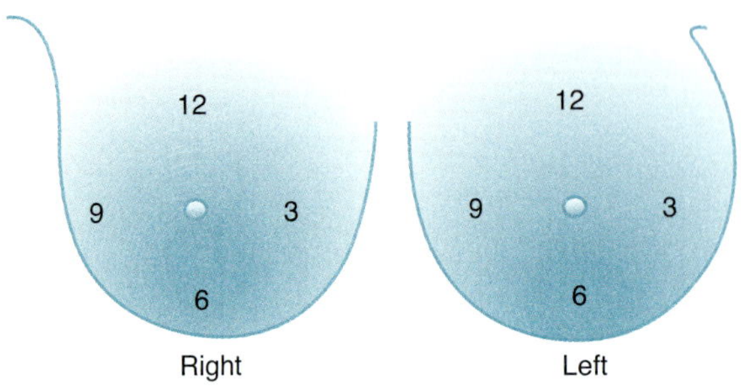

FIG. 76-2 Breast lesions are described in a clock-face manner. The lateral left breast is at the 3-o' clock position and the lateral right breast is at the 9-o' clock position.

Spot compression views maximally compress and immobilize an area of interest; this minimizes superimposition and geometric blurring. It is important to ensure that the area of interest is included in the field of view. Indications for spot compression views include evaluation of questionable mammographic densities, evaluation of masses, inclusion of tissue excluded from routine screening, correction of technical issues, and localizations.

Magnification views are obtained by moving the breast away from the image receptor, thereby increasing object to image receptor distance by generating an air gap. Grids are not utilized because scatter radiation is eliminated in the air gap. As the object to image receptor distance increases, the magnification factor increases. A magnification factor of 1.5× to 1.8× is common. Magnification is associated with a loss of resolution from the increasing penumbra effect, but this is overcome to a certain degree by utilizing a small focal spot of 0.1 mm. However, a small focal spot increases exposure time, and this may lead to increased motion artifact. Exposure may be increased to decrease exposure time. Indications for magnification views include evaluation of masses, evaluation of calcifications, evaluation of architectural distortion, ductography, and specimen imaging.

Rolled views are performed with lateral or medial rotation of the breast and are helpful in establishing the presence of a lesion or determining the location of a lesion. Rolled views can be utilized to move a lesion away from surrounding glandular tissue to allow for better evaluation. Additionally, rolled views may provide localization information if a lesion is seen only in one view. For example, if a lesion is seen only in the CC view and the superior breast is rotated medially with the inferior breast rotated laterally, a superior breast lesion will move medially as opposed to an inferior lesion which would move laterally. Central breast lesions do not move significantly on rolled views.

Tangential views can be helpful in the evaluation of palpable masses, postsurgical changes, postradiation therapy changes, and in the localization of lesions or calcifications to the skin.

BREAST ULTRASOUND

Sonography is a valuable tool in further characterization of mammographic lesions, clinically palpable breast abnormalities, or for guidance during interventional procedures. Minimal equipment requirements include a linear array transducer with a center frequency of 7.5 MHz and broad bandwidth. Higher frequency transducers are becoming more routinely used, resulting in increased near-field resolution. A stand-off pad may also increase visualization of superficial structures in the breast. When scanning, the patient should be in the supine, posterior oblique, or lateral decubitus position with the ipsilateral arm raised above the head for optimal visualization. Findings should be evaluated in two orthogonal planes. Color Doppler imaging can be helpful in assessing lesion vascularity and in evaluating the course of surrounding blood vessels for interventional planning. The use of the vocal fremitus technique may also aid in distinguishing true masses from hypoechoic fat lobules. Sonographic images should be labeled in a consistent manner and must include the patient's name, breast laterality, the clock-face position, scan plane (radial, antiradial, transverse, longitudinal), and the distance of the lesion from the nipple. When lesions are present, images with and without measuring calipers are necessary.

A sonographic examination of breast tissue should demonstrate a thin echogenic skin layer (1–2 mm). Fat lobules are hypoechoic, however, fat in the hila of lymph nodes is echogenic. Fibroglandular tissue is hyperechoic with ducts appearing as hypoechoic cylinders or round structures (depending on scanning plane) and Cooper ligaments as echogenic lines. The deep pectoral fascia is a thick echogenic line that separates the breast from the chest wall. Ribs appear as oval or thick linear shadowing hypoechoic structures in the deep portion of the image. The pectoral muscle appears hypoechoic with parallel echogenic lines.

Benign sonographic characteristics include round or oval shapes with thin, well-defined echogenic margins. Benign lesions are anechoic or homogeneously hyperechoic and may have posterior acoustic enhancement. Malignant characteristics include spiculated margins, taller than wide, angular margins, posterior acoustic shadowing, branching pattern, hypoechogenicity, calcifications, duct extension, and microlobulation.

Current indications for breast ultrasound are (1) assessment of palpable mass, (2) assessment of mammographic mass or density, (3) initial evaluation in symptomatic women 30 years or younger, (4) guidance for interventional procedures, and (5) evaluation of the postoperative breast (including implant assessment). A targeted ultrasound examination is performed after palpation of the area. The lesion can be fixed between two fingers to ensure that a palpated lesion correlates with the ultrasound examination. In young patients, an ultrasound examination is performed initially. However, if there is a suspicious finding or no corresponding sonographic finding, a mammogram may be performed as suspicious microcalcifications and subtle areas of architectural distortion may be detected mammographically. Implant rupture may be identified sonographically and will be further discussed in Chapter 81.

Ultrasound has been proven to be a useful adjunct to mammography especially in the high-risk population. The use of ultrasound as a screening tool is still being investigated. Sensitivities for the detection of nonpalpable cancers are increased from 68% with mammography alone to 88% with the addition of sonography in breast tissue of all densities. Cancers detected by ultrasound examination alone have been shown to be similar in size to small (approximately 1 cm) cancers found mammographically.

MAGNETIC RESONANCE IMAGING OF THE BREAST

Magnetic resonance imaging (MRI) of the breast is performed with a 1.5 Tesla magnet, utilizing a dedicated breast coil. The patient is placed in the prone position with the breasts suspended in the coil. Generally, a diagnostic protocol includes a localization sequence; a T1-weighted sequence, which is valuable in evaluating breast and axillary anatomy; a T2-weighted fat-saturated sequence, which is used for characterization of lesions; and postcontrast dynamic imaging, which is used in calculating the signal intensity curves and evaluating lesion enhancement. Two-dimensional (2D) and three-dimensional (3D) imaging has been utilized. The 2D technique acquires images slice by slice, where 3D imaging acquires a tissue volume that provides high resolution with thin slice thickness and allows for manipulation of images into any plane. Postprocessing can include a subtraction series that serves as an additional fat suppression tool. Maximum intensity projection (MIP) images can help localize lesions within the breast and illustrate their relationship to the skin, nipple, and chest wall. Both the morphology and kinetic curves of lesion enhancement are important features in interpretation. Kinetic analysis observes the immediate uptake of contrast within the lesion and the postcontrast phase. Rapid initial uptake, as compared to surrounding normal breast tissue, with plateau or washout of contrast in the late phase suggests a vascular malignant lesion. A slower initial uptake of contrast with a persistent increase in contrast signal suggests a benign process. Morphologic analysis of lesions by MRI is essential for diagnosis including shape, margins, and distribution. Lesions that are round or oval with smooth margins and homogeneous enhancement tend to be benign. An irregular, spiculated mass with heterogeneous, rim or central enhancement or enhancing internal septations is likely malignant. Ductal involvement may be inferred by linear, ductal, or segmental enhancement patterns. Evaluation of the nipple, skin, pectoral muscle, chest wall, lymph nodes, and visualized lung fields completes the interpretation.

Indications for breast MRI include screening high-risk patients, assessment of extent of ipsilateral disease in newly diagnosed breast cancer patients, assessment of chest wall or pectoralis muscle involvement, evaluation of the contralateral breast, surveillance for residual/recurrent disease after breast conservation surgery, evaluation of response to chemotherapy, further evaluation of mammographic or palpable abnormality, evaluation of axillary carcinoma with unknown primary, and assessment of silicone implant integrity.

A typical imaging protocol for silicone implant rupture would include a localizer sequence, T2-weighted sequence in sagittal and axial planes, and a "silicone bright" STIR with water saturation sequence.

IMAGE-GUIDED BREAST PROCEDURES

CYST ASPIRATION

The indications for cyst aspiration include symptomatic cysts and complex or complicated cysts. Under ultrasound guidance after prep and drape, a needle (22 or 20 gauge) is inserted through the skin adjacent to the transducer and its tip is placed in the center of the cyst. The cyst contents are aspirated. For simple cysts, if they aspirate completely, the fluid may be discarded. Simple cyst fluid may appear straw-colored, yellow, blue, or black. In cases of complex or complicated cysts, bloody aspirate, incomplete aspiration, or intramural nodule, the aspirate is sent for cytology analysis and a core biopsy is obtained from any residual solid component identified. After aspiration, a small bandage may be placed over the entry site and the patient may leave the department without any activity restrictions. Postprocedure complications include pain and bruising. Breast abscesses may also be aspirated if there is poor response to antibiotic therapy and a bacterial culture may provide assistance in selection of antimicrobial therapy or provide acute symptomatic relief. A larger gauge needle may be required (12–14 gauge).

ULTRASOUND CORE NEEDLE BIOPSY

Ultrasound-guided core needle biopsy is a safe, simple, and effective means of sampling any suspicious lesion demonstrable by ultrasound. After ultrasound localization of the lesion, the area is prepped and draped. After local anesthesia (lidocaine with and without epinephrine), a 3-mm dermotomy is made with a scalpel, slightly away from the transducer (approximately 1 cm) to allow for the shortest biopsy needle trajectory that is still parallel to the chest wall. There are two main types of biopsy devices in use: (1) the 14-gauge automated spring-loaded biopsy gun and (2) the 8- or 11-gauge vacuum-assisted directional biopsy device. The biopsy device is then inserted through the dermotomy, to the periphery of the lesion under ultrasound guidance. "Pre-" and "postfire" images are obtained with the needle adjacent to and subsequently through the lesion. Multiple samples are taken, placed in formalin, and sent to pathology for histologic analysis. At the conclusion of the biopsy, a small metallic marker clip is placed in the biopsy site. Postbiopsy mammogram will reveal the lesion's location.

Firm pressure is held at the biopsy site. The dermotomy is approximated with steri-strips or Dermabond. An icepack is placed on the breast and the patient is cautioned not to engage in strenuous activity or heavy lifting for the next 2 days. Complications include pain, bruising, hematoma, and infection. Patients that are taking anticoagulants are asked to discontinue aspirin 1 week before the procedure and to discontinue warfarin 3 to 4 days before the biopsy. In the latter group, laboratory tests for coagulation factors including INR obtained on the day of the procedure may be helpful. The patient may resume anticoagulation 2 days after the biopsy. For patients who are unable to discontinue their prescribed medication and have a crucial need for biopsy, preprocedure application of ice to the area and a smaller gauge biopsy needle, such as an 18-gauge spring loaded device can be utilized. Additionally, fewer passes can be made and firm pressure held for a longer period of time to ensure hemostasis.

The biopsy results are correlated with imaging. If concordant and benign, a 6-month follow-up may be scheduled. If concordant and malignant, a surgical consult is recommended. If the pathology results and the imaging are discordant, surgical excision is recommended to further evaluate possible sampling error.

STEREOTACTIC CORE NEEDLE BIOPSY

The indication for stereotactic core needle biopsy is a lesion that is best seen on mammogram. The majority of these lesions are calcifications; however, asymmetric mammographic densities and subtle isoechoic masses may also fall into this category. The prebiopsy mammogram aids in locating the lesion and determining the approach. The patient is placed prone on the stereotactic table. A single direct view and two angled views separated by 30 degrees are taken. The lesion is marked on the two angled views and its position is calculated. After prep and drape, local anesthesia is injected and a dermotomy is made. Subsequently, the tip of the biopsy needle is inserted through the skin. "Prefire" and "postfire" images are obtained. On the "postfire" view, the collecting trough of the needle should be through the lesion. Multiple samples are taken. Specimen radiographs are taken to demonstrate the targeted calcifications within the biopsy tissue. The sampled tissue is placed in formalin and sent to pathology for histologic assessment. A marker is placed at the biopsy site in the event that surgical excision is recommended. Post-biopsy and postmarker placement stereotactic images are taken demonstrating the biopsy cavity and satisfactory placement of the clip. Patient management after the procedure is the same as discussed under ultrasound-guided biopsy.

MRI-GUIDED CORE NEEDLE BIOPSY

MRI-guided core biopsy is utilized when lesions are identified on MRI but not seen on other modalities. Before the patient is placed prone in the breast coil, the initial MR examination demonstrating the lesion is reviewed carefully to determine nearby landmarks. The patient is then imaged with a fenestrated grid providing slight compression to immobilize the breast during the procedure. After contrast is injected, lesion conspicuity worsens with time, with the best visualization occurring within the first 2 minutes after injection. Once the location of the lesion is determined on postcontrast imaging, the biopsy needle is inserted through the grid and samples are taken, placed in formalin, and sent to pathology for histologic analysis. Free-hand biopsy, without grid placement may also be performed, however, it is more challenging because of the mobility of the breast. A marker is placed in the biopsy site after samples are obtained. Management after the procedure is the same as discussed under ultrasound-guided biopsy.

MARKER PLACEMENT

Marker placement within a lesion is necessary to provide localization of a lesion for subsequent surgery or for correlation with the mammogram. Markers are made of various metals including stainless steel and titanium. They are also composed of Gelfoam,™ collagen or polyethelen glycol, to enable visualization under ultrasound. Since breast MRI is used more often in staging patients prior to lumpectomy, facilities prefer to use markers with fewer artifacts so not to obscure the lesion.

PREOPERATIVE NEEDLE LOCALIZATION

Preoperative needle localization is utilized to identify a nonpalpable lesion for surgical excision. This is commonly performed with mammographic or sonographic guidance; however, free-hand, stereotactic-guided and MRI-guided localizations are also performed.

For mammographic localization, the shortest distance to the lesion and the length of needle necessary are predetermined. For example, if the lesion is in the superior aspect of the breast, placing the patient in the CC projection will be the initial grid image. Using the alphanumeric grid, the lesion coordinates are determined. The needle is placed through the skin, to the lesion. An orthogonal view is then taken, demonstrating the needle has gone through the lesion approximately 1.0 to 1.5 cm past the targeted lesion. The wire is deployed and a unilateral mammogram is taken with the wire in place for intraoperative use.

For sonographic localization, the needle is placed through the lesion and the wire is deployed under real-time sonographic imaging. A unilateral mammogram is obtained for intraoperative use.

The unilateral mammogram consists of CC and straight lateral views with the lesion clearly marked. A postoperative specimen radiograph is taken to confirm the targeted lesion has been excised. Surgical specimen radiographs document excision of targeted lesion, document removal of localization wire, mark the location of the lesion for the pathologist, detect unsuspected lesions, and give information about the proximity of the lesion to the margins. Specimen radiography is performed with compression and magnification. If the targeted lesion is not identified on the specimen radiograph, additional tissue may be obtained if the procedure has not concluded. Alternatively, a postoperative mammogram should be obtained to evaluate for residual lesion.

DUCTOGRAPHY

Ductography is performed to evaluate spontaneous, unilateral discharge from a single duct. Physical examination can elicit the discharge to assist in guiding the cannula. A 30- or 32-gauge, blunt-tipped cannula is inserted into the discharging duct and approximately 0.5 mL of undiluted, iodinated, water-soluble contrast is injected. Magnification views of the subareolar region are taken in orthogonal planes. Rolled views may also be obtained to separate the ducts for better visualization. Filling defects may be due to ductal debris, hematoma, or mass. Air bubbles may also present as filling defects, but they are sharply circumscribed and mobile. Fibrocystic change will display multiple cystic dilations at the ends of ducts, while dilated ducts that resume normal caliber away from the nipple represent duct ectasia. Ductography may be useful in localizing intraductal papillary lesions for surgery.

Suggested Reading

Eklund GW et al. The art of mammographic positioning. *Radiol Clin North Am.* 1992;30:21-53.

Pearson KL et al. Efficacy of step-oblique mammography for confirmation and localization of densities seen on only one standard mammographic view. *AJR Am J Roentgenol.* 2000;174:745-752.

Sickles EA. Practical solutions to common mammographic problems: tailoring the examination. *AJR Am J Roentgenol.* 1988;151:31-39.

QUESTIONS AND ANSWERS

1. A density in the inferior aspect of the MLO view is not seen on the CC view, but the density is seen more inferiorly on a true lateral view. In what quadrant is the density located?
   A. Upper inner
   B. Lower inner
   C. Upper outer
   D. Lower outer

   ANSWER: D. Lower outer. Lateral lesions are seen more inferiorly on a true lateral as compared with an MLO view, whereas medial lesions are seen more superiorly (Medial lesions = muffins rise; lateral lesions = lead sinks).

2. During ultrasound-guided aspiration, the aspirate from a cystic lesion is bloody. What is the next step in patient management?
   A. Discard aspirate and follow up in 1 year.
   B. Send aspirate for cytology, mark lesion, and recommend excisional biopsy.
   C. Discard aspirate and follow up in 6 months.
   D. Send aspirate for microbiologic evaluation and place patient on antibiotics.

   ANSWER: B. Bloody aspirates should be sent for cytology and excisional biopsy is recommended. A marker may be placed to aid in wire localization for excisional biopsy.

3. There is a spiculated mass in the right breast at the 9-o'clock position. In what aspect of the left breast should one place the transducer for evaluation of an equivalent location?
   A. Medial
   B. Superior
   C. Inferior
   D. Lateral

   ANSWER: D. Lesions are described in a clock-face location as if the examiner were facing the patient. Left lateral breast lesions are at 3-o' clock position and right lateral breast lesions are at 9-o' clock position.

4. What is the appropriate position of the localization wire tip relative to the targeted lesion?
   A. Immediately proximal to the lesion
   B. 3 cm past the lesion
   C. 1 to 1.5 cm past the lesion
   D. Within the lesion

   ANSWER: C. The localization wire tip should be 1 to 1.5 cm past the targeted lesion.

5. What is the optimum prefire position for an ultrasound-guided core needle biopsy?
   A. Core biopsy needle entirely through the lesion
   B. Core biopsy needle perpendicular to the chest wall and 5 cm proximal to the lesion
   C. Core biopsy needle perpendicular to the transducer and at the lesion
   D. Core biopsy needle parallel to the chest wall and transducer with core biopsy needle tip just proximal to the lesion

   ANSWER: D. The optimum prefire core needle biopsy position for an ultrasound-guided biopsy is just proximal to the targeted lesion with the needle parallel to both the transducer and the chest wall.

6. A cluster of amorphous calcifications is seen in the medial breast on CC view but not seen on the MLO view. What additional view would help localize the calcifications?
   A. Lateral–medial view
   B. Medial–lateral view
   C. Cleavage view
   D. Spot compression

   ANSWER: A. A lateral medial view would be optimal as the calcifications would be closer to the image receptor and this view would assist in localization of the calcifications. A cleavage view is a modified CC view that improves visualization of medial and posterior breast tissue. A spot compression view may provide additional information about the character of calcifications but would not improve knowledge of calcification localization.

7. Which of the following is an indication for breast MRI?
   A. High-risk patient screening
   B. Evaluation of silicone breast implants
   C. Evaluation of extent of disease
   D. Evaluation of response to neoadjuvant therapy
   E. All of the above

   ANSWER: E. Indications for breast MRI include screening high-risk patients, assessment of extent of ipsilateral disease in newly diagnosed breast cancer patients, assessment of chest wall or pectoralis muscle involvement, evaluation of the contralateral breast, surveillance for residual/recurrent disease after breast conservation surgery, evaluation of response to chemotherapy, further evaluation of mammographic or palpable abnormality, evaluation of axillary carcinoma with unknown primary, and assessment of silicone implant integrity.

8. Which of the following statements is *false*?
   A. Magnification views are obtained by moving the breast away from the image receptor, thereby increasing object to image.
   B. Grids are utilized to eliminate scatter radiation.
   C. A magnification factor of 1.5× to 1.8× is common.
   D. A small focal spot increases exposure time, and this may lead to increased motion artifact.

   ANSWER: B. Grids are not utilized in magnification views because scatter is eliminated through the air gap.

9. The terminal duct lobular unit is the site of origin for all of the following *except:*
   A. Fibrocystic change
   B. Ductal carcinoma in situ
   C. Papillary neoplasm
   D. Infiltrating ductal carcinoma

   ANSWER: C. Papillary neoplasms arise within the main lactiferous duct and its major branches.

10. A round mass is palpated in the axillary tail, which mammographic view is optimal for lesion evaluation?
    A. XCCL view
    B. CC view
    C. Cleavage view
    D. XCCM

    ANSWER: A. An XCCL view optimally images the axillary tail. Cleavage and XCCM views increase visualization of medial breast tissue.

77 BREAST SCREENING AND BREAST IMAGING REPORTING AND DATABASE SYSTEM (BI-RADS) LEXICON

Heidi R. Umphrey, Cheryl R. Herman, and David E. Hogg

BREAST SCREENING

Breast cancer is a leading cause of cancer death, second only to lung cancer in women. Women have a lifetime risk for developing breast cancer of approximately 12.5% (one in eight women). The incidence of breast cancer is approximately 110 cases per 100 000 women. The American Cancer Society (ACS) projects 182 460 new cases of breast cancer in women in 2008 and 1990 cases in men. Several randomized controlled trials have shown a survival benefit for women undergoing screening mammography as compared with control groups. Although mammography has shown proven benefit, it is not a perfect screening test with false-negative rates ranging from 7% to 15%, emphasizing the importance of self-breast examination and annual breast physical examination by a health care professional. Risk factors for breast cancer are listed in Table 77-1.

The ACS recommends annual screening mammography for all women starting at 40 years of age, monthly self-breast examination beginning at 20 years of age,

TABLE 77-1 Risk Factors for Breast Cancer

Gender
Age
Personal or family history of breast cancer
Prior breast biopsy with certain histology (atypical ductal hyperplasia (ADH) or LCIS)
BRCA1 or BRCA2 mutations
History of high-dose chest radiation therapy
Implicated factors
Early menarche
Late menopause
Late first-term pregnancy
Nulliparity
Postmenopausal obesity
Reported associations
Oral contraceptive use
Alcohol intake
Exogenous steroids (after 10 y of use)
Dietary fat intake

and an annual physical breast examination by a health care professional every 3 years (ages 20–39) and annually starting at age 40. The baseline study is no longer part of ACS screening guidelines.

MAMMOGRAPHIC SCREENING

A screening mammography examination usually consists of MLO and CC views of each breast; however, technologists utilize appropriate views to ensure complete imaging of all breast tissue. A marker can be utilized to localize prominent skin lesions. Surgical scars should be documented on an intake history form. In women with breast implants, at least four views are obtained of each breast including CC and MLO views with the implants in view in addition to CC and MLO views with the implants displaced. Usually, kilovolt peak (kVp) ranges from 24 to 32 for molybdenum targets and 26 to 35 kVp for rhodium targets. The average glandular breast tissue dose to an average breast cannot exceed 3 mGy per view for screen–film image receptors. Mammographic images must be labeled appropriately to include patient name, a unique patient identification number, date of examination, radiopaque laterality and projection marker placed closest to the axilla, facility name, facility location, technologist identification, cassette and screen identification number, and mammography unit identification number. Imaging receptors, compression paddles, and cassettes are available in two sizes (18 × 24 and 14 × 30 cm) to accommodate breasts of various sizes.

The angle of obliquity for MLO varies for different patients and is determined by the orientation of the fibers of the pectoralis muscle. The breast tissue in the lateral and inferior quadrants of the breast is mobile, whereas the upper inner breast has little inherent mobility. An adequate MLO view should show the widest aspect of the pectoralis muscle at the axilla, pectoralis muscle extending inferiorly to the level of the nipple, a convex shape to the anterior margin of the pectoralis muscle, an open inframammary fold, and a small amount of upper abdomen. Positioning may be limited because of physical disabilities or absence of the pectoralis muscle termed Poland syndrome.

The pectoralis muscle should be visualized on the CC view in approximately 30% to 40% of patients. Adequate medial breast tissue on the CC view is confirmed by visualization of the pectoralis muscle or cleavage. If neither is seen, the posterior nipple line (PNL) should be measured. The PNL is utilized to determine the adequacy of posterior tissue on a CC view. The distance from the anterior edge of the pectoralis muscle to the nipple is measured. The PNL should be within 1 cm as measured on MLO and CC views. If tissue extends to the posterolateral aspect of the image on the CC view, then an exaggerated craniocaudal (XCCL) view should be considered. The two indications for XCCL views are when tissue extends to the edge of the image on a CC view or when tissue is seen extending over the upper aspect of the pectoralis muscle in the MLO view.

Image quality must be excellent for adequate mammographic screening. Maximal compression is essential for optimal image quality. As breast tissue is thinned, optimal exposure with lower radiation dose and decreased scatter radiation is obtained. Immobilization of breast tissue minimizes geometric blurring; and as tissue is compressed, superimposition is decreased thereby improving lesion conspicuity. The size of the focal spot for screening mammography is 0.3 mm with smaller focal spot of 0.1 mm utilized in magnification mammography as previously discussed in Chapter 76. High-contrast images are essential for the identification of small breast cancers and malignant calcifications. Final contrast is a function of both subject and image receptor contrast. Subject contrast reflects differences in the radiation absorption of tissues being imaged (malignant masses, glandular tissue, calcifications, or fat) and varies by the quality of radiation beam and the amount of scatter radiation. Film contrast is dependent on subject contrast, scatter radiation, film and screen type used, film orientation in cassette, processing, and photographic density and fog. Screen–film cassettes utilized in mammography have a spatial resolution of 20 line pairs/mm. This high resolution is achieved when a single emulsion film is placed emulsion side down against an image-intensifying screen that is facing upward toward the breast in the film cassette. Most of the screen–film systems have relative speeds of 100 to 270 to produce an OD of 1.0 above base plus fog. Hurter and Driffield curves are plots of the film's optical density as a function of the log of exposure and demonstrate the low exposure latitude of screen–film mammography. However, screen–film mammography has higher resolution and higher film contrast when compared to conventional radiography. Glandular tissue needs to be adequately exposed; therefore, the photocell should be positioned correctly under glandular tissue. As discussed screen–film detectors have a limited dynamic range (25:1), and a highly glandular breast can have an exposure latitude exceeding 200:1 resulting in inappropriately exposed regions of the film. Digital detectors have dynamic ranges exceeding 1000:1 yielding an advantage to digital mammography over screen–film mammography. This advantage overcomes the limited resolution of digital mammography, which is on the order of 6 to 8 line pairs/mm.

MAMMOGRAPHY QUALITY STANDARDS ACT

The Mammography Quality Standards Act (MQSA) was enacted by Congress to ensure women quality mammography that enables the detection of early breast cancers. The MQSA was initially implemented in 1992, with final regulations issued in 1997. Under the Food and Drug Administration (FDA), the MQSA certifies breast-imaging facilities as capable of providing quality mammography. A breast-imaging facility must be accredited by an FDA-approved accreditation body, which includes the American College of Radiology and several states. The Veteran's Administration Facilities are exempt from the MQSA, but have their own mammography quality program whose standards are as strict as those required by the MQSA.

In order to become accredited by an FDA-approved accrediting body, the facility must comply with the following regulations. The physicians who read the mammograms, the mammography technologists who perform the studies and the medical physicists who survey the mammographic units must be properly trained and have adequate experience. This is established by maintenance of copies of diplomas, licensure, certificates, numbers of studies read or performed per period of time, and a log of continuing medical education credits. Specifically, MQSA requirements for interpreting physicians are outlined in Table 77-2. Each facility must have and be able to demonstrate an effective quality control program and must be able to keep certain records including the mammogram films, examination reports to the referring physicians, and the lay letters to the patient. The facility must demonstrate its ability to follow up on significant findings on the mammograms and must have a system in place for tracking biopsy findings that result from abnormal studies. Additionally, a medical audit is performed to evaluate accuracy of mammography and interpretation. Information derived for a medical audit includes the following: true-positive rate, true-negative rate, false-negative rate, false-positive rate, sensitivity, specificity, positive predictive value, and cancer detection rate. A true positive is defined as breast cancer diagnosed within 1 year after a biopsy recommendation for an abnormal mammogram. A true negative is no known breast cancer diagnosis within 1 year of a normal mammogram. A false positive is no breast cancer diagnosis within 1 year of a biopsy recommendation for an abnormal mammogram (Breast Screening and Breast Imaging Reporting and Database System [BI-RADS] categories 4 or 5), no breast cancer diagnosis within 1 year of an abnormal mammogram, or biopsy with benign findings within 1 year of a biopsy recommendation for an abnormal mammogram (BI-RADS categories 4 or 5). A false negative is a breast cancer diagnosis within 1 year of a normal mammogram. Sensitivity is defined as the probability of detecting cancer when it is present with a goal of better than 85%. It is the number of true positives divided by the sum of the true positives and false negatives. Sensitivity = TP/(TP + FN). Specificity is defined as the probability of a normal mammogram when there is no breast cancer present with a goal of better than 90%. Specificity = TN/(TN + FP). The PPV of abnormal findings at screening mammogram is the percentage of screening studies with abnormal findings that results in a diagnosis of breast cancer. The PPV of biopsies performed is the percentage of all biopsies performed that resulted in a diagnosis of breast cancer. The PPV of recommendations for biopsy is the percentage of patients with a biopsy recommendation that resulted in a diagnosis of cancer. Cancer detection rate is the number of cancers detected per 1000 patients evaluated with mammography. Cancer detection rate is approximately 6 to 8 per 1000 patients for initial screening examination and 2 to 4 per 1000 patients for repeated screening examinations. Interval breast cancers are described as cancers that become clinically apparent after a negative mammogram but prior to the next screening mammogram.

TABLE 77-2 MQSA Requirements for Interpreting Physicians

Licensure to practice in the state
Certification by an FDA-approved body to certify interpreting physicians or 3 mo full time training in mammographic interpretation, radiation physics, radiation effects, and radiation protection
Completion of 60 h of documented mammography continuing medical education (CME) and 8 h of training in each modality
Read at least 240 examinations in the preceding 6 mo under supervision or have read mammograms under the supervision of a fully qualified physician
Read 960 mammograms over a period of 24 mo
Completion of at least 15 category 1 CME credit in mammography over a 36-mo period, with 6 credits in each modality used

Additionally, the facility must undergo annual inspections by an FDA or State inspector who has completed the required training in the FDA mammography evaluation program. Under the Quality Control requirement, there are many tests that must be performed by the technologist or physicist to ensure optimal performance of equipment and image quality. The schedule of quality control tests performed by the technologists is outlined in Table 77-3.

MAMMOGRAPHIC SCREENING EVALUATION

Evaluation of screening mammograms like any radiologic examination should be performed in a standard

TABLE 77-3 Technologists Quality Control Test Schedule for Film-Screen Mammography

TEST	PERFORMED
Darkroom cleanliness	Daily
Processor QC	Daily
Screen cleanliness	Weekly
Phantom images	Weekly
View box cleanliness and viewing checklist	Monthly
Repeat analysis	Quarterly
Fixer retention	Quarterly
Darkroom fog	Semiannually
Screen–film contact	Semiannually
Compression	Semiannually

TABLE 77-4 BI-RADS Assessment Categories

Category 0	Assessment incomplete, need additional evaluation and/or prior mammograms for comparison
Category 1	Negative
Category 2	Benign finding(s)
Category 3	Probably benign, but initial short interval follow-up of 6 mo with 2-y stability (<2% malignancy)
Category 4	Suspicious abnormality, biopsy should be considered (>2% risk of malignancy)
Category 5	Highly suggestive of malignancy, appropriate action should be taken
Category 6	Known biopsy proven malignancy, appropriate action should be taken

fashion so that one is prepared to consistently identify abnormalities. First, the images should be assessed for overall quality with criteria previously set forth in this chapter. If the images are of appropriate quality, then the images should be evaluated for overall glandular tissue component. Subsequently, magnification viewing should be performed to evaluate for calcifications. The breasts should be divided into thirds with right to left comparison to evaluate for asymmetry or focal lesions. Specific attention should be directed to the posterior breast tissue. Finally, comparison should be made to previous mammographic images to evaluate for interval change.

MAMMOGRAPHY REPORTING BI-RADS LEXICON

The BI-RADS lexicon is a vocabulary used to describe various mammographic findings in a standardized fashion to ensure effective communication, thereby optimizing patient care. Breast composition is characterized as adipose, small, moderate, and dense. Adipose describes a breast that is predominately composed of fat tissue with a less than 25% glandular component. Small breast density implies a 25% to 50% component of glandular tissue. Moderate breast density implies 51% to 75% glandular tissue, and dense breasts are predominately composed of glandular tissue greater than 75%. Masses are space-occupying lesions that are by definition seen in two different views. Masses are further characterized by shape, margin, and density. Calcifications are further characterized as typically benign, suspicious, and higher probability of malignancy with distribution descriptors. A screening and diagnostic mammogram report should include an assessment category (Table 77-4). Screening mammogram report assessments are usually limited to BI-RADS categories 0, 1, or 2. BI-RADS assessment category 0 (additional evaluation needed) is referred to as a call back as the patient will return for additional imaging evaluation. A call back rate of 10% is ideal and will vary with experience. Lesions ascribed a category 3 (probably benign) reportedly have a less than 2% chance of malignancy.

HIGH-RISK BREAST CANCER SCREENING

The ACS describes three strategies to determine women at high risk for breast cancer including evaluation of family history, genetic testing, and review of clinical history. Breast screening in high-risk women is initiated at 30 years of age or 5 years prior to the earliest age of diagnosis of breast cancer in a first-degree relative. Annual MRI screening is recommended in women with a lifetime breast cancer risk of greater than or equal to 25% as predicted by models: women who underwent chest radiation between the ages of 10 and 30 years at dosages above 4 Gy such as for Hodgkin disease, and women who have a hereditary breast cancer syndrome such as Li Fraumeni, Cowden, or Bannayan-Riley-Ruvalcaba. Women with cancer predisposing mutations in either BRCA1 or BRCA2 have an increased risk of both breast and ovarian cancer. Risks of breast cancer in patients with BRCA1 and BRCA2 are 65% and 45% by age 70, respectively. Lobular carcinoma in situ and atypical lobular hyperplasia are both in the spectrum of lobular neoplasia and are associated with an increased risk of the subsequent development of breast cancer with lifetime estimates of increased risk from 10% to 20% (six- to tenfold increased risk). Atypical ductal hyperplasia (ADH) is along the continuum of ductal proliferative lesions ranging from ductal hyperplasia to ADH to ductal carcinoma in situ. ADH is associated with four- to fivefold increased risk of the development of a subsequent invasive breast cancer. The absolute risk of the development of a contralateral breast cancer in women with a personal history of breast cancer is estimated to be 5% to 10% in the 10 years following diagnosis, which is significantly higher than the general population.

SUGGESTED READING

American College of Radiology. *Illustrated Breast Imaging Reporting and Data System (BI-RADS)*. 3rd ed. Reston, VA: American College of Radiology; 1998.

Kuhl CK. MR Imaging for surveillance if women at high familial risk for breast cancer. *Magn Reson Imaging Clin N Am*. 2006;14:391-402.

Linver MN et al. The mammography audit: a primer for the mammography quality standards act (MQSA). *AJR Am J Roentgenol*. 1995;165:19-25.

Sickles EA. Management of probably benign lesions. *Radiol Clin North Am*. 1995;33:1123-1130.

Saslow D et al. American Cancer Society guidelines for breast screening with MRI as an adjunct to mammography. *CA Cancer J Clin*. 2007;57:90-104.

The Federal Register. http://www.fda.gov/cdrh/mammography/ 2009.

QUESTIONS AND ANSWERS

1. Which of the following quality control tests are performed weekly for film–screen mammography?
   A. Darkroom cleanliness
   B. Phantom images
   C. Processor QC
   D. Darkroom fog

   ANSWER: B. Phantom image testing is performed weekly (Table 77-3).

2. Which of the following locations is most likely to show motion artifact?
   A. Medial aspect of the CC view
   B. Central aspect of the CC view
   C. Inferior aspect of the MLO view
   D. Superior aspect of the MLO view

   ANSWER: C. Breast tissue in the inferior and lateral aspects of the breast is mobile. Motion artifact is secondary to inadequate compression, which is more likely to occur in the more mobile aspects of the breast.

3. A patient has a negative screening mammogram and 7 months later develops a palpable mass that is biopsied to reveal infiltrating ductal carcinoma. This is termed a:
   A. False-positive screen
   B. True-positive screen
   C. True-negative screen
   D. False-negative screen

   ANSWER: D. A breast cancer that is diagnosed within a year of a negative screening mammogram is a false negative.

4. All of the following are *true* with respect to film–screen mammography versus conventional radiography, *except*:
   A. Film–screen mammography has higher resolution.
   B. Film–screen mammography has greater exposure latitude.
   C. Film–screen mammography has higher film contrast.
   D. Film–screen mammography utilizes single emulsion film.

   ANSWER: B. Screen–film mammography has narrow exposure latitude. All the other answer choices are correct.

5. What is the expected number of cancers if interpreting 1000 initial screening mammograms?
   A. 20–30
   B. 1–2
   C. 6–10
   D. None

   ANSWER: C. The approximate number of expected breast cancers per 1000 initial screening examinations is 6 to 10. The expected number of breast cancers per 1000 follow-up routine breast screening examination is 2 to 4.

6. Over a year, 100 cancers are identified, 92 of these were identified based on biopsy recommendations from screening mammograms and an additional 8 cancers developed after a negative screening mammogram. What is the sensitivity in this population?
   A. 8%
   B. 80%
   C. 91%
   D. 92%

   ANSWER: D. Sensitivity is defined as a positive test in the presence of true disease. Sensitivity = TP/(TP + FN). TP = 92 and FN = 8. Sensitivity = 92/(92 + 8) = 92/100 = 0.92

7. A spiculated mass is identified in the left upper outer quadrant on screening mammogram. What is the BI-RADS assessment?
   A. BI-RADS 0
   B. BI-RADS 1
   C. BI-RADS 2
   D. BI-RADS 6

   ANSWER: A. BI-RADS assessment categories 0, 1, and 2 are utilized in screening mammography. BI-RADS category 0 is incomplete assessment requiring additional evaluation. This finding should be further evaluated with additional mammographic views, ultrasound and biopsy. BI-RADS category 1 is a negative assessment. BI-RADS 2 assessment is benign finding. BI-RADS 6 assessment designates known malignancy utilized in evaluation of response to neoadjuvant therapy or in second opinion cases.

8. What is the typical kVp used in screening mammography?
   A. 5–15 kVp
   B. 24–30 kVp
   C. 120–140 kVp
   D. 70–90 kVp

   ANSWER: B. Kilovoltage peak (kVp) varies dependent on breast size; however, the typical kVp range for mammography is 24 to 30.

9. Which of the following is a risk factor for development of breast cancer?
   A. Early menopause
   B. Early first-term pregnancy
   C. Late menarche
   D. Cowden syndrome

   ANSWER: D. There are numerous syndromes that increase risk for breast cancer, Cowden, Li Fraumeni, Bannayan-Riley-Ruvalcabe. Early menarche (not late) and late menopause (not early), as well as late first-term pregnancy are also risk factors.

10. The posterior nipple line measures 11 cm on the MLO view. What is an acceptable PNL measurement on the CC view?
   A. 10 cm
   B. 6 cm
   C. 8 cm
   D. 9 cm

   ANSWER: A. The PNL measurements should differ no more than 1 cm when comparing MLO and CC views if there is adequate tissue exposure.

78 EVALUATION OF BREAST MASSES

Heidi R. Umphrey, Cheryl R. Herman, and David E. Hogg

BREAST MASSES

Diagnostic evaluation of breast masses may be initiated from findings discovered on screening mammography or from abnormalities identified on self-examination or on annual physical examination by a health care professional. Each diagnostic evaluation should include a detailed review of patient history with particular attention to presentation and a complete review of patient images. A thorough evaluation is essential to determine the best approach for adequate characterization of breast masses.

Palpable abnormalities should be evaluated with routine mammographic views if the patient is older than 30 years of age and not pregnant. Patients younger than 30 years of age and/or pregnant patients should undergo ultrasound (US) evaluation initially. Masses, architectural distortion, or densities identified on screening mammography should undergo appropriate additional mammographic views and/or US as indicated.

A mass is defined by the BI-RADS lexicon as a space-occupying lesion that is seen in two different projections. The BI-RADS lexicon is employed to describe features of masses including shape, margins, and density. Additional features to consider include associated calcifications, effects on surrounding tissue, architectural distortion, "halo" sign, satellite lesions, multiple lesions, and stability. The characterization of associated calcifications may be helpful in determining benignity or malignancy and are further discussed in Chapter 80. An associated desmoplastic response in adjacent tissue is evidenced mammographically by spiculations and is associated with malignancy. The "halo sign" is a narrowly defined sharp lucency surrounding a mass and is most often associated with benign lesions. Multiplicity is usually associated with benignity; however, breast cancers and metastatic disease may be multifocal and multicentric in nature. Compression, rolled, and magnification views are utilized to further define shape, margins, and density of breast masses. US is useful in further evaluating lesion content and morphology. Additionally, US guidance for core biopsy is a valuable tool.

Mammographic mass shape descriptors include round, oval, lobular, and irregular. The probability of malignancy increases as mass shape progresses from round to irregular. Descriptors for mass margins include circumscribed, microlobulated, obscured, indistinct, and spiculated. The density of a mass may be fat containing or low, equal, or high density as compared to adjacent breast glandular tissue.

US mass shape descriptors include oval, round, and irregular. Margins are described as circumscribed, angular, indistinct, microlobulated, and spiculated. The mass boundary may reveal an abrupt interface or echogenic halo. Internal echogenicity may be anechoic, hyperechoic, complex, isoechoic, or hypoechoic. Posterior acoustic features may be seen and if present may show enhancement, shadowing, or a combination of both. Benign and malignant US features are listed in Table 78-1.

TABLE 78-1 Sonographic Features of Solid Masses

MALIGNANT FEATURES	BENIGN FEATURES
Hypoechoic	Intense homogenous hyperechogenicity
Angulated margins	Four or fewer gentle lobulations
Acoustic shadowing	Thin echogenic pseudocapsule
Microcalcifications	Oval shape
Duct extension	Absence of malignant characteristics
Taller than wide	Parallel to chest wall
Spiculation	
Branch pattern	

When describing masses, the following characteristics should be reported: size and location, mass type and descriptors, presence of associated calcifications, presence of associated findings, interval change, and BI-RADS assessment. Associated findings include nipple retraction and skin thickening. Differential diagnoses for various mass findings are listed in Table 78-2.

BENIGN BREAST MASSES

SKIN LESIONS

Skin masses include nevi, accessory nipples, squamous papillomas, epidermal inclusion (sebaceous) cysts, and neurofibromas. These lesions can often be differentiated from intraparenchymal lesions by partial or complete outline by air. Placement of skin markers and/or tangential views may also be useful in localizing these lesions to the skin.

TABLE 78-2 Differential Diagnoses of Masses

Spiculated masses	
Invasive ductal carcinoma	Invasive lobular carcinoma
Tubular carcinoma	Postbiopsy scar
Radial scar	Fat necrosis
Sclerosing adenosis	
Round masses	
Cysts	Fibroadenoma
Invasive ductal carcinoma	Medullary carcinoma
Mucinous carcinoma	Papillary carcinoma
Metastasis	Phyllodes tumor
Papilloma	Lactating adenoma
Epidermal inclusion cyst	
Solid masses with indistinct margins	
Invasive ductal carcinoma	Invasive lobular carcinoma
Lymphoma	Sarcoma
Focal Fibrosis	Pseudoangiomatous stromal hyperplasia (PASH)
Masses containing fat	
Lymph node	Hamartoma
Oil cyst	Lipoma
Liposarcoma	

EPIDERMAL INCLUSION CYSTS

Epidermal inclusion cysts are common, palpable, well-marginated intradermal lesions that may contain calcifications. Mammographically, these lesions are well circumscribed, localized to the skin on tangential views and may contain lucent centered calcifications. Sonographically, epidermal inclusion cysts are hypoechoic round to lobulated lesions localized to the dermis with well- to partially circumscribed margins. Careful sonographic evaluation may reveal a linear hypoechoic tract to the skin surface. A linear transducer may be beneficial in evaluation because of the superficial location. Inflamed epidermal inclusion cysts may have spiculated margins on mammography.

FAT-CONTAINING LESIONS

Fat-containing lesions in the breast are usually benign; masses may be completely fatty and appear radiolucent or have a mixed density. Fat density masses include lipomas and oil cysts. Mixed density masses include intramammary lymph nodes, hamartomas, fat necrosis, galactoceles, and postoperative or posttraumatic fluid collections.

LIPOMAS

Lipomas can be asymptomatic or present as a palpable mass. Mammographically, a well-circumscribed radiolucent mass with a thin capsule is seen. Sonographically, these well-circumscribed masses are oval to round. Histologically, these lesions are composed of mature adipose tissue with a thin-defined capsule.

OIL CYSTS

Oil cysts can be multiple or solitary. Oil cysts are radiolucent, variable in size, round with a radiodense rim, and evolve over time. Most oil cysts develop mural calcifications resulting in eggshell calcifications. On US, oil cysts are hypoechoic or isoechoic with increased through transmission; they may contain internal echoes. Most are asymptomatic but some may present as palpable lesions.

LYMPH NODES

Intramammary and axillary lymph nodes vary in number, shape, density, and location. Lymph nodes are usually round to oval masses with well-circumscribed margins located in upper outer quadrants. The presence of a fatty hilum seen centrally or peripherally on US or mammography is essential for confirmation. Sonographically, lymph nodes are well-circumscribed, oval hypoechoic masses with an area of hyperechogenicity either centrally or peripherally. Color Doppler can highlight vessels entering this echogenic region also known as the hilum. On MRI, lymph nodes are oval masses with rapid enhancement and washout postcontrast administration; the presence of a fatty hilum on the non–fat-suppressed T1 sequence is important for identification. Benign causes of axillary or intramammary lymphadenopathy include lymphoid hyperplasia, collagen vascular disorders, granulomatous disease, HIV infection, dermatopathic adenopathy, silicone adenopathy, or cat-scratch disease. Interval change is an important tool in the evaluation of lymph nodes particularly in patients with a history of cancer. Interval increase in lymph node size may warrant US-guided biopsy or fine needle aspiration if the patient has a history of malignancy or if the node enlarges by greater than 100%. Spiculated adenopathy may represent extracapsular extension of tumor.

HAMARTOMAS

Hamartomas also termed fibroadenolipomas are characterized by the presence of a pseudocapsule surrounding adipose, glandular, and fibrous elements. Sonographically, these lesions can be distinguished from surrounding breast tissue and are heterogeneous in echotexture. Since these lesions contain glandular tissue, parenchymal changes should always be assessed as elsewhere in the breast.

FAT NECROSIS

Fat necrosis may result from trauma or surgical intervention. In the acute setting, architectural distortion is seen which can be associated with overlying skin thickening and skin retraction. Calcifications associated with fat necrosis are usually dystrophic appearing coarse or lucent centered. Over time, the distortion evolves by decreasing in density, remaining stable to decreasing in size, and occasionally foci may develop into oil cysts. Fat necrosis rarely increases in size or density 1-year posttrauma or surgery, and this change warrants biopsy to exclude malignancy. Sonographic findings include an area of hyperechogenicity that ranges from well- to ill-defined, with associated cystic spaces or small round areas of hypoechogenicity. Fat necrosis has similar imaging features as malignant lesions, which may prompt biopsy in some cases.

SOFT-TISSUE MASSES

Benign soft-tissue density masses include cysts, adenomas, papillomas, fat necrosis, pseudoangiomatous stromal hyperplasia (PASH), focal fibrosis, sclerosing adenosis, abscess, postoperative fluid collections, vascular lesions, granulomatous disease, radial scar, and granular cell tumor.

CYSTS

Cysts are common breast lesions that occur in women of all ages with some predilection in the perimenopausal years. Without hormone replacement therapy, many cysts resolve or decrease in size after menopause. Patients with cysts can present clinically with one or several palpable abnormalities, focal tenderness, or less often nipple discharge. Cysts are frequently noted in asymptomatic patients on screening mammogram. Mammographically, cysts vary in number, laterality, size, and density. Most cysts are well-circumscribed but can have ill-defined or obscured borders. Calcifications can develop within cyst fluid termed milk of calcium or within the walls of cysts. In the absence of milk of calcium, further sonographic evaluation of internal matrix is necessary to exclude solid mass. Sonographically, cysts are well-circumscribed, anechoic lesions with posterior acoustic enhancement and thin edge shadows. Occasionally, internal echoes are seen within cysts that show mobility. Clusters of cysts can be seen in acini with thin septations and may represent the early stage of cyst development. Although, if there is any question concerning the complexity of a lesion, US-guided biopsy is recommended. Usually, simple cysts decrease dramatically after the first biopsy pass with histology revealing fragments of epithelial and apocrine lined cysts. Cyst aspiration is discussed in Chapter 77.

FLUID COLLECTIONS

Other fluid collections within the breast include galactoceles, postoperative or posttraumatic seromas and hematomas, and abscesses. These lesions may be round, oval, or lobular masses with variable cystic components and occasionally solid components. Clinical history and presentation are helpful in the diagnosis. Hematomas are related to trauma, and sonography reveals an echogenic mass with cystic evolution and regression at follow-up.

GALACTOCELES

Galactoceles develop in women who are pregnant or lactating. Fluid-fluid levels are often seen.

ABSCESSES

Mastitis and abscesses are commonly seen during the first 6 weeks of lactation or during weaning, but can affect any woman of any age. Patients present clinically with breast erythema, induration, and pain. Initial treatment is with antibiotics; and if interval improvement is not seen, US may be useful to evaluate for abscess. A complex cystic mass is seen on US. US-guided aspiration can prove therapeutic and diagnostic providing material for microbiologic cultures, which can be useful for antibiotic selection.

FIBROADENOMA

Fibroadenomas are common lesions, particularly in women aging from 20 to 30 years, that show regression postmenopause, resulting in hyalinization with coarse calcifications. Mammographically, these are well-circumscribed, lobulated, or oval masses. Clustered microcalcifications or coarse popcornlike calcifications may be seen within the mass. Sonographically, a well-circumscribed, oval, homogeneous hypoechoic mass is seen that is usually wider than tall or parallel to the skin. On MRI, fibroadenomas have the classic appearance of an enhancing oval or lobulated mass with well-circumscribed borders that contain nonenhancing internal septations with a gradual lesional enhancement pattern. Fibroadenomas are multiple approximately 20% of the time. Complex fibroadenomas contain superimposed fibrocystic changes including cysts greater than 3 mm, sclerosing adenosis, epithelial calcifications, and papillary apocrine changes.

TUBULAR ADENOMAS

Tubular adenomas are seen in women of age 20 to 30 years presenting as palpable mobile masses. Mammographically, a well-circumscribed, round, or oval mass is seen. Sonographic findings include a well-defined, oval, homogeneous, hypoechoic mass. These masses are indistinct from fibroadenomas. Small closely packed tubular structures with scant surrounding stroma are seen microscopically. The tubules are lined by a single layer of epithelial cells and by a discontinuous layer of myoepithelial cells.

LACTATIONAL ADENOMAS

Lactational adenomas typically occur with pregnancy and may present as a palpable mobile mass that exhibits rapid growth. Sonographically, these masses are lobulated, well-circumscribed, hypoechoic masses with posterior acoustic enhancement. Occasionally, fibrous bands or a cyst may be seen within the mass. Aspiration reveals milky fluid.

PHYLLODES TUMOR

Phyllodes tumors are fibroepithelial neoplasms that are rare and usually benign but metastases have been reported in 3% to 12% of patients. The mean age of presentation is 45 years, and most patients present with a palpable mass. Mammographically, a well-circumscribed, oval, or lobulated dense mass is seen. Increased size and a cystic component may suggest a malignant etiology but no definite imaging features differentiate benign from malignant variants of this tumor. Histologically, the epithelial elements of phyllodes tumors are similar to that of fibroadenomas; however, the stromal cells are monoclonal. Histologic criteria used to differentiate cytologically malignant phyllodes tumors include invasive margins, areas of stromal overgrowth, stromal hypercellularity with atypia, and prominent mitotic activity. Wide local excision is required as recurrence rate is high. Metastatic spread occurs hematogenously, not requiring axillary node dissection.

PAPILLOMAS

Solitary papillomas develop in subsegmental ducts. Women usually present with unilateral spontaneous serous or bloody nipple discharge. Bilateral nipple discharge is usually benign and may be endocrine in nature. Ductography (described in Chapter 77) may reveal round filling defects delineating the number and extent of ductal involvement, and ductography may be useful in surgical planning. Mammographic findings can include a dilated subareolar duct, a well-circumscribed, round, or oval mass possibly with an associated cluster of microcalcifications or coarse, curvilinear calcifications. Intraductal lesions can be identified on US with ease if the lesion is more proximal to the nipple or associated with ductal dilation. Papillomas are small friable tumors with an epithelial lining that is contiguous with that of the ducts and is differentiated from ductal hyperplasia by the presence of a fibrovascular core. Multiple papillomas can develop in terminal ducts and are similar histologically to solitary papillomas. Mammographic findings include a lobulated mass, multiple peripheral masses of varying sizes, or clusters of punctate calcifications. US reveals multiple solid masses or a combination of intraductal solid masses. These patients may be at an increased risk for breast cancer but data is limited.

GRANULAR CELL TUMOR

A granular cell tumor is a benign tumor likely originating from Schwann cells. US and mammographic findings are similar; a spiculated round mass is seen.

FIBROSIS

Focal fibrosis is usually seen in premenopausal women presenting with a hard palpable mass. Mammographic findings include an oval or round mass with well-circumscribed to ill-defined margins or less commonly asymmetric density, architectural distortion, or spiculated mass. US findings include a hypoechoic mass with well-circumscribed, lobulated, or ill-defined margins. These lesions are frequently biopsied and the histologic diagnosis is congruent with findings when biopsy targeting was accurate. Histologically, a proliferation of stromal tissue is noted with decreased or obliterated ductal and lobular elements. Etiologies include postinflammatory change, involutional change, or hormonal stimulation of fibroelastic tissue.

GRANULOMATOUS MASTITIS

Granulomatous mastitis is a rare disease affecting young premenopausal women. It has been associated with breast-feeding, oral contraceptive use, and may have a possible autoimmune component. Women may present with breast inflammation, mass, induration, or galactorrhea. The mammographic appearance may be highly variable including asymmetric density, focal asymmetry, ill-defined masses, or the absence of findings. US shows focal areas of hypoechogenicity or ill-defined masses with posterior acoustic shadowing. Evaluation for systemic symptoms should be included in patient history as sarcoid can rarely involve the breast. The malignant imaging findings usually prompt biopsy, which reveals chronic inflammatory cells and granulomas.

BREAST EDEMA

Breast edema is seen as diffuse bilateral or unilateral increased density on mammogram with overlying skin thickening. US imaging may reveal distended hypoechoic dermal lymphatics and subcutaneous edema. Breast edema may have many etiologies and correlation with patient history and additional findings is recommended. For example, breast edema with an enlarged heart and lower extremity edema may be related to congestive heart failure. Diffuse increased breast density may be related to cyclical change associated with hormone replacement therapy but there is no associated skin thickening. Increased breast density may be related to superior vena cava syndrome, but if unilateral changes are present mastitis or inflammatory breast cancer should also be considered.

DIABETIC MASTOPATHY

Diabetic mastopathy is an uncommon entity in premenopausal diabetic women and also in men. Clinically, these patients have a history of juvenile onset insulin-dependent diabetes with other related diabetic complications. Dense tissue is noted mammographically and an intense posterior acoustic shadowing is seen at US. Histologically, dense fibrosis is seen with thick bundles of collagen.

PSEUDOANGIOMATOUS STROMAL HYPERPLASIA (PASH)

PASH can be an incidental finding on breast biopsy or a clinically apparent mass. Symptomatic patients present with a firm, mobile, nontender mass in premenopausal or postmenopausal women on hormone replacement therapy. A noncalcified mass with well- to ill-defined margins is seen mammographically. A hypoechoic mass is noted on US. Microscopically, collagen fibers are noted in an intralobular stroma with slitlike channels that are lined by spindle myofibroblasts that are reactive for CD34 and muscle-specific actin but not factor VIII (an endothelial specific marker).

RADIAL SCARS AND COMPLEX SCLEROSING LESIONS

Radial scars and complex sclerosing lesions are similar histologically differing by size with radial scars being less than 1 cm and complex sclerosing lesions greater than 1 cm. Mammographically, architectural distortion with central fat is seen. The management of these lesions is controversial but most institutions follow a conservative approach with excisional biopsy after core biopsy diagnosis, as adequate sample size is needed to differentiate histologically between radial scar and tubular carcinoma.

GYNECOMASTIA

Gynecomastia is common, occurring in over 50% of men older than 44 years. Gynecomastia is the enlargement of the male breast with secondary branching of the ducts and proliferation of associated stromal tissue. Patients usually present with a palpable subareolar mass. Mammographically, a nodular pattern is characterized by increased tissue focally in the subareolar region. The fibrous pattern shows retroglandular tissue with fibrous extensions projecting into the fatty tissue. Diffuse glandular gynecomastia is similar to a dense glandular pattern seen in the female breast. On US, normal glandular tissue is seen in the subareolar region. Gynecomastia may be idiopathic, secondary to drugs, systemic disorders, estrogen excess, androgen deficiency, or physiologic reasons.

MALIGNANT BREAST MASSES

INVASIVE DUCTAL CARCINOMA

The most common malignant lesion of the breast is invasive ductal carcinoma (IDC) comprising 65% to 75% of breast cancer. Patients may present with a hard, fixed, palpable mass that may cause overlying skin thickening and retraction. If the cancer develops in the subareolar region, nipple retraction may also occur. Infiltration of tumor cells into the dermal lymphatic vessels produces inflammatory skin changes such as pea d'orange. Rarely, patients present with nipple discharge or with an isolated axillary metastasis without evidence of breast lesion. With the advent of screening mammography, patients with IDC are detected prior to clinical presentation. Mammographically, the most common finding is a spiculated mass. However, other mammographic findings include architectural distortion, a round or oval mass with well-circumscribed to ill-defined margins, focal parenchymal asymmetry, or diffuse increased density with associated malignant-type calcifications. The density of malignant breast lesions is highly variable as well but is usually greater than that of surrounding breast parenchyma. It is important to thoroughly evaluate for malignant calcifications associated with IDC, as an extensive intraductal component has been associated with increased recurrence rate, which may be related to incomplete resection. Sonographic findings include an irregular, ill-defined hypoechoic mass with posterior acoustic shadowing that is taller than wide. Extension of tumor into adjacent ducts can also be seen. When evaluating a suspected IDC, evaluation of both breasts and the ipsilateral axilla by US is essential for defining extent of disease and for staging. Patients with breast cancer are at an increased risk for additional lesions. Multicentric lesions are additional lesions within the same breast but in different quadrants, while multifocal lesions are seen within the same quadrant as the original lesion. Bilateral cancers identified within 6 months of the original diagnosis are synchronous lesions. Metachronous lesions are identified in the contralateral breast more than 6 months after the original diagnosis. MRI findings of IDC include an ill-defined mass with rapid enhancement and early washout; however, other enhancement patterns may be seen.

Infiltration of the epidermis of the nipple or areolar complex by malignant cells resulting in an eczematous reaction on physical examination is known as Paget disease.

Male breast cancer represents less than 0.5% of all breast cancers. Risk factors for breast cancer in men include advanced age, previous chest radiation, cryptorchidism, testicular injury, mumps after age 20, Klinefelter syndrome, family history of breast cancer, Jewish descent, and exogenous estrogen use. Patients usually present with a painless hard mass. Mammographic evaluation reveals a retroareolar, noncalcified round to oval mass with indistinct margins. Sonographically, a hypoechoic mass is seen with variable margins and posterior acoustic shadowing. Ipsilateral axillary nodal evaluation and contralateral breast evaluation is essential to evaluate extent of disease and staging.

INVASIVE LOBULAR CARCINOMA

Invasive lobular carcinoma (ILC) represents less than 10% of breast cancers. Bilateral breast involvement is seen in approximately 20% of patients emphasizing the need for contralateral breast evaluation. The mammographic appearance of ILC is variable. Imaging findings include noncalcified spiculated mass, unilateral breast atrophy, asymmetric density, or architectural distortion. Sonographic findings include significant posterior acoustic shadowing in large lesions and hypoechoic masses with angular or spiculated margins. The diffuse nature of this lesion is likely related to the single file infiltration of malignant cells through dense adjacent stroma. On MRI, ILC may exhibit early enhancement with washout in a segmental distribution. MRI may be valuable in evaluating the contralateral breast in patients with ILC.

TUBULAR CARCINOMA

Tubular carcinoma is a well-differentiated, slow growing IDC. Mammographically, a small spiculated, round mass is often seen which may be associated with pleomorphic calcifications. These cancers can be multifocal and bilateral and may show stability over time. Sonographically, a vertically oriented hypoechoic mass with irregular margins is seen with posterior acoustic shadowing. Histologically, these lesions may be difficult to distinguish on core biopsy from sclerosing adenosis and radial scars.

MEDULLARY CARCINOMA

Medullary carcinoma constitutes approximately 2% of breast cancers. Medullary carcinomas present clinically as palpable masses with rapid growth rates in young women usually younger than 50 years of age. Occasionally, these cancers present as interval cancers likely secondary to rapid growth rate. Mammographically, round to oval, moderate density masses are seen with well-circumscribed to ill-defined margins. Sonographic findings include hypoechoic masses with microlobulated to irregular margins and variable amounts of posterior acoustic enhancement. Histologically, malignant epithelial cells with pleomorphic nuclei and high mitotic rates are noted with an associated lymphoplasmacytic infiltrate.

MUCINOUS CARCINOMA

Mucinous carcinoma can present at any age but is more commonly seen in postmenopausal women. Typical mammographic presentation is a round mass with well-circumscribed to ill-defined margins. These lesions grow slowly over time. Sonographically, well-defined hypoechoic to isoechoic lesions are seen with variable amounts of posterior acoustic enhancement or shadowing.

PAPILLARY CARCINOMA

Papillary carcinoma is more common in older patients who present with a palpable mass. The mass is often subareolar in location and skin or nipple retraction may be seen. Mammographic findings include an oval, round, or lobulated mass with well-circumscribed margins. Sonographic findings include an isoechoic mass with microlobulations and variable cystic foci. Histologically, these lesions are difficult to differentiate from benign papillary lesions requiring adequate sampling; however, increased nuclear pleomorphism and increased mitotic rate are seen.

LYMPHOMA

Lymphoma can be primary to the breast when extramammary disease is excluded, but the breast is more often involved secondarily. Patients present with single or multiple well-circumscribed to ill-defined masses on mammogram. Occasionally, diffuse increased breast density may be seen. Calcifications are not usually seen. Axillary nodes may be involved. Burkitt-type lymphoma can present during pregnancy or lactation with bilateral breast involvement. Large B-cell lymphoma shows unilateral involvement in a wider age spectrum.

SARCOMA

Breast sarcomas are rare malignant tumors of stromal cells and include malignant phyllodes tumor, sarcoma, fibrosarcoma, malignant fibrous histiocytoma, carcinosarcoma, angiosarcoma, leiomyosarcoma, and liposarcoma. Patients usually present with a palpable mass. Mammographically, a well-defined, round mass is usually seen. On US, a heterogeneous solid mass is seen with variable posterior acoustic features. Axillary nodes are usually not involved as these lesions spread hematogenously.

METASTATIC DISEASE TO THE BREAST

The most common metastatic lesion to the breast is contralateral breast cancer. Extramammary breast metastases spread hematogenously, and lymphoma, leukemia, melanoma, ovarian, colon, renal, stomach, lung, bladder, and cervical carcinoma metastases have been reported. Mammography reveals solitary to multiple, well-defined, round lesions. US reveals hypoechoic lesions with variable posterior acoustic features.

Suggested Reading

American College of Radiology. Illustrated breast imaging reporting and data system (BI-RADS). 4th ed. Reston, VA: American College of Radiology; 2003.

Berg WA. Lessons from mammographic-histologic correlation of large-core needle breast biopsy. *AJR Am J Roentgenol*. 1996; 16(5):1111-1130.

Harvey JA. Finding early breast cancers: a practical approach. *Radiology*. 2008;248(1):61-76.

Kuhl CK. Concepts for differential diagnosis in breast MR imaging. *Magn Reson Imaging Clin N Am*. 2006;14(3):305-328.

Sabate JM et al. Radiologic evaluation of breast disorders related to pregnancy and lactation. *Radiographics*. 2007;27:S101-S124.

Sickles EA. Breast masses: mammographic evaluation. *Radiology*. 1989;173(2):297-303.

QUESTIONS AND ANSWERS

1. All of the following are *true* regarding tubular carcinoma *except*:
   A. Can present as a spiculated mass on mammography
   B. A well-differentiated slow-growing tumor
   C. Multicentric
   D. Large rapidly growing mass in young women

   ANSWER: D. Tubular carcinoma is a well-differentiated breast cancer that is slow growing and is more often seen in older women. Mammographically, it most commonly presents as a spiculated mass. Tubular carcinoma may be multicentric and bilateral.

2. Which of the following enhancement characteristics is most likely associated with a malignant mass on dynamic breast MRI?
   A. Early enhancement washout
   B. Nonenhancing internal septations
   C. Progressive enhancement with delayed imaging
   D. Slow gradual enhancement

   ANSWER: A. Malignant lesions may show early enhancement with rapid washout or early enhancement that plateaus. Nonenhancing internal septations are seen in fibroadenomas, benign lesions. Slow gradual enhancement is more suggestive of benignity.

3. What pathologic finding is responsible for the mammographic appearance of inflammatory breast cancer?
   A. Tumor cells invading the dermal lymphatics
   B. Inflammatory cells infiltrating the skin
   C. Tumor cells infiltrating epidermis of the nipple
   D. None of the above

   ANSWER: A. Malignant cells invading dermal lymphatics results in overlying skin changes seen in inflammatory breast cancer. Tumor cells infiltrating the epidermis of the nipple are seen in Paget disease.

4. An MRI reveals an oval lesion in the right upper outer breast with increased T1 signal centrally and low signal in this region on T2 fat-saturated images. What is the most likely diagnosis?
   A. Cyst
   B. Fibroadenoma
   C. Lymph node
   D. Invasive ductal carcinoma

   ANSWER: C. The loss of fat signal in the hilum on fat-suppressed sequence is helpful in the diagnosis of lymph node.

5. Which MRI finding is most often associated with breast cysts?
   A. Increased T2 signal
   B. Increased T1 signal
   C. Diffuse enhancement
   D. Decreased T2 signal

   ANSWER: A. Increased T2 signal is seen in most cysts consistent with internal fluid content.

6. What disease is characterized by eczematous skin changes around the nipple secondary to tumor cells infiltrating underlying epidermis?
   A. Inflammatory breast cancer
   B. Paget disease
   C. Lobular carcinoma in situ
   D. Atypical ductal hyperplasia

   ANSWER: B. Paget disease is secondary to infiltration of the areolar epidermis with tumor cells.

7. Which of the following lesions is the *least likely* to present as a round mass?
   A. Cyst
   B. Invasive ductal carcinoma
   C. Invasive lobular carcinoma
   D. Papillary carcinoma

   ANSWER: C. Invasive lobular carcinoma may present as an increased density, architectural distortion, or a spiculated mass.

8. Which of the following is *false* regarding phyllodes tumor?
   A. Mean age of presentation is greater than 60 years of age.
   B. Fibroepithelial tumor
   C. Malignancy is rare but can occur.
   D. Sonographic findings similar to fibroadenomas

ANSWER: A. The mean age of presentation for phyllodes tumors is 45 years.

9. A patient has a palpable mass on physical examination. What is the *least likely* diagnosis?
   A. Hematoma
   B. Cyst
   C. Papillary carcinoma
   D. Lobular carcinoma in situ

   ANSWER: D. LCIS is usually an incidental finding on biopsy that is associated with an increased risk for breast cancer. Hematoma, cyst, and papillary carcinoma can all present as a palpable abnormality.

10. A well-circumscribed solid mass with fat and soft-tissue density is seen in the inferior right breast on mammogram. What is the next step in management?
   A. 3-month follow-up
   B. 6-month follow-up
   C. Excisional biopsy
   D. Routine 1-year screening mammogram

   ANSWER: D. A well-circumscribed mass with both fat and soft-tissue density is a benign lesion. Differential diagnosis includes hamartoma, intramammary lymph node, fat necrosis, galactocele, and lipoma.

79 EVALUATION OF BREAST CALCIFICATIONS

Heidi R. Umphrey, Cheryl R. Herman, and David E. Hogg

INTRODUCTION

Breast calcifications are highly variable and develop secondary to various etiologies. The majority of calcifications seen on screening mammograms are benign in etiology; however, it is essential to identify malignant calcifications to detect early in situ disease. Calcifications conform to the surrounding tissue. For example, calcifications that form within ducts are rodlike following the distribution of the duct. The calcifications will be larger in subsegmental ducts, smaller in terminal ducts, and round or punctate in acini. Proliferative lesions may indent or truncate calcifications resulting in pleomorphism.

Calcifications identified on screening mammography may require additional imaging evaluation. Additional mammographic views are performed to better define the calcifications and identify any associated mass lesion. Magnification views provide additional detail about the form, size and density of calcifications. Distribution is usually evaluated on MLO and CC views. Tangential views may also be of assistance in determining the presence of skin calcifications. A lateral 90-degree view may demonstrate calcium suspended in fluid producing a meniscus or teacup appearance.

The ACR BI-RADS lexicon uses several descriptive terms for calcifications organized by the level of concern for malignancy including typically benign, suspicious, or higher probability for malignancy. The distribution of calcifications is an additional important descriptor in evaluation of breast calcifications. Scattered or diffuse calcifications are distributed throughout the breast randomly. Calcifications scattered in a large volume of breast tissue not conforming to a ductal distribution constitute a regional distribution. Five or more calcifications occupying a volume of less than 1 cm^3 of breast tissue are termed grouped or clustered. Calcifications distributed in a line are suggestive of ductal deposition but may also be vascular calcifications. A segmental distribution of calcifications is suggestive of extensive ductal involvement, which could be secondary to benign or malignant etiologies.

TYPICALLY BENIGN CALCIFICATIONS

Typically benign calcifications include skin, vascular, coarse, popcorn-like, large rodlike, round, lucent-centered, eggshell or rim, milk of calcium, suture, dystrophic, and punctate calcifications.

Skin or dermal calcifications form in dermal sebaceous glands associated with inspissated sebaceous material. Skin calcifications are round, lucent-centered and may be solitary or clustered. A common location for skin calcifications is posteromedial, projecting over the pectoral muscle on the MLO view and medially in the CC view. Tangential views can localize calcifications to the skin. Calcifications may also develop in association with nevi or other skin lesions. High-density products such as zinc oxide or talc may simulate dermal calcifications.

Calcium can be deposited in the media of arterial walls resulting in dense, linear, tram-track calcifications most commonly seen in postmenopausal women with atherosclerotic disease. Arterial calcifications may be associated with diabetes mellitus when seen in younger women. Discontinuous vascular calcifications may simulate ductal carcinoma in situ (DCIS).

Rarely, tortuous calcifications associated with a venous structure may be seen as sequela of Mondor disease or infection. Mondor disease is an uncommon self-limiting thrombophlebitis involving a superficial vein of the breast. Patients usually present with palpable tenderness corresponding to a prominent vein. This condition usually resolves spontaneously with supportive care. Mammograms demonstrate a cordlike density that may be associated with subcutaneous thickening. Ultrasound shows a superficial tubular structure with or without Doppler flow in the acute setting.

Dystrophic calcifications are found in stromal fibrous tissue and are variable in size and shape. They are coarse, dense, large, and irregular with associated areas of lucency. These calcifications are associated with benign conditions including fat necrosis, burns, surgery, radiation therapy, and previous trauma or infection. Dystrophic calcifications can also be seen delineating the fibrous capsules of breast implants.

Popcornlike calcifications are dystrophic calcification forming within the hyalinizing fibrous stroma of a fibroadenoma. These calcifications are dense and coarse seen within an associated mass. Ultrasound may confirm an associated oval mass. In benign fibroadenomas, calcifications are usually superficial in location in counterpoint to central calcifications in necrotic malignancies.

Ductal calcifications are the result of the precipitation of calcium salts in entrapped secretions within subsegmental ducts resulting in calcium casts of dilated ducts. These calcifications are cigar-shaped, coarse, smooth bordered, diffuse, and bilateral. These ductal calcifications are directed toward the nipple and central lucencies may be seen. Differential diagnosis includes duct ectasia, secretory disease, and plasma cell mastitis. Histologically, dilated ducts contain amorphous debris, foamy macrophages, and lipid-laden crystals with an associated plasmacytic infiltrate. Ductal epithelial lining is flattened and atrophic.

Round to punctate tightly clustered calcifications may be within acini. These lobular calcifications, when tightly clustered, may reflect sclerosing adenosis. Perilobular stromal proliferation seen in sclerosing adenosis and fibroadenomas may deform acinar spaces causing pleomorphic calcifications, which can be indistinguishable from DCIS and warrant a biopsy.

Lucent centered or eggshell calcifications can be seen within the walls of cysts, oil cysts, and silicone granulomas. Peripheral calcifications less than 1 mm thick are termed rim or eggshell calcifications. Calcium may also be present as a suspension within microcysts termed milk of calcium. These calcifications show characteristic variability on orthogonal views. Milk of calcium has a smudgy, amorphous appearance on CC views; however, this calcium layers in the dependent aspect of the cysts on a 90-degree lateral or MLO view producing curvilinear calcifications with a meniscus or teacup appearance. Microcysts and milk of calcium can be mutlifocal and bilateral.

Suture calcifications are coarse and can assume the shape of suture material, knots, or loops. These are more frequently seen in irradiated, postsurgical breast.

Parasites are rare but can localize to the breast and appear as calcifications involving the subcutaneous tissue or skeletal muscle. Trichinosis larvae can enter skeletal muscle such as intercostal muscles or the pectoralis muscle and subsequently encyst and calcify. Mammographically, calcified larvae may appear as linear 1 mm calcifications along the pectoralis muscles. Additionally, parasites reported to involve the breast include hydatid disease, shistosomiasis, and loiasis.

HIGHLY SUSPICIOUS CALCIFICATIONS

Linear, casting, branching, and pleomorphic calcifications are highly suspicious and warrant biopsy. Interval change in calcifications may also prompt biopsy. The differential diagnosis for these type calcifications includes DCIS, early stages of fat necrosis, dystrophic calcifications, fibrosis, and autoimmune disorders. There are several types of DCIS including micropapillary, cribriform, and solid types. DCIS grading is based on nuclear pleomorphism, with higher grades associated with the presence of central necrosis or comedo necrosis. The presence of central necrosis or comedo necrosis is associated with higher grade. It is important to evaluate extent of DCIS. Suspicious calcifications are best seen on mammography and stereotactically biopsied unless an associated mass is seen sonographically. It is essential to confirm the presence of targeted calcifications in specimen radiographs. Documentation of the identification of calcifications in the pathology specimen is important. If targeted calcifications are not documented microscopically by the pathologist, polarized microscopy should be performed. Calcifications composed of calcium phosphate appear basophilic on hematoxylin and eosin staining. Calcifications composed of calcium oxalate are not seen on routine hematoxylin and eosin staining but birefringement crystals can be seen under polarized microscopy. If polarized microscopy is negative, then the paraffin blocks containing the residual biopsy tissue should be radiographed to identify calcifications. It is important to determine concordance of biopsy results with imaging findings. Discordant results may reflect sample error and additional tissue should be obtained. DCIS can have a variable appearance on MRI but washout enhancement patterns following a ductal distribution are suspicious and may prompt MRI-guided biopsy.

Suggested Reading

D'Orsi CJ et al. Unusual lesions of the breast. *Radiol Clin North Am.* 1983;21:67-80.

Holland R et al. Microcalcifications associated with ductal carcinoma in situ: mammographic-pathologic correlation. *Semin Diagn Pathol.* 1994;11:181-192.

Kopans DB et al. Dermal deposits mistaken for breast calcifications. *Radiology.* 1983;149:592-94.

Sickles EA. Mammographic detectability of breast microcalcifications. *AJR Am J Roentgenol.* 1982;139:913-918.

Tabar L et al. Early detection of breast cancer: large section and subgross thick-section histologic correlation with mammographic appearances. *Radiographics.* 2007;27:S5-S35.

QUESTIONS AND ANSWERS

1. Which of the following is the highest-grade DCIS?
   A. Solid type with comedo necrosis
   B. Micropapillary
   C. Cribriform
   D. Medullary type

   ANSWER: A. Comedo necrosis is associated with higher-grade DCIS. Micropapillary and cribriform types are usually low to intermediate nuclear grade. There is no medullary-type DCIS.

2. Which BI-RADS lexicon descriptors of calcifications are most associated with malignant pathology?
   A. Milk of calcium
   B. Lucent centered
   C. Popcornlike
   D. Fine linear branching

   ANSWER: D. Fine linear branching or pleomorphic calcifications have a higher probability of malignancy. Milk of calcium is calcium suspended in microcysts that shows variability on orthogonal views. Lucent-centered calcifications are usually benign and can frequently be seen in skin calcifications. Popcornlike calcifications develop within the hyalinizing stroma of a fibroadenoma.

3. Large, coarse rodlike calcifications are seen throughout both breasts without interval change over 2 years. What BI-RADS assessment category is most appropriate?
   A. BI-RADS 6
   B. BI-RADS 2
   C. BI-RADS 4
   D. BI-RADS 5

   ANSWER: B. This is a typical mammographic presentation of secretory disease or plasma cell mastitis, which is benign.

4. Calcifications are seen in the subareolar breast on a CC view and are amorphous or smudgy. A true lateral view demonstrates high-density curvilinear calcifications in the subareolar breast with a teacup appearance. What do these calcifications most likely represent?
   A. DCIS
   B. Tubular carcinoma
   C. LCIS
   D. Microcysts

   ANSWER: D. The calcifications are milk of calcium seen in microcysts.

5. A cluster of pleomorphic calcifications in the left upper outer quadrant is biopsied stereotactically. Biopsy results include LCIS without calcifications. What is the next appropriate step in management?
   A. Request polarizing microscopy to evaluate for calcium phosphate.
   B. Request specimen radiographs to assess for calcifications.
   C. Follow-up 1-year mammogram
   D. Follow-up 6-month mammogram

   ANSWER: B. Perform radiographs of paraffin blocks to assess for calcifications. Polarizing microscopy should be requested to assess for calcium oxalate as calcium phosphate is seen on routine H&E staining.

6. A spiculated mass with associated pleomorphic calcifications is biopsied under US guidance. Biopsy findings are fibrocystic change with associated microcalcifications. What is the next appropriate step in management of this patient?
   A. Follow-up routine mammogram in 1 year
   B. Follow-up 6-month mammogram
   C. Biopsy results are discordant suggesting sampling error; excisional biopsy is recommended.
   D. Breast MRI

   ANSWER: C. Malignant findings at ultrasound and mammogram are discordant with the benign biopsy results, which likely reflect sampling error. Additional tissue is required to exclude malignancy.

7. Punctate clustered calcifications are seen in the left upper inner quadrant that show interval increase in number on screening mammogram. Stereotactic biopsy is performed and fibrocystic changes with birefringent crystals on polarizing microscopy. Which of the following is *true*?
   A. Calcifications are likely composed of calcium oxalate.
   B. US should be performed.
   C. Excisional biopsy is recommended.
   D. No calcifications were identified; paraffin blocks should be radiographed.

ANSWER: A. Calcifications composed of calcium oxalate are not seen on routine hematoxylin and eosin staining like calcium phosphate but require polarizing microscopy. Calcifications composed of calcium oxalate are seen within benign processes such as fibrocystic changes. Imaging findings are concordant with biopsy results.

8. An oval mass is seen in the left lower inner quadrant with associated coarse popcornlike calcifications. What is the most likely diagnosis?
   A. LCIS
   B. ILC
   C. Hyalinized fibroadenoma
   D. IDC

   ANSWER: C. The findings are consistent with hyalinized fibroadenoma.

9. Lucent centered calcifications are newly seen near the areola. What view would be best for localization to the skin?
   A. Cleopatra views
   B. Tangential views
   C. True lateral view
   D. Craniocaudal view

   ANSWER: B. Tangential views are utilized to localize lesions to the skin.

10. What distribution of calcifications is most likely to be benign?
    A. Diffuse
    B. Linear
    C. Clustered
    D. Grouped

    ANSWER: A. Diffuse or scattered calcifications are randomly distributed throughout the breast and are likely benign.

80 THE SURGICALLY ALTERED BREAST

Heidi R. Umphrey, Cheryl R. Herman, and David E. Hogg

BREAST BIOPSY

Advances in image-guided biopsy have decreased sampling error over time, reducing the rates of diagnostic excisional biopsies. Mammographic findings after image-guided needle biopsy may include round to spiculated masses in the immediate postbiopsy period, secondary to seroma, hematoma, or fat necrosis. Over time, minimal residual effect is seen mammographically with the exception of biopsy clip markers. Excisional biopsies contain an increased volume of tissue compared to core needle biopsy. Excisional biopsies are performed when there is discordance between the histologic and mammographic findings, suggesting sampling error, or when core biopsy histology reveals a high-risk lesion for breast cancer, such as atypical ductal hyperplasia and even LCIS at certain institutions. Finally, excisional biopsies may be necessary to further define a pathologic condition or exclude a malignant lesion such as radial scar versus tubular carcinoma. Mammographic findings after excisional biopsy include increased density, spiculated to round masses, architectural distortion, and dystrophic calcifications can be seen. High-density lesions can be further evaluated with US to determine if it is a fluid-filled lesion or solid tissue. Fluid collections may include hematoma, seroma, and abscesses. Many of these changes either resolve or evolve over time. If the mammogram reveals interval increase in size or density of postsurgical findings longer than 1 year after surgery, further evaluation with tissue diagnosis is required.

BREAST CONSERVATION THERAPY

The goal of breast conservation therapy is to achieve adequate local control of breast cancer via lumpectomy and radiation therapy with the additional benefit of a good cosmetic result. Mammographic findings after lumpectomy and radiation therapy are variable and evolve over time. In the acute posttherapy period, mammographic changes include increased edema as manifested by skin thickening and prominent trabeculae, usually seen as increased density. Sonographically, dilated dermal lymphatic, skin thickening, and increased echogenicity are seen. Skin thickening may be seen up to 2 years postradiation therapy. Fat necrosis is seen in the lumpectomy site and evolves over time. Initially, fat necrosis may be seen as a spiculated mass or architectural distortion mammographically. Over time, there may be a decrease in the size of distortion or spiculated mass with possible complete resolution over time. With evolution of fat necrosis, oil cysts or dystrophic calcifications may develop within the biopsy site. Fluid collections are seen frequently in postoperative patients within 4 weeks of lumpectomy. A round or oval mass is usually seen on mammogram with well-defined to spiculated margins, which can have variable densities. Sonographically, complex cystic masses are seen with cystic and solid components. Occasionally, fluid collections are slow to resolve but they usually resolve over 2 years. If the patient is asymptomatic, aspiration is not indicated as many of these collections reaccumulate postaspiration. Follow-up mammography after lumpectomy and radiation therapy varies among institutions. Some protocols require a mammogram immediately before radiation therapy to evaluate for residual calcifications and then perform diagnostic mammography at 6-month intervals for 2 years after breast conservation therapy. However, other facilities may obtain preradiation therapy mammography and instead obtain diagnostic mammograms at 12-month intervals for a longer period of time.

In the first 7 years after breast conservation therapy, recurrences are likely to arise close to the lumpectomy site. After 7 years, recurrences or secondary primary lesions can arise anywhere in the breast. Malignant-type calcifications at a prior lumpectomy site warrant biopsy. Developing masses, increased density, or increased size of distortion within a lumpectomy site also warrant biopsy.

MASTECTOMY

Mastectomy may be performed when there is extensive disease, chest wall involvement, personal choice, or prophylactically. After mastectomy, the chest wall is more easily palpated and recurrences are usually identified on a thorough physical examination. Palpable abnormalities can be further evaluated with US, which can also provide guidance for biopsy if indicated.

BREAST RECONSTRUCTION

Breast reconstruction can be performed at the time of mastectomy. Implants or autologous tissue may be used for reconstruction. Autologous tissue reconstructions are most commonly achieved via a transverse rectus abdominis myocutaneous (TRAM) flap. Mammographic findings after transverse rectus abdominis myocutaneous flap include increased areas of density superiorly and inferiorly. The rectus muscle is seen as a triangular or round density posteriorly. Over time, superior and inferior densities decrease in size. Similar changes of fat necrosis are seen including oil cysts and dystrophic calcifications.

REDUCTION MAMMOPLASTY

Hypertrophic breasts can lead to significant medical as well as psychosocial concerns for women. Medical morbidity includes postural issues, back pain, breast pain, and intertriginous infections at the mammary folds. Mammographic findings, after reduction mammoplasty include altered distribution of glandular tissue, elevation of the nipple, a swirling pattern of tissue inferiorly on MLO views, fibrotic bands in the subareolar region, distortion, oil cysts, and dystrophic calcifications.

BREAST AUGMENTATION

Breast augmentation is performed with saline, silicone, and dual lumen implants. Implants can be placed between the glandular breast tissue and the pectoralis muscle termed prepectoral or subglandular or they may be positioned posterior to the pectoralis muscle termed retropectoral or subpectoral. The type of implant and position of implant can usually be determined by mammography. Saline implants are less radiodense than silicone implants allowing visualization of wrinkles and valves. As foreign bodies, implants incite an inflammatory response that includes fibrosis and calcifications, producing a capsule. Implant rupture may result from trauma or secondary to aging of the implant and breakdown of the implant shell. While implant ruptures may be either intracapsular or extracapsular; most ruptures are intracapsular. Extracapsular implant rupture results from extrusion of the implant contents outside the capsule. When this occurs in a silicone implant, high-density amorphous material can be seen surrounding the implant or focal protrusion of the implant is seen on mammography. In cases of long-standing implant rupture, silicone may be seen extending into the superior chest wall and taken up by axillary lymph nodes. Sonographically, extravasated silicone may be visualized as specular echoes termed "snowstorm" deep to an echogenic line or as a hyperechoic mass. Extracapsular rupture of saline implants results in deflation of the implant, which can usually be determined by physical examination. Intracapsular rupture of an implant is the disruption of the implant shell with containment of the implant contents by the capsule. Intracapsular rupture is best seen on MRI, although US may demonstrate short linear hyperechoic bands in the central anechoic region of the implant, which are known as the "strairstep sign". Fat- and water-saturated series reveal silicone as high signal. Fragments of low signal implant shell are seen floating in the contents of the implant also known as the "linguini sign." Another finding is the "keyhole" sign, which is a single-layer loop of implant envelope within the lumen.

TABLE 80-1 Imaging Findings Associated with Silicone Implant Rupture

MODALITY	INTRACAPSULAR RUPTURE	EXTRACAPSULAR RUPTURE
Mammography	Negative	Silicone in breast tissue
		Silicone in axilla
		Contour deformity of implant
Ultrasound	Stairstep sign	Snowstorm sign
MRI	Linguini sign	Free silicone

This may represent a partial rupture or possible silicone or gel bleed. This must be differentiated form a "radial fold," which is a double-layer loop of envelope protruding into the lumen and represents normal infolding or wrinkling of the implant envelope (Table 80-1).

Suggested Reading

Dershaw DD et al. Mammographic findings after breast cancer treatment with local excision and definitive irradiation. *Radiology*. 1987;164(2):455-461.

Ganott MA et al. Augmentation mammoplasty: normal and abnormal findings with mammography and US. *Radiographics*. 1992;12(2):281-295.

Hogge JP et al. Mammography of autologous myocutaneous flaps. *Radiographics*. 1999;19:S63-S72.

Ikeda DM et al. Silicone breast implant rupture: pitfalls of magnetic resonance imaging and relative efficacies of magnetic resonance, mammography, and ultrasound. *Plast Reconstr Surg*. 1999;104(7):2054-2062.

Mendelson EB. Evaluation of the postoperative breast. *Radiol Clin North Am*. 1992;30(1):107-138.

Sickles EA et al. Mammography of the postsurgical breast. *AJR Am J Roentgenol*. 1981;136(3):585-588.

Steinbach BG et al. Mammography: breast implants–types, complications, and adjacent breast pathology. *Curr Probl Diagn Radiol*. 1993;22(2):39-86.

QUESTIONS AND ANSWERS

1. Which of the following mamographic findings can be seen after reduction mammoplasty?
   A. Dystrophic calcifications
   B. Oil cysts
   C. Elevated nipple
   D. All of the above

   ANSWER: D. All of the statements are true.

2. Extracapsular silicone breast implant rupture can be recognized on US by which of the following?
   A. Keyhole sign
   B. Linguini sign
   C. Snowstorm sign
   D. Highway sign

   ANSWER: C. The snowstorm sign on ultrasound is seen with extracapsular rupture. The linguini sign is low signal implant shell fragments floating in high signal silicone seen on MRI in cases of intracapsular rupture. The "keyhole" sign is a single layer loop of implant envelope within the lumen that may represent a partial rupture or possible silicone or gel bleed.

3. What is a contraindication to breast conservation therapy for newly diagnosed invasive ductal carcinoma (IDC)?
   A. Previous excisional breast biopsy with benign findings
   B. Previous augmentation
   C. Previous reduction mammoplasty
   D. Previous radiation therapy

   ANSWER: D. Previous radiation therapy is a contraindication for breast conservation therapy.

4. Mammography 2 years after right breast conservation therapy for IDC demonstrates interval increased density in the RUO architectural distortion with fine linear and pleomorphic calcifications. What is the BI-RADS assessment?
   A. BI-RADS 0
   B. BI-RADS 1
   C. BI-RADS 2
   D. BI-RADS 3

   ANSWER: A. Interval change in lumpectomy site at 2 years is suspicious for recurrence. Additional magnification views, ultrasound, and core biopsy should be considered.

5. A patient had a right mastectomy 4 years ago for ILC. She now reports a newly palpable mass at the mastectomy site. What is the next appropriate step?
   A. US and physical examination
   B. Mammogram
   C. Follow-up in 6 months
   D. MRI

   ANSWER: A. The most appropriate next step would be to perform a physical examination and targeted US.

6. What is the most common type of breast cancer?
   A. Invasive lobular carcinoma
   B. Invasive ductal carcinoma (IDC)
   C. Tubular carcinoma
   D. Phylloides tumor

   ANSWER: B. IDC is the most common histologic type of breast cancer.

7. The linguini sign of intracapsular silicone breast implant rupture is seen on which imaging modality?
   A. US
   B. MRI
   C. Mammography
   D. All of the above

   ANSWER: B. The Linguini sign is seen on MRI. Intracapsular silicone implant rupture cannot be seen on mammography. Extracapsular rupture of silicone implant is seen as the snowstorm on US.

Section 9
INTERVENTIONAL RADIOLOGY

81 DIAGNOSTIC ARTERIOGRAPHY

Heidi R. Umphrey and
Baljendra S. Kapoor

DIAGNOSTIC ARTERIOGRAPHY

Diagnostic arteriography is an established, safe, and accurate method of evaluating vascular disease. However, imaging of the arterial system is no longer limited to invasive techniques by conventional or digital subtraction angiography (DSA). CT angiography (CTA) and MR angiography (MRA), as well as Doppler ultrasound (US) have largely replaced DSA for diagnostic evaluation of the vascular system. Because of its invasive nature, DSA is now mainly utilized for the confirmation of uncertain findings on CTA, MRA, or vascular US and management of various diseases affecting the vascular system.

CATHETER-BASED ARTERIOGRAPHY: CONVENTIONAL VERSUS DSA

Improvement in the technique of DSA has significantly replaced the conventional film–screen angiography. DSA subtracts images obtained preiodinated-contrast injection "mask" from postiodinated-contrast injection images. DSA provides better contrast resolution, decreased examination time, and lower-contrast dose. Conventional angiography utilizes film–screen imaging in combination with rapid film changers and has the advantage of superior spatial resolution 6 line pairs/mm versus 2 line pairs/mm with DSA. Both angiographic techniques provide information pertaining to the vascular lumens with little information in regard to extraluminal pathology.

CONTRAST AGENTS

Most commonly, iodinated-contrast media is utilized for CTA or DSA. Low-osmolar contrast agents cause less discomfort and have lower incidence of mild allergic reactions such as itching and rashes. No study has demonstrated any significant difference in the incidence of major allergic reactions between low- and high-osmolar contrast agent. Low-osmolar contrast agents should be used in patients who are being treated for severe allergies or asthma and in patients with severe cardiac disease. Patients with previous history of allergic reaction to iodinated-contrast agent should be treated prophylactically prior to angiography, typically with methylprednisolone. Concurrent use of histamine blocker such as diphenhydramine has also been recommended. Patients with preexisting renal failure are more susceptible to nephrotoxicity by the iodinated-contrast agent and this risk is further compounded by coexisting diabetes mellitus, increasing age, and higher volume of contrast agent. Patients with paraproteinemias such as multiple myeloma are at increased risk of renal failure because of precipitation of proteins in the renal tubules. Adequate hydration, limiting the volume of contrast, and use of low-osmolar contrast agent are some of the strategies that can be utilized to decrease the renal function compromise. Although there is no convincing evidence of their effectiveness, acetylcysteine or fenoldopam have also been utilized to prevent the deterioration of renal function.

Mild reactions such as urticaria are treated by intramuscular or intravenous diphenhydramine, usually in the dose of 25 to 50 mg. For severe reactions, such as anaphylaxis (characterized by hypotension and tachycardia), maintenance of airway and circulation by intravenous fluids are extremely important. Pharmacologic agent of choice is epinephrine 0.3 mL of 1:1000 dilution subcutaneously or 1 to 3 mL of 1:10 000 dilution intravenously. For vasovagal reaction, characterized by bradycardia and hypotension, treatment of choice is atropine 0.6 to 2.0 mg intravenously.

An alternative to iodinated intravenous contrast is carbon dioxide (CO_2) in DSA imaging, as CO_2 dissolves rapidly in blood and is completely eliminated in a single pass through the lungs. This contrast agent may be utilized in patients with chronic renal insufficiency or in patients with severe iodinated-contrast allergy history. CO_2 should not be used for arterial imaging in the chest and head and neck secondary to potential neurotoxicity.

TECHNIQUE

For conventional angiography, the most common and safest approach is via the common femoral artery. The common femoral artery is palpated at the level of femoral head with the skin puncture site near the inferior margin of the femoral head to provide a means of compression. After sterile preparation and draping, a local anesthetic (usually lidocaine 1%) is injected in the skin and subcutaneous tissues and a small skin incision is made superficial to the common femoral artery.

While palpating the artery, the opposite hand is used to puncture the artery passing the needle at a 45-degree angle to the skin surface. With the double wall technique, the needle is passed through both walls of the artery. The stylet is removed and the cannula is withdrawn until pulsatile flow is obtained. The single-wall technique involves puncturing the wall with a hollow needle through the anterior wall only.

After brisk pulsatile flow is obtained, a guidewire is carefully passed though the needle and utilized to advance dilators, sheaths, and eventually catheters into the artery. Fluoroscopy is utilized to safely advance guidewires and catheters as to prevent subintimal injury. A test hand injection of contrast through a newly positioned catheter is important to ensure intraluminal position of the catheter within the desired vessel. Catheters are carefully flushed with heparinized saline throughout the procedure to prevent thrombus formation within the catheter. After the procedure is complete, the catheter and sheaths are removed and hemostasis is obtained at the puncture site via manual pressure. Retrograde common femoral puncture is the standard approach for the evaluation of thoracoabdominal aorta and its branches. Retrograde common femoral approach is also utilized for angiographic evaluation of contralateral iliofemoral arteries and lower extremity runoff. Less commonly utilized, antegrade common femoral approach is particularly suited for evaluation and endovascular treatment of infrapopliteal vasculature in the event contralateral approach is not technically feasible. A pulseless femoral artery can be punctured under ultrasound guidance or under fluoroscopy. Presence of calcification and anatomic location of the common femoral artery at the level of medial and middle third of the femoral head are useful in localizing the common femoral artery.

Advances in axial imaging yield excellent visualization of vessels as well as their relationship to adjacent structures by CT and MR. CTA depicts the vessel lumen accurately and with helical acquisition, multiple reconstructions can be performed from the axial data set without additional contrast or radiation. MR can be utilized to evaluate vascular pathology with or without administration of intravenous contrast. MRA utilizes the inherent contrast produced by nonsaturated protons within flowing blood relative to the stationary saturated protons within soft tissues during time of flight imaging. Additionally, phase-contrast imaging utilizes the property of flowing blood as it interacts with specialized gradients imposed on the main magnetic field. Data can be obtained in the 2D mode (slice mode) or in the 3D mode (slab mode). This data is subsequently postprocessed using maximum intensity pixel algorithms for display in multiple planes. Limitations of MRA include motion artifact, scan time, flow artifacts (which may occur at severe stenoses), and methemoglobin in thrombosed vessels that produces bright signal that could falsely simulate flow. US is an invaluable tool in vascular assessment particularly in the evaluation of the carotid arteries and peripheral arterial system of lower extremities. Additionally, US is a valuable tool for vascular access guidance for interventional procedures.

PREPROCEDURE EVALUATION

Preprocedure evaluation includes clinical history and physical examination of the patient. Prior imaging studies including US, CT, MRI, and so on should be reviewed. Coagulation profile (prothrombin time [PT], partial thromboplastin time [PTT], platelets) and renal function tests (blood urea nitrogen, creatinine) should also be reviewed before angiography. In a heparinized patient, heparin infusion is stopped approximately 4 hours prior to the arterial puncture and heparin may be restarted within 4 to 6 hours after the procedure. A PTT of 1.2 times control is acceptable in the absence of other bleeding abnormalities. If patient is on warfarin sodium (Coumadin), Coumadin should be stopped 5 to 7 days prior to the procedure. Aim is to achieve an INR level below 1.4; however, in certain emergency situations such as acute gastrointestinal bleeding in a patient with coagulopathy, a higher level of INR may be acceptable. Fresh frozen plasma and vitamin K (25–50 mg approximately 4–5 hours prior to the procedure) may be utilized to correct the INR. The platelet count should be greater than 50 000 μL.

POSTPROCEDURE MANAGEMENT

Traditionally, manual compression of the common femoral artery for 10 to 15 minutes just proximal to the arterial puncture site has been the mainstay of hemostasis. If bleeding recurs, another 10 to 15 minutes of manual compression should be applied. In last few years, the use of arterial closure devices has increased significantly.

Vascular closure devices such as perclose and angioseal can significantly shorten the time to ambulation. These devices utilize a collagen plug or suture.

POSTCATHETERIZATION COMPLICATIONS

Iatrogenic complications from femoral arterial catheterization include hematoma, dissection, thrombosis, pseudoaneurysms, distal embolization, and arteriovenous fistula. Risks factors include anticoagulation, large catheters or sheaths, inadequate compression, or poor access technique. Sonographic evaluation is the imaging study of choice. Hematoma is a mass of varying echogenicity without Doppler flow. A pseudoaneurysm (PSA) communicating with the femoral artery is seen on color Doppler as swirling flow "yin-yang." Color Doppler can also demonstrate high velocity "to-and-fro" flow at the site of the communication. US-guided thrombin injection is now the preferred mode of managing post-catheterization PSAs. Rarely, US-guided compression of the PSA neck by US transducer is used for thrombosis of the PSA. An AVF is more common after inferior entries, where the artery may lie just superficial to the vein. Arterialized flow is seen within the vein, and there is loss of high resistance triphasic arterial waveforms and low resistance flow (accentuated diastolic flow) within the artery proximal to the AVF.

NONSELECTIVE AORTOGRAPHY

Nonselective arteriography is usually performed with multiple side hole 5F or 4F catheters such as pigtail or omni flush catheter. In pediatric population, a 3F or 4F catheter is usually sufficient. Nonselective arteriography of the arch is routinely performed prior to evaluation of the major arteries arising from the arch in elderly patients because of atherosclerotic disease and potential complication of stroke because of dislodgement of plaque from catheter and guidewire manipulation.

The left anterior oblique (LAO) view provides information about the origins of left subclavian, left common carotid, and the brachiocephalic arteries. The right anterior oblique (RAO) view is utilized for the evaluation of right common carotid, right subclavian, and origins of both the vertebral arteries.

Abdominal aortography is used to evaluate the abdominal aorta and visceral branches. An approximately 30-degree LAO view provides the best view of origin of renal arteries. The position of the catheter depends on the clinical indication for the procedure. For the evaluation of mesenteric arteries, the catheter is placed at the level of T12 to include origin of the celiac artery. However, for evaluation of renal arterial or infrarenal disease, the catheter is typically placed at L2 to avoid unnecessary filling of the mesenteric circulation. Prior to power injection of the contrast, one must ensure that the pigtail is freely moving in the aorta to avoid injection into a side branch and to minimize the risk of atheroembolism. The most common access for evaluation of the thoracic aorta is via a common femoral artery approach with left axillary or translumbar arterial approaches providing access but is less desirable. For imaging of the thoracic aorta, a pigtail catheter is utilized and placed 1 to 2 cm distal to the aortic valve or within the descending aorta depending on the area of interest. The 45-degree LAO projection best displays the arch and great vessel origins; however, optimum positioning should be individualized with each patient. Contrast is injected at the rate of 20 to 30 mL/s for 2 seconds with rapid filming (frame rate 4–6/s). Extended filming may be necessary for patients with slow flow or suspected dissection. For abdominal aortography, the injection rate is 20 to 25 cm^3/s at 4 to 6 frames/s in AP and lateral projections. For the evaluation of atherosclerotic disease involving the pelvic arteries, angulation for the oblique views is individualized in each patient as tortuosity of these arteries varies in every patient; however, as a general rule contralateral oblique opens the ipsilateral internal iliac ostium; and ipsilateral oblique opens ipsilateral common femoral bifurcation.

SELECTIVE ARTERIOGRAPHY

Selective arteriography is performed by selective catheterization of the artery of interest by endhole catheters. Intravascular position of the catheter should be confirmed by aspiration of the catheter or by hemodynamic assessment of the waveform to avoid inadvertent injury to the vessel wall or dislodgement of clot formed at the tip of the catheter.

RENAL ANGIOGRAPHY

Renal arteries typically arise at the level of L2. Occasionally, there may be multiple renal arteries arising from the abdominal aorta. The most frequent indications for renal arteriography are evaluation of trauma, tumors and renovascular hypertension, and vascular anomalies. Diagnostic, nonselective abdominal aortography is useful to evaluate the orifice and multiplicity of the renal arteries. Catheter selection for renal arteriography includes cobra, SOS, VS1/2, and sidewinder and typical injection rate is 5 to 6 mL/s for a total of 12 to 14 mL. AP or slightly LAO views are usually sufficient to evaluate proximal renal arteries.

MESENTERIC ANGIOGRAPHY

Typical catheter choice is a visceral catheter such as Cobra, RC1/2, or VS1/2. Injection is continued through the venous phase to evaluate patency of portal vein. Some angiographers prefer to start from diagnostic arteriogram in lateral projection to evaluate origins of the mesenteric arteries. This can be particularly useful in elderly patients because of potential stenosis of the ostia by underlying atherosclerotic disease. Intravenous injection of 0.5 to 1.0 mg glucagon before superior mesenteric angiography decreases bowel motility and associated artifact. A typical injection rate for celiac/SMA is 6 to 7 cm^3/s for a total volume of 40 to 50 cm^3 and for IMA, it is 3 to 4 cm^3/s for a total volume of 18 to 20 cm^3.

CAROTID AND CEREBRAL ANGIOGRAPHY

Arch aortography with a nonselective pigtail or omni flush catheter optimizes catheter selection for selective carotid and vertebral arteriography. Evaluation of the origins of the major arteries from the aortic arch is particularly important when a patient is being evaluated for underlying atherosclerotic disease. For the carotid arteries, the catheter tip is placed just proximal to the bifurcation and contrast is injected at the rate of 5 to 6 cm^3/s with a total volume of 8 to 10 cm^3. Provided there is no significant carotid bifurcation disease, the external and internal carotid arteries can be selectively catheterized.

For internal carotid arteries, contrast is injected at the rate of 4 to 5 cm^3/s for a total volume of 7 to 8 cm^3. Imaging is performed in an AP projection with 10- to –15-degrees cranial angulation, lateral, and 45-degree LAO or RAO views. For evaluation of vertebral arteries, the catheter is placed in the proximal subclavian artery and a test injection is performed. If the origin of the artery is unremarkable, the vertebral artery is selected and contrast is injected at the rate of 5 to 6 cm^3/s for a total of 10 cm^3. Reflux of contrast into the opposite vertebral artery and filling of its posterior inferior cerebellar artery (PICA) branch is usually desired while evaluating intracranial circulation to avoid catheterization of opposite vertebral artery. Commonly used catheters for intracranial angiography include the following: 5F-angled glide headhunter (H1, H3, H1 H), Berenstein, vertebral, glide JB-1, JB-2, JB-3, SIM1, SIM2, and SIM3.

UPPER EXTREMITY ANGIOGRAPHY

Common indications for upper extremity angiography are trauma, tumor, atherosclerotic disease, vasculitis, and arteriovenous malformations. A 4F to 5F headhunter or an angled glide catheter is utilized to select the subclavian or axillary artery. Contrast is injected at the rate of approximately 5 to 6 cm^3/s with a total volume of approximately 10 to 12 cm^3.

LOWER EXTREMITY ANGIOGRAPHY

The most common indication for lower extremity angiography is evaluation of atherosclerotic disease. Pelvic arteriography is performed by placing the pigtail catheter in the distal aorta. AP and both oblique views are obtained by injecting contrast at approximately 10 cm^3/s for a total volume of 18 to 20 cm^3. Most of the angiographic tables are equipped for bilateral lower extremity runoff. For bilateral lower extremity run off (bolus chase), the typical volume injected is 6 to 10 cm^3/s for 10 to 12 seconds. Selective single limb angiography can be performed by crossing over to the opposite side utilizing a 4F or 5F RIM catheter and exchanging it to 4F to 5F Berenstein or JB1 catheter. Angiography is performed by stationary DSA runs at 5 to 6 cm^3/s for a total volume of 10 to 12 cm^3 of contrast.

ANATOMY AND CONGENITAL VARIANTS

Arteries are composed of three layers including a thin, endothelial lined layer called the intima, a variably thick muscular layer known as the media, and an outer fibrovascular layer termed the adventitia.

THORACIC AORTA

The thoracic aorta extends from the aortic valve to the diaphragmatic hiatus and is divided into three segments: the ascending aorta, aortic arch, and descending aorta. The ascending segment extends from the aortic valve to the origin of the brachiocephalic artery. Proximally, three sinuses correspond to the three aortic cusps; the coronary arteries arise from two of these sinuses. The left coronary artery arises from the left coronary sinus and the right arises from the right aortic sinus. The ascending aorta has a diameter of 2.5 to 3.5 cm in adults and is normally larger than the diameter of the descending aorta. The aortic arch extends from the origin of the brachiocephalic artery to the attachment of the ligamentum arteriosum with a normal right-to-left course. The arch gives rise to the brachiocephalic, left common carotid, and left subclavian arteries in most individuals. The most common variation in arch anatomy is a common trunk for the brachiocephalic and left common carotid arteries (approximately 20%). The isthmus is the arch between the left subclavian artery origin and the ligamentum arteriosum and is a focus of aortic narrowing. The descending thoracic aorta comprises the remainder of the thoracic aorta and usually gives rise to nine pairs of intercostal arteries. The two upper intercostals spaces are supplied by the superior intercostal artery arising from the costocervical trunk. Bronchial arteries vary but most often arise from the level of T4-7 with the most common pattern consisting of one right and two left arteries.

COLLATERAL CIRCULATION

Obstructive lesions involving the thoracic aorta result in activation of the collateral circulation. The most common obstructive lesion involves the proximal descending thoracic aorta and is seen in coarctation of the aorta. The obstruction at this level results in hypertrophy of the subclavian arteries and their muscular branches, bilaterally. Just distal to the obstruction, there is reversal of flow in the intercostal arteries toward the descending aorta. These intercostal arteries are supplied by the internal mammary arteries. Both internal mammary arteries also provide flow to the lower extremities via the epigastric arteries.

The most frequent arch anomaly is left aortic arch with aberrant right subclavian artery seen in approximately 1% of individuals. The right subclavian artery arises as a fourth branch of the aortic arch, most commonly crossing posterior to the esophagus. Dilation at the origin of the aberrant vessel is termed diverticulum of Kommerell. This anomaly is rarely symptomatic but patients can present with dysphagia (dysphagia lusoria). Associated cardiac anomalies are seen in 10% of patients with coarctation of the aorta and tetrology of Fallot being most common.

A right arch with mirror image arterial branching occurs in approximately 60% of individuals with right arch anatomy and has no retroesophageal impression. It has a high association with congenital heart disease, most commonly tetrology of Fallot. A right aortic arch with aberrant left subclavian artery is seen less often and either the arch or aberrant vessel may cause posterior impression on the esophagus. Associated congenital heart disease is seen in a small percentage of patients with tetrology of Fallot, including atrial septal defect and coarctation seen most frequently.

Coarctation is a narrowing of the aortic lumen with two classic forms described. An "infantile" form consists of focal distal arch obstruction at the level of the ductus arteriosum with proximal hypoplasia of the aortic arch. This is symptomatic in childhood. The "adult" form is a discrete infolding of the aorta opposite the ligamentum arteriosum. It is seen more often in males and often associated with other anomalies including bicuspid aortic valve, patent ductus arteriosus (PDA), ventricular septal defect (VSD), as well as circle of Willis aneurysms. Coarctation is frequently seen in Turner syndrome (XO) patients.

Clinically, patients may exhibit hypertension of the upper extremities and diminished pulses in the lower extremities. In the young infants, radiographs show enlarged heart because of cardiac failure. In the young child, the chest radiograph demonstrates an enlarged heart with dilated descending aorta distal to the level of coarctation. In the older children and adults, characteristic "3" sign formed by dilatation of the proximal left subclavian artery proximally, an indentation in the contour of the descending thoracic aorta just inferior to the aortic knob in the frontal projection representing the area of coarctation and poststenotic dilatation. Tortuous, dilated intercostal arteries may produce rib notching (ribs 3–9). Acquired coarctation can result from idiopathic inflammatory conditions, radiation vasculitis, rubella syndrome, and neurofibromatosis. MR is the imaging modality of choice for coarctation. Angiography provides extent of aortic involvement and allows for measurement of pressure gradients.

ABDOMINAL AORTA

The abdominal aorta originates at the diaphragmatic hiatus and extends to bifurcate into common iliac arteries at the level of L4. The abdominal aorta normally measures 2.5 cm in diameter proximally tapering to 1.5 to 2.0 cm distally. The major branches of the abdominal aorta include the celiac axis at T12-L1, the superior mesenteric artery at L1-2, and the inferior mesenteric artery at L3-4 arising from the ventral aorta. Paired main renal arteries arise laterally at the level of L2 in most patients. Paired phrenic, adrenal, and gonadal arteries as well as four pairs of lumbar arteries arise from the lateral or posterolateral aorta.

In the event of obstructive aortoiliac disease, there are multiple collateral pathways present in the abdomen and pelvis to maintain arterial flow distally. Activation of a particular collateral pathway depends upon the site of arterial obstruction. These pathways include the following:

- Superior epigastric to common femoral artery via inferior epigastric artery.
- Lumbar arteries to external iliac arteries via iliolumbar and internal iliac and to common femoral artery via iliac-circumflex artery.
- Inferior mesenteric artery to external iliac artery via hemorrhoidal and internal iliac artery.
- Median sacral artery to external iliac artery via lateral sacral and internal iliac artery branches.
- Internal iliac artery provides collateral flow to opposite internal iliac artery via free anastomosis between the branches of anterior division of internal iliac arteries and lateral sacral artery.
- Internal iliac artery to ipsilateral common femoral artery via iliac circumflex artery and profunda femoris artery.

UPPER EXTREMITY

The right subclavian artery arises from the brachiocephalic artery, and the left subclavian artery arises from the aortic arch. The branches of the subclavian artery include (in order): vertebral artery, internal mammary artery, thyrocervical trunk, and costocervical trunk. The axillary artery extends from the lateral aspect of the first rib and gives rise to the anterior and posterior circumflex arteries. The brachial artery courses along the medial aspect of the upper arm branching into the radial and ulnar arteries just proximal to the elbow. Just distal to the origin of the ulnar artery, it gives rise to the common interosseous artery that usually terminates in the distal forearm; however, continuation of this artery into the hand is termed a persistent median artery and is a common variant. The radial and ulnar arteries form the deep and superficial palmar arches in the hand respectively.

LOWER EXTREMITY

The common iliac arteries originate at the bifurcation and extend to the pelvic brim, subsequently branching into external and internal iliac arteries. The internal iliac artery (hypogastric artery) gives rise to the anterior trunk (branches: superior and inferior vesicle, middle hemorrhoidal, internal pudendal, obturator, inferior gluteal, and prostatic or uterine arteries as well as branches to ductus deferens and seminal vesicles) and the posterior trunk (branches: iliolumbar, lateral sacral, and superior gluteal arteries). The external iliac arteries course to the inguinal ligament giving off the deep circumflex iliac and inferior epigastric arteries. The common femoral artery bifurcates into the profunda femoris and the superficial femoral artery (SFA) near the inferior margin of the femoral head. The SFA courses in the anteromedial thigh to the adductor canal. The popliteal artery is the continuation of the SFA at the level of the adductor canal coursing through the knee.

The popliteal artery divides inferior to the knee into the anterior tibial (AT) artery and a short tibioperoneal trunk that in short order divides into the peroneal and posterior tibial (PT) arteries. The AT artery passes over the interosseous membrane below the knee descending into the anterior compartment of the leg continuing into the foot as the dorsalis pedis artery. The peroneal artery terminates above the ankle and the PT continues into the foot posterior to the medial malleolus into the plantar aspect of the foot giving off medial and lateral plantar arteries. A persistent sciatic artery is a rare congenital variant seen as an enlarged inferior branch (inferior gluteal) of the internal iliac artery exiting the pelvis posteriorly through the lower portion of the greater sciatic foramen providing dominant inflow to the leg as the proximal SFA may be hypoplastic or absent. This is usually a bilateral finding. Because of its superficial location, this artery is prone to injury and aneurysm.

ATHEROSCLEROSIS

Atherosclerotic plaques are intimal lesions that protrude into vascular lumens producing luminal obstruction, which can be concentric or eccentric in nature. Dystrophic calcification may be seen in the chronic plaques. Risk factors for atherosclerosis include age (more than 60 years), sex (male greater than female), diabetes, hypertension, cigarette smoking, genetic predisposition, and hyperlipidemia. Atherosclerosis can lead to ischemic symptoms that vary based on the artery involved and severity of disease. Associated complications include plaque ulceration, acute thrombosis, and distal embolization. Sudden changes in symptomatology usually indicate an acute complication with clinical findings including diminished pulses, claudication, hair loss or skin changes, rest pain, and gangrene.

Atherosclerosis is a systemic disease and multiple arterial beds can be involved simultaneously. It is usually symmetric and commonly affects arterial bifurcations and ostia secondary to increased turbulence. Imaging shows concentric or eccentric luminal narrowing with occasional poststenotic dilatation. In the lower extremities, the most common artery involved is the SFA followed by the iliac, tibial, popliteal, and common femoral arteries. Arteriography plays a valuable role in preoperative planning and percutaneous intervention including percutaneous angioplasty, stent placement, and atherectomy. Findings indicating a significant stenosis include greater than 50% luminal narrowing, presence of collateral flow, and peak systolic gradient across the lesion of greater than 10 mm Hg.

Thromboembolism is a common cause of acute arterial occlusion with emboli originating from the heart, proximal aneurysms, or proximal atherosclerotic lesions. The characteristic angiographic appearance is abrupt vessel occlusion with a superior convex meniscus, multiple lesions with emboli at bifurcations, lack of collateral flow, and vasospasm. Arterial thromboembolism results in acute arterial occlusion and threatened ischemia. Clinical presentation includes pain, pulselessness, pallor, paresthesias, and paralysis. Minimizing time from diagnosis to intervention is crucial to prevent tissue or even limb loss.

ANEURYSMS

Aneurysms are localized abnormal dilation of vessel walls and are classified as true aneurysms with all three layers intact or false aneurysms with one or more layers disrupted and containment provided by adjacent extravascular connective tissue. Most thoracic aneurysms are asymptomatic but patients can present with chest pain, stridor, dysphagia, SVC syndrome, and hoarseness. Important risk factors for the development of aneurysms are age, sex (male greater than female), and cigarette smoking.

Chest radiographs demonstrate contour abnormality with aortic tortuosity and vessel wall calcifications. Axial imaging may differentiate aneurysms from other posterior mediastinal masses. CTA and MRA demonstrate wall diameter, mural thrombus, wall calcifications, degree of luminal patency, and mass effect on adjacent mediastinal structures. Ruptured or leaking aneurysms reveal increased soft-tissue density, resulting form mediastinal hematoma and associated left pleural effusion. MR shows signal intensities of blood products within the mediastinum. Angiography is typically reserved for operative planning when it is vital to establish the relationship of the aneurysm to the great vessels, coronary arteries, and vascular supply to the spinal cord. Imaging of the abdominal aorta may also be needed. Angiography is unreliable in evaluation of aneurysms size in the presence of mural thrombus.

Atherosclerotic aneurysms are the result of mild-to-moderate inflammation involving the aortic wall and degradation of structural components of the aorta by matrix metalloproteases. This is combined with impairment of the vasovasorum blood supply to the vessel wall resulting in loss of muscular fibers within the media. Fusiform irregular walls are noted secondary to mural thrombus. Discontinuous curvilinear and plaquelike calcifications are seen. Syphilitic aneurysms are the late sequelae of untreated syphilis resulting from obliterative endarteritis of vasovasorum. Subsequent scarring and retraction of the vessel wall produces wrinkling of the intima known as "tree barking." Syphilitic aneurysms predominately affect the ascending aorta and aortic arch. Mycotic aneurysms result from weakening of vascular wall from bacterial infection. Patients with bacterial endocarditis, intravenous drug use, aortic surgery, and immunocompromised state are predisposed to these types of aneurysms. These may arise from a septic embolus from endocarditis, vascular wall infection from bacteremia, or direct infectious spread from adjacent structures. These are saccular aneurysms occurring in the ascending and descending aorta. Clinical presentation may include sudden onset pulsatile abdominal mass and fever. CT demonstrates a noncalcified saccular aneurysm with periaortic fluid, gas, or vertebral osteomyelitis. The most common organisms are *Staphylococcus* and *Salmonella* species. Indium-labeled white cell radionuclide imaging is useful in differentiating this from other types of aneurysm. Rupture occurs in as many as 80% of mycotic aneurysms.

Connective tissue disorders such as Marfan and Ehler-Danlos syndrome are associated with abnormal collagen production resulting in cystic medial necrosis and ascending aortic aneurysm formation. The characteristic symmetrical dilation of the sinuses of Valsalva is termed "tulip bulb aorta" and differentiates Marfan from atherosclerotic aneurysms. Ankylosing spondylitis, Reiter syndrome, and relapsing polychondritis are other causes that are associated with thoracic aortic aneurysms.

An abdominal aortic aneurysm (AAA) is defined as dilation of the abdominal aorta greater than 3 cm. They occur in 2% to 6% of the targeted population, most commonly in white males older than 60 years. Most AAA are asymptomatic and are detected on physical examination as a pulsatile mass or incidentally on imaging studies. Clinical presentations can include abdominal pain, abdominal mass, and distal embolic events. Most are infrarenal and are secondary to atherosclerosis. Progressive mural thrombus within the aneurysm may result in occlusion of branch vessels. They tend to be fusiform and enlarge at a rate of 2 to 4 mm per year. Extension into the iliac arteries is common. Complications of AAA include rupture, peripheral embolization, thrombosis, and infection. The incidence of AAA rupture is directly related to increasing aneurysm size (Table 81-1).

US is the imaging modality of choice for initial evaluation, screening, and follow up of AAA. Asymptomatic AAA less than 4 to 5 cm in diameter are followed with serial US until intervention is needed. US can detect

TABLE 81-1 Aortic Aneurysm Diameter and Risk of Rupture

SIZE OF ANEURYSM	RISK OF RUPTURE (%)
<4 cm	10
4–7 cm	25
7–10 cm	45
>10 cm	60

intramural thrombus, accurately size the aneurysm, and detect extension into the iliac arteries. US is limited by patient body habitus, overlying bowel gas, and in evaluation of renal arterial involvement. CTA surpasses US in defining the relationship of the aneurysm to the renal arteries and surrounding structures. CTA with 3D reconstruction is useful for treatment planning. CT is the modality of choice for evaluation of suspected rupture, leaking aneurysm, and perianeurysm fibrosis. Aneurysms are repaired with either endograft or open graft placement procedures. CTA is extremely valuable in evaluation of postendograft repair of AAA particularly in assessment of endoleak and migration of the endograft.

There are five types of endoleak (Table 66-1). A type I endoleak develops secondary to inadequate or ineffective seal at the proximal or distal aspect of the graft thereby allowing a persistent perigraft inflow. A type II endoleak is secondary to persistent collateral retrograde blood flow into the aneurysm sac, commonly from lumbar arteries, the internal iliac artery, or other collateral vessels. A type III endoleak arises when there is a defect within the graft fabric or between segments of a multisegmental graft. A type IV endoleak is secondary to "bleed-through" or inflow across the pores of a graft. Type V endoleak is endotension; there is no visible contrast or flow in the aneurysm sac but continued expansion. Popliteal artery aneurysms occur in approximately 4% to 10% of patient population with AAA. Imaging of the patients suspected with popliteal artery aneurysm should include the abdominal aorta and popliteal arteries as these aneurysms are bilateral in over 50% of the patient population and approximately 62% of the patients with popliteal aneurysms will also have concomitant AAA. The most common presentation is ischemia because of embolization and rupture is rare. US is 100% sensitive in diagnosing the popliteal artery aneurysm. All symptomatic aneurysms should be repaired and treatment is recommended for asymptomatic aneurysms larger than 2 cm in diameter.

The splenic artery is a common site of visceral artery aneurysm. Most are solitary and localized to the distal two-thirds of the splenic artery. Patients are usually asymptomatic. These are more common in women and have an increased rupture rate during pregnancy accompanied by a 25% mortality rate. Symptomatic aneurysms, enlarging aneurysms, association with pregnancy or childbearing women, or size greater than 2 cm are indications for intervention.

AORTIC DISSECTION

An aortic dissection is defined as a separation of the layers of the vessel wall creating a false lumen with blood dissecting between and along the laminar planes of the media. The media defect can be acquired or congenital as in the case of Marfan syndrome. Predisposing factors to dissection include hypertension, bicuspid aortic valve, coarctation, pregnancy, scoliosis, pectus excavatum, trauma, prior aortic surgery, and intra-aortic balloon pump. Mortality is usually associated with retrograde dissection into the pericardium causing tamponade, massive aortic regurgitation, or pleural space hemorrhage. Aortic dissection is more common in men between the ages of 40 and 60. Patients may present with sudden severe substernal pain with radiation to the back. Asymmetrical pulses in the upper extremities are often seen when there is such involvement.

There are two classification systems to describe aortic involvement in dissection. The Debakey classification describes three types of dissection (Table 81-2). The Stanford classification is composed of two types of dissections. Type A is the most common type and involves the ascending aorta with variable involvement of the arch and descending aorta. Type B is limited to the arch and descending aorta. Aortic dissection involving the ascending aorta is usually repaired surgically on an emergent basis because of involvement of the aortic root and coronary arteries and a high risk of rupture into pericardial and pleural cavities. A dissection involving the descending aorta is usually managed by conservative medical treatment with aggressive blood pressure control.

CT is excellent for evaluation of dissection with accuracy greater than 90%. The intimal flap is seen as a linear filing defect within the aortic lumen. The true and false lumens may be opacified; although the false lumen may exhibit delayed opacification and late filling of branch vessels arising from the false lumen. The false lumen may compress the true lumen appearing larger and may also contain thrombus. Aortography is rarely

TABLE 81-2 Debakey Classification of Dissection

Type I	Ascending aorta, arch, and variable portions of the descending thoracic aorta
Type II	Ascending aorta, worst prognosis
Type III	Originates near the isthmus distal to the left subclavian artery, does not involve the ascending aorta or the aortic arch, most common type

necessary unless an intervention is planned. The common femoral approach usually allows access to the true lumen as dissections rarely involve the external iliac arteries. Contrast opacification of both the true and false lumens is very important particularly in the cases involving the ascending aorta to determine involvement of the aortic root and coronary arteries. The classic finding is a "double barrel" sign with an interposed intimal flap. The intimal flap usually originates in the anterolateral ascending aorta and spirals to the left posterolateral aspect of the descending aorta to the abdomen. Visceral arteries may be supplied by true or false lumen. The left renal artery is frequently supplied by the false lumen. Symptomatic occlusive complications of aortoiliac dissection can be effectively managed with minimally invasive techniques such as percutaneous fenestration, stent placement, or stent graft placement.

VASCULITIDES

The term "vasculitis" refers to pathologic inflammation and necrosis of the blood vessel wall. Vasculitides are classified based on the vessel size involved. Large vessel vasculitis includes temporal arteritis and Takayasus arteritis. Medium vessel vasculitis includes polyarteritis nodosa and Kawasaki disease. Small vessel vasculitis includes Churg-Strauss syndrome, hypersensitivity vasculitis, Wegeners granulomatosis, and Behcet syndrome.

TAKAYASU DISEASE

Takayasu disease is a granulomatous vasculitis of the medium- and large-sized arteries. The etiology is idiopathic and it primarily affects young (20–40 years) Asian women. It is characterized by marked weakening of the upper extremity pulses known as "pulse less disease." Fibrous thickening and narrowing of the aorta including aortic arch is classically seen, but branch involvement can also be seen with marked narrowing of arteries supplying the upper body and viscera. The acute stage is characterized by fever, myalgia, arthralgia, and malaise. The fibrotic stage is characterized by pulse deficits, claudication, bruits, and renovascular hypertension. Chest radiographs may show calcifications in the aortic wall. Arteriography shows long or short segment smooth narrowing of the aorta or branch arteries.

GIANT CELL ARTERITIS

Giant cell or temporal arteritis is the most common form of systemic vasculitis in adults. This is more common in women than men. This is a granulomatous arteritis primarily affecting the temporal arteries but vertebral, ophthalmic arteries, as well as the aorta may also be involved. On clinical examination, patients are generally older than 50 and may also exhibit polymyalgia rheumatica, jaw claudication, and visual loss. Affected arteries may be tender and demonstrate nodular thickening, erythema, and swelling. Laboratory investigation may reveal elevated erythrocyte sedimentation rate and elevated C–reactive protein. On US, a hypoechoic halo with scattered areas of increased peak systolic velocity may be useful in diagnosis. CT, MR, or arch angiography can demonstrate large artery involvement.

POLYARTERITIS NODOSA

Polyarteritis nodosa is a systemic necrotizing vasculitis affecting small- or medium-sized muscular arteries in young adults. Histopathologically, there is transmural inflammation. Inflammatory destruction of the media leads to aneurysm formation. The renal and visceral arteries are frequently affected with relative sparing of the pulmonary vessels. Clinical presentation may include malaise, fever, weight loss, hypertension, and abdominal pain. Hepatitis B infection is reported in approximately 7% of the patients. Diagnosis is based on arteriographic documentation of mesenteric or renal artery aneurysms or biopsy.

KAWASAKI DISEASE (MUCOCUTANEOUS LYMPH NODE SYNDROME)

Kawasaki disease or mucocutaneous lymph node syndrome is an arteritis primarily affecting the coronary arteries seen in infants and young children. Coronary artery involvement results in coronary artery aneurysm formation, which can be seen on echocardiography. It is associated with an acute self-limiting illness including fever, palm, and sole erythema, desquamative rash, conjunctivitis, and cervical lymph node enlargement. Uncommonly, other large, medium, or small arteries may also be involved.

SMALL VESSEL VASCULITIS

Angiography plays a limited role in the diagnosis of small vessel vasculitis. Diagnosis is primarily based on clinical and laboratory findings. Churg-Strauss syndrome or allergic granulomatous angitis usually involves small muscular arteries with eosinophilia and extravascular granulomas in a patient with a history of allergic rhinitis, asthma, or both. Hypersensitivity vasculitis includes serum sickness, Henoch-Schonlein purpura, and drug hypersensitivity reaction. Wegeners granulomatosis involves a necrotizing granulomatous process of the respiratory tract and kidneys. Laboratory tests are positive for ANCA test but are negative for antinuclear antibody test. Behcet syndrome is a multisystem inflammatory disorder characterized by recurrent oral aphthous ulcers, genital ulcers, uveitis, and skin lesions.

BUERGER DISEASE (THROMBOANGITIS OBLITERANS)

Buerger disease is secondary to acute and chronic inflammation of small- and medium-sized arteries characterized by segmental thrombosis. The etiology is unknown with venous involvement occurring occasionally. Nearly all patients are smokers and the great majority are young males. The erythrocyte sedimentation rate and serum C-reactive protein are usually normal. Claudication is a common clinical presentation. The arteries supplying the calf and foot are most commonly affected; however, upper extremity involvement may also occur affecting ulnar or radial arteries. Arteriographic findings include bilateral distal extremity arterial occlusions, intervening normal appearing arteries, multiple corkscrew collaterals, and sparing of larger inflow arteries without any evidence of atherosclerosis.

COLLAGEN VASCULAR DISEASES

Collagen vascular diseases including rheumatoid arthritis, systemic lupus erythematosus, and scleroderma affect the small- and medium-sized arteries of the distal upper extremities. Involvement is typically bilateral and symmetrical with progressive concentric vessel narrowing leading to occlusion with poorly developed collaterals. The vasospastic disorder Raynaud phenomenon is frequently associated.

RADIATION VASCULITIS

Endothelial injury caused by radiation can result in subintimal fibrosis and arterial stenosis or occlusion. The extent of vascular injury corresponds to the area irradiated.

TRAUMA

Aortic transection results from sudden deceleration injury usually in a high-speed motor vehicle collision or penetrating injuries as well as iatrogenic injuries during endovascular or surgical procedures. The laceration may involve one or more layers of the aortic wall. The most common site for injury is the aortic isthmus near the attachment of the ligamentum arteriosum, followed by aortic root and diaphragmatic hiatus injuries. This injury has more than 90% mortality prior to reaching the hospital and 85% mortality within 24 hours of hospital admission; therefore, prompt diagnosis is essential. Chest radiographs demonstrate widened mediastinum, indistinct aortic knob, abnormal aortic contour, and rightward displacement of the nasogastric tube and/or trachea. CT findings include mediastinal hemorrhage (may be because of bony trauma or disruption of venous structures), abrupt aortic or branch vessel contour change, aortic PSA, intimal flap, pseudocoarctation, and contrast extravasation. Conventional angiography findings include subtle intimal tears, complete transection, traumatic PSA, and posttraumatic coarctation.

Blunt abdominal injury is most often associated with acute deceleration injuries usually related to motor vehicles (seat belt injuries). Injuries to major branch vessels such as renal arteries are commonly associated. Clinical symptoms can be obscured by other intra-abdominal or musculoskeletal injuries; however, absent or decreased pulses as well as embolic events are signs of possible aortic injury. If peritoneal lavage or CT abdomen and pelvis demonstrate intraperitoneal hemorrhage, the patient is sent to operating room for the repair of intra-abdominal injuries. Bleeding in the pelvic retroperitoneum is very difficult to control surgically and surgical decompression of hematoma usually leads to increased blood loss. If the patient remains hemodynamically unstable, emergency angiography and possible embolization of the bleeding artery are required. CT and angiographic findings of arterial injury include initimal irregularity, dissection, laceration with PSA, retroperitoneal hematoma, and thrombosis. Penetrating trauma increases the risk for arteriovenous fistula.

Peripheral vascular injury is usually caused by blunt or penetrating trauma. Patients may present with normal physical examination or reveal a cold, pulseless, ischemic extremity, and/or an expanding pulsatile hematoma suggesting arterial injury. Angiographic findings of peripheral vascular injury include intimal tear, spasm, extrinsic compression, contrast extravasation, occlusion, PSA, and arteriovenous fistula. Posterior knee dislocation should proceed to arteriography, as there is an increased incidence of popliteal artery injury and thrombosis.

TUMORS

Primary vascular tumors are rare and can be classified as benign or malignant. Benign vascular tumors produce vascular channels lined with endothelium without cellular atypia. Hemangiomas are predominately superficial in location but may be found within solid organs. Hemangiomas vary in size from a few millimeters to several centimeters in diameter. Capillary hemangiomas are the most common subtype of hemangioma and are usually seen in the superficial tissues of children. Most of capillary hemangiomas resolve by age 7. On angiography, pooling of contrast within the vascular spaces of a cavernous hemangioma demonstrates "cotton wool" appearance. Usually, hemangiomas are dark on T1 and very bright on T2 MR imaging. Glomus tumors are benign tumors that are extremely painful. Glomus tumors arise from the modified smooth muscle cells of the glomus body. The glomus body is a specialized arteriovenous anastomosis that is involved in thermoregulation. These tumors usually arise in the distal aspects of the digits most often under the fingernails. Intermediate grade vascular tumors include Kaposi sarcomas (KS) and hemangioendotheliomas. KS have a variable presentation with most tumors being asymptomatic. There is a frequent occurrence of KS in AIDS patients. While many of these lesions are superficial, these tumors may also arise within the viscera and lymph nodes. Hemangioendotheliomas are vascular tumors occurring around medium-sized and large veins in the soft tissues of adults. The differential diagnosis includes metastatic carcinoma, melanoma, and other sarcomas.

The most common primary malignant vascular neoplasms are venous leiomyosarcoma. More than half of the cases of leiomyosarcoma involve infrarenal inferior vena cava (IVC). Other malignant vascular tumors include angiosarcomas and hemangiopericytomas. Angiosarcomas are malignant endothelial neoplasms that occur more often in older adults. While these tumors may occur anywhere in the body, they are more likely to occur in the skin, soft tissue, breast, and liver. Hepatic angiosarcomas are associated with exposure to certain carcinogens including arsenic, thorotrast, and polyvinyl chloride. Angiosarcomas may also arise in the setting of postmastectomy lymphedema for breast cancer. Angiosarcomas show local spread and distant metastases. Hemangiopericytomas are derived from pericytes arranged along capillaries and venules. These tumors may arise in the pelvic retroperitoneum or extremities but can also arise within the CNS extra-axial tissues as well. Approximately two-thirds of hemangiopericytomas have a benign course with the remaining third exhibiting aggressive behavior.

Secondary vascular involvement by a neoplasm is more common than primary vascular tumors. Invasion of veins is more common than the arteries and IVC is particularly prone to invasion by tumor thrombus. IVC involvement is frequently seen with renal cell carcinoma. Vascular invasion is also frequently seen with hepatomas. Diagnosis is usually made by CT or MRI and current CTA and MRA protocols are very sensitive in identifying the vascular invasion by the tumor. Angiography is primarily performed with the intent of embolizing the tumor, if clinically warranted.

Vascular encasement, invasion, and vascular mass are highly suspicious features for malignant neoplasm. Vascular encasement by the malignant tumors tends to be irregular in appearance. Smooth encasement can be caused by malignant neoplasms but can also be seen in benign process such as inflammation. Other common features seen on angiography include distorted angioarchitecture, neovascularity, or tumor blush and arteriovenous shunting. The arteriovenous shunting is characterized by filling of the veins within the mass during the opacification of the arteries in the other areas. Most common hypervascular tumors are leiomyosarcoma, renal cell carcinoma, melanoma, carcinoid, and islet cell tumor. Adenocarcinomas and squamous cell carcinomas tend to be hypovascular.

ARTERIOVENOUS MALFORMATION

Arteriovenous malformations are high flow congenital lesions. These lesions are characterized by one or more tangles of interconnected arterioles and venules representing the "nidus" without normal capillaries. Majority of the AVMs are found in the lower limbs. Large AVMs can clinically present with symptoms of congestive heart failure because of left-to-right shunt, limb hypertrophy, and hemorrhage. Superficial lesions are usually pulsatile. Mainstay of treatment is transcatheter embolization using absolute alcohol, glue, coils, and/or particles. Surgical resection carries a high risk of recurrence.

Venous malformations are congenital low flow lesions, which clinically present with pain and/or swelling because of thrombosis, mass effect, infiltration of soft tissues such as muscle and hemorrhage. These lesions are nonpulsatile. These lesions are comprised of large venous/vascular spaces, which demonstrate slow and delayed filling on angiography. Most commonly these lesions are managed by direct puncture and sclerosis using sclerosing agents such as absolute alcohol and sodium tetradecyl sulfate. Venous malformations can be associated with Klippel-Trenaunay syndrome, a complex usually involving the lower extremities and associated with limb hypertrophy. Hereditary hemorrhagic telangiectasia (Osler-Weber-Rendu) is an autosomal dominant disorder characterized by arteriovenous malformations affecting lung, liver, brain and spinal cord, as well as skin and gastrointestinal telangiectasias.

ARTERIOVENOUS FISTULAS

Arteriovenous fistulas are acquired lesions and they usually arise as a result of trauma including iatrogenic trauma, or inflammation/infection. These lesions represent direct connections between arteries and veins bypassing the capillary network. These lesions can result in high output cardiac failure. Arteriography demonstrates arteriovenous shunting as a result of direct communication of artery with vein without intervening capillary phase. Both the feeding artery and the draining vein are usually hypertrophied. Treatment is usually occlusion of the shunt by endovascular approach (covered stent or coils, if possible) or surgical ligation. Arteriovenous fistulas are also surgically developed for chronic hemodialysis access.

HEMOPTYSIS

Bronchial arteriography is indicated in patients with hemoptysis usually in patients with tuberculosis, cystic fibrosis, and carcinoma. Hemoptysis of more than 300 mL of blood in 24 hours is usually considered as massive hemoptysis. Bronchoscopy is sometimes helpful in localizing the area of interest. Arteriography is performed for the purpose of diagnosis and management of the hemoptysis. A descending aortogram is obtained as a road map. Bronchial arteries typically arise between T4 and T7. Bronchial arteries demonstrate wide variation in their number and origin. The most common variation is two left and one right bronchial artery. Selective injections of the subclavian, intercostal, and internal mammary arteries as well as thyrocervical trunk may be necessary if no clear source of hemoptysis is identified on bronchial arteriography. Hypertrophied bronchial arteries are usually identified on descending thoracic aortogram. There may be abnormal lung parenchymal blush and shunting to pulmonary artery branches and veins. Selective catheterization of the bronchial arteries with a Mickelson, Cobra or Simmons catheter is performed. Typically, embolization is performed using 300 to 700 μm particles. Complications are uncommon. Most dreadful complication includes inadvertent embolization of artery of Adamkiewicz (arises from the aorta between T8 and L4) resulting in motor spinal cord injury.

Thoracic outlet syndrome is the compression of the brachial plexus or subclavian vessels at the thoracic outlet is usually produced at one of three sites: scalene triangle, costoclavicular space, or pectoralis minor tunnel. The etiologies include cervical ribs, scalenus minimus muscle, anterior scalene muscle, and anomalous first rib resulting in brachial plexus compression causing neurologic symptoms and subclavian artery compression causing ischemic symptoms from distal emboli, claudication, and subclavian vein thrombosis. Acquired lesions include fractures involving clavicle or first rib with large callus formation or nonanatomic alignment and supraclavicular mass. Cross-sectional imaging with CT or MR is useful for evaluating the arteries and surrounding structures. Angiography is performed with arm in neutral as well as the position that causes symptoms. Angiography may demonstrate stenosis, aneurysm formation with arteriographic evidence of distal emboli, and presence of thrombus.

Hypothenar hammer syndrome results from chronic repetitive trauma to the hand, at the hook of the hamate where the ulnar artery crosses; this may result in aneurysm formation, occlusion, and distal embolization.

SUGGESTED READING

Beckman JA, Creager MA. Aortic aneurysms. In: Rooke TW, ed. *Vascular Medicine & Endovascular interventions*. Hoboken, NJ: Blackwell Futura; 2007:187.

Bettman MA. Angiographic contrast media. In: Kandarpa K, Aruny JE, eds. *Handbook of Interventional Radiologic Procedures*. Hagerstown, MD: Lippincott Williams & Wilkins; 2002:526.

Caridi JG, Hawkins IF, LeVeen RF, Klioze SA. Carbon dioxide angiography. In: Kandarpa K, Aruny JE, eds. *Handbook of Interventional Radiologic Procedures*. Hagerstown, MD: Lippincott Williams & Wilkins; 2002:536-537.

Ebert EC, Hagspiel KD, Nagar M, Schlesinger N. Gastrointestinal involvement in polyarteritis nodosa. *Clin Gastroenterol Hepatol*. 2008;6:960-966.

Greckens U, Cattlaens N, Lampe EG, et al. Management of arterial puncture site after catheterization procedures: evaluation of a suture mediated closure device. *Am J Cardiol*. 1999;83:1658-1663.

Henke PK. Popliteal artery aneurysms: tried, true, and new approaches to therapy. *Semin Vasc Surg*. 2005;18:224-230.

Hessel SJ, Adams DF, Abrams HL. Complications of angiography. *Radiology*. 1981;138:273-281.

Kadir S. Arteriography of the thoracic aorta. In: Sadoon K, ed. *Diagnostic Angiography*. St. Louis MO: W.B. Saunders Company; 1986: 126-129.

Kaufman JA. Thoracic aorta. In: Kaufman JA, Lee MJ, eds. *Vascular & Interventional Radiology: The Requisites*. St. Louis MO: Mosby; 2004:222-223, 249.

Lasser EC, Berry CC, Talner LB, et al. Pretreatment with corticosteroids to alleviate reactions to intravenous contrast material. *N Engl J Med*. 1987;317:845-849.

O'Sullivan GJ, Buckenham TM, Belli AM. The use of the angioseal hemostatic puncture closure device in high risk patients. *Clin Radiol*. 1999;54:51-55.

Phillips RR, Culham JAG. Coarctation of the aorta. In: Stanley B, ed. *Abram's Angiography*. Boston, MA: Little Brown; 1997: 434.

Spies JB, Bakal CW, Burke DR, et al. Standard for diagnostic arteriography in adults. *J Vasc Interv Radiol*. 1993;4:385-395.

QUESTIONS AND ANSWERS

1. How is DSA superior to conventional angiography?
   A. Better contrast resolution
   B. Decreased examination time

C. Lower-contrast dose
D. All of the above

ANSWER: D. DSA provides better contrast resolution, decreased examination time, and lower-contrast dose than conventional angiography.

2. Which of the following is the most common complication of a popliteal artery aneurysm?
A. Thrombosis/embolism with limb ischemia
B. Rupture
C. Popliteal vein thrombosis
D. None of the above

ANSWER: A. The most common complication of popliteal artery aneurysm is distal ischemic from thrombosis/embolism.

3. What is the etiology of a type II endoleak?
A. Retrograde collateral flow from a patent arterial branch
B. Porosity of graft
C. Tear in the graft fabric
D. None of the above

ANSWER: D. A type II endoleak is secondary to persistent collateral retrograde blood flow into the aneurysm sac, commonly from lumbar arteries, the internal iliac artery, or other collateral vessels.

4. The left bronchial artery most commonly arises from which of the following?
A. Pulmonary artery
B. Thoracic aorta
C. Intercostals artery
D. Subclavian artery

ANSWER: B. Bronchial arteries vary but most often arise from the thoracic aorta at the level of T4-7 with the most common pattern consisting of one right and two left arteries.

5. What is the most common site of aortic injury?
A. Diaphragmatic hiatus
B. Aortic root
C. Aortic isthmus
D. Descending aorta

ANSWER: C. The most common site for injury is the aortic isthmus near the attachment of the ligamentum arteriosum, followed by aortic root and diaphragmatic hiatus injuries.

6. Concerning Buerger disease, which of the following statements is *false*?
A. More common in females
B. Patients are frequently smokers.
C. Patients most commonly present with claudication.
D. Secondary to inflammation of small- and medium-sized arteries

ANSWER: A. Buerger disease is more common in males than females.

7. What is the etiology of a type I endoleak?
A. Ineffective seal at the proximal or distal aspect of the graft
B. Persistent collateral retrograde blood flows into the aneurysm sac.
C. Defect within the graft fabric or between segments of a multisegmental graft
D. Endotension

ANSWER: A. A type I endoleak is secondary to an inadequate seal at the proximal aspect of the graft thereby allowing a persistent perigraft inflow.

8. Concerning Kawasaki disease, which of the following is *false*?
A. Arteritis that primarily affects the coronary arteries
B. Adults older than 70 years
C. Fever, desquamative rash, and cervical adenopathy
D. Coronary artery aneurysm formation

ANSWER: B. Kawasaki disease is mainly seen in children and infants.

9. Behcet syndrome is a vasculitis characterized by all of the following *except:*
A. Oral aphthous ulcers
B. Uveitis
C. Genital ulcers
D. *H. pylori* infection

ANSWER: D. Behcet syndrome is a multisystem inflammatory disorder characterized by recurrent oral aphthous ulcers, genital ulcers, uveitis, and skin lesions. There is no association with *H. pylori*.

10. What is Giant cell (temporal) arteritis?
A. Most common form of systemic vasculitis in adults
B. More common in women than men
C. Granulomatous arteritis
D. All of the above are true.

ANSWER: D. Giant cell or temporal arteritis is the most common form of systemic vasculitis in adults. It is more common in women than men. It is a granulomatous arteritis.

82 ARTERIAL INTERVENTIONS

Anne F. Fitzpatrick and Souheil Saddekni

PATHOPHYSIOLOGIC BASIS OF BALLOON ANGIOPLASTY

Since the first angioplasty was performed in 1964, the use of imaging to perform a variety of minimally invasive arterial procedures has grown exponentially. Advantages include diminished pain and recovery time when compared with open procedures. Currently, arterial interventions can generally be divided into two major categories: revascularization (angioplasty, stenting, thrombolysis) and embolization.

ANGIOPLASTY

The majority of cases of arterial occlusive disease are secondary to atherosclerosis. The importance of the effects of atherosclerosis cannot be overestimated, as it is the leading cause of death in the developed world. Risk factors include age, male gender, and genetic predisposition. While these risk factors cannot be reduced by behavior modification, multiple other risk factors can be reduced or eliminated, including hyperlipidemia, hypertension, smoking, and diabetes mellitus.

Vascular injury by any of the above insults causes endothelial dysfunction, which allows smooth muscle cells from the media to migrate into the intima, proliferate, and elaborate extracellular matrix. The result is intimal thickening. In addition, lipids accumulate within the intima. The combination of the thickened intima with lipid deposits gives rise to the characteristic feature of atherosclerotic disease, the fibrofatty plaque, or atheroma. Atheromas have a core composed of cholesterol and cholesterol esters, fibrin and thrombus, as well as lipid-filled monocytes and smooth muscle cells known as foam cells. Overlying this core, there is a fibrous cap, which contains smooth muscle cells, macrophages, lymphocytes, extracellular matrix, as well as small vessels supplying the periphery of the lesion.

The basic atherosclerotic lesion can be complicated by additional changes, including calcification and hemorrhage into the plaque from the small vessels feeding the periphery of the plaque. This hemorrhage, in turn, can induce rupture or ulceration of the plaque. Rupture of the plaque may release thromboemboli of the lipid core contents into the blood stream, while ulceration can expose a thrombogenic surface of the plaque. This thrombogenic surface may induce platelet deposition and clot formation, which can occlude the lumen of the vessel.

Atherosclerosis affecting the lower extremity vessels may produce chronic lower extremity ischemia, manifested as intermittent claudication. Patients typically present with pain, which is constant in terms of location and relationship to physical activity. This pain resolves with cessation of the inciting activity. Pain location depends on the site of vascular compromise. For example, patients who have mainly distal aortic and/or common/internal iliac artery disease present with pain involving the buttocks, whereas patients who have superficial femoral artery or popliteal artery disease present with calf claudication. Signs of peripheral vascular disease include diminished or absent peripheral pulses, as well as atrophy of the subcutaneous tissues and hair loss on the affected extremity. Patients with suspected peripheral arterial disease are often initially evaluated with measurement of the pressures in their ankle arteries, compared to the pressures in their arms, known as the ankle to brachial index (ABI). A diminished ABI indicates a hemodynamically significant vascular lesion between the heart and the ankle, and the lower the ABI value, the more severe the lesion. An ABI less than or equal to 0.90 in a patient at rest is diagnostic of peripheral arterial disease. More comprehensive noninvasive laborotory testing incorporates ultrasound with Doppler, plethesmography, segmental pressures, and pulse volume recordings and evaluation ABI at rest and after exercise. These tests provide a more specific idea of the severity and location of abstruction.

As the atherosclerotic disease progresses, patients may develop rest pain, described as burning or aching pain localized to the forefoot, which begins after the patient reclines. The pain can usually be relieved by placing the affected extremity in a dependent position. The diagnosis can be confirmed using measurements of pressures in the ankle and toe, with rest pain occurring with an ankle pressure of less than 50 mm Hg or a toe pressure of less than 30 mm Hg. Further progression of the disease leads to ulceration and gangrene. In this clinical setting, an ankle pressure of less than 70 mm Hg or a toe pressure less than 50 mm Hg indicates that the patient's ulceration is because of ischemia (rather than to other etiologies, such as neuropathy). Both rest pain and ulceration indicate that the patient is at risk for limb loss, and because arterial disease in the extremities is often accompanied by generalized atherosclerosis, rest pain and ulceration can also indicate that the patient is also at much higher risk for myocardial infarction and stroke.

Chronic lower extremity ischemia may be managed in several ways. Nonoperative management is acceptable for patients not at risk for limb loss; that is, those without rest pain or ulceration. Tenets of nonoperative management include smoking cessation and modification of other risk factors, such as hypertension, hyperlipidemia, and hyperglycemia. Exercise is also encouraged, as it not only improves the symptoms of claudication, but also may help in improving cardiovascular health. The importance of improving cardiovascular fitness cannot be emphasized enough, as more than 50% percent of patients with peripheral vascular disease may also have concomitant coronary artery disease. Finally, a variety of pharmacologic agents have been used to improve the symptoms of chronic lower extremity ischemia, including antiplatelet agents and vasodilators. Currently, only pentoxifylline, a methylxanthine derivative which decreases the viscosity of blood and increases the deformability of erythrocytes, and Cilostazol, a phosphodieterase III inhibitor which results in vasodilation and decreased platelet aggregation, have been approved by the FDA for the treatment of intermittent claudication. However, only cilostazol appears to have a clinically significant effect over placebo in increasing symptom-free walking distance.

Chronic lower extremity ischemia, which results in disabling claudication, meaning that it limits the patient's ability to participate in daily activities or that threatens the limb, is an indication for invasive treatment. Invasive options include percutaneous transluminal angioplasty or surgical bypass.

The first percutaneous transluminal angioplasty was performed in 1964 by Charles Dotter, who dilated a stenosis of the popliteal artery. Expanding the lumen using the "Dotter" procedure relied on passing a large catheter through the stenotic lumen. Therefore, it was limited by the size of the percutaneously introduced dilating catheter approaching the size of the artery itself. This procedure remained in very limited use in the United State. However, some investigators in Europe continued to explore this new technique, which ultimately resulted in Gruentzig introducing a simple modification to the dilating procedure in 1974. Gruentzig's innovation involved using a balloon to dilate the superficial femoral artery, a technique which he then applied to other arteries in the body. Four years after his superficial femoral artery procedure, he published reports of renal and coronary artery balloon dilatation, as had been previously predicted by Dotter. Thus, the Swiss cardiologist's innovation has ignited a remarkable revolution in the treatment of cardiovascular disease, which has continued unabated into the present day. The popularity of the angioplasty technique has prompted major research and development in atherosclerotic disease pathophysiology, plaque formation, and mechanism of action of angioplasty. Additional research has been aimed at eliciting the reasons for success or failure of angioplasty, as well as in developing stents to reduce the risk of angioplasty failure. As a result, percutaneous angioplasty currently plays a major role in the treatment of occlusive vascular disease.

The improved cross-sectional diameter of the lumen of the vessel achieved with angioplasty was initially believed to be secondary to compression of the plaque along the wall of the vessel. Since that time, however, investigators have determined that the most important contributing factor is actually the disruption of the intima, with extension of the plaque into expanded media. An additional contributing factor (although not as important as the plaque fracture) is stretching of the media.

Much was learned in the first decade of angioplasty. It became clear that not all peripheral atherosclerotic lesions are well-suited to angioplasty. Factors such as lesion morphology, technical constraints, and comorbidities have been reported to influence outcome. This knowledge was helpful in establishing general guidelines, based mainly upon the anatomic location, length of the lesion, and associated calcification. The Society of Cardiovascular and Interventional Radiology (SCVIR, now known as SIR) proposed guidelines including four categories from ideal lesions to those nonsuitable for angioplasty. These evolved over a period of more than a decade to a consensus known as the TASC standards, the Trans-Atlantic Inter-Society Consensus Document on Management of Peripheral Arterial Disease, the result of a collaboration between multiple medical societies in Europe and North America. The original document was published in 2000 and was subsequently revised in 2007. Briefly summarized, percutaneous therapy is the standard treatment for TASC A lesions (single stenosis less than 3 cm in length), while TASC D lesions (long complete occlusion of the entire artery) should be treated with surgical intervention. Therapy for category B and C lesions is not quite as structured, although the current recommendation is for percutaneous therapy for B lesions and surgery for C lesions if the patient is a good operative candidate. The Society of Interventional Radiology has established standards of practice governing the evaluation of patients for angioplasty, as well their care, both during and after the procedure.

In general, percutaneous angioplasty is a safe and effective procedure in selected patients, but it does carry certain risks. Major complications are usually related to vascular injury and include hematoma, pseudoaneurysm, or arteriovenous fistula at the access site; distal embolization; occlusion and/or rupture of the angioplastied vessel.

The use of angioplasty is not just limited to treatment of peripheral vascular disease or coronary artery disease. It has also been well-documented in the treatment of vascular disease affecting the renal arteries. Renal artery angioplasty has been used for the treatment of

TABLE 82-1 Atherosclerotic Versus Fibromuscular Dysplasia Stenosis

DISEASE PROCESS	PATIENT POPULATION	LESION LOCATION	DIAGNOSIS	TREATMENT
Atherosclerosis	>50 y, male > female	Primarily ostial	US or MRA/CTA first	Angioplasty and stenting
Fibromuscular dysplasia	Third–fifth decades, female > male	Distal main renal artery	Angiography	Angioplasty alone

renovascular hypertension as well as renal insufficiency secondary to renal artery stenosis. The two most common causes of renal artery stenosis are atherosclerosis and fibromuscular dysplasia (FMD), with the majority of FMD lesions being of the medial fibroplasia with aneurysm subtype. Other causes include Takayasu arteritis, neurofibromatosis, abdominal aortic coarcation, and compression of the renal artery by a mass or hematoma. However, these etiologies are far less common. While both diseases may cause renal artery stenosis, atherosclerotic renal stenosis and FMD differ substantially in affected patient populations, lesion location, diagnosis, and treatment.

Renal artery stenosis, secondary to atherosclerosis typically affects older male patients, in contrast to FMD, which typically affects younger female patients. The two pathologies also differ in their locations. Atherosclerotic lesions are usually ostial lesions, arising from aortic plaque extension into the proximal renal artery. In contrast, FMD is usually located within the mid-to-distal renal artery, with extension into the anteroposterior divisions. Atherosclerosis is also more likely to cause renal insufficiency, uncommon in FMD (Table 82-1).

Diagnosis of renovascular hypertension can be difficult, as it accounts for only 5% of all causes of hypertension. However, certain elements in the patient's hypertensive history are suggestive such as young age, sudden onset (particularly in a woman), severe, hypertension refractory to optimal medical therapy, no family history, abdominal bruit, and the development of renal insufficiency while on an ACE-inhibitor. When renovascular hypertension is suspected, further evaluation is indicated.

Suspected atherosclerotic renal artery stenosis is initially evaluated noninvasively. Workup may include radionuclide renogram with angiotensin-converting enzyme challenge, renal vein sampling to check for renin secretion on the affected side with suppression of secretion on the uninvolved side, or ultrasound. Ultrasound provides anatomic information and renal morphology, evaluating for congenital or acquired medical or surgical renal diseases affecting the kidneys. Ultrasound criteria for greater than 60% stenosis of renal artery stenosis include a peak systolic velocity greater than or equal to 180 cm/s and renal artery peak systolic velocity to aortic peak systolic velocity ratio of greater than or equal to 3.5. The resistive index is also important in the evaluation of renal artery stenosis, as a resistive index of less than 80 suggests that the lesion will be amenable to invasive therapy. MRA and CTA can also be used in the initial evaluation of renal artery stenosis secondary to atherosclerosis. Atherosclerotic renal artery stenosis, which involves the ostium or the proximal renal artery can be reliably depicted in CTA especially with the new generation multidetector CT with postprocessing.

Nonatherosclerotic renal artery stenosis should be suspected in young patients and children with hypertension. Neurofibromatosis, abdominal aortic dysplasia, or midaortic syndrome can involve the aorta and the renal ostia. Main, distal, and branch renal arteries are narrowed in a variety of FMD entities. The desire for less invasive testing in the young is often mitigated by the difficulty in imaging and lack of resolution of the small intrarenal vessels, which frequently necessitate the need for selective arteriography.

The angiographic signs for hemodynamically significant renal artery stenosis include greater than 75% decrease in luminal diameter, poststenotic dilatation, collateral circulation from adjacent lumbar arteries, and ultimately diminished renal mass. When these signs are not clearly seen, a pressure gradient of more than 10 mm Hg across the lesion could be used as an indicator for hemodynamic significance. Renal insufficiency secondary to renal artery stenosis can be diagnosed when there are bilateral significant renal artery stenoses with rapidly deteriorating renal function or loss of renal mass.

Options for revascularization include surgery and percutaneous therapy. Technical success rates for percutaneous therapy are very high, ranging from 80% up to 100%. However, the degree of clinical improvement varies, depending upon the pathology of the lesion (FMD responds better than atherosclerotic ostial lesions) as well as the indication for intervention (i.e., hypertension versus renal insufficiency). In general, outcomes for renovascular hypertension are better than those for azotemia. However, there are certain predictors of success with percutaneous therapy in patients with azotemia, such as bilateral lesions within the proximal renal artery proper (not ostium), serum creatinine less than 3.0 mg/dL. Ostial atherosclerotic lesions traditionally have not been as successful with balloon angioplasty, with significant residual stenosis at the ostium in the majority of cases. Technical success has improved with the advent of stenting, and in fact, many ostial lesions are primarily stented. However, this did not necessarily result in a similar clinical benefit, because of the multifactorial etiology of hypertension and renal insufficiency in mostly older patients. On the other hand, percutaneous less invasive therapy is a better option than surgery in a patient with diffuse atherosclerotic disease and multiple comorbidities.

Complications of angioplasty include puncture site injuries, such as hematoma, pseudoaneurysm, or arteriovenous fistula formation; flow-limiting dissection; arterial rupture; emboli either to the distal renal artery or the extremities; and renal failure.

STENTING

Despite the many successes of angioplasty alone, some lesions may develop recurrent stenoses or demonstrate a persistent gradient following angioplasty. In addition, angioplasty itself may damage the vessel, causing a flow-limiting dissection. For these lesions, a transcatheter-deployed vascular stent was developed. There are two basic types of stents: balloon-expandable and self-expanding. Balloon-expandable stent diameter is dependent upon the dilating balloon. These stents are less flexible than self-expanding stents, and thus should be avoided across joints (knee or hip). However, they do tend to maintain their diameter better as compared to self-expanding stents. Self-expanding stents, as their name implies, do not require a balloon dilatation for deployment. While they are more flexible than expandable stents, they can also be more difficult to position and less precise.

Stent deployment has become the standard for treating stenoses of the coronary, carotid, subclavian and renal arteries, and has also been described both for celiac and superior mesenteric artery stenoses, particularly ostial lesions, as well as aortic stenoses.

Although, angioplasty alone can be successful in treating short focal stenoses of the iliac and peripheral arteries, it appears that stenting has largely replaced balloon angioplasty. Current indications for iliac artery stent deployment include persistent transstenotic gradient following angioplasty, dissection of the angioplastied artery, stenosis length greater than 3 cm, and following recanalization of a chronically occluded arteries. While stents have been deployed in the femoral and popliteal arteries, the patency rates for these vessels are not as optimal as those with the iliac arteries.

THROMBOLYSIS

Acute thrombosis of a blood vessel results in ischemia in the tissue supplied by that vessel and can have devastating effects upon that tissue. Virchow triad describes the three factors contributing to pathologic thrombosis: endothelial injury, stasis or turbulent blood flow (as seen with ulcerated atherosclerotic lesions), or hypercoaguable states. Thrombolysis is the delivery of a plasminogen activator to dissolve thrombus and restore blood flow. Prior to the advent of thrombolysis, acute thrombosis of an ischemic limb was treated with surgical mechanical thrombectomy. Thrombolysis, however, not only offers the advantage of restoring perfusion to the affected extremity, but can also help identify any preexisting lesion predisposing to thrombosis.

The pharmacologic basis of thrombolysis is the use of tissue plasminogen activator (t-PA). Tissue plasminogen activator, as its name implies, is an endogenous substance secreted by vascular endothelial cells, which converts plasminogen to plasmin. Plasmin both breaks down the fibrin, which combines with red blood cells and platelets to form thrombus, as well as prevents the propagation of thrombin.

Thrombolytic agents such as streptokinase, urokinase, and t-PA were initially used in clinical settings for treatment of acute large pulmonary embolism and acute myocardial infarction via intravenous systemic delivery. This nontargeted approach with associated major bleeding complications gave way to the more targeted and more effective, rt-PA (Activase) catheter-delivered thrombolytic therapy. Other derivatives such as Retavase and TNK-tPA are less commonly used, while Streptokinase and Urokinase are no longer in use.

Because of the potentially devastating side effects of thrombolytic therapy, careful patient selection is warranted. Of note, when evaluating for intervention in a patient with acute limb-threatening ischemia (critical limb ischemia or CLI), it is important to establish that the extremity is still viable. Patients who have no sensation or movement in an extremity with no arterial or venous Doppler signals may not have a salvageable limb, no matter what the type of intervention. Absolute contraindications to thrombolysis for peripheral vascular occlusive diseases include cerebrovascular accident (CVA) within the past 2 months, neurosurgery within the past 3 months, or gastrointestinal bleeding within the past 10 days. Relative contraindications include pregnancy, coagulopathy, severe uncontrolled hypertension, and recent major surgery.

There are two basic techniques for thrombolysis pharmacologic and mechanical. Catheter-directed infusion thrombolysis involves crossing the occluded segment with a guidewire, and then placing a catheter with multiple sideholes across the length of the lesion, thus "bathing" the lesion with a continuous infusion of t-PA. This infusion may last from 8 to 24 hours, and the patient will usually require observation in an intensive care unit during this time. An additional mechanical component has been added in the majority of cases in an effort to

TABLE 82-2 Emobolization Agents

AGENT	OCCLUSION TIME	VESSEL SIZE	POTENTIAL USES
Coils	Permanent	Any	Trauma, varicocele
PVA particles/Acrylic spheres	Permanent	Small	Tumors
Gelatin sponge (Gelfoam)	Temporary absorbed over 4–6 wk	Small/medium	Trauma
Glues	Permanent	Any	AVM
Ethidiol	Permanent	Small	Hepatic chemoembolization
Thrombin	Permanent	Any	Aneurysm, persistent flow following embolization with another agent
Sotradecol	Permanent	Small/medium	Varicose veins
Ethanol	Permanent	Any	AVM, tumor

shorten the length of therapy and enhance the lytic effect by disrupting the clot. Pulse-spray thrombolysis involves positioning a catheter with multiple side holes in the thrombus, and then injecting short bursts of t-PA through the catheter, with the intent to both mechanically disrupt the clot, as well as deliver the t-PA. Power driven mechanical devices use fragmentationa and aspiration such as the Amplatz thrombectomy device. The Angiojet and the Trellis are routinely used in conjunction with lytics to achieve thrombolysis within 4 to 6 hours.

The success of thrombolytic therapy in peripheral vascular occlusive disease can be as high as 85% to 95%. Patients who respond within 2 hours of thrombolysis tend to have better outcomes, as do patients with acute occlusions. Patients with chronic occlusions have better long-term results with surgery. Regardless of which treatment modality used, careful search and correction of predisposing underlying stenoses should be corrected to prevent rethrombosis.

The most common complication associated with thrombolysis is bleeding at the puncture site. The risk of this complication is also increased by the simultaneous usage of heparin and/or aspirin, and the risk also increases with the duration of the procedure. Distal embolization is another potentially serious complication. In most cases, the embolus can be resolved with continued infusion. Other complications include pericatheter thrombosis (unusual when the patient is also given systemic heparin), compartment syndrome, renal failure, and infrequent but serious hemorrhage potentially anywhere in the patient.

EMBOLIZATION

In some pathologic states, such as hemorrhage or hypervascularity resulting from a neoplasm, inflammation, or an arteriovenous malformation, the goal of therapy is to disrupt blood flow. While these conditions are not as common as occlusive vascular disease, percutaneous embolotherapy is a well-established and safe method for addressing these potentially lethal problems. Percutaneous transcatheter embolization involves delivering one or more of various agents via a catheter to a selected vessel in order to induce thrombosis. The agents include metal coils; particulate agents, such as polyvinyl alcohol (PVA) particles, acrylic spheres, and gelatin sponge; and liquids, such as glues, ethidiol, sotradecol, thrombin, and ethanol. The agent chosen depends upon the indication for the procedure, velocity of flow, the size of the vessel to be embolized, and the desired occlusion time (permanent versus temporary) (Table 82-2).

SPECIFIC INDICATIONS FOR EMBOLIZATION

The use of embolization was first described in the treatment of posttraumatic hemorrhage from a pelvic fracture. Retroperitoneal hemorrhage in the trauma patient with pelvic fractures may result from fractures of cancellous bone, exacerbated by coagulopathy from hypothermia and blood transfusions. In these patients, resuscitation, reduction of the fractures, and external fixation may be sufficient therapy, as these measures can tamponade the bleeding source. However, pelvic fractures can also result in bleeding from the injury to large vessels in the pelvis, in which case, the patient may not respond to external fixation. Patients who remain hemodynamically unstable may benefit from percutaneous embolization. CT usually identifies the general location while a CTA may identify the specific site. Angiography should be performed expeditiously to identify the source of bleeding. Extravasation of contrast from a specific arterial branch identifies the bleeding site, which then can be readily selectively or super-selectively catheterized and the bleeding branch embolized. Appropriately sized coils are commonly used to stop the flow of blood. However, even if no source is identified, bilateral internal iliac embolization should be performed in desperate situation if the patient remains unstable. Bilateral embolization is performed, as cross-pelvic vascular communication can result in continued hemorrhage if only one side is selected.

Embolization has also been widely used in the treatment of splenic injury. While a hemodynamically stable patient with a splenic laceration or hematoma without a large hemoperitoneum may be managed with observation, patients with more severe splenic injury require either splenectomy or splenic artery embolization. While the spleen is not essential to life, it does have an important function in protecting the body from opsonized, encapsulated bacteria. Splenic artery embolization offers the advantage of stopping or preventing further splenic hemorrhage while preserving splenic tissue, although it can result in splenic infarction and/or splenic abscess. Distal embolization is typically performed using coils or PVA particles superselectively into the site of extravasation. More proximal splenic artery embolization may be necessary when distal catheterization is impossible because of tortuosity of the splenic artery, in which case, midsplenic artery embolization is reported to be as effective.

Embolization has also been described in the management of liver injuries. Initially, a hemodynamically unstable patient with a known hepatic laceration is managed with exploratory laparotomy with suture ligation of bleeding vessels and/or packing. This will commonly control both arterial and hepatic or portal venous bleed. However, if bleeding persists, or if the patient is hemodynamically stable with a known hepatic artery pseudoaneurysm, hepatic angiography with embolization is indicated. Because of the extensive hepatic collateral arterial supply, embolization should be as selective as possible, with occlusion of the artery both proximal and distal to the injury. Coils and/or particles may be used. Hepatic infarction is less likely than splenic infarction because of the dual blood supply of the liver.

Angiography with embolization can be used in the diagnosis and treatment of acute gastrointestinal bleeding, which is classified by location of the source: upper (proximal to the ligament of Treitz) or lower (distal to the ligament of Treitz). Upper GI bleeding is more common and is usually secondary to either peptic ulcer disease or gastritis. The initial workup of upper GI bleeding (following stabilization of the patient) is endoscopy, which is both diagnostic and therapeutic. If endoscopy fails, is not available, or is contraindicated, arteriography can be performed. Angiography can detect bleeding of 0.5 mL/min in the upper GI tract. Lower GI bleeding is usually colonic in origin, with diverticulosis and angiodysplasia being the most common causes in patients older than 50 years. The rate of bleeding must be at least 0.5 to 1.0 mL/min before it is detectable by angiography. As a result, only about 50% of angiograms are positive in acute lower GI bleeding. A tagged red blood cell scan is more sensitive in this setting, detecting bleeds of 0.1 mL/min. Therefore, hemodynamically stable patients are better served by initial evaluation with either endoscopy or a tagged red blood cell scan. In contrast, massive hemorrhage may make endoscopy difficult, so arteriography with embolization or intraarterial vasopressin infusion is the procedure of choice in the hemodynamically unstable patient with active lower GI bleeding.

Depending upon the source of the bleeding, either intraarterial vasopressin infusion or embolization can be performed. Vasopressin, or antidiuretic hormone, is synthesized within the hypothalamus and is normally secreted in response to hyperosmolality or diminished circulating blood volume. It results in water retention and vasoconstriction. Administered intra-arterially, it can relieve diffuse mucosal hemorrhage or bleeding from small vessels. It is most commonly used for diverticulosis in the lower GI tract. Because of its effects on diffuse mucosal hemorrhage, it can be used for gastritis as well, although if the patient has a known gastric source of bleeding, embolization of the left gastric artery is usually performed, as the left gastric artery is the source of bleeding in 85% of these patients. Branches of the gastroduodenal artery are a common site of bleeding from duodenal ulcers or complications of pancreatitis. If prior endoscopy has identified bleeding in the duodenum, embolization with particles or coils can be performed imperically even if arteriography fails to demonstrate extravasation. Rich duodenal collaterals prevent ischemic complications. The major contraindication to intraarterial vasopressin is ischemia; either coronary, gastrointestinal, or peripheral arterial, as the vasoconstriction can worsen ischemia in these vascular beds. The length of therapy and frequent hemodynamic side effects have made intra-arterial vasopressin infusion less desirable and infrequently used intervention.

Embolization, in contrast, is better suited to bleeding from identified extravasated arteries, as with peptic ulcer disease or even colonic bleed if used selectively, as it achieves diminished enough flow to achieve hemostasis without actually inducing ischemia.

Massive hemoptysis is the expectoration of 200 to 600 mL of blood or frankly bloody sputum within a 24-hour period. It has a high mortality rate (up to 75%), with the most common cause of death being asphyxiation, as the blood is very irritating to the airway. As a result, it is a medical emergency and should be managed expeditiously. Initial bronchoscopy is helpful to identify the involved lung or lobe, as well as allow for placement of an intrabronchial balloon tamponade. Intubation may also be necessary for airway protection. While surgical resection of the affected area was traditionally the therapy for hemoptysis, it can be very technically difficult because of the vascularity of the lesions.

Ninety percent of cases of hemoptysis involve the bronchial arteries, with the pulmonary arteries acting as the source only 10% of the time. While normal bronchial arteries are typically diminutive and difficult to select, bronchial arteries involved in massive hemoptysis are often hypertrophied, usually secondary to chronic inflammation, with tuberculosis and aspergillosis being the most common etiologies worldwide, while bronchiectasis is the most common cause in the United States. The bronchiectasis can occur with sarcoid and cystic fibrosis. Pulmonary arterial hemoptysis is usually caused by pseudoaneurysms that develop in the setting of destructive lung disease, such as cavitary aspergillosis or tuberculosis. It should be suspected if an initial bronchial artery embolization is technically successful, but the patient continues to bleed.

The hypertrophied bronchial arteries may be seen on the original arteriogram. However, if patients have a history of prior embolizations or surgery, evaluation of additional arteries, such as the subclavian artery, thyrocervical trunk, and internal mammary artery, is also suggested to eliminate these vessels as potential sources of bleeding.

Embolization is usually performed with particles, as up to 30% of patients have recurrent episodes of hemoptysis. Since coils block the proximal portions of the bronchial arteries, they would preclude further reembolization. The goal of therapy is to reduce flow enough to induce hemostasis, while not causing ischemia. The initial embolization is usually the most technically successful, as smaller, less accessible arteries are recruited in successive episodes of hemoptysis. The most feared complication of bronchial artery embolization is spinal cord injury, as a result of embolization of the anterior spinal artery, so special care is taken for its identification.

While the most common malignant liver lesion in the United States is metastatic colorectal cancer, worldwide, the most common hepatic malignancy is hepatocellular carcinoma. Embolization of both of these lesions with a particulate or liquid can be performed in conjunction with delivery of a chemotherapeutic agent directly to the tumor. The therapy has two mechanisms of action: tumor necrosis because of flow obstruction of the vessel feeding the tumor, as well as the direct delivery of a chemotherapeutic agent to the lesion, at a much higher dose than could be administered systemically. This therapy is possible without causing ischemic necrosis because of the dual blood supply from the hepatic artery and the portal vein, with many malignancies preferentially deriving their blood supply from the hepatic artery.

While surgical resection is the gold standard for treatment of resectable hepatocellular carcinoma, chemoembolization is the therapy of choice for nonresectable lesions and those not amenable to percutaneous ablation therapy. It can also be used to reduce tumor bulk prior to tumor resection or radiofrequency ablation, or to control tumor growth prior to transplantation. Absolute contraindications to the procedure include tumor resectability, infection, or advanced liver disease, in which case, chemoembolization may lead to hepatic failure. Relative contraindications include marginal liver function, encephalopathy, renal insufficiency, thrombocytopenia, as well as portal tumoral thrombosis, as embolization of the hepatic artery could then result in liver infarction. However, if hepatopedal collateral flow is still present, the procedure may still be performed.

The usual chemotherapeutic agent to treat hepatocellular carcinoma is Doxorubicin, although it may also be combined with Cisplatin or Mitomycin C. The agent is then combined with Ethidiol (iodized oil), which is taken up by tumoral cells, and/or particles. The goal of therapy is stasis of flow, thus preventing washout of the chemotherapeutic agent. Therefore gelfoam or PVA particles are often injected with or after the chemo-oil mixture. Postprocedure, the patient may develop the so-called postembolization syndrome, which is associated with abdominal pain, fever, nausea, malaise, and elevated liver function tests. This syndrome usually spontaneously resolves. Other complications include nontarget embolization, hepatic arterial injury, liver failure, gall bladder infarction, as well as complications at the access site.

UTERINE ARTERY EMBOLIZATION

The most common indication for uterine artery embolization is symptomatic uterine leiomyomas (fibroids), although it has also been used for postpartum hemorrhage and palliation of gynecologic malignancies. Leiomyomas are the most common tumors in women (occurring in at least 25% of women), and they respond to estrogen. As a result, involution typically occurs following menopause. However, in a woman of reproductive age, they may lead to menorrhagia (most common indication for embolization), pelvic pain, dyspareunia, bladder outlet obstruction, and miscarriage. Patients can be treated medically with gonadotropin releasing hormone, but have recurrence of symptoms following cessation of the hormone. Symptomatic fibroids can also be treated surgically, either with hysterectomy or myomectomy. However, uterine artery embolization offers the advantages of preserving the uterus, while treating all fibroids at the same time. Embolization can also be an adjunct to surgery, reducing tumor bulk prior to resection.

Initial evaluation should include pelvic ultrasound and/or MRI, as well as a full gynecologic workup to assess for other causes of bleeding. Uterine artery embolization is not recommended for women with pedunculated or mainly submucosal tumors. MRI helps differentiate between adenomyosis, the extension of endometrial glandular tissue into the myometrium, and leiomyomas, although uterine artery embolization can be used for certain cases of adenomyosis. Contraindications to the procedure include pregnancy, active pelvic inflammatory disease, prior radiation to the pelvis, history of severe anaphylactic contrast reaction, and renal insufficiency.

The procedure is performed with particles. Leiomyomas are well-suited to embolization as they are hypervascular and preferentially receive flow from the uterine artery, with the goal of embolization to diminish flow within the uterine arteries and reduce tumoral hypervascularity. Results vary slightly with the indication for the procedure, with menorrhagia improving in up to 90% of patients. Uterine artery embolization performed for mass effect is slightly less efficacious. Most women report postembolization syndrome, with severe pelvic cramping, which improves over subsequent week. Other complications include premature menopause (more common in women older than 45 years) and infection requiring hysterectomy.

Suggested Reading

Becker GJ, Katzen BT, Dake MD. Noncoronary angioplasty. *Radiology*. 1989;170:921-940.

Bero CJ, Cardella JF, Reddy K, et al. Recombinant tissue plasminogen activator for the treatment of lower extremity peripheral vascular occlusive disease. *J Vasc Interv Radiol*. 1995;6: 571-577.

Bosch JL, Hunink MGM. Meta-analysis of the results of percutaneous transluminal angioplasty and stent placement for aortoiliac occlusive disease. *Radiology*. 1997;204:87-96.

Castaneda-Zuniga WR, Formanek A, Tadavarthy M, et al. The mechanism of balloon angioplasty. *Radiology*. 1980;135:565-571.

Coldwell DM, Stokes KR, Yakes WF. Embolotherapy: agents, clinical applications, and techniques. *Radiographics*. 1994; 14:623-643.

Dawson DL, Cutler BS, Hiatt WR, et al. A comparison of cilostazol and pentoxifylline for treating intermittent claudication. *Am J Med*. 2000;109:523-530.

Dotter CT, Judkins MP. Transluminal treatment of arteriosclerotic obstruction. Description of a new technique and a preliminary report of its application. *Circulation*. 1964;30:654-670.

Drooz AT, Lewis CA, Allen TE, et al. Quality improvement guidelines for percutaneous transcatheter embolization. *J Vasc Interv Radiol*. 2003;14:S237-S242.

Gruntzig A, Senning A, Siegenthaler WE. Non-operative dilation of coronary artery stenosis. *N Engl J Med*. 1979;301:61-68.

Henry M, Amor M, Ethevenot G, et al. Palmaz stent placement in iliac and femoropopliteal arteries: primary and secondary patency in 310 patients with 2–4 year follow-up. *Radiology*. 1995;197:167-174.

Kandarpa K, Aruny JE. *Handbook of Interventional Procedures*. Philadelphia, PA: Lippincott Williams & Wilkins; 2002.

Kandarpa K, Becker GJ, Ferguson RDG, et al. Transcatheter interventions for the treatment of peripheral atherosclerotic lesions: part II. *J Vasc Interv Radiol*. 2001;12:807-812.

Kandarpa K, Becker GJ, Ferguson RDG, et al. Transcatheter interventions for the treatment of peripheral atherosclerotic lesions: part I. *J Vasc Interv Radiol*. 2001;12:683-695.

Kaufman JA, Lee MJ. *Vascular and Interventional Radiology: The Requisites*. Philadelphia, PA: Mosby; 2004.

Kinney TB, Chin AK, Rurik GW, et al. Transluminal angioplasty: a mechanical-pathophysiological correlation of its physical mechanisms. *Radiology*. 1984;153:85-89.

Kitamura Y, Ascher SM, Cooper C, et al. Imaging manifestations of complications associated with uterine artery embolization. *Radiographics*. 2005;25:S11-S132.

LaBerge JM, ed. *Interventional Radiology Essentials*. Philadelphia, PA: Lippincott Williams & Wilkins; 2000.

Liapi E, Georgiades CC, Hong K, Geschwind JFH. Transcatheter arterial chemoembolization: current technique and future promise. *Tech Vasc Interv Radiol*. 2007;10:2-11.

Norgren L, Hiatt WR, Dormandy JA, et al. Inter-society consensus for the management of peripheral arterial disease (TASC II). *Eur J Vasc Endovasc Surg*. 2007;33:S1-S70.

Pelage JP. Bronchial artery embolization: anatomy and technique. *Tech Vasc Interv Radiol*. 2007;10:274-275.

Pentecost MJ, Criqui MH, Dorros G, et al. Guidelines for peripheral percutaneous transluminal angioplasty of the abdominal aorta and lower extremity vessels. *J Vasc Interv Radiol*. 2003;14:S495-S515.

Semba CP, Murphy TP, Bakal CW, et al. Thrombolytic therapy with use of alteplase (rt-PA) in peripheral arterial occlusive disease: review of the clinical literature. *J Vasc Interv Radiol*. 2000;11:149-161.

Spies JB, Bakal CW, Burke DR, et al. Angioplasty standard of practice. *J Vasc Interv Radiol*. 2003;14:S219-S221.

Standards of Practice Committee of the Society of Cardiovascular and Interventional Radiology. Guidelines for percutaneous transluminal angioplasty. *Radiology*. 1990;177:619-626.

Veith FJ, Abbott WM, Yao JST, et al. Guidelines for development and use of transluminally placed endovascular prosthetic grafts in the arterial system. *J Vasc Interv Radiol*. 2003;14: S405-S417.

Working Party on Thrombolysis in the Management of Limb Ischemia. Thrombolysis in the management of lower limb peripheral arterial occlusion- a consensus document. *J Vasc Interv Radiol*. 2003;7:S337-S349.

QUESTIONS AND ANSWERS

1. Which of the following is *not* a risk factor for arterial occlusive disease?
   A. Smoking
   B. Age
   C. Female gender
   D. Diabetes mellitus
   E. Hypertension

   ANSWER: C. Cigarette smoking, increasing age, diabetes mellitus, and hypertension are all risk factors for arterial occlusive disease. Female gender does not incur an increased risk for arterial occlusive disease, although male gender does.

2. What is the ABI at or below which peripheral arterial disease is diagnosed?
   A. 1.00
   B. 0.90
   C. 1.20
   D. 1.40

   ANSWER: B. An ABI less than or equal to 0.90 in a patient at rest is diagnostic of peripheral arterial disease. However, more comprehensive noninvasive laboratory testing involves the use of ultrasound with Doppler, plethesmography, segmental pressures, and pulse volume recordings and evaluation ABI at rest and after exercise. These tests give a more specific idea of the severity and location of obstruction.

3. What is the mechanism of action of Cilostazol?
   A. Decreased blood viscosity
   B. Increased erythrocyte deformability
   C. Antiplatelet effect
   D. Vasodilation and decreased platelet aggregation

   ANSWER: D. Cilostazol is a phosphodieterase III inhibitor, which results in vasodilation and decreased platelet aggregation. Cilostazol has a clinically significant effect when compared to placebo in increasing symptom-free walking distance.

4. What is the *most* important factor in successful percutaneous transluminal angioplasty?
   A. Compression of the plaque along the vessel wall
   B. Stretching of the media
   C. Disruption of intima with extension of the plaque into the media
   D. Displacement of platelet

   ANSWER: C. Investigators have determined that the most important contributing factor in the improvement of cross-sectional diameter of the lumen of the vessel is disruption of the intima, with extension of the plaque into expanded media. Other, much less important factors include compression of the plaque along the wall of the vessel and stretching of the media.

5. What is the therapy of choice for hypertension secondary to renal artery stenosis caused by the medial fibroplasias subtype of fibromuscular dysplasia?
   A. Angioplasty alone
   B. Angioplasty with renal artery stent placement
   C. Surgical revascularization

   ANSWER: A. FMD lesions typically respond well to percutaneous angioplasty alone and usually do not require stent placement unless there is a complication associated with the procedure, such as dissection. In contrast, atherosclerotic ostial lesions often require stenting in addition to angioplasty, because the narrowing is usually secondary to extension of aortic plaque into the proximal renal artery, rather than a discrete lesion of the renal artery itself. Surgical revascularization, because of the associated higher morbidity and mortality, is rarely used for the treatment of FMD affecting the renal arteries. Of note, management of the patient with hypertension secondary to FMD should include pharmacologic therapy as necessary to control the patient's blood pressure.

6. What is an absolute contraindication to thrombolysis?
   A. Acutely ischemic extremity with profound motor and sensory loss
   B. CVA within past 2 months
   C. GI bleed within past 10 days
   D. All of the above

   ANSWER: D. An acutely ischemic extremity with profound motor and sensory loss is not viable, and cannot be salvaged, no matter what type of revascularization therapy is chosen. Additional contraindications include GI bleeding within 10 days prior to contemplated thrombolysis, as well as cerebrovascular accident within 2 months of possible thrombolysis, and neurosurgery or intracranial bleed within 3 months of possible thrombolysis.

7. What is the initial treatment of an unstable patient with pelvic fractures?
   A. Immediate angiography with prophylactic embolization
   B. Resuscitation, reduction of the fracture, and external fixation
   C. Emergent operative exploration

   ANSWER: B. The initial treatment of an unstable patient with pelvic fractures is resuscitation, reduction of the fracture, and external fixation. If the patient remains unstable despite resuscitation and fixation, and no other source of intraabdominal or intrapelvis hemorrhage is present, angiography with possible embolization may be performed. If no source of bleeding is identified by angiography in a hemodynamically unstable patient, the procedure should be terminated, and the patient taken to the operating room for emergent exploration of the retroperitoneal hematoma.

8. What is the initial diagnostic workup for hematemesis?
   A. Upper endoscopy
   B. Lower endoscopy
   C. Tagged red blood cell scan
   D. Angiography

   ANSWER: A. The initial workup of upper GI bleeding (following stabilization of the patient) is endoscopy, which is both diagnostic and therapeutic. A stable patient with lower GI bleeding may be evaluated first with a tagged red blood cell scan or endoscopy. An unstable patient with lower GI bleeding should proceed directly to angiography, as heavy bleeding may make endoscopy technically difficult.

9. What is the most common cause of bronchial artery hypertrophy leading to massive hemoptysis?
   A. Lung cancer
   B. Lung abscess
   C. Chronic inflammation within bronchiectasis
   D. Pulmonary pseudoaneurysm

   ANSWER: C. The most common cause of bronchial artery hypertrophy is chronic inflammation resulting in bronchiectasis. This chronic inflammation can result from chronic infection, including tuberculosis, as well as diseases like cystic fibrosis and sarcoidosis. Lung abscesses and lung cancer are less frequent causes of bronchial artery hypertrophy causing massive hemoptysis, and pulmonary pseudoaneurysms from cavitary lung lesions can cause bleeding from *pulmonary* arterial hemoptysis.

10. What is (are) the mechanism(s) of action of hepatic chemoembolization?
   A. Tumor necrosis secondary to disruption of hepatic arterial blood flow
   B. Direct delivery of chemotherapeutic agent
   C. Tumor necrosis secondary to disruption of portal vein flow
   D. A and B only
   E. B and D only
   F. All of the above

   ANSWER: D. Hepatic chemoembolization is possible because of the dual blood supply of the liver, with many malignancies preferentially deriving their blood supply from the hepatic artery (not the portal vein). Thus, the tumor's blood supply can be embolized, while the liver itself continues to receive blood from the portal vein. In addition, chemoembolization directly delivers chemotherapeutic agents to the tumor, at much higher doses than would be possible if systemically administered.

83 VENOUS DISEASE

Karthikram Raghuram, Kay M. Hamrick, and Jeffery R. White

VENOUS ANATOMY

UPPER EXTREMITY VEINS

The superficial venous system drains the upper extremities into the deep venous system. There are three major superficial veins: (1) cephalic (radial side), (2) basilic (posterior medial side), and (3) median (anterior forearm). At the level of the cubital fossa, the median cubital vein connects the cephalic, basilic, and median veins.

Veins of the arm drain via the basilic or cephalic system. The basilic vein, embryologic remnant of the postaxial vein, is continuous with the axillary vein. The basilic vein is located along the medial border of the biceps muscle. The brachial artery, accompanying venae comitantes, and brachial plexus lie deep to this vein, under the brachial fascia. The basilic vein pierces the brachial fascia to join the deep veins (brachial veins) at the distal two-thirds of the arm.

The cephalic vein runs between the biceps and brachialis muscles. Proximally, it lies between the pectoralis major and deltoid muscles. The cephalic vein arches deep and drains into the axillary vein deep to the medial border of the pectoralis minor muscle.

The paired brachial veins accompany the brachial artery and are closely related to the median and radial nerves. These veins empty into the basilic vein at the lateral border of the pectoralis major muscle.

The axillary vein lies inferior and anterior to the axillary artery with the brachial plexus between these two vessels. At the lateral edge of the first rib, the axillary vein becomes the subclavian vein.

The subclavian vein lies anterior to the scalenus anterior and unites with the internal jugular vein to form the brachiocephalic vein. The subclavian vein does not contain any valves.

The left brachiocephalic vein (4–6 cm long) runs obliquely downward behind the cranial sternum to the first right costal cartilage where it unites with the right brachiocephalic vein forming the superior vena cava (SVC). In its course, it crosses anterior to the pleura over the left lung. Rarely, the left brachiocephalic vein may take a vertically downward course in the mediastinum before it joins the right brachiocephalic vein. The right brachiocephalic vein (2–3 cm long) begins behind the sternal end of the right clavicle and passes directly inferiorly to join the left brachiocephalic vein.

The internal jugular veins extend from the jugular foramen, enter the carotid sheath coursing lateral to the common carotid artery and anterior to the vagus nerve.

SUPERIOR VENA CAVA

The SVC, remnant of the right anterior cardinal vein, is 7 cm long and 2 cm in diameter. It extends from the level of the first right costal cartilage to the third right costal cartilage. The pericardial reflection/insertion ranges from 1.0 to 5.0 cm and the carina is always located at or above the pericardial reflection and the azygos vein drains into the SVC just above the reflection. A persistent left SVC is the most common anomaly (0.3%) and usually drains into the coronary sinus. A bridging innominate vein may or may not be present.

INFERIOR VENA CAVA

The inferior vena cava (IVC) is formed at approximately the level of L5 by the union of the two common iliac veins, coursing superiorly in the retroperitoneum to the right of the midline anterior to the lumbar and lower thoracic spine. The IVC exits the abdomen through the diaphragmatic hiatus and drains into the inferior and posterior wall of the right atrium. There is some variation to the size of the IVC, which does not contain valves.

Embryology of the Inferior Vena Cava

Three pairs of fetal veins are located in the lower chest and abdomen that ultimately form the IVC. These are the posterior cardinal, subcardinal, and supracardinal veins. The posterior cardinal veins disappear completely, however, persistence on the right side can result in a retrocaval right ureter. IVC duplication results from persistence of the left supracardinal vein and regression of the right supracardinal vein results in a left-sided IVC. Unless there is an associated subcardinal vein (suprarenal IVC) anomaly, normal anatomy is restored above the level of the renal veins in all these variations.

The major contributors to the IVC are the hepatic, renal, gonadal, and common iliac veins. Additionally, small lumbar, right adrenal, and phrenic veins drain to it.

RENAL VEINS

Commonly, there is a single renal vein on either side. The left renal vein typically passes anteriorly between the aorta and the superior mesenteric artery and joins the IVC opposite the right renal vein at the L2 vertebral body level. The right renal vein drains directly into the IVC. Up to 40% of individuals may have variations in renal vein anatomy, including multiple right renal veins (28%), circumaortic left renal vein (5%–7%), and retroaortic left renal vein (3%).

ILIAC AND FEMORAL VEINS

The femoral vein accompanies the femoral artery and receives the profunda femoris vein just below the inguinal ligament along with the great saphenous vein. Above the inguinal ligament, the femoral vein continues as the external iliac vein. At the level of the sacroiliac joint, the external iliac vein joins the hypogastric vein to form the common iliac vein. At the level of the L5 vertebral body, the two common iliac veins unite with each other to form the IVC. The right common iliac vein is nearly vertical and the left iliac vein is longer than the right. The right common iliac artery can course over the origin of the left common vein as it traverses to the right, significantly narrowing the vein under certain circumstances (May Thurner syndrome).

LOWER EXTREMITY VEINS

The dominant superficial veins of lower extremity include the greater saphenous and the lesser saphenous veins. The greater saphenous vein begins from the medial marginal vein on the dorsal aspect of the foot and drains into the femoral vein approximately 3 cm below the inguinal ligament. It ascends in front of the medial malleolus and along the medial side of leg, where it is related to the saphenous nerve. At the knee, it is located posterior to the medial condyle of the femur. It passes upward medially in the thigh. Its dominant tributary is the accessory saphenous vein in the thigh. Just before its entry into the deep femoral vein, it receives the superficial epigastric vein and the superficial circumflex iliac vein. The superficial epigastric vein communicates with the thoracoepigastric vein, an important communication between the femoral and axillary veins.

The lesser saphenous vein is formed behind the lateral malleolus as a continuation of the lateral marginal vein. It ascends along the lateral margin of the Achilles tendon to reach the midline in the back of the leg. The vein runs directly superiorly and perforates the deep fascia in the lower part of the popliteal fossa and drains into the popliteal vein between the two heads of the gastrocnemius muscle. Just before it penetrates the deep fascia, it gives off collaterals that connect to the greater saphenous vein. In the lower part of the leg, the vein is closely related to the sural nerve; in the upper two-thirds, it is closely related to the medial cutaneous nerve of the calf.

The deep veins accompany the arteries and have multiple valves. The posterior and anterior tibial veins are paired veins that accompany the posterior and anterior tibial arteries. The popliteal vein is formed by the union of the anterior and posterior tibial veins. It receives the lesser saphenous vein just behind the knee joint.

TEMPORARY VENOUS ACCESS

Indications for placing temporary venous access include acute renal failure, failure of permanent graft or fistula in a patient on hemodialysis, chemotherapy infusion, and additional procedures in a patient with difficult venous access. Arteriovenous fistulas (AVFs) require at least 1 month to mature and AV grafts require at least 3 weeks; therefore, obtaining a temporary access for hemodialysis is critical for patients with renal failure. The National Kidney Foundation Dialysis Outcomes Quality Initiative (NKF-DOQI) states that <10% of chronic hemodialysis patients be on temporary access while their permanent access matures. Catheters are designed to achieve 400 to 600 mL/min flow rates. Polyurethane catheters dominate the market over the previously used silicone catheters because of their high tensile strength.

Typical sites for central venous placement include internal jugular veins, subclavian veins, femoral veins, and on rare occasions IVC via translumbar approach. The subclavian vein should be reserved for emergent cases only because subclavian vein stenosis and thrombosis occur at a higher rate than other access sites.

Temporary access can be divided into nontunneled and tunneled. Nontunneled catheters are designed for short periods (no longer than 3 weeks) and have a higher infection rate than tunneled catheters. NKF-DOQI states that a femoral catheter cannot be in place for longer than 5 days. Nontunneled catheters have the advantages at being able to be placed at the bedside and can be placed in a septic individual.

Tunneled catheters are designed for longer time use. The only contraindication is sepsis. Patient must be afebrile and have negative blood cultures for preceding 48 hours. Tunneled catheters have an increased incidence in central vein stenosis and thrombosis.

Complications of placing these catheters include pneumothorax, air embolus, hemothorax, dislodgement of catheter, introduction of infection, and injury to vascular structures. If a catheter is proven to be infected, it should be removed. Another rare complication is formation of fibrin sheath occluding the distal ports. In these cases, the fibrin sheath can be removed by placing a snare around the catheter and gently scraping the sheath away from the catheter tip or by angioplasty. If the catheter becomes thrombosed, injection of tissue plasminogen activator has a high success rate.

Maintenance of these catheters requires a minimal daily heparin flush and heparin infusion into the ports. Problems with these catheters include inadequate flow rate, infection, leaking, and pain. NKF-DOQI states that no more than 5% tunneled catheters should fail on first dialysis after the procedure. Inadequate flow rates can be treated with exchange of the catheter, repositioning at the atriocaval junction, snaring/stripping fibrin sheath, or thrombolytics.

PERMANENT VENOUS ACCESS

ARTERIOVENOUS FISTULAS

Fistulas account for approximately 20% of the permanent dialysis access. AVFs are favored over AV grafts because of lower incidence of infection, thrombosis, and need for intervention. Some believe that AVFs actually function longer than grafts, but this is controversial. AVF requires at least 1 month to mature before it can be used for hemodialysis.

AVFs are placed surgically and have many different possible locations. The locations can be divided into three general categories: (1) upper extremity (usually radial artery and cephalic vein), (2) upper extremity with transplanted venous return, and (3) lower extremity using femoral artery and saphenous vein.

The preferred location is the radiocephalic (also known as the Brescia-Cimino). As a general rule, the fistula should be made at the most distal possible connection based on the presurgical sonographic examination. Additional possible upper extremity locations include snuffbox (between extensor pollicis longus and brevis tendons), ulnar artery to basilic vein, brachial artery to antecubital vein, and brachiobasilic (Dagher). If the upper extremity vessels do not meet the criteria for fistula creation, then a lower extremity AVF can be created (although a graft is preferred at this location) or, rarely, an anterior chest AVF (axillary/subclavian artery to ipsilateral or contralateral axillary/jugular vein).

Care must be taken in maintaining a functional AVF. On physical examination, a thrill should be palpable along the entire length of the fistula. If the venous limb is occluded, a pulse should be palpable on the arterial limb of the fistula. If a thrill is persistent during the occlusion of the venous limb, then there is flow through large side-branches, which need to be ligated or embolized, usually surgically.

A dysfunctional graft can fall into two major categories: (1) failure to mature and (2) poor function. The NKF-DOQI states that if a radiocephalic fistula fails to support hemodialysis (blood flow >300 mL/min) after 4 months, another type of permanent access needs to be established. AVF failure to mature can be further divided into two categories: (1) inadequate flow and (2) too low

TABLE 83-1 Complications of AVF Intervention

Vein rupture during angioplasty resulting in loss of access	Bleeding can be controlled with external manual compression or an occlusive balloon
Ischemia of the hand	Requires immediate surgical intervention or distal thrombectomy to salvage the hand
Intracranial hemorrhage secondary to thrombolysis	
Myocardial infarction or pulmonary edema	Because these patients have ESRD and are already volume overloaded, care must be taken not to give too much fluids during the procedure
Sepsis	

venous resistance. Inadequate blood flow is most likely secondary to a stenosis either within the native artery proximal to the anastomosis or within the anastomosis itself. These are usually treated with angioplasty; however, care must be taken with the native artery because a dissection, thrombosis, or embolus can be devastating requiring immediate surgery. Inadequate venous resistance causes the venous limb to fail to "arterialize." This is invariably due to large venous branches, which need to be ligated/embolized.

A poorly functioning AVF (like a graft) is most likely secondary to venous outflow stenosis. A low *Kt*/*V* (where, *K* is total urea clearance of the dialyzer, *t* is time, *V* is volume), high recirculation calculation, or elevated venous pressures all indicate venous stenosis. Venous stenosis is treated with angioplasty.

Thrombosed AVF can be treated with either thrombolysis or mechanical thrombectomy. Again, care must be taken since these are the native vessels and not a graft (especially with the arterial limb). Also, the majority of the mechanical thrombectomy devices are FDA approved for grafts and not native vessels. There are several potential major complications when treating a dysfunctional AVF (Table 83-1).

ARTERIOVENOUS GRAFTS

Grafts are more commonly placed than AVF (80%). AV grafts have the advantage over AVF; they can have variable lengths making connection between the arterial and venous limb easier. Originally, there were two different types of grafts: saphenous vein graft (not used anymore) and prosthetic graft. There are two main categories of prosthetic grafts: (1) fabric (Dacron) and (2) synthetic polymers (PTFE). The latter are favored over the fabric grafts, which can fray after multiple needle punctures. In addition, the PTFE grafts are supported by external rings, thereby, decreasing external compression and kinks. Both types allow ingrowth of tissue, incorporating the graft into the viable tissue.

Grafts can be further subdivided into straight and loop grafts. Originally, loop grafts were thought to be superior to straight grafts; however, over time this topic has become controversial. The locations of the grafts are similar to AVFs, however, extensive repositioning of the native vessels is not necessary. When a graft is placed, it is best to have a wide loop, permitting easier passage of percutaneous catheters and mechanical thrombectomy devices. In addition, if arterial and venous anastomosis are in close proximity to each other, determining the arterial versus the venous limb may be more difficult, especially if the graft is completely thrombosed.

Unique to grafts is a condition called ischemic (or arterial) steal syndrome. This occurs when there is a reversal of the arterial blood flow distal to the graft. This occurs in approximately 2% of the grafts but is not seen with AVF. The symptoms range from a cool sensation of distal extremity to limb-threatening ischemia. Ischemic steal syndrome may be due to diseased native artery proximal or at the anastomosis. Treatment includes angioplasty of proximal arterial stenosis or surgery with ligation of the graft, intentionally narrowing (or banding) the arterial inflow or distal artery ligation (or revascularization) depending on the location of the graft.

Maintenance of a graft is critical to avoid thrombosis. The inflow rate of a graft needs to be at least the same as dialysis pump rate (300 mL/min). On physical examination, the graft (like AVF) should have a thrill in its entirety. If there is a stenosis, the thrill is replaced with a pulse proximal to the stenosis. There will be a thrill or bruit at the stenosis with diminished or no pulse distally. Venous pressure during hemodialysis is the best indicator for graft dysfunction. A venous pressure of greater than 125 mm Hg (via 15-gauge needle at 200–225 mL/min at dialysis) indicates graft dysfunction. Additionally, if the normalized pressure ratio (venous pressure/systolic pressure) is greater than 0.4 mm Hg, this indicates there is a stenosis. If the arterial inflow pressure does not sustain a rate greater than 300 mL/min, then an arterial stenosis is likely. The actual blood flow rate is a poor indicator of graft dysfunction. Sonographic investigation is an excellent modality in detecting stenoses; however, it is not cost effective for routine surveillance. Early thrombosis (less than 6 weeks) is considered a technical or mechanical error while later thrombosis is considered to be secondary to intimal hyperplasia resulting in venous stenosis at the venous anastomosis.

The NKF-DOQI guidelines state that there should be less than 0.5 thrombotic episodes in a graft per patient per year. In addition, graft patency rates should be 70% at 1 year, 60% at 2 years, and 50% at 3 years. There are many causes of graft dysfunction, which include thrombosis (most common), infection (the only contraindication for percutaneous intervention), pseudoaneurysm, atherosclerosis of arterial inflow vessels (poor graft thrill), and lymphoceles. Thrombosis, resulting in a decrease in blood flow and increase in graft pressures, most commonly occurs because of a stenosis at the venous outflow anastomosis (80% of dysfunctional grafts). Other causes of thrombosis include altered platelet function, hypercoagulable state, and external compression of the graft.

A pseudoaneurysm is usually caused by a defect in the prosthetic graft, usually due to poor cannulation technique and venous hypertension. These rarely resolve spontaneously and have a risk of spontaneous rupture. Treatment involves covered stent, or thrombin injection directly into the pseudoaneurysm.

A lymphocele is a perigraft collection of ultrafiltrate that weeps across the graft pores, usually near the arterial anastomosis. This collection can develop into a fistula with skin breakdown. Fistulogram will demonstrate no communication with the collection; this allows differentiation from pseudoaneurysm.

Treatment options for dysfunctional graft include both surgical and percutaneous intervention. Patients with a history of right ventricular failure, pulmonary hypertension, right-to-left shunt, or cardiac dysrhythmia are not optimal candidates for percutaneous intervention and should be referred for surgical thrombectomy. In addition, patients should have a satisfactory hematocrit level because mechanical thrombectomy may further decrease the blood volume by mechanical destruction of the red blood cells and too much aspiration.

There are four common steps involved with all percutaneous thrombosed graft treatments. Initial venogram is performed. As stated earlier, the most common site of abnormality for a thrombosed graft is at the venous anastomosis. Secondly, thrombus within both the venous and arterial limbs is removed. Prior to starting, 2000 to 5000 units of heparin are injected. The venous limb is usually cleared of all the thrombi before inserting another sheath and clearing the arterial limb. Then, venous and arterial stenoses are treated. There are two schools of thought about the timing of venous intervention. Traditionally, correction of the venous stenosis is left for the end of the procedure, so the potential pulmonary thrombosis burden will be less, as the stenosis will prevent the emboli from entering the systemic circulation. Others believe addressing the stenosis first, which will decrease intragraft pressure and thereby decrease the risk for arterial emboli. The diameter of the balloon should be 10% to 20% greater than vessel diameter. Finally, the arterial plug, composed of fibrin and packed red blood cells, is dislodged. A compliant balloon (Fogarty) is typically used with care not to injure the native artery or dislodge emboli into the arterial circulation.

Both mechanical thrombectomy and thrombolysis are common techniques used to declot a graft. There are many different types of mechanical thrombectomy devices on the market. Some have a rotating driveshaft, which makes operating at acute angles difficult. Thrombolysis usually uses a combination of heparin with either urokinase or streptokinase. A "lyse and wait" technique is used when a lytic agent is injected a certain time period prior to the procedure. Complications with percutaneous intervention include arterial emboli, vessel rupture, and arterial rupture. To date, no clinically significant pulmonary embolus has been encountered with these techniques, however, the theoretical risk remains.

VENOUS THROMBOEMBOLIC DISEASE

Venous thromboembolic disease comprises deep venous system thrombosis (DVT), pulmonary thromboembolism (PTE), and venous insufficiency. There are approximately 20 million new cases of lower-extremity and 200 000 to 6 000 000 of upper-extremity DVT yearly. The most critical consequence is a large pulmonary embolism resulting in death. Pathophysiology of venous thrombosis is complex, as described by the Virchow triad (Table 83-2).

Extremity DVT commonly presents with unilateral extremity edema, pain, and warmth. Sometimes, the first presentation is pulmonary embolism. Occasionally, massive DVT involving the entire venous system of the extremity presents as phlegmasia in the extremities with congestion, massive edema, and limb-threatening compartment syndrome. Dilated and prominent collateral veins are sometimes noted. History of antecedent inciting causes such as trauma, prolonged immobilization, and exercise (Paget-Schroetter syndrome in upper extremity) can be useful.

Doppler ultrasound is the mainstay of diagnosis. CT venography in concert with a CT pulmonary angiogram can be performed as a single study to assess for DVT and PTE at the same sitting. MRI has a problem-solving role in lower extremity DVT and is more useful in upper extremity DVT to assess the central veins. Conventional venography is rarely performed, restricted to specific scenarios in-

TABLE 83-2 Virchow Triad

Slow venous flow	External compression, prolonged immobilization
Disruption in vein wall	Trauma from catheters, previous DVT
Hypercoagulable state	Cancer, polycythemia vera, antithrombin III deficiency, protein S or C deficiency, estrogen therapy

cluding evaluation of central DVT in the upper extremities prior to intervention for thrombolysis/thrombectomy, prior to upper extremity permanent dialysis access placement, or prior to placement of a vena cava filter.

Complications of DVT include PTE, phlegmasia cerulea dolens, and postthrombotic syndrome with chronic venous insufficiency. The main principles underlying management are the prevention of PTE and progression of the DVT, both achieved by anticoagulant therapy. An IVC filter addresses only the issue of a possible PTE and does not affect the progression of DVT. Thrombolysis in concert with IVC filter placement addresses both and is the only method that decreases the risk of postphlebitic syndrome and restores venous patency.

The mainstay in the prevention of PTE in a patient with known DVT is the use of anticoagulants, either warfarin or heparin. Warfarin (Coumadin) is the drug of choice for management on an outpatient basis; however, there are certain risks associated with the use of warfarin and maintaining a therapeutic international normalized ration (2.0–3.0). These include bleeding risks related to preexisting conditions such as ulcer disease, bleeding from minor trauma, hematuria, and intracranial hemorrhage in patients with hypertension. Approximately 20% of patients on Coumadin therapy develop complications that necessitate discontinuing therapy, which often mandates filter placement. There are several indications for filter placement (Table 83-3).

IVC filters are best positioned, with the superior tip exposed to the wash in of blood from both renal veins, thereby reducing the risk of IVC occlusion and maintaining renal vein outflow even if there is a large embolus trapped in the filter. A good quality IVC venogram is mandatory before placing filter. In addition, review of prior cross-sectional imaging studies may help detect unexpected venous variant anatomy. Some of the important variations that could affect the placement include IVC diameter greater than 28 mm (requires OptEase, Bird's nest filter, or the presence of anatomical variations in renal veins [40%]). These variations include multiple renal veins (28%)—usually not an issue as long as they are in close proximity, circumaortic renal vein (5%–8.7%), and retroaortic left renal vein (3%). For the latter two, filter needs to be placed above the renal veins in most cases. Bird's nest filters are not recommended in a suprarenal location because of the increased risk of prolapse of the coils into the heart. If there is enough distance, the filter could be placed in the IVC below the entry of the circumaortic component.

TABLE 83-3 Indications for Caval Filter Placement

Contraindication to Coumadin therapy
Patient is considered unable to maintain the rigorous follow-up required when on Coumadin therapy
Free floating iliofemoral or IVC thrombus
Temporary IVC filtering in patients with increased risk of DVT in the preoperative setting (trauma, gynecologic surgery, etc.)
Patients who have had a prior massive PE or have DVT with limited cardiopulmonary reserve

There can also be caval variations, such as duplicated IVC. Usually the infrarenal segment is duplicated and the left IVC drains into the left renal vein. Filters may be placed in both infrarenal IVCs or in a suprarenal location. There are multiple filters marketed with varying shapes without significant difference in their effectiveness.

RETRIEVABLE FILTERS

The long-term outcomes of filter placement are unknown, and there is risk of caval thrombosis. Also, comparative studies between filter placement alone and anticoagulation demonstrate there is comparable decrease in risk of PTE with greater risk of progressive DVT. Filters are most commonly placed when there is a contraindication to anticoagulation. Retrievable filters are of two types: temporary and optional. Temporary filters are not approved in the United States and consist of the filter attached to a wire or retrievable device that can be left in situ and removed when filtration is no longer desired. Optional filters can be removed either using a snare or an appropriate retrieval device.

These filters are best suited for patients who are at high risk for venous stasis and thromboembolism, such as trauma patients with orthopedic injury and patients undergoing gynecologic surgery.

SUPERIOR VENA CAVA FILTERS

The proposed indications for SVC filter are analogous to those for IVC filter. Contraindications include the following: (1) extensive SVC thrombus; (2) SVC diameter greater than 28 to 30 mm; (3) uncorrectable, significant coagulopathy; and (4) venous pacemaker.

FILTERS CHOICE

Because of the long-term experience with the Greenfield filter, some physicians choose this filter for younger patients. The bird's nest filter is needed for patients with a large vena cava (approved up to 40 cm in diameter). When there is only a short segment of usable IVC, such as when there is a low insertion of a renal vein, placing a Greenfield filter or Gunther Tulip (which can be secured in a small length of cava) may be preferable.

Knowing the characteristics of each filter will help in choosing the optimal filter for each clinical scenario.

COMPLICATIONS

Complications of filter placement include access site complications such as hematoma, AV fistula, and access vein thrombosis. Complications related to the filter include acute complications such as caval perforation, malposition of the filter, and migration of the filter. Chronic complications include filter migration, fracture, low-grade caval perforation, and IVC occlusion. Additional risks to a jugular/subclavian approach include pneumothorax, air embolism, arrhythmias, and SVC injury with mediastinal/pericardial hemorrhage.

VENOUS THROMBOLYSIS

Catheter-directed thrombolysis is the only method of DVT management that restores venous patency and decreases the risk of postphlebitic syndrome. However, it is underused and is typically reserved for patients with massive acute DVT in the lower extremity (phlegmasia cerulea dolens) or effort thrombosis in the upper extremity (Paget-Schroetter syndrome). There is a relative lack of data from randomized controlled trials comparing catheter-directed therapy with anticoagulation therapy.

Patients with symptomatic acute iliofemoral DVT (less than 10 days) or phlegmasia, diagnosed by conventional venography and/or color Doppler ultrasound who are eligible for thrombolytic therapy and long-term anticoagulation are candidates for this therapy. This subset of patients are often otherwise healthy and may have an underlying obstructive venous lesion such as May Thurner syndrome. The presence of active internal bleeding, history of a cerebrovascular accident, recent intracranial or intraspinal surgery (less than 1 year), pregnancy, and/or coagulopathy are contraindications. Phlegmasia can also occur in patients with pelvic carcinomatosis or diffuse malignancies, and these patients have limited survival and may not represent ideal candidates for thrombolysis.

There are three general categories of upper extremity DVT. Primary or spontaneous upper extremity DVT occurs in young patients and is due to an underlying mechanical lesion in the costoclavicular space or interscalene triangle. The presence of an anomalous bone, muscle slip, or musculotendinous insertion leads to chronic subclavian vein narrowing. When recurrent occupational or exertional stress is superimposed, intimal damage occurs that results in thrombosis. This is also known as Paget-Schroetter syndrome.

Secondary DVT in the upper extremity results from an identifiable underlying disease processes such as malignancy or hypercoagulable state. Also, mechanical compression by mass or lymph nodes or local invasion by malignancy result in thrombosis.

A third and growing cause of upper extremity DVT is the placement of indwelling central venous catheters. Venous thrombosis in the upper extremity is often clinically silent and may affect up to 30% of patients with central catheters. Symptomatic upper extremity DVT occurs in approximately 3% to 4% of patients. Presenting symptoms include arm pain, swelling, cyanosis, facial edema, and rarely pulmonary embolism.

MANAGEMENT

In the setting of acute primary DVT, anticoagulation and thrombolysis have been used, with the latter method gaining in popularity as it allows the reestablishment of venous patency. A combination of mechanical thrombectomy and thrombolytic infusion have been used with good results. However, there are no randomized controlled trials comparing systemic and catheter-directed thrombolysis. In the case of effort thrombosis, the culprit compressive lesion is best treated by surgery, as the mechanical component of the compression cannot be addressed by endovascular methods. May-Thurner syndrome is treated by stent placement at the left iliac vein stenosis with good long-term success. The incidence of DVT caused by central venous catheters can be reduced by administration of low-dose heparin in selected patients considered to be at a higher risk.

MISCELLANEOUS

SUPERIOR VENA CAVA SYNDROME

SVC syndrome refers to obstruction or occlusion of the SVC with impaired venous return from the upper extremities, head, and neck to the right atrium. Symptoms include facial edema, cough, dyspnea, orthopnea, hoarseness, nausea, headache, plethora, and distention of superficial veins. Life-threatening complications may include cerebral or laryngeal edema. However, mortality is usually secondary to the underlying cause of the venous occlusion. SVC syndrome may result from lung or mediastinal cancer encasing or invading the SVC (80%), mediastinal fibrosis, or from indwelling catheters or cardiac pacer leads causing occlusion. Treatment options for SVC syndrome include surgery, radiation therapy, chemotherapy, and angioplasty with or without stenting. Endovascular therapy has become the mainstay of treatment for SVC syndrome with stent placement for malignant disease and angioplasty for benign disease. Complications include arrhythmia, acute right heart failure or pulmonary edema from fluid overload, intracerebral hemorrhage secondary to procedural thrombolysis, and acute pericardial effusion and tamponade.

INFERIOR VENA CAVA OCCLUSION

Causes of IVC occlusion include thrombus (extending from an iliac vein, filter placement, trauma, surgery, or placement of an indwelling catheter) or external compression (retroperitoneal mass, pregnancy, adenopathy, or retroperitoneal fibrosis). Tumor infiltration of the IVC is also a culprit.

Acute occlusion presents as bilateral lower extremity edema with or without phlegmasia. More commonly, the occlusion is chronic with development of collaterals. The presence of dilated abdominal wall veins and bilateral lower extremity edema suggests IVC occlusion. Ultrasound, CT, and MRI help in the diagnosis of IVC obstruction and allow identification of an etiology in most cases. Treatment includes thrombolysis in the acute setting and angioplasty with or without stent placement if there is an underlying stenosis.

GONADAL VEIN EMBOLIZATION

Gonadal vein embolization is performed in males for testicular varicocele and in female patients for pelvic congestion syndrome. Varicoceles are encountered in 20% to 40% of male patients with infertility. Treatment is by embolization using coils and sclerosing agents. Technical success rate ranges from 83% to 96%. There is a 12% to 16% rate of recurrence, which is treated surgically.

Veins from the mediastinum testis form the pampiniform plexus, which arises in the scrotum and extends into the spermatic cord. The plexus coalesces into the internal spermatic vein, which passes through the inguinal canal and ascends through the retroperitoneum. Ultimate venous drainage is to the IVC on the right and the renal vein on the left. Ureteric, lumbar, perirenal, and retroperitoneal veins empty into the gonadal veins.

Pelvic congestion syndrome in women represents noncyclic pelvic pain in the absence of menstruation that is severe enough to cause functional disability. Causes include endometriosis versus pelvic adhesions. This condition usually affects women in the age group of 20 to 30 years. The symptoms are typically exacerbated by standing or lifting and may improve on lying supine. Etiology is considered to be ovarian vein reflux. Ultrasound is usually used for detection and quantification of the dilated veins. Treatment includes embolization using coils and sclerosing agents. Technical success rates and potential complications are the same as for varicoceles in men.

ADRENAL VEIN SAMPLING

Adrenal vein sampling localizes a hyperfunctioning adrenal adenoma, secreting either aldosterone or cortisone, when cross-sectional imaging has failed. This procedure differentiates unilateral adrenal adenoma from bilateral adrenal hyperplasia. Simultaneous catheterization of both adrenal veins is performed and samples are obtained concurrent with peripheral venous samples, before and after stimulation with ACTH. The aldosterone–cortisol ratio remains high before and after ACTH stimulation on the abnormal side. On the normal side, the aldosterone–cortisone ratio does not change with ACTH stimulation and remains similar to that in the peripheral femoral vein. In the case of Cushing's syndrome, ACTH stimulation is not required. The treatment for unilateral adenoma is resection. Bilateral adrenal hyperplasia is usually treated medically.

VENOUS INSUFFICIENCY

Venous insufficiency affects 25% of all women (72% of those older than 60 years) and 15% of all men. Risks factors for developing venous insufficiency include hereditary (25% with one afflicted parent; 25% for men and 60% for women with two afflicted parents), lifestyle (27% increased risk with sedentary lifestyle and 36% increased risk with prolonged standing), body habitus (increased BMI for females and increased height for males), and prior history of DVT (50%–60% of the cases).

The pathophysiology of developing venous insufficiency can be divided into three general categories: valvular insufficiency (most common), venous obstruction (DVT or external compression such as pregnancy), and muscle pump dysfunction.

Gravity helps with arterial circulation in the sense that the primary vector of gravity pushes the blood to the distal extremities. This is reverse for venous flow and alternate mechanisms are needed to propel the blood against gravity. This is accomplished first by muscle pump action. As a muscle contracts, the deep vein within that muscle is externally compressed by its surrounding muscle. When this occurs the blood is propelled from that vessel. Valves within the veins are present to prevent the blood from being propelled in the wrong direction. So, any disruption in this mechanism can result in venous insufficiency.

TABLE 83-4 Venous Perforators List

Hunter	Medial thigh
Dodd	Distal thigh
Boyd	Medial knee
Cockett	Posterior tibial

Anatomy specific for venous insufficiency include superficial veins (lesser saphenous, greater saphenous), perforators (connect deep veins to the superficial), reticular veins (tributaries to the saphenous), and capillaries (cause spider veins and telangiectasia). Twenty percent of the population has duplicated saphenous veins. Identifying which vein is dilated will help isolate which valve is incompetent (Table 83-4).

Besides cosmetic appearance, venous insufficiency can result in a various array of symptoms including pain, pruritus, night cramps, fatigue, heaviness, and leg restlessness. Advanced changes include edema, hyperpigmentation, dermatitis, lipodermatosclerosis, and ulceration. There is specific terminology used for the dilated vein. A varicose vein is a dilated, protruding, tortuous, saccular superficial vein in the subcutaneous tissues. A reticular vein is a dilated, tortuous, nonprotruding superficial vein in the subcutaneous tissues. A telangiectasia is a spider appearing, tortuous nonprotruding or dilated vein in the dermis.

Ultrasound evaluation is the modality of choice for evaluating venous insufficiency and etiology of disease. Indication for sonographic examination includes symptomatic or asymptomatic visible varicose veins, symptoms of venous hypertension, or recurrent varicose veins after surgery. Generally, ultrasound is not indicated for telangiectasia. On sonographic examination, incompetent valves, DVT, extent of dilated veins, and reversal of blood flow can be visualized.

Treatment for venous insufficiency can be categorized into four groups: (1) conservative, (2) surgical, (3) sclerotherapy, and (4) endovascular thermal ablation. Conservative therapy includes compression stockings, improve calf muscle function, good skin hygiene, losing weight, regular exercise, and avoiding prolonging periods of standing or sitting.

Surgical option for venous insufficiency involves groin surgery to expose and ligate the diseased great saphenous vein and surrounding tributaries. A stripping tool is inserted at the groin, threaded through the great saphenous vein exiting through the skin just below the knee; the saphenous is then tied to the stripping tool and pulled from below the knee.

Sclerotherapy involves refluxing a sclerosing agent into the saphenous vein. This may be an isolated treatment method or used in conjunction with surgery. There is a high rate of recanalization and symptom recurrence compared to the other modalities of treatment. Typically, the procedure is performed with ultrasound guidance. Common sclerosing agents include sodium tetradecyl sulfate (Sotradecol), polidocanol, 23.4% saline, 25% dextrose with 10% saline, and sodium morrhuate. Anaphylactic reactions, toxic reactions, hemolysis, and skin necrosis/ulceration are some of the complications associated with sclerotherapy.

Endovascular thermal ablation can involve using a radiofrequency probe, a laser (most common), or cryotherapy probe (poorer results). There is a 98% successful procedure rate with a 93% persistent saphenous vein occlusion. Contraindications to the procedure include dermatitis, cellulitis, severe edema, and allergies to local anesthetics.

Avoiding tight-fitting undergarments and clothing, crossing legs, and sitting and standing for long periods of time will decrease the recurrence of venous insufficiency. In addition, regular exercise, weight loss, and elevating legs at least twice a day will also decrease the rate of recurrence.

Suggested Reading

Aruny J. Maintaining native arteriovenous fistulas for dialysis access. *Tech Vasc Interv Radiol.* 1999;2(4):199-207.

Bittles MA, Hoffer EK. Gonadal vein embolization: treatment of varicocele and pelvic congestion syndrome. *Semin Interv Radiol.* 2008;25(3):261-270.

Gelbfish G. Surgical care of the arteriovenous graft: issues for the interventionalist. *Tech Vasc Interv Radiol.* 1999;2(4):179-185.

Gray RJ. Angioplasty and stents for peripheral and central venous lesions. *Tech Vasc Interv Radiol.* 1999;2(4):189-198.

Greenstein S, Patel V, Kim D. Surgical creation of fistulas and grafts. *Tech Vasc Interv Radiol.* 1999;2(4):174-178.

Kaufman JA. Retrievable vena cava filters. *Tech Vasc Interv Radiol.* 2004;7(2):96-104.

Kinney TB. Inferior vena cava filters. *Semin Interv Radiol.* 2006;23(3):230-239.

Lautin JL, Cynamon J. Declotting grafts with thrombolysis. *Tech Vasc Interv Radiol.* 1999;2(4):217-220.

Lorenz JM. Unconventional venous access techniques. *Semin Interv Radiol.* 2006;23(3):279-286.

Murphy DK. Superior vena cava filters. *Tech Vasc Interv Radiol.* 2004;7(2):105-109.

O'Horo SK, Soares GM, et al. Acute pericardial effusion during endovascular intervention for superior vena cava syndrome: case series and review. *Semin Interv Radiol.* 2007;24(1):82-86.

Roberts A, Valji K. Screening and assessment of dialysis graft function. *Tech Vasc Interv Radiol.* 1999;2(4):186-188.

Savader SJ, Trerotola SO. *Venous Interventional Radiology with Clinical Perspectives.* 2nd ed. New York, NY: Thieme; 2000.

Vesely TM. Techniques for using mechanical thrombectomy devices to treat thrombosed hemodialysis grafts. *Tech Vasc Interv Radiol.* 1999;2(4):208-216.

Wahl S, Cynamon J. Central dialysis catheters. *Tech Vasc Interv Radiol.* 1999;2(4):221-227.

QUESTIONS AND ANSWERS

1. Which of the following steps would *not* be performed initially during an AV graft declot?
   A. Angioplasty the venous stenosis
   B. Mechanical thrombectomy
   C. Dislodgement of arterial plug
   D. Injection of thrombolytics

   ANSWER: C. You would never dislodge the arterial plug first as this would increase risk of the embolization into the systemic circulation, possibly resulting in limb-threatening ischemia.

2. If a patient has a duplicated IVC, where is an IVC filter usually placed?
   A. Infrarenal right IVC
   B. Suprarenal IVC
   C. Infrarenal left IVC
   D. Filter is contraindicated and thrombolysis should be performed.

   ANSWER: B. With a duplicated IVC, a suprarenal filter or infrarenal filter in both IVCs is recommended.

3. In a circumaortic renal vein, which IVC filter *cannot* be used?
   A. Gunther Tulip
   B. OptEase
   C. Internal jugular vein approached filter
   D. Bird's nest

   ANSWER: D. With a circumaortic renal vein, IVC filter needs to be placed usually in a suprarenal location. A bird's nest filter has increased risk of prolapse of the coils into the heart.

4. What is the standard treatment of malignant SVC syndrome?
   A. Stenting
   B. Surgery
   C. Angioplasty
   D. Endovascular treatment is only undertaken with benign disease.

   ANSWER: A. In general, stent placement is used for malignant SVC syndrome, as it is permanent. Angioplasty is used for benign disease.

5. A perforator vein of the medial thigh, which is fairly consistent in location, is also known as
   A. Dodd
   B. Boyd
   C. Cockett
   D. Hunter

   ANSWER: D. Hunter (medial thigh), Dodd (distal thigh), Boyd (medial knee), and Cockett (posterior tibial) are names given to perforators.

6. What is a dilated, tortuous, nonprotruding superficial vein in the subcutaneous tissues?
   A. Varicose vein
   B. Telangiectasia
   C. Reticular vein
   D. Deep vein

   ANSWER: C. A varicose vein is a dilated, protruding, tortuous, saccular superficial vein in the subcutaneous tissues. A reticular vein is a dilated, tortuous, nonprotruding superficial vein in the subcutaneous tissues. A telangiectasia is a spider appearing, tortuous nonprotruding or dilated vein in the dermis.

7. What causes Paget-Schroetter syndrome?
   A. Presence of an anomalous bone, muscle slip or musculotendinous insertion leading to chronic subclavian vein narrowing
   B. Recurrent occupational or exertional stress causing intimal damage resulting in thrombosis
   C. Hypercoagulable state secondary to heredity condition
   D. Thrombosis secondary to underlying malignancy

   ANSWER: B. This is the definition of Paget-Schroetter syndrome.

8. Where is the cephalic vein located?
   A. Medial border of the biceps muscle
   B. Between the biceps and brachialis muscles
   C. Lateral border of pectoralis major muscle
   D. Pierces the brachial fascia to join the deep veins (brachial veins) at the distal two-thirds of the arm

   ANSWER: B. The cephalic vein courses between biceps and brachialis muscles. The basilic vein is continuous with the axillary vein and is located along the medial border of the bicep.

9. On physical examination of AVF, where should a thrill be palpable?
   A. On the arterial limb only
   B. On the venous limb only
   C. Throughout the entire graft
   D. Only when the venous or arterial limb is occluded.

   ANSWER: C. The thrill should be felt throughout the entire graft. With occlusion of the venous side, and pulse should be felt on the arterial side.

10. When are temporary nontunneled catheters contraindicated?
    A. Sepsis
    B. When patient has a nonfunctioning AV graft
    C. Hypercoagulable state
    D. None of the above

    ANSWER: D. Temporary nontunneled catheters are for short-term use (less than 3 weeks). Unlike tunneled catheters, sepsis is not a contraindication.

84 ABDOMEN AND LIVER

Kok C. Tan and Souheil Saddekni

VASCULAR ANATOMY

The liver parenchyma is made up of lobules consisting of sinusoids around a central draining vein, bounded by the portal triad of branches from the bile duct, portal vein, and hepatic artery at the periphery. The liver is mainly composed of hepatocytes, which perform the main metabolic function of the liver and Kupffer cells that form part of the reticuloendothelial system. The liver receives approximately two-thirds of its blood supply from the portal vein and one-third from the hepatic artery. Blood drains via the hepatic veins into the inferior vena cava, and then into the heart.

PORTAL HYPERTENSION

Portal hypertension refers to abnormally high pressure in the portal vein. It is defined as a portal pressure greater than 10 mm Hg, (normal 5–10 mm Hg). Alternatively, it can be defined by the gradient between the wedge hepatic venous pressure (which is an indirect measurement of the pressure in the sinusoids and hence the portal vein) and the free hepatic venous or the inferior vena cava pressure. The normal gradient is less than 5 mm Hg. This gradient is also called corrected sinusoidal portal pressure. Because of great variations of intra-abdominal pressures reflected in a baseline increase of the pressure in the portal vein and inferior vena cava, a more accurate measurement of true portal hypertension is to use the gradient rather than absolute pressures.

Portal hypertension is most commonly encountered in patients with cirrhosis. The common conditions leading to cirrhosis and portal hypertension are alcoholic liver disease and chronic viral hepatitis. Patients in whom a cause cannot be identified are said to have cryptogenic liver cirrhosis. Not all patients with portal hypertension have cirrhosis. Cirrhosis refers to a specific histologic finding of diffused fibrosis and abnormal liver nodularity, resulting from chronic hepatocellular injury.

The causes of portal hypertension can be organized into several categories based upon the level of obstruction: prehepatic, intrahepatic, and posthepatic. Pathologists have further divided the intrahepatic causes into presinusoidal, sinusoidal, and postsinusoidal causes on the basis of histologic findings depending on the predominant location of the fibrosis with regard to the sinusoids (Table 84-1).

Portal hypertension is caused by an increased resistance to blood flow through the liver. Fibrotic changes in the hepatic parenchyma increase the portal pressure by causing an increase in intrahepatic resistance. On a cellular level, the increased pressure results from a combination of deposition of collagen in the spaces of Disse and hepatocyte swelling, both of which increase the sinusoidal pressure and cause a relative resistance to sinusoidal flow.

Resistance to hepatopetal flow through the higher pressure portal system toward and through the liver with increased pressure leads to a backflow and compensation by shunting blood away from the liver (hepatofugal) in a retrograde fashion into the lower pressure systemic circulation. This may occur spontaneously in the form of numerous characteristic collateral venous pathways called varices.

Varices are large, thin-walled veins, which dilate gradually and at a certain point they bleed. Bleeding appears at highest risk in larger varices and with high PV–IVC gradients (greater than 12 mm Hg). Gastroesophageal varices (coronary veins and esophageal

TABLE 84-1 Causes of Portal Hypertension

PREHEPATIC	INTRAHEPATIC, PRESINUSOIDAL	INTRAHEPATIC, SINUSOIDAL	INTRAHEPATIC, POSTSINUSOIDAL	POSTHEPATIC
Arterioportal fistulas	Schistosomiasis	Cirrhosis	Budd-Chiari syndrome	Right heart failure
Portal vein thrombosis	Sarcoidosis	Gauchers disease	Venoocclusive disease	IVC obstruction
Splenic vein thrombosis	Toxins	Alcohol abuse		Constrictive pericarditis
	Chronic hepatitis			
	Primary biliary cirrhosis			
	Feltys syndrome			

TABLE 84-2 Types of Varices Seen with CT in Portal Hypertension

TYPE OF VARICES	FREQUENCY (%)
Coronary veins	80
Esophageal	45
Paraumbilical	43
Abdominal wall	30
Perisplenic	30
Retrogastric	27
Paraesophageal	22
Omental	20
Retroperitoneal/paravertebral	18
Mesenteric	10
Splenorenal	10
Gastrorenal	7

Permission granted for use by RadioGraphics Cho KC, Patel YD, Wachsberg RH, Seeff J. Varices in portal hypertension: evaluation with CT. *Radiographics.* 1995;15:609-622.

veins) are most commonly seen at CT. Gastrorenal varices are least commonly seen (Table 84-2).

The spontaneous pathways are often insufficient to decrease portal pressures to normal levels. When variceal bleeding occurs it is considered a medical emergency and the patient should be hospitalized and medically treated to control the bleeding. Supportive measures and vasoactive drugs are used immediately, followed by endoscopy as soon as possible. Endoscopic sclerotherapy is the first line of invasive treatment, which can be effective in the majority of cases. However, recurrence is common and the underlying cause of portal hypertension remains untreated. This can be addressed by the creation of percutaneous transhepatic portosystemic shunt (TIPS) or one of several surgical portosystemic shunt operations.

Ascites is a common and serious complication of cirrhosis and the 2-year survival after ascites develops is approximately 50%. Sinusoidal hypertension is felt to be responsible to a large degree of ascites development. When ascites becomes refractory to medical treatment requiring frequent paracentheses, TIPS should be considered.

TRANSJUGULAR INTRAHEPATIC PORTOSYSTEMIC SHUNT

TIPS decompresses the portal system by the percutaneous transjugular intrahepatic creation of a low resistance portosystemic shunt in the liver between the portal vein and the hepatic vein. A stent or stent-graft is placed across the shunt tract in the liver to maintain it open. Self-expanding metal stents were used for almost a decade. Despite the initial success, malfunction of bare metal stents was reported to occur at a high rate (17%–73% in the first 6 months) requiring frequent revision. Covered e-PTFE stent-graft (Viatorr, W. L. Gore & Associates, Flagstaff, AZ) has practically replaced bare stents and have shown much higher patency rates (80%–84% at 1 year) and lower rebleeding.

The TIPS procedure is usually indicated in patients with variceal bleeding and ascites refractory to medical management. Absolute contraindications to TIPS placement include biliary sepsis, severe hepatic failure, and occluded portal venous system.

A patent portal vein should be documented before TIPS is attempted. This is usually performed with ultrasound interrogation of the liver and a Doppler study of the hepatic and portal venous system. Cross-sectional imaging such as MRI or CT may also provide similar information. Sometimes such imaging may reveal the presence of a mass lesion along the anticipated tract of the shunt, which can alter management decisions.

Prior to TIPS, appropriate blood work should be performed. As general guidelines, platelet counts should be above 50 000 and the international normalized ratio should preferably be below two. In some patients, intubation may be required for airway control. Otherwise, TIPS may also be performed under conscious sedation in experienced hands (fentanyl, midazolam, droperidol). Standard hemodynamic monitoring including ECG, oxygen saturation, and blood pressure should be performed throughout the procedure.

The presence of ascites, especially around the liver, can complicate the TIPS procedure by altering the angle the portal vein makes with the hepatic vein. Therefore, drainage of ascites prior to performing the TIPS procedure is advised.

TECHNICAL CONSIDERATION

The necessary equipment is put together by vendors in special "kits" to facilitate the procedure. The two most commonly used kits for TIPS are the Rosch-Uchida and Ring sets (Cook, Bloomington, IN). The preferred access route is via the right internal jugular vein. The 10F 40-cm-long vascular sheath is then advanced and pressure readings in the right atrium and inferior vena cava are recorded.

A curved multipurpose A (MPA) catheter is then used to select a hepatic vein. The preferable hepatic vein to access is the right hepatic vein, which lies posterior to the right portal vein. Occasionally, tips is performed from the middle hepatic vein and directed posteriorly to the right portal vein. A free hepatic pressure and venogram is obtained. This catheter can also be used to do a wedge hepatic venous pressures and venogram; however, an occlusion balloon catheter such as a Fogarty balloon catheter is preferable. The balloon is inflated and wedged and hepatic venous pressure is then measured. The intrahepatic portal pressure is expressed as the hepatic vein pressure gradient or the difference between the wedged hepatic venous pressure and the free hepatic or IVC venous pressure. The normal gradient is equal to or less than 5 mm Hg. A gradient larger than 5 mm Hg is indicative of portal hypertension and a gradient above 12 mm Hg is associated with the development of variceal hemorrhage. A wedge hepatic venogram will most likely show reflux of contrast through the sinuses into the portal vein to various degrees depending on the degree of postsinusoidal fibrosis and hepatofugal flow in the portal vein. This reflux is essential to mark the location of the target portal vein in relation to the hepatic vein to be bridged. A wedge venogram using CO_2 rather than iodated contrast is very useful in this regard as CO_2 is much more likely to reflux much further than iodinated contrast and landmark the location of the portal vein.

The diagnostic MPA catheter is removed and exchanged for a guiding cannula and sheath, which is placed in the hepatic vein. A syringe partly filled with contrast is then attached to the needle hub. When using a right hepatic vein approach, the needle is rotated anteriorly and advanced. The length of the needle pass depends largely on the size of the liver and the relative location of the portal vein. As a general guide, the needle should be advanced approximately 1 cm beyond the expected location of the portal vein. Aspirate the contrast syringe during slow needle withdrawal, and when blood is aspirated, gently inject contrast to identify the vascular structure entered. Once a suitable portal branch is punctured, a glide wire is then manipulated through the portal vein into the splenic vein. The needle is removed and a 5F diagnostic catheter advanced into the splenic vein. Portography is then performed and portal pressures are measured directly.

The entire sheath is then advanced and the parenchymal tract is dilated with 10 mm angioplasty balloon. This is generally the most painful part of the procedure for the patient, and added analgesics are recommended when performing the procedure under conscious sedation. Typically two focal indentations are present on the balloon, which represent the more resilient fibrous tissue of the portal and hepatic veins walls.

An 8- to 12-mm e-PTFE covered stent-graft is then deployed across the newly created transhepatic tract. The first 2 cm is placed in the portal vein are bare (noncovered), while the section that is positioned within the liver tract up into the hepatic vein is covered with impermeable material to prevent bile leaks from entering the shunt tract. Once deployed, we generally use a 10-mm balloon to expand the stent in the tract. For large portal veins and/or treatment of ascites, the use of 12-mm stent grafts and expanding them to full 12 mm with balloon angioplasty may be necessary to reduce the gradient to recommended levels. However, this may increase the incidence of hepatic encephalopathy.

A venogram is performed to document satisfactory positioning of the stent and the pressure gradient across the newly created shunt is determined. Flow in the splenic and portal vein should be antegrade up through the shunt and into the IVC. Significant reduction or cessation in retrograde flow in varices should occur. The portogram may show little or no antegrade flow into right and left portal vein branches indicating reversal of flow (hepatofugal) from the intrahepatic portal veins. Liver perfusion becomes largely hepatic artery dependent.

When TIPS is performed to control variceal bleeding, embolization of the varices should be performed after the TIPS has been created. Coils in the main trunk of the varices may suffice. More distal embolization can be achieved with sclerosing agents.

Following TIPS procedure, the generally desired end point is reduction of the portosystemic gradient to below 12 mm Hg for esophageal variceal bleeding and 8 mm Hg or lower for refractory ascites.

The complication rate from TIPS in experienced hands is less than 5% with a mortality rate of less than 2%. The most serious and potentially lethal complications of TIPS are almost always related to transhepatic puncture. Peritoneal exsanguination can occur from perforation of an extrahepatic portion of the portal vein or from hepatic arterial injury with associated perforation of the hepatic capsule (Table 84-3). Worsening of hepatic encephalopathy after TIPS occurs in 30%. This is believed to be caused by ammonia, a neurotoxin that

TABLE 84-3 Complications of TIPS

	REPORTED RATE (%)
Major complications	**3**
Hemoperitoneum	0.5
Stent malposition	1
Hemobilia	2
Radiation skin burn	0.1
Hepatic infarction	0.5
Renal failure requiring dialysis	0.25
Death	1
Minor complications	**4**
Transient contrast induced renal failure	2
Encephalopathy controlled by medical therapy	15–25
Hepatic artery puncture causing clinically apparent injury	1
Fever	2
Entry site hematoma	2

precipitates hepatic encephalopathy, from the gastrointestinal tract. The intact liver normally clears almost all of the portal vein ammonia, converting it into glutamine and preventing entry into the systemic circulation. The increase in blood ammonia following TIPS is a consequence of blood shunting through the TIPS, bypassing the normal liver metabolism.

The technical success rate for TIPS approaches 95%. There is improved survival of patients with refractory ascites when treated with TIPS. Shunt failure in the first 30 days is almost always secondary to acute thrombosis because of improper stent placement or bile duct injury with leakage of bile and mucus into the shunt. Beyond 30 days, intimal hyperplasia can produce narrowing of the stent. Postprocedure TIPS sonography should be performed prior to discharge to serve as a baseline study for outpatient shunt follow-up.

Ultrasound surveillance is recommended and performed routinely periodically by many authors. However, given the infrequent stenosis associated with covered stents, clinical surveillance with elective ultrasound when stent malfunction is suspected could be used effectively especially with the covered stent-grafts.

Based on duplex Doppler findings, shunt stenosis should be suspected and catheterization should be recommended if any of the following direct criteria are present:

- Increase or decrease in peak flow velocity in a similar location within the stent of greater than 50 cm/set relative to the initial baseline study, or
- Absolute peak flow within the stent that is less than 60 cm/s. This has been shown to be greater than 95% sensitive and specific for significant shunt stenosis, or
- Presence of a velocity transition point within the stent through which the velocity is accelerated by a factor of two or more.

Indirect findings that may suggest shunt malfunction and the need for interventional follow-up include the following:

- Decrease in peak velocity in the main portal vein of greater than 33% from baseline
- Reversal of blood flow in the main, right, or left portal vein, or segmental portal vein branch after the initial post-TIPS baseline study
- Reversal to hepatofugal flow in a portosystemic collateral vein, such as a coronary vein or paraumbilical vein, from one study to the next
- Development of retrograde flow in the right hepatic vein, which has been described in the presence of stenosis of the right hepatic venous outflow tract (*Note*: This no longer applies for covered stents and applies only for noncovered stents in the hepatic vein segment. Covered stents are occlusive to antegrade flow in the right hepatic vein from the time of placement.)
- Developing or worsening ascites or splenomegaly.

Venography combined with pressure measurements represents the gold standard for assessing TIPS patency. This should be performed whenever the screening ultrasound suggests a stenosis or when the patient experiences recurrent ascites or bleeding.

PERCUTANEOUS TRANSHEPATIC CHOLANGIOGRAM AND PERCUTANEOUS TRANSHEPATIC BILIARY DRAINAGE

Percutaneous transhepatic cholangiogram (PTC) is the radiographic examination of the liver and bile ducts done by inserting a thin needle through the skin into the liver and injecting contrast medium (cholangiography) in order to visualize the bile ducts. If and when obstruction is documented, percutaneous transhepatic biliary drainage (PTBD) is followed in order to drain the biliary tree and relieve obstruction. The procedure involves placement of a self-retaining tube, which remains in the liver. Bile drains through the tube into the small intestine or into a collection bag outside the body or both.

DUCTAL ANATOMY

Intrahepatic ductal anatomy is modeled after the segmental anatomy of the liver by Couinaud (Fig. 50-1). At the hilum, there are two main hepatic ducts, the right and left, which join to form the common hepatic duct. The right hepatic is formed by the right posterior duct (RPD) and the right anterior duct (RAD). The RAD drains segments 5 and 8 (the anterior segments) and the RPD drains segments 6 and 7. The RPD has a more horizontal course than the RAD, which has a more vertical course. Normally, the RPD courses behind the RAD and joins the RAD on its medial side to form the right hepatic duct. The left hepatic duct courses horizontally and drains segments 2 to 4. It joins the right hepatic duct to form the common hepatic duct and exits the liver at the biliary hilum together with the portal vein and the hepatic artery. The common hepatic duct is joined by the cystic duct to form the common bile duct. The common bile duct measures approximately 8 mm in diameter in normal individuals.

This standard anatomy is present in approximately 57% of patients. Many variations exist but these remain outside the scope of this chapter.

PATIENT PREPARATION

Patient preparation is similar for all transhepatic biliary interventional procedures. Antibiotic prophylaxis is mandatory and in our institution, ciprofloxacin is administered.

Coagulation parameters must be checked carefully and any bleeding tendency must be corrected. Intravenous fluids are started especially for patients with malignant obstruction who have not been eating or drinking well prior to arrival at the hospital. Even when they do arrive at the hospital, they are frequently fasted for a variety of tests and procedures.

TECHNIQUE

Percutaneous Transhepatic Cholangiogram

PTC is performed predominantly from the right side of the patient. The patient is placed supine on the fluoroscopy table. The right flank and right hypochondrium is sterilely prepared. Usually a combination of midazolam and fentanyl is used for conscious sedation.

Under direct fluoroscopy, the patient is asked to inhale deeply and the inferior most point of lung descent is marked. This is to avoid transgressing the pleura.

A suitable location is marked along the mid-axillary line and a 15 cm 22 G Chiba needle is passed from the right flank parallel to the rib toward the vertebral bodies. This should be performed in one smooth motion. The inner stylet is then withdrawn and a syringe containing full strength contrast material is then attached to the needle hub via an extension tubing. The needle is then slowly withdrawn and small aliquots of contrast are injected every 1 to 2 mm until a bile duct is entered.

If a bile duct is not entered on the first pass, successive passes are made in a fan shape down through the liver toward the biliary hilum. It would be prudent not to withdraw the needle fully outside the liver capsule, so that only one hole in the liver capsule is made. This helps to reduce bleeding complications.

When a duct is entered, contrast is injected to outline the biliary system. If stone disease is suspected contrast is diluted down to approximately 200 to 250 mg/mL iodine concentration to avoid obscuring filling defects. Radiographs are obtained in multiple projections in order to delineate ductal anatomy and identify the level of obstruction as well as localize the presence of any filling defects, which may represent stones, debris, or tumor material. Care should be taken not to forcefully inject the biliary system since this can result in an increase in back pressure and reflux into blood circulation causing biliary sepsis.

Success rates for PTC lie between 97% and 100% in experienced hands. As many as 15 to 20 passes can be safely made, but after this, if a bile duct has not been entered, then the procedure is best terminated.

Complications are minimal and occur in some 1% to 2% of patients. These include hemorrhage, sepsis, and bile leak leading to biliary peritonitis.

Percutaneous Transhepatic Biliary Drainage

Percutaneous biliary drainage is usually performed to relieve biliary obstruction. The majority of distal CBD obstructions are diagnosed and successfully studied and stented endoscopically. The role of PTC and PTBD is currently indicated for cases where ERCP and endoscopy has technically failed and/or not possible owing to prior surgical operation (Roux-en-Y).

It is prudent to obtain preprocedure imaging prior to undertaking this procedure. An ultrasound study, CT study, or MRCP may be performed in order to diagnose and ascertain the level of obstruction, to detect the presence of malignant disease, confirm intrahepatic ductal dilatation, and to rule out the presence of ascites.

A right-sided approach is most commonly used. A right-sided PTC is performed as described. When a bile duct is entered, contrast material is injected to opacify the biliary system. If a favorable duct is entered by the initial needle puncture, a 0.018-in guidewire is placed through the needle and manipulated toward the hepatic hilum. If the initial entry was unfavorable, then a second needle would be used to puncture an opacified duct with a more favorable orientation. Once the 0.018-in guidewire has gained reasonable purchase within the duct, a coaxial set (Neff set, Cook, Bloomington, IN) consisting of a 22-gauge metallic cannula inside a tapered 4F dilator inside a 7F dilator is advanced over the wire into the biliary duct. Once good purchase is obtained, the 0.018-in guidewire and inner cannula are removed and a 0.035-in hydrophilic glidewire passed through the outer dilator (which acts as a sheath) into the biliary tree. A 4F catheter is inserted through the sheath and the glidewire is then manipulated across the biliary stricture into the duodenum, followed by the catheter.

Once both catheter are wired safely in the small bowel, the hydrophilic glidewire may be exchanged for a stiff Amplatz wire. The percutaneous track can then be serially dilated to accommodate a biliary catheter with multiple side holes positioned above and below the level of obstruction. All effort should be made to cross the obstruction initially to allow locking the pigtail loop of the catheter in the bowel to avoid dislodgement, which commonly occurs if the catheter is left in the bile ducts above the obstruction for external drainage. An internal–external biliary catheter is also preferred since drainage can occur both percutaneously into an external bag and internally into the small bowel.

A left-sided approach is technically a little more challenging and is usually done if there is a hilar stricture, which does not allow the left and right ducts to communicate. In general, a segment 3 duct is chosen because it courses inferiorly toward the margin of the left lobe. Again a 22G Chiba needle is used and contrast material used to outline the biliary system. A 0.018-in guidewire is manipulated toward the biliary hilum followed by the Neff set. A hydrophilic wire and catheter are again used to cross the stricture and placed in the small bowel. Once in place a left-sided catheter is actually better tolerated by the patient since it does not go between the ribs and is less likely to dislodge.

Percutaneous Cholecystostomy

Percutaneous cholecystostomy is a valuable technique for the management of patients with cholecystitis who are critically ill or unfit for surgery. This procedure is a temporizing measure, which buys the patient some time so that definitive surgery can be carried out when the patient has recovered from an acute illness.

Preprocedure workup includes a detailed history and physical examination, baseline studies of serum bilirubin, amylase, lipase, and alkaline phosphatase. A CBC and coagulation profile should also be obtained.

Because bile in disease gallbladders is commonly infected, a broad-spectrum antibiotic such as ciprofloxacin is commonly administered. Ideally, this should be administered 1 to 4 hours prior to the interventional procedure and continued for several days in the presence of cholecystitis or cholangitis.

Percutaneous cholecystostomy can often be performed under conscious sedation. In general, two approaches may be employed—the transperitoneal and transhepatic access routes. Many operators prefer the transperitoneal approach since it is more direct and avoids the necessity of going through the liver. One of the main drawbacks to this approach is that the catheters and wires often buckle outside of the gallbladder because of gallbladder mobility. This could lead to loss of access and bile leak into the peritoneal cavity.

A transhepatic approach can be used to avoid this problem since the entry of the catheter is closer to the attachment of the gallbladder to the liver where the gallbladder is relatively fixed in position.

Using a needle, the gallbladder is punctured under ultrasound guidance. The gallbladder is then opacified with contrast to confirm position. A guidewire is then inserted through the needle under fluoroscopic guidance. The tract is subsequently dilated and an 8F to 10F self-retaining pigtail catheter is then positioned within the gallbladder lumen. It should be remembered that a mature cholecystostomy tract takes 4 to 6 weeks to develop in debilitated patients and 2 to 3 months in patients who are immunocompromised.

Technical success rates are in excess of 95%. Bile leakage is a feared complication, and cases of massive biliary ascites and chemical peritonitis have been reported. Other complications include intraperitoneal hemorrhage, gallbladder perforation, sepsis, hemobilia, and pneumothorax. The rate of major complication is approximately 6% to 8% while the mortality rate from this procedure is less than 2%.

Suggested Reading

Carr C, Tuite C, Soulen M, et al. Role of ultrasound surveillance of transjugular intrahepatic portosystemic shunts in the covered stent era. *J Vacs Interv Radiol*. 2006;17:1297-1305.

Dib N, Oberti F, Cales P. Current management of the complications of portal hypertension: variceal bleeding and ascites. *CMAJ*. 2006;174(10):1433-1443.

McIntyre N, Burroughs AK. Cirrhosis, portal hypertension, and ascites. In: *Concise Oxford Textbook of Medicine*. chap 5.36.

QUESTIONS AND ANSWERS

1. Which of the following is the normal portal venous pressure?
   A. 0 to 5 mm Hg
   B. 5 to 10 mm Hg
   C. 10 to 20 mm Hg
   D. None of the above

   ANSWER: B. 5 to 10 mm Hg is the normal portal venous pressure. Any value above 12 mm Hg is considered to be portal hypertension. This reflects the noncorrected, absolute pressure. When systemic venous pressures are elevated a corrected sinusoidal pressure or a gradient of PV–IVC is more accurate and 5 mm Hg is the upper limit of normal for gradient.

2. All the following represent causes for intrahepatic presinusoidal portal hypertension *except:*
   A. Chronic hepatitis
   B. Myelofibrosis

C. Felty syndrome
D. Budd-Chiari syndrome

ANSWER: D. Budd Chiari is a cause of intrahepatic postsinusoidal portal hypertension. All the others are causes of intrahepatic presinusoidal portal hypertension. Felty syndrome is a complication of rheumatoid arthritis. It is the triad of seropositive (rheumatoid factor positive) rheumatoid arthritis, neutropenia, and splenomegaly.

3. Which of the following is the first diagnostic study of choice for evaluating upper GI bleeding for varices?
   A. Esophagoduodenoscopy (EGD)
   B. Esophagography
   C. Diagnostic portal venography
   D. Nuclear medicine tagged red blood cell scan

   ANSWER: A. EGD is the first-line study for evaluation of upper GI bleeding, regardless of etiology. It is both diagnostic and potentially therapeutic.

4. Which of the following is the approximate risk of encephalopathy after TIPS?
   A. 5% to 10%
   B. 10% to 20%
   C. 20% to 30%
   D. >50%

   ANSWER: C. The rate of encephalopathy after TIPS is 23% to 29%. Most cases respond to medical therapy. However, 3% to 5% of patients undergoing TIPS have encephalopathy that is refractory to medical treatment.

5. Which of the following Doppler findings suggest TIPS stenosis?
   A. Change in velocity of greater than 20 cm/s in a similar location within the stent compared to baseline
   B. Maximum velocity within the stent of less than 60 cm/s
   C. No flow in the TIPS shunt
   D. All the above

   ANSWER: B. A change in velocity of greater than 50 cm/s in a similar location within the stent compared to baseline, and retrograde flow in the right hepatic vein are suggestive of TIPS stenosis. No flow in the TIPS shunt suggests TIPS occlusion.

6. The following are *all* indications for a percutaneous transhepatic biliary drainage *except*:
   A. Relief of biliary obstruction
   B. Diversion of biliary flow in cases of bile leak
   C. Provide access for biliary intervention
   D. Sphincterotomy

   ANSWER: D. PTBD is performed for the relief of biliary obstruction, diversion of biliary flow in cases of bile leak as well as to provide access for biliary manipulation such as brush biopsy. Sphincterotomy is usually performed during an ERCP.

7. Factors that predispose a patient to cholangiocarcinoma include *all* the following *except*:
   A. Inflammatory bowel disease
   B. Sclerosing cholangitis
   C. Clonorchis sinensis infection
   D. Rheumatoid arthritis

   ANSWER: D. Inflammatory bowel disease, sclerosing cholangitis, Caroli disease, and clonorchis sinensis infection are the top four factors that predispose an individual to cholangiocarcinoma. Rheumatoid arthritis is not known to be associated with cholangiocarcinoma.

8. What is the incidence of pancreatitis following a PTC procedure?
   A. 1%
   B. 5%
   C. 10%
   D. 15%

   ANSWER: A. The incidence of pancreatitis following a PTC procedure is approximately <1%. Other complications include death (<1%), bleeding (<3%), sepsis (<3%), and peritonitis (<2%). Overall major complication rate is approximately ≤8%.

9. Hepatic lobar atrophy caused by cholangiocarcinomas is caused *primarily* by compression of which of the following structures?
   A. Hepatic arteries
   B. Portal veins
   C. Biliary ducts
   D. Hepatic veins

   ANSWER: C. The primary cause of parenchymal atrophy is the obstruction of biliary ducts. Cholangiocarcinomas are known to cause segmental atrophy of the liver parenchyma, including, in some cases, entire lobar (left or right) atrophy.

10. *All* the following are indications for a dedicated left hepatic PTC approach *except*:
    A. Extensive neoplastic involvement of the right hepatic lobe by primary or secondary tumor
    B. Diversion of bile flow in cases of bile leak from the common duct

C. As part of a combined drainage procedure of both the right and left lobes in cases of hilar obstruction
D. Obstruction of the main left hepatic duct with no communication between the left- and right-sided ducts

ANSWER: B. All the rest are indications for a left hepatic PTC approach in order to adequately decompress the biliary system. PTCD for diversion of CBD leak can be performed from either right or left approach.

85 GASTROINTESTINAL AND BILIARY DISEASE AND INTERVENTION

Kay M. Hamrick and Emily R. Norman

GASTROINTESTINAL BLEEDING

Gastrointestinal (GI) bleeding is the most frequent indication for the angiography of mesenteric vessels. GI bleeding results in approximately 300000 hospital admissions each year. In approximately 75% of cases of upper GI bleeding and 80% of cases of lower GI bleeding, bleeding will spontaneously cease. However, when bleeding persists or is recurrent, angiography plays an important role in both evaluation and treatment.

The first step in the treatment of GI bleeding is accurate characterization as acute or chronic. This can be usually determined through a detailed history or review of the patient's clinical symptoms and laboratory findings. Tachycardia and hypotension occur when acute blood loss exceeds 500 mL, and hypovolemic shock occurs with a blood loss of 15% or more of the circulating blood volume. The effects of acute blood loss can manifest as failure of multiple systems including cardiac, renal, neurologic, and pulmonary systems, especially in patients in whom bleeding does not cease spontaneously. Most deaths attributable to GI bleeding occur in elderly patients and patients with multiple comorbid conditions exacerbated by blood loss. Probably the most important benefit of arteriography is that it allows minimally invasive intervention such as embolization.

It is important to differentiate between upper and lower sources of blood loss prior to intervention when possible. Nearly 90% of acute GI bleedings occurs in the upper GI tract, which is defined as proximal to the ligament of Treitz (esophagus, stomach, and duodenum). It is usually suspected in the setting of positive gastric aspirate and melanotic stool, though hematochezia can be seen as well. Upper GI bleeding leads to hospitalization in approximately 0.1% of patients each year and carries a mortality rate of approximately 10%. Lower GI bleedings occur distal to the ligament of Treitz (small bowel, colon, and rectum). Lower GI bleeding is less common than upper GI bleeding—approximately 30% of all GI bleeding cases and up to 0.02% of hospital admissions each year. It carries a mortality rate of 3.6%.

Scintigraphy is also used to detect GI bleeding. This method is more sensitive than arteriography and can detect active bleeding at rates as low as 0.05 to 0.1 mL/min. Drawbacks to this technique include poor spatial resolution of scintigraphic images and occasional false-positive results. False-positive results can be minimized using the in vitro technique for erythrocyte labeling.

To diagnose ongoing hemorrhage with arteriography, bleeding must occur at a rate of at least 0.5 to 1.0 mL/min. Angiography has a sensitivity of 63% to 90% and 40% to 86% for upper and lower gastrointestinal bleeding, respectively, with a specificity of up to 100% for both. In case the initial arteriogram is nondiagnostic, a second arteriogram is warranted if bleeding recurs. Extravasation of the contrast material into the bowel lumen is pathognomonic for active gastrointestinal hemorrhage. A "pseudovein" occurs when contrast collects in the dependent portion of the bowel lumen between linear mucosal folds. Extravasation can also be seen as an amorphous contrast collection that persists through the venous phase.

TECHNIQUES

Treatment of GI bleeding, particularly lower GI bleeding, is more frequently using superselective embolization with microcoils or particles.

Particulate embolic agents used in the setting of acute hemorrhage include polyvinyl alcohol (PVA) and absorbable gelatin sponge (Gelfoam). Trisacryl microspheres (Embospheres) are now available in multiple sizes for use in different vascular territories. These must be combined with an iodine-contrast agent for fluoroscopic visualization and then injected through a catheter or more commonly a microcatheter. PVA is available in particle sizes ranging from 100 to 1200 μm. An appropriate range of particle size must be chosen based on the size of the vessels to be occluded. Smaller particles will reach more distal vessels, and it is important to note that this increases the likelihood of necrosis. Generally, particles smaller than 300 μm are not used. Care should be taken not to reflux the particle–contrast mixture beyond the intended area of embolization. PVA and Embosphere particles are permanent occlusive agents, as are coils, PVA, and collagen spheres.

For more temporary occlusion, Gelfoam can be used, although it can incite an inflammatory response and eventually achieve permanent thrombosis. Once injected, Gelfoam acts as both a mechanical occlusive agent and a thrombogenic agent, occluding the vessel. Gelfoam is available as a sponge, which can either be cut into small pieces called pledgets or from which a slurry can be made.

UPPER GASTROINTESTINAL BLEEDING

The most common cause of nonvariceal upper GI bleeding is ulcer disease. Other causes of upper GI hemorrhage include hemorrhagic gastritis, Mallory-Weiss tear, vascular lesions, neoplasms, and variceal bleeding. Variceal bleeding is discussed in Chapter 84. The number of cases of upper GI bleeding increases with patient's age. In a study performed in the United States, approximately 44.5% of all patients with upper GI bleeding were aged 60 years or older. Morbidity and mortality rates also increased with age; 73.2% of deaths occurred in patients older than 60 years. First-line therapy for upper GI bleeding usually consists of endoscopy with intervention when a bleeding is directly visualized. Transendoscopic treatments of acute bleedings include thermal coagulation, banding, or injection of vasopressin at the bleeding site. Vasopressin injection controls blood loss in approximately 70% of patients. Endoscopy is especially helpful given that gastritis is a condition that is notoriously difficult to evaluate and treat with arteriography given its diffuse nature. However, the more focal lesions of the upper GI tract, such as chronic gastric ulcers, stress-induced gastric ulcers, and Mallory-Weiss tears, are better treated by arterial embolization.

Gastric Ulcer Disease

As previously stated, ulcers are the most common source for upper GI bleedings. Embolization is the preferred method of treatment for hemorrhage from the pyloroduodenal region. Vasopressin can be problematic as its effects are often dampened by the inflammatory changes associated with some duodenal ulcers, which renders nearby vessels. The rich collateral network supplying the duodenum from the celiac and superior mesenteric arteries reduces the risk of infarction following embolization. Some controversy exists as to the best method for upper GI embolization, but Gelfoam is the generally preferred embolic material in most patients with gastrointestinal hemorrhage. It is associated with a low risk of infarction and does not present the many complications seen with the use of vasopressin. Combinations of different embolic agents may be more effective than embolization with a single agent, and combining Gelfoam with microcoils is often successful and permanent.

Hemorrhagic Gastritis

Infusion of vasopressin directly into the left gastric artery is effective in 82% of patients with diffuse hemorrhagic gastritis. Vasopressin acts to constrict vascular smooth muscle, particularly at the arteriolar and capillary levels. Vasopressin infusion is begun at a rate of 0.2 U/min for 20 minutes. If bleeding persists, the rate can be increased to 0.4 U/min for another 20 minutes. If this fails, vasopressin infusion is stopped. If, however, the bleeding stops after the 20-minute infusions, vasopressin is continued at the effective rate for 24 hours and then slowly tapered to avoid rebound hyperemia.

Although often successful, this method of treatment may cause serious complications in 8% to 43% of patients. Vasopressin-induced constriction of branches of the inferior phrenic artery can cause ventricular arrhythmias. The antidiuretic effect of vasopressin also limits its use in patients with congestive heart failure, and urine output should be monitored in patients receiving 24 hour drips. More importantly, prior gastrointestinal embolization is a contraindication to the use of vasopressin because of a heightened risk of bowel infarction due to the previous occlusion of some of the arteries that normally serve the area of hemorrhage.

Mallory-Weiss Tear

Mallory-Weiss tears are most often seen in the clinical setting of binge drinking followed by repeated vomiting; however, any condition that leads to a sudden rise in gastric pressure may be a cause. Hiatal hernia is a predisposing factor and is seen in as many as 30% to 100% of patients with tears. Bleeding is due to longitudinal lacerations (intramural dissections) at the gastroesophageal junction or cardia. In the majority of cases of (80%–90%), bleeding spontaneously stops and emergency intervention is not needed. When intervention is required, it is usually performed endoscopically. However, when endoscopic treatments fail, vasopressin injection or embolization following subselection of the left gastric artery are valid options, with vasopressin injected more frequently.

Neoplasm

Carcinoid is a neoplasm of the small bowel, which can occasionally result in upper GI hemorrhage. Patients are most likely to present with chronic, unexplained GI hemorrhage. Carcinoid syndrome (flushing of the head and neck, asthma-like attacks, and diarrhea) occurs in less than 10% of those patients in whom the disease has spread to the liver. Carcinoid tumors are usually ileal in location and may be seen via barium contrast fluoroscopy, enteroclysis, or CT. The arteriographic features of small bowel carcinoid tumor can also be characteristic. Mesenteric nodal metastasis from primary bowel tumor creates a mesenteric desmoplastic process, which can result in kinking, straightening, and retraction of the mesenteric arteries. Classically, the arteries in the affected mesentery radiate outward from a central nidus of tumor in a stellate or "sunburst" pattern.

LOWER GASTROINTESTINAL BLEEDING

The most common cause of lower GI hemorrhage is diverticulosis (20%–55%). Other causes include angiodysplasia (3%–40%), neoplasms (8%–26%), colitis (6%–22%), and benign anorectal lesions (9%–10%). Lower GI bleeding is much more commonly seen in the elderly patient population.

For evaluating lower GI bleedings, colonoscopy is often the first step. However, if the bleeding is severe, colonscopic identification of the source of the blood loss may be impossible because of the large amount of blood in the colon. Colonoscopy is most effective in patients with intermittent hematochezia who are clinically stable. Arteriography of lower GI bleedings has been found to identify the source in 40% to 50% of patients when performed while there are clinical signs of active bleeding.

Diverticulosis

Diverticulosis is a common acquired condition in Western societies. The disease is caused by lack of fiber in the diet. It occurs in approximately 50% of adults older than 60 years. Diverticula are most commonly located in the sigmoid and descending colon, though the source of diverticular bleeding is more often found to be the right colon near the splenic flexure. Diverticular bleeding originates from vasa rectae located in submucosa, which can rupture at the dome or the neck of the diverticulum. Up to 20% of patients with diverticular disease experience bleeding, and the bleeding stops spontaneously approximately 80% of the time. When bleeding does not stop spontaneously, the initial treatment is vasopressin injection using the same technique as described for hemorrhagic gastritis. However, vasopressin injection is associated with all of the aforementioned complications and is also associated with a high rate of rebleeding. Therefore it is used primarily for temporary stabilization prior to a more definitive treatment.

In rare cases, diverticulosis can cause massive lower GI bleeding, which is defined as the requirement of greater than six units of packed red blood cells replaced in 24 hours. Massive bleedings have an overall incidence of approximately 20.4 per 100 000 patients, with an overall mortality rate of 10%. Once the source of bleeding has been located, the standard of therapy has been surgical intervention with possible bowel resection. Increasingly, however, super-selective embolization of the mesenteric vessels is an alternative treatment. Because of the lack of collateral vessels in the distal bowel, there is an increased risk for ischemia following embolization. Therefore, to prevent this complication, embolization should be performed beyond the marginal artery as close as possible to the bleeding point in the terminal mural arteries.

Angiodysplasia

Angiodysplasia is the most common vascular abnormality of the GI tract. It is second after diverticulosis as a source of lower GI hemorrhage. The prevalence of angiodysplasia is 0.8% in healthy patients older than 50 years who are undergoing screening colonoscopy. Angiodysplasia is a degenerative lesion composed of a small tangle of abnormally communicating arteries and veins in the mucosa and submucosa of the bowel. Seventy-seven percent of angiodysplasias are located in the cecum and ascending colon, 15% are located in the jejunum and ileum, and the remainder are distributed throughout the alimentary tract. These lesions typically are nonpalpable, small (less than 5 mm), and are typically located on the antimesenteric border of the bowel.

Patients with bleeding angiodysplasias usually present with maroon-colored stool, melena, or hematochezia. Bleeding is usually low grade but can be massive in approximately 15% of patients. Chronic iron deficiency anemia and stools that are intermittently positive for occult blood may occasionally be the only manifestations of angiodysplasia. Bleeding stops spontaneously in more than 90% of cases but is often recurrent.

Arteriography does not usually demonstrate active bleeding. However, the arteriographic appearance of angiodysplasia is pathognomonic, and arteriography is often performed while the patient is asymptomatic. A small tangle of tortuous vessels is visualized during the late arterial and capillary phases. The most diagnostic feature on angiography is the appearance in the arterial phase of a densely opacified vein draining the lesion, appropriately called the "early draining vein." Arteriographic injections to evaluate for angiodysplasia should not last longer than 4 seconds in order to minimize the overlap between arterial and venous opacification. Angiodysplasias are usually treated by various endoscopic methods including electrocautery and sclerotherapy, and more severe cases are treated with surgical resection of the affected bowel. Selective mesenteric artery embolization is rarely performed as it has a high complication rate. Therefore, the role of angiography in treatment of angiodysplasias is usually in preoperative localization of small bowel lesions before surgical resection.

Inflammatory Bowel Disease

Inflammatory bowel disease is another fairly common cause of lower GI bleeding and subsequent anemia. Diagnosis is often made via endoscopy or barium contrast studies, but when bleeding occurs before diagnosis has been made, arteriography can play an important role. Most commonly, angiography demonstrates increased contrast staining and early venous return when compared with adjacent bowel loops. This often is accompanied by an increase in caliber of the supplying arteries, and bowel may be affected in the typical "skip pattern." The two angiographic signs considered to be diagnostic of Crohn disease include the presence of mesenteric neovascularity and the "zoning" sign. The "zoning" sign refers to a double-layer appearance of the bowel wall with a densely staining inner wall representing a hypervascular submucosa and mucosa and a thickened but relatively avascular outer muscle layer. No single finding is thought to be diagnostic of ulcerative colitis. Acute bleedings can be treated by superselection and either vasopressin infusion or coiling.

GASTROSTOMY AND GASTROJEJUNOSTOMY TUBES

Gastrostomy and gastrojejunostomy (G-J) tubes are indicated in patients requiring long-term nutritional support. Gastrostomy tubes have been placed by surgeons since the late 1800s. It was not until 1983 that the technique of percutaneous gastrostomy was described in the radiologic literature. Since that time, numerous papers have described the methods of ultrasonographic and fluoroscopic placement of various types of percutaneous gastrostomy tubes.

Clinical presentations and goals of treatment define the kind of tube that should be placed as well as whether a gastrostomy or gastrojejunostomy should be placed. Patients usually present with inability to swallow, dysfunctional swallowing, or obstruction and are neurologically impaired because of cerebral vascular accident, degenerative CNS disease, or chronic neurologic disorders such as cerebral palsy. Other conditions include head and neck tumors, esophageal carcinoma, and chronic esophageal strictures. Gastric outlet obstruction from tumors necessitate placement of the tube via the stomach into the jejunum. Diabetic patients with gastroparesis also require gastrojejunostomy tubes.

Prior to performing the procedure the patient must be evaluated and any prior imaging must be reviewed. There are few absolute or relative contraindications to gastrostomy and gastrojejunostomy (Table 85-1).

Some patients have a large left lobe of the liver that crosses the midline and may require ultrasonographic marking prior to performing the procedure. As with all procedures, informed consent must be appropriately maintained. A nasogastric tube is placed. Some patients may have difficult nasogastric intubation because of obstructing lesions or severe neurologic dysfunction. A small arterial catheter such as a 5F Berenstein placed with the aid of a hydrophilic wire may be used to intubate the stomach in these patients. Some authors advocate the placement of oral barium contrast agent on the evening prior to the procedure to better image the colon. Intravenous access is necessary so that sedation and analgesia may be performed.

The patient should be fasting for at least 8 hours prior to the procedure. While the patient is in the supine position, the relationship of the stomach to the liver, spleen, large and small bowel must be determined. This is usually possible with the aid of fluoroscopy, and rarely ultrasound is required to mark the left lobe of the liver. Care must be taken to avoid the superior epigastric artery, which runs in the mid portion of the abdominous rectus muscle. Distention of the stomach with air via the nasogastric tube serves to outline the stomach and push the anterior wall to the abdominal wall allowing ready access for percutaneous puncture with a 5F trocar needle. Approximately 600 to 1000 mL of air is instilled in order to decrease the compliance of the stomach wall and to bring it closer to the abdominal wall. The patient is instructed to try to hold the air in the stomach; however, some are unable to cooperate because of comorbid conditions. A dose of 1 mg of glucagon may be given to

TABLE 85-1 Contraindications to Gastrostomy or Gastrojejunostomy Tubes

Absolute	Extensive gastric varices
	Total gastrectomy
	Uncorrectable coagulopathy
Relative	Overlying viscera
	Ascites
	Ventriculoperitoneal shunt

decrease the peristalsis of the stomach thereby aiding in gastric distention. This must be given immediately before the procedure because of the short half-life of glucagon: 3 to 5 minutes. Intragastric location of the sheathed needle is confirmed with the placement of water-soluble contrast material. Care must be taken to avoid aspiration since the risk is increased with the nasogastric tube and gastric distension. A stiff guidewire is placed with subsequent dilation of the tract with Teflon dilators so that the desired gastrostomy catheter may be placed. The catheter is secured in place and placed to gravity drainage for 24 hours. Feeds may be ordered at one-half strength after the initial 24 hours to be advanced as tolerated after 12 hours.

There has been controversy in the literature regarding the placement of T-fasteners. It is generally accepted that they may be helpful but are not necessary when placement of a gastrostomy is desired. The incidence of complications in percutaneous gastrostomy placement may be increased if with no T-fasteners are used. However, there may be increased pain and skin breakdown associated with the use of T-fasteners. T-tube fasteners must also be used when patients are on steroids in that there is delayed formation of a fibrous tract. Because of the lack of a mature fibrous tract, they are indicated when placement of a jejunal tube via the stomach is desired. Gastrojejunostomy tubes are generally more difficult to place and require increase radiation exposure relative to simple gastrostomy procedures. There may be difficulty crossing the pylorus. These tubes are longer in length and smaller in diameter in the jejunal lumen and therefore more prone to blockage. It is important to determine if gastric decompression is desired so that a double lumen G-J may be placed rather than a single lumen.

Complications include peritonitis, aspiration pneumonia, bleeding, infection, and injury to the liver and spleen. Rarely vasovagal reaction and hypotension may be seen. Complication rates of percutaneous gastrostomy placement of 5.9% have been reported by Wollman et al.—lower than the rates reported by gastroenterologists and surgeons. The use of prophylactic antibiotics is controversial. The incidence of infection is greater for those placed by gastroenterologists, and antibiotics are warranted in these cases. As tubes may occlude, patient and caretaker education is very important. Once occluded, things such as meat tenderizer, cola, and guidewires may be used to re-establish patency. Tube replacement is often necessary.

The technique of direct percutaneous jejunostomy has been described and is indicated in rare cases. These include previous gastric surgery or resection, abnormal stomach position, and duodenal or gastric outlet obstruction. Various techniques have been described. These include using previously placed tube as has a fluoroscopic target. This can be placed transnasally or via a percutaneous gastrojejunostomy. In either situation, distension of the jejunum with air and the use of T-fasteners is necessary. CT fluoroscopy has also been described as a method of localization. Results compare favorably with those placed via laparoscopy and surgery.

Cecal perforation carries a high mortality. The risk of perforation increases when the diameter is greater than 12 cm. Percutaneous cecostomy is an alternative to traditional surgical techniques for cecal decompression. T-fasteners are used and the technique is similar to that of percutaneous gastrostomy.

Enteric catheters placed radiographically offer the advantage of less sedation and analgesia requirement. Many of these tubes can be placed with local anesthesia only. This is helpful in patients with cardiac and respiratory dysfunction. Costs are also less than those generated in the endoscopy and surgical suites.

PERCUTANEOUS BILIARY INTERVENTION

Percutaneous biliary interventions include percutaneous transhepatic cholangiogram (PTC) with or without external or external–internal drainage, and placement of expandable metallic stents for internal drainage in patients with unresectable malignant disease. PTC has a diagnostic role in patients with failed endoscopic retrograde cholangio-pancreatography (ERCP) or anatomy unfavorable to performing ERCP. Percutaneous cholecystostomy tubes are placed in patients who are not surgical candidates with calculous and acalculous cholecystitis. Retained stones may also be removed percutaneously with or without the aid of lithotripsy; however, T-tube tracts must mature for at least 6 weeks before doing surgery.

PTC has been used for diagnosis and definition of biliary anatomy in patients with biliary obstruction. Presently, definition of anatomy is readily achieved with ultrasound, CT, and MRI. Diagnosis is also made possible with endoscopic techniques. Plastic internal stents can be placed and biopsies performed for tissue diagnosis. In cases of failed ERCP, percutaneous techniques are useful in providing drainage in patients with symptomatic jaundice; patients with prior surgery including biliary enteric anastomosis are not candidates for ERCP.

Prior to performing percutaneous cholangiogram, the patient's history and pertinent laboratory results must be reviewed and informed consent must be obtained. Risks including infection, bleeding, bile leak with possible biliary peritonitis, and pneumothorax must be discussed.

There is a 5% to 10% risk of significant complications associated with this procedure with mortality rate as high as 1% to 2.5%. The patient should be fasting for at least 8 hours prior to the procedure. Intravenous access should be in place for administration of sedation and analgesia. Antibiotics should be given at least 1 hour prior to the procedure, and should be broad-spectrum and provide for gram-negative as well as anaerobic coverage. The risk of infected bile increases in patients with prior surgery. The bile is infected in approximately one-third of patients with malignant disease and two-thirds of patients with benign stricture or stone disease. Once a biliary tube is in place, the bile becomes colonized, thereby making sepsis a possible complication even with simple tube exchanges.

Contraindications for percutaneous biliary intervention include uncorrectable coagulopathy, known vascular tumors, and cystic liver disease. Cirrhosis, ascites, and multiple liver metastases are relative contraindications. Patients should be able to cooperate during the procedure by performing breath holds during passage of the needle.

There is no difference in complication rate regarding a left- or right-side approach. The right approach is from the right midaxillary line. The left is a subxiphoid approach. The most commonly used system is the Neff set (Cook, Bloomington, IN). This consists of a 22-guage needle, a 5F sheath system and a 0.018-in guidewire. Once the 5F sheath has been placed in the biliary system, a 4F angled catheter such as a Kumpe may be used with a 0.035 in angled glidewire to negotiate the catheter into the duodenum. It is important to fill the biliary tree prior to passage of the level of obstruction as much as possible to avoid pitfalls in diagnosis. Common pitfalls include air bubbles, lack of filling of the left side, (more anteriorly/nonclepent located), and false level of obstruction. If the contrast material is too dense, a stone or filling defect may be obscured.

Knowledge of intrahepatic ductal anatomy is necessary when performing percutaneous cholangiogram. Normally the right posterior duct and right anterior duct join together to form the right hepatic duct, which joins the left hepatic duct at the hilum. This is present in 57% of cases. The right posterior duct is more horizontally oriented compared to the right anterior duct. Variations occur with the drainage of the right posterior duct and right anterior duct. Most commonly the right posterior duct may drain into the left hepatic duct, in approximately 21% of cases. The right posterior duct may also drain directly into the main hepatic duct. Rarely the right anterior duct may drain into the left. There may be a confluence of the right anterior duct, right posterior duct, and left duct at the hilum.

Abnormalities seen on cholangiograms may be due to benign disease such as stones or stricture secondary to inflammation. Stones are seen as persistent filling defects. They must be differentiated from blood clots, biliary debris, and polypoid tumors. Patients with sclerosing cholangitis may have extrahepatic or intrahepatic involvement. Most commonly it is diffuse. Appearance may include "beading" or a "shaggy" appearance of the ducts. Primary cholangitis is associated with inflammatory bowel disease, retroperitoneal fibrosis, and cholangiocarcinoma. There is a 70% predominance in the male population. These patients present with chronic or intermittent obstructive jaundice, abdominal pain, and may have fever. Dilatation will usually be present in patients with cholangiocarcinoma. However, because of the different presentations any patient with rapid decline should be considered to have cholangiocarcinoma. Since biopsy is difficult, this diagnosis often remains elusive. Secondary cholangitis may be due to chronic bacterial infection, AIDS cholangitis, and bile duct ischemia. The organisms associated with biliary infection in patients with AIDS are cytomegalovirus and *Cryptosporidium* species.

Tumors affecting the biliary tree produce obstruction by ductal compression either by hilar nodes or hepatic metastases. Evaluation of the distal duct at the ampula can often be difficult, since inflammatory change and tumor can often have a similar appearance. Biopsy is helpful for further evaluation.

The presence of self-expanding metallic stents has been instrumental in decreasing length of hospital stay. Many institutions place these at the same setting as the initial PTC in patients with known unresectable malignant disease. The currently available 7F delivery systems require no significant additional tract dilatation. Patients with hilar obstruction may be treated with dual stents, one from the right and one from the left. These should be placed simultaneously to avoid the inability to place the contralateral stent. If a safety stent is not left in place, the stent should be balloon dilated. In cases where clot is left in the system, a safety stent should be left in place until bleeding clears.

When long-term internal–external drainage is desired, it is important to secure the tube to minimize movement. Movement occurs with respiratory motion; however, securing the tube decreases the likelihood that a side hole will slip and communicate with a vascular structure or cause a bile leak. Side holes must be proximal to the level of obstruction to allow adequate drainage. If the tube is securely attached at the skin a loop may form between the skin and the liver with respiratory movement. It is advisable to leave a 2 cm distance when suturing the catheter to the skin to avoid this problem.

Tubes must be followed by the interventional team. It is important to perform daily rounds on these patients while in the hospital. Care includes flushing the catheter with 5 mL of sterile saline every shift for the first 48 hours. Antibiotics in coordination with the referring service must be continued for at least 2 to 3 days. If these tubes are to be left in long-term, it is important to educate caretakers with instructions to flush the tube daily and to attach a bag if fever develops. The catheter should be capped prior to patient discharge to ensure this will be tolerated. Catheters must be replaced every 2 to 3 months, sooner if problems develop. Initially an 8F biliary catheter is placed. Once the tract is dilated from respiratory movement, it is best to exchange for a 10 or 12F tube.

Other uses for internal–external biliary drainage catheters include conduits for brachytherapy and a guide for the biliary surgeon when there is a high hilar obstruction. Surgical morbidity and mortality are also decreased with decreasing the bilirubin prior to surgery. PTC also has a role in cases with biliary leak postlaparoscopic cholecystectomy. PTC can define the level of the leak and is often necessary to divert draining bile until the leak has healed. Patients who have had biliary enteric surgery may develop benign structures. PTC with balloon dilation is often helpful in resolving these strictures. However, these patients must be stented for approximately 6 to 12 months in order for the stricture to resolve.

GALLBLADDER INTERVENTION

Beginning in the 1980s, gallbladder intervention and percutaneous biliary stone retrieval became accepted medical practice. Diagnostic aspiration of the gallbladder in cases of infection has been performed in the past but has been largely abandoned because of the lack of sensitivity. Gallbladder biopsy in cases with gallbladder mass or metastatic disease have been successful in more than 90% of cases. This is performed with a 20- or 22-gauge needle. Currently the most useful gallbladder intervention is that of drainage in patients with cholecystitis.

Patients may present with either calculous or acalculous cholecystitis. Many of these patients have comorbidities, which preclude emergent surgery. In most instances of acalculous cholecystitis drainage with the appropriate antibiotics is satisfactory treatment. Placement of a drainage catheter in patients with calculous cholecystitis may serve as a temporizing measure to surgery. However, once the tract has matured, generally about 6 weeks, stones can be removed percutaneously.

There is controversy concerning the approach for the placement of cholecystostomy tubes. Some prefer to go directly into the gallbladder through the peritoneal cavity while others advocate traversing the liver bare area, where the gallbladder abuts the liver. Both approaches require the use of ultrasound. If the Seldinger technique it used, fluoroscopic guidance is also necessary for wire placements and subsequent dilatations. A Neff system can be used. If the procedure is done at the bedside in the intensive care unit because a patient is too unstable to be transferred, the trocar method may be advantageous. Advantages of going through the bare area of the liver include decreased mobility of the gallbladder and decreased incidence of bile leak into the peritoneal cavity. Disadvantages include an increased risk of bleeding if dilatation is necessary for stone removal. The main advantage of the transperitoneal approach is for subsequent percutaneous stone removal. Disadvantages include the increased mobility of the gallbladder fundus and the possibility of colonic interposition. Technical success rates with both approaches are approximately 100%.

As with any other tube placed by the interventional team, daily rounds must be made. The catheters must be irrigated every shift. Tubes must be left in for a minimum period of 2 to 3 weeks to make sure that a mature tract has formed. A cystocholangiogram must be performed prior to removal to ensure that there is no peritoneal leakage and that the cystic duct is patent.

Complications of percutaneous cholecystostomy are rare, 0% to 8%. Surgical complications are reported as high as 24%. Complications associated with percutaneous treatment include bleeding, hypotension, and biliary peritonitis.

SUGGESTED READING

Barkmeier JM, Trerotola SO, Wiebke EA, et al. Percutaneous radiologic, surgical endoscopic, and percutaneous endoscopic gastrostomy/gastrojejunostomy: comparative study and cost analysis. *Cardiovasc Intervent Radiol.* 1998;21(4): 324-328.

Barnacle AM, Aylwin AC, Jackson JE. Angiographic diagnosis of inflammatory bowel disease in patients presenting with gastrointestinal bleeding. *AJR Am J Roentgenol.* 2006;187:976-985.

Belaiche J, Louis E, D'Haens G, et al. Acute lower gastrointestinal bleeding in Crohn's disease: characteristics of a unique series of 34 patients. *Am J Gastroenterol.* 1999;94:2177-2181.

Bell SD, Carmody EA, Yeung EY, et al. Percutaneous gastrostomy and gastrojejunostomy additional experience in 519 procedures. *Radiology.* 1995;194(3):817-820.

Bezzi M, Zolovkins A, Cantisani V, et al. New ePTFE/FEP-covered stent in the palliative treatment of malignant biliary obstruction. *J Vasc Interv Radiol*. 2002;13(6):581-589.

Clark RA, Colley DP, Eggers FM. Acute arterial gastrointestinal hemorrhage: efficacy of transcatheter control. *AJR Am J Roentgenol*. 1981;136(6):1185-1189.

Coons H. Metallic stents for the treatment of biliary obstruction: a report of 100 cases. *Cardiovasc Intervent Radiol*. 1992;15(6): 367-374.

Cope C, Davis AG, Baum RA, et al. Direct percutaneous jejunostomy: techniques and applications—ten years experience. *Radiology*. 1998;209(3):747-754.

Darcy M. Treatment of lower gastrointestinal bleeding: vasopressin infusion versus embolization. *J Vasc Interv Radiol*. 2003;14(5):535-543.

Giuliano AW, Yoon HC, Lomis NN, Miller FJ. Fluoroscopically guided percutaneous placement of large-bore gastrostomy and gastrojejunostomy tubes: review of 109 cases. *J Vasc Interv Radiol*. 2000;11(2 Pt 1):239-246.

Hastings GS. Angiographic localization and transcatheter treatment of gastrointestinal bleeding. *Radiographics*. 2000;20: 1160-1168.

Kandarpa K, Aruny JE. *Handbook of Interventional Radiologic Procedures*. 3rd ed. Philadelphia, PA: Lippincott Williams & Wilkins; 2001.

Khanna A, Ognibene SJ, Koniaris LG. Embolization as first-line therapy for diverticulosis-related massive lower gastrointestinal bleeding: evidence from a meta-analysis. *J Gastroint Surg*. 2005;9:343-352.

Kiyosue H, Mori H, Matsumoto S, Yamada Y, Hori Y, Okino Y. Transcatheter obliteration of gastric varices: part 1. anatomic classification. *Radiographics*. 2003;23:911-920.

Lee MJ. Biliary intervention. In: Kaufman JA, Lee MJ, eds. *Vascular and Interventional Radiology the Requisites Series*. Philadelphia, PA: Mosby; 2004.

Mueller PR, Ferucci JT Jr., Teplick SK, et al. Biliary stent endoprosthesis: analysis of complications in 113 patients. *Radiology*. 1985;156(3):637-639.

Rose SC. Biliary system. In: Valji K, ed. *Vascular and Interventional Radiology*. 2nd ed. Philadelphia, PA: Elsevier; 2006.

Saad WE. Hepatobiliary intervention. In: Waldman D, Patel N, Saad W, eds. *Interventional Radiology Secrets*. Philadelphia, PA: Hanley & Belfus, Inc.; 2004.

Turner MA, Cho S, Messmer JM. Pitfalls in cholangiographic interpretation. *Radiographics*. 1987;7(6):1067-1105.

Wollman B, D'Agostino HB, Walus-Wigle JR, et al. Radiologic, endoscopic, and surgical gastrostomy: an institutional evaluation and meta-analysis of the literature. *Radiology*. 1995; 197(3):699-704.

QUESTIONS AND ANSWERS

1. Which of the following is an appropriate indication for TIPS?
   A. Definitive treatment of cirrhosis and portal HTN
   B. Treatment of ascites prior to medical intervention
   C. Bleeding esophageal varices refractory to sclerotherapy
   D. Prevention of variceal bleeding

   ANSWER: C. TIPS is indicated for variceal bleeding refractory to sclerotherapy. It often serves as a bridge to liver transplantation, which is the definitive treatment for cirrhosis and portal hypertension. The first-line treatment of ascites is medical intervention. Sclerotherapy should be attempted to control variceal bleeding prior to TIPS.

2. Which of the following vessel is most commonly affected with Mallory-Weiss tear?
   A. Left gastric artery
   B. Coronary vein
   C. Short gastric artery
   D. Phrenic vein

   ANSWER: A. A Mallory-Weiss tear occurs at the gastroesophageal junction, which is supplied by the left gastric artery.

3. Which of the following is *true*?
   A. Angiography is more sensitive to occult bleeding than TcRBC-labeled scan.
   B. In vivo labeling of RBCs is usually used.
   C. In vitro labeling of RBCs decreases false-positive rates.
   D. Scintigraphy can detect bleeding rates as low as 0.5 to 1.0 mL/min.

   ANSWER: C. TcRBC-labeled scan is ten times more sensitive than angiography for the detection of GI bleeding. Rates as low as 0.05 to 0.1 mL/min can be detected. In vitro labeling decreases false-positive rates.

4. Which of the following procedure is appropriate in the setting of hematemesis?
   A. Endoscopy
   B. Angiography
   C. Abdominal CT with contrast
   D. Upper GI examination

   ANSWER: A. The first-line evaluation of patients with upper GI bleeding is endoscopy. Often a source will be identified that may be treated with sclerotherapy.

5. Which of the following is the most common angiographic finding in angiodysplasia of the colon?
   A. Angiography does not usually show evidence of bleeding.
   B. Minimal bleeding
   C. Moderate bleeding
   D. Massive bleeding

ANSWER: A. Angiodysplasia is more often found in elderly patients and patients with hereditary hemorrhagic telangiectasia. These lesions present on the antimesenteric border of the GI tract and demonstrate an early draining vein. These lesions bleed intermittently and are rarely identified by acute hemorrhage.

6. All of the following are *absolute contraindications* to G-tube placement, *except*
   A. Uncorrectable coagulopathy
   B. Portal hypertension with gastric varices
   C. Ascites
   D. Recent ventriculoperitoneal shunt

   ANSWER: C. Uncorrectable coagulopathy, anterior gastric wall tumor, gastric varices as well as a recently placed ventriculoperitoneal shunt are contraindications to placement of a gastrostomy tube. Ascites is a *relative* contraindication.

7. What is (are) the advantage(s) of a left-sided PTC via the left lobe of the liver?
   A. Less painful location
   B. Decreased possibility of pleural complications
   C. Improved visualization of the entire biliary tree
   D. A and B
   E. B and C

   ANSWER: D. The advantages of a left-sided approach for a PTC are less likelihood of pleural involvement due to the subxiphoid approach and increased patient comfort due to the placement of the tube anteriorly. Often intercostal pain results from a right-side approach. In addition because of the pleural reflection, the pleural may be crossed.

8. What is the first intervention to try in a patient with persistent hemobilia following placement of a PTC?
   A. Visceral arteriogram
   B. PTC to look for vascular communication
   C. Upsize the biliary catheter and flush regularly to clear thrombus
   D. Remove the catheter and have the patient lay in the right lateral decubitus position

   ANSWER: C. The initial treatment in a patient with persistent hemobilia following internal–external drainage is to upsize the tube with the hope that bleeding will tamponad. Once this is done, a cholangiogram may be performed to confirm there is no vascular communication. A visceral arteriogram should not be performed until other measures are exhausted.

9. How are benign biliary enteric strictures best managed?
   A. Balloon dilation and stenting for 4 weeks
   B. Expandable metallic stent
   C. Self-expanding metallic stent
   D. Internal–external drainage for 6 to 12 months

   ANSWER: D. Benign biliary strictures require internal–external or plastic tube stenting for 6 to 12 months. Metallic stents are not indicated in patients with a long life expectancy since they eventually become occluded.

10. Which of the following is the most common cause of AIDS cholangiopathy?
    A. *Enterococcus*
    B. *Cryptosporidium*
    C. *Escherichia coli*
    D. Toxoplasmosis

    ANSWER: B. The most common causes of biliary tract infection in patients with HIV are CMV and *Cryptosporidium* species.

86 GENITOURINARY

Rachel F. Oser

INTRODUCTION

Interventional radiology techniques can apply to a wide array of renal and ureteric pathologies. In the past, percutaneous nephrostomy (PCN) for relief of acute obstruction was the most commonly performed intervention. Although PCN is still commonly performed, it has been joined by a host of newer indications and procedures. This chapter will provide a brief overview of techniques and indications.

ANATOMY

An understanding of relevant anatomy is key to the safe and effective performance of any interventional procedure.

Kidneys are paired organs that lie, surrounded by fat, in the retroperitoneal space on either side of the vertebral column between the twelfth thoracic and third lumbar vertebra. Typically, the left kidney is located 1 to 2 cm higher than the right. The axis of the kidney parallels the psoas muscles, with the upper pole located medial and anterior to the lower pole. The pleura attaches to the tenth rib laterally and the twelfth rib medially, and typically overlaps the upper renal poles increasing the risk of pneumothorax or hydrothorax when upper pole access is required.

The renal hilum contains the renal pelvis, renal artery(ies), and renal vein(s). The renal artery is located posterior to the renal vein and the renal pelvis is located posterior to both the artery and vein. The renal artery divides into anterior and posterior divisions at the renal hilum and then further divides into segmental branches. The segmental renal arteries in turn give rise to the interlobar arteries. The interlobar arteries course around the renal pyramids and give rise to the arcuate and then interlobular arteries. These arteries supply the renal cortex. Renal venous anatomy is more variable. Typically, there are two or three main venous trunks that join to form the renal veins in the renal hilum.

The Brodel line is a relatively avascular plane lying along the posterolateral aspect of the kidney between the anterior and posterior vascular territories. Because of the relative paucity of vessels in this region of the kidney, it is the safest approach for percutaneous interventions. Although, this plane cannot easily be determined on imaging, a posterolateral oblique approach is typically used to minimize bleeding complications. Also, entry into a peripheral calyx or infundibulum rather than the renal pelvis ensures that any vessels crossed are small branches, not a main renal artery or vein.

The ureter courses inferiorly from the renal pelvis along the anteromedial surface of the psoas muscle. At the level of the common iliac artery, it angles medially and then swings posterolaterally into the pelvis. It then courses medially to join the bladder at the ureterovesicular junction. The ureter may have areas of physiologic narrowing at the ureteropelvic junction, the midureter at the level of the common iliac artery, and at the ureterovesicular junction. Vascular supply to the ureters is from ureteral branches of the renal artery; these typically arise from the renal artery in the hilum and appear as fine spiraling vessels that follow the course of the ureters.

The bladder is located in the pelvis behind the symphysis pubis. The dome of the bladder is draped by the peritoneum; the remainder of the bladder is extraperitoneal. Vascular supply to the bladder is from branches of the anterior division of the internal iliac artery, and enters through the posterior and lateral aspects of the bladder.

PATIENT PREPARATION

Any interventional procedure should begin with a thorough review of the patient's past medical history, previous imaging, allergies, and medications. Review of previous imaging can be especially helpful. Attention should be paid to the level of the kidneys and their relationship to adjacent structures such as colon, liver, and spleen, as well as the diaphragm and pleural reflections. Appropriate laboratory studies, including a coagulation panel and serum creatinine, are obtained. Any coagulation abnormalities should be corrected prior to intervention. Preprocedure antibiotics are indicated if there is a history of infection or pyonephrosis. Specific antibiotics are subject to operator preference. The author typically uses cefazolin (Ancef) 1 g intravenous.

Percutaneous renal interventions are often painful and conscious sedation is almost always indicated. Prior to procedure, airway assessment must be performed and a history of prior pain medication obtained. Patients on chronic pain medications may be difficult for the interventional radiologist to safely sedate. For PCN, the patient will be placed in the prone position. This may create difficulties on ventilation for some obese patients. Positioning can also be problematic in pregnant patients and patients with recent abdominal surgery. If a patient is difficult to sedate or there are airway issues, anesthesia should be consulted for assistance in sedation and airway management.

ANTEGRADE PYELOGRAPHY

Antegrade pyelography is the process of inserting a needle or catheter percutaneously into the renal collecting system and injecting contrast to image the pelvicalyceal system and ureters. Although it was widely used as a diagnostic imaging test in the past, it has been largely replaced by cystoscopy and retrograde urography. Currently, antegrade pyelography is used to guide percutaneous interventions and, less frequently, for performance of the Whittaker test.

TECHNIQUE

The patient is placed in the prone position on the fluoroscopy table. If the goal of the procedure is antegrade pyelography alone, the needle can be directed into the renal pelvis under either fluoroscopic or sonographic guidance. More typically however, antegrade pyelography is a prelude to intervention. In these cases, an approach via a posterior calyx is preferred. The most common landmark for the renal pelvis is the lateral margin of the paraspinal muscles at the level of the L2 transverse process. However, if a direct pelvic access is desired, ultrasound (US) guidance may be simpler.

A 20- to 22-gauge trocar needle is then advanced into the kidney. The author typically uses a 22-gauge

15-cm Chiba needle. A longer or stiffer needle may be needed in obese patients or patients with scarring because of previous interventions. The trocar is then removed from the needle. The needle is slowly withdrawn until urine is aspirated. Contrast is then injected and imaging performed. A tilt table may be helpful in visualizing the distal ureter. It is important to not overfill the collecting system as this may lead to bacteremia and sepsis in patients with infected or colonized urine.

WHITTAKER TEST

The Whittaker test is a ureteral stress test, which is used to assess renal function and determine whether or not a chronically dilated collecting system is obstructed. In the past, this test was used as the gold standard for determining whether or not a ureteropelvic junction (UPJ) obstruction needed treatment. In recent years, nuclear medicine studies such as Lasix renography have replaced the Whittaker test despite a 10% to 15% false-positive rate.

The patient is prepared and positioned as for antegrade pyelography. A needle is placed in the renal pelvis and a Foley catheter is placed in the bladder. Water manometers are attached to the needle in the collecting system as well as the Foley catheter. Opening pressures are obtained in the collecting system and bladder. The ureter is infused with dilute contrast media (20%) at a flow rate of 10 mL/min for 5 minutes. Pressures are rechecked—if no evidence of obstruction is present, the flow rate can be increased to 15 to 20 c^3/min and pressures checked again in 5 minutes. The differential pressure is determined by subtracting the bladder pressure from the ureteral pressure (Table 86-1). Finally, the test should be repeated with a full bladder to assess the effect of bladder pressure on the upper collecting system. This may be important with bladder outlet obstruction or bladder dysfunction.

The Whittaker test should be stopped if the urine appears infected or pressure in the kidney is higher than 35 cm H_2O or if the patient experiences pain during the procedure.

TABLE 86-1 Whittaker Test: Normal and Abnormal Pressures Differentials

FLOW RATE (c^3/min)	PRESSURE DIFFERENTIAL (cm H_2O)	DEGREE OF OBSTRUCTION
10	<13	Normal
10	14–22	Mild
10	23–35	Moderate
10	>35	Severe (stop the test)

PERCUTANEOUS NEPHROSTOMY

PCN refers to the insertion of a tube through the skin and renal parenchyma to the collecting system of the kidney. PCN placement is widely used for relief of obstruction, diversion of urine, and accessing the collecting system in preparation for other procedures such as percutaneous nephrolithotomy or stent placement.

Obstruction of the collecting system may be the end result of many disease processes. This includes stone disease, tumor, retroperitoneal fibrosis, surgical mishap, and others (Table 86-2). The end result is complete or parietal obstruction of flow from the renal pelvis to the bladder. Important clinical consequences of renal obstruction are sepsis, with or without shock, pain, impaired renal function, and ultimately renal failure. Sepsis is an indication for emergent PCN as septic shock can be fatal. Impaired renal function necessitates urgent, but not emergent, PCN. Renal dysfunction is usually reversible after relief of obstruction.

Diversion of urine is usually indicated to allow healing of renal, ureteral, or bladder leaks or fistulas. Typically urine is diverted as completely as possible away from the area of injury. Usually this involves a combination of PCN, drainage of any fluid collections, and often either an indwelling Foley catheter or suprapubic catheter for bladder drainage.

Percutaneous access to the renal collecting system is often the initial step in many endourologic procedures. Although many of these are primarily performed by the urologist, interventional radiologists are often primary operators in some stent placement, stone removal, and other procedures.

In addition to understanding the indications for nephrostomy placement, the interventionalist should understand when placing a PCN is not indicated.

TABLE 86-2 Causes of Ureteral Obstruction

Intrinsic	Calculi
	Clot
	UPJ
	TB
	Postoperative
	UVJ
	Tumor
Extrinsic	Lymphadenopathy
	Pelvic malignancy
	Pregnancy
	Trauma
	Iatrogenic
	Retroperitoneal fibrosis
	Prostate cancer
	Bladder cancer

True contraindications to PCN are few. Most contraindications are relative and can be corrected over a period of hours to days. Potential contraindications include bleeding diathesis, untreated infection, neoplasia, anatomic variations, and moral/ethical considerations. Because of the vascularity of the kidneys, bleeding is always a serious risk with PCN. Therefore, normal coagulation parameters are imperative prior to PCN. In patients with abnormal coagulation profiles, this should be corrected before proceeding. Patients with acute infection should be treated with antibiotics prior to PCN to decrease the risk of urosepsis. Anatomic considerations such as horseshoe kidney, pregnancy, obesity, scoliosis, colonic interposition, and renal transplant will affect technique and approach. Review of any relevant prior imaging such as CT or US is critical. In patients with an irreversibly obstructed kidney, the nephrostomy catheter cannot be removed without developing a urine leak that may not resolve over time. Therefore, PCN in terminal inoperative cancer patients essentially commits the patient to PCN and routine exchanges for the remainder of their lives. This should be discussed with the patient and family prior to placement.

Preprocedure evaluation is similar to that for antegrade nephrostogram. In addition, the question of what procedure is in the patient's best interest should be considered. In many cases, retrograde drainage (performed by urology) is a better and safer option.

TECHNIQUE

Many different modalities have been successfully used for accessing the renal collecting system. The most commonly used is fluoroscopy, either using bony landmarks or intravenous contrast opacification of the collecting system. US guidance is also popular and is especially helpful with renal transplants and in thin patients. Typically, real-time US guidance is used for the initial access into the system, and the remainder of the procedure is performed under fluoroscopic guidance. Both CT- and MR-guided access have also been described, but both modalities are more cumbersome to use than US and fluoroscopy.

When using either osseous landmarks or real-time US as a guide, the first step is to access the collecting system with a 21- or 22-gauge Chiba needle. The system is then opacified with contrast media and an antegrade nephrostogram performed. Once the collecting system is opacified, the appropriate calyx for intervention is chosen.

Ideally a lower pole posteriorly oriented calyx is chosen as the site of entry. A 20 to 30 degrees posterolateral oblique approach is most likely to keep the entry to the kidney along Brodel avascular zone and minimize the risk of bleeding complications. By choosing a lower pole calyx and not entering laterally, the risks of pneumothorax and bowel perforation are minimized; however, planned intervention may require a riskier approach. Direct entry into the renal pelvis without passing through renal parenchyma should be avoided, as this approach leads to higher incidence of bleeding and urine leak.

Once an appropriate entry site is chosen, fluoroscopy is used to guide a 21- or 22-gauge Chiba needle into the calyx. Position is confirmed by aspiration of urine and injection of contrast. Only small amounts of contrast should be injected until secure positioning within the collecting system is confirmed to avoid extravasation of contrast around the collecting system, which may obscure the calyces and make subsequent intervention more difficult.

A 0.018-in guidewire is then manipulated through the needle and into the renal pelvis. A conversion system, such as Neff or Accustick system, is then used to upsize the access to allow for placement of a 0.035- or 0.038-in guide wire in the renal pelvis. The wire should then be advanced down the ureter. At our institution, we prefer to use an Amplatz extra-stiff wire for catheter placements. The stiff wire provides good support for interventions and minimizes complications.

The tract is serially dilated and a catheter, typically an 8F or 10F self-retaining pigtail, is placed with the curl in the renal pelvis. Care should be taken during manipulations to not override the wire and perforate the collecting system, as this may lead to catheter malposition and urine leak. There are many brands of catheters available and choice is based on operator preference.

OUTCOMES

PCN is a safe and effective therapy. Success rate is typically more than 98%. In patients with urosepsis, PCN and adequate drainage usually results in clinical improvement within 24 to 48 hours. Patients with obstructive renal dysfunction will demonstrate prompt diuresis and decrease in creatinine. Pain related to obstruction is also usually promptly improved.

COMPLICATIONS

Complication rates for PCN vary widely between published series (Table 86-3). Larger-bore catheters and catheters placed for percutaneous stone removal generally are associated with higher complication rates. On average, complication rates of 4% to 6% are reported. Major complications, such as bleeding requiring surgery or embolization (1%–2%), sepsis (1%–2%), and pneumothorax/hydrothorax (1%), are relatively rare. Minor infection, tube-related issues such as dislodgement,

TABLE 86-3 Complications for Percutaneous Nephrostomy

TYPE	INCIDENCE (%)
Bleeding	
Requiring transfusion	1–3
Associated with vascular injury	0.5–1
Adjacent organ injury	
Bowel	0.1
Pneumothorax/hydrothorax	0.1–0.3
Sepsis	1–3
Mortality	0.05–0.3
Catheter "problems"	2–18

kinking, obstruction and leaks, minor infections, and bleeding not requiring therapy may occur in up to 20% of cases. Arterial injury resulting in pseudoaneurysm or arteriovenous fistula formation can occur in 1% of cases and is usually successfully treated with endovascular therapy such as coil embolization.

As with any major intervention, the key to minimizing complications is good technique and patient selection combined with prompt recognition of complications when they occur. Bloody urine is common after PCN placement. It usually clears within 24 to 48 hours and should not be confused with the rapid bleeding associated with arterial injury. Flank pain is common within the first day after catheter placement and usually abates over time. Adequate pain therapy is critical. A local nerve block may be helpful in patients with persistent catheter-related pain, especially in those patients with intercostal catheters.

CATHETER MAINTENANCE

Self-retaining pigtail-type catheters are most commonly used for PCN. Many manufacturers have designed catheters specifically for this purpose and the choice of brand is dependent on operator and hospital preference. Urologists will often leave a Foley or Council catheter, both of which have a balloon retention system, in place as a PCN catheter. This catheter type is more difficult to place and exchange over a wire and is less favored by interventional radiologists. Typically, catheters should be flushed regularly and have regular dressing changes even after the patient is discharged. The interventional radiology team, including physicians, nurses, residents, and physician assistants, should be available to provide training in catheter care to the patient and family. A printed instruction sheet with contact numbers should be given to the patient and family. Because urine tends to crystallize on and in the tube as well as on the pigtail-retention sutures, routine exchanges are necessary for maintenance of long-term PCN catheters. Patients will require catheter exchange every 2 to 3 months. Pregnant patients and other patients who form stones quickly may need to be scheduled for more frequent catheter exchanges. Exchanges should be performed over a wire under fluoroscopic guidance, usually in an outpatient setting.

PERCUTANEOUS NEPHROSTOLITHOTOMY

Percutaneous nephrostolithotomy (PCNL) is a treatment option used for removal of renal calculi. Other options include surgery and extracorporeal shockwave lithotripsy. PCNL is most often used for patients with staghorn calculi, unusual anatomy (e.g., horseshoe kidney, calyceal diverticula), or stones limited to the upper collecting system, which are difficult to reach with an ureteroscope. Open stone surgery, once the standard for stone removal, is now rarely performed.

For PCNL, an access is obtained percutaneously in the upper collecting system as for PCN. The entry site is chosen in conjunction with the urologist to maximize access to the stone for subsequent removal. Because of this, the site is often in the upper pole and the risk of complications is substantially higher than with a standard PCN. The initial access is obtained and a wire and catheter are manipulated past the stone to the bladder. Patients with complex anatomy, multiple stones, or staghorn calculi may require more than one access for optimal results.

In patients with large staghorn calculi, maneuvering past the stone may be challenging. In our practice, the urologist places a retrograde ureteral catheter before the patient arrives in interventional radiology. This allows us to identify the best access for intervention and guide our PCN more accurately.

A wire is then placed in the bladder and the tract is dilated to 28F to 34F to allow for placement of a nephroscope directly in the upper collecting system. The stone is then fragmented using ultrasonic or laser lithotripsy. At the conclusion of the procedure, a PCN is left in place, usually a large-bore Council catheter. Although the entire procedure can be performed in the operating room using a C-arm fluoroscopy unit, we prefer to place the access in the radiology department and send the patient to the OR with a percutaneous catheter extending from the access site to the bladder. The tract dilation and stone removal are then performed in the OR under general anesthesia by the urologist.

URETERAL STENTS

Ureteral stents allow for the treatment of many of the same conditions as PCN without the discomfort of an external drainage catheter. They are most frequently placed for treatment of ureteral obstruction, leaks, before or after lithotripsy for stone disease, and prior to complex pelvic surgery. Although ureteral stents are most frequently placed in a retrograde fashion by a urologist during cystoscopy, they can also be placed in an antegrade fashion either in conjunction with PCN or as primary therapy.

As with PCN, contraindications to ureteral stent placement are most often relative. Untreated urinary tract infections and urosepsis should be treated first with PCN and intravenous antibiotics. Ureteral stent placement can be performed after the initial infection has been treated. When a bladder fistula or leak is present, urinary diversion is required for healing. As ureteral stents drain the urine into the bladder, they are not appropriate in this instance. Ureteral stents are, however, the first line of treatment for ureteral injury or leak. Because the distal end of the stent rests in the bladder, it can cause irritation. Therefore, stents are not recommended for patients with bladder irritability.

TECHNIQUE

The first step in antegrade ureteral stent placement is percutaneous access to the upper collecting system. Preparation and positioning is the same as for PCN. If a previously placed PCN is present, this can be used as access. Otherwise, a new access should be obtained as for PCN placement. A catheter and guidewire are then manipulated across the UPJ, down the ureter, and into the bladder under fluoroscopic guidance. Once access is obtained, extending from the skin to the bladder, stent placement can be performed.

Two types of ureteral stents are available for percutaneous placement. The first is an internal/external stent, which has an external component, a pigtail loop in the renal pelvis, and a second loop in the bladder. The external component can either be left to drainage or capped, allowing for entirely internal drainage with no need for a drainage bag. The advantage to this type of catheter is that it can be exchanged in the interventional radiology suite, without the need for cystoscopy.

Internal stents are favored by patients because they obviate the need for an external catheter and drainage bag; 8F or 10F double-J ureteral stents are the most frequently used sizes. These are manufactured in a range of lengths, although the 26-cm length is generally acceptable in most adults. As for any catheter, several different manufacturers make systems designed for antegrade ureteral stent placement, and the choice of design is left to operator preference. Like external stents, they also need to be exchanged every 2 to 3 months to maintain patency. Unlike external drains or stents, exchange must be performed in the cystoscopy suite by the referring urologist.

Patients with ileal conduit placement after cystectomy can develop stenosis and occlusion at the junction of the ureter and ileal conduit. If untreated, this can lead to hydronephrosis and renal dysfunction. Reoperation is difficult in these patients, and ureteral stenting is often the treatment of choice. Because of the postoperative anatomy, placing a ureteral stent in this group of patients is challenging. Cystoscopy and retrograde stent placement is difficult because of the redundancy of the ileal conduit and variability in location of the implanted ureters. These patients are usually referred to the interventional radiologist for stenting.

Ureteral stenting begins in these patients as in any PCN, with the patient in the prone position. Access is gained percutaneously into the collecting system. The catheter and wire are then manipulated down the ureter and into the ileal conduit under fluoroscopic guidance. In patients with normal anatomy, the ureteral stent is then placed. In patients with an ileal conduit, however, the distal end of the stent will quickly be obstructed with secretions if it is left in the conduit. Because of this, the stent is ideally placed with one end in the upper collecting system and the other end extending outside the patient's conduit with the distal pigtail draining into the ostomy bag. To achieve this, the patient is rolled on their side. The catheter and wire are then manipulated to the ileostomy and pulled outside the patient. This leaves a wire extending from the initial access site in the patient's back and out the patient's front. A double-J ureteral stent can then be passed along the wire in a retrograde fashion and positioned as desired. The wire is then removed. Like any stent, these need to be exchanged under fluoroscopic guidance every 2 to 3 months. Because the stent extends outside the body, this can be done easily in a retrograde fashion, in an outpatient setting with minimal patient discomfort.

SUPRAPUBIC CYSTOSTOMY

Suprapubic cystostomy is typically used to acutely decompress an obstructed bladder or for long-term urinary diversion in patients with chronic bladder outflow obstruction, neurogenic bladder, bladder fistulae, or bladder or urethral injury. Although often performed by urologists, suprapubic cystostomy can be easily and safely performed in the interventional radiology suite.

TECHNIQUE

The procedure is performed in a fluoroscopy suite. Although bony landmarks can be used, we prefer to use US guidance for the puncture. Either trocar or Seldinger technique can be used. Once in the bladder, contrast should be injected to confirm catheter placement. For initial drainage, a self-retaining 10F pigtail all-purpose drainage catheter is adequate. For long-term drainage, the initial access can be upsized exchanged for a larger Foley catheter once the tract is mature. The Foley catheter can be exchanged by the referring urologist, home health, or a nursing home as needed.

Complications associated with suprapubic cystostomy are minimal, especially with US guidance. Attention should be paid to stick low, just above the symphysis pubis to avoid the peritoneal cavity and overlying bowel loops. A midline puncture will ensure avoiding the inferior epigastric arteries.

SCLEROTHERAPY FOR RENAL CYSTS

Benign renal cysts, either cortical or parapelvic, are found in more than 50% of all people older than 50 years. Typically, these cysts are asymptomatic; however, large, infected, or hemorrhagic cysts may require therapy. Large enough cysts may rarely cause obstruction of the collecting system, urine stasis with stone formation, and renin-dependent hypertension.

Asymptomatic cysts do not require treatment. Symptomatic cysts can be managed with a combination of percutaneous drainage and sclerotherapy. Drainage alone may relieve initial symptoms, but 30% to 80% will quickly reaccumulate fluid. To prevent recurrence, sclerotherapy aims to destroy the epithelial lining of the cysts, following drainage, thus preventing reaccummulation of fluid. A variety of agents have been used as sclerosants including Betadine, absolute alcohol, tetracycline, and sodium morrhuate, among others. Absolute alcohol is the most commonly used agent.

Techniques for cyst sclerosis vary between operators, but the major steps are similar. Initially, the cyst is punctured under US guidance. A small drainage catheter is then placed and fluid aspirated. Contrast should be injected to assess the volume of the cyst and to ensure that there is no communication between the cyst cavity and the collecting system. Contrast is then aspirated and 25% to 50% of the cyst volume replaced with sclerosing agent. The sclerosant is left in place for 15 to 30 minutes. The patient should be encouraged to change position frequently while the sclerosant is in place to allow for maximal contact between the sclerosant and the walls of the cyst. Overdistension of the cyst should be avoided to prevent infiltration of sclerosant into adjacent tissues and vascular structures.

After 15 to 30 minutes, the sclerosant is aspirated. For small cysts, this may be adequate and the catheter can be removed. For larger or recurrent cysts, the catheter is left to drainage. The procedure may need to be repeated several times until the amount of fluid is less than 5 to 10 cm^3. The catheter is then removed.

If the cyst communicates with the collecting system, sclerosant should *not* be injected to avoid formation of strictures. In cases of infected cysts, the infection should be drained and treated with antibiotics before sclerosing. Infection has a strong sclerosing effect, and these cysts may resolve on their own after drainage. Hemorrhagic cysts should be drained and the fluid assessed for possible malignancy. Sclerosis can be performed after the fluid clears.

Outcomes of sclerotherapy for renal cysts are good, with reported success rates of 75% to 100%. Serious complications are rare, but include bleeding, infection, and vascular injury. The sclerosing agents can also be associated with adverse effects, especially if they contact notargeted tissues. Effects may include local inflammation, fat necrosis, and retroperitoneal fibrosis. Fortunately, these complications can be avoided with careful technique.

BIOPSY

Percutaneous biopsy is indicated both to make a specific diagnosis for renal parenchymal disease in native and transplanted kidneys and to diagnose some tumors. For diffuse parenchymal disease, US is generally used for real-time needled guidance. A 16- to 18-gauge core biopsy gun with a short needle excursion is placed within the periphery of the kidney and several cores obtained. By keeping the biopsy area away from the renal hilum, large blood vessels are avoided minimizing bleeding complications. US performed after removal of the biopsy needle is performed to look for persistent bleeding. If an arterial bleed is seen after biopsy, the patient is referred to angiography for possible embolization of the bleeding artery.

Renal tumors may also be biopsied percutaneously. Most solid renal masses require surgical removal. However, biopsy may be required in debilitated patients, or patients with suspicion for lymphoma, metastases, or other unusual pathologies. Although in the past biopsy of renal masses was not in favor because of concern over tumor seeding of the tract, this appears to not be a major concern. Real-time US guidance and biopsy with an 18- to 22-gauge core biopsy gun is most frequently used. CT guidance is also possible, but is generally more cumbersome in the kidney than US.

Transabdominal or endoluminal US or CT can also guide the biopsy of ureteral or bladder masses. Brush biopsy of ureteral masses can be performed from a percutaneous access as well. However, most masses within the collecting system are biopsied by an urologist under direct visualization at cystoscopy.

For any biopsy, complications are similar to those seen with any percutaneous access at that site. Bleeding is the most commonly seen complication, especially for renal biopsy. Vascular injury may occur with larger-gauge needles, and is readily treated with selective embolization of the injured artery. If untreated, vascular injury that is due to biopsy may lead to pseudoaneurysm or arteriovenous fistula formation. These complications are also readily treated with endovascular therapy. Bleeding complications are minimized by avoiding the larger vessels in the central kidney.

Suggested Reading

Castaneda-Zuniga WR. *Interventional Radiology*. Vol 2. 3rd ed. Baltimore, Maryland: Williams and Wilkins; 1997.

Kaufman JA, Lee MJ. *Vascular and Interventional Radiology: The Requisites*. Philadelphia, PA: Mosby; 2004.

Laberge J, Gordon Roy, Kerlan R, Wilson M. *Interventional Radiology Essentials*. Baltimore, Maryland: Lippincott Williams & Wilkins; 2000.

QUESTIONS AND ANSWERS

1. Which of the following is *not* an indication for PCN?
   A. Renal calculi
   B. UPJ obstruction
   C. Ureteral obstruction in pregnancy
   D. Renal cell carcinoma

   ANSWER: D. PCN placement is widely used for relief of obstruction, diversion of urine, and accessing the collecting system in preparation for other procedures such as percutaneous nephrolithotomy or stent placement. Renal cell carcinoma is usually treated with surgical removal.

2. Which of the following is an indication for ureteral stenting?
   A. Bladder rupture that is due to trauma
   B. Ureteral leak after surgery for UPJ obstruction
   C. Vesicovaginal fistula
   D. Urethral injury

   ANSWER: B. When a bladder fistula or leak is present, urinary diversion is required for healing. As ureteral stents drain the urine into the bladder, they are not appropriate in this instance.

3. Renal biopsy is required before treating any patient with a solid renal mass.
   A. True
   B. False

   ANSWER: B. Most solid renal masses require surgical removal. However, biopsy may be required in debilitated patients, or patients with suspicion for lymphoma, metastases, or other unusual pathologies.

4. Which of the following is the ideal location for accessing a kidney percutaneously?
   A. Renal pelvis
   B. Any anterior calyx
   C. Upper pole posterior calyx
   D. Lower pole posterior calyx

   ANSWER: D. Ideally a lower pole posteriorly oriented calyx is chosen as the site of entry. A 20 to 30 degrees posterolateral oblique approach is most likely to keep the entry to the kidney along Brodel's avascular zone and minimize the risk of bleeding complications. By choosing a lower pole calyx and not entering laterally, the risks of pneumothorax and bowel perforation are minimized.

5. Which of the following is the Brodel line?
   A. Most vascular portion of the renal parenchyma
   B. Dividing line between the upper and lower ureter
   C. Relatively avascular plane between the anterior and posterior vascular divisions of the kidney
   D. Most direct access between the skin and the renal parenchyma

   ANSWER: C. The Brodel line is a relatively avascular plane lying along the posterolateral aspect of the kidney between the anterior and posterior vascular territories. Because of the relative paucity of vessels in this region of the kidney, it is the safest approach for percutaneous interventions. Although, this plane cannot easily be determined on imaging, a posterolateral oblique approach is typically used to minimize bleeding complications.

6. Which of the following is the most commonly used sclerosing agent for renal cysts?
   A. Absolute alcohol
   B. Sodium morrhuate
   C. Tetracycline
   D. All of the above

   ANSWER: A. A variety of agents have been used as sclerosants including Betadine, absolute alcohol, tetracycline, and sodium morrhuate, among others. Absolute alcohol is the most commonly used agent.

7. The renal pelvis is located posteriorly to the renal artery and vein at the hilum.
   A. True
   B. False

ANSWER: A. The renal hilum contains the renal pelvis, renal artery(ies), and renal vein(s). The renal artery is located posterior to the renal vein and the renal pelvis is posterior to both the artery and vein.

8. Which of the following is an indication for suprapubic cystostomy?
   A. Neurogenic bladder
   B. Bladder outlet obstruction
   C. Vesicovaginal fistula
   D. All of the above

   ANSWER: D. Suprapubic cystostomy is typically used to acutely decompress an obstructed bladder or for long-term urinary diversion in patients with chronic bladder outflow obstruction, neurogenic bladder, bladder fistulae, or bladder or urethral injury.

9. Which of the following is a complication of PCN?
   A. Sepsis
   B. Pneumothorax
   C. Bleeding
   D. All of the above

   ANSWER: D. Overall complication rates of 4% to 6% are reported. Major complications, including bleeding requiring surgery or embolization (1%–2%), sepsis (1%–2%), and pneumothorax/hydrothorax (1%), are relatively rare.

10. Concerning PCN drainage catheters, which of the following is *true*?
    A. Typically 6F or smaller
    B. Do not require exchanges because urine is a liquid
    C. Best long-term option for most patients
    D. Ideal for relief of acute renal obstruction

    ANSWER: D. PCN placement is widely used for relief of obstruction, diversion of urine, and accessing the collecting system in preparation for other procedures such as percutaneous nephrolithotomy or stent placement.

87 PULMONARY ANGIOGRAPHY AND INTERVENTION

Ahmed Kamel Abdel Aal and Bao T. Bui

INTRODUCTION

With great technological advancement in CT angiography (CTA) and the development of multidetector CT (MDCT) that is greatly expanding in speed and detection, conventional pulmonary angiography (PA) has slowly fallen to the wayside, relegated to problematic and difficult cases in which CT and other techniques have not shown a definitive cause. PA involves the injection of contrast into the pulmonary arteries to obtain radiographic evidence of different pathological processes, and therefore is quite invasive compared to standard CTA techniques. CT is also less operator dependent than angiography and requires less technical expertise. While multidetector helical CTA has steadily become the first test ordered by clinicians to evaluate for patients with symptoms of acute pulmonary thromboembolism (PTE), conventional PA remains the gold standard.

ANATOMY

Pulmonary arterial circulation begins in the heart at the level of the pulmonary valve. The main pulmonary artery arises from the conus arteriosus of the right ventricle extending superiorly and to the left for approximately 5 cm. It is initially anterior to the ascending aorta, and then passes to the left of the ascending aorta as it continues superiorly, to lie in the concavity of the aortic arch.

The main pulmonary artery divides into the right and left pulmonary arteries. The left pulmonary artery is slightly smaller and shorter than the right. It passes anterior to the descending aorta and superior to the left main bronchus. As such, it has a slightly higher position in the chest than the right pulmonary artery. It is attached to the concavity of the aortic arch by the ligamentum arteriosum. It divides into the upper and lower lobar branches.

The right pulmonary artery is slightly larger and longer than the left. It passes anterior to the right bronchus and posterior to the ascending aorta and superior vena cava (SVC). It subsequently divides into two branches: a larger lower branch to the middle and lower lobes and a smaller branch to the upper lobe.

The pulmonary lobar arteries divide into segmental, subsegmental, and lobular branches. Lobular arteries are at the center of the secondary pulmonary lobules, the functional unit of the lung.

There is usually one pulmonary vein from each lobe of the lungs with the right middle and upper lobes uniting to form a common trunk. Four trunks, two from each lung, empty into the left atrium. On both sides, the pulmonary veins are inferior to the pulmonary arteries, except at the level of the hilum where the superior pulmonary veins lie anterior to the right and left pulmonary arteries. The left pulmonary vein is anterior to the descending thoracic aorta. The right pulmonary vein is posterior to the SVC. Anomalous pulmonary venous drainage can be total or partial and is often associated with congenital heart disease.

The bronchial arteries provide a much smaller portion of the total pulmonary blood flow. They are generally of minor clinical significance and only important in diseases that cause their enlargement, such as cystic fibrosis. In such cases, erosion of these dilated bronchial arteries by the disease process will produce hemoptysis that is often life threatening. Bronchial artery anatomy is very variable and is classified into four types. The most common pattern is two left and one right bronchial artery (type 1). The left bronchial arteries usually arise from the anterolateral surface of the thoracic aorta below the ligamentum arteriosum, while the right bronchial artery usually arises from a common trunk with an intercostals artery (intercostobronchial trunk). However, it is not uncommon to find bilateral single bronchial arteries (type 2), two left and two right bronchial arteries (type 3), or a single left and two right bronchial arteries (type 4). The origins of the bronchial arteries can also be quite variable with some arising from the brachiocephalic, subclavian, or internal mammary artery. It is important to emphasize that, in approximately 5% of the population, the right intercostobronchial trunk contributes to or arises with the artery of Adamkiewicz, which supplies the anterior spinal artery, and needs careful consideration when performing bronchial artery embolization.

TECHNIQUE

PULMONARY ANGIOGRAPHY

INDICATIONS

The main indication for PA is to evaluate for PTE. Classically, pulmonary angiograms are obtained whenever there is an intermediate or high clinical index of suspicion supported by a ventilation/perfusion (V/Q) scan that is interpreted as intermediate or high probability. However, this practice has changed in many institutions, and the standard is to initially obtain a pulmonary CTA for those patients if there is reasonable clinical suspicion. With the advent of MDCT, the entire thorax can be imaged during the first pass of contrast in the pulmonary circulation. This can be acheived during a single breath hold, even in patients with PTE who suffer from dyspnea related to their disease. Pulmonary CTA can detect thrombus in the pulmonary artery up to the third-order branch with optimal technique and contrast timing. CTA also has the advantage of entertaining other diagnoses that can be the cause of the patient's symptoms.

Pulmonary arteriograms are reserved for those cases in which CTA cannot be performed or in cases of massive or central PTE causing significant hemodynamic compromise and in patients who are potential candidates for thromboembolectomy. Less commonly, pulmonary arteriogram is performed prior to inferior vena cava (IVC) filter placement if documentation of deep venous thrombosis cannot be achieved.

CONTRAINDICATIONS

There is no absolute contraindication to pulmonary arteriograms. The most important relative contraindications are as follows:

- Severe pulmonary hypertension leading to high right ventricular pressure: Systolic pressure more than 70 mm Hg and diastolic pressure more than 20 mm Hg are associated with increased mortality as high as 2% to 3%. In these cases, if pulmonary arteriogram is still indicated, nonionic isoosmolar contrast agents (Visipaque 320 or 270) can be used. Furthermore, subselective-targeted angiograms should be performed to minimize contrast load.
- Left bundle branch block (LBBB): The manipulation of the catheter across the right heart might lead to right bundle branch block. This might lead to complete heart block if the patient had preexisting LBBB. This can be avoided by performing pulmonary arteriogram with the tip of the catheter placed in the distal IVC or SVC to avoid manipulations in the right heart and right bundle branch block. Alternatively, a transvenous pacer can be placed before the procedure.
- Congestive heart failure: This should be preferably treated prior to pulmonary arteriogram.

PROCEDURE

PA is usually performed through a transfemoral approach and occasionally through a transjugular or transbrachial approach. A large pigtail catheter, usually 7F or 8F, is advanced from the puncture site through the right heart and pulmonary valve into the main pulmonary artery. We found that a 5F-angled pigtail catheter allows easy manipulation in the right heart with the aid of a J-wire. The small French size also provides less risk of postprocedure bleeding from the access site. Right ventricular and pulmonary artery pressures should be obtained first, since elevated pressures may influence the performance of subsequent angiograms (see contraindications given in the previous paragraph). PA with the catheter in the main pulmonary artery is then performed. Selective catheterization and angiography of the right or left pulmonary artery can also be performed. Approximately 30 to 50 mL of low-osmolar or isoosmolar nonionic contrast is injected at a rate of 15 to 25 mL/s with filming usually at 4 frames/s. The different projections depend on clinical suspicion, but often an AP and right and left posterior oblique views of the lung base are performed. Other views are supplemental to the above standard views. Every effort should be made to obtain images during maximum inspiration. Magnified superselective views are sometimes needed to demonstrate a more peripheral thrombus. In this case, balloon occlusion catheters may be used. The balloon should not produce complete occlusion of the catheterized branch and should be deflated immediately at the end of the angiogram.

COMPLICATIONS

Although invasive, the morbidity and mortality of PA are generally low. Complications are mostly related to access technique or contrast-induced nephropathy, ranging from 1% to 5%. Other more serious but less common complications reported include significant arrhythmia, endocardial stain, and right ventricular perforation. Mortality from pulmonary arteriogram is less than 0.5% and is related to acute right ventricular failure in most patients.

BRONCHIAL ANGIOGRAPHY

INDICATIONS

By far the most common indication for bronchial angiogram is hemoptysis. Mild-to-moderate hemoptysis usually requires only clinical monitoring. Massive hemoptysis is defined as more than 300 to 600 mL/24 h, although it varies from 200 to 1000 mL/24 h, according to different authors. The more common causes for hemoptysis include cystic fibrosis and infections such as tuberculosis, bronchiectasis, and bronchogenic carcinoma. Other less common indications for bronchial angiogram include evaluation of bronchial arteries in case of congenital heart disease with interruption of the pulmonary circulation and evaluation of bronchial arteries following lung transplant.

PROCEDURE

The procedure is usually performed through a transfemoral approach. The level of the bronchial arteries is quite variable and ranges from T4 to T9. However, approximately 90% of bronchial arteries arise at the level of T5-6, and the carina acts as a convenient fluoroscopic landmark. In cases of iliac or aortic tortuosity, a long sheath may be used to enhance catheter manipulation. A variety of catheters may be used; the most common and convenient are Mikelson, Simmons I, and shepherd's hook catheters. However, H1, Cobra, and RC2 catheters can also be used. The catheter tip should be directed to a lateral to anterolateral position during the search for the bronchial arteries. Occlusion of the bronchial arteries, especially the intercostobronchial trunk, should be avoided since this may result in cord ischemia. Angiograms are usually performed through hand injection of 3 to 10 mL of contrast material. Hand injections have the advantage of adjusting the pressure and flow of contrast in the bronchial arteries by the operator to avoid injury and rupture of the small distal diseased branches.

PULMONARY ARTERIAL HYPERTENSION

CLINICAL PRESENTATION AND CONSIDERATION

The mean pulmonary artery pressure ranges from 12 to 16 mm Hg. Pulmonary arterial hypertension (PAH) is defined as mean pulmonary artery of more than 25 mm Hg during rest or more than 30 mm Hg during exercise, although some authors define it as systolic pulmonary artery pressure exceeding 30 mm Hg.

Patients with PAH often present with nonspecific signs and symptoms including dyspnea, fatigue, and chest pain. The clinical findings are nonspecific, frequently requiring catheterization and pressure measurements for accurate diagnosis.

Classically, there are two types of PAH: primary and secondary. In primary PAH, the cause is unknown and the disease mostly occurs in middle-aged women. Secondary PAH may be caused by a variety of underlying pulmonary or arterial abnormalities and can be subdivided into four types: pulmonary thromboembolic disease, intra- or extracardiac shunts, chronic lung disease, and left heart failure. The increase flow or obstruction leads to vasoconstriction and remodeling of the pulmonary arterial walls resulting in fibrosis. Elevated right heart pressure is required to pump blood through stiffer pulmonary arteries eventually leading to right ventricular failure.

IMAGING FEATURES

Imaging findings of PAH include enlarged central pulmonary arteries, elevated pulmonary arterial pressure, and marked tapering and attenuation of the peripheral branches. PA is often unable to determine the exact cause or differentiate between the types of PAH and other tests are frequently necessary.

ACUTE PULMONARY EMBOLISM

CLINICAL PRESENTATION

Acute pulmonary embolus is a very common clinical problem and is one of the primary indications for PA. The clinical presentation for acute pulmonary embolism is quite nonspecific, with the minority of patients presenting with classic dyspnea, pleuritic chest pain, and cough. Other nonspecific symptoms include tachypnea and tachycardia. The workup for chest pain, therefore, often involves the exclusion of pulmonary embolus. It frequently requires a high degree of clinical suspicion. Although clinicians are quite aware of its presence and clinical impact, it is often underdiagnosed.

Patients respond to acute pulmonary embolism differently, depending on their cardiopulmonary reserve. Patients with normal pulmonary and cardiac functions tolerate large emboli well without much morbidity. However, with underlying cardiac or pulmonary disease, small embolus can cause much morbidity and sometimes even death.

The most common source of acute pulmonary embolism arises from lower extremities and pelvic deep venous thrombosis, with the latter occurring more in postpartum patients. The deep veins of the upper extremities are increasingly becoming a cause of embolus, especially in relation to intravenous drug abuse. Superficial veins of the extremities are not known to cause thromboembolic disease to the lungs. Large emboli often break apart as they travel into the central systemic veins and pulmonary arteries, showering smaller emboli into the pulmonary arterial circulation. Pulmonary infarction however is rare, because of dual supply of the pulmonary parenchyma and the fact that most pulmonary emboli lodge more centrally, allowing for collateral flow. Therefore, pulmonary infarction is more commonly associated with peripheral embolus. Large or saddle emboli cause the most significant morbidity and can lead to acute right heart failure secondary to pulmonary hypertension or even death.

Imaging Features

The most specific signs for pulmonary embolus in any imaging technique whether CT, MR, or conventional PA is intraluminal filling defect, abrupt arterial cutoff, or both. Intraluminal filling defects usually occur at branching points. Suspicious lesions and filling defects should be more carefully examined with different projections and magnification views. A true filling defect should be constant on multiple views. Secondary less specific signs on conventional PA include slow flow or regional oligemia, which are suggestive but not definitive in the diagnosis of acute PTE. Most pulmonary emboli tend to be multiple and bilateral with smaller emboli involving multiple vessels, particularly of the lower lobes.

An advantage of conventional PA over CT includes better visualization of more peripheral embolus. Pulmonary CTA is comparable to conventional angiography in central embolus, and its ability to detect small pulmonary emboli has significantly improved with the development of MDCT. The main limitation remains in its reliable detection of small subsegmental peripherally located pulmonary emboli, although the clinical significance of such small emboli remains debatable. Another advantage of CTA includes its less invasive nature and the ability to visualize other intrathoracic structures and suggest an alternative diagnosis when available. It is quicker to perform and requires less technical expertise, and therefore is favored by most emergency departments in triaging those patients with clinical presentation suspicious for PTE. Conventional PA currently is reserved for problem solving in patients with clinical suspicion of acute pulmonary embolus but with negative CTA or V/Q scans.

Treatment and Prognosis

The mortality rate for acute pulmonary embolus remains high, reaching approximately 20% in some studies. The classic treatment includes anticoagulation with heparin and long-term warfarin therapy for 6 months or more, while maintaining INR between 2.0 and 3.0. Some patients require lifelong anticoagulation therapy. Anticoagulation will lyse the current thrombus and will prevent recurrence. Most acute emboli will lyse with standard medical therapy; however, a minority of patients will develop chronic pulmonary embolus and PAH, requiring more invasive surgical thromboembolectomy. Patients in whom anticoagulation is contraindicated, placement of an IVC filter to prevent further emboli is necessary.

Sometimes, acute relief of clot burden is required to improve the hemodynamic status of patients on the verge of right ventricular failure. This can be achieved using systemic or catheter-directed thrombolysis. It is important to emphasize that a small decrease in the degree of pulmonary artery obstruction leads to dramatic clinical improvement in most cases. However, thrombolytics are not without side effects and contraindications, and should be used in carefully selected patients to avoid adverse outcomes.

Embolectomy is the last resort for patients with fulminant PE, who failed or have a contraindication for thrombolysis. Surgical embolectomy has very high morbidity and mortality rates. Alternatively, percutaneous embolectomy carries a more favorable outcome in most cases. The catheter-based devices can be divided into those that remove the thrombus versus those that fragment the thrombus into smaller pieces that lodge more peripherally, thus decreasing the pulmonary vascular resistance in the main pulmonary artery. The latter may be followed by catheter-directed thrombolysis.

CHRONIC PULMONARY EMBOLISM

Clinical Presentation

Chronic pulmonary embolic disease is often due to recurrent episodes of emboli in patients with underlying disease or condition that predisposes to stasis. Less often, it can occur because of failure of lysis of acute pulmonary emboli. Clinically, these patients present with nonspecific symptoms of progressive exertional dyspnea, hemoptysis, or fatigue. These patients rarely present emergently, and the workup is often due to other causes.

Imaging Features

As chronic and unresolved emboli damage and obstruct the pulmonary circulation, remodeling of the pulmonary arterial walls occurs giving rise to the imaging features of chronic pulmonary embolism. The remaining normal pulmonary circulation is diminished leading to increase in pulmonary artery and right heart pressures. Most patients have evidence of PAH during pressure measurements, and show enlarged central pulmonary arteries on chest radiographs and CT with pruning of the peripheral arterial branches. Conventional PA often demonstrates multiple segmental and lobar perfusion deficits consistent with infarcts. Pulmonary artery dilatation and pruning of the peripheral pulmonary arterial branches, irregularities, webs, and stenoses can be seen. Residual linear filling defects resulting from recanalization of prior thrombus can also be seen.

Treatment and Prognosis

Chronic pulmonary emboli do not respond to medical treatment and require surgical thromboembolectomy in most cases. Anticoagulation, however, is still required to prevent further showering of emboli, especially in patients who are clinically unstable. IVC filters are also used for the same purpose.

PULMONARY ARTERY THROMBOSIS

Thrombosis of the main pulmonary artery and its branches can occur in association with parenchymal lung disease, congenital heart disease, thoracic trauma, or because of systemic diseases such as polycythemia vera or sickle cell disease.

On pulmonary arteriograms, the involved vessel will be occluded, yet without the leading edge sign of an embolus. There is usually no peripheral filling beyond the thrombus suggesting intrinsic thrombosis rather than an ill-fitting embolus.

PULMONARY ARTERY ANEURYSM AND PSEUDOANEURYSM

Clinical Presentation and Consideration

Pulmonary arterial aneurysms are uncommon compared to aneurysms in the systemic circulation. True aneurysms may be congenital or acquired, and PAH plays an important role in its pathogenesis and formation. Pulmonary artery pseudoaneurysms may be iatrogenic, infectious, or traumatic in etiology. Other less common etiologies include vasculitis, syphilis, tuberculosis (Rasmussen aneurysm), bilharziasis, neoplasms, mycotic emboli, and connective tissue disorders. Patients with pulmonary artery aneurysms or pseudoaneurysms are usually asymptomatic or present with symptoms of their underlying illness. Massive hemoptysis is a common presenting symptom in patients with acute aneurysm rupture and can be life threatening.

In the vasculitis category, Behçet is a landmark. It is a multisystem disease most often seen in men of Mediterranean and Southeast Asian descent who present with oral and genital ulcers, skin lesions, orbital and CNS inflammatory changes, and GI inflammatory symptoms. Hughes-Stovin syndrome is a less well-known cause of pulmonary artery aneurysm and recurrent thrombophlebitis. Iatrogenic perforation of the pulmonary artery during placement of Swan-Ganz catheter is a frequent cause of pulmonary arterial pseudoaneurysms. Conventional PA is both diagnostic and therapeutic in cases of pulmonary aneurysms and pseudoaneurysms.

Imaging Features

Pulmonary artery aneurysm is easily recognized on both contrast-enhanced CT and PA. Infectious causes including disseminated bacterial infections and tuberculosis tend to be multiple and often peripherally distributed. Syphilitic and vasculitic pseudoaneurysms tend to be more centrally distributed.

Treatment and Prognosis

The treatment for pulmonary artery aneurysm and pseudoaneurysm involves coiling of the lesion itself or the artery feeding the lesion. Pseudoaneurysms are less easily handled since the fragile pseudoaneurysm is prone to rupture during manipulations and coil placement. Ideally, the feeding pulmonary artery should be embolized with coils or Amplatzer vascular plugs.

In certain cases, coils may be gently deployed inside the cavity of the pseudoaneurysm. Even with modern endovascular treatment modalities, the prognosis is often poor owing to the patient's multiple underlying conditions and illnesses.

PULMONARY ARTERIOVENOUS MALFORMATION

Clinical Presentation and Consideration

Pulmonary arteriovenous malformations (PAVM) are abnormal communications between the pulmonary arteries and veins without intervening capillaries. They are considered functional extracardiac shunts with blood flowing from the right to left heart without oxygenation or filtration in the lungs. They can occur either as isolated entities or in association with Osler-Weber-Rendu syndrome (otherwise known as hereditary hemorrhagic telangiectasia). In Osler-Weber-Rendu syndrome, patients have arteriovenous malformations in the GI tract, liver, and CNS. Approximately 5% to 15% of Osler-Weber-Rendu syndrome patients have PAVM, while 50% to 60% of patients with PAVM have Rendu-Osler-Weber syndrome. PAVM are multiple in 30% to 50% and bilateral in 30% of cases.

These patients often present primarily with hemoptysis. The resulting right-to-left shunt can cause serious complications related to systemic embolization, such as stroke, transient ischemic attack, and cerebral abscess, reported in up to 40% of patients.

PAVM are classified according to their angioarchitecture as simple and complex. The simple malformations are recognized to have a single segmental artery feeder and include up to three subsegmental arteries. Complex PAVM by definition have two or more different segmental arteries supplying the malformation. Approximately 80% of PAVM are simple and the malformations are usually located in the lower lobes.

Imaging Features

Contrast-enhanced CT is the preferred imaging modality for PAVM because of its ability to visualize small peripheral lesions. Both lungs should be studied to ensure that small AVM are not missed. PAVM typically appear as multilobulated intensely enhancing masses, with large vessels extending from the mass to the hilum, representing enlarged feeding arteries and draining veins. Volume-rendered three-dimensional reformatted images and multiplanar reformatted images are helpful in planning for percutaneous transcatheter embolization. It must be emphasized that great care should be taken during insertion of intravenous lines and during contrast administration, to avoid introduction of air bubbles.

PA is usually performed to confirm the diagnosis and when percutaneous transcatheter embolotherapy is indicated. Because of the right-to-left shunt, PA in patients suspected with PAVM must be performed with extra care. Careful attention must be paid to the technique to ensure no air embolus will occur. Similar attention should be paid to intravenous line insertion, and the use of filters in these lines is highly recommended. Heparin is often required to prevent thrombus formations around the catheters and guidewires. Pulmonary angiograms will demonstrate enlargement of the feeding artery, with early shunting of contrast during the arterial phase into an enlarged draining vein through an aneurysmal sac. Pulmonary angiogram has the advantage of delineating the angioarchitecture of the PAVM and the feeding arteries. The size of the feeding artery should be measured since PAVM with feeding artery diameter of more than 3 mm should be treated to avoid paradoxical systemic embolization.

Treatment and Prognosis

In the last decade, percutaneous transcatheter embolotherapy has become the mainstay for most patients with PAVM. Its advantages are that it is less invasive, can be easily repeated in case of recurrence, and a variety of materials are available for embolization. Significant improvements have occurred in catheter techniques, making interventional management simpler and safer. Detachable balloons are historical and were abandoned because of the risk of deflation and paradoxical embolization. Fibered coils are currently used and their diameter should be at least 20% larger than the feeding artery, to avoid paradoxical embolization. The scaffold and anchoring techniques, during placement of coils, have been described in literature to avoid coil embolization into the systemic circulation. More recently, the Amplatzer vascular plug has been used for the treatment of PAVM. The Amplatzer vascular plug is a detachable self-expandable cylindrical device made from a nitinol wire mesh that allows the device to compress inside a delivery catheter and then return to its intended shape to occlude the target vessel. It is recommended to oversize the device by approximately 30% to 50% of the feeding artery diameter to prevent device migration after deployment. The limitation of the Amplatzer vascular plug device is that it requires distal placement of a 5F to 8F guiding catheter, depending on the diameter of the feeding artery to be occluded, which can be technically challenging. Also, the delivery wire of the Amplatzer vascular plug is quite stiff and maneuvering it through tortuous anatomy may be slightly difficult. Recurrence is secondary to recanalization of occluded vessels or interval growth of accessory vessels. Recurrence rates range from 5% to 57%. Recanalization is the most common cause of recurrence, accounting for approximately 90% of recurrent cases. CTA is an excellent modality for follow-up of patients after embolotherapy to evaluate for recurrence. Some patients may need repeat sessions of embolization.

PULMONARY VARIX

Pulmonary varices are focal dilatations of the pulmonary veins that may occur in association with congenital and acquired heart disease or in asymptomatic patients without cardiac abnormality. These lesions are seen as well-defined enhancing structures on CT in relation to a vessel, and frequently produce a diagnostic dilemma since they have a similar appearance to PAVM. However on pulmonary angiograms, the varix shows delayed-contrast filling on the pulmonary venous phase as opposed to early shunting and venous filling in PAVM.

PULMONARY ARTERY STENOSIS

Pulmonary artery stenosis (PAS) is usually a disease of children and usually associated with congenital heart disease. Children with pulmonary arterial stenosis typically present with dyspnea, fatigue, tachypnea, or tachycardia. In adults, PAS is rare, and vasculitis is the most common etiology. Other causes include chronic PE, post–lung transplant, and extrinsic compression by masses, granulomatous disease, adenopathy, fibrosing mediastinitis, or other intrathoracic processes.

PAS is easily diagnosed with a contrast-enhanced CT of the chest. The main, right, or left pulmonary artery may be small. Conventional PA is rarely required for the diagnosis of PAS, except for documentation of peripheral disease beyond the resolution of axial imaging.

The management of PAS includes angioplasty with possible stent placement or surgery, depending on the anatomy and location of stenosis. Angioplasty is sometimes preferred over stent placement, especially in children where potential mismatch between the deployed stent and the size of the stenosed artery after somatic growth is a concern. Generally the prognosis depends on the underlying congenital heart disease and other associated conditions.

VASCULITIS

Clinical Presentation and Consideration

Takayasu arteritis is systemic vasculitis affecting large and medium-sized arteries, most commonly involving the aorta and its proximal branches. Pulmonary arterial involvement can occur mostly in the form of arterial occlusion, stenosis, and aneurysm formations. These patients are typically middle-aged women of all racial backgrounds, although it was initially described in Japanese women. Common presenting symptoms can be nonspecific, such as fever, fatigue, and weight loss, or specific symptoms relating to the distribution of the arteries involved. Patients can present with light-headedness or loss of vision because of involvement of the carotid arteries, arm weakness because of involvement of the subclavian arteries, or hypertension because of involvement of the renal arteries. A classic symptom, which gives rise to a more common name of Takayasu arteritis, is "pulseless disease" that is due to subclavian artery occlusions.

Imaging Features

During PA, pulmonary arterial involvement ranges from stenosis to complete occlusion, although aneurysmal dilatation can also occur. There is no predilection for any side or lobe involvement, and there is no correlation between pulmonary arterial disease and systemic disease. A characteristic feature of active Takayasu's arteritis is wall enhancement on CT and MRI examinations following administration of contrast.

Treatment and Prognosis

The mainstay of treatment for Takayasu's arteritis is to control the systemic inflammatory changes using steroids and immunosuppressive drugs. Complications of the disease can be managed as they arise. Long-term prognosis is not known.

HEMOPTYSIS AND BRONCHIAL ARTERY EMBOLIZATION

Clinical Presentation and Consideration

Mild-to-moderate hemoptysis usually requires only clinical monitoring. Massive hemoptysis, defined as more than 300 to 600 mL in 24 hours, generally requires treatment. In most cases, severe hemoptysis results from a systemic arterial source, rather than from the pulmonary circulation. The most common causes of hemoptysis requiring therapy include cystic fibrosis, bronchiectasis, infections such as tuberculosis, and bronchogenic carcinoma.

Significant bleeding from pulmonary arterial origin is quite rare, usually associated with systemic arterial source, and is commonly seen in cases of destructive pulmonary parenchymal lesions. Examples of such lesions include cavitary tuberculosis, invasive aspergillosis, pyogenic abscesses, and large necrotic tumors. However, it may also occur in case of pseudoaneurysms of various etiologies and in case of PAVM.

CT studies are helpful in determining the probable site of bleeding. Bronchoscopy may show the site of bleeding, especially when performed early in management, and may guide selective intrabronchial balloon tamponade. However, in most cases, bronchoscopy provides no additional information over radiographic studies and should only be reserved for patients in whom radiographic studies failed to localize the site of bleeding. Selective intubation or double-barrel endotracheal tube may be necessary to protect the non-bleeding lung.

Imaging Features

Bronchial angiography is performed for patients with massive hemoptysis or hemoptysis requiring therapy, as it can be both diagnostic and therapeutic. The technique of bronchial angiography is described earlier in this chapter. The bronchial artery supplying the source of hemoptysis is usually hypertrophied and tortuous, measuring more than 3 mm. Other angiographic signs suggestive of bronchial arterial source are parenchymal staining, hypervascularity, bronchial-pulmonary shunting, and bronchial artery aneurysms. An important feature that differentiates hemoptysis from acute gastrointestinal hemorrhage is that hemoptysis rarely demonstrates contrast extravasation on bronchial angiograms even if massive or clinically apparent. Collateral pathways to the bronchial arteries from the internal mammary, intercostals, and branches of the subclavian arteries should be clearly delineated, as they can be the source of bleeding in some cases. Pulmonary angiograms are performed if no source is found on bronchial angiogram, and there is strong evidence for pulmonary arterial cause such as pseudoaneurysm or PAVM.

Treatment and Prognosis

The treatment of choice for hemoptysis is embolization. Before embolizing the bronchial artery culprit, a careful search for collateral pathways between the bronchial artery and the anterior spinal artery must be performed. If there is a collateral pathway, extra care must be taken so that spinal cord infarction can be avoided. This is done by superselective catheterization of the bronchial artery using a microcatheter and placing the microcatheter as distal as possible within the artery before injection of embolic material. Spinal cord infarction is a rare complication in the hands of an experienced interventionalist; however, it is a potential significant risk that patients should be aware of and accept prior to performing the procedure. Another potential complication of bronchial angiogram is transverse myelitis manifesting with paraplegia. This is also a rare complication (less than 1%) and the cause is unknown.

Embolization of the bronchial artery is usually accomplished with polyvinyl alcohol (300–900 μm) or Gelfoam pledgets. This is delivered as distal as possible, preferably through a microcatheter. Coils can be used very distally, but not at the orifice of the bronchial artery since it may need to be accessed again in cases of recurrent hemorrhage. If the bronchial artery gives collateral branches to the spinal artery or other critical branches to the trachea and esophagus, embolization should be performed distal to these arteries and using particle size that is essentially larger than 250 μm to prevent nontarget embolization of these critical branches. Follow-up angiograms are performed intermittently during embolization to determine the progress and search for any complication.

The prognosis for patients undergoing bronchial artery embolization is generally good. Complications such as spinal cord infarction, pulmonary infarction, tracheal and esophageal necrosis are rare. Surgically, therapy is considered if bronchial artery embolization is ineffective. In some patients in whom bronchial artery embolization is used to control acute massive hemorrhage, definitive surgical therapy may be necessary to correct the underlying abnormality.

PULMONARY ARTERY TUMORS AND ENDOVASCULAR PULMONARY ARTERY CATHETER-BASED BIOPSY

Primary pulmonary artery tumors are very rare, accounting for less than 15% of thoracic tumors. The most common are sarcomatous tumors, such as leiomyosarcoma and spindle cell sarcoma. Primary tumors commonly have a central location; however multifocal tumors can also occur. Secondary tumors are mostly because of invasion of the pulmonary artery by mediastinal and lung tumors, with bronchogenic carcinoma being the most common.

CT and MRI can clearly demonstrate the tumor and suggest whether it is primary or secondary. Both can show the extent of obstruction of the pulmonary artery lumen. However, the most important aspect of CT and MRI is their ability to distinguish these enhancing tumors from a nonenhancing thrombus. During angiography, pulmonary artery tumors are seen as filling defects in the main pulmonary artery or its branches. Endovascular biopsy of these tumors can be performed using various devices that were originally used for ventricular biopsy, but can also be used in the pulmonary arteries. Forceps are commonly used and can remove a tissue sample of 2 to 5 mL depending on the forceps caliber.

FOREIGN BODY RETRIEVAL

Percutaneous retrieval of intravascular foreign bodies has become the standard of treatment. The majority of cases are due to separated catheter fragment or lost wires during catheter insertion by inexperienced personnel. Foreign bodies may lodge in the SVC, right heart, or pulmonary circulation. Retrieval is usually accomplished using a variety of snares; the most famous and commonly used is the gooseneck snare. Other devices that can be used include a retrieval basket, pigtail catheter and tip-deflecting wire, and grasping forceps. If the foreign body migrates to the distal pulmonary artery, a pigtail catheter may be used to dislodge it into a more proximal position where it can be snared.

Suggested Reading

Arcasoy SM, Kreit JW. Thrombolytic therapy in pulmonary embolism: a comprehensive review of current evidence. *Chest*. 1999;115:1695-1707.

Auger WR, Fedullo PF, Moser KM, et al. Chronic major-vessel thromboembolic pulmonary artery obstruction: appearance at angiography. *Radiology*. 1993;182:393-398.

Castaner E, Gallardo X, Rimola J, et al. Congenital and acquired pulmonary artery anomalies in the adult: radiologic overview. *Radiographics*. 2006;26:349-371.

Engelke C, Schaefer-Prokop C, Schirg E, et al. High-resolution CT and CT angiography of peripheral pulmonary vascular disorders. *Radiographics*. 2002;22:739-764.

Goldhaber SZ. Pulmonary embolism. *N Engl J Med*. 1998;339: 93-104.

Gossage JR, Kanj G. Pulmonary arteriovenous malformations: a state of the art review. *Am J Respir Crit Care Med*. 1998;158: 643-661.

Johnson MS. Current strategies for diagnosis of pulmonary embolus. *J Vasc Interv Radiol*. 2002;13:13-23.

Lee EW, Grant JD, Loh CT, et al. Bronchial and pulmonary arterial and venous interventions. *Semin Respir Crit Care Med*. 2008;29:395-404.

Pelage JP, Hajjam ME, Lagrange C, et al. Pulmonary artery interventions: an overview. *Radiographics*. 2005;25:1653-1667.

Ray CE, Kaufman JA, Geller S, et al. Embolization of catheter-induced pulmonary artery pseudoaneurysm. *Chest*. 1996;110: 1370-1373.

QUESTIONS AND ANSWERS

1. From which of the following arteries does the bronchial arteries most commonly arise?
   A. Thoracic aorta
   B. Pulmonary artery
   C. Subclavian artery
   D. Internal mammary artery

   ANSWER: A. The bronchial arteries most commonly arise from the thoracic aorta—the most common pattern of bronchial arteries is two left and one right bronchial artery. They less likely arise from the subclavian, internal mammary, or intercostal arteries, and they are not branches of the pulmonary artery.

2. Which of the following is an absolute contraindication to pulmonary angiography?
   A. Systolic pressure more than 70 mm Hg and diastolic pressure more than 20 mm Hg
   B. Congestive heart failure
   C. LBBB
   D. None. There is no absolute contraindication to PA.

   ANSWER: D. There is no absolute contraindication to PA. Congestive heart failure, LBBB, and severe PAH are all relative contraindications to PA.

3. Which of the following is the most specific sign of acute pulmonary embolus on any imaging modality?
   A. Regional oligemia
   B. Pulmonary arterial stenosis or web
   C. Pulmonary infarction
   D. Intraluminal filling defect

   ANSWER: D. The most specific signs for pulmonary embolus in any imaging technique are intraluminal filling defects, abrupt arterial cutoff, or both.

4. Which of the following is the most common cause of pulmonary pseudoaneurysm?
   A. Congenital etiology
   B. Iatrogenic
   C. Neoplasms
   D. Vasculitis

   ANSWER: B. Most pulmonary arterial pseudoaneurysms are iatrogenic or traumatic in etiology. The other causes are less common.

5. Which of the following is the typical clinical presentation of PAVM?
   A. Cerebral abscess
   B. Stroke
   C. Pulmonary abscess
   D. Hemoptysis

   ANSWER: D. They can present with cerebral abscess and stroke because of right-to-left shunting, which bypasses the filter function of the lung. They almost never present with pulmonary abscess.

6. Which of the following is the definition of PAH?
   A. Increase right heart pressure
   B. There are no accepted criteria—the condition is diagnosed by clinical symptoms
   C. Mean pulmonary artery of more than 25 mm Hg during rest or more than 30 mm Hg during exercise
   D. Systolic pressure of more than 70 mm Hg or diastolic pressure of more than 20 mm Hg

   ANSWER: C. Choice D qualifies as severe PAH.

7. Which of the following is the conventional treatment for PAVM?
   A. Coils
   B. Particles
   C. Glue
   D. Amplatzer vascular plug

   ANSWER: A. Embolization cannot be performed using particles because of the risk of paradoxical embolization. The Amplatzer vascular plug is an emerging treatment for PAVM. Glue is not used in the treatment of PAVM.

8. Which of the following is the definition of pulmonary varix?
   A. Focal dilatations of the pulmonary veins
   B. Focal dilatation of pulmonary arteries
   C. Abnormal communication between pulmonary artery and vein without an intervening capillary bed
   D. Abnormal communication between pulmonary artery and bronchial artery

   ANSWER: A. Focal dilatation of pulmonary arteries are pulmonary arterial aneurysms. Abnormal communication between pulmonary artery and vein without intervening capillaries are PAVM.

9. Which of the following is a specific imaging characteristic of Takayasu arteritis?
   A. Pulmonary arterial stenosis or occlusion
   B. Wall enhancement on postcontrast CT and MRI
   C. Aneurysmal dilatation of the pulmonary arteries
   D. Multiple AVM

   ANSWER: B. Takayasu arteritis typically occurs in middle-age women. There is no correlation between pulmonary arterial disease and systemic disease.

10. Which of the following are etiologies for hemoptysis that may require bronchial artery embolization?
    A. Cystic fibrosis
    B. Bronchiectasis
    C. Neoplasms
    D. Infections
    E. All of the above

    ANSWER: E. All of the above are causes of massive hemoptysis requiring bronchial artery embolization. Cystic fibrosis is the most common cause.

88 SPINE INTERVENTION

Shyamsunder B. Sabat and Edgar S. Underwood

PERCUTANEOUS VERTEBROPLASTY

Percutaneous vertebroplasty (PV) is a minimally invasive procedure in which medical grade bone cement is injected into a severely osteolytic or already collapsed vertebra under image guidance (usually under fluoroscopy or CT) to strengthen the bone and/or for pain relief.

Vertebroplasty has been performed for several decades as an open procedure to augment purchase for pedicle screws and to fill voids from tumor resection. PV was first performed in 1984 in France on a 54-year-old woman who had severe pain from an aggressive C2 hemangioma and her pain was permanently cured. PV was introduced to the United State in 1993.

According to the Osteoporosis Foundation, 10 million people have osteoporosis (Table 88-1), including 45% of white women older than 50 years. An estimated 700 000 osteoporosis-related vertebral compression fractures occur annually (which is higher than the incidence of hip fractures), resulting in 150 000 hospitalizations. Twenty-five percent of women aged 75 years and 50% of women aged 80 years have at least one fractured vertebra. With each osteoporotic vertebral compression fracture, there is a 9% loss in forced vital capacity and 23% increase in mortality.

Size of vertebral bodies varies in direct proportion to overall patient size. Volume of a cervical vertebral body in an average individual is about 7 mL for C5 and 23 mL for L3. Only half of this is fillable volume and with collapse, the volume decreases proportionately. Cement is injected into the intertrabecular spaces of the vertebral body avoiding the large para- and intervertebral veins, and even small volumes of cement can provide relief of symptoms.

Bone mass peaks at 30 years and remains without significant loss till advanced age or menopause. Axial load in the thoracic spine leads to fracture because of natural kyphotic curve in that region. In the cervical and lumbar spine, axial load leads to burst-type fracture. A vertebral compression fracture is defined as 20% or 4 mm reduction of individual vertebral body height. Vertebral compression fracture is generally anterior wedge compression since 75% of body weight is borne by anterior two-thirds of the spine. Posterior cortex is typically maintained in osteoporotic fractures. Single vertebral fracture is more common at any one presentation than multiple fractures. Most fractures are around T12-L1, T7, and T8 being next common location.

TABLE 88-1 Predisposing Factors for Osteoporosis

Advanced age
Menopause
Chronic steroid therapy
Prolonged immobilization
Disuse from muscular atrophy
Drugs (phenytoin)
Malabsorption
Malnutrition
Osteogenesis imperfecta

TABLE 88-2 Fractures Likely to be Unresponsive with Standard Therapy

Burst fracture
Osteonecrosis
Fractures at dorsolumbar junction
Progressive collapse
Compression fractures more than 30 degrees
Advanced age
Malnutrition
Malignant fracture

Rest, analgesics, and bracing are the mainstay of treatment for osteoporotic fractures. For persistently painful fracture, PV can be used. Certain types of fractures are more likely to be refractory to conventional treatment (Table 88-2). Indications for surgical treatment include cord compression with neurologic deficit, progressive deformity like kyphosis/scoliosis leading to pulmonary compromise, and progressive spinal deformity with imbalance. Relative indications for surgery include pain even after percutaneous therapy or cosmesis. Now even progressive deformity can be treated with vertebroplasty or kyphoplasty, with goals of treatment being pain relief and vertebral body stabilization.

Most vertebral compression fractures occur spontaneously (46%) or after only minimal trauma (36%). Because of lack of a clear history of trauma, correct diagnosis is made in only 43% of first visits to a physician. History and physical examination should be performed to correlate the location of pain and tenderness with the level of the compression fracture and to exclude the presence of focal neurologic deficit or myelopathy. Imaging is an essential part of the workup (Table 88-3). Conventional radiographs are often the first study and may show diffuse osteopenia and often multiple collapsed vertebrae of different ages. MRI is the single best evaluation option; it helps differentiate fractures of varying ages. Acute and subacute fractures less than 30-days-old show characteristic bone marrow edema pattern: hypointense on T1-weighted images and hyperintense on T2-weighted images and STIR sequences. There is a band of T2 hyperintensity adjacent to the fracture endplate in approximately 50%. Additional subacute blood products may be seen in and around the endplate. Healed fractures may show normal marrow signal or can be hypointense on T1-weighted images and T2-weighted images because of sclerosis. If MRI is contraindicated, bone scintigraphy can also be used to differentiate acute from chronic fracture. MRI and bone scintigraphy also have prognostic value and patients with typical MRI findings of acute fracture or positive bone scan have excellent pain relief. CT can demonstrate extension of the fracture line to the endplates or posterior vertebral body, as this increases chances of cement leak and subsequent complications. Otherwise, CT may not be routinely done before percutaneous intervention.

TABLE 88-3 Goals of Imaging

Confirmation of diagnosis
Determination of age of fracture
Extent of collapse
Presence of spinal canal or foraminal stenosis
Intactness of posterior cortex
Extent of involvement of the pedicles
Normal variants of pedicles (short, narrow, absent)
Associated pathologies

Imaging may also help in differentiating osteoporotic from malignant collapse. In difficult cases tissue can be obtained for diagnosis through the cannula during the procedure. Other preprocedure routine laboratory studies include CBC, PT/INR/PTT. If there is plan to do a venogram prior to the procedure, BUN and serum creatinine levels are needed, although some do not consider it necessary given the small volume (3–5 cm^3) of contrast. Preanesthetic workup is essential if general anesthesia is to be used, but this is rarely needed.

There are several indications for PV (Table 88-4), including painful osteoporotic vertebral compression fractures refractory to conventional medical therapy. This indication is also applicable for young patients with osteoporosis because of predisposing metabolic abnormalities such as prolonged steroid use, secondary to inflammatory bowel disease, rheumatoid arthritis, systemic lupus erythematosus, asthma, and prior transplantation. Failure of medical therapy is defined as minimal or no pain relief with administration of physician prescribed analgesics or achievement of adequate pain relief only with narcotic dosage that induces excessive and intolerable sedation, confusion, or constipation. At least 2 weeks of conservative treatment is tried before consideration as medical failure. Best results are obtained

TABLE 88-4 Clinical Indications for Percutaneous Vertebroplasty

Painful compression fracture unresponsive to conservative medical management, including long-term steroid use
Malignant compression fracture (metastases; multiple myeloma)
Benign compression fracture (hemangioma)
Painful compression fracture with osteonecrosis (Kummell disease)
Unstable compression fracture (movement)
Multiple compression fractures with risk of pulmonary or GI compromise or spinal deformity increasing risk for fall
Preoperative before surgical stabilization
Chronic fracture(s) with nonunion or internal cystic changes
Traumatic burst fracture with refractory pain (not widely accepted; role for future use of resorbable cements)

TABLE 88-5 Characteristics of Aggressive Hemangioma

Involvement of entire vertebral body
Thoracic location
Irregular honeycomb trabeculation
Expanded cortex with indistinct margins
Soft-tissue component
Low fat content
Extension to neural arch
Bony collapse

when vertebroplasty is not delayed beyond 6 months. After this period the efficacy of the procedure in relieving pain decreases. However, there have been reports of intervention after several years of vertebral fracture with good clinical outcome, especially if MRI or bone scan is positive.

Fracture or severe osteolysis from painful metastasis or multiple myeloma with or without adjuvant radiation or surgical therapy is another indication for intervention. Although, there is a theoretical possibility of the injected cement dislodging tumor cells into the vertebral venous system promoting metastasis, there are no reports of this. Because of this theoretical risk, vertebroplasty should be performed after radiation therapy. There are no studies on efficacy of vertebroplasty before or after radiation therapy. Maximal doses of therapeutic radiation do not have an impact on the mechanical or chemical properties of bone cement.

Fracture or severe osteolysis caused by painful benign tumors like vertebral body hemangiomas unresponsive to conservative treatment is a third indication for PV. With aggressive lesions with destruction of the posterior cortex, there is increased risk of cement leak. Eosinophilic granuloma, fibrous dysplasia, and vertebral hemangioma weaken the vertebral body and hence may benefit from PV, hemangioma being the most common benign indication (Tables 88-5 and 88-6). Osteoid osteoma and aneurysmal bone cyst do not need structural reinforcement and hence are not indications for PV.

TABLE 88-6 Indications for Percutaneous Vertebroplasty for Hemangioma

CLINICAL AND RADIOGRAPHIC FINDINGS	VERTEBROPLASTY
Asymptomatic without radiologic signs of aggressiveness	Not indicated
Severe back pain without radiologic signs of aggressiveness	Indicated
Asymptomatic with radiologic signs of aggressiveness	Periodic follow-up; indicated if follow-up not possible
Symptomatic with radiologic signs of aggressiveness (epidural extension or severe pain)	Indicated

TABLE 88-7 Patient Criteria for Vertebroplasty (Must Meet All)

Focused pain in region of fracture
Tenderness on palpation
Absence of radicular pain or cord compression
Acute or subacute fractures less than 1-y-old; older fractures up to 2 y can also be treated in select cases with positive MRI or bone scan indicating incomplete healing
Fracture unresponsive to medical therapy (analgesics, bed rest, immobilization)
Fracture with activity on bone scan or edema on MRI
Pain from fracture negatively impacting mobility and other day-to-day activities

Specific clinical criteria must be met if percutaneous intervention is to be performed (Table 88-7).

There are several absolute contraindications to PV (Table 88-8). Radicular pain or radiculopathy caused by a compressive syndrome unrelated to vertebral body collapse is a relative contraindication. This type of pain is generally not caused by an uncomplicated compression fracture and warrants a thorough search for the cause of pain before attempting vertebroplasty. Retropulsed fragment with greater than 30% spinal canal compromise is also a relative contraindication. Cement injection in such cases can further push the fragments backward and aggravate the cord or root compression; however, this has been done carefully with good results. Tumor extension into epidural space with significant spinal canal compromise is not very amenable to treatment unless accompanied by planned surgical decompression of the spinal canal. Another relative contraindication includes severe vertebral body collapse greater than 80% to 90% (vertebra plana), although a small series of patients with 65% to 70% vertebral body collapse in the lower thoracic/upper lumbar level were treated using the bilateral transpedicular approach with partial or complete pain relief in almost all patients. However, incidence of cement leak was substantial, luckily without any consequence. Stable fractures that do not

TABLE 88-8 Contraindications

Absolute contraindications
Asymptomatic stable fracture
Healed fracture
Patient clearly improving on medical therapy
Prophylaxis in osteopenic patients with no evidence of acute fracture. Currently there is no role for prophylactic vertebroplasty for osteoporotic vertebrae at high risk for collapse
Osteomyelitis of target vertebra
Presence of discitis, epidural abscess, or sepsis
Untreated coagulopathy/hemorrhagic diasthesis
Acute traumatic fracture of healthy vertebra
Allergy to any required component

cause pain, fractures greater than 1 year old, and osteoblastic metastasis are also relative contraindications.

The mechanism by which PV relieves pain is not well understood and is at present mostly hypothetical. It is thought that mechanical stabilization of the vertebral body reduces micromotions between the fractured fragments and reduces nerve fiber irritation. Additionally, mechanical injury to tumor tissue, chemical cytotoxic effects of methylmethacrylate (MMA) monomer, and thermal damage to the pain nerve fibers may also contribute to pain relief. The volume of cement needed for PV is much less than the vertebral body volume; as little as 2 to 3 mL of cement in the thoracic and 3 to 5 mL in the lumbar region can provide moderate-to-complete pain relief in most individuals. Stiffness and strength are two important mechanical parameters. The former is associated with pain relief and the latter reduces tendency to refracture. Injection of the appropriate volume of cement is more important than unipedicular versus bipedicular injections. Vertebroplasty generally does not result in significant height restoration, only about 1 or 2 mm, the upper limit being obtained by hyperextending the spinal segment during the procedure. For height restoration, inflatable balloons (kyphoplasty) are used.

EQUIPMENT

PV can be performed under fluoroscopic or CT guidance, the former is the most common. CT is useful especially for severely osteoporotic patients with limited visualization of the bony landmarks, in cases where pedicles are destroyed beyond recognition, in patients with short pedicles (many have advocated biplane fluoroscopy in all above circumstances). In treatment of cervical, high thoracic vertebrae and sacrum, CT is preferred over fluoroscopy. While CT gives good contrast resolution, drawbacks of CT include lack of real-time needle guidance. Single fixed plane fluoroscopy is inadequate; single plane or biplane C-arm fluoroscopy is required.

Needles used for PV are the same ones as those for bone biopsy. They have 11-G trocar and cannula system. Thinner 13-G needles can be used if pedicles are thin. Needles are usually 10 cm long, but if patient is large, a 15-cm needle is recommended. If concomitant bone biopsy is contemplated, a 17-G needle is used. They all have fixed handles that can be introduced by direct hand pressure or by tapping with a mallet.

Ideally, cement should have following properties: easy handling, injectability, high radiopacity, adapted viscosity, nontoxic, nonclotting, and have a relatively long setting time (approximately 15 minutes). Polymethylmetacrylate (PMMA) cements are the most widely used. Many FDA-approved cements are available for PV and kyphoplasty. Barium sulphate is the most common radiopaque agent and added 20% to 30% by weight. Zirconium dioxide, strontium carbonate, and other metals (titanium, tantalum, and tungsten) can also be used as radio-opacifiers.

All patients are routinely given IV antibiotics 30 minutes before the procedure. Adding antibiotics to the cement mixture is disputed. Although it is routinely used in orthopedic cements, infection in PV is far less common, and routine use is justified only in immunocompromised patients. Tobramycin or vancomycin are typically added to the cement mixture in such cases but may adversely affect cement-handling properties.

PV and kyphoplasty are usually performed as outpatient procedures. Conscious sedation administered by a trained nurse is usually sufficient for the procedure. Local anesthesia is also used using lidocaine mixed with 1% sodium bicarbonate liberally and skin, subcutaneous tissue, muscles, as well as the periosteum are infiltrated. General anesthesia is limited to patients who cannot lie flat or prone and agitated patients who cannot lie still. Patients who cannot lie prone can sometimes be managed by lateral positioning with as much prone tilt as possible.

There are several approaches for vertebroplasty (Table 88-9), but transpedicular route is the most common. Most occur from T6 to L5 and pedicles in these regions provide an adequate route. Osteoporotic fractures generally do not involve the cervical spine and most cervical vertebroplasties are done for tumor.

There are several fundamental principles of cement deposition:

- Complete coverage of a vertebral body by cement is not necessary for a good clinical outcome.

TABLE 88-9 Approaches for Percutaneous Vertebroplasty

Cervical	Anterolateral	Lateral approach is not used to avoid injury to the vertebral artery. C2 approach should be behind the angle of mandible. Transoral route is avoided for fear of bacterial contamination
Thoracic	Transpedicular (first choice) or parapedicular (costovertebral)	Transpedicular route can be used from T6 inferiorly. In upper thoracic level, anterolateral or parapedicular approach is used similar to cervical. The costovertebral route can be used if pedicles are absent, not visualized because of severe osteoporosis, or destroyed by tumor
Lumbar	Transpedicular*	
Sacral	Posterior oblique†	

*Transpedicular is the safest approach here.
†Posterior oblique approach is necessitated by sacral anatomy.

- There should be cement in both halves of the vertebral body. In practice however, any cement across the midline is usually sufficient.
- Once cement is distributed across the midline, there is no improvement in clinical outcome in using a bipedicular approach.
- Avoid cement accumulation at the posterior margin of the vertebral body.
- A small amount of cement extravasation into the disc space is frequently unavoidable and is usually asymptomatic.
- Cement extravasation into the disc space theoretically increases the chances of fracture of the adjacent vertebra and hence disc space extravasation should be minimized.
- Cement extravasation into the adjacent perivertebral venous plexus is often inevitable but injection must stop at this point at least temporarily so that a cement embolus is not produced.

Patients are usually monitored for up to 2 hours postprocedure. After this the patient can bear weight with assistance and can be discharged home. Oral analgesics should be satisfactory for pain in the postprocedure pain. If there is severe pain, radiating pain, numbness, bowel bladder dysfunction CT scan should be advised to exclude cement leak and cord or root compression. If there is severe dyspnea, CT angiography or ventilation–perfusion scan of the lungs is recommended to evaluate for pulmonary embolism.

When performed by experienced operators, complication rate is usually low and is around 1% to 3% for osteoporotic fractures, while complication rate for malignant fractures is higher at approximately 7% to 10%. Most significant complications occur from cement leakage, although most leakage is asymptomatic. Other complications most commonly include transient back pain, soreness, and fever. These usually responds well to nonsteroidal anti-inflammatory agents and resolve within 24 hours. Infection is extremely rare, but vertebral osteomyelitis following vertebroplasty or kyphoplasty has high mortality in elderly patients and requires surgical corporectomy and weeks of intravenous antibiotics. Cement or marrow fat emboli can form during PV but are generally asymptomatic because emboli are small. In patients with poor pulmonary reserve, this can result in respiratory compromise. Stroke can occur in patients with right-to-left shunts. Visualization of perivertebral venous plexus is very common during PV and is not a matter of deep concern but rather caution. Injection should be suspended momentarily for cement to solidify. Cord nerve compression is more common following treatment of pathologic fractures resulting from metastasis. Radicular pain caused by cement compression usually responds to analgesics with local steroid and anesthetic injections. Motor deficits like bowel or bladder dysfunction, which are caused by large volume leaks should prompt immediate CT scan and surgical consult. Pneumothorax is a complication that can occur with procedures at the thoracic level. Death occurs in 1:50 000 cases of vertebroplasty or kyphoplasty. It is either caused by severe allergic reaction to bone cement or pulmonary embolism by fat or cement. The risk increases with the number of vertebrae treated at each session. It is prudent not to treat more than three vertebrae in a single session. There have been no reports of true cement failure but two cases of fracture progression, which were because of inadequate cement filling. Cement increases the stiffness of the vertebral body. Earlier reports indicated increased risk of fractures around the treated vertebral body. But later, investigators have refuted this claim. It appears that the same osteoporotic mechanism, which caused collapse of the previous vertebrae, causes collapse of the adjacent vertebra also. However, some controversy still remains.

Pain relief is often immediate but may take 72 hours. In most studies approximately 80% to 90% patients with age-related or steroid-induced osteoporosis experience excellent pain relief. Pain relief is less dramatic with malignant fractures, although at least one-half of patients experience some degree of relief. For optimum outcome, further bone loss should be minimized. Also, modifications in lifestyle are advocated to prevent excess mechanical stress on the spine and further fractures.

KYPHOPLASTY

Vertebroplasty only addresses pain and stability of the vertebral body but does not affect the spinal deformity associated with vertebral compression fracture. Also, cement leak remains a problem. It was thought that if a cavity could be created within the vertebral body and cement was injected into it, cement leak could be reduced. Kyphoplasty (balloon-assisted vertebroplasty) was conceived to address these problems.

Kyphoplasty is a recent modification of vertebroplasty in which usually two balloons are inflated within the vertebral body and a space is created into which cement injection is performed. Indications include the following:

- Spinal canal stenosis because of vertebral body collapse in which height restoration may potentially relieve the symptoms of stenosis.
- Traumatic fracture in which repositioning of the endplate is attempted.
- Difficult vertebroplasties for tumorous indications in which creation of an intravertebral cavity may help in cement injection.

TABLE 88-10 Kyphoplasty Versus Vertebroplasty

Greater restoration of height of the vertebral body
Injection of a more viscous cement
Decreased incidence of extravasation
Lower risk of recurrent fracture

Contraindications for kyphoplasty are usually the same as for vertebroplasty and include extreme vertebral collapse (vertebra plana) in which the superior endplate is below the level of pedicles making it technically difficult/unsuitable for kyphoplasty and carrying the risk of segmental artery injury.

A transpedicular route is used from T10 to L5 level. In the thoracic vertebral bodies from T9 and above the pedicles are narrow and laterally directed, hence an extrapedicular approach is used. Using the posterolateral technique, only one balloon can be placed within the vertebral body but less height is finally achieved than with the double balloon technique. Kyphoplasty is rarely done in the cervical vertebrae, but there are reports of kyphoplasty in the lower cervical vertebrae using an anterolateral approach.

Kyphoplasty can be performed in both acute, 1- to 2-week-old, and chronic fractures. According to some authors, the percentage of height restoration is nearly 100% when fractures are treated within the first 2 weeks. After this the fracture reduction is less predictable. There is considerable controversy as to the definite benefits of kyphoplasty over vertebroplasty (Table 88-10).

Kyphoplasty is more costly and complex than vertebroplasty. Additionally, kyphoplasty is often performed in the operating room with general anesthesia. The patients are commonly kept overnight in the hospital. Thus, total cost of kyphoplasty is approximately 10 to 20 times more than vertebroplasty. Additionally, there is no objective evidence that it is safer or more effective for pain relief.

LORDOPLASTY

A limitation of kyphoplasty is the loss of correction when the balloons are deflated before injection of cement. Lordoplasty is another technique to restore vertebral height by indirect fracture reduction as with an internal fixateur. The fractured and the adjacent vertebrae are cannulated bipediculary and the adjacent vertebrae are augmented with cement. After injecting cement, the fractured vertebra is reduced by applying a lordotic moment via the cannulas. The pretension is maintained by connecting the cannulae with a bar or fixation clamps, and the fractured vertebra is reinforced with cement in a manner similar to vertebroplasty. Only after the cement has set, are the connections between the cannulas released. Thus, in lordoplasty in addition to the fractured vertebra, the adjacent vertebrae are also augmented with cement. Lordoplasty can be performed along with kyphoplasty.

SACROPLASTY

Sacral insufficiency fractures can be caused by osteoporosis or by tumor. Patients often complain of low back or buttock pain. Because of the nonspecific nature of symptoms, they are often misdiagnosed or have delayed diagnosis. Conventional imaging is often nondiagnostic, but CT and MRI are excellent. Traditional treatment has been rest and narcotic analgesics. Sacroplasty, analogous to vertebroplasty, was developed to address this use of only fluoroscopy is not optimal as it is often difficult to visualize the sacrum and the fracture precisely resulting in improper needle placement. Likewise, using conventional CT is risky as there is no real-time guidance during actual cement injection, raising the risk of cement extravasation into sacral foramina and nerves and vessels therein. The procedure is best done under CT-fluoroscopy, or if CT is used for used for needle placement, fluoroscopy should be used for cement injection.

SUGGESTED READING

Berlemann U, Franz T, Orler R, et al. Kyphoplasty for treatment of osteoporotic vertebral fractures: a prospective non-randomized study. *Eur Spine J*. 2004;13(6):496-501.

Butler CL, Given CA II, Michel SJ, et al. Percutaneous sacroplasty for the treatment of sacral insufficiency fractures. *AJR Am J Roentgenol*. 2005;184:1956-1959.

Deramond H, Depriester C, Galibert P, Le Gars D. Percutaneous vertebroplasty with polymethylmethacrylate. Technique, indications, and results. *Radiol Clin North Am*. 1998;36:533-546.

Gangi A, Kastler BA, Dietemann JL. Percutaneous vertebroplasty guided by a combination of CT and fluoroscopy. *AJNR Am J Neuroradiol*. 1994;15(1):83-86.

Jensen ME, Dion JE. Percutaneous vertebroplasty in the treatment of osteoporotic compression fractures. *Neuroimaging Clin N Am*. 2000;10(3):547-568.

Jensen ME, Evans AJ, Mathis JM, Kallmes DF, Cloft HJ, Dion JE. Percutaneous polymethylmethacrylate vertebroplasty in the treatment of osteoporotic vertebral body compression fractures: technical aspects. *AJNR Am J Neuroradiol*. 1997;18:1897-1904.

Mathis JM, Barr JD, Belkoff SM. Percutaneous vertebroplasty: a developing standard of care for vertebral compression fractures. *AJNR Am J Neuroradiol*. 2001;22:373-381.

Melton LJ III. Epidemiology of spinal osteoporosis. *Spine*. 1997; 22:2S-11S.

Wong W, Reiley MA, Garfin S. Vertebroplasty/kyphoplasty. *J Womens Imaging*. 2000;2(3):117-124.

QUESTIONS AND ANSWERS

1. What is the most common indication for percutaneous vertebroplasty?
   A. Osteoporosis
   B. Metastasis
   C. Vertebral body hemangioma
   D. Multiple myeloma

   ANSWER: A. Osteoporosis is by far the most common and most important indication for percutaneous vertebroplasty. It is an important treatment option for pain from osteoporotic fractures resistant to conservative treatment like bracing, rest, and moderate doses of narcotic analgesia. It is not done prophylactically to prevent osteoporotic collapse.

2. Bone cement may contains all *except*:
   A. PMMA
   B. Barium sulphate
   C. Zirconium dioxide
   D. Powered Iron

   ANSWER: D. PMMA is polymethylmethacrylate. It is supplied in powder form and is mixed with liquid methyl methacrylate (MMA) monomer. It has doughlike consistency and is very biocompatible. But MMA is a tissue irritant. PMMA has a setting time of 15 to 20 minutes. PMMA cements have low intrinsic radiopacity, so exogenous substances are added. The most common is barium sulphate. Others are zirconium dioxide (has minimum interference on properties of cement), strontium carbonate, tantalum, tungsten, and titanium. Iron is not used and would be incompatible with MRI.

3. What percentage of patients will experience, in the near term, pain relief after vertebroplasty for acute osteoporotic fractures?
   A. 10%–20%
   B. 50%–60%
   C. 80%–90%
   D. Erratic

   ANSWER: C. Approximately 80% to 90% patients with acute osteoporotic fractures experience pain relief after vertebroplasty. Pain relief is slightly less in patients with fractures from malignant disease and other causes (approximately 50% to 80%). Pain relief in hemangioma is higher than metastatic fractures but less than osteoporotic fractures.

4. What is the approach used for vertebroplasty of the cervical spine?
   A. Transpedicular
   B. Interspinous
   C. Lateral
   D. Anterolateral

   ANSWER: D. In the cervical and sometimes upper thoracic vertebra, the best approach is anterolateral. The transpedicular is used from T6 to L5. Lateral approach is not used in cervical spine to avoid injury to vertebral vessels. Interspinous approach is never used at any level.

5. What is the single best preprocedure evaluation for vertebroplasty of osteoporotic collapse?
   A. CT
   B. DEXA
   C. MRI
   D. Bone scan

   ANSWER: C. MRI is the single best modality of investigation, as it can differentiate between acute and chronic fractures. This is important because acute fractures respond best to vertebroplasty. Also, it aids in diagnosing other causes of back pain. A bone scan can be performed in patients in whom MRI is contraindicated. It can also differentiate acute from chronic fractures. CT should be used when there is a suspicion of posterior cortex breach or to evaluate complex fractures. Irrespective of these advanced tests, all patients should frontal and lateral radiography of the spine.

6. What is the best modality to direct sacroplasty?
   A. CT
   B. MRI
   C. Fluoroscopy
   D. CT-fluoroscopy

   ANSWER: D. Use of fluoroscopy alone is not optimal as it is often difficult to visualize the sacral fracture precisely, resulting in improper needle placement. Likewise using conventional CT is risky as there is no real-time guidance during actual cement injection. The procedure is best done under CT-fluoroscopy. MRI is not typically used.

89 PRINCIPLES OF TUMOR ABLATION

Clinton R. Smith and
Edgar S. Underwood

INTRODUCTION

Numerous advances have occurred in the oncologic application of interventional radiology techniques. Catheter-based therapies for primary and metastatic neoplasms of the liver, as well as percutaneous imaging–guided chemical and thermal ablative therapies have seen growth and show promising results.

Hepatocellular carcinoma (HCC) is the fifth most common cancer worldwide, related to the increasing number of patients with hepatitis B and C. It is an aggressive tumor, which frequently occurs in those patients who have developed cirrhosis, although it can occur in noncirrhotic livers as well. Hepatic resection and transplantation are the primary treatments in appropriately selected patients; however, a majority of patients are poor surgical candidates (because of medical comorbidities, limited hepatic reserve, or hepatic lesions too numerous or too large), and there are a limited number of organs available for transplant.

Metastasis to the liver from colorectal carcinoma and other neoplasms is also a significant clinical problem. Surgical resection is considered the treatment of choice for isolated hepatic metastasis. As with HCC, few patients meet criteria for resection.

Renal cell carcinoma (RCC) accounts for approximately 85% of renal tumors. Promising results have been demonstrated with radiofrequency ablation (RFA) and cryoablative therapies in patients who are poor candidates for nephron-sparing surgery. Percutaneous treatment of RCC is also proving beneficial in patients with hereditary syndromes such as von Hippel-Lindau, as well as nontraditional indications such as palliation and pain control, transfusion-dependent hematuria, post-biopsy bleeding, and transitional cell carcinoma.

Primary lung cancer is the most common cause of cancer death in the United States and accounts for approximately 29% of all cancer deaths. For early-stage non–small cell lung carcinoma, surgical resection is the treatment of choice. The lungs are the second most common organs for metastasis of solid organ malignancies. Minimally invasive percutaneous therapy has become an option in patients with primary or metastatic lung cancer who are not surgical candidates or have failed chemotherapy and external-beam radiation.

TRANSARTERIAL CHEMOEMBOLIZATION

HEPATOCELLULAR CARCINOMA

Only 30% to 40% of patients with HCC are candidates for curative therapy (resection, transplantation, or percutaneous ablation); therefore, most patients are only suitable for palliative or locoregional therapy. Improved survival (as compared to optimal supportive care) with chemoembolization has been shown in recent trials. This is related to the fact that approximately 80% of the blood supply to HCC and liver metastases is derived from the hepatic artery. About three-fourths of blood supply to normal liver is portal venous. Therefore, therapeutic agents infused or injected directly into the hepatic artery preferentially target tumor rather than normal hepatic parenchyma.

The most commonly used chemotherapeutic agents are doxorubicin alone, or a mixture of doxorubicin, mitomycin C, and cisplatin. This cocktail is mixed with Lipiodol, an iodized ester derived from poppy seeds that acts as a carrier. This mixture is selectively taken up and retained by HCC and some metastatic liver lesions. With addition of embolic particles or gelatin foam as well as Lipiodol, arterial inflow is reduced, leading to decreased drug washout. Concentrations of chemotherapy drugs of up to 100 times that of systemic intravenous administration can be achieved.

A variety of embolic agents have been described in combination with the Lipiodol/chemotherapeutic cocktail (Gelfoam powder or pledgets, embospheres, starch and glass microspheres, and polyvinyl alcohol particles). Despite the tumor necrosis expected after particle embolization when combined with the cytotoxic effect of the chemotherapeutic agents, many tumors do not develop extensive necrosis. This raises the question of whether the embolization stimulates upregulation of certain molecular factors, which could inhibit cell death and stimulate vascular growth.

For unresectable HCC not amenable to percutaneous ablation (usually because of large size), transarterial chemotherapy (TACE) is currently the favored treatment. It is considered palliative, but can be an adjunctive therapy to resection or a bridge to transplantation or combined with ablation for palliation. However, many patients are not suitable candidates for TACE because of poor liver function. In patients with reduced hepatic reserve, this therapy may accelerate liver failure and negate the desired antitumoral effect or survival benefit.

Absolute contraindications include tumor resectability, severe hepatic disease (Child-Pugh, class C), and intractable infection. Relative contraindications include, but are not limited to, serum bilirubin more than 2 mg/dL, LDH more than 425 U/L, AST more than 100, tumor burden more than 50% of the liver, portal vein thrombosis, uncorrectable coagulopathy or thrombocytopenia, cardiac or renal insufficiency, ascites or recent variceal bleeding, poor performance status, extrahepatic metastases, encephalopathy, and extensive arteriovenous shunting through the tumor. Patients with functional compromise of the sphincter of Oddi (prior hepaticojejunostomy, sphincterotomy, or biliary stent) are at increased risk of hepatic abscess after TACE.

The technique involves preprocedural care including hydration, broad-spectrum antibiotics, and antiemetics.

A prolonged arteriogram of the superior mesenteric artery evaluates for variant anatomy and portal vein patency. A celiac axis injection is then performed followed by selection of the desired hepatic artery branch.

The chemotherapeutic agent(s) with Lipiodol is then injected followed by an embolic agent. A chemotherapy-resistant (metallic) three-way stopcock is required. Embolization should occur beyond the gastroduodenal artery, and attention should be given to other regional arteries to avoid nontarget embolization, usually performed with distally placed microcatheters. However, if there are multiple tumors in one lobe, hepatic lobar chemoembolization can be performed. Whole liver chemoembolization should be avoided to reduce risk of severe liver injury.

Postprocedural care includes hospital admission with continued aggressive intravenous hydration, analgesia with PCA pump, antiemetics, and continued antibiotics. Patients are usually discharged within 2 days when pain is controlled and oral intake is sufficient. Some authors recommend continued outpatient antibiotics of up to 5 days.

Follow-up imaging and laboratory evaluations should be performed after at least 4 to 6 weeks and at 3-month intervals thereafter. Reduction in tumor size is the optimal result of any chemoembolization according the World Health Organization and Response Evaluation Criteria in Solid Tumors (RECIST). Assessment of size alone may not be reliable because of initial increase in size from necrosis with edema and/or hemorrhage. In addition to contrast-enhanced CT, some authors recommend a perfusion-diffusion MRI to evaluate for free water content (indicating cell death). Also, MRI can overcome the limited ability to discern true enhancement versus retention of Lipiodol within the tumor on CT.

Complications from TACE include postembolization syndrome (pain, nausea, fatigue, fever, and/or leukocytosis), liver abscess, tumor rupture, irreversible liver failure, hepatorenal syndrome, septicemia and nontarget embolization including gallbladder infarction.

One recent meta-analysis found that no chemotherapeutic agent or combination of agents was significantly superior. Also, there is no evidence of benefit with Lipiodol. Gelatin foam is the most commonly used embolic agent, but polyvinyl alcohol may be better; bland transarterial embolization appears as good as transarterial chemoembolization for metastases but chemoembolization is better than bland for HCC.

Other variations of TACE include drug-eluting microspheres and radiation-emitting microspheres. The drug-eluting microspheres can be loaded with doxorubicin, and the sustained release over a longer period is potentially an advantage over standard TACE. ^{90}Yttrium-labeled microspheres are also available for treatment of HCC and liver metastases. For this treatment, the gastroduodenal artery and sometimes other regional arteries are embolized to prevent reflux, which could cause severe radiation-induced gastrointestinal ulceration. Also, hepatopulmonary shunting must be excluded prior to administrating the ^{90}Y-bearing spheres. This is done by an initial angiogram and ^{99m}Tc-labeled MAA injection followed by nuclear medicine lung scan to calculate a hepatopulmonary shunt fraction.

HEPATIC METASTASES

In similar fashion, liver metastases from colorectal carcinoma and neuroendocrine tumors can be embolized with or without chemotherapeutic agents. There is much less experience with TACE for colorectal carcinoma metastases than for HCC. Most trials for colorectal metastasis involve a surgically placed hepatic artery infusion pump, that is, infusional hepatic intraarterial chemotherapy. For neuroendocrine tumors, the benefit of TACE over bland transarterial embolization is not certain. One recent study suggests that adding chemotherapeutic agents to transarterial embolization is not beneficial in patients with carcinoid tumor, but does improve outcome in patients with islet cell tumors.

PERCUTANEOUS ETHANOL/ACETIC ACID INJECTION

ETHANOL

Percutaneous ethanol injection (PEI) is probably still the most widely used method for HCC tumor ablation worldwide. PEI is a highly effective, inexpensive, and easy-to-perform method for treatment of small HCC. PEI can easily be performed in areas of the world where HCC is endemic and health care resources are limited. Its mechanism involves small vessel thrombosis, denaturation of cellular proteins, and cytoplasmic dehydration. The resulting coagulative necrosis is not distinguishable from thermal ablation.

Chemical ablation works better for HCC than for liver metastatic disease. The ethanol injection into the tumor has a more uniform distribution for HCC ("soft" tumor in a "hard" cirrhotic liver). For metastatic disease, the ethanol distribution is less favorable (hard tumor in a soft normal liver). However, local recurrence is more common in tumors larger than 5 cm in diameter. As a result, PEI is not recommended for large lesions. Ideally, PEI is used for tumors smaller than or equal to 3 cm in diameter and adjacent to thermally sensitive areas such as central bile ducts and bowel. Other selection criteria include unresectability, no extrahepatic disease, and poor surgical candidates. Patients with advanced liver disease (Child-Pugh class C) are poor candidates for PEI, as no survival benefit has been demonstrated. Other contraindications include portal vein thrombosis, tumor burden more than 30% of total liver volume, coagulopathy, and platelet count less than 40 000/mm^3.

Real-time ultrasound (US) or CT guidance can be used to perform PEI. This can be done as an outpatient for smaller lesions, but multiple separate injection sessions may be necessary. Alternatively, a "one-shot" method with general anesthesia and hospital admission can be performed. Under US visualization, slow injection is done with a multiside hole needle. The area of ethanol injection becomes echogenic, and the injection should be stopped if bile ducts, hepatic vessels, or gallbladder fills. Historically, a tumor volume calculation was performed to estimate the amount of ethanol needed for ablation. In general, 1 to 8 mL of 95% ethanol is injected for a staged approach for four to twelve sessions. The one-shot technique involves injecting 60 to 150 mL in multiple injections over 30 minutes.

Complications are infrequent and usually well-tolerated using the staged approach, including ethanol intoxication, local pain, and transient fever. Rarely, severe hemorrhage has been reported, as has seeding of the needle tract. For the one-shot method, complications can be more frequent and severe, including portal venous thrombosis, hemoperitoneum, variceal bleeding, liver failure, and transient renal insufficiency.

PEI has shown similar survival rates as surgical resection in small lesions. Tumor size more than 3 cm has been shown to be most predictive of local recurrence. Histologic grade, Child-Pugh score, and size/number of lesions are the most important factors related to survival after PEI for HCC. RFA has been compared with PEI, with the results of one study showing fewer treatment sessions to achieve the same degree of tumor necrosis, and a slightly higher complication rate with RFA.

ACETIC ACID

Percutaneous acetic acid injection (PAI) is also an effective method for ablation of small HCC. A 50% solution of acetic acid and sterile water is prepared and injected in similar fashion as PEI. The advantage of PAI is that the septa and capsule of tumors can be infiltrated to a greater degree than with PEI. A smaller volume and fewer treatment sessions are needed to achieve the same ablative effect as ethanol. Only one-third of the volume of acetic acid is needed as compared to 95% ethanol. In one randomized prospective trial, significant and substantial differences in cancer-free and overall survival rates were observed favoring PAI. Side effects and complications unique to PAI include metabolic acidosis with renal toxicity as well as transient hemoglobinuria.

RADIOFREQUENCY ABLATION

RFA creates thermal injury by depositing electromagnetic energy within the patient. A high-frequency alternating current moves from an electrode tip into surrounding tissue. Because of high resistance of the tissue, the ions attempt to follow the alternating current and create frictional heat by their movement. The tissue temperature and duration of heating are important factors related to tissue necrosis. Tissue heated to 50°C to 55°C for 4 to 6 minutes causes irreversible cellular damage. Between 60°C and 100°C, near-instantaneous tissue coagulation is produced with irreversible damage to mitochondrial and cytosolic enzymes. At 100°C to110°C, tissue carbonizes and vaporizes, which actually acts as an insulator and reduces efficacy. Therefore, the goal of RF ablation is to achieve and maintain approximately 50°C to 100°C for 4 to 6 minutes. In reality, longer applications must be used because of relatively slow thermal conduction through tissues.

To increase the volume of tissue ablated, multitined probes have been developed, which allow for destruction of the tumor and an acceptable margin (usually defined as 360 degrees, 1 cm surrounding each tumor). An important concept is that of heat efficacy (optimized heat deposition and minimized heat loss) and the bio-heat equation described by Pennes, and simplified by Goldberg and colleagues (coagulation = energy deposited × local tissue interactions − heat loss). Tissue heterogeneity and regional blood flow causing tissue cooling ("heat sink" effect) are therefore important causes of incomplete coagulation.

RFA can be performed with percutaneous CT, MR, or US guidance, and can be done under conscious sedation, but general anesthesia is sometimes required. Open or laparoscopic RFA with US guidance is also used for liver lesions. In tumors larger than 2 to 3 cm, multiple overlapping spheres or cylinders of ablation are needed to treat the tumor with an acceptable margin. In addition to larger and multitined probes, other methods have been developed to increase the ablation volume and decrease number of overlapping sections. These include internally cooled electrodes, cluster electrodes, more powerful electric generators, perfusion or injection of liquid agents (saline, ethanol or acetic acid), and reduction of blood flow with preablation transcatheter embolization.

LIVER

Selection of patients for RFA includes nonresectable HCC with a single tumor smaller than 5 cm or up to three lesions, each smaller than 3 cm. Additionally, there can be no evidence of extrahepatic disease, vascular invasion, severely impaired liver function (Child-Pugh class C), or a performance status test of 0. For nonresectable colorectal carcinoma liver metastasis, lesions must be confined to the liver or have limited pulmonary metastatic involvement. Most centers prefer to treat patients with four or fewer hepatic lesions, but excess of this number is not an absolute contraindication. The tumor size is the most important factor in predicting outcome, and for metastatic lesions, the tumor should not exceed 3 to 4 cm in greatest diameter.

Most authors agree that the heat sink phenomenon is most significant adjacent to vessels 3 mm and more in diameter. In the liver, this offers some protection for lesions adjacent to large hepatic vessels; however, subcapsular lesions adjacent to gastrointestinal structures should be avoided for percutaneous treatment. The colon appears to be at greater risk than the stomach or small bowel. Laparoscopic approach or use of hydrodissection (percutaneous injection of 5% dextrose in water to displace adjacent structures) should be used. Central bile ducts and gallbladder are also at risk for lesions ablated near the liver hilum. Needle tract seeding is also a concern, particularly for subcapsular lesions, but some devices offer a "track ablation" mode for coagulation at the time of withdrawal of the probe.

RFA is relatively well-tolerated, but severe and fatal complications have been reported. These include liver failure, portal vein thrombosis, GI perforation, liver abscess, pneumothorax, pleural effusion, skin burns, subcapsular hematoma or hemoperitoneum, acute renal insufficiency, and needle tract seeding. Also, a postablative syndrome of pain, fever, and malaise has been reported and is self-limited and reportedly less common than with TACE.

For treatment of HCC, RFA has essentially supplanted PEI because of several recent studies showing superior long-term survival and recurrence rates. As previously mentioned, some studies showed a higher complication rate with RFA, but this did not result in increased mortality. Although resection remains the gold standard in patients meeting criteria for resection, two recent reports showed comparable overall and disease-free survival rates for RF compared to resection in solitary HCC less than 5 cm in diameter. Although recurrence rates after RFA are higher than resection, this does not appear to change long-term survival.

For patients with resectable metastatic liver disease from colorectal carcinoma, surgical resection remains the gold standard. However, RFA has become the most widely accepted ablative technique for treatment of nonresectable colorectal carcinoma metastases. There is indirect evidence that RFA is preferred over chemotherapy regimens and improves survival in selected patients with limited liver metastatic disease. Local recurrence and intrahepatic progression appear to affect long-term survival with unresectable CRC metastasis, unlike with HCC. Recurrence rates appear to increase dramatically with increase in tumor size between 2.5 and 3.0 cm.

Combined therapies: Several studies have been conducted regarding a combination of the previously described therapies (TACE, PEI and/or RFA), the most common combination of which includes TACE and RFA. The most recent of these studies has data to suggest that in selected patients, a combination of TACE/RFA was significantly better than either alone. Benefit was seen in patients with unifocal and multifocal disease. Median survival and tumor response were superior in the combined therapy group, and benefit was not offset by adverse effects on liver function.

KIDNEY

The greatest success in RFA of renal lesions has been reported in tumors less than 3 to 4 cm in greatest dimension. Patients who are not candidates or choose not to have nephron-sparing surgery typically belong to one of two categories. One group has sporadic RCC (solitary tumor of 3 to 4 cm and otherwise normal renal function) and can be treated more aggressively with a wider tumor margin in hopes of preventing recurrence. The other group has hereditary syndrome (such as VHL) predisposing to multiple recurrent RCC. These patients are at long-term risk of renal impairment, and as such, a less aggressive approach is recommended to extend good renal function for as long as possible.

There are several unique technical aspects of performing RFA of renal lesions as compared to liver RFA. Placing the patient in lateral decubitus or semiprone positioning helps shift bowel loops out of the way, and the use of hydrodissection can be quite useful. Adjacent bowel, ureters, adrenal gland, and several nerves and muscles are at increased risk for thermal injury. Acute hypertensive crisis can result from injury to the adrenal gland.

Also, cortical lesions are more amenable than medullary lesions because of less heat sink effect, as well as some proposed "oven effect" of surrounding fat for exophytic lesions. There is considered to be more of a heat sink effect in the kidney as compared to the liver, given that the kidney has five times greater blood flow per gram of tissue. However, since the kidney is an end organ without the dual blood supply as in the liver, this can be advantageous by first ablating the more central portion of larger lesions. This "deep first" technique can significantly decrease peripheral blood flow.

Complications of renal RFA include infection, hemorrhage, and tumor seeding. Since a postablation abscess can mimic tumor recurrence, some authors advocate prophylactic antibiotics. As described previously for the liver, tract ablation can be performed to minimize risk of tumor seeding. Although hemorrhage is a complication of RFA, the risk of significant bleeding is less than that of partial nephrectomy. In fact, RFA has been used to treat life-threatening transfusion-dependent hematuria and hemorrhage after partial nephrectomy.

LUNG

In addition to primary lung cancer and metastatic lung disease, thermal ablation can be used for treatment and/or palliation of chest wall masses or other thoracic skeletal metastases. Currently, RFA and other thermal ablative methods are most useful for early-stage lung cancer in nonsurgical candidates, small and favorably located pulmonary metastatic disease, and for symptomatic palliative treatment of late-stage malignancies. Patient selection for lung RFA is therefore directed by the ultimate goal, whether for potential cure, prolongation of survival, or palliation of symptoms.

Most patients who are candidates for percutaneous lung biopsy are able to undergo lung RFA. There are few absolute contraindications, including bleeding disorders and recent anticoagulant use. In fact, pulmonary RFA can be done safely in patients with only one lung. Caution should be used in patients with emphysema and pulmonary fibrosis, and some authors recommend pulmonary function testing prior to the procedure with a threshold FEV_1 more than 400 mL. Many patients also have cardiac pacemakers and defibrillators which are susceptible to energy interference in the RF and microwave frequencies. Coordination with cardiac electrophysiologists or use of an alternative ablative therapy such as laser or cryoablation should be considered.

Complications include postablation syndrome (pain, fever, chills, anorexia and/or malaise), pneumothorax, sympathetic pleural effusion, hemoptysis, bronchopleural fistula, hemorrhage, skin burns (because of inappropriate grounding pad placement), injury to adjacent mediastinal organs/nerves, infection/abscess formation or acute respiratory distress syndrome. Pneumothorax is most common and typically occurs in 30% to 60% of cases, but requires aspiration or tube placement only in approximately 20% of patients. Creative methods to avoid some of these complications have been developed, including the previously discussed hydrodissection technique, as well as intentional pneumothorax creation to separate peripheral lung lesions from the parietal pleura and mediastinal structures. One unique risk of pulmonary RFA is systemic embolization with possibility of stroke that is due to microbubbles from tissue heating at "roll-off" temperatures.

To date, no randomized and controlled clinical trial exists comparing thermal ablation techniques alone, or in combination, to established therapy for lung malignancies. Preliminary data suggest that RFA may prolong survival in patients with medical comorbidities who have a resectable lesion but are not able to undergo surgery. It is clear that complete ablation is most likely in tumors ≤ 3 cm.

CRYOABLATION

Cryoablation is another effective thermal ablative modality that has been studied in liver (HCC and metastasis) and RCC primarily, but also shows promise for treatment of other cancers. Because of the large size of the initial cryoprobes, this technique was usually done via an open or laparoscopic approach. However, with development of argon gas–based units and much smaller probes (11–17 gauge), percutaneous approach with imaging guidance is gaining popularity and showing safety and efficacy comparable to surgical approaches. The mechanism of tumor ablation involves rapid expansion of argon gas at the probe tip resulting in temperatures reaching −100°C over a few seconds. This freezing initially causes extracellular ice formation with subsequent movement of intracellular water, changes in pH, protein denaturation, and mechanical disruption of cell membranes; also, local microvascular injury leads to diminished perfusion and delayed cell death.

For percutaneous approaches, imaging guidance with US, CT, and MRI are all feasible options, although the first two are most commonly used because of more availability. The technique used for ablation is similar whether for treatment of nonresectable primary or metastatic liver and lung tumors, renal neoplasms, or other lesions such as prostate cancer or skeletal metastases. Patient selection for cryoablation in the setting of HCC is similar to that of RFA (single mass less than 5 cm or up to three masses less than or equal to 3 cm in diameter); however, larger tumors might possibly be treated more effectively with cryoablation, as discussed later in the chapter. For hepatic metastases, some authors recommend treating up to five lesions with diameter of approximately 4 cm. In patients with RCC, cryoablation is considered for a single tumor less than

4 cm in diameter, but multiple lesions can be treated in a single session for hereditary syndromes such as VHL.

After appropriate patient selection and preprocedure preparation, including correction of any coagulation or platelet abnormality, percutaneous cryoablation can usually be performed with conscious sedation. If needed, a biopsy can be performed prior to the ablation, but caution should be exercised because bleeding from the biopsy can occasionally obscure the lesion for cryoprobe placement. Because of relatively small ablation volume per probe, multiple probes are often needed to cover the entire lesion with an acceptable surgical margin. A commonly used guideline is the "2 to 1 rule," in which probes are positioned within a given lesion no more than 2 cm apart and no more than 1 cm from the margin of the lesion. This allows for optimal temperatures between −20°C and −40°C to ensure tumor killing, and the synergistic effect of multiple probes leads to much colder isotherms centrally within large ice balls. The outer edge of the ice ball should extend several millimeters beyond a lesion because the outer isotherm (0°C) is not absolutely cytotoxic.

Similar to the heat sink effect seen with RFA, a "cold sink" effect occurs with cryoablation adjacent to larger vessels, and this should be considered for probe placement. Injury to collagenous structures of blood vessels is unlikely with cryoablation, and the 2 to 1 rule can be modified adjacent to vascular structures. One author recommends placing a probe within 5 mm of the lesion edge on the vessel side, with no more than 1 cm between probes. Also, thermodissection methods such as injection of air, carbon dioxide, water, or balloon placement can be used to separate adjacent critical structures. For renal cryoablation, circulation of warm saline through retrograde ureteral stents has been described to offer some protection to the ureter and central renal collecting system.

Once the cryoprobes are adequately positioned, the ablation is usually performed in a double freeze-thaw cycle of 8 to 12 minutes each. This double cycle causes more complete and confluent cell death with synergistic cytotoxic effect as compared to a single freeze cycle. Active thawing can be achieved performed if needed by instillation of helium rather than argon gas through the probes.

A comparison of percutaneous cryoablation and RFA reveals several relative advantages and disadvantages of these modalities. Compared to RFA, cryoablation is much less painful and able to be done with conscious sedation on an outpatient basis more frequently. Better visualization of the ice ball by CT allows for more precision and confidence that the lesion has been adequately covered; however, if US is used, the far side of the ice ball cannot be completely visualized because of acoustic shadowing. Another advantage described for cryoablation is that it may be safer to treat central lesions, whether hepatic or renal. Animal studies suggest less damage to the renal collecting system than the heat-based modalities. Larger areas (up to 8–10 cm) can be treated because of simultaneous placement of multiple probes, and the size and shape of the ablation zone can be modeled to some degree, because of adjustable settings for each probe.

A disadvantage of cryoablation includes the lack of cauterization effect seen with the heat-based techniques. This may put patients at a slightly higher risk of bleeding immediately post procedure, although the majority of these will stop with conservative management, and few patients have clinically significant bleeding requiring further intervention. Also, compared to RFA, the zone of ablation for each cryoprobe is smaller (approximately 2 cm diameter), thus requiring multiple probes be placed.

Two complications unique to cryoablation of liver lesions also have been described, but are fortunately uncommon. One is that of liver "cracking," which can result in rapid and massive hemorrhage. This usually occurs during the thawing phase and was previously thought to be due to the air-ice interface encountered in open procedures, but has been seen with percutaneous treatments as well. Another unique complication is "cryoshock," which is a severe systemic response similar to tumor lysis syndrome, which results in severe coagulopathy, thrombocytopenia and DIC, and multiorgan failure. This has been reported after RFA and cryoablation, but more frequently with the latter. This possibly occurs because of the lack of immediate coagulative effect seen with RFA and the absorption of necrotic debris during reperfusion of the ablated zone after cryotherapy.

Other complications of liver and renal cryoablation include postablation syndrome, tumor seeding, injury to adjacent structures (or central biliary structures in the case of liver cryoablation), abscess formation (rare unless compromise of sphincter of Oddi), arteriovenous fistulas, or pneumothorax.

Regarding treatment of small renal masses, there is question as to whether a surgical or percutaneous approach is preferable. The percutaneous route is relatively newer because of the recent advent of small probes with the argon gas–based systems. One recent meta-analysis concluded that percutaneous ablation is safer and equally effective as a surgical approach, but more than one session may be necessary for complete treatment. Also, there has been no definitive conclusion regarding whether RFA or cryoablation of small RCC is preferable. Another recent meta-analysis suggested that cryoablation results in better local tumor control, less need for treatment, and may be associated with a lower risk of progression to metastatic disease as compared with RFA. However, in this report, it was noted that the differences in metastatic progression were marginally significant and that most of the cryoablations were performed laparoscopically rather than percutaneously.

MICROWAVE ABLATION

Microwave ablation (MWA) for HCC causes tissue death by coagulation necrosis using electromagnetic energy with frequencies greater than or equal to 900 MHz. Dipole water molecules oscillate billions of times per second at the same frequency as the microwave electric field which causes friction and heat. The MWA system is composed of a microwave generator, flexible coaxial cable, and microwave antenna (probe). This can be performed with open or laparoscopic surgery, or percutaneously with US, CT, or MR imaging. Patient selection criteria and technique are similar to RFA for HCC.

There are several theoretical advantages of MWA as compared to RFA. MWA can provide larger tumor ablation volumes, faster ablation times, and more complete tumor kill. Also, the heat sink effect is less than that for RFA. MWA tissue heating is primarily active (rather than passive) as seen with RFA. This gives a larger zone of active heating and does not rely on electrical conduction (no grounding pads). Tissue desiccation and charring is not a major concern with MWA; therefore, consistently high temperatures can be achieved within a tumor. Another advantage is the ability to create complete necrosis despite presence of fibrous tissue or a septum. The majority of experience with MWA for HCC is from Asia, and comparable long-term survival rates with surgery have been reported for tumors less than or equal to 4 cm in selected patients.

LASER INTERSTITIAL THERMAL THERAPY

Optical range or near-infrared wavelength light emitted from a bare 400-μm laser fiber can be conducted into a targeted lesion causing heat and coagulative necrosis. An Nd:YAG laser is used most frequently, and this laser has also been used to treat lesions in the esophagus, colon, stomach, and bronchial tree. The laser interstitial thermal therapy system consists of multiple optical fibers placed into a tumor through cannulated needles positioned under US, CT, or MR imaging guidance. Although there have been promising results for treatment of HCC, experience is limited and no clear advantage over other ablative techniques has been documented.

SUGGESTED READING

Callstrom MR, Charboneau JW. Technologies for ablation of hepatocellular carcinoma. *Gastroenterology*. 2008;134(7):1831-1835.

Clark TW. Chemical ablation of liver cancer. *Tech Vasc Interv Radiol*. 2007;10(1):58-63.

Curley SA, Stuart KE, Schwartz JM, et al. Nonsurgical therapies for localized hepatocellular carcinoma. Up-To-Date Online Resource; updated June 13, 2008.

Dodd GD, Soulen MC, Kane RA, et al. Minimally invasive treatment of malignant hepatic tumors: at the threshold of a major breakthrough. *Radiographics*. 2000;20:9-27.

Garrean S, Hering J, Saied A, et al. Radiofrequency ablation of primary and metastatic liver tumors: a critical review of the literature. *Am J Surg*. 2008;195(4):508-520.

Goldberg SN, Gazelle GS, Mueller PR. Thermal ablation therapy for focal malignancy: A unified approach to underlying principles, techniques, and diagnostic imaging guidance. *Am J Roentgenol*. 2000;174:323-331.

Hinshaw JL, Lee FT Jr. Cryoablation for liver cancer. *Tech Vasc Interv Radiol*. 2007;10:47-57.

Hui GC, Tuncali K, Tatli S, et al. Comparison of percutaneous and surgical approaches to renal tumor ablation: meta-analysis of effectiveness and complication rates. *J Vasc Interv Radiol*. 2008;19:1311-1320.

Kalva SP, Thabet A, Wicky S. Recent advances in transarterial therapy of primary and secondary liver malignancies. *Radiographics*. 2008;28:101-117.

Kunkle DA, Uzzo RG. Cryoablation or radiofrequency ablation of the small renal mass: a meta-analysis. *Cancer*. 2008;113:2671-2680.

Lencione R, Crocetti L. Radiofrequency ablation of liver cancer. *Tech Vasc Interv Radiol*. 2007;10(1):38-46.

Liang P, Wang Y. Microwave ablation of hepatocellular carcinoma. *Oncology*. 2007;72(suppl 1):124-131.

Liapi E, Georgiades CC, Hong K, et al. Transcatheter arterial chemoembolization: current technique and future promise. *Tech Vasc Interv Radiol*. 2007;10:2-11.

Marelli L, Stigliano R, Triantos C, et al. Transarterial therapy for hepatocellular carcinoma: which technique is more effective? A systematic review of cohort and randomized studies. *Cardiovasc Intervent Radiol*. 2007;30:6-25.

Maybody M, Solomon SB. Image-guided percutaneous cryoablation of renal tumors. *Tech Vasc Interv Radiol*. 2007;10:140-148.

McTaggart RA, Dupuy DE. Thermal ablation of lung tumors. *Tech Vasc Interv Radiol*. 2007;10(2):102-113.

Pennes HH. Analysis of tissue and arterial blood temperatures in the resting human forearm. *J Appl Physiol*. 1948;1:93-122.

Rose SC, Thistlethwaite PA, Sewell PE, et al. Lung cancer and radiofrequency ablation. *J Vasc Interv Radiol*. 2006;17:927-951.

Steward MJ, Warbey VS, Malhotra A, et al. Neuroendocrine tumors: role of interventional radiology in therapy. *Radiographics*. 2008;28:1131-1145.

Stone MJ, Venkatesan AM, Locklin J, et al. Radiofrequency ablation of renal tumors. *Tech Vasc Interv Radiol*. 2007;10:132-139.

Venook AP. Nonsurgical treatment strategies for colorectal cancer liver metastases. UpToDate Online Resource; updated March 14, 2008.

QUESTIONS AND ANSWERS

1. Why is transarterial chemoembolization a safe and viable palliative therapy for liver tumors?
   A. Most tumors are supplied by the hepatic artery, and a normal liver has its main blood supply from the portal vein.
   B. Doxorubicin mixes well in Lipiodol.
   C. Tumor necrosis is induced by embolization with microspheres.
   D. Embolization may stimulate upregulation of factors which can stimulate vascular growth.

   ANSWER: A. As the normal liver receives most of its blood from the portal vein embolization of the hepatic artery will not cause liver necrosis of normal parenchyma. The other statements are true as well but not unique to hepatic artery embolization.

2. What is the best clinical indication for tumor ablation using chemical injection (alcohol or acetic acid)?
   A. Tumors >5 cm in diameter
   B. Colon cancer metastases in an otherwise normal liver
   C. Primary HCC in a cirrhotic liver
   D. Endocrine metastasis

   ANSWER: C. These tumors frequently have a "pseudocapsule," which acts to contain the chemical agent in the tumor allowing greater and more localized tumor necrosis. Tumors larger than 5 cm in diameter are not optimally treated with ablation, and local injection should not be done for neuroendocrine tumors. Also, metastases in an otherwise normal liver may allow diffusion of the chemical agent with less tumor necrosis and more damage to surrounding structures.

3. Regarding RFA versus cryoablation, which of the following is *true*?
   A. Cryoablation is safer because there is less chance of postprocedure bleeding.
   B. RFA is preferred because it causes less pain.
   C. RFA is easier to monitor with CT guidance.
   D. Cryoablation is less painful than RFA, and, therefore, can usually be done without general anesthesia.

   ANSWER: D. There is less pain during the ablation process using cryoablation. There may be a higher incidence of bleeding with cryoablation. The ablation zone is harder to define on CT during RFA but will be demarcated during cryoablation.

4. What is the advantage of using MWA over RFA?
   A. It causes tumor necrosis without thermal energy.
   B. It is faster than RFA and can ablate a larger area.
   C. There is no risk to surrounding structures with microwave.
   D. There is no postablation syndrome with microwave.

   ANSWER: B. Ablation can be accomplished in less time and to one larger area with microwave than with RFA. All ablative procedures can cause postablation syndrome and can damage surrounding structures. Also, microwave causes ablation by the generation of heat.

5. Which of the following is the most common *severe* complication of ablative therapy?
   A. Hemorrhage
   B. Postablation syndrome
   C. Infection
   D. Stroke

   ANSWER: A. Bleeding is the most common severe complication though it is rarely life threatening. Postablation syndrome occurs but is usually easily manageable. Infection can be severe but is usually easily treated. Stroke has been rarely reported with lung ablation because of microbubbles, but is very uncommon.

Section 10
NUCLEAR RADIOLOGY

90 RADIATION SAFETY, INSTRUMENTATION, AND QUALITY CONTROL

Jon A. Baldwin and Kok C. Tan

INTRODUCTION

Imaging in nuclear medicine is significantly different than those in most other imaging modalities in radiology. Rather than passing a beam of energy through a patient and measuring its attenuation, radioactivity is injected into a patient, and the distribution of that radioactivity is captured by a specialized imaging system. Many of the radioactive substances in use in nuclear medicine are composed of two substrates: the radionuclide and a ligand to which the radionuclide is "tagged" to, creating a radiopharmaceutical. Occasionally, the radionuclide in its "native" chemical and physical state is the radiotracer used (e.g., $Na^{123}I$, $Na^{131}I$, ^{133}Xe, $Na^{99m}TcO_4$). Radiotracers each have a unique biodistribution and imaging appearance, which is then altered in particular disease processes. As such, nuclear medicine imaging is more about the imaging of physiology or function, rather than that of anatomy. In this chapter, we will begin by reviewing some basic physics, such as characteristics of radioactive decay, including production of commonly used radionuclides, and how their decay affects image quality and patient dose. We will then discuss how images are generated, and what type of quality control is performed, and when to assure proper image reconstruction. Finally, some of the basic Nuclear Regulatory Commission (NRC) guidelines pertinent to diagnostic and therapeutic nuclear medicine are reviewed.

PHYSICS OF NUCLEAR MEDICINE

Radioactivity is a random process by which unstable atoms emit energy and/or particles in an attempt to become more stable. The way a particular atom will decay at a particular instant cannot be known for certain, but can be expressed by a percentage based on observational evidence. For the purposes of this review, there are essentially two forces at work in a nucleus—the electromagnetic, which is repulsive between protons, and the strong nuclear force, which is attractive between nucleons (protons and neutrons) over small distances. In stable (nonradioactive) isotopes of lighter elements, the proportion of protons to neutrons is 1:1. As elements get larger, the repulsive force from the large numbers of protons present needs to be counteracted by the strong nuclear force. The proportion of protons to neutrons approaches 1:1.5. To move toward this proportion, the atom can undergo decay. Alpha (α) decay, beta minus ($\beta-$) decay, positron decay ($\beta+$), or electron capture decay (EC) are processes that look to balance the electromagnetic and strong forces (Table 90-1).

α DECAY

This form of decay tends to occur in heavier unstable atoms. A charged (+2) α particle, which in reality is a helium nucleus (^4He), is emitted. The daughter's mass (A) is decreased by four, and the atomic number (Z) is decreased by two. Photonic energy, in the form of a gamma (γ) ray, is also usually emitted as part of this process. Currently, radionuclides that decay by α decay are not used in nuclear medicine.

TABLE 90-1 Radionuclides and Their Modes of Decay

TYPE OF DECAY	RADIONUCLIDES
$\beta-$ emitter, no imageable γ produced	^3H, ^{14}C, ^{32}P, ^{89}Sr, ^{90}Y
$\beta-$ emitter, imageable γ produced	^{99}Mo, ^{131}I, ^{133}Xe, ^{153}Sm
$\beta+$ emitter	^{11}C, ^{13}N, ^{15}O, ^{18}F, ^{68}Ga, ^{82}Rb
Electron capture	^{67}Ga, ^{111}In, ^{123}I, ^{201}Tl
Isomeric transition	^{99m}Tc, ^{113m}In

β− DECAY

In this form of radioactive decay, a β− particle, which is in essence a nuclear-formed electron (e^-), is emitted from the nucleus. One can think of it as a neutron being "transformed" to a proton. The daughter's mass is unchanged, but the atomic number is increased by one. This decay occurs in "neutron rich" radionuclides. The β− particle will travel a short distance, and then come to rest. This particle has the potential to damage DNA, and is the basis of radionuclide therapy with ^{32}P, ^{89}Sr, ^{90}Y, ^{131}I, and ^{153}Sm. Certain radionuclides also have γ photonic emissions that occur and can be imaged.

β+ DECAY

In positron decay, a β+ particle, which is a nuclear-produced "positive" electron, is emitted from the nucleus. A proton is thus "transformed" into a neutron. The daughter's atomic mass is unchanged, and the atomic number is decreased by one. This decay occurs in "proton rich" radionuclides, but only when enough energy (1.02 MeV) is available for positron decay. The particle will travel a short distance before it comes to rest, at which time it will contact a "negative" electron and annihilate, giving off two 511 keV γ photons approximately 180 degrees apart. These emissions are imaged in positron emission tomography (PET). Radionuclides important to nuclear medicine that decay by positron emission are usually produced by a cyclotron (the exception being ^{82}Rb, a cardiac PET perfusion agent produced in a generator system). β+ decay often competes with electron capture decay, even when enough energy is available for positron emission. For example, ^{18}F decays by β+ 87% of the time, and by EC 13% of the time.

ELECTRON CAPTURE DECAY

This form of decay occurs in "proton rich" radionuclides, when there is not enough energy available for positron decay. The atom captures an orbital electron, "transforming" a proton into a neutron. The daughter's atomic mass is unchanged, and the atomic number is decreased. γ Photons can also be emitted and imaged. In addition, the orbital electron vacancies will be filled by electrons from adjacent orbits, resulting in either characteristic x-ray emissions or Auger electron emission. Sometimes it is the characteristic x-rays that are more abundant or advantageous for imaging, as is the case in decay of ^{201}Tl; it is the characteristic x-rays of the ^{201}Hg daughter that are imaged. These radionuclides are also cyclotron produced.

ISOMERIC TRANSFORMATION

A radionuclide in an excited state (an "isomer") will get rid of excess energy by emitting γ photon. These isomers are generally of very short duration, except in the case of a metastable radionuclide. These have a measurable interval before emitting their photon. These radionuclides are designated with an "m" by their atomic mass number (e.g., ^{99m}Tc). This process competes with internal conversion, in which the excess energy is transferred to an orbital electron, which is then ejected from its orbit. Orbital vacancies will be filled by electron from adjacent orbits, resulting in characteristic x-rays or Auger electron emission.

It is important to remember that radioactive decay is a random process. One cannot know for sure how a particular atom in a sample will decay, and what the energies of the resultant particles/photons will be. β− and β+ particles will have a E_{max} and a mean E. Energy is "randomly" distributed among the particles, γ photon and the antineutrino or neutrino. The average energy of a particle is approximately one-third of its maximum energy ($E_{ave} = 1/3\ E_{max}$). Also remember that internalized particulate emissions are much more damaging to biologic structures, and contribute more to patient dose than do internalized or externalized photonic emissions. β+ and β− particles do not travel far before they deposit their energy and "do their damage"; they can be shielded against with plastic or plexiglass (in fact, it is important to avoid using lead shielding with β− emitters, as penetrating bremsstrahlung x-rays will be produced). Photon emissions are much more penetrating, and must be shielded with denser materials such as tungsten or lead. Of the five processes by which photons interact with matter (coherent scattering, photoelectric absorption, Compton scattering, pair production, and photodisintegration), the two that are important in nuclear medicine are photoelectric absorption and Compton scattering. The end result of either of these processes is the production of an ion pair: an ejected electron from the atom, and a positive ion (due to the loss of the electron), which will then ultimately interact with tissue and potentially damage it. Additionally, photoelectric absorption will result in either characteristic x-rays or Auger electron emission as the inner electron shell is filled. Compton scatter will have a "scatter photon," the γ photon with decreased energy resulting from its interaction with an outer shell electron. Tables 90-1 and 90-2 summarize radionuclide decay and production.

RADIONUCLIDES AND RADIOPHARMACEUTICALS

With an understanding of how different radionuclides decay, it is possible to use that information to under-

TABLE 90-2 Sources of Radionuclides

SOURCE OF RADIONUCLIDE	RADIONUCLIDE
Reactor	^{99}Mo, ^{131}I, ^{133}Xe, ^{137}Cs
Cyclotron	^{11}C, ^{13}N, ^{15}O, ^{18}F, ^{111}In, ^{123}I, ^{67}Ga, ^{201}Tl
Generator	^{68}Ga, ^{82}Rb, ^{99m}Tc ^{113m}In

stand some of the properties of radiopharmaceuticals used in diagnostic and therapeutic nuclear medicine. Several factors go toward making an ideal *diagnostic* radiopharmaceutical. First, the photons emitted have to be within a range that lends itself to being recorded onto a usable image. The ideal range of photon energy for nuclear medicine camera systems is between 100 and 200 keV. Although energies above or below this can be imaged, the image quality and resolution is not ideal. Second, the radionuclide should have no particle emissions, as this increases the dose to the patient, without contributing to the image. Third, the half-life of the radionuclide has to be such that there is adequate time for the radiopharmaceutical to localize in the organ of interest. Unnecessary long half-lives, however, will generally result in larger doses to the patient (assuming the activity is not removed from the body by some biologic process). The chemical properties of the radionuclide are also important. If the radionuclide is not going to be used in its natural form, but rather "tagged" to a ligand that will allow proper localization, its chemistry must be such that it will permit it to be incorporated stably within the radiopharmaceutical. The radiopharmaceutical itself should be nontoxic to the patient, and be sufficiently resistant to degradation for the duration of the diagnostic study. Therapeutic radiopharmaceutical criteria share some of these criteria, but $\beta-$ particle emission is required. Half-life of the radiopharmaceutical can vary, but should be long enough to treat the condition in question, but not to cause excessive harm to normal structures. A few therapeutic agents (e.g., ^{131}I, ^{153}Sm) can be imaged, so as to observe areas being treated and discover unsuspected disease. Other therapeutic radionuclides do not emit photons that can be imaged (Table 90-1).

The workhorse radionuclide of diagnostic agents in nuclear medicine is ^{99m}Tc. It fulfills the majority of the criteria cited above. An additional factor that makes ^{99m}Tc appealing is that it is obtained from a generator system, enhancing its availability. Radionuclide generators consist of a radionuclide with a relatively long half-life, with a relatively short-lived daughter. The daughter typically can be easily removed from the parent due to different chemical properties. Examples include the ^{99}Mo/^{99m}Tc generator system, in which ^{99}Mo (T ½ = 67 hours) decays to ^{99m}Tc (T ½ = 6 hours); the ^{82}Sr/^{82}Rb generator system, in which ^{82}Sr (T ½ = 25 days) decays to ^{82}Rb (T ½ = 75 seconds); and the ^{113}Sn/^{113m}In generator system, in which ^{113}Sn (T ½ = 115 days) decays to ^{113m}In (T ½ = 1.7 hours).

^{99}Mo/^{99M}Tc GENERATOR

In this system, ^{99}Mo is adhered to an alumina column. As it decays, the daughter ^{99m}Tc is not bound as tightly to the column. Physiologic saline is washed across the column, and ^{99m}Tc is eluted from the column in the form of sodium pertechnetate (Na^{99m}TcO$_4$). Na^{99m}TcO$_4$ is in a +7 valence state, and must be reduced to a suitable form to label the chelates. This is usually accomplished with stannous ions. If there are errors in the reduction process, insoluble impurities may be introduced. In addition, before it is injected into the patient, the radiopharmaceutical should be sterile and pyrogen free. All of these steps require quality control testing to ensure that the radiotracer is in compliance with set guidelines.

Radionuclide Purity

Radionuclide purity is expressed as the percentage of activity present that is due to the radionuclide of interest. ^{99}Mo is a long-lived nuclide with particle emission and high energy photons. These factors can increase the dose to patient and degrade the patient's images. To test for the presence of ^{99}Mo, the sample is shielded with lead, with the test based on the different photopeaks of the radionuclides. It is important that the ^{99}Mo be assayed first, and in the special lead shield supplied by the manufacturer of the dose calibrator. ^{99m}Tc is then assayed directly in a plastic sleeve. The basis of the test is that the high energy ^{99}Mo photons will not be attenuated by the lead, but the 140 keV ^{99m}Tc photons will be attenuated. Activity of ^{99}Mo (in µCi) is divided by activity of ^{99m}Tc (in mCi) to obtain a ratio. The NRC allows no more than 0.15µCi of ^{99}Mo per 1 mCi of ^{99m}Tc *at the time of administration*. As a rule of thumb, if the ratio is less than 0.038 at the time of elution, the material will be suitable for injection for at least 12 hours.

Chemical Purity

The column inside the generator is made of aluminium oxide (Al_2O_3). For this reason, alumina can be eluted from column. This can form colloids with ^{99m}Tc, which would show up as liver activity, or can cause sulfur colloid aggregation, which would lead to lung uptake on a liver-spleen scan. The test performed is similar to the colorimetric test performed with pH paper; excessive alumina will change the color of the paper. The permissible amount is 10 mg Al^{3+} per 1 mL ^{99m}Tc eluate.

Radiochemical Purity

The assessment of the radiochemical purity of the ^{99m}Tc radiopharmaceutical is determining the degree of successful tagging of the ^{99m}Tc to the biological component contained in the kit. The $Na^{99m}TcO_4$ obtained from the generator is added to the reaction vial. This vial contains stannous chloride ($SnCl_2$, the reducing agent), the pharmaceutical to be tagged, preservatives, and is purged with N_2 gas (to prevent reduction of Sn by O_2 in the air). Instant thin layer chromatography (TLC) is usually performed to assess the chemical purity of the radionuclide. To check for the presence of free pertechnetate, the radiopharmaceutical is placed on the chromatographic strip and acetone solvent is used; acetone will move with the solvent front. To check for insoluble impurities, such as hydrolyzed reduced technetium, saline is used. The insoluble impurity will not move with the solvent front. If the radiotracer is itself insoluble, there is no test available to check for the presence of hydrolyzed reduced technetium in that sample, so the possibility that it is present is ignored. The United States Pharmacopeia (USP) has limits of acceptability for radiochemical purity. The limits are 95% for $Na^{99m}TcO_4$, 92% for ^{99m}Tc sulfur colloid, and 91% for all other ^{99m}Tc radiopharmaceuticals.

Particle size of certain compounds may also be checked by a hemocytometer as part of the quality control procedure.

Miscellaneous Testing

The USP maximum diameter recommendation for macroaggregated albumin (MAA) is 150 μm, with 90% of the particles between 10 and 90 μm. The sterility of a compound must also be tested, either by incubating the radiopharmaceutical on agar media, or by the Bactec system. This system uses ^{14}C labeled glucose, and in the presence of bacteria, $^{14}CO_2$ is released. If the radiopharmaceutical is to be used for cisternography, it must also be pyrogen free. Endotoxins may be evaluated by the limulus amoebocyte lysate test. This material is derived from the amoebas present in the tail of the horseshoe crab, which in the presence of an endotoxin, will form an opaque gel.

Once the radiopharmaceutical is made and meets NRC and USP standards, it is ready to be administered to the patient. The route of administration is typically intravenously, but some are administered subcutaneously, and some are ingested. One now needs an imaging system that can localize and record the distribution of the radiotracer. This system is the gamma scintillation camera.

BASIC INSTRUMENTATION

The gamma scintillation camera converts photons emitted by the radionuclide in the patient's body into a light pulse, which is then subsequently converted into a voltage signal, which is then used to form an image. This is true for both "conventional" nuclear medicine scintigraphy, as well as for imaging with positron emitting radionuclides. In this section, we will first discuss non-PET imaging. The basic components of a gamma camera system are the collimator, the scintillation crystal, the photomultiplier tube array, the pulse height analyzer (PHA), and the control console with computer integration. Each of these components contributes to the accurate localization of the radiotracer distribution within the patient. The radiopharmaceutical used and its time to desired/optimized biodistribution will determine some image parameters—the timing of the image acquisition, the type of collimator used, and the photopeak window setting.

COLLIMATOR

Ideally, the concentration of photons arriving at a radiation detector would be proportional to the number of photons emitted in the respective body part being imaged. However, unwanted photons can arise from background activity in tissues in front, behind, or to the side of the body part being imaged. These photons reduce image contrast and may distort the data analysis. Secondly, photons arising from the organ of interest may travel "off axis" since radiation is given off equally in all directions. Thirdly, Compton scatter can degrade the image. Recall that Compton scatter arises from photons that originate in or adjacent to the organ of interest and then interact with a loosely bound orbital electron resulting in image degradation. The collimator is the first portion of the gamma camera system that the emitted photon encounters. It is made of perforated lead and is interposed between the patient and the scintillation crystal. It is designed to reduce scatter and allows the gamma camera to correctly localize radionuclide events in the patient's body. It does this by discriminating against unwanted photons on the basis of their direction of travel. The collimator cannot, however, distinguish between photons of different energy. This is done by the PHA (discussed later). A *parallel hole collimator* is the workhorse collimator in clinical practice. It consists of thin lead dividers interspersed by thousands of uniformly distributed gaps or holes. The choice of parallel hole collimator would depend on the photon energy level of the isotope being imaged, and the sensitivity or resolution desired. The thickness of the lead septa and the interspace distance between the lead dividers determines the optimized photopeak for the collimator. A low-level energy collimator is conventionally used for radiotracers with photon energies of 1 to 200 keV (e.g., ^{99m}Tc, ^{123}I, ^{133}Xe, ^{201}Tl). Medium energy collimators are designed for radiotracers with maximum photon energies of 200 to 400 keV (e.g., ^{67}Ga, ^{111}In) by having thicker lead septa than the low energy collimators. Photons with lower energies are unlikely to pass through the thicker lead septa. High-energy collimators have been designed for radiotracers with maximum photon energies more than 400 to 600 keV. ^{131}I falls into this category; even though the principle imaged photon is "medium energy," there are 19 possible different γ rays emitted, some of which (7% abundance) have a 637 keV photon. Sensitivity and resolution of an image, in regard to the collimator, is related to the length of the lead septa. There is an inverse relation between these two parameters, and improving one comes at the cost of worsening the other. High-resolution collimators have long septa. This significantly reduces the chance that a photon coming at an oblique angle will strike the crystal face. This, however, means that fewer photons will strike the crystal face and the sensitivity suffers. Put another way, if the length of the septa is increased, the count rate decreases and the resolution increases. The difference between a general collimator and a high sensitivity collimator of the same energy (low, medium, or high) is that high sensitivity collimators may allow approximately twice as many counts to be imaged, but the spatial resolution will also be degraded accordingly. High-sensitivity collimators are important in the use of dynamic acquisitions, for example, in the flow phase of a bone scan, and in other instances when a low count density is expected. It should be noted that in parallel hole collimators the distance of the patient from the camera face will not affect the sensitivity. As the distance between the two increases, counts reduced by the effect of the inverse square law are compensated for by the increased field of view the increased distance affords. The net effect is that count rates are unchanged. Resolution, however, is significantly decreased as the distance between patient and collimator increases. The septa are no longer able to eliminate photons coming from an oblique angle to the crystal face. A *pinhole collimator* behaves in much the same way as a pinhole camera. As such, the field of view increases with distance and the resulting image is magnified and inverted. Its main clinical purpose is to image small parts objects such as the thyroid and the bones of the hands and feet. *Converging hole collimators* are used to magnify the image, without image inversion as in pinhole collimators. These collimators have holes that converge toward a point approximately 50 cm in front of the collimator. As the patient moves away from the collimator up to the focal point, sensitivity increases. Beyond the focal point, however, sensitivity decreases. Resolution decreases with distance. A *diverging collimator* is one whose holes and lead septa point away from the crystal surface, minimizing the image. They permit imaging of a larger area of the body on a small crystal face than is possible with a simple parallel hole collimator. The diverging collimator can increase the area to be imaged by approximately 30%. Resolution and sensitivity both decrease as the patient is moved away from the collimator. An important thing to remember about nonparallel hole collimators is that since they are magnifying or minimizing a three-dimensional object, image distortion can occur.

SCINTILLATION CRYSTAL

Once the photon emerges from the patient, and gets past the collimator, it will interact with the crystal. This crystal is made of sodium iodide doped with thallium. The photon interacting with the iodide will cause an ejection of an orbital electron, producing a pulse of fluorescent light. The amount of light produced varies directly with the energy of the photon striking the crystal. Photomultiplier tubes (PMT) behind the crystal surface detect the light and amplify it. The likelihood of a photoelectric event and consequent complete energy absorption in the sodium iodide crystal is greater at low energies and decreases at higher energies, because the probability of Compton interaction increases at higher energy levels. Approximately 30% of the light from each event reaches the PMTs. The thickness of the crystal will affect the efficiency of gamma ray detection and spatial resolution of the image. The thicker the crystal, the more likely events are to be captured. However, with a thicker the crystal, the spatial resolution worsens, as the PMTs are further away from scintillation event. The relationship of crystal thickness and energy of the photon emitted from the patient also has an impact on sensitivity and resolution. The higher the photon energy, the more likely the photon will pass through the crystal without producing a scintillation event. For example, there is near-100% efficiency of detection for ^{99m}Tc, ^{123}I, ^{133}Xe, and ^{201}Tl photons with a ½-in crystal. That same crystal has only about a 25% efficiency for detecting ^{131}I photons. As with collimators, sensitivity is sacrificed for spatial resolution. For thinner crystals, sensitivity decreases ~10% as more photons pass through, but there is ~30% increase in spatial resolution. This is due to the PMTs being closer to the scintillation event, and the light pulse can be localized more accurately. Thicker crystals do better for detecting higher energy photons.

PHOTOMULTIPLIER TUBES

PMTs detect light pulses produced by the crystal, amplifies them and converts them into an electrical signal of measurable magnitude. Usually, an array of PMTs are aligned behind the crystal for event localization. The number of PMTs used affects the ability of the system to localize where the pulse originated from; therefore, more PMTs will increase resolution. A scintillation event in the crystal is invariably recorded by one or more PMTs, and the final image is determined by the amount of light sensed by each tube, thus affecting the pattern of PMT voltage output. For each event, the summation signal is then formed by weighing the output from each tube. Two kinds of signal processing take place. The summed pulse typically called the Z pulse is related to intensity of the output. This is used to determine if the detected event falls within the desired energy range and should be accepted into the formation of the image. If it does not fall into the desired energy range, it will be rejected by the PHA. Simultaneously, the signal from each scintillation event is localized spatially to an x and y coordinates in a Cartesian plane. It should be noted that a potential source of image degradation lies within the circuits of the PMTs. The electronics of the PMTs are such that there may be variations in how an individual PMT perceives a light impulse of specific intensity. This can result in an inhomogeneous distribution of activity across the image. This can be corrected for through the use of computer correction factors. This parameter, called field uniformity, will be discussed in more detail below in the quality control section.

PULSE HEIGHT ANALYZER

The basic principle of the PHA is to discard unwanted signals, so that only photons with the photopeak of the radiotracer used in the study are being imaged. The photopeak is the characteristic energy of photons emitted by a particular radionuclide. Imagine a plot was made of the photon energy (*x*-axis) versus number of counts (*y*-axis) for ^{99m}Tc, as imaged with gamma camera system. ^{99m}Tc emits a gamma ray with an energy of 140 keV when it decays to ^{99}Tc, so one might expect all of the counts to be located at that energy. In fact, when imaged by the scintillation camera, the highest number of counts would have a Gaussian distribution on either side of this main photon energy of the radiotracer. Other peaks would be found as well, however, as a result of the different interactions of the 140 keV photons with other components of the imaging system. These include the iodine escape peak, the backscatter peak, lead x-ray peak, and Compton edge. The iodine escape peak is the result of the interaction of a ^{99m}Tc photon with the K shell electron of the iodine near the edge of the sodium iodine crystal. The energy of that ejected electron is then lost, shifting the peak to the left (140 keV – 28 keV = 112 keV). Another peak results from the interaction of the ^{99m}Tc photon with the K shell electrons of the lead in the collimator. The characteristic x-rays produced from this interaction produce a peak in the range of 75 to 88 keV. A third peak occurs when a ^{99m}Tc gamma ray first undergoes 180 degrees scatter and is subsequently absorbed by the sodium iodide crystal. The resulting loss of energy from the scatter event results in the backscatter peak (140 keV – 50 keV = 90 keV). Finally, the effect of Compton scatter of the 140 keV photon within the crystal gives a peak from 0 to 50 keV (Fig. 90-1).

The above mentioned peaks are seen if one considers only a source of ^{99m}Tc interacting with the camera system. The plot of counts versus energy are different when the ^{99m}Tc photons are escaping from a patient who has been injected with a ^{99m}Tc radiopharmaceutical. There is still a sharp peak at 140 keV with a Gaussian distribution; however, to the left of the peak there is a large broad peak resulting from Compton scatter of the 140 keV photons within the patient. These scattered photons will then strike the crystal with energies from approximately 90 keV to just less than 140 keV. These energies will mask the iodine escape peak and backscatter peaks (Fig. 90-2). Compton scatter from the patient significantly degrades the images obtained from the patient.

Other radiotracers will have distinct "plots" based on the energies of the photons they emit and their interactions with the camera system. In addition, there may be multiples of these photopeaks in radiotracers that have several abundant photon energies (^{67}Ga and ^{111}In being the most important in nuclear medicine). Finally, unwanted photons can arise from background activity, from scattered radiation, or radiation from interfering isotopes. The PHA determines which events occurring in the crystal will be displayed and which will be rejected. It is able to do this because the energy deposited by a scintillation event in the crystal bears a linear rela-

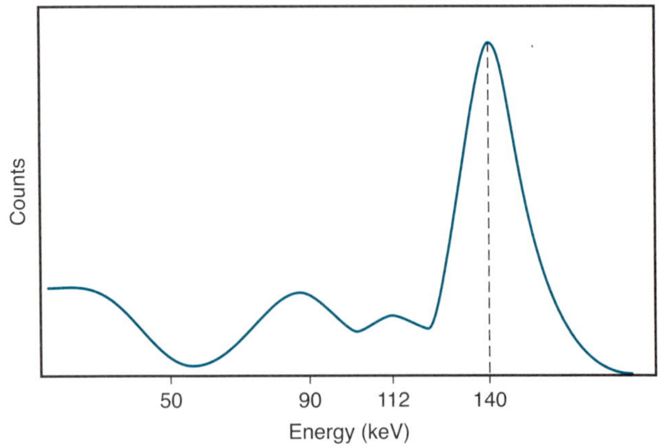

FIG. 90-1 Plot of a point source ^{99m}Tc photon energy, as imaged by a gamma camera system. The peak at 140 keV is the energy resulting from the decay of ^{99m}Tc to ^{99}Tc. The peak at 112 keV is the iodine escape peak. The peak at 90 keV is a combination of the backscatter and Pb x-ray peaks. The Compton edge is at 50 keV, with Compton scatter seen from 0 to 50 keV.

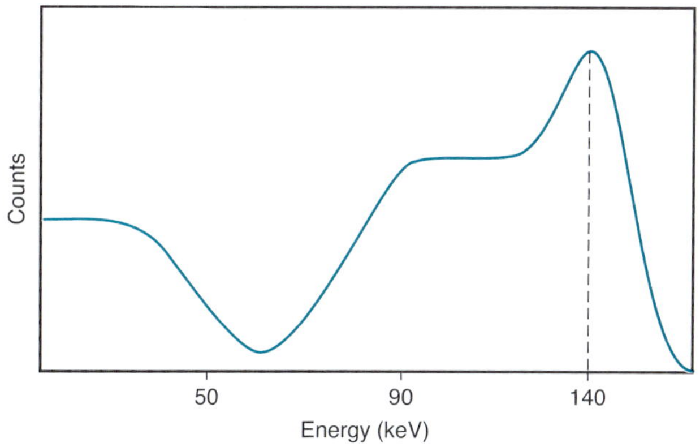

FIG. 90-2 Plot of ^{99m}Tc photon energy emitting from a patient, as imaged by a gamma camera system. Compton scatter occurring within the patient accounts for the broad peak from 90 to 140 keV.

tionship to the voltage signal emerging from the PMT. Signal intensity information is then matched against a voltage discriminator otherwise known as a "window." The window has an upper and lower limit that defines the window width. This allows energy related to the desired isotope photopeak to be recorded. Any signal higher or lower than this range will be rejected. Some cameras have several PHAs, which allow several photopeaks to be used at once. This is useful for radionuclides with multiple photopeaks such as ^{67}Ga and ^{111}In, or in doing dual tracer studies, where two radiopharmaceuticals with different energies are imaged at the same time. A classic example of this is performing a ^{99m}Tc bone scan and an ^{111}In tagged WBC to assess for osteomyelitis. One can simply change the window setting to see if there is congruent or noncongruent uptake at a suspected site. This cannot be accomplished with all radiotracer combinations, however, because of a phenomenon called "downscatter." More energetic photons can spill into a window of a less energetic photon emitter, especially when Compton scatter within a patient is occurring. Some clinical examples are performing a V/Q scan with ^{133}Xe and ^{99m}Tc MAA, or a bone scan with ^{99m}Tc MDP followed by a ^{67}Ga scan for suspected vertebral osteomyelitis. ^{133}Xe has a photopeak of 81 keV. Recall that Compton scatter of ^{99m}Tc within a patient has an approximate range of 90 to 140 keV, which is close to the ideal window of ^{133}Xe. If the ^{99m}Tc MAA portion of the V/Q scan was performed first, when the ^{133}Xe was imaged, there would be interference in image quality from scattered ^{99m}Tc photons. A similar phenomenon occurs with ^{99m}Tc and ^{67}Ga (^{67}Ga has photopeaks of 93, 184, 300, and 393 keV). In both cases, the portion of the study that uses the lower energy photon must be done first to avoid downscatter. This is especially important when using ^{67}Ga, which has a half-life of 78 hours; if done first, one would have to wait at least a week for activity from the ^{67}Ga (physical half-life, 78 hours; effective half-life ~50 hours) to clear sufficiently to perform the ^{99m}Tc study! Also in regard to ^{67}Ga, an astute observer would no doubt have discerned that part of the reason that ^{67}Ga has poor imaging characteristics is the downscatter phenomenon that is present even when used by itself, because of its multiple photopeaks.

Once the impulses from the PMT have been processed by the PHA, depending on voltage signal it is either accepted or rejected based on the window setting selected by the technologist. Once sufficient accepted signals, with their x and y coordinate information, have been obtained, this data is then used to assemble a diagnostic image. The image can then be recorded by photographic or electronic means.

TYPES OF IMAGE ACQUISITIONS

Nuclear medicine images acquired by a gamma camera system can be obtained as a "static" image for a predetermined number of counts, or for a set time. In addition, a dynamic acquisition can be acquired, with the camera capturing and recording the distribution of radiotracer as it moves through the patient over short time intervals. When improved spatial resolution is needed to make the proper diagnosis, a SPECT acquisition can be performed. A camera or cameras are rotated either 180 or 360 degrees around the patient, typically moving 3 to 6 degrees at a time. Orbits can be circular or elliptical. The more projections obtained, for a longer period of time, the better the image quality. However, as patients often cannot tolerate remaining motionless for long periods of time, compromises must be made. Patient motion can severely degrade image quality. Combinations of number of camera stops and time per stop that result in acquisition times less than 30 minutes are favored. Another important imaging parameter is image matrix size—the number of pixels over the imaging surface. A matrix size of 128 × 128 has better resolution than a matrix size of 64 × 64, but comes at a cost of increased acquisition time, increased processing time, and reduced count density per pixel, which adversely impacts image contrast. Once the study is acquired, the data can be processed to construct a three-dimensional image of the organ or body part scanned. This is done by mathematical techniques called filtered back projection or iterative reconstruction. Mathematical filters are used before or after image reconstruction to help eliminate noise in the image, smooth the image, and improve resolution. These filters will allow predetermined frequencies to "pass" through—contribute to the final image—while disregarding other frequencies. Images can be degraded by attenuation from within the patient. This can be corrected for by passing a photon through the patient (whether from a radionuclide like ^{153}Gd or a CT scanner) and measure its attenuation through the patient. This attenuation map can then be used to "reassign" counts based on the probability of their being attenuated. This method is most commonly used in SPECT myocardial perfusion imaging. The final reconstructed image can be viewed in a rotating three-dimensional view and can be sectioned into the three orthogonal planes for review.

QUALITY CONTROL FOR GAMMA CAMERAS

As seen from the above discussion, there are numerous components involved in generating a diagnostic quality image. If any of these fails, image quality may suffer. Several parameters are tested at specified intervals to ensure that the camera system is working properly (Table 90-3). Of the listed parameters, window setting, uniformity, spatial resolution, and linearity are checked most frequently.

FIELD UNIFORMITY

This parameter requires daily assessment and measures the uniformity of the response of the gamma camera across its entire field of view. As discussed previously, individual PMT can assign slightly different voltages to the same photon energy because of differences in their internal electronics, as well as slight variations in crystal thickness. To make certain that the computer corrections are functioning to ensure that uniformity remains within accepted percentages (2%–5%; as low as 1% if SPECT is to be performed). If measurements are made with the collimator in place, extrinsic uniformity is being tested. Measurements without the collimator are testing intrinsic uniformity. For extrinsic field uniformity, most nuclear medicine facilities use either a phantom filled with a uniform solution of $Na^{99m}TcO_4$ in water or a permanent disk source of uniformly distributed ^{57}Co (half-life of 270 days). ^{99m}Tc flood sources have the advantage of being easily available and relatively cheap. However, with its half-life of 6 hours, it has to be refilled daily. Thorough mixing is imperative, so that uniform distribution of radiotracer is presented to the crystal face (watch out for air bubbles!). Contamination of a department by ^{99m}Tc from a dropped flood source has ruined many a nuclear medicine technologist's morning. The ^{57}Co sheet source avoids this complication by being uniformly distributed throughout a plastic matrix. Sheet sources cost more, and do eventually have to be replaced. The ^{57}Co photopeak (122 keV) approximates that of ^{99m}Tc. The image obtained should be inspected carefully. A highly uniform appearance is expected, although very minor mottling from the PMTs is acceptable. A failure of a PMT can be recognized as an area of decreased activity. Cracked crystals are also readily identified, and damage to the collimator system can be detected (when performing an extrinsic test). For testing uniformity, one does not have to do *both* extrinsic and intrinsic tests daily, either check is sufficient. However, it is wise to do the check that is not performed daily

TABLE 90-3 Quality Control for Gamma Cameras

PARAMETER	FREQUENCY OF TESTING	METHOD OF TESTING
Window setting	Each patient	Verify correct energy window setting for radionuclide used
Uniformity, extrinsic	Daily, before first patient	^{99m}Tc flood/ ^{57}Co sheet source, collimator in place
Uniformity, intrinsic	Daily, before first patient	^{99m}Tc point source at the proper distance from crystal face; collimator removed
Spatial resolution	Weekly	^{99m}Tc flood/ ^{57}Co sheet source covered by bar phantom
Linearity	Weekly	^{99m}Tc flood/ ^{57}Co sheet source covered by bar phantom
SPECT calibration floods	Per manufacturer, usually monthly	High activity ^{99m}Tc flood source
Center of rotation (SPECT)	Per manufacturer, usually monthly	SPECT acquisition of a ^{99m}Tc point source
Tomographic resolution (SPECT)	Quarterly	Obtain ^{99m}Tc line source SPECT and planar acquisition and compare resolution; cannot exceed 10% of planar value
Tomographic uniformity (SPECT)	Quarterly	Image cylindrical tomographic phantom
Collimator performance	Annually*	^{99m}Tc flood/ ^{57}Co sheet source, collimator in place, for 1 million counts
Energy resolution	Annually*	Various radionuclides used, FWHM calculated
Count rate capability	Annually*	Two sources of ^{99m}Tc counted, one higher in activity than the other. Look for count rate that causes a 20% data loss (while using a 20% window)
Sensitivity	Annually*	Count rate for per μCi (using 20% window), for each collimator

*Parameters that are checked annually can be checked more frequently if a problem is suspected.

periodically to assure that parameter is within specifications (i.e., if intrinsic uniformity is checked daily, extrinsic uniformity could be checked weekly). If the camera being tested for uniformity performs SPECT acquisitions, a much higher count image (at least 30 million counts instead of 1 million) is acquired at least quarterly. Nonuniform fields can lead to "bull's eye" or ring artifacts on acquired images.

WINDOW SETTING

This should be checked before the acquisition of each patient. If the improper window setting is used, image degradation can occur from improper photopeaks being accepted by the camera system. The most common approach to this is to use a symmetrical window centered at the energy peak of the radionuclide label being used in the imaging process. For ^{99m}Tc, the recommendation is to use a 20% window centered around a 140 keV photopeak. Using a narrower window of 10% to 15%, or an asymmetric window (i.e., centered slightly more than 140 keV) will improve resolution.

SPATIAL RESOLUTION AND LINEARITY

Bar phantoms containing lines with differing degrees of interspacing are routinely used to evaluate image resolution and linearity in the clinical setting. With modern imaging equipment, a weekly assessment is sufficient. Resolution is defined as the ability to discriminate between two distinct points. It is expressed subjectively in terms of the smallest bar pattern visible on the image. All groups in the bar phantom should also appear straight and parallel (linearity). Some distortion at the edge of the field of view is acceptable. The spatial resolution of a gamma camera is expressed quantitatively as the full width at half maximum (FWHM) of a line spread function. A narrower FWHM indicates better spatial resolution. In modern cameras, intrinsic resolution approaches 3 mm FWHM.

POSITRON EMISSION TOMOGRAPHY IMAGING

PET imaging shares many of the same principles as imaging with non-PET radiotracers. In fact, before the advent of PET-specific imaging systems, PET studies were (and occasionally still are) imaged with the standard gamma camera. Even with a thicker crystal and high energy collimator, image quality is poor, as the 511 keV photon is not optimally imaged with a NaI crystal. Cameras are now available that utilize the characteristics of positron emitters to reconstruct high quality, high resolution images. As discussed earlier, positron emitters decay by releasing a positron—a positive electron—that travels a short distance before it comes to rest. When it does so, and comes in contact with a negative electron, an annihilation reaction occurs, giving off two 511 keV photons approximately 180 degrees apart. Using a full ring of detectors (or in the case of the gamma camera, two rotating camera heads), one can detect these "coincidence" events striking the camera face at the same time, and use that line of response to ultimately generate an image. PET-specific imaging devices typically incorporate a full ring of crystals, so that events will less likely be lost. The crystals have been designed to more effectively harness the energy of the 511 keV photon to cause a scintillation event. These crystals are denser than NaI, with a higher effective Z (atomic number) for better "stopping power." The most commonly used crystals are bismuth germinate oxide (BGO), lutetium oxyorthosilicate (LSO), and gadolinium oxyorthosilicate (GSO), with effective Z of 74, 66, and 59, respectively. The last two crystals have superior light output and time resolution compared to BGO. Light from the photoelectric interaction of the 511 keV photon and the crystal is taken up by PMTs that are optically coupled to the crystals. Using the properties of the annihilation event, if there are two scintillation events that occur in paired detectors (detectors that share an arc across from a particular detector) that are recorded within a brief time window (10 nanoseconds), these are recorded as a true event. This effectively represents collimation, not by a physical lead device, but by electronics. This leads to excellent sensitivity (since photons are not physically lost). A few imaging systems do include collimation in the form of removable septa that can slide in and out between detectors to shield against "crosstalk" from activity outside the plane of interest. When the septa are inserted, it is called a two-dimensional acquisition. When the septa are not in place, it is referred to as a three-dimensional acquisition. The three-dimensional acquisition has the benefit of increased sensitivity, but suffers from increased misregistered events. Spatial resolution is much better than in SPECT, on the order of 7 mm in clinical imaging. Some resolution is lost because of the fact that a positron will travel a short distance (approximately 6 mm for the cardiac perfusion agent, ^{82}Rb; approximately 2 mm for ^{18}F) before it comes to rest and annihilates, leading to uncertainty as where the decay actually occurred. In addition, because of the kinetic energy of the positron, not all annihilation events result in photons that are 180 degrees; this noncolinearity can lead to loss of resolution on the order of 1 to 2 mm. Other problems include misregistered events owing to Compton scatter of photons or false events from two single events that strike the crystal within the 10 nanosecond window. Images are typically corrected for attenuation by either a ^{153}Gd transmission scan or with CT.

OTHER RADIATION DETECTORS

There are several other instruments that are commonly used in nuclear medicine departments. Some of these have direct clinical applications, whereas some are used to detect radiation in a sample or the environment. The Geiger-Mueller (GM) counter is a device used to detect small amounts of radioactive contamination. The probe is a gas-filled chamber wherein the enclosed gas becomes ionized when exposed to radiation. There is a high voltage between the anode and cathode of the detector, such that a single ionization event causes a propagation of additional electrons, amplifying the effect. The result is a device that is extremely sensitive for the detection of even small amounts of radiation. The drawback to using this device is that it is easily overwhelmed in high radiation fields—it takes some time for the charge in the detector chamber to dissipate, leading to "dead time" before it can detect another event. The maximum exposure rate reliably detected with a GM counter is 100 mR/h. Ionization chambers are used when higher dose rates are expected. They solve the dead time problem by applying a lower voltage across the anode to the cathode, so there is no large propagation of electrons as in the GM counter. Ionization chambers can detect exposure rates of 0.1 to 100 R/h. The dose calibrator used in nuclear medicine departments to assay the radiopharmaceutical activity is an ionization chamber. When a dose is placed in the chamber, and the radionuclide being measured is input into the selector (i.e., the reading will change depending on if the radiotracer being measured is ^{99m}Tc versus ^{67}Ga or ^{131}I), a readout of the activity is made in mCi. The range that can be measured is from 30 μCi to 2 Ci. Periodic quality control to determine constancy (dose is within 5% of computed activity; checked daily), linearity (accurate readout for activities over the whole range of potentially encountered activities; checked quarterly), accuracy (radiotracer standard measured and compared to what the activity should be; performed at installation and annually), and geometry (the correction for different positioning/sample size of the dose in the chamber; performed at installation). A third device that is commonly found in nuclear medicine departments is a sodium iodide well counter. In essence, this is a small gamma camera with a single PMT and PHA. In this case, the scintillation crystal surrounds the sample; a hole is present in a block of NaI crystal (hence the name well counter), which is encased in shielding material. Surrounding the sample with detector increases the efficiency of detection of radiation manifold. However, this efficiency leads to a problem with dead time. If the activity in the sample exceeds approximately 5000 counts per second (much less activity than a μCi), the reading will likely be significantly underreported. A modified version of a NaI well counter is the thyroid probe used to calculate thyroid uptake values. The probe also has NaI crystal surrounded by shielding, a PMT and a PHA. The opening in the shielding is pointed at the patient's neck at a precise constant distance, and readings are taken. A summary of selected radiation detectors is listed in table (Table 90-4).

RADIATION SAFETY AND NRC REGULATIONS

There is no safe dose of radiation, as in theory it takes only a single photon or particle to cause damage to DNA resulting in a genetic alteration. Of course, we know that the higher the dose of radioactivity one is exposed to, the more likely biological harm is to occur. With that in mind, efforts have been made to assure both the general public and workers that may be exposed to radiation that any exposure they may receive is *a*s *l*ow *a*s *r*easonably *a*chievable—the basis of the ALARA program that will be found at any medical facility that utilizes radiation for clinical and research uses. Most of these directives can be found in the Code of Federal Regulations (CFR) part 19 (deals with inspections and instructions to workers), part 20 (deals with radiation protection standards), and part 35 (deals with human use of radioisotopes). The NRC is the governing body that has been charged with the enforcement of these directives. Individual States can reach an agreement with the Federal government to regulate directives regarding use of radioactivity in their state. The directives of these "Agreement States"

TABLE 90-4 Summary of Ancillary Nuclear Medicine Devices for Detection and Quantification of Radioactivity

DEVICE	DOSE RATE RANGE RELIABLY DETECTED	COMMENT
GM counter	<100 mR/h	Dead time a factor at high dose rates
Ionization chamber	0.1 mR/h–100 R/h	Dose calibrator is a type of ionization chamber (range 30 μCi–2 Ci)
Well counter	<1 μCi	Dead time a factor at high dose rates

can be more strict than those of the NRC, but cannot be less so.

Radiation Safety Radioactive Contamination

No matter how much care is taken to ensure that radiopharmaceuticals do not end up contaminating objects in a department, accidents do occur from time to time. It is important to remember that if a spill or contamination event occurs while a patient is in distress, the needs of the patient outweigh containment concerns. Once the patient has been stabilized and is no longer in danger, then containment procedures become the priority. When it is first realized that a spill has or potentially has occurred, efforts should be made to confine the spill to the area. Gloves and shoe covers (if available) should be worn. Absorbent materials should be placed over the area where the spill took place. The radiation safety officer (RSO) should be notified as soon as possible, to help manage and coordinate efforts. The location should be "cordoned off" to help prevent accidental tracking and spreading of material to uncontaminated areas. It would be best if the RSO were the one to clean the spill, but if that is not possible, use damp absorbent materials to clean the spill, working inwards toward the center of the spill. Use of tongs or forceps is preferred to handle the absorbent material, if available. Proper protective equipment should be worn (gloves, shoe covers, and face shield/mask), as should be a personal dosimeter/film badge. When the cleanup is completed, and counts have fallen to a few times of background or less, items used during the cleanup will need to be either surveyed or presumed to be contaminated, and held with other contaminated objects until they have decayed to safe levels (as a rule of thumb, 10 half-lives of the radionuclide). After this time they can be returned or discarded as regular trash.

Those individuals who were in the area at the time of the spill and are potentially or known to be contaminated will need to be surveyed by the RSO in a different area (to avoid counting interference from the spill itself). Because of the inverse square law, this does not have to be a large distance away. Care should be taken to make sure contamination is not present on their shoes before they are moved to a different area. If there is contamination on an individual, its location is noted. If it is an article of clothing that is contaminated, that clothing is removed and (usually) will be held by the RSO in a safe area until the activity has decayed to safe levels. If the skin of an individual is contaminated, the area is washed thoroughly with soap and water, taking care to not damage the skin (abrasions may allow the contamination to enter the body).

Radioiodine Therapy

^{131}I therapy for nonmalignant and malignant thyroid disease is both safe and efficacious. Many precautions must be taken, however, to protect the patient, their family and friends, and the general public from unnecessary radiation exposure. Whether a patient must be confined to a hospital room for his/her therapy is dependent on the measured activity at a specified distance from their chest. Some agreement States have the limit as 5 mR/h at 1 m from chest (which equates to approximately 30 mCi of activity of ^{131}I). The NRC has the limit as 7 mR/h at 1 m from chest (which equates to approximately 33 mCi of residual activity of ^{131}I). Activities that exceed these limits will necessitate confinement of the patient to a hospital room until these rates are achieved. The precautions that a patient need to take related to the fact that they are being made radioactive with an energetic long-lived (physical half-life, 8 days; effective half-life varies with thyroid uptake and renal function, but is usually quoted as 7.6 days), and the ways that the body seeks to eliminate the ^{131}I that is not taken up by the thyroid gland/thyroid malignancy. ^{131}I is eliminated from the body mainly through urine, but is also excreted in feces, saliva, sweat, and breast milk. In terms of radioactivity emitting from a source, exposure to individuals is reduced through three main factors: time, distance, and shielding. We do not send patients home with lead shielding, so time and distance are utilized to mitigate exposure. Patients are encouraged to increase the distance between themselves and other individuals, particularly pregnant women and children. The amount of time the patient spends around any one particular individual should also be limited. This is of course easy to control while the patient is in a private hospital room—visitors are discouraged or not allowed, and nursing staff are instructed to limit time spent in the room. Once the patient is discharged, or if they have received an outpatient therapy, they are told to sleep alone for the first 3 days after treatment or release. During this period, they should avoid kissing, sexual intercourse, and prolonged physical or intimate contact. When considering the ways ^{131}I is eliminated from the body, the remaining precautions will make sense. The patient is encouraged to drink plenty of fluids and to urinate frequently. This will hasten the elimination of ^{131}I not taken up by the thyroid or malignancy. Good bathroom hygiene is critical. Ideally, the patient should have sole use of a bathroom. Toilets should be flushed twice to assure that potential contamination is removed. Males are encouraged to be seated during urination to limit splashing of urine. Washing hands thoroughly with soap and water after urinating or defecating will help prevent spreading contamination. When eating, some recommend that disposable utensils and plates be used; if they are not, utensils and plates should not be shared and washed separately. Clothes and linens used by the patient should also be washed thoroughly and separately. The majority of the above precautions should be observed for at least 3 days after release from the hospital or after administration of an outpatient therapy. Lactating mothers should NOT receive ^{131}I therapy, unless there is an absolute medical necessity—there would be an increased radiation burden to the breasts because of the hyperemia from the breast-feeding; breast-feeding will need to be discontinued at any rate to prevent radioiodine being passed to the nursing child. Because of an increased risk of miscarriage after ^{131}I therapy, female patients should not attempt to become pregnant for 6 to 12 months after therapy.

Precautions also have to be taken for the administrators of the therapy, as well as the facility where high-dose recipients will be confined. The administrator must keep distance from the patient to minimize personal radiation dose. Everyone involved with patient must wear personal dosimeter/film badge. Gloves must be used by the dose administrator. A mask to prevent inhalation of aerosolized ^{131}I is sometimes worn by the patient, the administrator, or both. Every participant in therapy must have his/her thyroid counted 24 hours after the therapy is performed. The room in which the patient stays will have to be prepared before the patient arrives. Signs informing the public and staff that the room is a radiation area must be posted. Absorbent material is taped to the floor, around the commode in the bathroom at a minimum, but usually throughout the room. This is very important, as iodine binds very well to many floor surfaces, particularly linoleum, making it difficult to remove contamination. Many facilities will wrap in plastic items like a phone, remote control or other device that a patient will frequently handle. Alternatively, a patient can wear gloves to handle these devices. Once the patient has been released, the RSO will have to survey the room before housekeeper can enter it to clean it, and before it can be used by another patient.

Regulations General Public

According to the CFR part 20, each licensee shall conduct operations so that there is an annual dose limit of 100 mrem for members of the public, and that the dose in any *unrestricted area* does not exceed 2 mrem in any 1 hour. General radiation safety rules (no smoking, eating, drinking, etc.) must be posted in each laboratory in which radioactive materials are used. In addition, State/NRC regulations and telephone numbers must be posted conspicuously in each nuclear medicine department. In addition, signage must be placed indicating which type of radiation area one may expect to encounter: "Radiation Area"—an accessible area where an individual could receive a dose equivalent in excess of 0.005 rem (0.05 mSv) in 1 hour at 30 cm from the radiation source or from any surface that the radiation penetrates; "High Radiation Area"—an accessible area where an individual could receive a dose equivalent in excess of 0.1 rem (1 mSv) in 1 hour at 30 cm from the radiation source or from any surface the radiation penetrates; "Very High Radiation Area"—an accessible area where an individual could receive an absorbed dose in excess of 500 rads (5 grays) in 1 hour at 1 m from a radiation source or from any surface that the radiation penetrates.

OCCUPATIONAL EXPOSURE DOSE LIMITS

According to the CFR part 20, the licensee shall control the occupational dose to individuals older than18 years to 5 rem total body effective dose equivalent per year, 15 rem to the lens of the eye per year, 50.0 rem total organ dose equivalent per year, and 50 rem to the extremities per year. Additionally, the Licensee shall reduce the dose that an individual may be allowed to receive in the current year by the amount of occupational dose received while employed by any other person or facility (i.e., these doses are inclusive for *all* facilities where an individual works at). Additional limits apply to the embryo/fetus of a declared pregnant woman. This declaration consists of formally notifying the employer of the pregnancy *in writing*, and providing an estimated date of conception. The limit of the dose to the embryo/fetus over the entire 9-month period of gestation is 0.5 rem. This dose should be delivered at a fairly uniform rate over the entire gestation period and not delivered in a few large doses. The dose equivalent to the embryo/fetus is the sum of the deep-dose equivalent to the declared pregnant woman, and the dose equivalent to the embryo/fetus resulting from radionuclides in the embryo/fetus and radionuclides in the declared pregnant woman. This rule permits additional 0.05 rem if the declared pregnant worker has greater than 0.45 rem at the time of notification. Monitoring of employees is required if an individual is likely to receive a dose greater than10% of limits (500 mrem/y), receive an intake greater than10% of the annual limit on intake (ALI: the derived limit for the amount of radioactive material taken into the body of an adult worker by inhalation or ingestion in a year), and/or an individual is entering a high or very high radiation area. Summation of internal and external doses is necessary if both internal and external doses are required to be monitored. Every employer is responsible for informing each employee on an *annual basis* of the worker's cumulative radiation dose.

Recordable and Reportable Events

There have been a few changes in recent years regarding misadministration terminology and definitions. The NRC no longer requires that administered doses be within 10% of the prescribed dose; this has now changed to 20%. Many states still have the 10% rule in place, however. In addition, the NRC has changed its terminology in regards to diagnostic reportable events, and it is in now termed a "Medical Event." The corresponding criteria are incorrect radiopharmaceutical administered to patient, diagnostic dose differing from prescribed dose by greater than 20%, or administration of radiopharmaceutical by an unprescribed route. The difference between a diagnostic recordable event and a diagnostic medical event essentially is governed by the amount of dose that a patient receives as a result of the error. A recordable event is one in which the whole-body dose is *less than* 5 rem and any single organ dose is less than 50 rem. In a diagnostic medical event, the whole-body dose exceeds 5 rem and any single organ dose is greater than 50 rem. A therapeutic medical event occurs if the administered dose was not within 20% of prescribed dose. Medical events/reportable events require documenting the details of the error and notifying the NRC/state in writing of the misadministration, its effect, if any, on the individual(s) who received the misadministration, and that the referring physician and affected individual was notified of the error. Also to be included are what actions, if any, have been taken or are planned to prevent a recurrence. This should be reported to the NRC no later than the next calendar day after discovery of the medical event. Recordable events require documenting details of the event as above and keeping a record of it for 3 years.

Receiving, Storing, and Disposing of Radioactive Materials

Most nuclear medicine departments have their radiopharmaceuticals delivered to them. These packages must be received and surveyed according to NRC regulations. In addition, every package containing radioisotopes must be logged in appropriately. This includes recording the radionuclide, the product name, the chemical form, the physical form, and the lot number. The time, date, and activity at time of calibration also needs to be recorded, as does the time, date, and activity at time of receipt, shipper's package identifying number, and initials of person receiving the package. These packages need to be monitored for contamination if the package bears DOT radioactive material labels, or the package is crushed, damaged, or leaking. The recipient must immediately notify final delivery carrier and the NRC regional office if removable contamination limits are exceeded and/or external radiation exposure rate limits are exceeded. If your license requires you to survey every package received by your department, results of this monitoring must be recorded in a logbook. Radiation surveys are conducted both with a GM counter and via wipe tests. The GM counter tests are performed at the surface of the package and at 1 m above the surface. Wipe surveys are performed on all sides of the container. Security of nuclear medicine departments is a focus of inspectors. Areas that store radioactive materials must employ some sort of security (locked doors, keycard access, etc.) to prevent theft or access to unauthorized individuals. Items that are contaminated with or have residual amounts of radioactivity on them can be held behind lead shielding until they decay to background levels (generally 10 half-lives of the radionuclide), at which time they can be thrown away as regular trash.

Suggested Reading

Chandra R. *Nuclear Medicine Physics: The Basics*. Lippincott Williams & Wilkins; 2004.

QUESTIONS AND ANSWERS

1. A patient is suspected to have multinodular goiter of the thyroid gland. Which of the following radionuclides is best suited to image the thyroid gland?
   A. 5 mCi $Na^{131}I$
   B. 5 mCi $Na^{123}I$
   C. 5 mCi $Na^{99m}TcO_4$
   D. 5mCi ^{201}Tl Chloride

   ANSWER: C. $Na^{99m}TcO_4$. ^{131}I is not used for routine diagnostic imaging of patients with a thyroid gland. The imaging characteristics of ^{131}I are poor, due to its 364 keV photon. More importantly, if the dose listed in choice A was administered, it would have resulted in a dose of approximately 5000 rads to the thyroid gland (1000 rad per mCi of ^{131}I). Although it can be used to image the thyroid gland, ^{123}I is not used at this dose in a routine diagnostic scan, as it would also give a high dose to the thyroid gland, albeit less than ^{131}I (10 rad per mCi of `^{123}I). The 159 keV photons emitted by ^{123}I are ideal for the gamma camera imaging system, and a thyroid uptake can also be performed with the same dose. The usual dose of ^{123}I for imaging of the thyroid gland is 200 to 400 μCi. $Na^{99m}TcO_4$ results in the lowest dose to the thyroid gland of the thyroid imaging agents (1 rad per 5 mCi of $Na^{99m}TcO_4$), and also has excellent imaging characteristics. It is technically challenging to do a thyroid uptake with $Na^{99m}TcO_4$, so a small amount of ^{131}I or ^{123}I is used for the uptake portion of the study (if performed). It should be noted that dose to the thyroid per unit of activity quoted above assumed a normal thyroid uptake. ^{201}Tl is not used to image the thyroid, although it is sometimes used in parathyroid adenoma imaging.

2. The patient in the prior question is indeed diagnosed with multinodular goiter. The ordering clinician asks that you treat the patient with a therapeutic dose of radioactive iodine. Which of the following is the correct dose rate and distance to avoiding having the patient confined to the hospital?
   A. 5 mR/h at 1 m from chest
   B. 10 mR/h at 1 m from the chest
   C. 5 mR/h at 3 m from the chest
   D. 10 mR/h at 3 m from the chest

   ANSWER: A. 5 mR/h at 1 m from chest.

3. A technologist asks you to review at a bone scan. The image quality is severely deficient, with poor resolution and contrast. Which of the following is the *least* likely explanation for the described appearance?
   A. Nonfunctional PMT
   B. Patient too far away from collimator
   C. Incorrect collimator used

   ANSWER: B. A solitary nonfunctional PMT would give a focal round (or possibly hexagonal) defect within the field of view. All other choices can result in "diffuse" poor image quality.

4. What is the allowable limit of ^{99}Mo in an eluate of ^{99m}Tc at the time of administration?
   A. 10 mg per 1 mL of ^{99m}Tc
   B. 10 mCi per 1 mCi of ^{99m}Tc
   C. 0.15 μg per 1 mL of ^{99m}Tc
   D. 0.15 μCi per 1 mCi of ^{99m}Tc

   ANSWER: D. 0.15 μCi per 1 mCi of ^{99m}Tc. The permissible amount of Al^{3+} is 10 mg per 1 mL of ^{99m}Tc.

5. Which of the following parameters is tested with a point source of ^{99m}Tc?
   A. Extrinsic uniformity
   B. Intrinsic uniformity
   C. Spatial resolution
   D. Linearity

   ANSWER: B. Intrinsic uniformity is performed with the collimator removed from the imaging system, and a point source located a predetermined distance from the crystal face (on the order of 1–2 m). All other choices use a sheet/flood source.

6. Which of the following is an acceptable amount of radiation exposure in 1 hour for an area declared as an unrestricted area?
   A. 10 mrem
   B. 5 mrem
   C. 2 mrem
   D. 1 mrem

   ANSWER: C. 2 mrem in 1 hour.

7. You are preparing to perform an ^{89}Sr therapy on a patient with painful osseous metastases from prostate carcinoma. A helpful colleague recommends that you shield the ^{89}Sr dose with lead shielding. You respond.
   A. Lead shielding is not necessary, as β− particle emissions from the radiopharmaceutical are not very penetrating.
   B. Lead shielding is not necessary, as it may increase the dose of radiation that you will receive.
   C. Thank you very much, that is very thoughtful of you. Lead shielding is just what I was looking for.
   D. How could you possibly have made partner before me?

   ANSWER: B. Lead shielding is in fact not desired, as it can cause penetrating bremsstrahlung x-rays to be produced. Although D may be a valid observation, it is not the best choice for this question.

8. A V/Q scan has been ordered for a patient suspected of having pulmonary thromboembolism. As the patient has severe COPD, you opt to use ^{133}Xe as your ventilation agent. Which of the following statements is *true*?
   A. Vents should be positioned at or near the ceiling.
   B. Ventilation portion of the study should be performed first.
   C. Ventilation portion of the study should be performed in a positive pressure room.

D. Ventilation portion of the study is best imaged in the anterior projection.

ANSWER: B. The ventilation portion of the study should be performed first. If the perfusion portion was performed first, the downscatter phenomenon would degrade the ^{133}Xe ventilation images. ^{133}Xe studies should be performed in a *negative* pressure room (to keep a spill from exiting the room). Because ^{133}Xe is heavier than air gas, vents for "cleaning up" a spill are best situated close to the floor. ^{133}Xe ventilation studies are acquired in the posterior projection, as pulmonary thromboembolisms are more likely to go posteriorly. Attenuation of ^{133}Xe's 81 keV photon from overlying breast or chest wall also lessens the utility of the anterior projection.

9. Concerning adult workers, which of the following is correct regarding occupational dose limits?
   A. 50 rem total body effective dose equivalent per year
   B. 50 rem to the lens of the eye per year
   C. 50 rem to the extremities per year
   D. 50 rem total body effective dose per year at each facility they work

   ANSWER: C. Adult workers are allowed 50 rem to the extremities per year. In addition, adult workers are allowed 5 rem total body effective dose equivalent per year, 15 rem to the lens of the eye per year, and 50 rem total organ dose equivalent per year. These doses are for inclusive for ALL facilities that an individual works at.

10. A patient presents to your clinic for a stress myocardial perfusion study. When the patient reaches peak stress, the technologist administers the radiotracer, and the stress portion of the study is completed as per the protocol. When the patient is imaged 1 hour later, no cardiac activity is seen but solely osseous structures. Which of the following steps do you now need to take?
    A. Document details of the occurrence
    B. Notify the NRC/state in writing of the misadministration
    C. Notify the NRC/state of plans for preventing recurrence
    D. All of the above

    ANSWER: A. Document details of the occurrence. This is a recordable event, not a medical event (the former "reportable event"); the wrong radiopharmaceutical was administered, but the whole-body dose would be less than 5 R and single organ dose would be less than 50 R.

91 SKELETAL NUCLEAR MEDICINE

Pradeep G. Bhambhvani

INTRODUCTION

Bone scan has been available and used for decades to image the skeletal system. It is very sensitive for pathology; but lacks specificity. It can image the entire skeletal system at a relatively low cost and therefore, remains popular for skeletal imaging. Bone scinntigraphy the normal bone response to pathology and not the disease itself.

RADIOPHARMACEUTICALS

The radiotracer most commonly used for bone scan is Tc-99m methylene diphosphonate (MDP), where technetium-99-m is the radioactive component and MDP the biological component. MDP binds to the hydroxyapatite present in the osteoid matrix. Tc-99m MDP can be prepared from a simple kit, where free pertechnetate is added to a vial containing MDP, stabilizers and stannous ion, the latter helps with reducing the valence state of technetium and thereby helps binding of technetium-99m with MDP. Free pertechnetate results when there is inadequate stannous ion available to reduce technetium and is evident as tracer activity in the salivary glands, thyroid gland, and stomach. This results in poor quality images and therefore reduces the sensitivity of the bone scan. After IV injection, the Tc-99m MDP is taken up by the osteoid matrix of the bone and also at other sites of calcification. Approximately 50% of the dose is taken up by bone and the remaining gets excreted by the kidneys. Peak bony uptake occurs 1 hour after injection, and imaging is usually done 2 to 4 hours after tracer injection for optimal skeletal-to-background ratios. Tracer uptake is directly proportional to the amount of osteoid matrix and blood flow. Additional radiotracers are available for imaging the skeletal system including Gallium-67, Samarium-153, and F-18, the latter is used in PET imaging.

IMAGING PROTOCOL

Typical bone scan done for evaluation of skeletal metastases involves IV injection of radiotracer and subsequent delayed imaging 2 to 4 hours later. An average dose for adult is 20 mCi (740 mBq). Patients are encouraged to keep themselves well hydrated and void frequently to minimize radiation to the urinary bladder. Whole-body scan and planar images are obtained for suspicious or symptomatic regions. Additional SPECT (single photon emission computed tomography) can be obtained of specific areas of interest to improve image contrast resolution, and accurate lesion localization, as in imaging of the spine and facial bones. In instances where skeletal infection, trauma, prosthesis loosening and RSD are clinical concerns, a three-phase bone scan can be done. The "flow" phase involves the first minute of imaging after tracer injection over the area of concern. The "pool" phase involves imaging the soft tissues in the regions of interest 5 to 15 minutes after tracer injection and the "delayed" phase is conventional delayed imaging of the osseous structures done 2 to 4 hours after tracer injection.

NORMAL AND ABNORMAL BIODISTRIBUTION

In a normal bone scan, the radiotracer uptake is essentially symmetrical. Careful patient positioning is necessary to avoid apparent asymmetry. Most pathological states involving the bone invoke an osteoblastic response, seen on a bone scan as increased uptake of Tc-99m MDP. This is usually seen as sclerotic lesions on radiographs, although the scintigraphic findings frequently precede the radiographic findings. Diminished uptake can be seen in areas of bone destruction associated with aggressive metastases, although usually even with lytic lesions, there is increased blood flow and attempt at reactive bone repair, seen as areas of increased radiotracer uptake.

In a child, intense uptake is seen in the growth plate complex, which diminishes with advancing age until fusion of the epiphyseal plate occurs. Frequently child immobilization is required to obtain satisfactory images. Attention to the region of the growth plate is necessary as there is a tendency of infection and metastasis to favor the metaphysis. The growth plate complex appears globular in infants and as the child begins to walk, it appears more linear. Metabolic dysfunction resulting from chronic kidney disease and chronic steroid therapy may result in decreased growth plate uptake.

The sacroiliac joints appear to have increased uptake, thought to be due to weight bearing. Altered weight bearing and stress patterns may result in abnormal tracer accumulations in the asymptomatic extremity. Correlation with history is necessary in such instances.

The skull is very variable in appearance. Persistent visualization of the skull sutures in adult life may be normal, however when marked, can be seen in renal osteodystrophy. Diffuse uptake in the calvarium, especially in the frontal region can be seen in benign hyperostosis frontalis interna. In infants, the base of the skull has increased uptake.

Focal uptake at the sternal manubrial junction is a normal finding and does not indicate pathology. Sternal foramina described in the lower sternum appear as uniform circular regions of radiotracer activity surrounding an area of central photopenia is also a normal variant.

In the lower thoracic and lumbar spine, the vertebrae are better identified, when compared to the cervical, upper and mid-thoracic vertebrae. Also the normal curvature of the spine causes portions of the spine closer to the detector to appear hotter than other regions.

Increased uptake in the patellae is commonly seen in the bone scan and usually ascribed to degenerative change.

In women, mild and diffuse uptake in breasts and uterus may be normally seen, although focal uptake may be indicative of pathology.

Arthritic changes involving the weight-bearing joints in the lower extremities and also the sternoclavicular and acromioclavicular joints can be seen.

External artifacts from metallic and other objects, like belts, coins, breast implants, pacemakers may appear as regions of decreased uptake/photopenia.

Renal and urinary bladder activity is normally seen, as the tracer is excreted by the kidneys. Reduced kidney activity and persistent background activity may be an indication of kidney disease, although more often poor visualization of the kidneys is a result of increased tracer accumulation in the skeletal system, associated with the "superscan," seen in diffuse skeletal metastatic disease, or metabolic bone disease such as renal osteodystrophy, severe thyrotoxicosis, or acromegaly. In some instances, the kidneys may be low lying or pelvic in location, as after renal transplant or with horseshoe-shaped kidneys. Prominent radiotracer pelvicaliceal accumulation in the upright position may be an indication of obstructive uropathy. If the renal cortical activity is greater than or equal to the lumbar spine, consider drug therapy or iron overload, as in hemachromatosis or after multiple blood transfusions.

Significant bladder activity will limit complete evaluation of the pelvis and therefore voiding is a must prior to imaging.

External urinary contamination is usually evident on imaging without much difficulty.

SPECT imaging of the pelvis may result in streaking artifacts because of increasing urinary bladder activity during image acquisition.

Bisphosphonates therapy results in diffusely decreased skeletal uptake of Tc-99m MDP.

Radiation therapy is also associated with decreased radiotracer uptake at the site of skeletal radiation. Knowledge of radiation history is necessary in such cases.

Soft tissue accumulation of Tc-99m MDP is well reported in various disease entities, like neoplasms, hematomas, heterotopic bone formation or myositis ossificans, in the myocardium in amyloidosis, in splenic infarcts, pleural effusions, ascites, and at sites of dystrophic and metastatic calcification. Diffuse uptake can be seen in normal breasts and gynecomastia; however focal regions of activity in the breast can be associated with benign and malignant etiologies. Tracer uptake in visceral organs, like in the lungs and stomach is seen in metabolic disorders like hyperparathyroidism.

EVALUATION OF METASTATIC BONE DISEASE

Bone metastases are commonly associated with several malignancies. Malignancies involving breast, prostate, lung, and kidneys represent the source of approximately 80% of all osseous metastases. Patients present without symptoms or with bone pain, fractures and sometimes as spinal cord compression. Bone metastases occur via direct, lymphatic or hematogenous dissemination. Batson's plexus is a mesh of vertebral veins that connect with veins of the brain, skull, ribs, viscera and the vertebral column; they have been implicated in skeletal metastases associated with breast and prostate cancer.

Bone scan is much more sensitive than radiographs in detecting skeletal metastases, with the reported sensitivity between 62% and 100%. Bone scan can detect as little as 5% to 15% in bone turnover, whereas it requires a 50% loss in bone mineral content before the lesion can be seen on radiographs. The sensitivity is lower in detection of purely osteolytic cancers like multiple myeloma and other osteolytic skeletal metastasis. Lytic lesions associated with multiple myeloma are detected approximately half the time on bone scan, as compared to 80% detection on skeletal survey. Therefore, skeletal surveys are preferred in evaluation of osseous involvement in patients with multiple myeloma. This is a reflection of relative absence of reactive bone repair, possibly due to the production of an osteoblast inhibitory factor in this condition. Patterns of uptake in multiple myeloma would include normal, cold or photopenic areas or occasionally focal areas of increased uptake. Bone scan may also be normal in instances where the metastases are localized to the bone marrow. Occasionally in cases of aggressive tumors, there may be an absence of a reparative response and a cold or photopenic lesion is noted. Approximately 90% of patients with skeletal metastases present with multiple lesions of varying size, shape, and intensity. Only 10% of patients with cancer present with a solitary bone metastasis. The percentage increases to 35% when two new lesions were detected, and reaches 100% when five new lesions were identified. Specifically a solitary rib lesion has approximately a 10% probability of representing a metastasis in a patient with known malignancy. Approximately 80% of all osseous metastatic lesions are in the axial skeleton. In the spine, sensitivity of lesion detection increases with use of SPECT, which may also be helpful in distinguishing benign from malignant processes, based on patterns of uptake on bone scan, specifically with uptake in the body itself favoring malignancy.

FLARE PHENOMENON

The flare phenomenon, which indicates a good response of bone metastases to treatment, is associated with increasing intensity and/or number of lesions on bone scan. It can be seen with bone scan as well as F-18 PET scan. Patients are typically asymptomatic and corresponding radiographs usually show sclerosis of the lesions. The phenomenon is usually seen between 2 weeks to 3 months following treatment, but can occasionally be seen as late as 6 months after treatment. Continued increase in the number and intensity of lesions beyond 6 months after treatment completion is usually indicative of disease progression. In general, it is appropriate to wait for approximately 3 months following completion of treatment regimen prior to repeating the bone scan. The diagnosis of flare phenomenon requires two criteria:

1. Increased intensity and/or number of lesions on bone scan (thought to be secondary to increased osteoblastic activity associated with healing of bone metastasis) and
2. Subsequent decreased uptake in these lesions on repeat bone scan after 3 months.

PROSTATE CANCER

Bone metastases are commonly seen in prostate cancer, and occur in up to 85% of patients dying of prostate cancer. Also patients who have bone metastases on scintigraphy at presentation have a higher mortality than those without. Bone metastases are uncommon (less than 1%) in patients with PSA less than 10 ng/mL and proportionally increase in incidence with rising PSA values, although PSA values are unreliable for assessment of metastases in those patients who have undergone androgen deprivation therapy. The incidence of osseous metastasis is also directly proportional to increasing Gleason histological grades, as all patients with a "superscan" appearance of widespread metastases have high histological grades.

LUNG CANCER

Many patients with lung cancer present with disseminated metastatic disease including skeletal metastases, especially those with small cell and anaplastic cancer. Interestingly arterial metastases are more commonly seen with lung cancer, as these tumors can easily invade the vasculature. Thus involvement of the appendicular skeleton is more commonly seen in lung cancer.

In addition to the focal lesions noted in bone scan associated with osseous metastases, lung cancer may be notable for hypertrophic osteoarthropathy (HOA). Hypertrophic osteoarthropathy occurs in up to 10% of patients with lung cancer and involves clubbing of the fingers and toes, and periostitis of the long bones. Patients may have pain and swelling about the wrists and less commonly the ankles and knees. Radiographs may reveal periosteal new bone formation. Bone scan is notable for increased activity along the periosteum of long bones ("tramline sign"). Hypertrophic osteoarthropathy tends to resolve following tumor resection. It can also be seen in other chronic illnesses including, bronchiectasis, cystic fibrosis, mesothelioma, pneumoconiosis, cyanotic heart disease, and inflammatory bowel disease.

BREAST CANCER

The skeleton is the most common site of distant metastases in breast cancer. Detection of skeletal metastasis with bone scintigraphy precedes radiographic detection, by an average of 4 to 6 months. In breast cancer patients, there is a low positive yield for the bone scan in patients with asymptomatic stage I disease and those with small primary tumors (less than 2 cm), therefore the routine use of preoperative bone scanning in these patients is probably unnecessary. Approximately 5% of patients present with stage IV disease (distant metastases), and those with only bone metastases have a significantly better survival when compared to those with bone and extraskeletal metastases. Women with breast cancer, present with bone metastasis at the time of diagnosis, have a markedly worse prognosis. In patients with breast cancer, 21% of patients relapsed with a solitary bone metastasis, the most common location being the spine. However, an isolated sternal lesion, which is usually a benign finding in the setting of breast cancer, has a 75% to 80% likelihood of being an osseous metastasis.

NEUROBLASTOMA

It is one of the most common extracranial solid tumors in children and is frequently associated with skeletal metastasis. Frequently the primary tumor is seen on the bone scan. Lesions are typically multifocal in the metaphysis, commonly in the proximal humeri, distal femurs, and proximal tibiae, although involvement of the skull, vertebrae, ribs, and pelvis is also commonly seen. Imaging with I-123 or I-131 MIBG is more sensitive than bone scan for metastatic evaluation, though a combination of both imaging is complementary

OTHER TUMORS

There is decreased sensitivity in detection of bone metastases from kidney tumors, as they are associated with "cold or photopenic" lesions, and are therefore better assessed with skeletal survey or MRI.

Focal or diffuse uptake may be seen in Hodgkin's lymphoma, although presently lymphomas are best evaluated with F-18 FDG PET-CT.

Focal or diffuse abnormalities may be seen in systemic mastocytosis, a condition associated with tissue mast cell infiltration. Patients complain of bone pain, abdominal pain, flushing, diarrhea, and skin rashes.

A spectrum of scintigraphic findings are seen in histiocytosis, including focally increased uptake noted in unifocal eosinophilic granuloma, negative scans, and cold lesions, some with a peripheral rim of activity.

PRIMARY BONE TUMORS

There is a limited role of bone scintigraphy in evaluation of primary bone tumors, as MRI provides additional information regarding soft tissue involvement and tumor margins. Bone scan is useful in evaluating skeletal metastatic spread and response to therapy in these instances.

OSTEOGENIC SARCOMA

It is the most common primary malignant bone tumor. It occurs most commonly in the second decade of life, in the metaphysis of long bones, with 50% of cases occurring about the knee. Tracer accumulation is increased with patchy areas of decreased uptake within the overall increased region of activity. The major use of bone scintigraphy is in detection of skip lesions in the medullary bone adjacent to the primary tumor and detection of distant skeletal metastases. Local evaluation after limb amputation is important, as increased activity in the stump after 6 months may indicate local recurrence.

EWING SARCOMA

It is the second most common primary bone tumor after osteogenic sarcoma. More than 80% of the Ewing sarcomas occur in patients younger than 20 years, and interestingly blacks are rarely affected. The tumor usually arises in the diaphysis of a long bone (humerus, femur, tibia, or fibula), but 20% arise in the pelvis and lesions in the pelvis are associated with a worse prognosis. The most common presenting symptoms are pain and swelling. Patients may complain of systemic symptoms such as fever, anorexia, weight loss, and fatigue, and the clinical presentation may be confused with chronic osteomyelitis. The lesion usually produces a "moth-eaten" pattern of bone destruction on plain film radiographs and the lesion is typically "hot" on blood flow, pool, and delayed bone scan images. Bone scan is useful to assess for skeletal metastasis and monitoring therapy. The incidence of distant metastasis at the time of presentation ranges from 10% to 40%, most commonly to the lungs and bone. On follow-up, the skeleton is the first site of metastatic disease in approximately 25% of patients.

OSTEOID OSTEOMA

Osteoid osteoma is a benign bone tumor that occurs most commonly in adolescents and young adults, with 90% of cases seen in patients younger than 25 years. The osteoma is most commonly cortical but can be medullary, periosteal, or intracapsular in location. Typical clinical presentation is localized bone pain, worse at night and relieved with aspirin. The proximal femur and tibia account for a majority of the cases. When the lesion occurs in the spine (10% of cases), it nearly always occurs in the posterior elements (50%) and is frequently associated with a painful scoliosis with the convexity of the curve oriented away from the side of the lesion. The most common location of a spinal lesion is the lumbar spine.

On plain films, the very vascular nidus of the osteoid osteoma is lucent and is surrounded by dense, reactive sclerosis. MRI demonstrates decreased signal intensity because of the reactive bony sclerosis, but the nidus may produce a brighter signal.

On bone scan, the lesion is hot on all three phases. On delayed images, the nidus may be seen as a focal area of even greater activity within the diffuse abnormality. A normal bone scan virtually excludes the diagnosis of an osteoid osteoma. Bone scan is also useful in the follow-up of these patients after treatment, as persistent scintigraphic abnormality may be indicative of residual disease. SPECT is very useful for precise localization. Intraoperative localizing probes and monitoring radioactivity of removed bone fragments have been used during surgery.

FIBROUS DYSPLASIA

Usually there is intense tracer activity associated with monostotic or polyostotic fibrous dysplasia.

HETEROTOPIC OSSIFICATION

This is also referred to as "myositis ossificans," which is usually seen after trauma, other etiologies of heterotopic ossification include after paralysis or spinal cord injury, or hip joint replacement. Serial bone scans are useful to evaluate the maturity or the degree of inflammatory activity in myositis ossificans. Recurrence of heterotopic ossification is decreased when mature calcification is excised. Decreasing MDP uptake is seen as the heterotopic ossification matures. Three-phase bone scanning is very sensitive for the early detection of myositis ossificans.

OSTEOMYELITIS

Osteomyelitis is infection localized to bone or the bone marrow. It can occur as a result of hematogenous seeding, contiguous spread of infection to bone from adjacent soft tissues and joints, or direct inoculation of infection into the bone as a result of trauma or surgery. In long bone hematogenous osteomyelitis, the most common site of infection is in the metaphysis. The major blood vessel to long bones usually penetrates the midshaft of the bone and then travels toward both ends, forming metaphyseal vascular loops just before it hits the epiphyseal plates. Slowed blood flow in these loops along with the absence of basement membranes predisposes the metaphysis to osteomyelitis. For the same reason osteomyelitis involving the epiphysis is uncommon. In the setting of osteomyelitis, inflammatory exudate in the marrow leads to increased intramedullary pressure, with subsequent extension of exudate into the bone cortex where it can rupture through the periosteum. If this occurs, the periosteal blood supply is interrupted, leading to necrosis. The resulting pieces of separated dead bone are known as "sequestra." New bone formation in regions of periosteal damage is known as an "involucrum." Acute osteomyelitis is infection in bone prior to development of sequestra, whereas after the formation of sequestra, the infection is considered to be chronic. In children the femur and tibia are the most common sites of osteomyelitis.

Hematogenous osteomyelitis is usually monomicrobial, while contiguous osteomyelitis may be either polymicrobial or monomicrobial. *Staphylococcus aureus*, coagulase-negative staphylococci, and aerobic gram-negative bacilli are the most common organisms; other pathogens implicated include streptococci, enterococci, anaerobes, fungi, and mycobacteria. Acute osteomyelitis typically presents with dull pain at the involved site, with or without movement, local tenderness, warmth, erythema, swelling, and fever. Acute osteomyelitis can also present as septic arthritis. Chronic osteomyelitis presents with pain, erythema, or swelling, sometimes in association with a draining sinus tract. If exposed bone is present, osteomyelitis is very likely.

Establishing an accurate and early diagnosis of osteomyelitis is critical, since the infection can require prolonged antibiotic therapy and/or aggressive surgical intervention. The gold standard for diagnosis is isolation of bacteria from a bone biopsy sample obtained via sterile technique, and histological findings of inflammation and osteonecrosis. Laboratory tests are usually nonspecific. Radiographs are limited by their sensitivity and specificity. In early infection, radiographs may be normal, whereas in chronic osteomyelitis; typical findings include cortical erosion, periosteal reaction, mixed lucency and sclerosis. MRI is very sensitive for the detection of acute osteomyelitis. It is useful in delineating the extent of cortical destruction and evaluating the bone marrow and associated soft tissue inflammation, as in the setting of cellulitis or myositis. Additionally it can also demonstrate sinus tracts, fistulas, and abscesses.

Scintigraphy is especially useful early on when radiographic abnormalities are not evident, and initiation of early treatment prevents irreversible bone damage. Sensitivity greater than 90% is described in several series for diagnosis of osteomyelitis. Characteristic finding in a "three-phase bone scan" is increased activity in the blood flow and pool phases and intense focal uptake in the involved bone in the delayed phase. However, these findings are not specific for infection as similar findings have been described in neuropathic joints, fractures, including stress fractures, gout, rheumatoid arthritis, etc. SPECT is very useful in evaluating the skull or the spine. In the absence of underlying bone disease, the overall sensitivity for a three-phase bone scan is 94% and the specificity 95% for detection of osteomyelitis. In instances where bone remodeling may be present, the sensitivity is 95%, but the specificity declines to 33%. In an adult a negative bone scan essentially rules out infection.

In children symptoms can be unreliable and infection could be multifocal, therefore it is important to perform a whole-body scan. Subperiosteal pus/edema, joint effusion, or vasospasm can decrease vascularity to the infected area. Therefore, in a child, increased blood flow may be absent, even when there is a clear abnormality on delayed images. Positioning is extremely important especially in children, as activity in the growth plates may mask the focus of infection in the neighboring metaphysis, if the camera is not perpendicular to the physis and subtle asymmetric activity may be the only indicator of an early osteomyelitis. Photopenic (cold) defects on delayed images are uncommon but may be seen particularly in the very early stages of the infection. Therefore in children, if the bone scan is normal initially and if there is sufficient clinical suspicion, a repeat examination should be repeated in 2 to 3 days, or a gallium examination may be performed. As the condition evolves into the sub acute phase, hyperemia rather than ischemia becomes the dominant finding.

MRI is probably the modality of choice when evaluating patients for suspected vertebral osteomyelitis. Gallium scan combined with bone scan, has a 86% accuracy in the detection of vertebral osteomyelitis, can be done in those patients who cannot tolerate MR. Indium 111 leukocyte imaging is not as sensitive for infection of the spine as for other musculoskeletal infections and may be falsely negative in up to 80% of cases.

NEUROPATHIC FOOT

Neuroarthropathy develops most commonly in the tarsal and tarsometatarsal joints (60%) followed by the metatarsophalangeal joints (30%) and tibiotalar joints (10%). The most common cause of Charcot joints is diabetes mellitus. It predisposes these patients to infection because of underlying neuropathy, vasculopathy, and leukocyte dysfunction. Loss of pain sensation and proprioception, facilitated by vasculopathy and WBC dysfunction, leads to repeated trauma, ulceration, and infection. The most frequent sites of infection are pressure points over bony prominences, including the metatarsal heads, phalanges, and the calcaneus. Diagnosis of osteomyelitis complicating the neuropathic joint is very challenging, as the combination of arthropathy, ulceration, and soft tissue infection results in increased activity on all phases of the bone scan, resulting in low specificity. Radiographs are poorly sensitive in this situation. Combined tagged WBC and Tc-99m sulfur colloid marrow imaging is the procedure of choice for the evaluation of patients with Charcot joints, as it can better identify those patients with true osteomyelitis, where one would typically see accumulation of labeled WBCs and lack of or decreased marrow activity. MRI complements scintigraphy in evaluation of suspected osteomyelitis in the Neuropathic foot.

PROSTHESIS EVALUATION

Approximately 500 000 hip and knee arthroplasties are performed annually in the United States. Complications can arise after surgery, including infection, aseptic loosening, joint dislocation, heterotopic ossification, and fracture. Differentiating infection from aseptic loosening, the most common complication of arthroplasty is challenging. Because the treatment of these entities is radically different, accurate differentiation is very important. Treatment of loosening is usually a single step revision arthroplasty, whereas for infection, treatment involves removal of hardware, prolonged antibiotic therapy, and eventual revision arthroplasty.

Bone scan finding of periprosthetic activity is very nonspecific. The increased periprosthetic activity reflects increased bone mineral turnover, which can be seen in infection as well as other conditions like aseptic loosening. Up to 1 year after hip arthroplasty, patterns of periprosthetic uptake are variable, beyond 1 year in case of cemented hip prosthesis, most asymptomatic patients have a normal scan; however, up to 10% of asymptomatic patients will have some periprosthetic uptake despite no complications. In case of cementless or porous coated hip arthroplasty, where bony in growth occurs into the porous coating applied to the prosthesis surface, persistent uptake beyond 1 year is even more prevalent. Similar observations have been made with knee arthroplasty. Although not commonly done, a baseline study done with serial imaging would be more useful in following these patients. Typically, there is diffusely increased periprosthetic activity associated with infection, as opposed to aseptic loosening in which there is a focal uptake noted around the prosthesis. However, these findings are not specific and significant overlap of findings exists in infection and loosening. Conventional bone scan has a sensitivity of 65%, specificity of 70%, and an accuracy of 70% for the diagnosis of infected prosthesis. However bone scan is useful as a screening examination because a normal scan essentially rules out a prosthesis complication. Combined leukocyte–marrow imaging is helpful to overcome issues created by variable marrow distribution postoperatively and should be used regularly in evaluating a painful arthroplasty. It is based on the observation that infection stimulates the accumulation of tagged WBC and suppresses the uptake of sulfur colloid in the bone marrow. The reported sensitivity, specificity and accuracy with combined imaging are greater than 90%.

BONE MARROW SCINTIGRAPHY

This procedure is performed with Tc-99m sulfur colloid in patients with sickle cell anemia, to demonstrate marrow expansion and marrow infarctions. It is however unable to differentiate between acute and chronic marrow infarction. In infection, it is used along with labeled WBC to evaluate osteomyelitis and in evaluation of a painful prosthesis to differentiate infection from aseptic loosening.

METABOLIC BONE DISORDERS

HYPERPARATHYROIDISM

Primary hyperparathyroidism in most patients will have a normal bone scan. In general, only severe cases of the disorder demonstrate findings on the bone scan. Scintigraphic findings include increased activity on delayed images can be seen in the axial skeleton, the long bones, the mandible, the skull, the acromioclavicular joints, hands, and the sternum (areas which frequently demonstrate demineralization on plain film). Focal abnormalities may be seen with Brown tumors, or compression fractures. Soft tissue tracer activity has been reported in sites of metastatic calcification (often the lungs, kidneys, and stomach).

In secondary hyperparathyroidism, unlike primary hyperparathyroidism, the bone scan is usually abnormal. There is diffusely increased skeletal activity, with decreased renal activity producing a "superscan" appearance in severe renal osteodystrophy. This is due to the generalized increase in bone turnover and not just tracer retention caused by renal failure. Absence of bladder activity makes it more likely that the superscan appearance is from renal osteodystrophy rather than metastatic disease or other metabolic diseases. Additional findings seen include the beading of activity along the costochondral junctions ("rosary bead appearance"), diffuse calvarial uptake, mask-like periorbital accumulation, uptake in the maxilla, mandible, and sternum. Brown tumors may also produce focal abnormalities.

OSTEOMALACIA

The bone in this condition is inadequately mineralized. It results from dietary insufficiency of calcium, phosphorus, and/or Vitamin D, GI malabsorption or inadequate Vitamin D synthesis. Bone scan is reliable in detection of Looser zones or pseudofractures, seen frequently and symmetrically in the ribs.

PAGET DISEASE OF BONE

Paget disease or osteitis deformans is a benign disorder of bone remodeling and affects between 3% and 4% of the population older than 40 years and up to 10% to 11% after age 80 years. The exact cause of Paget disease is not known; a viral etiology has been postulated. Pathologically, there is an increased osteoclastic resorption of bone followed by intense osteoblastic activity and increased vascularity. The most commonly involved bones are of the axial skeleton, spine (30%–75%), skull (25%–65%), pelvis (30%–75%), and proximal long bones (25%–35%, femur and tibia). Monostotic disease occurs in 10% to 35% of patients and is more often seen in the axial skeleton. Polyostotic disease (65%–90%) occurs more commonly. Paget disease can be asymptomatic, and is often found incidentally when working up increased serum alkaline phosphatase or abnormal radiographs done for other reasons. Clinical features include local pain, tenderness, bowing deformities, kyphosis of the spine, and bone expansion.

Classically, there are three phases to this disorder—lytic phase, mixed phase, and blastic phase. Initially, intense osteoclastic activity produces the lytic or incipient active phase. The scintigraphic appearance is fairly typical with intense radiotracer accumulation throughout the affected bone, with the exception of the lytic phase more commonly seen in the skull, where the uptake is mainly noted at the margins of pagetic involvement (osteoporosis circumscripta) and also after therapy. In the long bones, the process begins in the subchondral region of the epiphysis and extends along the shaft in a characteristic V shaped ("flame" or "blade of grass") appearance. Additional patterns and signs have been described including the "Mickey Mouse sign," in a pagetic vertebra, with a typical pattern of an inverted triangle of three dots indicating involvement of the transverse processes and the "Abe Lincoln sign" with monostotic mandible involvement, etc. Differential diagnosis on bone scan includes malignancy, where typical uptake is more focal and circular, without bony expansion, although sometimes differentiation between Paget disease and skeletal metastasis is very difficult. Scintigraphy is more sensitive than plain films for disease detection during the lytic phase. Scintigraphy is also useful to monitor disease progression while on therapy, where response is associated with regression of scintigraphic abnormalities, although changes in alkaline phosphatase and urinary hydroxyproline and N-terminal telopeptide better monitor response to treatment.

Sarcomatous degeneration occurs in less than 1% of patients with Paget disease. Patients with severe polyostotic disease and males have an increased risk for degeneration. New focal pain and swelling are the most common clinical complaints. The most common location is the hip, pelvis, and shoulder. The most common neoplasm is an osteosarcoma (50%–60% of cases), but pleomorphic sarcoma, chondrosarcoma, fibrosarcoma, giant cell tumor, and malignant fibrous histiocytomas have all been reported. Radiographs may show a new, enlarging lytic lesion. Bone scan commonly reveals decreased uptake of tracer within the lesion in comparison to the adjacent Pagetoid bone, however, increased activity may also be seen. Increased gallium accumulation associated with relatively decreased Tc-99m MDP activity suggests malignant degeneration.

AVASCULAR NECROSIS

There are several etiologies for avascular necrosis, including trauma (most common), idiopathic, steroids, ETOH abuse, sickle cell disease, caisson disease, vasculitis (SLE), pancreatitis, bisphosphonate use, radiation therapy, polycythemia, and Gaucher disease. In children, Legg-Calve-Perthes disease results in avascular necrosis of the femoral head epiphysis. Bone scan findings depend on the time since the vascular insult. With acute interruption of blood flow, infarcted bone is seen as a cold or photopenic region. Once bone repair begins, increased tracer uptake is initially noted at the margin of infarction, which progressively increases into the infarcted zone and eventually normalizes once healing is complete.

COMPLEX REGIONAL PAIN SYNDROME OR REFLEX SYMPATHETIC DYSTROPHY

Complex regional pain syndrome includes a spectrum of motor, sensory, and autonomic findings predominantly affecting the extremities. Clinical findings include pain, swelling, vasomotor changes, functional impairment, and muscle wasting. It can occur after trauma, CVA and other acute illnesses. The classic finding in bone scintigraphy includes increased uptake in the blood flow and blood pool phases reflecting increased vascularity and periarticular uptake in the delayed phase. However, abnormality in all the three phases is seen in less than 50% of patients. The periarticular uptake in the delayed phase has very high sensitivity (greater than 95%), but specificity is decreased in patients with diabetes and foot infections. Bone scan findings vary depending on the time of onset of the syndrome, with the classic findings seen in the initial 5 months. Thereafter the increased flow is not seen and the periarticular uptake may be decreased, normal, or persistently increased.

SKELETAL TRAUMA

Bone scan has an important application in detection of occult skeletal trauma in both children and adults. It allows for detection of trauma at a very early stage predating the radiological findings. Approximately 80% of bone scans will show increased activity at the site of fracture by 24 hours, and 95% by 72 hours, although the elderly and debilitated patients may not show activity for several days. In the latter instances repeat imaging approximately 7 days later is recommended. The time a fracture takes to heal to result in a normal bone scan is variable. Approximately 60% to 80% of nondisplaced and uncomplicated fractures revert to a normal bone scan in 1 year and greater than 95% in 3 years. However in cases where the joint is involved, posttraumatic arthritis can confound or result in indefinite increased uptake on a bone scan.

STRESS FRACTURES

Stress fractures occur because of repetitive activity applied on normal bone. The involved bone reacts to the repetitive stress by internal osseous remodeling, which strengthens the bone to withstand the particular stress. However during the remodeling process, there is a period when bone resorption exceeds bone formation, which temporarily weakens the cortex. Microfractures can result if the stress is continually applied to the bone and eventually an overt fracture may result if these micro fractures are not allowed to heal. Bone scan is very sensitive in these instances and will typically show increased activity, 1 to 2 weeks before radiographic abnormality is apparent. The sensitivity of bone scan for the diagnosis of stress fracture approaches 100%. Typically, increased activity is seen in the blood flow, pool, and delayed images. The metatarsals and the posterior medial cortex of the tibia are the most common locations for stress fractures.

In the sacrum, stress fractures are associated with osteoporosis or prior radiation therapy to the pelvis. This characteristic sacral insufficiency fracture has a "butterfly" or "Honda sign" appearance with fracture lines running vertically through the left and right sides of the bone just medial to the sacroiliac joints, and a transverse fracture just below the level of the sacroiliac joints. Radiographs are typically normal, but may show sclerosis in sacral ala.

Shin splints (stress periosteal reaction) are characterized by abnormal linear (nonfocal) tracer activity along the posteromedial tibial cortex. It is usually seen in runners and results from tearing of muscle fibers anchoring the muscle to the periosteum, resulting in a periosteal reaction. Patients present with exercise-induced pain in the posteromedial distal leg. The radionuclide uptake is usually superficial and mild to moderate in intensity along the distal and posteromedial tibial cortex. No significant increase in blood flow is seen with shin splints, unlike stress fractures.

OSTEOPOROSIS

Osteoporosis is a skeletal condition characterized by low bone mass, which is associated with reduced bone strength and an increased risk of fractures, particularly at the spine, hip, wrist, humerus, and pelvis. Osteoporosis is commonly identified in postmenopausal women most likely related to the decrease in estrogen secretion. Other causes of osteoporosis include corticosteroid use, Cushing's disease, prolonged inactivity, and nutritional deficiencies. Skeletal scintigraphy has very limited role in detection and follow-up of osteoporosis. Bone mineral density is the most important determinant of bone fragility and risk of fracture. Quantitative assessment of bone mineral density (BMD) using Dual energy x-ray absorptiometry is the most common clinically used modality in evaluation of osteoporosis. The normal value for BMD is within one standard deviation of the young adult reference mean (T-score). The WHO has defined osteopenia as a BMD T-score between 1 and 2.5 standard deviations below the young adult reference mean. Osteoporosis is defined as a T-scores, 2.5 standard deviations below the young adult mean.

SUGGESTED READING

Brown ML. Bone scintigraphy in benign and malignant tumors [review]. *Radiol Clin North Am.* 1993;31(4):731-738.

Even-Sapir E. imaging of malignant bone involvement by morphologic, scintigraphic, and hybrid modalities. *J Nucl Med.* 2005;46:1356-1367.

Jacobson AF, Stomper PC, Jochelson MS, Ascoli D, Henderson IC, Kaplan WD. Association between number and sites of new bone scan abnormalities and presence of skeletal metastases in patients with breast cancer. *J Nucl Med.* 1990;31: 387-392.

Love C, Din AS, Tomas MB, Kalapparambath TP, Palestro CJ. Radionuclide bone imaging: an illustrative review. *Radiographics.* 2003;23:341-358.

Palestro CJ, Love C, Tronco GG, Tomas MB, Rini JN. Combined labeled leukocyte and technetium 99m sulfur colloid bone marrow imaging for diagnosing musculoskeletal infection. *Radiographics.* 2006;26:859-870.

Shehab D, Elgazzar AH, Collier BD. Heterotopic ossification. *J Nucl Med.* 2002;43: 346-353.

Smith SE, Murphey MD, Motamedi K, Mulligan ME, Resnik CS, Gannon FH. Radiologic spectrum of Paget disease of bone and its complications with pathologic correlation. *Radiographics.* 2002;22:1191-1216.

Tumeh SS, Beadle G, Kaplan WD: Clinical significance of solitary rib lesions in patients with extraskeletal malignancy. *J Nucl Med.* 1985;26:1140-1143.

QUESTIONS AND ANSWERS

1. In nuclear imaging of the musculoskeletal system, what advantages does SPECT offer over planar imaging?
   A. Better spatial resolution
   B. Faster imaging time
   C. Better image contrast resolution

   ANSWER: C. SPECT imaging offers the advantage of improved image contrast resolution and accurate lesion localization in the three planes over planar imaging. Target to background ratio is improved by removing the overlying tissues, which is not possible in planar imaging. Spatial resolution is degraded with SPECT imaging.

2. Superscan can be seen in all the following conditions *except*:
   A. Osseous metastases
   B. Renal osteodystrophy
   C. Bisphosphonate therapy
   D. Hyperparathyroidism

   ANSWER: C. Diffusely increased skeletal uptake is a unique scintigraphic pattern referred to as "superscan." The renal activity/kidneys are not clearly seen or absent in a superscan. They can be seen in diffuse skeletal metastatic disease, primary hyperparathyroidism, and renal osteodystrophy. Poor skeletal uptake of tracer may be an indication of chronic bisphosphonate therapy.

3. Presence of gastric activity in a whole-body bone scan is suggestive of free pertechnetate, if the following is also seen:
   A. Pulmonary activity
   B. Thyroid activity
   C. Renal and urinary bladder activity
   D. Cerebral activity

   ANSWER: B. Free pertechnetate results when there inadequate stannous ion available to reduce the technetium ion. The free technetium is evident as activity in the salivary glands, thyroid gland, and the stomach. Technetium tagged to MDP is the isotope used in bone scintigraphy. It is predominantly excreted via the kidneys and as a result renal and urinary bladder activity is normally seen in bone scans. Pulmonary, gastric, and renal uptake can be seen in metabolic disorders such as hyperparathyroidism.

4. What is the most common complication following primary joint replacement surgery?
   A. Aseptic joint loosening
   B. Infection
   C. Fracture
   D. Heterotopic ossification

   ANSWER: A. By 10 years after arthroplasty, 50% of prostheses have radiographic evidence of loosening and 30% require revision. Its pathogenesis includes pseudomembranous structure made of histiocytes, giant cells, lymphocytes, plasma cells, and sometimes neutrophils, which develops at the cement bone interface, and osteolysis induced by unsuccessful attempts at phagocytosis induced by particulate debris from component degradation and secretion of cytokines and enzymes. These damage the bone and cartilage leading to osteolysis and prosthesis loosening. The rate of infection following primary joint replacement surgery is approximately 1% for hip prosthesis and 2% for knee joint prosthesis. Following revision surgery, the rates of infection are higher, approximately 3% for hip replacements and 5% for knee joint replacements. Differentiating aseptic loosening, the most common complication of arthroplasty, from infection is challenging.

5. The combined WBC/bone marrow scintigraphy protocol performed for evaluation of osteomyelitis is based on the fact that infection:
   A. Is associated with accumulation of tagged WBC and decreased accumulation of the Tc-99m sulfur colloid in the bone marrow scan

B. Stimulates accumulation of Tc-99m sulfur colloid and decreases accumulation of tagged WBC
C. Stimulates accumulation of both tagged WBC and Tc-99m sulfur colloid
D. Decreases accumulation of both tagged WBC and Tc-99m sulfur colloid

ANSWER: A. Leukocyte imaging may be false-positive because of normal WBC activity in the bone marrow or healing bone, in evaluations of osteomyelitis. Therefore it is used in combination with marrow imaging, where congruent uptake in leukocyte and marrow imaging is consistent with physiologic marrow uptake, but incongruence, where there is WBC uptake and corresponding absence of marrow uptake, is suggestive of infection.

6. What is the most likely etiology for a solitary rib focal lesion on bone scan?
A. Solitary skeletal metastasis
B. Rib fracture
C. Infection
D. Osteoid osteoma

ANSWER: B. Approximately 90% of patients with skeletal metastases present with multiple lesions. Only 10% of patients with cancer present with a solitary bone metastasis. The most common etiology in this instance is related to trauma. In a published trial evaluating solitary focal rib lesions in extraskeletal cancer, only 12% of patients were attributed to have solitary bone lesion on bone scan, the remaining 88% were from benign reasons. Ribs are an unusual location for osteoid osteomas, which are usually seen in the femurs.

7. Which of the following entities is *least likely* to show uptake on bone scan?
A. Bone island
B. Osteoid osteoma
C. Osteomyelitis
D. Paget disease.

ANSWER: A. All the above except bone island are associated with increased flow and bone repair and therefore increased activity on a bone scan. Mild focal uptake may be occasionally seen in bone islands, reflecting the mild metabolic activity of the bone island, usually associated with larger and metabolic bone islands.

8. Which of the following joints is most commonly involved with Charcot arthropathy?
A. Knees
B. Tibiotalar
C. Tarsal and tarsometatarsal
D. Metatarsophalangeal

ANSWER: C. Neuroarthropathy develops most commonly in the tarsal and tarsometatarsal joints (60%) followed by the metatarsophalangeal joints (30%) and tibiotalar joints (10%). The most common cause of Charcot joints is diabetes mellitus. It predisposes these patients to infection because of underlying neuropathy, vasculopathy, and leukocyte dysfunction. Loss of pain sensation and proprioception, facilitated by vasculopathy and WBC dysfunction, leads to repeated trauma, ulceration, and infection. The most frequent sites of infection are pressure points over bony prominences, including the metatarsal heads, phalanges, and the calcaneus. Diagnosis of osteomyelitis complicating the neuropathic joint is very challenging, as the combination of arthropathy, ulceration, and soft tissue infection results in increased activity on all phases of the bone scan, resulting is low specificity. Radiographs are poorly sensitive in this situation. Combined radio labeled WBC and Tc-99m sulfur colloid marrow imaging is the procedure of choice for the evaluation of patients with Charcot joints as it can better identify those patients with true osteomyelitis, where one would typically see accumulation of labeled WBC and lack of or decreased marrow activity. MRI complements scintigraphy in evaluation of suspected osteomyelitis in Charcot arthropathy.

9. What is the most common organism responsible for prosthetic joint infection?
A. *S. aureus*
B. *Staphylococcus epidermidis*
C. *E. Coli*
D. *Pseudomonas aeruginosa*

ANSWER: B. *S. epidermidis* (30%) and *S. aureus* (20%) are the most common offending organisms implicated for prosthetic joint infections. Approximately one-third of joint infections occur within 3 months of the arthroplasty, a third occur within 1 year of implantation and the remainder after 1 year of surgery.

10. Vertebral uptake in a bone scan with SPECT is suggestive of bone metastases when there is involvement of the:
A. Vertebral body
B. Lamina
C. Articular facets
D. Spinous process

ANSWER: A. More than 50% of all skeletal metastases are found in the vertebral column; however, several other benign entities can cause increased uptake in the spine on bone scan, for example, arthritis and confound interpretation. Patterns of uptake in the vertebral column, seen on SPECT can help distinguish between benign and malignant etiologies. It is a well-known fact that skeletal metastases have a tendency to localize in the marrow containing axial skeleton. A majority of the spine metastases will therefore initially lodge in the bone marrow contained in the vertebral body prior to extension into the surrounding bone. Uptake in the posterolateral elements, like the lamina and spinous processes and the anterolateral aspect of the vertebral body with substantial sparing of the vertebral body usually indicate a benign process.

92 PULMONARY SCINTIGRAPHY

Pradeep G. Bhambhvani

PULMONARY EMBOLISM

Acute pulmonary embolism (PE) is a common and frequently fatal condition. It is obstruction of the pulmonary artery or one of its branches by thrombus that originated elsewhere in the body. Other materials such as tumor, air, or fat are also well-known causes of PE. Its clinical presentation is variable and nonspecific, which makes accurate diagnosis difficult. It can be classified as acute or chronic. Patients with acute PE typically develop symptoms and signs immediately after obstruction of the pulmonary vessels. In contrast, those with chronic PE tend to develop slowly progressive dyspnea over a period of years because of pulmonary hypertension. PE is associated with a mortality rate of approximately 30% without treatment, primarily the result of recurrent embolism. However, accurate diagnosis followed by effective therapy with anticoagulants decreases the mortality rate to between 2% and 8%.

Risk factors for PE include immobilization, surgery within the last 3 months, stroke, prior history of venous thromboembolism, malignancy, central venous instrumentation within the last 3 months, chronic heart disease, obesity, and heavy cigarette smoking (more than 25 cigarettes per day).

In the Prospective Investigation of Pulmonary Embolism Diagnosis II (PIOPED II), the most common symptoms associated with PE were dyspnea at rest or with exertion (73%), pleuritic pain (44%), cough (34%), greater than 2-pillow orthopnea (28%), calf or thigh pain (44%), calf or thigh swelling (41%), and wheezing (21%). The most common signs were tachypnea (54%), tachycardia (24%), rales (18%), decreased breath sounds (17%), an accentuated pulmonic component of the second heart sound (15%), and jugular venous distension (14%). Circulatory collapse was uncommon (8%). Massive PE may be accompanied by acute right ventricular failure. Symptoms or signs of lower extremity deep venous thrombosis (DVT) were common (47%).

The radiological diagnostic tests commonly employed in the evaluation of a patient with suspected PE include chest radiography, radionuclide ventilation–perfusion (V/Q) scan, pulmonary CT arteriography (CTA), and pulmonary angiography. Pulmonary angiography is the definitive diagnostic modality or reference standard in the diagnosis of acute PE; it has a sensitivity of 98% and a specificity of 97%. However, it is infrequently done as it is invasive and expensive compared to other modalities.

Chest radiographic abnormalities are common in patients with PE; however, they are not helpful diagnostically, because they are also seen in patients without PE. In a large prospective study, atelectasis and/or a pulmonary parenchymal abnormality was noted in 69% and 58% of patients with and without PE, respectively, Pleural effusion was detected in 47% and 39% of patients with and without PE, respectively, and approximately 12% of the chest radiographs in patients with pulmonary emboli were interpreted as normal. Various signs described including Westermark sign (attenuation of the pulmonary vessels distal to the embolus), the Fleischner sign (prominence of the proximal pulmonary artery from the embolus), and Hampton hump (pleural-based density resulting from infarction) are rare radiographic findings in acute PE.

Because of its widespread availability, pulmonary CTA is being increasingly used to diagnose patients with suspected PE. The benefit of CTA in addition to faster scan times is the ability to detect alternative etiologies that may explain the patient's clinical presentation. Reported data suggests that CTA is not inferior to V/Q scanning for ruling out PE. However, CTA requires concomitant pretest clinical probability assessment (Table 92-1) to be an effective diagnostic tool for confirming or excluding PE. Discordant CTA and clinical findings should prompt additional testing. Conventional pulmonary angiography is often required in this setting to definitively exclude pulmonary embolism. The PIOPED II trial concluded that there was increased sensitivity in diagnosis of suspected PE when CTA was combined with CT

TABLE 92-1 Clinical Probability of PE (Well Criteria)

CLINICAL FEATURES	SCORE (POINTS)*
Clinical signs and symptoms of DVT (objectively measured leg swelling and pain with palpation)	3.0
Heart rate >100 beats/min	1.5
Immobilization ≥3 consecutive days (bed rest except to access bathroom) or surgery in previous 4 wk	1.5
Previous objectively diagnosed PE or DVT	1.5
Hemoptysis	1.0
Malignancy (cancer patients receiving treatment within 6 mo or receiving palliative treatment)	1.0
PE as likely as or more likely than alternative diagnosis (based on history, physical examination, chest radiograph, electrocardiogram, and blood tests)	3.0

DVT, deep venous thrombosis; PE, pulmonary embolism.
*<2.0 Low probability; 2.0–6.0 Moderate probability; >6.0 High probability.

venography to assess the iliac, femoral, and popliteal veins for acute DVT with similar specificity when compared with CTA alone. Compression sonography has been reported elsewhere to be similarly accurate for evaluation of DVT. It is worthwhile to note that CTA is associated with significantly greater radiation burden to the body (absorbed radiation dose is between 8 and 10 mSv), particularly to the female breast as compared to the V/Q scan (absorbed radiation dose is approximately 2 mSv), although in a pregnant woman the consensus evidence points toward a lower fetal radiation dose with shielded CTA as compared to the V/Q scan. V/Q scan is the modality of choice in instances of renal insufficiency and contrast allergy, which preclude use of CTA.

The diagnostic accuracy of CTA appears to vary widely between institutions, which may be due to differences in the experience of radiologists interpreting the images and also image quality. Clinicians should consider their institution's experience and the pretest probability of PE when deciding whether to use CTA and/or whether to pursue other additional diagnostic testing.

VENTILATION–PERFUSION SCINTIGRAPHY

V/Q scintigraphy involves use of radioactive tracers, which map the ventilation and perfusion of the lung fields. The perfusion scan uses microscopic radioactive particles that are trapped in the pulmonary capillary system, whereas the ventilation examination uses an inhaled radiopharmaceutical.

Normal pulmonary ventilation (V) and perfusion (Q) are matched, with a normal gradient, that is, the lung apices are less ventilated and perfused compared to the lung bases. In PE, a thrombus occludes the pulmonary artery or one of its branches and reduces distal pulmonary arterial perfusion. The lung parenchyma in this setting usually remains perfused from the bronchial artery circulation, usually preventing pulmonary infarction. This results in a state where the pulmonary perfusion is reduced coupled with normal ventilation, resulting in a V/Q mismatch, the hallmark finding of pulmonary embolic disease.

RADIOPHARMACEUTICALS

Perfusion Radiotracers

Tc-99m macroaggregated albumin (Tc-99m MAA) is the radiotracer most commonly used today. The radioactive label is technetium-99m and the biological component is macroaggregates of albumin particles. The particles range in size from 10 to 100 μm. The diameter of the pulmonary capillaries ranges from 7 to 10 μm. Withdrawal of blood into the syringe with the radiotracer, prior to injection should be avoided to avoid clumping of the Tc-99m labeled MAA particles. After intravenous injection, the Tc-99m MAA particles travel to the right heart and are eventually trapped in the pulmonary capillaries. Regions of decreased perfusion are seen as photopenic or cold areas. It is important to note that not only absent but also diminished activity can be a pattern seen in PE. The MAA particles have a biological half-life of approximately 4 to 6 hours.

In general, the perfusion scan is safe examination. A minimum of 100 000 particles are required for a satisfactory adult perfusion scan. In clinical practice, between 200 000 and 500 000 particles are usually administered. The number of particles is reduced in pulmonary hypertension, pregnancy, right-to-left shunts, neonates, and children younger than 5 years. Decreasing the number of particles is not synonymous with decreasing the level of radioactivity, and this has to be kept in mind when formulating the radiotracer.

Ventilation Radiotracers

Two different classes of radiotracers are available for ventilation imaging: the radioactive gases (xenon 133, xenon 127, and krypton 81 m) and the radio aerosols (Tc-99m DTPA and Technegas). Xenon 133 and Tc-99m DTPA are presently available in the United States.

Xenon 133

Xenon 133 is the only radioactive gas available commercially in the United States. It is very sensitive for detection of chronic obstructive pulmonary disease. It has a physical half-life of 5.3 days and a biological half-life of 30 seconds during washout; therefore, only one view (usually posterior) can be obtained using a single detector. With dual detectors, an anterior view can be also obtained. Additionally, images with xenon-33 are of poor resolution owing to its low photopeak of 80 keV, which mandates that it be done before the Tc-99m MAA (photopeak 140 keV) perfusion study. Phases of the procedure include wash-in (single maximal inspiration of xenon 133 and breath hold), equilibrium (normal breathing of xenon 133 and room air) and washout (normal breathing of room air). Decreased uptake in any of these phases is considered to be abnormal. Persistent pulmonary xenon activity in the washout phase is indicative of air trapping. Abnormal accumulation of xenon in the right upper quadrant can be seen in patients with hepatic steatosis because of its fat solubility.

Tc-99m DTPA

Aerosol ventilation with Tc-99m DTPA is widely used in the United States. It requires patient cooperation because of the need of breathing via a mouthpiece with a nose clamp in place for several minutes. Like with xenon 133, ventilation examination with Tc-99m DTPA should be completed before the perfusion study, as the counts achieved are much lower than the perfusion examination. Multiple images are obtained as with the perfusion study, these include anterior, posterior, right and left lateral, right and left posterior, and anterior obliques, to enable complete visualization of the lung fields. With radioaerosols, activity may be seen in the mouth, pharynx, large airways, and the stomach (from swallowed activity). Clumping in the central airways most commonly occurs in bronchial asthma, chronic obstructive pulmonary disease, or in patients who are unable to comply with deep breathing.

INTERPRETATION

Normal V/Q scan should have homogenous distribution of tracer throughout the bilateral lung fields. Areas of normal attenuation include the hilar structures, cardiac silhouette, spine, sternum, pacemakers, and other implanted devices. Images obtained should be preferably in the same position for the ventilation and the perfusion components of the examination. Correlation with a recent chest radiograph is necessary. The sine qua non of acute PE in a V/Q scan is multiple, moderate-to-large, wedge-shaped perfusion defect(s) in area(s) of normal lung ventilation. However, several other etiologies including prior or unresolved PE, fat, air, septic embolism, vasculitis, may result in unmatched V/Q defects. The probability of PE increases with increasing number of mismatched perfusion defects. Infrequently in PE there may be pulmonary infarction, which will result in a ventilation defect that is usually smaller than the perfusion defect along with a corresponding radiographic abnormality (triple match).

Perfusion defects are described in terms of their size and location. Defects are considered large if they involve more than 75% of the lung segment, moderate if involve between 25% and 75% of the lung segment (counted as being approximately half of a large defect), and small if involvement is less than 25% of the lung segment. The defects are additionally described in terms of being segmental and nonsegmental, that is, corresponding to one or more bronchopulmonary segments. A nonsegmental defect is one that does not conform to the segmental anatomy and is less likely to be a consequence of an acute PE, for example, defects secondary to pneumonia, pacemaker artifact, tumor, adenopathy, and cardiomegaly. Often the defects are difficult to characterize on the basis of their segmental anatomy.

Many patients, especially those with chronic obstructive pulmonary disease and bronchial asthma, have multiple perfusion and ventilation abnormalities that are usually matched. The perfusion abnormality in these instances is a consequence of compensatory vasoconstriction in response to hypoxia. "Reverse mismatch" refers to a state where there is ventilation abnormality accompanied by normal perfusion or a perfusion abnormality, which is smaller than the ventilation abnormality. Reverse mismatched defects are seen in pleural effusions, lobar pneumonia, lung atelectasis, gross cardiomegaly, acute exacerbation of chronic obstructive pulmonary disease, and acute partial bronchial obstruction. In these conditions, the hypoxia driven vasoconstriction fails or is incomplete.

The PIOPED study, a multi-institutional study, funded by the National Institutes of Health has been the most comprehensive study evaluating the accuracy of V/Q scintigraphy. V/Q scans are essentially reported as normal or abnormal. Abnormal scans are in turn reported based on size, number, matched/unmatched ventilation and perfusion defects, and the findings of chest radiographs. The abnormal scans are categorized as being very low probability, low probability, intermediate probability, or high probability for an acute PE (Table 92-2).

A normal perfusion scan irrespective of the ventilation scan and radiographic findings effectively excludes pulmonary embolism (likelihood of PE less than 5%). A low probability scan carries a likelihood of 10% to 20% of acute PE. Usually this results when the perfusion defect is less than 25% of the segment, irrespective of the appearance of the ventilation scan or the chest radiograph or when the V/Q defects are matched or when the radiographic abnormality is larger than the corresponding perfusion defect. The high probability scans, in the appropriate clinical setting, carry a high likelihood of

TABLE 92-2 Modified PIOPED Criteria for Diagnosis of Pulmonary Embolism

High probability (>80% likelihood for PE)	Greater than or equal to 2 large mismatched segmental perfusion defects or the arithmetic equivalent in moderate or large defects with a normal chest radiograph
	Any perfusion defect substantially larger than the radiographic abnormality
Intermediate probability (20%–80% likelihood for PE)	One moderate to less than two large mismatched perfusion defect(s) or the arithmetic equivalent in large and/or moderate defects
	Single moderate to large matched ventilation–perfusion defect with normal chest radiograph
	Triple matched defect in the lower lung field
	Difficult to categorize as low or high probability
Low probability (< 20% likelihood for PE)	Any perfusion defect with a substantially larger chest radiographic abnormality
	Any number of small perfusion defects with a normal chest radiograph
	Nonsegmental perfusion defects (e.g., cardiomegaly, enlarged or ectatic aorta, enlarged hila, elevated diaphragm)
	Multiple matched V/Q abnormalities, with a normal chest radiograph
Normal	No perfusion defects or perfusion exactly outlines the shape of the lungs seen on the chest radiograph (note that hila and aortic impressions may be seen and the chest radiograph and/or ventilation study may be abnormal).

acute PE (greater than 80%) and include either two or more large unmatched perfusion defects with a normal chest radiograph or a combination of defects that add up to two or more large defects, with at least one of the defects being moderate or large. The intermediate probability scan carries a 20% to 80% probability for an acute PE, includes those that do not meet the criteria of low or high probability scans. Typically these include a single unmatched perfusion defect of at least moderate size or a triple matched defect in the lower lung fields where there are corresponding abnormalities in the V/Q scans and the chest radiograph. Triple matched defects in the upper and midlung fields are categorized as being low probability. The updated PIOPED II recommendations have introduced the very low probability category (Table 92-3), which carries a likelihood of less than 10% for acute PE, and includes nonsegmental defects, perfusion defect smaller than radiographic defect, stripe sign, etc.

Special Signs and Situations

"Stripe sign" refers to presence of stripe of radiotracer activity at the periphery or base of the wedge-shaped perfusion defect, representing perfused lung tissue between the perfusion defect and the adjacent pleural surface. It usually indicates a very low probability for an acute PE.

TABLE 92-3 Criteria for Very Low Probability of PE in PIOPED II

Nonsegmental perfusion abnormalities. These include enlargement of the heart or hilum, elevated hemidiaphragm, linear atelectasis, or costophrenic angle effusion with no other perfusion defect in either lung
Perfusion defect smaller than corresponding radiographic lesion
≥2 matched V/Q defects with regionally normal chest radiograph and areas of normal perfusion elsewhere in the lungs
1–3 small segmental perfusion defects (<25% of a segment)
Solitary triple matched defect (defined as a matched V/Q defect with associated matching chest radiographic opacity) in the middle or upper lung zone confined to a single segment
Stripe sign, which consists of a stripe of perfused lung tissue between a perfusion defect and the adjacent pleural surface (best seen on a tangential view)
Pleural effusion equal to one-third or more of the pleural cavity with no other perfusion defect in either lung

"Fissure sign" refers to the curvilinear perfusion defects representing pleural fluid in the interlobar pulmonary fissures; it usually indicates the presence of a pleural effusion but can also be seen in the presence of fissural pleural thickening and also in chronic obstructive pulmonary disease. In the supine position, pleural fluid layers dependently, resulting in an appearance where one lung is diffusely hypoperfused in case where the pleural effusion is unilateral.

Solitary lobar or solitary whole-lung perfusion defects are unusual findings associated with acute PE and can be associated with hilar mass, hypoplastic pulmonary artery, and mediastinal fibrosis. A large saddle embolus could result in unilateral diffuse hypoperfusion, but is very uncommon.

A perfusion defect with a corresponding substantially larger radiographic abnormality is suggestive of low probability, while perfusion abnormality with a similar or smaller radiographic abnormality is referred to as intermediate probability when in the lower lung fields and low probability when in the upper and midlung fields.

Pleural effusions may produce reverse mismatched defects or triple matched defects. According to the PIOPED data, matched defects caused by small pleural effusions (blunting of the costophrenic angle) should be classified as "intermediate" probability, while defects caused by larger effusions should be classified as low probability; however, it is important to note that PE is associated with pleural effusions of all sizes, and thus all pleural effusion–related triple matches should be assigned an intermediate probability. It is worth remembering that a pleural effusion in acute PE is rarely seen without other perfusion defects.

In chronic obstructive pulmonary disease, both segmental and nonsegmental matched ventilation and perfusion defects can be seen, while in pulmonary hypertension, V/Q scan may be normal or notable for multiple, small, and unmatched, usually nonsegmental perfusion defects. In contrast, acute PE causes multiple large unmatched, segmental perfusion defects. Mucous plugs in the airways usually result in matched V/Q defects.

In small and medium vessel pulmonary vasculitis, V/Q scans may show focal matched defects or evidence of pulmonary infarctions, unless the patient has known pulmonary thromboembolism like in systemic lupus erythematosus associated with antiphospholipid antibodies. Large and medium vessel vasculitis such as Takayasu's arteritis can result in scans indistinguishable from acute PE. Depending on the anatomic location, bronchogenic carcinoma may compress a major pulmonary artery resulting in a unilateral nonperfused lung or lobe of the lung with associated normal ventilation.

ACCURACY OF V/Q SCAN

In the PIOPED trial, the sensitivity of a high probability V/Q scan was only 41%, while the specificity was 97%. This means that a majority of patients with PE had a low or intermediate probability V/Q scan and those with a high probability V/Q scan almost always have a PE. Another finding of the PIOPED trial and many others is the low likelihood of adverse clinical outcomes in patients with normal and low probability V/Q scans (less than 1%).

FOLLOW-UP V/Q SCAN IN ACUTE EMBOLISM

One of the most common causes of a false-positive V/Q scan is an unresolved prior PE. Usually the perfusion defects become smaller or may disappear altogether. Sometimes new defects appear from fragmentation of larger, central thrombi that move distally. However, up to 35% of acute emboli do not completely resolve; these are usually larger defects and seen in the elderly. After a high-probability V/Q scan, a follow-up V/Q scan in 3 months after the initial scan is recommended to establish a new baseline and allow time for resolution of the initial defects. Perfusion defects that persist at 3 months are likely to remain unresolved.

QUANTITATIVE V/Q SCAN

Ventilation and perfusion scintigraphy can provide estimation of the extent of pulmonary parenchymal disease and therefore help predict the consequences of lung resection and radiation therapy. It is useful in the preoperative evaluation prior to planned lung surgery for pulmonary malignancy, lung volume reduction surgery in chronic obstructive pulmonary disease and prior to lung transplantation. Differential right and left lung function is obtained by acquiring anterior and posterior images of both lung fields and drawing regions of interest around each lung field and calculate the geometric mean which is the square root of anterior counts times the posterior counts to correct for attenuation. Additional calculations can be made by dividing each lung into upper, middle, and lower lung zones.

SUGGESTED READING

Freeman LM, Krynyckyi B, Zuckier LS. Enhanced lung scan diagnosis of pulmonary embolism with the use of ancillary scintigraphic findings and clinical correlation. *Semin Nucl Med.* 2001;31:143-157.

Goodman LR, Stein PD, Matta F, et al. CT venography and compression sonography are diagnostically equivalent: data from PIOPED II. *AJR Am J Roentgenol.* 2007;189:1071-1076.

Gottschalk A, Stein PD, Sostman HD, Matta F, Beemath A. Very low probability interpretation of V/Q lung scans in combination with low probability objective clinical assessment reliability excludes pulmonary embolism. *J Nucl Med.* 2007;48:1411-1415.

Gottschalk A, Sostman HD, Coleman RE, et al. Ventilation-perfusion scintigraphy in the PIOPED study. Part II. Evaluation of the scintigraphic criteria and interpretations. *J Nucl Med.* 1993;34:1119-1126.

Gottschalk A, Stein P, Goodman LR, Sostman HD. Overview of PIOPED II. *Semin Nucl Med.* 2002;32:173-182.

Sostman HD, Stein PD, Gottschalk A et al. Acute pulmonary embolism: sensitivity and specificity of ventilation-perfusion scintigraphy in PIOPED II study. *Radiology.* 2008;246:941-946.

Stein PD, Fowler SE, Goodman LR, et al. Multidetector computed tomography for acute pulmonary embolism. *N Engl J Med.* 2006;354:2317-2327.

The PIOPED Investigators. Value of the ventilation/perfusion scan in acute pulmonary embolism: results of the prospective investigation of pulmonary embolism diagnosis (PIOPED). *JAMA.* 1990;263:2753-2759.

Wells PS, Anderson DR, Roger M, et al. Excluding pulmonary embolism at the bedside without diagnostic imaging: management of patients with suspected pulmonary embolism presenting to the emergency department by using a simple clinical model and D-dimer. *Ann Intern Med.* 2001;135:98-107.

Worsely DF, Alavi A. Comprehensive analysis of the results of the PIOPED study. *J Nucl Med.* 1995;36:2380-2397.

Worsely DF, Alavi A, Aronchick JM, Chest radiographic findings in patients with acute PE observations from the PIOPED study. *Radiology.* 1993;189:133-136.

QUESTIONS AND ANSWERS

1. Which of the following chest radiographic findings is most commonly seen in patients with an acute pulmonary embolism?
   A. Pleural effusion
   B. Normal
   C. Atelectasis
   D. Westermark sign

   ANSWER: C. Radiographic abnormalities are commonly seen in patients with PE; however, they are not helpful diagnostically because they are also found in patients without PE. In the reported literature, atelectasis and/or a pulmonary parenchymal abnormality was noted most commonly in patients with PE. Approximately 12% of the chest radiographs in patients with pulmonary emboli were interpreted as normal. Various signs described including Westermark sign (attenuation of the pulmonary vessels distal to the embolus), the Fleischner sign (prominence of the proximal pulmonary artery from the embolus), and Hampton hump (pleural-based density resulting from infarction) are rare findings in acute PE.

2. Quantitative Lung Perfusion scan done for a patient with idiopathic pulmonary fibrosis, prior to lung transplant, is reported as

   Right lung anterior = 22 000 counts/min
   Right lung posterior = 16 000 counts/min
   Left lung anterior = 28 000 counts/min
   Left lung posterior = 22 000 counts/min

   Using the geometric mean technique, what is the percentage perfusion to the right and left lungs, respectively?
   A. 43% and 57%
   B. 38% and 62%
   C. 35% and 65%
   D. 45% and 55%

   ANSWER: A. Geometric mean is the square root of anterior counts multiplied by posterior counts. In this case, it is 18 762 for the right lung field and 24 819 for the left lung field. The sum of both the right and left lung field geometric mean would be 43 581. On dividing the geometric mean of the right lung field by the sum of the geometric means of both lung fields, the differential perfusion of the right lung field is 43%, while for the left lung field is 57%. Quantification of differential lung ventilation and perfusion can help predict the consequences of lung resection and radiation therapy and is useful in the preoperative evaluation prior to planned lung surgery for pulmonary malignancy, lung volume reduction surgery in chronic obstructive pulmonary disease, and prior to lung transplantation.

3. What is the most common cause of false-positive V/Q mismatches for acute pulmonary embolism?
   A. Vasculitis
   B. Tumor
   C. Previous pulmonary embolism
   D. Bronchial asthma

   ANSWER: C. Of the potential causes of false-positive V/Q scans, previous PE or unresolved PE is the most common cause. After a high probability V/Q scan, a follow-up V/Q scan in 3 months after the initial scan is recommended to establish a new baseline and allow time for resolution of the initial defects.

4. Visualization of the kidneys on a lung perfusion image is more likely due to an anatomic right-to-left shunt if activity is also seen in which of the following other organ?
   A. Stomach
   B. Liver
   C. Brain
   D. Thyroid

   ANSWER: C. Nuclear perfusion study using macro aggregates of albumin demonstrates the presence of right-to-left shunt, as presence of cerebral and renal activity. Scintigraphy cannot distinguish between intracardiac and intrapulmonary shunt. After injection the MAA particles enter the systemic circulation, evident as visualization of the brain and kidney activity. Renal activity can also be seen in instances of free pertechnetate or following absorption of Tc-99m after the ventilation study. However in neither of these instances is cerebral activity seen, which is a typical finding of a systemic right-to-left shunt. Free pertechnetate is notable for presence of gastric, salivary glands, thyroid, and renal activity.

5. What is the most appropriate Tc-99m labeled radiopharmaceutical for a right-to-left shunt study?
   A. Macroaggregates of albumin (MAA)
   B. Sestamibi
   C. DTPA
   D. Sulfur colloid

   ANSWER: A. MAA particles attached to a radioactive label, Tc-99m are used most commonly for perfusion lung scan, evaluation of a right-to-left shunt, and to determine shunt severity. Scintigraphy cannot distinguish between intracardiac and intrapulmonary shunt. The MAA particles, which vary in size between 10 and 100 μm, normally get trapped in the pulmonary capillary bed and give an image of distribution of blood flow in the lung fields. In instances of right-to-left shunts, these particles are able to enter the systemic circulation evident as visualization of the brain and kidney activity. Renal activity can also be seen in instances of free pertechnetate or following absorption of Tc-99m after the ventilation study. However, in neither of these instances is cerebral activity seen, which is a typical finding of a systemic right-to-left shunt. Free pertechnetate is notable for presence of gastric, salivary glands, thyroid, and renal activity.

6. When correlating the V/Q scan with chest radiograph, which of the following statements is true?
   A. When the size of the defect in the lower lung field equals that of the radiographic abnormality, the probability of PE is low.
   B. When the size of a perfusion defect in the lower lobe is larger than the radiographic abnormality, the probability of PE is low.
   C. When the size of the lower lung field perfusion defect is less than the size of the radiographic abnormality, the probability of PE is intermediate.
   D. When the perfusion scan is normal and the radiograph has evidence of bilateral pulmonary infiltrates, it essentially excludes the diagnosis of an acute pulmonary embolism.

   ANSWER: D. Any perfusion defect with a substantially larger chest radiographic abnormality is considered low probability. On the other hand, a perfusion defect that is much larger than the radiographic abnormality is high probability. Matched ventilation, perfusion and radiographic findings are referred to as a triple match. A triple match in the upper and mid lung fields is said to represent a low probability for an acute PE, whereas a triple match in the lower lung field is considered to indicate an intermediate probability for an acute PE.

   A "normal" perfusion scan essentially rules out an acute PE, irrespective of the radiographic findings.

7. Which of the following can cause platypnea-orthodeoxia?
   A. Hepatopulmonary syndrome
   B. Hepatorenal syndrome
   C. Cirrhosis
   D. Ischemic cardiomyopathy

   ANSWER: A. "Platypnea" is defined as an increase in dyspnea induced by the upright position and relieved by recumbency, whereas "orthodeoxia" refers to arterial oxyhemoglobin desaturation upon assuming an upright posture, which is also improved by recumbency. Orthodeoxia in patients with liver disease is strongly suggestive of hepatopulmonary syndrome, although it can be seen in a number of other diseases, including postpneumonectomy, recurrent pulmonary emboli, atrial septal defects (including patent foramen ovale), and chronic lung disease. In general, the diagnosis of hepatopulmonary syndrome is confirmed when the following exist: liver disease, an elevated alveolar-arterial gradient while breathing in room air, and intrapulmonary vascular dilations, latter resulting in a large right-to-left shunt. Intrapulmonary vascular dilations are presently detected using contrast-enhanced echocardiography, technetium-99m-labeled MAA scanning (perfusion lung scan), and pulmonary arteriography. Nuclear perfusion scan using Macroaggregates of albumin demonstrates the right-to-left pulmonary shunt, evident as presence of cerebral and renal activity. Scintigraphy is used to quantify the shunt, but cannot distinguish between intracardiac and intrapulmonary shunt. Liver transplantation is presently considered the most effective treatment in hepatopulmonary syndrome associated with severe hypoxemia.

8. Regarding perfusion scintigraphy with Tc-99m MAA particles, which of the following statements is *true*?
   A. Patients with one lung are at increased risk of complications from the test.
   B. Renal activity is highly suggestive of a right-to-left shunt.
   C. If 50 000 particles of MAA are administered in an adult, the image quality will likely be poor.
   D. Normally the ratio of administered particles to the number of pulmonary capillaries is 1:50.

   ANSWER: C. Tc-99m labeled MAA particles is the most commonly used radiopharmaceutical in perfusion scintigraphy today. Approximately 200 000 to 500 000 particles are injected IV for the perfusion scan. There are approximately 280 billion pulmonary capillaries, which normally result in a particle-to-capillary ratio of approximately 1:1 million. A minimum of 100 000 particles are required in adults to obtain a satisfactory examination. In certain conditions such as pulmonary hypertension, pregnancy, right-to-left cardiac shunt, and in children, the number of particles given for the scan is reduced. In general the perfusion scan is safe examination, even in right-to-left cardiac shunts, where the MAA particles enter the systemic circulation, evident as visualization of the brain and kidney activity.

9. Geometric mean is calculated using the following formula, where A = Anterior Counts and B = Posterior Counts.
   A. (A + B) (A + B)
   B. Square root of A × B
   C. Square root of A + B
   D. Square root of (A + B) (A + B)

   ANSWER: B. Geometric mean = Square root of A × B is applied in quantification of differential lung ventilation and perfusion, which is useful in the preoperative evaluation prior to planned lung surgery for pulmonary malignancy, lung volume reduction surgery in chronic obstructive pulmonary disease, and prior to lung transplantation. Anterior and posterior images of bilateral lung fields are obtained, regions of interest are drawn around both lung fields and geometric mean is calculated for attenuation correction.

10. Your obstetrician colleague calls for advice regarding choice of imaging in a 22-year-old female patient in her second trimester of pregnancy with normal kidney function and complains of shortness of breath. There is clinical concern of an acute pulmonary embolism. What would be your recommendation?
    A. Ventilation and perfusion lung scan
    B. Chest radiography
    C. Pulmonary CTA
    D. Ultrasound duplex Doppler of the lower extremities

    ANSWER: C. Pregnant women have a fivefold increased risk for venous thromboembolism including acute PE and DVT. Clinical examinations are unreliable, and imaging the patient is essential. An evaluation to rule out PE during pregnancy is especially challenging because of concerns regarding fetal radiation exposure. Radiographic abnormalities are commonly seen in patients with PE; however, they are not helpful diagnostically, because they are also found in patients without PE. V/Q scanning has traditionally been associated with less radiation exposure to the fetus than CTA. However, there is published evidence suggesting CTA is actually associated with a lower average fetal radiation dose than V/Q scanning during all trimesters. One drawback, however, of CTA is that it exposes maternal breast tissue to relatively high doses of radiation, much higher than that associated with V/Q scanning. Ultrasound examination of the lower extremity venous system is helpful in diagnosis of DVT and not acute PE, although the both entities are sometimes seen together and often managed similarly.

93 NUCLEAR MEDICINE: GASTROENTEROLOGY

Sibyll Goetze

GASTROINTESTINAL MOTILITY

GASTRIC EMPTYING STUDIES

Introduction

Gastric emptying studies (GES) using radionuclides are performed to evaluate gastric motor function. They are often considered the "gold standard," and "most physiologic" examinations, because of their noninvasive nature, use a physiologic liquid or solid meal, and the resultant quantitative information. Radionuclide GES are very reproducible and serial examinations after therapeutic interventions can help establish their effectiveness. Typical indications for GES are evaluation of symptoms such as (postprandial) nausea, vomiting, or abdominal pain, gastroesophageal reflux disease, difficult glycemic control in diabetic patients, suspected or known gastroparesis, and assessing response to therapy.

Technique

Patient preparation includes a fast of at least 4 hours prior to the procedure. Some experts recommend performing GES in premenopausal women on day 1 to 10 of the menstrual cycle to prevent possible effects of hormonal variation on gastric emptying.

GES can be performed using a solid (solid gastric emptying studies [SGES]) or liquid (liquid gastric emptying studies [LGES]) meal. In addition, dual phase/dual isotope studies with different radionuclides for the solid and liquid meal have also been used for the simultaneous evaluation of both liquid and solid emptying. The current consensus is that SGES are more sensitive than LGES. Therefore, patients should undergo SGES if possible when evaluation of gastric motility is warranted. Nevertheless, there is emerging data that a number of patients may have normal solid and abnormal liquid gastric emptying. The radiopharmaceuticals used to label (solid or liquid) meals most commonly are 99mTc sulfur colloid (0.2–0.5 mCi) and, less frequently, Indium 111 (0.1–0.3 mCi) (Table 93-1). There is a variety

TABLE 93-1 Radiation Dosimetry for GI/Hepatobiliary Imaging Agents in Adults

RADIOPHARMACEUTICAL	ADMINISTERED ACTIVITY (mCi)	RADIATION DOSE TO TARGET ORGAN (rad/mCi)	EFFECTIVE DOSE (rem/mCi)
99mTc sulfur colloid po (gastric emptying)	0.2–0.5	0.41 (large intestine)	0.089
In 111 po (gastric emptying)	0.2–0.5	2.0 (large intestine)	0.3
99mTc sulfur colloid IV	4–6 mCi (liver spleen scan), 10 mCi (GI bleeding study)	0.27 (spleen)	0.052
Tc99m RBC	20–30 mCi	0.085 (heart)	0.031
Tc-99m pertechnetate (Meckel scan)	8–12	0.23 (large intestine)	0.048
Tc-99m disofenin			
Tc-99m mebrofenin	1.5–5.0	0.41 (gallbladder)	0.089

Data modified from the Society of Nuclear Medicine Procedure Guidelines. www.snm.org.

of (especially solid) GES protocols, including different approaches to meal composition, patient positioning, and imaging protocol. It is important that normal gastric emptying rates are established for each specific protocol. In addition, the stability of the radiolabel of a solid meal in gastric juice must be established. For liquid gastric emptying studies, almost any liquid can be used, such as water, orange juice, or milk (usually 300–500 mL). Solid meals may consist of eggs (scrambled, whole, egg whites, or egg substitute), or beef stew, or liver, and/or toast. The radiolabeled solid meal should be ingested promptly, ideally within 5 to 10 minutes. The technologist should record any deviation from the standard procedure, such as any portion of the meal that was not eaten or if it took longer than 10 minutes to finish the meal. Imaging should begin immediately after ingestion of the meal. Images may be obtained standing, sitting, or supine, but should not change during the study. Planar images should include the distal esophagus, the stomach, and the proximal small bowel in the field of view. To account for movement of the meal from posterior to anterior (gastric fundus to antrum) and differences in attenuation, imaging in the anterior and posterior view and subsequent calculation of the geometric mean (square root of the product of counts in the anterior and posterior region of interest [ROI]) is recommended. Alternatively an LAO view may be used (especially for LGES). The exact type of imaging (continuous dynamic, intermittent data acquisition) and duration varies per specific protocol, nevertheless the study usually takes at least 30 minutes for LGES and at least 90 minutes for SGES (often longer [2–4 hours]). Continuous dynamic imaging (i.e., at a rate of 30–60 s/frame) is more useful for LGES and, when used for solid emptying studies, has the advantage of more accurately determining the gastric emptying half times and lag phase. For SGES, intermittent imaging that determines the percent retention (or emptying) at certain time points may be more efficient. Follow-up studies should always be done under the same conditions as the baseline study. Of note, a most recent procedure guideline from the society of Nuclear Medicine makes specific recommendations of a standard meal based on consenses guideline.

Interpretation

A region of interest is drawn around the radiotracer activity in the stomach and time activity curves are obtained. Solid gastric emptying usually demonstrates a so-called "lag phase" (a period during which food is grinded to small particles in the stomach and no emptying into small bowel occurs) followed by emptying in a constant, linear fashion. Liquid gastric emptying begins immediately after ingestion (no lag phase) and usually has a (mono)exponential characteristic.

Gastric emptying can be measured and quantified in several ways, for example, as half emptying time (the time it takes to reach half the maximum counts), or emptying rate (%/min), or percent emptying (or retention) at specific time points (e.g., 1–4 hours; end of study). Gastric emptying data obtained is compared to normal values (again, normal values must be established and validated for each specific protocol). Normal values for SGES vary, depending on the protocol. A normal halftime for liquid emptying is approximately less than 10 to 20 minutes. There are a variety of factors that may affect gastric emptying (Table 93-2). Sources of error include poor labeling of the solid meal, nonstandard meal or procedure, significant variation in the environment (noise, temperature, etc.), vomiting, fasting status less than 4 hours, esophageal retention, gastroesophageal reflux, overlap of small bowel and stomach in the ROI, and meal not eaten entirely or over a prolonged period of time (greater than 10 minutes). Review of (dynamic) images should be done to assess for incidental findings such as gastroesophageal reflux and for quality control (correct ROI, overlap of small bowel, and stomach in the ROI).

TABLE 93-2 Selected Factors Affecting Gastric Motility

Meal		Volume
		Composition (fat, protein, salts/nutrients)
		Acidity
		Caloric content
		Particle size
Environment		Time of day
		Ambient (temperature, noise, lighting)
Patient	Demographics	Gender (hormonal status in females)
		Age
	Concurrent conditions	Stress/anxiety
		Trauma
		Gastroenteritis
		Metabolic disorders (hyperglycemia, acidosis...)
		Diabetes mellitus
		Thyroid disorders
		Connective tissue disorders (systemic sclerosis...)
		Peptic ulcer disease
		Amyloidosis
	Medication	Anticholinergic medication
		Opiates
		Beta agonists
		Antidepressants
		Estrogen/progesterone
		Alcohol
		Nicotine
		Metoclopramide
		Erythromycin
Procedure		Patient position
		Camera position (anterior, anterior/posterior/LAO)
		Attenuation correction
		Single/dual isotope studies

ESOPHAGEAL TRANSIT SCINTIGRAPHY

Esophageal transit scintigraphy may be useful in the evaluation of esophageal motility disorders. Although esophageal manometry is the main diagnostic tool for the diagnosis of esophageal motility disorders and barium radiography can provide qualitative assessment of (impaired) motility, the scintigraphic technique provides quantitative information. This could be particularly useful in the evaluation of therapeutic interventions. Esophageal transit scintigraphy is noninvasive, quantitative, and relatively easy to perform. After an overnight fast, the patient consumes a radiolabeled (Tc-99m sulfur colloid) liquid or semisolid meal in the upright or supine position (protocols vary). Dynamic imaging is performed while the patient is eating and continued for a period of time thereafter (15–30 minutes), ROI are drawn around the radiotracer activity in the esophagus (as well as the stomach) and time activity curves can be derived. Esophageal transit time and/or residual esophageal activity can be quantified.

GASTROINTESTINAL BLEEDING

INTRODUCTION

Gastrointestinal (GI) bleeding can be divided into upper or lower GI bleeding depending on its origin (proximal or distal to the ligament of Treitz). Causes of upper GI bleeding include esophageal varices, gastric or duodenal ulcers, gastritis or duodenitis among other. Lower GI bleedings are caused by diverticula, neoplasm, angiodysplasia, and inflammatory bowel disease. Both endoscopy and angiography may be able to identify the cause of bleeding; in addition, they may also be able to provide therapeutic control. The goal of GI bleeding scintigraphy is to localize the source of GI bleeding with the hope that the patient can be triaged to the appropriate therapeutic intervention (angiography, endoscopy, surgery) or next diagnostic test. With radionuclide techniques, GI bleeding with bleeding rates as low as 0.1 mL/min may be detected (or 2–3 mL of blood total). Radionuclide studies for the evaluation of GI bleeding are usually performed using Tc-99m labeled red blood cells (RBC), although Tc99m sulfur colloid may be used as well.

GASTROINTESTINAL BLEEDING SCINTIGRAPHY USING TC-99M LABELED RBC

There are essentially three techniques of RBC labeling with Tc-99m pertechnetate (Table 93-3): the so-called in vivo, modified in vitro, and in vitro techniques. The techniques vary not only in technical complexity but also labeling efficiency (which relates to image quality). In vitro labeling is recommended for GI bleeding scintigraphy, although a modified in vitro technique may also be acceptable. In vivo labeling is not recommended. When RBCs are used, strict adherence to procedures such as correct patient identification and handling of blood products is mandatory to prevent administration of one patient's blood into another patient.

Imaging is begun after injection of the radiotracer (an initial "flow" or "radionuclide angiography" phase is optional). Because movement of a GI bleeding can be fast (due to stimulation of peristalsis), frequent dynamic images (10–60 s/frame) are recommended to accurately localize the site of bleeding. Duration of initial imaging is usually 60 to 90 minutes. The field of view should include the entire abdomen and pelvis in the

TABLE 93-3 Methods for Red Blood Cell Labeling with Tc-99m Pertechnetate

	IN VIVO	MODIFIED IN VITRO	IN VITRO (UltraTag©)
	Inject tin IV	Inject tin IV	Draw blood
	Wait	Wait	Label blood according to UltraTag© Red Blood Cell kit instructions (tin and Tc-99m pertechnetate)
Technique	Inject pertechnetate IV	Withdraw venous blood into syringe	Readminister labeled blood to patient.
		Add pertechnetate to blood in syringe and mix	
		Reinject labeled blood	
Simplicity of procedure	+++	++	+
Labeling efficiency	75%–80%	85%–90%	98%
Image quality	+	++	+++
Cost			(More costly)

anterior view. Additional views such a lateral view of the pelvis or a postvoid image may be helpful to avoid misinterpretation due to overlying bladder activity. Delayed (dynamic and/or static) images (2–24 hours after initial radiotracer injection) may be useful if no bleeding is detected on initial images. These images should be viewed with caution as they may (more often then initial studies) result in incorrect localization of bleeding site. If the patient continues to show signs and symptoms of active GI bleeding, starting a new study by injecting labeled RBC again may be more useful than just obtaining delayed images. Pharmacologic interventions such as glucagons or heparin administration are not widely used.

Normal RBC biodistribution includes the vascular space of the heart/great vessels, liver, spleen, and kidneys. Some of the radioactivity is excreted into the urine, and the bladder is usually seen.

RBCs that extravasate into the bowel lumen are identified as radiotracer activity that appears rather suddenly, increases in intensity over time, and/or that moves in a pattern consistent with lumen of the small or large bowel (this may be antegrade or retrograde). Small bowel bleeding can be distinguished from large bowel bleeding by its swift serpiginous movement. To definitely distinguish small bowel from large bowel bleeding or accurately localize the bleeding, it may be necessary to continue imaging after the bleeding was detected scintigraphically—until a distinctive pattern of movement is noted.

Sources of error include intermittent nature of bleeding (bleeding stopped by the time the scan was acquired), technical error such as failure to image the entire abdomen/pelvis or insufficient frame rate of dynamic images. In addition, blood pool activity in (abdominal) vessels (especially if abnormal such as ectatic aorta or varices), hemangiomas or genitalia, or radiotracer accumulation in a hydronephrotic kidney or hydroureter or transplant kidney may be mistaken for an area of active bleeding. A full urinary bladder may obscure a lower (rectal) bleeding. If excess free pertechnetate is present, gastric mucosal activity may be very prominent and may mimic bleeding. If this is suspected, extra views of the thyroid/salivary glands can confirm the presence of free pertechnetate.

Gastrointestinal Bleeding Scintigraphy Using TC-99M Sulfur Colloid (SC)

The usual dose of Tc-99m sulfur colloid is 10 mCi. Because of the short residence time within blood pool (serum half-life of 3 minutes), dynamic imaging of the entire abdomen and pelvis (similar to the RBC technique) is obtained for only 20 to 30 minutes. Normal biodistribution includes the liver, spleen and bone marrow. Similar to the labeled RBC technique, the hallmark of GI bleeding is a new site of abnormally increased radiotracer uptake that demonstrated motion in an intraluminal pattern. Fixed areas of uptake may be related to ectopic spleen, or asymmetric bone marrow.

Disadvantages of the sulfur colloid technique compared to RBC imaging are related to the fast clearance by the reticuloendothelial system: bleeding must be active at the time of injection, as imaging for greater than 30 minutes or delayed images are not useful. In addition, bleeding sites in the upper abdomen (e.g., stomach, hepatic and splenic flexures) may be obscured by physiologic uptake in the liver and spleen. On the other hand, the shorter preparation and acquisition time may be advantageous since reinjection and reimaging is an option. The fast blood pool clearance results in an excellent target to background ratio for the mid and lower abdomen if a bleeding is visualized. Overall, Tc-99m sulfur colloid is nowadays rarely used.

MECKEL SCAN

A Meckel diverticulum is a remnant of the omphalomesenteric duct located in the ileum, approximately 50 to 80 cm proximal to the ileocecal valve. Approximately 50% of Meckel diverticula contain gastric mucosa. Bleeding secondary to Meckel diverticula may be secondary to ulceration of the adjacent small bowel mucosa. Because one of the properties of Tc-99m pertechnetate is to accumulate in gastric mucosa (particularly in the mucin cells), it is used in patients (typically young children) having unexplained GI bleeding due to a suspected Meckel diverticulum. Meckel scintigraphy should be performed when the patient is not actively bleeding. If active bleeding is present, the most appropriate radionuclide technique is a GI bleeding scintigraphy (using labeled RBC). Prior to the procedure, the patient should fast for 6 hours. Pharmacologic pretreatment is not considered mandatory when performing Meckel scintigraphy, nevertheless it may be considered (especially if there is continued clinical suspicion despite a negative study result). Pretreatment with pentagastrin, H2 (histamine) blockers, and/or glucagons has been reported to improve the accuracy of Meckel scintigraphy. Pentagastrin for example enhances the uptake of pertechnetate by the gastric mucosal cells and has been shown to increase rapidity, intensity, and duration of pertechnetate uptake. On the other hand, it also stimulates GI motility, which could potentially reduce the activity at ectopic sites. H2 blockers such as cimetidine and ranitidine block the secretion of pertechnetate from the gastric cells and increase uptake in gastric mucosa leading to more intense and prolonged uptake. Oral cimetidine (300 mg qid × 2 days in adults) is the preferred choice of histamine blockade. Glucagon, an antiperistaltic agent, relaxes the smooth muscles of the GI tract and may delay or prevent washout from pertechnetate both from the stomach and from the ectopic site. Other interventions reported to improve accuracy of the examination is placing the patient in a left lateral decubitus position during imaging and nasogastric tube suction (both may prevent secretions from the stomach to enter the small bowel). With the patient supine (or left lateral decubitus), dynamic planar images of the anterior abdomen and pelvis (30–60 s/frame) are obtained for 30 to 60 minutes. Additional oblique, lateral, or posterior projections including a postvoid image may be helpful. Radiotracer uptake in the ectopic gastric mucosa generally appears as a distinct focus that is seen at the same time as the normal gastric mucosa (usually within the first 5–10 minutes). The diverticulum may be located anywhere in the abdomen, although the right lower quadrant is the typical location. Sources of error are radiotracer activity in the kidneys, ureter, or bladder; or radiotracer excreted by normal gastric mucosa that enters the small bowel. False-positives may be caused by bowel irritation from recent endoscopy or laxatives. In addition, any lesion with increased blood pool, such as ulceration, inflammation, tumor, or intussusceptions may be confused with the Meckel diverticulum. On the other hand, Meckel diverticula that are small in size or those that have an ischemic or necrotic component may appear later than the normal gastric mucosa or are not visualized at all. False-negative examinations may also be caused by attenuation from recent barium study, recent in vivo labeling of RBC, or perchlorate.

HEPATOBILIARY IMAGING

Introduction

Hepatobiliary scintigraphy described radionuclide studies that evaluate the function and integrity of the hepatobiliary system by visualizing the production and flow of bile from the liver through the biliary system into the intestinal tract. Common indications are suspected acute cholecystitis, common bile duct obstruction, chronic cholecystitis (also sometimes called biliary dyskinesis), bile leak, postcholecystectomy syndromes, and congenital abnormalities of the hepatobiliary tree.

Patient Preparation

The patient should be fasting for 4 to 24 hours for gallbladder visualization. If the patient has been fasting for greater than 24 hours, the gallbladder may not be able to fill (in this circumstance, the patient may be treated with sincalide, see below). To avoid effects of opioid medication, the scan should be delayed by more than 4 hours after the last opioid medication dose.

Radiotracers

Tc-99m labeled IDA (iminodiacetic acid) analogs are used for hepatobiliary scintigraphy. They have similar uptake (carrier mediated), transport (active membrane transport), and excretion mechanisms as bilirubin. Nevertheless IDA are neither conjugated nor metabolized. Tc-99m labeled disofenin (DISIDA) or mebrofenin (BRIDA) are the radiopharmaceuticals of choice. They are injected intravenously at a dose of 1.5 to 5 mCi for adults. Higher doses (up to 10 mCi) may be necessary in hyperbilirubinemia. Mebrofenin may also have an advantage over disofenin in this circumstance because of its higher hepatic extraction. Dynamic images of the anterior abdomen are performed immediately after the radiotracer administration. An initial blood flow phase is optional. If performed, the liver is typically visualized several seconds after other abdominal organs (spleen or kidney) are seen because the blood supply of the liver is predominantly by the portal vein (and not arterial). Images are generally obtained for 60 minutes (or less if gallbladder and bowel are clearly visualized). Additional views, especially a right lateral and left anterior oblique views, may be helpful to clarify anatomy and confirm gallbladder visualization. When the gallbladder is not visualized at 60 minutes, 4 hour delayed images or images after morphine augmentation may be performed. Delayed images (up to 24 hours) may be necessary in patients who have severe hepatocellular dysfunction, suspected common bile duct obstruction or biliary atresia. Delayed images at 2 to 4 hours (along with patient positioning maneuvers) can also be helpful if bile leak is suspected. Any drainage catheters and bags ought to be included in the field of view.

Interventions

Sincalide

Sincalide, a synthetic C-terminal octapeptide of cholecystokinin (CCK), stimulates gallbladder contraction and relaxes the sphincter of Oddi. It is given in doses of 0.01 to 0.02 μg/kg body weight over 30 to 60 minutes. Faster injections (3–10 minutes) can be used but may result in gallbladder spasm and more frequent side effects. Sincalide can be given prior to the injection of the radiotracer if the patient is NPO > 24 hours. Other indications are the assessment of gallbladder ejection fraction (GBEF) and excluding common bile duct obstruction. The GBEF can be determined after gallbladder contraction stimulated by sincalide. For that purpose, sincalide is infused after the gallbladder has filled on initial imaging (usually at 60 minutes). Dynamic acquisition is continued for an additional 30 or 60 minutes. GBEF can be calculated using the immediate presincalide image and the postsincalide data. ROI are drawn around the gallbladder and GEBF is calculated as follows:

$$\text{GBEF (\%)} = [(\text{maximum GB count} - \text{minimal GB counts}) / \text{maximum GB count}] \times 100$$

Normal values of GBEF that have been established depend on the specific protocol (total dose, dose rate, length of infusion) and range from >0% to >40%. A normal GBEF excludes acute acalculous cholecystitis (if the gallbladder fills initially) and chronic Cholecystitis. Bowel visualization after sincalide administration helps to differentiate common duct obstruction from normal variant.

Fatty meal

Fatty meal stimulation may be performed to assess gallbladder contractility if sincalide is unavailable or cannot be given (lack of intravenous access for example).

Phenobarbital

Phenobarbital is given in infants suspected of having biliary atresia (5 mg/kg/d divided in two doses) for 3 to 5 days prior to hepatobiliary scintigraphy. This stimulates hepatic cells and may increase the excretion of radiotracer, decreasing the false-positive rate.

Morphine augmentation

Morphine sulfate (MSO_4), given at doses of 0.04 –to 0.1 mg/kg body weight, can be administered if acute cholecystitis is suspected and the gallbladder is not visualized at 1 hour as an alternative to delayed imaging. The thought is that morphine increases the tone of the sphincter of Oddi, thus "forcing" the radiotracer into the gallbladder if the cystic duct is indeed patent. Morphine should only be given if radiotracer is seen in the small bowel (patent common bile duct). If the liver and intra- and extrahepatic biliary tree have only minimal residual radiotracer present, a "booster dose" of radiotracer (1 mCi) may be given in conjunction with morphine. Imaging is continued for an additional 30 minutes following morphine administration. Attention to possible contraindications (allergy, respiratory compromise, acute pancreatitis) is important.

Imaging Findings

Normal

Normal hepatobiliary scintigraphy is characterized by prompt visualization of the liver, followed by transit of radiotracer activity into the intra- and extrahepatic biliary tree, gallbladder, and small bowel. Gallbladder and small bowel are seen within an hour in most normal studies.

Acute cholecystitis

Acute cholecystitis is scintigraphically characterized by gallbladder nonvisualization on (4 hour) delayed images or after morphine augmentation (nonvisualization at 60 minutes could be acute cholecystitis, chronic cholecystitis or normal variant). The so-called "rim sign" describes a band of increased radiotracer uptake in the hepatic tissue adjacent to the gallbladder fossa that is related to increased blood flow and inflammation. It is more often associated with severe gangrenous or phlegmonous cholecystitis and is associated with a higher frequency of complications and poorer prognosis. Overall sensitivities are reported to be 95% to 100% with specificities of 91% to 99%. Potential causes of false-positive results are insufficient fasting (less than 4 hours), prolonged fasting (greater than 24 hours), severe hepatocellular dysfunction or intercurrent illness, high grade common bile duct obstruction, rapid biliary to bowel transit, severe chronic cholecystitis, and previous cholecystectomy. False-negative examinations are extremely rare but may be encountered if radiotracer activity in or near the gallbladder fossa (overlying bowel loop, bile leak, congenital abnormalities, activity in the kidneys) is mistaken for gallbladder visualization.

Chronic cholecystitis

In chronic cholecystitis, the gallbladder is usually visualized within 1 hour after radiotracer administration. The hallmark of chronic cholecystitis is an abnormally reduced GBEF. A decreased GBEF may also be seen in acute acalculous cholecystitis, certain nonbiliary conditions (acute intermittent illness, diabetes mellitus, obesity, pancreatic insufficiency, sickle cell disease), and several medications (morphine, atropine, calcium channel blocker, progesterone, histamine blockers among other).

Common bile duct obstruction

Common bile duct obstruction is usually suspected when there is no or severely delayed (>60 minutes) biliary to bowel clearance. With acute, complete, or high-grade obstruction, there is usually prompt liver uptake, but no visualization of the biliary tree and gallbladder (because of "back pressure" from the obstruction preventing excretion of radiotracer from the liver). With prolonged obstruction, hepatocellular dysfunction is eventually seen, which makes interpretation of lack of small bowel activity more difficult. Nonvisualization of small bowel at 60 minutes may also be seen in up to 20% of normal individuals. In these cases, the gallbladder (if present) is usually seen, and administration of sincalide or delayed images should be obtained to differentiate normal variant from obstruction.

Biliary atresia

Hepatobiliary scintigraphy in infants can help differentiate between neonatal hepatitis (biliary to bowel clearance demonstrated) and biliary atresia (no biliary to bowel clearance). Both entities usually have persistent liver uptake due to poor hepatocellular function. Delayed images are often necessary and should be obtained for 24 hours if necessary. Premedication with phenobarbital to stimulate hepatic enzymes is recommended. If an initial scan was performed without premedication and is consistent for biliary atresia (bowel not visualized), a repeat study after appropriate premedication is recommended. Radiotracer activity in the urinary tract or diaper may be confused with bowel activity and can lead to false interpretation.

Bile leak

A biliary leak is likely present when radiotracer accumulates in locations other then the liver, biliary tree, gallbladder, bowel, or urine. Accuracy of detection by hepatobiliary scintigraphy depends on the severity and location of the leak. Delayed images, additional views, changes in patient positioning, and correlation to anatomic imaging (location of fluid collections, postsurgical (blind) bowel loops, etc.) are all useful.

Postcholecystectomy pain

There are several reasons for pain after cholecystectomy including sphincter of Oddi dysfunction which has the scintigraphic appearance of (partial) common bile duct obstruction. Pretreatment with sincalide to increase bile flow may improve accuracy of the study for that indication. Visual and (semi)quantitative parameters taking into account clearance of radiotracer form the liver parenchyma and common bile duct, timing of small bowel visualization, and appearance of intra- and extrahepatic ducts have been employed.

Other findings

Enterogastric (duodenogastric) reflux may be incidentally seen during hepatobiliary scintigraphy. It may possibly be an alternative explanation of the patient's symptoms (epigastric/abdominal discomfort).

HEMANGIOMA IMAGING

Liver blood pool imaging using 99mTc labeled RBCs is performed for the detection of hepatic hemangiomas. A typical clinical situation would be a liver lesion detected on anatomical imaging (ultrasound, CT, and MRI) that has some but not all typical characteristics of hemangioma, and clarification is felt necessary. Blood flow ("radionuclide angiography") and immediate blood pool images are optional for hepatic blood pool imaging. Delayed blood pool images at 30 minutes to 3 hours are mandatory. The study should be obtained in multiple views (anterior, posterior, and lateral) including the view most likely to reveal the lesion (based on anatomic imaging). When the lesion is small (less than 2 cm), or when multiple lesions are present, and/or when planar imaging is unrevealing, SPECT or SPECT/CT (if available) imaging is recommended. Markedly increased radiotracer activity on delayed blood pool of a hepatic lesion is very specific for a cavernous hepatic hemangioma (the lesions usually have no increased (arterial) blood flow or immediate blood pool uptake). Hemangiomas >2 to 3 cm are generally always identified on planar images, whereas SEPCT is useful for lesions smaller than that (lesions as small as 0.5 cm may be detected with SPECT imaging). Other tumors of the liver (i.e., angiosarcomas) could possibly also have increased uptake during the delayed blood pool phase (yet they also have increased flow). False-negatives may be encountered in hemangiomas with partial fibrosis or thrombosis. Lesion location (i.e., lesions adjacent to the heart, great vessels, and kidney) can also affect accuracy.

LIVER SPLEEN SCAN

Liver spleen scintigraphy is not frequently used nowadays, since most liver lesions can be characterized with newer types of imaging (ultrasound, CT, and MRI). Liver and spleen radionuclide imaging may still be used in selected liver lesions (e.g., suspected focal nodular hyperplasia), to assess for functioning splenic tissue (suspected asplenia, residual splenic tissue in patient with thrombocytopenia postsplenectomy, accessory spleen, and masses). For liver spleen scans, 4 to 6 mCi of 99mTc sulfur colloid (small colloid particles: 0.1–1.0 μm) is injected intravenously. After injection, sulfur colloid is quickly phagocytized by the reticuloendothelial system. Imaging is begun after more than 15 to 20 minutes when blood pool clearance has occurred. Planar images of the abdomen in the anterior, posterior, lateral, and oblique views are usually obtained. SPECT (or SPECT/CT) imaging may be useful. Extra views with (size) markers for measuring liver and spleen size and for identifying anatomical landmarks may also be helpful in certain circumstances. Normal biodistribution includes the liver (85%), spleen (10%), and bone marrow (5%). The so-called colloid shift describes increased radiotracer uptake in the spleen and bone marrow relative to the liver. This phenomenon can be observed in hepatic dysfunction and portal hypertension, hypersplenism, or bone marrow activation (i.e., cytopenia). Diffuse pulmonary activity is nonspecific and could be secondary to cirrhosis, infection, neoplasm, coagulopathy, estrogens, trauma, or excess aluminum in colloid. Sources of error may be related to anatomic variations, respiratory motion, and colloid size (i.e., smaller particles may be localizing preferentially in the bone marrow, larger particles in the spleen).

SPLENIC IMAGING USING HEAT DAMAGED RED BLOOD CELLS

Heat-damaged red blood cells are cleared by functioning splenic tissue. Therefore radionuclide (Tc-99m pertechnetate) labeled heat damaged RBC can also be used for splenic imaging. Heat damage is accomplished generally by heating RBCs in a waterbath at 49ºC to 50ºC for 20 minutes. Imaging is begun 30 minutes to 2 hours after reinjection of the heat damaged RBCs. If ectopic splenic tissue is suspected, images of the entire abdomen (or chest depending on the situation, i.e., prior trauma) are obtained. SPECT (or SPECT/CT) may be useful. Sources of error may be secondary to the degree of damage to the red blood cells.

OTHER IMAGING TECHNIQUES

HEPATIC PERFUSION STUDIES

Hepatic perfusion imaging following the injection of Tc-99m macroaggregated albumin through a hepatic artery catheter is performed to determine the biodistribution of agents to be administered via the catheter (i.e., chemotherapy, radiolabeled microspheres). This helps to assure that the catheter is correctly placed to deliver the therapeutic agent to the liver tumor and to avoid perfusion of normal extrahepatic tissue such as the lungs or GI tract. Multiple planar views of the abdomen as well as images of the lungs are obtained after radiotracer injection.

Images should be reviewed for the presence of radiotracer accumulation within the liver (masses) and uptake outside the liver (i.e., lung, stomach, small bowel). Significant lung uptake caused by right-to-left shunting can also be quantified.

SUGGESTED READING

Sandler MP, ed. *Diagnostic Nuclear Medicine*. 4th ed. Philadelphia, PA: Lippincott Williams & Wilkins; 2003.

Donohoe KJ, Maurer AH, Ziessman HA, Urbain J-L C, Royal HD, Martin-Cumin J. Society of Nuclear Medicine Procedure Guideline for Adult Solid Meal Gastric Emptying Study. http://interactive.snm.org/docs. Accessed May 6, 2009.

Royal HD, Brown ML, Drum DE, Nagle CE, Sylvester JM, Ziessman HA. Society of Nuclear Medicine Procedure Guideline for Hepatic and Splenic Imaging. http://interactive.snm.org/docs. Accessed May 6, 2009.

Balon HR, Bill DR, Fink-Bennett DM, et al. Society of Nuclear Medicine Procedure Guideline for Hepatobiliary Scintigraphy. http://interactive.snm.org/docs. Accessed May 6, 2009.

Ford PV, Bartold SP, Fink-Bennett DM, et al. Society of Nuclear Medicine Procedure Guideline for Gastrointestinal Bleeding and Meckel's Diverticulum Scintigraphy. http://interactive.snm.org/docs. Accessed May 6, 2009.

QUESTIONS AND ANSWERS

1. Which of the following statements about gastric emptying studies is *true*?
   A. Solid meals are usually labeled with Tc-99m DTPA.
   B. Liquid gastric emptying is typically exponential.
   C. Liquid gastric emptying is abnormal if solid emptying is impaired.
   D. Patient should ingest a nonlabeled test meal just prior to the radiolabeled meal to make sure he/she tolerates the meal.

   ANSWER: B. Solid (or liquid) meals are usually labeled with Tc-99m sulfur colloid (In 111 is an alternative). Liquid gastric emptying may be normal when solid gastric emptying is impaired. It is certainly not always abnormal. No test meal is necessary; in fact the patient needs to be fasting for at least 4 hours. It is nevertheless good practice to inform the patient about the procedure (including the meal) beforehand, and ensure there are no intolerances or dietary restrictions.

2. Differences between GI bleeding scintigraphy using labeled RBC and studies using Tc-99m sulfur colloid include.
   A. Studies with labeled RBCs are typically shorter.
   B. Radiation dose to the spleen is higher in labeled RBC studies.
   C. Sensitivity for bleedings in the upper abdomen is higher in sulfur colloid studies.
   D. False-positives studies from blood pool activity in abnormal vascular structures (abdominal varices) are not usually encountered with sulfur colloid imaging.

   ANSWER: D. Given the fast clearance of sulfur colloid from the blood pool, false-positives examinations from blood pool activity in abnormal vascular structures are not usually encountered with sulfur colloid imaging, although it is a problem with RBC scintigraphy. Studies with sulfur colloid are typically shorter because of the fast clearance. The radiation dose to the spleen is higher in sulfur colloid studies. Target organ for labeled RBC studies is the heart. The sensitivity for bleedings in the upper abdomen is lower in sulfur colloid studies because of the overlying intense uptake of the liver and spleen.

3. Regarding labeling of red blood cells with Tc-99m pertechnetate, which of the following statements is *true*?
   A. In vivo technique requires venous blood sampling.
   B. In vitro technique has the highest labeling efficiency.
   C. Image quality is not effected by the type of labeling technique.
   D. Labeling techniques are robust and not influenced by medications.

   ANSWER: B. The in vivo technique does not require venous blood sampling. The in vitro technique has the highest labeling efficiency, followed by the modified in vitro technique. The in vivo technique has the poorest labeling efficiency. Since image quality has to do with labeling efficiency, it is affected by the labeling technique. Labeling may be affected by multiple factors including medications (heparin, doxorubicin among other), iodinated contrast, antibodies (e.g., from transfusion), too much or not enough stannous ion used during labeling, or incorrect incubation time intervals during labeling.

4. All of the following medications have been used to enhance the accuracy of Meckel scintigraphy, *except*.
   A. Sincalide
   B. Pentagastrin
   C. Glucagon
   D. Cimetidine

   ANSWER: A. Sincalide has no role in Meckel scintigraphy. It is used in hepatobiliary imaging (see above). Pentagastrin enhances the uptake of pertechnetate by the gastric mucosal cells, resulting in a more rapid and intense and durable pertechnetate uptake. Cimetidine is a histamine blocking agent that blocks the secretion of pertechnetate from the gastric cells and increases uptake in gastric mucosa again leading to more intense and prolonged uptake. Ranitidine is another H2 blocker that can be used. Glucagon relaxes the smooth muscles of the GI tract and may delay or prevent washout from pertechnetate from the Meckel diverticulum.

5. Hepatobiliary scintigraphy using 99mTc mebrofenin is performed in a 50-year-old woman with right upper quadrant pain and gallstones visualized on ultrasound. After 60 minutes of imaging, the gallbladder and common bile duct is visualized, yet no radiotracer is seen in the small bowel. What is the most likely diagnosis?
   A. Acute cholecystitis
   B. Normal variant
   C. Acute complete common bile duct obstruction
   D. False-negative finding from prolonged fasting

   ANSWER: B. Visualization of the gallbladder implies a patent cystic duct and therefore, excludes acute cholecystitis with a high degree of certainty. The hallmark of acute complete common bile duct obstruction is nonvisualization of the intra-/extrahepatic biliary tree, gallbladder, and small bowel. Prolonged fasting status may affect visualization of the gallbladder (possibly leading to false-positive examinations); it has no influence on initial biliary to bowel clearance. The differential diagnosis for the above finding (nonvisualization of the bowel at 1 hour despite activity in the gallbladder and common bile duct) includes partial common bile duct obstruction and normal variant (may be seen in 20% of normal patients).

6. What would *not* be an appropriate next intervention in the patient described before?
   A. Infuse sincalide intravenous over 30 minutes and continue imaging
   B. Delayed images at 4 hours
   C. Imaging after having eaten a fatty meal
   D. Administer morphine sulfate intravenous and continue imaging for another 30 minutes

   ANSWER: D. To differentiate between obstruction and normal variant, sincalide infusion, which stimulates gallbladder contraction and relaxes the sphincter of Oddi, would be the best next step. Alternatively, imaging after stimulation with a fatty meal or just delayed images may also be an option. Morphine is not indicated. In fact, it is contraindicated if small bowel is not visualized. Morphine is used in suspected acute cholecystitis if the gallbladder is not visualized at 60 minutes as an alternative to delayed imaging.

7. A diabetic patient with postprandial abdominal discomfort underwent a solid phase gastric emptying study that demonstrated delayed gastric emptying. Possible sources of error or confounding factors for this result include all of the following *except*:
   A. Poor, unstable radiolabel of the solid meal
   B. Hyperglycemia
   C. Overlap of small bowel in the region of interest
   D. Patient did not eat the entire meal.

   ANSWER: A. Poor, unstable radiolabel of a solid meal may result in more rapid gastric emptying than expected (the Tc-99m sulfur colloid may bind to gastric secretions (fluids) resulting in mixed liquid/solid emptying characteristics). Diabetic patients may suffer from diabetic gastroparesis from autonomic dysfunction. In addition, acute hyperglycemia can cause delayed gastric emptying. It may be of value to have blood sugars monitored in patient with diabetes and instruct them to bring medication/insulin on the day of the study. Overlap of small bowel in the region of interest leads to overestimation of total counts (and therefore falsely prolonged gastric emptying). Gastric emptying depends on meal volume (larger meals empty faster than smaller meals), so if the patient did not eat the entire meal, gastric emptying may be prolonged compared to standard normal values for that meal.

8. A patient has a 1.5 cm liver lesion that demonstrates atypical characteristics for a hemangioma on contrast-enhanced CT. A labeled red blood cell study is requested for further evaluation. Which of the following statements is *true*?
   A. Increased early arterial flow and immediate blood pool images will confirm that the lesion is a hepatic hemangioma.
   B. If the lesion is "cold" on the RBC study, it will confirm that the lesion is malignant.
   C. SPECT imaging should be considered.
   D. Performing the scan with heat damaged red blood cells improves accuracy.

   ANSWER: C. Increased delayed blood pool (at 30 minutes–3 hours) is the hallmark of a hepatic hemangioma. Typically, the lesions do not have increased early arterial flow and immediate blood pool. A "cold" lesion on a RBC study is very nonspecific and is seen in most lesions, benign or malignant, other than hemangiomas. SPECT imaging should be considered since it improves lesion localization if the lesion size is less than 2 to 3 cm. Red blood cells used for hemangioma imaging are never heat damaged. Heat-damaged red blood cells have been used for imaging splenic tissue.

9. Which of the following statements regarding hepatobiliary scintigraphy for the evaluation of infants with persistent hyperbilirubinemia is *true*?
   A. Should never be performed without pretreatment with phenobarbital.

B. Imaging for up to 12 hours is sufficient.
C. Biliary atresia is excluded if radiotracer is seen in the intestinal tract.
D. Disofenin with a maximal dose of 0.1 for infants is the preferred radiopharmaceutical.

ANSWER: C. Biliary atresia is excluded if radiotracer is seen in the bowel. Careful inspection of dynamic and static images to ensure that other radiotracer activity (GU tract, contamination) is not mistaken for bowel activity is important. On the other hand, nonvisualization of bowel is consistent with biliary atresia, but may also be caused by severe hepatocellular dysfunction from any cause. The scan may be performed without pretreatment with phenobarbital. Nevertheless, if a scan performed without phenobarbital pretreatment does not show biliary to bowel clearance, the examination should be repeated after appropriate pretreatment (phenobarbital: 5 mg/kg/d divided in two doses, for 3–5 days). Although some experts suggest checking phenobarbital levels prior to HIDA scanning, this is not mandatory. Imaging for up to 12 hours may not be sufficient. Images up to 24 hours are often necessary. Mebrofenin is preferable to disofenin in this circumstance (hyperbilirubinemia) because of its higher hepatic extraction. The dose for infants and children is weight based (0.05–0.2 mCi/kg), with a minimum recommended activity of approximately 0.5 mCi.

10. Areas of focally or regionally increased radiotracer uptake within the liver during scintigraphic procedures can be seen in which of the following conditions?
    A. Liver hemangioma – HIDA scan
    B. Focal nodular hyperplasia – sulfur colloid scan
    C. Hepatic adenoma – labeled red blood cell scan
    D. Budd Chiari syndrome – quadrate lobe of the liver on sulfur colloid scan

ANSWER: B. There are only a few focal hepatic lesions that have somewhat typical appearance on certain radionuclide studies (most lesions are usually "cold" or have such variable patterns that scintigraphic examinations have very limited predictive value). The most important one is hepatic hemangioma, which is essentially the only liver lesion that would demonstrate increased delayed blood pool activity. Another hepatic lesion is focal nodular hyperplasia (FNH), which contains hepatocytes and Kupffer cells. FNH may demonstrate sulfur colloid uptake equal or greater than the liver in approximately 50% to 60%. Therefore, normal or increased sulfur colloid uptake in a liver lesion is very suggestive of FNH. Of note, a regenerative nodule in a cirrhotic liver may also have increased sulfur colloid uptake. There are also several vascular abnormalities that can lead to differences in regional hepatic perfusion and thus cause areas of increased radiotracer uptake (on either HIDA or sulfur colloid scan), such as Budd Chiari syndrome (hepatic outflow obstruction such as hepatic vein thrombosis), which leads to increased uptake in the caudate lobe (the caudate lobe has separate venous efferent blood flow directly to the inferior cava). Occlusion of the superior vena cava can lead to increased uptake (on HIDA, sulfur colloid, or other scans) in the quadrate lobe of the liver because of collateral venous pathways (if the tracer was injected in the upper extremity) (occlusion of the inferior vena cava may lead to the same pattern in the lower extremity were chosen for injection of the radiotracer).

94 GENITOURINARY NUCLEAR MEDICINE

Jon A. Baldwin

The primary role of nuclear medicine is in the functional analysis of the genitourinary system (Table 94-1).

RENAL IMAGING AGENTS

Selection of the renal radiopharmaceutical is dependent on the parameter one wishes to assess. Twenty percent of total renal function is the result of glomerular filtration; the remaining 80% is the result of tubular secretion. ^{99m}Tc diethylenetriamine penta-acetic acid (^{99m}Tc DTPA) is almost entirely filtered through the glomerulus, and therefore is an agent used to determine

TABLE 94-1 Indications for Radionuclide Study of GU Tract

Renal perfusion
Quantitative and differential function of native kidneys
Evaluation for obstruction (Lasix renography)
Screening for renovascular hypertension (captopril renography)
Quantitative and differential function of allograft kidneys
Radionuclide cortical imaging
Screening for and evaluation of vesicoureteral reflux
Evaluation of testicular torsion

glomerular filtration rate (GFR). Approximately 5% to10% of ^{99m}Tc DTPA is bound to plasma proteins once injected, which will result in a slight underestimation of GFR. ^{99m}Tc DTPA can demonstrate renal perfusion (radionuclide angiogram), renal parenchymal abnormalities, and assesses the renal collecting system and bladder for obstruction. It is not the ideal agent for assessment of the renal parenchyma itself, as it has a brief nephrogram phase; the cortical imaging agents described later in the chapter are superior for this task. In addition, the extraction fraction is approximately 10% to 20%, which somewhat limits the utility of ^{99m}Tc DTPA in patients with poor renal function or longstanding/high-grade obstruction, when compared to other radiopharmaceuticals with higher extraction fractions. Peak cortical uptake usually occurs by 3 to 5 minutes. One-half of the peak cortical activity is reached at 15 to 20 minutes. Bladder activity typically appears by 6 minutes at the latest. Ureter activity may not be seen in normal subjects.

Prior to 1986, the radiopharmaceutical that measured tubular secretion was ^{131}I orthoiodohippurate (^{131}I OIH). ^{131}I OIH is primarily (80%) cleared by tubular secretion, with the remainder filtered at the glomerulus. ^{131}I OIH is no longer commercially available in the United States. Tubular secretion and, by extension, the measurement of effective renal plasma flow (ERPF), is now primarily measured by the radiotracer ^{99m}Tc mercaptylacetyltriglycine (^{99m}Tc MAG3). Because the radionuclide label is ^{99m}Tc, a larger radiotracer dose may be used than with ^{131}I OIH. The 140-keV photons emitted are far superior to those of ^{131}I OIH for rendering images used to interpret morphology of the kidneys and generate time activity curves. ^{99m}Tc MAG3 is predominately cleared by the proximal tubules, with less than 5% filtration. The overall clearance of ^{99m}Tc MAG3 is approximately 60% that of ^{131}I OIH, because of slower plasma clearance and higher proportion of protein binding. In truth, ^{99m}Tc MAG3 measures the clearance of ^{99m}Tc MAG3, *not* ERPF; a correction factor is necessary to compute an ERPF when using this agent. It is a better agent to use in patients with renal dysfunction, as its extraction fraction (40%–50%) is superior to that of ^{99m}Tc DTPA.

Imaging of the renal cortex can be achieved with one of two agents. Both agents are fixed to proximal renal tubular cells via sulfhydryl group binding. The most commonly used radiopharmaceutical is ^{99m}Tc dimercaptosuccinic acid (^{99m}Tc DSMA). Approximately 40% of the dose is ultimately concentrated in the renal cortex. Because of its slow clearance rate, a delay of 1 to 3 hours is necessary for optimal imaging. Once this delay is met, however, the image quality is very good, with an excellent target-to-background ratio. ^{99m}Tc glucoheptonate (^{99m}Tc GH) is also used for cortical imaging. A radiolabeled carbohydrate, a smaller percentage of this radiotracer is bound to the cortex when compared to ^{99m}Tc DMSA. ^{99m}Tc GH is also filtered, so it can be imaged after injection to assess renal flow, the collecting system, and the bladder. Table 94-2 summarizes commonly used renal radiopharmaceuticals.

TABLE 94-2 Renal Radiopharmaceuticals Used in Renal Imaging

RADIONUCLIDE	DOSE (mCi)	PARAMETER ASSESSED	CRITICAL ORGAN
^{99m}Tc DTPA	10–20	GFR	Bladder
^{99m}Tc MAG3	5–10	ERPF	Bladder
^{99m}Tc GH	10–20	GFR and cortical	Bladder
^{99m}Tc DSMA	1–5	Cortical	Kidney

QUANTITATIVE AND DIFFERENTIAL RENAL FUNCTION

It should be noted that no imaging of the radiopharmaceutical need be performed to quantify either GFR or ERPF in certain circumstances. Some institutions use a plasma-sampling technique that generates a "superior" result in terms of accuracy and reproducibility than a camera-based technique. The drawback to this method is having to handle blood products, as well as additional laboratory training and credentialing. For the purposes of review, an outline of the plasma sample technique will follow. Before the patient is injected with the radiopharmaceutical, the dose is placed in a dose calibrator and the reading is recorded. The patient is injected with the radiopharmaceutical, and if imaging is to be performed, the camera is started. The syringe is again placed in the dose calibrator, and a "residual" is measured. This number is subtracted from the original reading, and the difference is the dose that the patient actually received. At a specific time, a blood samples will be taken from the patient. The time used is based on data beyond the scope of this discussion; suffice to say that it is approximately 45 minutes for ^{99m}Tc MAG3 and at 60 and 180 minutes ^{99m}Tc DTPA (because of its slower plasma clearance). The sample is spun in a centrifuge, and the plasma is subsequently placed in a well counter (along with a radiopharmaceutical standard) and counted. This result is then decay corrected. Knowing how much radiopharmaceutical was injected into the patient, and how much remains in the plasma at a fixed time period, one can use this information to calculate GFR or ERPF (depending on the radiopharmaceutical used). A critical assumption in this method is that the full dose was delivered intravascularly. The presence of a dose infiltration at the injection site could artificially increase or decrease the measured renal function parameter if the infiltration is relatively "loculated" (activity is not in the plasma because of it being sequestered, artificially inflating the result) or gradually reenters the circulation via the lymphatics, respectively.

Most facilities have found that a camera-based method of determining renal function is sufficiently accurate and reproducible for their needs. Care should be taken when using this method, however, as differences in positioning and processing can cause wide variations in results, as will be described. Before the patient is injected, the dose is imaged at a precise geometry and distance from the camera's collimator for a set time, usually 1 minute. Meticulous attention to detail is crucial when positioning the dose for reproducibility. The patient is then injected with the radiopharmaceutical, and sequential images are obtained for a set time (typically 6 minutes for ^{99m}Tc DTPA). These images are then processed, and regions of interest are drawn around the kidneys, as well as outside the kidneys for background correction. The background-corrected counts for each kidney can then be compared as a percentage to the injected dose. Attenuation must be corrected for by using the patient's weight and height using standardized formulae. Potential sources of error for this method include dose infiltration, imprecise positioning of the radiotracer syringe, inclusion of a blood pool structure (such as the liver or spleen) in the background correction region of interest (ROI), and imprecise "attenuation correction" because of variability in kidney depth in patients.

The majority of functional renal imaging performed in the United States is performed with ^{99m}Tc MAG3. The review in the remainder of this section will assume that ^{99m}Tc MAG3 is the radiopharmaceutical being used; if there are significant differences in normal values or pathologic findings when using ^{99m}Tc DTPA, they will be described.

For the purposes of the study of renal function, the patient and camera are positioned in such a way as to minimize attenuation from overlying structures and ensure that the kidney is centered in the field of view. The camera is situated posterior to the supine patient for the study of native kidney function, and the camera is situated anterior to the supine patient for the study of renal allograft function. Anterior camera positioning is also preferred for imaging of horseshoe kidneys. ROIs are drawn around the kidney(s), and time activity curves are produced. Once the patient is injected, the radiotracer transits through the kidney in three phases: vascular, concentration, and excretory (Fig. 94-1). The vascular phase represents renal perfusion. It begins approximately 15 to 20 seconds after injection, and within 4 to 6 seconds after aorta visualization. This peaks at

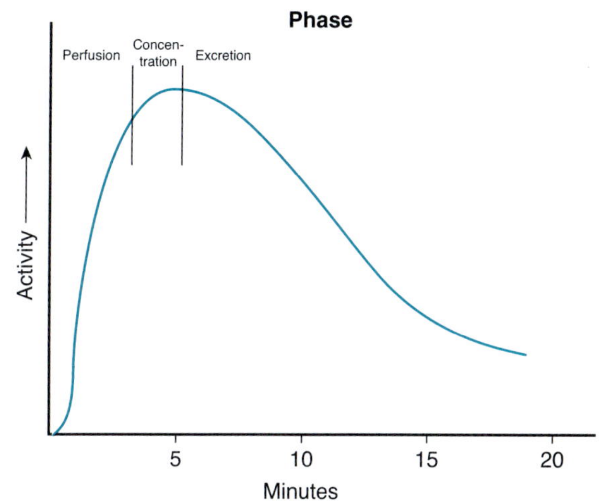

FIG. 94-1 Three phases of the renogram.

approximately 30 seconds and levels off. Because of the quick nature of this process, dynamic serial images are made for every 1 to 5 seconds for 1 minute. ROIs are drawn around both kidneys and the aorta, taking care not to include the spleen or liver (Fig. 94-2). Activity within the kidneys is ideally symmetric and approximately equal to slightly less intense compared to the peak of the aorta activity. An injection with a good bolus is imperative for reliable data. Table 94-3 lists common causes for patterns of altered perfusion, in addition to some pathologies which do not have an altered perfusion phase. The next phase of uptake is the cortical uptake phase, also known as the parenchymal phase. It typically lasts 1 to 5 minutes. In this phase, the tubular secretory accumulation of the radiopharmaceutical predominates. The slope of this uptake correlates with global renal function; a steep slope is indicative of good renal function, while a more gradual increase is indicative of poor renal function. It is during this phase that true differential function of the kidneys is best determined. If one waits much beyond 3 minutes, they run

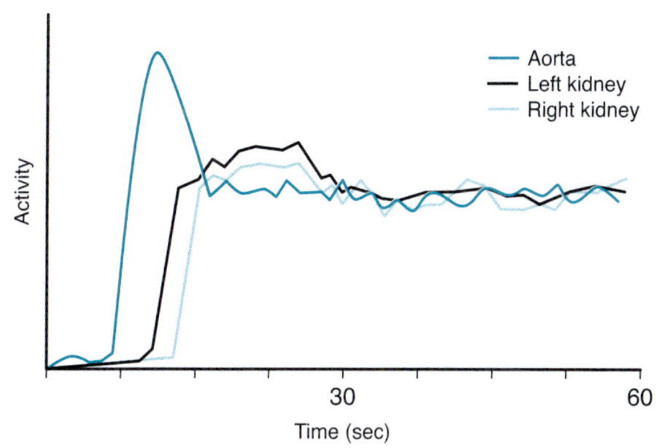

FIG. 94-2 Time-activity curve for renal perfusion.

TABLE 94-3 Renal Perfusion Findings

Symmetric decreased perfusion	Poor bolus/injection technique
Asymmetric decreased perfusion	Renal artery thrombosis
	Renal vein thrombosis
	Avulsion of renal artery
	Acute pyelonephritis
	Acute rejection (allograft)
	Longstanding high-grade obstruction
Asymmetric/focal increased perfusion	Renal artery aneurysm
Normal perfusion	Acute tubular necrosis
	Interstitial nephritis
	Cyclosporine toxicity

the risk of excreted radiotracer in the renal pelvis contributing to the counts within the ROI of the kidneys. Our facility has chosen 1 minute as the time at which differential function is determined. This, of course, presupposes that the injection was performed as a bolus, and that the camera was initiated at the time of injection. Improper timing of camera operation can alter not only differential function values, but peak time (typically 3–5 minutes) and 20/3 ratio values as well. As the study progresses, the final phase, the excretory phase, is entered, which lasts for the remainder of the study. During this phase, the excretion of radiotracer should exceed the uptake of radiotracer in normal patients. There is a gradual downsloping of activity, with radiotracer entering the renal pelvis and collecting systems on its way to the bladder. Approximately half of the peak counts is reached at approximately 7 to 10 minutes in normal patients. A way to quantify whether a patient has retention or not is to compare the number of counts within the ROI at 20 minutes to the number of counts at either peak activity, or at 3 minutes. This is called the 20/peak or 20/3 ratio, respectively. Please note that while these ratios are often used as a measure of cortical retention, the number would also be increased in obstruction, in which case the majority of the counts would be coming from the renal pelvis as opposed to the cortex. One must carefully inspect the images to attempt to conclude where the counts are coming from. Another potential source of error is the hydration status of the patient. If the patient is not adequately hydrated, this may lead to delays in excretion of radiotracer from the tubules. Table 94-4 summarizes normal ^{99m}Tc MAG3 findings.

TABLE 94-4 Summary of Normal ^{99m}Tc MAG3 Renal Scan Findings

PEAK TIME	DIFFERENTIAL FUNCTION	20/PEAK	20/3
3–5 min	50% + 6%	0.3	≤0.8

DIURETIC RENOGRAPHY

Intravenous-contrast urography and renal ultrasound provide excellent anatomic structural information in the evaluation of renal obstruction, but do not provide functional urodynamics. Renal scans performed without diuretics may demonstrate decreased perfusion to the affected kidney, the severity of which is dependent on the chronicity of the obstruction. The appearance of the concentration and excretory phases are also related to the chronicity of the obstruction, and the amount of preserved renal function. If the obstruction is indeed longstanding, the typical renogram appearance will reflect poor and asymmetric uptake, with a flattened renogram curve. An acute or subacute obstruction, however, will have continuously accumulating radiotracer, with a markedly delayed time to peak in the affected kidney (Fig. 94-3). This appearance can also be seen in a patient with a dilated collecting system as in nonobstructive hydronephrosis from a variety of causes: prior obstruction now reversed, vesicoureteral reflux (VUR), urinary tract infection, lax pelviureteral muscle, and congenital malformations.

The use of a diuretic such as Lasix will help differentiate between the conditions mentioned previously and mechanical obstruction. It is given intravenously over 1 to 2 minutes, and has a quick onset of action. Increasing renal flow by diuresis, radiotracer may be forced from the collecting system to the bladder. There are several variations as to how much and when to give the radiotracer. Most institutions will administer 40 mg of Lasix to its adult patients (1 mg/kg for the pediatric population, with maximum of 40 mg). If the patient has renal insufficiency, the dosage of Lasix can be increased to try to compensate for the decreased renal function. Likewise, as GFR is affected more by longstanding obstruction than is ERPF, ^{99m}Tc MAG3 should be used in patients will poor renal function. If renal function is

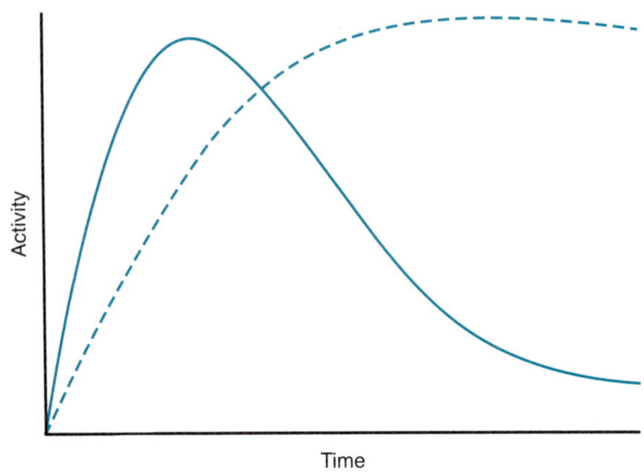

FIG. 94-3 Time-activity curve in an acutely obstructed kidney.

preserved, ^{99m}Tc DTPA will perform as well as ^{99m}Tc MAG3. Variations in timing of Lasix administration include prior to, at the time of, and after radiopharmaceutical injection. Administration prior to or at the radiopharmaceutical injection is preferred in patients with poor renal function, as this will give additional time for the Lasix to work. If given after the radiopharmaceutical, most institutions try to give it near peak activity, anywhere from 10 to 20 minutes after radiotracer injection. If there is no obstruction present, in less than 10 minutes there should be less than half of the counts remaining than were present at the peak. This is a normal time to half peak after Lasix administration. A transient slight upward deflection or plateau is not unusual in the renogram curve in normal patients. This represents diuretic-induced increased flow before clearance from the collecting system. When there is no response to Lasix, or there is continued accumulation of radiotracer within the renal pelvis, and the half peak has not been reached by 20 minutes after Lasix administration, the obstruction is present. Time to half peak between 10 and 20 minutes (15–20 minutes according to some authors) is indeterminate for obstruction. The most common cause for this finding is a very dilated renal pelvis with a subsequent reservoir effect. Numerous conditions can lead to a false positive for obstruction. In addition to the cause just listed, poor hydration status can contribute to a lack of response of Lasix; in this study, adequate hydration is imperative. Poor renal function can also lead to a poor response to Lasix administration. In these cases, the amount and timing of Lasix can be adjusted as listed to maximize the effect. Pressure from a full or neurogenic bladder may prevent the flow of radiotracer from the renal pelvis. In these cases, making sure the patient voids before the study (or self-catheterizes, in the case of neurogenic bladder) may help to prevent this phenomenon. In some cases, a Foley catheter may be needed in place during the study. Diuretic renography findings and false positives are summarized in Tables 94-5 and 94-6.

RENOVASCULAR HYPERTENSION

Only approximately 10% of patients with hypertension have a discernable cause for their high blood pressure; the majority of this population have "essential hypertension." Of those individuals who do not have essential hypertension, a significant number have renovascular hypertension (RVH). Risk factors for the presence of RVH include malignant/resistant hypertension, abrupt onset of hypertension, early or late onset of hypertension, and worsening renal function after initiation of angiotensin-converting enzyme (ACE) inhibitor therapy. The two main causes of RVH are atherosclerosis and fibromuscular dysplasia. The decrease in perfusion pressure in the afferent arterioles caused by the presence of either of these conditions is detected by the juxtaglomerular apparatus. In an effort to preserve perfusion pressure across the glomerulus, the cells of the juxtaglomerular apparatus release renin. Renin converts circulating angiotensinogen to angiotensin I, which is subsequently converted by ACE into angiotensin II, the active form. Angiotensin II increases perfusion pressure in the glomerulus and thereby GFR by preferential constriction of the efferent arteriole. Angiotensin II also increases sodium and water retention by decreasing peritubular hydrostatic pressure (as a consequence of efferent arteriole constriction) and by increasing aldosterone secretion from the adrenal gland. The administration of an ACE inhibitor would reduce these effects, and is the basis of radionuclide screening for RVH with an ACE inhibitor, such as captopril.

Several factors must be taken into account in regard to patient preparation. To increase the sensitivity of the study, the patient should stop ACE inhibitors prior to the renal study. The length of time to stop ACE inhibitor therapies varies with the duration of effect of the particular drug (3–5 days if the patient is taking captopril). Since patients with true RVH have high blood pressure that is difficult to control, this may not always be feasible; these patients may have the study using their dose of the ACE inhibitor as the pharmacologic agent. If the patient is to receive captopril as the pharmacologic agent for the renal scan, they should not have eaten for at least 4 to 6 hours to promote GI uptake of the drug (this precaution is unnecessary if an IV ACE inhibitor like enalapril is used). The patient should be well hydrated, however, dehydration can cause errors in interpretation. Before administration of the ACE inhibitor, it

TABLE 94-5 Diuretic Renography Findings

TIME TO HALF PEAK AFTER LASIX ADMINISTRATION	DIAGNOSIS
>10 min (15 min, some authors)	Not obstructed
Between 10 (15) and 20 min	Indeterminate for obstruction
>20 min	Obstructed

TABLE 94-6 Potential False Positives for Obstruction in Diuretic Renography

Inadequate patient hydration
Poor renal function
Massively dilated renal pelvis
Rigid/noncompliant renal pelvis
Full/neurogenic bladder
Neonate—(functionally immature kidneys)

is wise to review the patient's history and medications. This will help guide you as to the best dose of ACE inhibitor to use (usually 25–50 mg captopril PO; 5 mg enalapril IV). Using a lower dose may be more prudent on patients who are on large doses of other antihypertensive medications (to avoid inducing hypotension in the patient). Ideally, an IV should be placed before administration of the ACE inhibitor should the patient become hypotensive, and IV hydration become necessary. A baseline blood pressure should be checked, and periodic blood pressure measurements should be taken over the course of an hour to make sure the patient does not become hypotensive. After this uptake period, the patient will be ready to receive their radiopharmaceutical dose. Many facilities also administer IV Lasix at the time of radiopharmaceutical administration. This will promote collection system clearance, so as to not confound interpretation (i.e., counts emanating from renal pelvis retention rather than cortical retention).

The appearance of renal artery stenosis (RAS) will vary depending on the radiopharmaceutical chosen. If ^{99m}Tc DTPA, a GFR agent, is used, the affected kidney will demonstrate asymmetric decreased uptake and flow in that kidney because of the loss of perfusion pressure across the glomerulus along with a decrease in GFR of greater than 10%. However, ^{99m}Tc MAG3, a tubular agent, will have asymmetric marked cortical retention in the affected kidney. The curve has the appearance of the one given for renal obstruction (Fig. 94-3), with the counts in the ROI resulting from cortical retention as opposed to retention within the collecting system. If the study does not have the classic marked cortical retention appearance for RAS, a baseline study can be performed to compare to the ACE inhibitor study. Other findings that can be seen (compared to baseline) are a delay in time to peak of more than 2 minutes, delay in collecting system visualization by more than 2 minutes, and a 15% increase in cortical retention. If bilateral cortical retention is seen, it typically does not represent bilateral RAS, but rather the presence of hypotension or dehydration. Table 94-7 summarizes diagnostic criteria and the resulting interpretations. A "high probability for a hemodynamically significant RAS indicates there is a 90% chance that RAS is present. Low probability indicates the chance of RVH from RAS is less than 10%.

RENAL ALLOGRAFT FUNCTIONAL IMAGING

The study of allograft function is performed identically to that of the study of native kidney function, except that the camera is placed over the anterior pelvis for imaging. ^{99m}Tc MAG3 is typically used for imaging, although ^{99m}Tc DTPA can be used. ^{99m}Tc MAG3 is preferred because of its higher uptake and better target-to-background appearance. When used in conjunction with knowledge of the type of allograft implanted (cadaveric, living related, or living unrelated donor) and the time from implantation, a renal scan of the renal transplant is a good screening test to help differentiate conditions that can frequently occur in allografts, including accelerated acute rejection, acute rejection, chronic renal allograft nephropathy (chronic rejection), acute vasomotor nephropathy (AVN; less precisely referred to as acute tubular necrosis, ATN), and drug toxicity. Renal scans can also help detect surgical complications.

NONSURGICAL COMPLICATIONS

Hyperacute rejection is extremely rare, secondary to HLA immunologic screening. If preformed antibodies were present in the recipient's circulation, this type of rejection would result. This is an immediate response, typically too quick for imaging, and if imaging is performed, the allograft would appear as a photopenic area in the pelvis. The allograft cannot be saved.

Accelerated acute rejection can occur in patients who have had prior transplantations or other conditions that can cause increased antibodies in the circulation

TABLE 94-7 Summary of ACE Inhibitor Renal Study Findings and Interpretations

ACE INHIBITOR RENAL STUDY FINDING	STUDY INTERPRETATION
Unilateral decrease in uptake and clearance with ^{99m}Tc DTPA	High probability for a hemodynamically significant renal artery stenosis
Global decrease in GFR >10% when compared to baseline	
Unilateral marked cortical retention with ^{99m}Tc MAG3	
Change in function or symmetry present, but <10% compared to baseline	Intermediate probability for a hemodynamically significant renal artery stenosis
Bilateral cortical retention	
Baseline study changes/asymmetric poorly functioning kidney on both studies/baseline poor global renal function	
Symmetric function with normal renogram curves	Low probability for a hemodynamically significant renal artery stenosis

(e.g., multiple blood transfusions, pregnancy). This will typically occur as early as 3 days after implantation. If the patient had a normal baseline renal scan, one would expect an increase in time to peak and cortical retention (increased 20/3 ratio). As this is the scan appearance for acute vascular nephropathy, this can be differentiated on the basis of a normal baseline study and its early manifestation (3–5 days) after transplantation. If the initial study had the appearance of AVN, superimposed accelerated acute rejection or acute rejection can be suspected on the basis of renal function not improving over time (as typically occurs in AVN).

Acute rejection is more frequent in incidence than accelerated acute rejection. It has an imaging appearance similar to accelerated acute rejection (delayed time to peak, increased 20/3 ratio). Perfusion to the allograft will be delayed, if initial dynamic perfusion images are obtained. The time frame for the manifestation of acute rejection is longer than accelerated acute rejection, with its appearance typically occurring postoperative day 7 to 10. It is a common complication within the first 3 months of transplantation, although it can occur after this time frame in patients who have discontinued immunosuppressive therapy. AR can be mediated by either cell-mediated or humoral processes, although cell-mediated processes tend to predominate. Both accelerated acute rejection and AR often respond to medical therapy.

Despite the advances in immunosuppressive therapy, chronic allograft nephropathy/chronic rejection is the inevitable fate for a renal allograft. This manifestation can be delayed for many years with good therapy. The risk for hastened chronic rejection (appearing in 6–12 months) is increased if the allograft has had severe AVN, prior severe acute rejection, and immunosuppressive drug (cyclosporine and tacrolimus) toxicity. Imaging features include normal to mildly delayed time to peak, relatively decreased uptake, and minimal to no cortical retention. If measured, ERPF or GFR demonstrate a steady decline in function over time.

Acute vascular nephropathy, also referred to as ATN, is typically a complication of cadaveric donor kidneys, although living donor kidneys can have this complication if there is a long delay before implantation. Typically, there is a delay in uptake and time to peak, delay in appearance of radiotracer within the bladder and cortical retention leading to an increased 20/3 ratio. If dynamic renal allograft initial perfusion imaging is performed, it is usually normal. This condition is present in the baseline renal scan, and improves on subsequent studies. If the appearance does not resolve, superimposed acute rejection should be considered.

Cyclosporine and tacrolimus, although important for mitigating immune reactions that would lead to acute rejection, are known culprits for long-term decrease in allograft function, with longstanding use ultimately leading to chronic allograft nephropathy. Scintigraphic appearance of cyclosporine toxicity mimics the appearance of acute vascular nephropathy, with normal initial dynamic perfusion and cortical retention. Of course, the appearance of this cortical retention would not be present on the initial postoperative study, but only after weeks of therapy. Long-term use would lead to a chronic allograft nephropathy appearance. Given new immunosuppressive regimens, and lower doses of cyclosporine prescribed, this is now a less common complication.

SURGICAL COMPLICATIONS

Urine extravasation (urinoma) can be seen in both leakage from the ureterovesical anastomosis and damage to the transplant ureter. If present, this condition will lead to radiotracer outside the allograft or bladder, although delayed imaging may be necessary to demonstrate this. Care should be taken in interpretation of delay images when ^{99m}Tc MAG3 is used, as over time this is excreted into the bowel and may confound the picture for urinoma.

Ureteral obstruction can be the result of extrinsic compression from overlying hematoma or lymphocele or from ischemic scarring of the ureter and/or anastomosis. Diuretic renal scan, performed as described earlier in the chapter, can help detect this condition and differentiate it from a dilated collecting system. As the renogram curve can appear similar in obstruction, acute vascular nephropathy, and acute rejection, the images should be carefully scrutinized to determine whether the counts are coming from the cortex or the collecting system.

Lymphocele and hematoma will typically present as perinephric photopenic areas on a renal scan.

Arterial thrombosis is an extremely rare complication; this may be the result of difficulties related to implanting the allograft anastomosis into the patient's iliac artery. A renal scan of this condition would demonstrate no flow or function. If only a segmental arterial branch is obstructed, the scan may demonstrate an area of infarction within the allograft.

Venous thrombosis is usually a consequence of autoimmune complications, which occurs within the first few days to weeks of transplantation. This frequently will lead to loss of an allograft. As there are no collaterals within the allograft, the venous congestion will ultimately lead to a lack of flow in the allograft. Scintigraphic appearance is similar to arterial thrombosis, with a photopenic defect in the patient's pelvis surrounded by background activity.

RAS can occur in a transplanted kidney if there is constriction at the arterial anastomosis site (most commonly) or distal to the anastomosis site. An ACE inhibitor renal scan can be performed when this condition is suspected. When using ^{99m}Tc MAG3, if there is no cortical retention on the renal scan after ACE inhibitor, then there is a low probability that a hemodynamically significant RAS is present. If, however, there is marked cortical retention after ACE inhibitor administration, one should perform a baseline study without an ACE inhibitor, to eliminate the presence of acute vascular nephropathy or acute rejection, which would have similar scintigraphic appearance. If ^{99m}Tc DTPA is used, one would expect a marked decrease in flow and clearance in the presence of an ACE inhibitor. This would reverse on the baseline study without an ACE inhibitor.

RADIONUCLIDE CORTICAL IMAGING

The agents for renal cortical imaging are ^{99m}Tc DMSA and ^{99m}Tc GH. Although ^{99m}Tc DMSA results in a higher dose to the patient's kidney, the dose to the gonads is less than that of ^{99m}Tc GH, and for this reason, as well as its superior resolution, it is preferred for cortical imaging in the younger pediatric population. Renal cortical imaging is most often used to detect the presence of acute pyelonephritis in the pediatric population, in both symptomatic individuals, and in those with known VUR. ^{99m}Tc DMSA cortical imaging is more sensitive than ultrasound. An additional indication is differentiation of prominent column of Bertin from a malignant renal mass (a renal mass will not have ^{99m}Tc DMSA uptake, but column of Bertin will). The patient is imaged in the supine position at 1 to 3 hours after injection. A high-resolution parallel-hole collimator is used. A minimum of posterior planar views is acquired, although anterior and oblique views are preferred. Magnified views of the kidneys with a pinhole or converging collimator are recommended. SPECT images of the kidneys can also be performed, but this is sometimes difficult to accomplish in a nonsedated pediatric patient. If ^{99m}Tc GH is used, imaging is similar, but a flow phase is also acquired initially. Acute pyelonephritis can appear as a single focal ill-defined area of decreased uptake, multifocal areas of decreased uptake, or as diffuse decreased uptake in an otherwise normal-sized kidney. The first and second appearances can also be seen in tumors and scars as well. While a scar will typically have volume loss and contraction, leading to irregular contour, a mass may not. Correlation with ultrasound is recommended. The last appearance is indicative of a diffuse inflammatory process. Other "artifacts" that can cause inhomogeneous radiotracer distribution are overlying attenuation in the superior poles from liver and spleen, fetal lobulation, or relative decreased counts centrally from the collecting system. ^{99m}Tc DMSA is useful for following the course of the patient, and when the defect resolves or progresses to scar. It is recommended that there is an interval of 3 to 6 months between scanning.

RADIONUCLIDE CYSTOGRAPHY

The majority of cases of acute pyelonephritis in the pediatric population are the result of VUR of infected urine from the bladder into the kidneys. While radiographic-contrast cystography gives good anatomic information, and can detect the presence of posterior urethral valves in males, radionuclide cystography is the favored method for evaluation and follow-up for VUR. Radionuclide cystography is the more sensitive of the two modalities, being able to detect reflux volumes as low as 1 mL. In addition, the radiation dose to the gonads is substantially less than with the radiographic study, with anywhere from 50 to 150 times less exposure. The drawback is the loss of anatomical information because of resolution limitations; the usual radiographic system of grading cannot be applied.

The patient is placed in the supine position, with the camera posterior to the patient and positioned such that the bladder and kidneys will be in the field of view. The bladder is catheterized and connected to a 500-mL bag of normal saline 25 cm above the table; 0.5 to 1.0 mCi of ^{99m}Tc sulfur colloid (^{99m}Tc SC) is added to the bag of saline. ^{99m}Tc SC is preferred, because sodium pertechnetate ($Na^{99m}TcO_4$) or ^{99m}Tc DTPA may be absorbed by the bladder wall, especially in the presence of inflammation and excreted by the kidneys. The radiotracer is instilled into the bladder during a dynamic acquisition of images until the bladder is filled. Any reflux seen will be graded (Table 94-8). After bladder capacity is reached, the patient is preferably placed in the sitting position (with the camera posterior) as the patient voids. If the patient cannot void on request, supine positioning with the patient voiding into a diaper or towel can be performed. Dynamic imaging is performed during voiding as well, once again looking for the presence of reflux. A static postvoid image is also obtained, and can be used for the determination of postvoid residual volume. Given the amount of activity present in the bladder, it is possible that subtle reflux into the proximal ureter may be missed, but this is usually of little clinical consequence.

TABLE 94-8 Grading of Vesicoureteral Reflux

RADIOTRACER ACTIVITY	RADIONUCLIDE CYSTOGRAPHY "GRADE"	EQUIVALENT CONTRAST CYSTOGRAPHY GRADE
Confined to ureter	Mild/scintigraphic grade I	Grade I
Reflux into renal pelvis	Moderate/scintigraphic grade II	Grade II/III
Reflux into renal pelvis with clearly dilated collecting system/ureter	Severe/scintigraphic grade III	Grade IV/V

TESTICULAR IMAGING

The radionuclide imaging of testicular flow has almost entirely been relegated to historical interest with the availability, sensitivity, and specificity of ultrasound imaging. When performed, it is a good study for the differentiation of acute testicular torsion from other causes such as epididymitis. The radiotracer used is $Na^{99m}TcO_4$. The patient is imaged supine, with the camera anterior to the scrotum. The penis may be taped to the abdominal wall to keep it out of the field of view. A lead shield behind the testicles may help eliminate background activity from the thigh. It is helpful to have a marker placed on the affected side. A normal study will have symmetric low-level flow within the scrotum. The interpretation of abnormal studies will not only depend on the appearance, but also on clinical information, such as time from onset of pain and side of the pain.

Flow images may be normal in early acute testicular torsion. Abrupt termination of flow may be seen at the site of the torsion ("nubbin sign"). On the blood pool phase, focal absent activity can sometimes be seen at the affected testicle.

Delayed torsion: Although previously called "missed torsion," in these litigious times, delayed torsion has become the preferred term. For this condition, the torsion has been in place for some time, and the likelihood of testicle salvage is small. The most common appearance is a halo of increased activity (from hyperemia) around a central area of photopenia (testicle with no flow). While this is the typical appearance of delayed torsion, the appearance of testicular abscess is similar.

Findings in acute epididymitis include increased flow and blood pool activity to the painful side caused by the increased hyperemia of inflammation.

SUGGESTED READING

Blaufox MD, Aurell M, Bubeck B, et al. Report of the radionuclides in nephrology committee on renal clearance. *J Nucl Med.* 1996;37:1883-1890.

Dubovsky EV, Russell CD, Bischof-Elaloye A, et al. Report of the radionuclides in nephrology committee for evaluation of transplanted kidney (review of techniques). *Semin Nucl Med.* 1999;29:175-188.

QUESTIONS AND ANSWERS

1. Of the following appearances, which is *least* likely to represent a diagnosis of acute pyelonephritis in a ^{99m}Tc DMSA renal study?
   A. Focal cortical defect
   B. Irregular renal contour
   C. Multifocal cortical defects
   D. Diffusely decreased uptake unilaterally

   ANSWER: B. Focal cortical defect with irregular renal contour. Scarring from a previous infection usually results in volume loss and contraction, which can lead to an irregular renal contour. Admittedly, in practice this may be difficult to distinguish. All of the other appearances can be seen in the presentation of acute pyelonephritis.

2. A patient with suspected RVH has a baseline renal scan, which is reported as normal. A renal scan performed with captopril demonstrates marked asymmetry in function, with normal function on the right and marked decreased function on the left. Which of the following radiopharmaceuticals was used in this study?
   A. ^{99m}Tc DTPA
   B. ^{99m}Tc MAG3
   C. ^{99m}Tc DMSA
   D. $Na^{99m}TcO_4$

   ANSWER: A. ^{99m}Tc DTPA. The presence of RAS is associated with cortical retention in the affected kidney when ^{99m}Tc MAG3 is used as the radiotracer. ^{99m}Tc DTPA would demonstrate an asymmetric decrease in function in the affected kidney, because of the decrease in perfusion pressure across the glomerulus (^{99m}Tc GH—not listed—would likely demonstrate the same effect on the renogram portion of the study). ^{99m}Tc DMSA is a cortical imaging agent, not used for the detection of RAS. $Na^{99m}TcO_4$ is not used for functional renal imaging.

3. Which of the following statements regarding radionuclide cystography is *true*?
   A. $Na^{99m}TcO_4$ is the preferred radiopharmaceutical for this study.
   B. Reflux grading system is same as for contrast-voiding urethrocystography.

C. Dose to the patient's gonads is approximately 10–15 times less than received from a radiographic contrast-voiding urethrocystography.
D. Radionuclide cystography can detect reflux volumes as low as 1 mL.

ANSWER: D. Radionuclide cystography can detect reflux volumes as low as 1 mL. $Na^{99m}TcO_4$ is not usually used, as it can be absorbed through an inflamed bladder wall and excreted by the kidneys. $Na^{99m}Tc$ SC is the radiotracer of choice. Because of resolution limitations, scintigraphic grading of reflux is typically described as minimal (equivalent to radiographic grade I), moderate (equivalent to combined grades II and III), and severe (equivalent to combined grades IV and V). The dose to the gonads is substantially less than with the radiographic study, with anywhere from 50 to 150 times less exposure.

4. A pediatric patient has a prior history of vesicuoureteral reflux, pyelonephritis, and renal caliculi. The patient now presents with left flank pain and temperature of 100.1°F. The pediatrician has asked for a renal scan to narrow his differential. Assuming all of the following radiotracers are available at your facility, which of the following agents would give the most information about possible causes for the clinical appearance?
   A. ^{99m}Tc DTPA
   B. ^{99m}Tc MAG3
   C. ^{99m}Tc GH
   D. ^{99m}Tc DMSA

   ANSWER: C. ^{99m}Tc GH. The point of this question is to remind you that ^{99m}Tc GH has the ability to image flow of the kidneys, as well as to do delayed cortical imaging. With the history of prior renal caliculi and flank pain, the patient could be presenting with obstruction, which the flow phase of the study could assess for. With the histories of vesiculoureteral reflux and pyelonephritis, ^{99m}Tc GH can assess for the presence of pyelonephritis. All of the other listed radiotracers could only definitively investigated for one of these conditions, not both.

5. Your facility employs a plasma-sampling technique to determine global renal function (using ^{99m}Tc MAG3) in addition to imaging to determine differential function. When performing a renal scan on a patient, the technologist started the camera late, after the time of the radiotracer injection. Which of the following findings would still be accurate?
   A. Peak time
   B. Differential function
   C. ERPF
   D. GFR
   E. 20/3 ratio

   ANSWER: C. ERPF. All of the choices listed except for GFR are dependent on the computer analysis of the data obtained from the images obtained. Peak time would be delayed. As differential function is determined at a specific point in the renogram curve, this would also be inaccurate, as counts from the excretory phase would be in the ROI. 20/3 ratio would also be inaccurate because of the timing error. Plasma sampling is not affected by camera errors. GFR is not measured by ^{99m}Tc MAG3.

6. Which of the following findings is most consistent with a finding of acute testicular torsion?
   A. Asymmetric increased flow and blood pool to the painful side of the scrotum
   B. Asymmetric decreased flow and blood pool to the painful side of the scrotum
   C. Asymmetric increased flow with central photopenia to the painful side of the scrotum
   D. Symmetric flow and blood pool within the scrotum

   ANSWER: B. Asymmetric decreased flow and blood pool to the painful side of the scrotum. Increased flow and blood pool to the affected side is consistent with an inflammatory condition, such as epididymitis. Increased flow with central photopenia is the typical appearance of delayed torsion. Symmetric flow and blood pool will sometimes be seen in the earliest phases of acute testicular torsion, but more likely represents a normal study or torsion of a testicular appendage.

7. Which of the following agents has the highest dose to the kidneys?
   A. ^{99m}Tc DTPA
   B. ^{99m}Tc MAG3
   C. ^{99m}Tc GH
   D. ^{99m}Tc DMSA

   ANSWER: D. ^{99m}Tc DMSA. The critical organ for all other listed radiopharmaceuticals is the bladder.

8. Which of the following parameters is most useful in differentiating acute rejection of a renal allograft from acute vascular nephropathy (ATN)?
   A. Time from implantation
   B. Peak time
   C. ERPF
   D. 20/3 ratio

ANSWER: A. Time from implantation. Of the listed responses, this is the most helpful in differentiating acute rejection from ATN (acute vascular nephropathy). ATN is more likely to be present initially, with gradual improvement over time. Acute rejection typically begins to arise 10–14 days after transplantation. Renal perfusion (not listed) would also help differentiate these conditions. ATN has preserved perfusion, whereas acute rejection typically has decreased perfusion. Peak time is delayed in both conditions, and 20/3 is increased in both as well. ERPF may be low in both conditions.

9. Which of the following time to half peak after Lasix administration values is most consistent with obstruction?
   A. 8 minutes
   B. 10 minutes
   C. 15 minutes
   D. 20 minutes

   ANSWER: D. Time to half peak after Lasix administration less than 8 or 10 minutes is not compatible with obstruction; 15 minutes is indeterminate for obstruction.

10. In which of the following conditions would you expect the renal perfusion (vascular phase) to be normal?
    A. Acute pyelonephritis
    B. ATN of a cadaveric renal allograft
    C. Acute rejection of a cadaveric renal allograft
    D. Renal vein thrombosis

    ANSWER: B. ATN. Of the listed conditions, acute tubular necrosis is the only one, which is likely to have preserved perfusion.

95 CENTRAL NERVOUS SYSTEM SCINTIGRAPHY

Jon A. Baldwin

INTRODUCTION

Radionuclide imaging of the central nervous system (CNS) is one of function, rather than of anatomy. Most commonly requested studies are brain SPECT studies that assess regional cerebral blood flow (rCBF) and brain PET studies that assess glucose metabolism (with ^{18}F-FDG PET). Less commonly requested neurological studies include planar radionuclide angiography and cisternography. Diversionary shunt patency studies are also infrequently ordered. Table 95-1 lists radiopharmaceuticals used in nuclear medicine imaging of the CNS.

SPECT IMAGING OF THE BRAIN

One of the earliest agents used to image rCBF was ^{123}I iodoamphetamine (IMP). IMP is a lipophilic amine derivative able to cross the blood-brain barrier (BBB), and temporarily binds to amphetamine receptors. It is not fixed in the neurons and tends to wash out over time. This is a historical agent that is no longer clinically available in the United States. Another agent that can demonstrate rCBF is the noble gas ^{133}Xe. It also is readily diffusible across the BBB. It is quickly cleared, so the study can be repeated often. It is a technically challenging agent to use, and has poor imaging characteristics (the 81-keV photon is easily attenuated and scattered, and is below the ideal imaging window of 100–200 keV). ^{133}Xe has been

TABLE 95-1 CNS Radiopharmaceuticals

RADIOPHARMACEUTICAL	IMAGE ACQUISITION	APPLICATION IMAGED
^{99m}Tc diethylenetriaminepenta-acetic acid (^{99m}Tc DTPA)	Dynamic planar	Radionuclide angiography and cisternography; diversionary shunt patency
^{99m}Tc hexamethylpropyleneamine oxine (^{99m}Tc HMPAO)	Dynamic planar, SPECT	Radionuclide angiography and rCBF
^{99m}Tc ethyl cysteinate dimer (^{99m}Tc ECD)	Dynamic planar, SPECT	Radionuclide angiography and rCBF
^{133}Xe	SPECT	rCBF
^{15}O H_2O	PET	rCBF
^{201}Tl chloride	SPECT	Tumor imaging (tumor recurrence versus radiation changes)
^{18}F-fluoro-2-deoxyglucose (^{18}F-FDG)	PET	Glucose metabolism
^{18}F-fluoro-L-dopa (^{18}F-FDOPA)	PET	Presynaptic dopaminergic function
^{18}F-fluorothymidine (^{18}F-FLT)	PET	DNA synthesis/tumor imaging
^{18}F-misonidazole (^{18}F-MISO)	PET	Measure tumor hypoxia
^{111}In-DTPA	Dynamic planar	Radionuclide cisternography; diversionary shunt patency

mostly relegated to research applications. The workhorses of SPECT imaging of rCBF in clinical applications are the ^{99m}Tc radiotracers hexamethypropyleneamine oxime (^{99m}Tc HMPAO—Ceretec) and ethyl cysteinate dimer (^{99m}Tc ECD—Neurolite). Both are neutral and lipophilic, and are relatively fixed in the neuron; there is, however, slow washout of ECD over time (~6% per hour). Both also have a high first pass extraction (^{99m}Tc HMPAO ~80%, ^{99m}Tc ECD ~60%–70%). They accumulate in the cortex in proportion to blood flow, both slightly underestimating true rCBF. As they are essentially fixed in the neurons, SPECT imaging can be delayed with both radiotracers. Delay can be anywhere from 15 minutes to 2 hours with ^{99m}Tc HMPAO, without loss of image quality or information. Since blood clearance is faster with ^{99m}Tc ECD than ^{99m}Tc HMPAO, early ^{99m}Tc ECD images are superior to delayed ^{99m}Tc ECD images. Delayed ^{99m}Tc ECD images are also inferior to delayed ^{99m}Tc HMPAO images, because of the slow washout, resulting in considerable loss of activity from the cortex as time from injection increases. For both radiotracers, the uptake is predominately within the cortex. There is relative increased uptake in the caudate and lenticular nuclei, the thalami, and the cerebellum. White matter has much less uptake when compared to gray. Ventricles have near-absent to absent uptake. In addition, there are differences in normal biodistribution between the two radiopharmaceuticals: ^{99m}Tc HMPAO accumulates more in the frontal lobes, thalamus, and cerebellum; ^{99m}Tc ECD demonstrates slight preferential uptake in the parietal and occipital lobes. These slight differences can make comparison studies difficult between the two radiopharmaceuticals. The ^{99m}Tc rCBF radiotracers are used in numerous applications, including differentiating dementias, seizure localization, evaluation of vascular parameters, and tumor imaging. As the patterns of uptake in dementias and in seizure foci are similar regardless of whether ^{18}F-FDG or ^{99m}Tc rCBF radiotracers are used, those topics will be discussed after the section on PET imaging. The least common SPECT clinical application is for tumor imaging. The rCBF radiotracers typically are not used for this purpose. If tumors are evident at all, they may demonstrate nonspecific focal hypoperfusion (^{99m}Tc ECD can occasionally present as focal increased uptake). SPECT radiotracers used for imaging include ^{201}Tl chloride and ^{99m}Tc sestamibi. ^{99m}Tc sestamibi is uncommonly used. ^{201}Tl chloride is a potassium analog taken up by the Na^+/K^+ pump. Its distribution relates to blood flow, the presence of BBB breakdown, and the metabolic activity of the lesion. Although inflammatory conditions can also take up ^{201}Tl, tumors will have more intense uptake than infections. Abnormalities will have uptake greater than that of the scalp. Occasionally there may be a need to draw a region of interest around the abnormality and the contralateral normal side, and then compare intensities. Alternatively, one can compare the intensity to normal scalp activity; activity twice that of scalp activity is considered high. The main utility of this technique is differentiation of recurrent glioma from radiation therapy changes. A recurrence would have much higher uptake than radiation changes. ^{201}Tl can also help grade gliomas, but ^{18}F-FDG PET is preferred for this application.

SPECT IMAGING OF ^{99M}TC rCBF RADIOTRACERS IN VASCULAR APPLICATIONS

Two studies are used to evaluate vascular reserve and/or collateral blood flow in the brain: carotid artery balloon occlusion studies and the acetazolamide (Diamox) challenge study. Certain conditions (e.g., carotid body tumor, intracranial aneurysm) may call for the sacrifice/occlusion of one of the internal carotid arteries. Preoperative testing with ^{99m}Tc rCBF radiotracers has a very significant positive impact on patient morbidity and mortality. These patients are taken to the neurointerventional suite, and a balloon is temporarily inflated in the selected carotid artery. Radiotracer is injected while the balloon is inflated. SPECT images are performed after the patient is out of the recovery room. Images are compared for relative asymmetry in radiotracer distribution. If collateral flow from the circle of Willis is not sufficient, there will be significant asymmetry in rCBF. Markedly asymmetric patients are at increased risk of stroke after carotid artery sacrifice, and would benefit from carotid artery bypass. The second test can assess the presence of ischemia within the brain. Diamox is a carbonic anhydrase inhibitor that causes vasodilatation. After it is administered (1 g, intravenous), one can look for areas of decreased vascular reserve. It is convenient to think of the study as an adenosine stress test for the brain. Diseased vessels are already maximally dilated in an attempt to meet the vascular constraint, and cannot further respond to Diamox. Normal vessels, however, can respond by vasodilating. Ischemic areas will appear as relative defect at "stress," and are at risk for future infarction. When a baseline study without Diamox is performed, these areas would tend to be isointense to the Diamox intensity or demonstrate improvement. Portions of the cortex that have already infarcted will appear with absent or near-absent activity on both studies.

Accurate interpretation of cerebral flow studies requires an understanding of the relationship between perfusion and metabolism in regard to imaging with rCBF agents and ^{18}F-FDG. These two parameters are often matched or "coupled," which is to say that areas that are metabolically active require adequate perfusion. Instances in which this relationship is "uncoupled" occur during evolution of a stroke. Initially in the face of an insult, and lasting for approximately 48 to 72 hours, the metabolism of brain tissue will be preserved despite the decrease in perfusion. This is the so-called misery perfusion. The area of decreased perfusion (on SPECT images) may be greater than the lesion seen if the patient had a CT scan, indicating there is additional tissue that is at risk for infarction. If therapy can be initiated to relieve ischemia, some brain tissue may be salvaged. If no intervention is made, over time this mismatch cannot be maintained. Damage to the tissue vessels can result in excessive blood flow, or the so-called luxury perfusion (lasting approximately 1–3 weeks after onset). By this time, though, the ischemia is progressing to infarct and metabolism declines.

Crossed cerebellar diaschisis is another finding that can be seen in both SPECT rCBF and PET ^{18}F-FDG imaging. When a lesion with decreased uptake is present in the cerebral cortex, either from tumor, infarct/ischemia, or trauma, a decrease is often also seen in the contralateral cerebellar cortex. This is especially true if the cerebral supratentorial lesion involves the motor cortex. As the cerebellar neurons of the corticopontocerebellar pathways are not "stimulated" because of loss of cerebral cortical function, blood flow is shunted away from this area, leading to decreased metabolism as well.

PET IMAGING OF THE BRAIN

Depending on the radiotracer, PET imaging can assess perfusion as well (e.g., ^{15}O-H_2O), but usually evaluates metabolism of a particular substrate. Glucose metabolism is the most commonly used, but in reality, the potential for PET imaging is limitless in terms of metabolic pathways (Table 95-1). ^{18}F-FDG PET, a glucose analog, is ideally suited to assessing regional brain metabolism, as the brain is an obligate glucose user. ^{18}F-FDG crosses the BBB by glucose transporters and is phosphorylated in neurons, which effectively traps it so that the activity cannot redistribute. Peak uptake in brain is approximately 35 minutes. Renal clearance is rapid, giving good target to background ratio. The normal pattern of uptake is similar to that of the ^{99m}Tc rCBF radiotracers: relative increased uptake in the caudate and lenticular nuclei, the thalami, and the cerebellum. White matter has much less uptake when compared to gray, and ventricles have near-absent to absent uptake. Resolution is better with PET imaging (on the order of 5 mm) than SPECT (order of 7 mm). It is important to remember that distribution can be altered by external conditions (as is true for SPECT brain imaging as well). For instance, bright lights in the room at time of injection can increase occipital lobe uptake. It is better to have intravenous access before the injection of the dose to decrease painful stimuli, which may increase uptake in pain centers. When using a glucose analog like ^{18}F-FDG, it is best if the patient's glucose is less than 200 mg/dL; otherwise, competition from increased glucose pool may lead to less uptake of the radiotracer. Common indications for imaging with ^{18}F-FDG PET include dementia, seizure localization, and tumor imaging.

TUMOR IMAGING WITH ^{18}F-FDG PET

Most oncology patients are imaged from the skull base to midthigh, with the exception of head and neck cancers and melanoma. Part of the reasoning behind this is the variable uptake that ^{18}F-FDG can have with metastases. Because the brain is an obligate glucose user, background activity can obscure metastases. Metastases can appear hypermetabolic (usually an anaplastic or relatively dedifferentiated cancer), isointense, or hypometabolic (often the result of edema, although can represent glucose metabolism less than that of adjacent cortex). An application that has some utility is grading gliomas, as well as determination of recurrent gliomas versus radiation necrosis. High-grade gliomas typically have brisk ^{18}F-FDG uptake while radiation changes do not.

PATTERNS OF UPTAKE IN DEMENTIAS (TABLE 95-2)

One of the most common indications for SPECT or PET imaging of the brain is to evaluate dementia. Because of

TABLE 95-2 Dementia Pattern on SPECT and PET Imaging

PATTERN OF DECREASED UPTAKE	DEMENTIA
Frontal and temporal lobes	Frontotemporal dementia/Pick disease
Superior posterior parietotemporal lobes	Alzheimer disease
Frontal, parietal, and temporal lobes with motor strip and occipital sparing; parietotemporal decrease > frontal decrease	Advanced Alzheimer disease
Posterior parietotemporal and occipital lobes, slight relative sparing of mesial temporal lobe	Lewy body disease (Parkinson dementia has similar appearance)
Global rCBF decrease, frontal predominance; presence of scattered cortical defects and/or decrease in a vascular territory (such as ICA, MCA) aids in diagnosis	Vascular dementia
Heterogeneous appearance, with scattered cortical/subcortical decreased perfusion; focal increased perfusion possible	AIDS-dementia complex

the coupling of perfusion and metabolism, patterns of uptake in dementias are similar, whether the radiotracer is ^{18}F-FDG or one of the ^{99m}Tc rCBF radiotracers. Sensitivity and resolution of PET imaging is better than SPECT imaging; otherwise, the preference of whether to use PET or SPECT is based on availability and preference.

Symmetric decrease of uptake in the frontal and temporal lobes is seen in frontotemporal dementias: rare Pick disease, familial frontotemporal dementias, and primary progressive aphasia. Other conditions that can cause a symmetric frontal decrease include schizophrenia, depression, and progressive supranuclear palsy. The most commonly encountered dementia is Alzheimer dementia (also known as senile dementia, Alzheimer type). The classic appearance of Alzheimer dementia is symmetric decrease in uptake involving the cortex of the superior posterior temporal and parietal lobes. Variations on this appearance can occur. In early Alzheimer dementia, the decreased uptake can appear as asymmetric involvement of the posterior parietotemporal cortex. In advanced Alzheimer dementia, there is symmetric involvement of the frontal cortex as well, although the degree of decrease is still greater in the posterior parietal and temporal lobes. Typically there is sparing of the motor strip, occipital lobe, and basal ganglia, even in advanced Alzheimer dementia.

Lewy body dementia (LBD) has an appearance similar to Alzheimer dementia, with decreased uptake within the posterior parietal and temporal regions. In LBD, however, there is involvement of the occipital lobe as well. Some decrease can also be seen in the cerebellum. There may be relative sparing of the hippocampal regions in comparison to Alzheimer dementia. The pattern of uptake in Parkinson dementia is virtually the same as LBD.

Acquired immunodeficiency syndrome (AIDS)–dementia complex can have a heterogeneous pattern uptake, predominately with focal decreased uptake, although focal increased uptake can sometimes be seen. The defects are typically seen in frontal, temporal, and occipital lobes, as well as the basal ganglia.

Vascular dementia is typically a diagnosis of exclusion. There are various presentations, from a global decrease with a frontal predominance to scattered cortical defects (the result of thromboembolic disease) to a major vascular territory decrease. Combinations of these patterns can also be seen.

PATTERNS OF UPTAKE IN SEIZURE LOCALIZATION STUDIES (TABLE 95-3)

SPECT and PET imaging for localizing seizures play an important role in evaluating for and directing of surgical resection. At the very least, it can direct optimal placement of intracranial EEG leading to more discrete seizure localization prior to resection. The pattern of uptake is more dependent on the type of study performed rather than the radiotracer used. If radiotracer is injected while the patient was actively seizing, focal increase uptake would be seen at the seizure focus, using either a perfusion or metabolism agent. Because of complexity of timing of ictal seizure localization studies, these are usually performed at specialized centers. Antiseizure medications are typically discontinued, and the patient undergoes continuous video-monitored EEG. ^{18}F-FDG is usually not used because of shorter half-life and higher cost. ^{99m}Tc HMPAO or ECD is injected within seconds of seizure onset, although actual imaging can occur later. When the study is interpreted, it is important to know that the injection was performed at the correct time. Additional helpful information include clinical and EEG findings at the time of the seizure (lateralization and localization) and if it was "typical." A positive ictal study will appear as a focal area of increased uptake, most commonly the temporal lobes, since most seizures are the result of mesial temporal sclerosis. The ictal SPECT study is the most sensitive and specific of the nuclear medicine studies for seizure localization.

Since the majority of facilities do not perform ictal SPECT studies, most seizure localization is performed during the interictal state, with either ^{18}F-FDG or a ^{99m}Tc rCBF radiotracer. The findings for a positive study are the same regardless of the radiopharmaceutical: a focal area of relative decreased uptake. Of the two interictal studies, interictal PET with ^{18}F-FDG is more sensitive for the detection of the seizure focus,

TABLE 95-3 Summary of Seizure Localization Studies

STUDY	FINDINGS	COMMENT
Ictal SPECT with ^{99m}Tc rCBF agent	Focal increased uptake at seizure focus	Most sensitive study for seizure localization
Interictal PET with ^{18}F-FDG	Focal decreased uptake at seizure focus	Better sensitivity than interictal SPECT study
Interictal SPECT with ^{99m}Tc rCBF agent	Focal decreased uptake at seizure focus	

especially in cases of extratemporal epilepsy. Although unlikely, if a patient was injected with ^{18}F-FDG at or near the time of a seizure, it would appear the same as an ictal SPECT study.

PLANAR NUCLEAR MEDICINE CNS STUDIES

There are several nuclear medicine studies of the CNS that do not require SPECT or PET acquisitions. They include cerebral radionuclide angiography in cases of suspected brain death, radionuclide cisternography to assess for a suspected communicating hydrocephalus (such as normal-pressure hydrocephaly) or cerebral spinal fluid (CSF) leak, and diversionary shunt patency studies.

RADIONUCLIDE ANGIOGRAPHY

Although the diagnosis of brain death is primarily a clinical one, radionuclide angiography may aid in the diagnosis, especially when the EEG and clinical criteria are equivocal. Accuracy and speed in diagnosis is critical, especially when organ donation is being considered. Edema, softening, necrosis, and autolysis of brain tissue lead to increased intracranial pressure. As pressure rises, it prevents intracranial perfusion. Lack of blood flow to the brain on a radionuclide angiography study is diagnostic of brain death. Historically, this study was performed with ^{99m}Tc DTPA. It is cleared rapidly from blood, so repeat study can be performed if necessary. Interpretation can be difficult, however, as poor bolus technique and/or overlying scalp activity can confound the dynamic flow portion of the study. Scalp tourniquet was advocated to reduce interfering scalp activity, although use of a tourniquet is contraindicated in children, as it increases intracranial pressure, and has the potential for creating a false-positive study. With the newer ^{99m}Tc agents, use of a tourniquet has fallen out of favor. With ^{99m}Tc DTPA on delayed static images, the presence of the major venous sinus suggests of intracranial blood flow, but this is not reliable. Because of these difficulties, ^{99m}Tc HMPAO or ^{99m}Tc ECD are more commonly used. Positive blood flow can be determined on the initial flow images, as well as the delayed images, since both cross the BBB. Good bolus is important for an accurate flow study. A positive study will have no flow above the base of the skull. There may be increased focal increased uptake at the nose ("hot nose sign"), as flow is shunted to the external carotid artery because of increased intracranial pressure. Delayed static images will confirm no uptake within the cortex. It is prudent to image injection site and the liver for confirmation purposes. This ensures that decreased flow is not due to a dose infiltration or to a hypotensive state (i.e., liver uptake proves systemic perfusion is adequate), respectively.

CISTERNOGRAPHY (TABLE 95-4)

For evaluation of CSF dynamics, approximately 500 μCi of sterile and pyrogen-free ^{111}In DTPA is injected into the subarachnoid space via lumbar puncture. Imaging of the injection site is recommended to check for "loculation" and ensure assent of the radiotracer through the spinal canal. Anterior and lateral planar images of the head are obtained at 6, 24, 48, and 72 hours as needed. Activity usually reaches the basal cisterns at 1 to 4 hours in normal adults, shortly followed by the frontal poles and sylvian fissure and interhemispheric cisterns. At this point, the anterior images have a trident-like appearance. At 24 hours, there should be complete ascent over the cerebral convexities and the parasagittal region, with relative clearance from the basal cisterns. The presence of early and persistent radiotracer activity in the lateral ventricles is abnormal (communicating hydrocephalus) giving a heart-shaped appearance, although some investigators say transient entry at 4 hours that clears by 24 hours is a normal variant. Additional findings suggesting communicating hydrocephalus include a delay of more than 24 hours in the ascent of activity over the convexities, and delayed clearance of activity. Patients with significant cortical atrophy may have a delay in this ascent, although they will not have ventricular activity. In patients with a

TABLE 95-4 Scintigraphic Appearance of CSF Dynamics

SCINTIGRAPHIC APPEARANCE	POSSIBLE CAUSES
"Trident sign" at 1–6 h, radiotracer activity over the convexities at 24 h, good clearance of activity at 24 h	Normal dynamics Noncommunicating hydrocephalus
Delayed transit over the convexities, but no ventricular activity seen	Cerebral atrophy Evolving/early communicating hydrocephalus
Delayed transit over the convexities, presence of ventricular activity ("heart-shaped" appearance), poor clearance/persistent activity at more than 24 h	Communicating (normal-pressure) hydrocephalus

noncommunicating hydrocephalus, the pattern of uptake is typically normal.

Cisternography may also be used to localize intermittent rhinorrhea or otorrhea. When imaging a patient with a suspected CSF leak, one may use ^{99m}Tc DTPA instead of ^{111}In DTPA. Since the duration of imaging is likely to be less than in the investigation of suspected hydrocephalies, the shorter half-life of ^{99m}Tc DTPA should not be an issue. The better imaging characteristics of ^{99m}Tc DTPA may also aid in the detection of subtle leaks. The study is performed like cisternography examination, but imaging of the presumed site of leak is performed at 1 and 3 hours. Some advocate placing the patient in Trendelenburg position to aid the flow of activity to the basal cisterns. If a particular position is thought to promote leak, the patient should be placed accordingly. The use of pledgets in the nares or ears can significantly increase identification and localization (anterior vs. posterior rhinorrhea) of leaks. A blood sample, with plasma centrifuged out, can be placed in the well counter along with the pledgets. This will help determine if the pledget activity represents absorbed activity from the plasma versus a true leak. A true positive study will have a high ratio of activity when comparing pledget to plasma.

DIVERSIONARY SHUNT PATENCY

As these studies are also typically of short duration, one can use ^{99m}Tc DTPA ($\sim$1 mCi) as in the CSF leak studies. Injection is typically done by the neurologist or neurosurgeon with aseptic technique. Patient is imaged in the supine position, although upright positioning may be necessary if flow appears obstructed. Dynamic images are obtained of the injection site and reservoir, and activity is followed as it descends to its destination, which is frequently the peritoneum or right atrium, but could also be the pleural space. If it is a patent ventriculoatrial shunt, in addition to following the activity to the heart, one will see kidney and bladder activity, as ^{99m}Tc DTPA is a renal imaging agent. Patent ventriculoperitoneal and ventriculopleural shunts will demonstrate activity coating the peritoneum and pleura, respectively. If the shunt is not patent, activity will remain in the ventricles or may abruptly terminate at the obstruction. As it is difficult to gauge where the activity terminates within the patient, it is often helpful to place radioactive markers on anatomical landmarks (suprasternal notch, xyphoid process, etc) or place a sheet source behind the patient to outline the body habitus. Delayed static images for up to 24 hours may be beneficial.

APPROACH TO UNKNOWN BRAIN CASES (FIG. 95-1)

Distinguishing different radiotracers can be difficult, but there are a few defining concepts. Overall, ^{18}F-FDG images have relatively better resolution. Perfusion and metabolism patterns are often the same. ^{18}F-FDG assesses glucose metabolism in the brain and ^{99m}Tc HMPAO assesses rCBF; these processes are coupled such that the appearances of many disorders are similar. There are few conditions that demonstrate focal increased uptake; a focal unilateral hot spot in a temporal lobe usually indicates an ictal SPECT scan. Differential considerations for focal increased uptake outside the temporal lobe include an extratemporal seizure focus (if an ictal SPECT study), a hypermetabolic metastasis (if a FDG PET study), a recurrence of glioma (if a FDG PET study, or in a ^{201}Tl chloride study as well. In the latter case, image quality would be poor), and AIDS-dementia complex (SPECT uptake would be heterogeneous, with predominately focal areas of hypoperfusion, occasional focal hyperperfusion). If there are no focal areas of increased uptake, then look for areas of focal or regional decreased uptake. Focal unilateral decrease in the temporal lobe suggests a seizure focus on interictal SPECT or PET. A solitary focus of unilateral decreased uptake outside temporal lobe can represent an extratemporal seizure focus on an interictal SPECT or PET study, ischemia/infarct, or malignancy (remember, it has to be *very* FDG avid to be noticeably hot on PET). Focal scattered cortical defects suggest a thromboembolic phenomenon, such as multiinfarct dementia. If the decreases appear more "regional," assess if they are symmetric or asymmetric. Symmetric frontal and temporal decrease is consistent with frontotemporal lobe dementia or Pick disease. If the decrease involves the bilateral posterior parietal and temporal lobes, then consider Alzheimer dementia (realizing, of course, that early Alzheimer dementia can have some asymmetry in uptake). If there is bilateral frontal, parietal, and temporal lobe decrease with motor strip and occipital lobe sparing, this suggests advanced Alzheimer dementia. If, however, there is bilateral posterior parietal/temporal with occipital involvement, consider Lewy body disease or Parkinson dementia. When the "regional" decrease is asymmetric and confined to a vascular territory, consider a vascular ischemia (or dementia in the proper clinical setting), or a balloon occlusion study. Finally, the appearance of vascular dementia can vary, and is typically a diagnosis of exclusion. One can see a global rCBF decrease with a frontal predominance. Often there are scattered focal areas of hypoperfusion or an ICA/MCA regional defect to aid in the diagnosis.

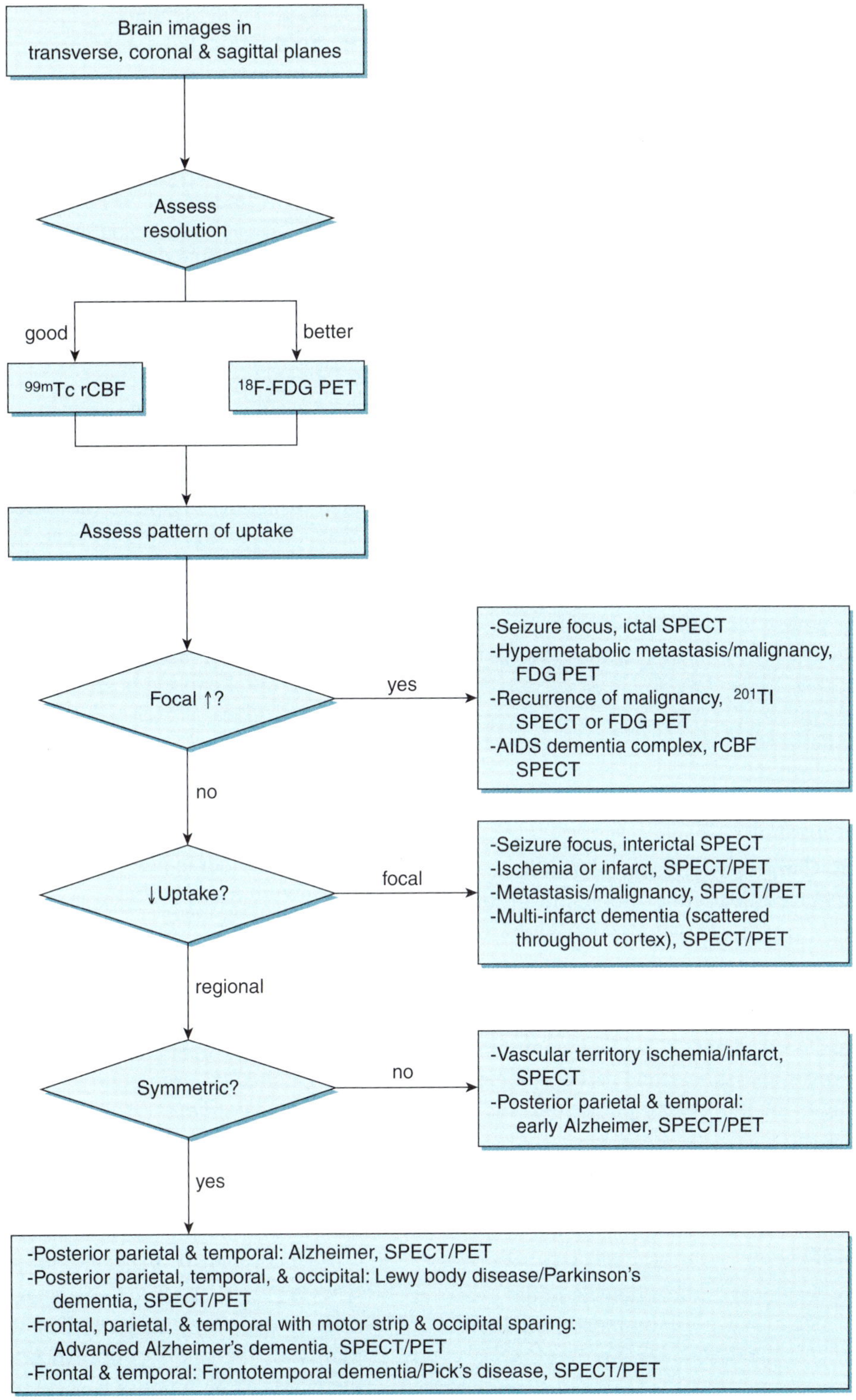

FIG. 95-1 Approach to unknown brain SPECT and PET image interpretation.

Suggested Reading

Bohnen NI. In: Wahl RL, ed. *Principles and Practice of Positron Emission Tomography*. Philadelphia, PA: Lippincott Williams &Wilkins; 2002:276.

Carmago EE. Brain SPECT in neurology and psychiatry. *J Nucl Med.* 2001;42:611-623.

Fulham MJ. In: Wahl RL, ed. *Principles and Practice of Positron Emission Tomography*.Philadelphia, PA: Lippincott Williams &Wilkins; 2002:137.

Mountz JM, et al. Neuroimaging in cerebrovascular disorders: measurement of cerebral physiology after stroke. *Semin Nucl Med.* 2003;33:56.

QUESTIONS AND ANSWERS

1. A patient undergoes SPECT imaging of the brain with ^{99m}Tc HMPAO. The images demonstrate symmetric relative decreased uptake in the frontal, temporal, and parietal lobes. You note that there is sparing of activity within the motor strip and occipital lobe. Which of the following is the most likely diagnosis?
   A. Pick disease
   B. Alzheimer dementia
   C. Lewy body disease
   D. Vascular dementia
   E. Seizure localization

   ANSWER: B. This constellation of findings is typical for advanced Alzheimer dementia (Table 95-2).

2. A patient undergoes SPECT imaging of their brain with ^{99m}Tc HMPAO. The images demonstrate global decreased cortical uptake, with bilateral scattered focal cortical and subcortical defects. Which of the following is the most likely diagnosis?
   A. Pick disease
   B. Alzheimer dementia
   C. Lewy body disease
   D. Vascular dementia
   E. Seizure localization

   ANSWER: D. Scattered cortical defects in the setting of global decreased rCBF is most consistent with vascular dementia (Table 95-2).

3. A patient undergoes PET imaging of the brain with ^{18}F-FDG. The images demonstrate symmetric frontotemporal lobe decreased activity. Which of the following is the most likely diagnosis?
   A. Pick disease
   B. Alzheimer dementia
   C. Lewy body disease
   D. Vascular dementia
   E. Seizure localization

   ANSWER: A. Symmetric frontotemporal lobe decrease is typical of a frontal lobe dementia such as Pick disease Table 95-2.

4. A patient undergoes SPECT imaging of the brain with ^{99m}Tc HMPAO. The images demonstrate focal increased uptake within the left mesial temporal lobe. Which of the following is the most likely diagnosis?
   A. Pick disease
   B. Alzheimer dementia
   C. Lewy body disease
   D. Vascular dementia
   E. Seizure localization

   ANSWER: E. A seizure focus appears as a focal area of increased uptake on an ictal SPECT study. Very few other conditions have focal increased uptake on ^{99m}Tc HMPAO imaging.

5. A patient undergoes PET imaging of the brain with ^{18}F-FDG. The images demonstrate relative decreased uptake in the posterior parietotemporal and occipital lobes. Which of the following is the most likely diagnosis?
   A. Pick disease
   B. Alzheimer dementia
   C. Lewy body disease
   D. Vascular dementia
   E. Seizure localization

   ANSWER: C. LBD and Parkinson dementia usually have occipital lobe involvement. Advanced Alzheimer dementia usually spares the occipital lobe.

6. Regarding the appearance of CSF flow dynamics in radionuclide cisternography, which of the following patterns is *normal*?
   A. Persistent intensity of activity at 24 hours
   B. Flow of radiotracer over the convexities at 24 hours
   C. "Trident-shaped" pattern of uptake at 24 hours
   D. "Heart-shaped" pattern of uptake at 24 hours

   ANSWER: B. Lack of clearance or no change in activity over time suggests that there is an abnormality in the reabsorption of CSF. By 24 hours, there should be migration of activity over the convexities. "Trident" pattern (delay in ascent, no ventricular activity) can be seen in cerebral atrophy. Persistent activity in the ventricles is not normal, and is seen in normal-pressure hydrocephalus.

7. Concerning radionuclide cerebral angiography for determining brain death, in which of the following

situations is the use of a scalp tourniquet *most* indicated?

A. Radionuclide cerebral angiography performed with ^{99m}Tc DTPA in a child
B. Radionuclide cerebral angiography performed with ^{99m}Tc HMPAO in a child
C. Radionuclide cerebral angiography performed with ^{99m}Tc DTPA in an adult
D. Radionuclide cerebral angiography performed with ^{99m}Tc HMPAO in an adult

ANSWER: C. Use of a tourniquet is contraindicated in a child, as there is fear that the tourniquet may raise intracranial pressure, leading to a false-positive study. A flow phase is not as critical when using ^{99m}Tc HMPAO, since it crosses the BBB. If intracranial flow is present, one need only look at the delayed images for confirmation. A tourniquet is not an absolute requirement when using a blood pool agent such as ^{99m}Tc DTPA, but as there is no crossing of the BBB, the flow images are more critical.

8. Which of the following choices listed below correctly lists the sensitivity and specificity of radionuclide studies for the detection of a seizure focus in descending order?

A. Ictal SPECT with ^{99m}Tc HMPAO, interictal PET with ^{18}F-FDG, interictal SPECT with ^{99m}Tc HMPAO
B. Interictal PET with ^{18}F-FDG, interictal SPECT with ^{99m}Tc HMPAO, ictal SPECT with ^{99m}Tc HMPAO
C. Interictal SPECT with ^{99m}Tc HMPAO, ictal SPECT with ^{99m}Tc HMPAO, interictal PET with ^{18}F-FDG

ANSWER: A. Ictal SPECT is the most sensitive and specific for seizure localization. If a facility cannot do ictal SPECT, ^{18}F-FDG interictal PET is the best study available, followed by interictal SPECT.

9. Which of the following situations is the *most* helpful in detecting a CSF leak in radionuclide cisternography?

A. Use of ^{111}In DTPA instead of ^{99m}Tc DTPA as the radiotracer
B. Use of pledgets
C. Imaging the patient in the supine position
D. Imaging the patient in Trendelenburg position

ANSWER: B. The use of pledgets may detect an occult leak as well as better localize the leak (i.e., anterior vs. posterior nose). There is no advantage in the use of ^{111}In DTPA instead of ^{99m}Tc DTPA in the setting of cisternography for CSF leak. The half-life of ^{99m}Tc DTPA is usually sufficient for detection of the leak, which is typically demonstrated in less than 4 hours. Many centers will place patients in Trendelenburg position after the intrathecal injection to promote movement to the basal cisterns, but once that occurs, the patient is positioned in such a way as to promote CSF leakage.

10. Which of the following statements is *true* regarding diversionary shunt patency studies?

A. Patient should be imaged in Trendelenburg position.
B. Imaging for up to 48 hours is recommended.
C. ^{111}In DTPA is the imaging agent of choice.
D. ^{99m}Tc DTPA is the imaging agent of choice.

ANSWER: D. Imaging is performed in the supine position, and if need be, in the upright position. Imaging in Trendelenburg position may actually impede flow. As the study is typically performed with ^{99m}Tc DTPA, imaging at 48 hours is not possible. One *could* use ^{111}In DTPA for the study, but the cost and imagining characteristics of ^{99m}Tc DTPA are better.

96 NUCLEAR CARDIOLOGY

Sibyll Goetze

MYOCARDIAL PERFUSION IMAGING

OVERVIEW

Myocardial perfusion can be evaluated with SPECT (most commonly performed) or PET perfusion tracers. Common indications include evaluation of chest pain, (re)evaluation of known coronary artery disease, heart failure, and preoperative testing. To differentiate between normal, ischemic, and scarred myocardium (Table 96-1), patients undergo stress testing, which can be achieved using physical exercise or pharmacologic intervention and will be described in this chapter.

TABLE 96-1 Pattern in Myocardial Perfusion Imaging

	STRESS	REST
Normal	Normal	Normal
Ischemia	Abnormal (↓)	Normal
Infarct	Abnormal (↓)	Abnormal (↓)

SPECT MYOCARDIAL PERFUSION IMAGING

Radiopharmaceuticals

Thallium-201

Thallium-201 (Tl-201) decays by electron capture with a physical half-life of 73 hours (the principal photon energy is 69–83keV [from mercury x-ray]). The usual dose is 2 to 4 mCi. Being a potassium analog, Tl-201 is taken up by myocardial cells via active transport (Na+/K+-ATPase). After injection, Tl-201 concentration in the myocardium reflects myocardial blood flow. The extraction fraction of Tl-201 is relatively high (approximately 85% at first pass during resting flow conditions) and proportional to myocardial blood flow over a wide range of flow rates. Over time, Tl-201 undergoes washout, with relatively rapid washout from normal myocardium and slower washout from abnormal (ischemic) myocardium. This phenomenon is called "redistribution," and may lead to normalization of myocardial perfusion defects over time (therefore, imaging needs to be performed no later than 5–10 minutes after injection of the radiotracer for stress imaging). Thallium is cleared though the kidneys (which is also the target organ).

Tc-99m Labeled Agents

Tc-99m-labeled agents include Tc-99m-sestamibi, Tc-99m tetrofosmin (which have similar properties), and Tc-99m-teboroxime. The use of the latter agent (Tc-99m teboroxime) in clinical practice is very limited because of rapid washout from the myocardium.

Tc-99m Methoxyisobutylisonitrile (Sestamibi)

Tc-99m sestamibi (an isonitrile) is a lipophilic cation, which enters the myocardial cells via passive diffusion. Within the cell, it localizes to mitochondria. The extraction fraction of sestamibi (40%–50% at first pass) is lower than that of thallium or teboroxime. Sestamibi practically does not redistribute. Imaging is usually delayed for at least 15 minutes (after exercise) to 30 to 90 minutes (at rest and after pharmacologic stress) to allow for liver washout and better target-to-background ratio. Clearance of sestamibi is via the hepatobiliary system. The target organ is the colon.

Tc-99m Tetrofosmin

Tc-99m tetrofosmin (diphosphine agent) has very similar characteristics compared to sestamibi, except for slightly higher heart/liver ratios allowing for relatively earlier imaging.

Tc-99m-Teboroxime

Tc-99m-teboroxime has the highest extraction fraction of all SPECT imaging agents (more than or equal to 90% at resting flow rates), but is not widely used in current practice.

Imaging Protocols

There are various imaging protocols, including 1- or 2-day; stress-only, rest-stress, or stress-rest; single- (i.e., Tc-99m-labeled agent at both stress and rest) or dual-isotope (Tl-201 at rest and Tc-99m-labeled agent at stress) protocols, which can be used depending on patient characteristics, imaging laboratory preference, and logistics. For same-day single-isotope protocols, a low dose (8–10 mCi of sestamibi) is used initially followed by a three times higher dose (24–30 mCi of sestamibi) for the second portion of the study. For 2-day protocols, full doses (24–30 mCi of sestamibi) can be administered each day.

Stress Testing

Exercise Stress

Physical exercise increases cardiac workload and thus myocardial oxygen demand. This may reveal areas of significant coronary artery stenosis, because these areas are not able to vasodilate to meet the increased oxygen demand. There are several methods for exercise stress testing, with a variety of treadmill exercise protocols (the Bruce protocol is commonly used) as well as supine and upright bicycle exercise. It is important to be aware of contraindications to and endpoints for exercise testing (Tables 96-2 and 96-3). Vasodilator stress testing can

TABLE 96-2 Contraindications to Exercise Testing

ABSOLUTE	RELATIVE
Acute myocardial infarction (within 2 d)	Left main coronary stenosis
High-risk unstable angina	Moderate stenotic valvular heart disease
Uncontrolled cardiac arrhythmias causing symptoms or hemodynamic compromise	Electrolyte abnormalities
Symptomatic severe aortic stenosis	Severe arterial hypertension (SBP >200 mm Hg and/or DBP >110 mm Hg)
Uncontrolled symptomatic heart failure	Tachyarrhythmias or bradyarrhythmias
Acute pulmonary embolus or pulmonary infarction	Hypertrophic cardiomyopathy and other forms of outflow tract obstruction
Acute myocarditis or pericarditis	Mental or physical impairment leading to inability to exercise adequately
Acute aortic dissection	High-degree atrioventricular block

Reprinted with permission from Gibbons RJ, Balady GJ, Bricker JT, et al; American College of Cardiology Foundation and the American Heart Association. ACC/AHA 2002 guideline update for exercise testing: a report of the American College of Cardiology/American Heart Association Task Force on Practice Guidelines (Committee on Exercise Testing). 2002. Available at: http://www.acc.org/ qualityandscience/ clinical/guidelines/exercise/exercise_clean.pdf.

TABLE 96-3 Indications for Terminating Exercise Testing

ABSOLUTE INDICATIONS	RELATIVE INDICATIONS
Drop in systolic blood pressure of >10 mm Hg from baseline blood pressure despite an increase in workload, when accompanied by other evidence of ischemia	Drop in systolic blood pressure of (≥10 mm Hg from baseline blood pressure despite an increase in workload, in the absence of other evidence of ischemia
Moderate to severe angina	ST or QRS changes such as excessive ST depression (>2 mm of horizontal or downsloping ST-segment depression) or marked axis shift
Increasing nervous system symptoms (e.g., ataxia, dizziness, or near-syncope)	Arrhythmias other than sustained ventricular tachycardia, including multifocal PVCs, triplets of PVCs, supraventricular tachycardia, heart block, or bradyarrhythmias
Signs of poor perfusion (cyanosis or pallor)	Fatigue, shortness of breath, wheezing, leg cramps, or claudication
Technical difficulties in monitoring ECG or systolic blood pressure	Development of bundle-branch block or IVCD that cannot be distinguished from ventricular tachycardia
Subject's desire to stop	Increasing chest pain
Sustained ventricular tachycardia	Hypertensive response (SPB >250 mm Hg and/or DBP >115 mm Hg)
ST elevation (≥1.0 mm) in leads without diagnostic Q waves (other than V_1 or a VR)	

Reprinted with permission from Gibbons RJ, Balady GJ, Bricker JT, et al; American College of Cardiology Foundation and the American Heart Association. ACC/AHA 2002 guideline update for exercise testing: a report of the American College of Cardiology/American Heart Association Task Force on Practice Guidelines (Committee on Exercise Testing). 2002. Available at: http://www.acc.org/qualityandscience/clinical/guidelines/exercise/exercise_clean.pdf

be considered if exercise is contraindicated. Adequate exercise is defined as reaching more than or equal to 85% of the maximal age predicted heart rate (220−age) and/or a "double product" (HR × SBP) of at least 25 000. Exercise can be continued further once a patient has reached at least 85% of age-predicted maximal heart rate if they remain asymptomatic and no other indications for terminating the test exist.

Although left bundle branch block (LBBB) is not a contraindication to exercise testing per se, it should be avoided in patients undergoing SPECT imaging. Perfusion defects can occur in approximately 50% of patients with LBBB if the heart rate increases (as it does with exercise). These patients should undergo vasodilator stress.

Pharmacologic Stress Testing

Vasodilator

Dipyridamole and adenosine are both vasodilators used for stress myocardial perfusion imaging if a patient is unable to undergo exercise testing.

Adenosine

Adenosine is an (nonselective) A2 receptor agonist. It is given via continuous infusion (140 μg/kg/min) over 5 or 6 minutes (radiotracer is injected at 3 minutes). Through activation of the A2 A receptor, it causes coronary vasodilation, increasing myocardial blood flow by three- to fourfold. Stenotic coronary arteries are less able to vasodilate, which results in less radiotracer uptake in regions of the myocardium supplied by the stenotic artery. Contraindications and indications for terminating the test early are presented in Table 96-4. Possible side effects are AV block, peripheral vasodilation (hypotension, headache), and bronchospasm. Chest pain is common (25%–30%) and not necessarily related to CAD. Because of the very short half-life of adenosine (less than 10 seconds), most side effects resolve after discontinuation of the infusion, and aminophylline is rarely required.

Dipyridamole

Dipyridamole (Persantine) increases the levels of adenosine by preventing reuptake and deamination of adenosine. It is administered as an IV infusion (0.56

TABLE 96-4 Contraindications and Indications for Early Termination of Vasodilator Pharmacologic Stress Testing

CONTRAINDICATIONS	EARLY TERMINATION CRITERIA
Asthma (with ongoing wheezing)	Severe hypotension (SBP <80 mm Hg)
Unstable acute MI/unstable angina less than 1 d	Development of symptomatic, persistent second-degree or complete heart block
AV block greater than first degree or sick sinus syndrome without PM	Wheezing
Recent (less than 24 h) of caffeine-containing products, dipyridamole-containing medications, theophylline, aminophylline	Severe chest pain associated with CT depression of ≥2 mm
SBP less than 90 mm Hg	Signs of poor perfusion (cyanosis or pallor)
Profound sinus bradycardia (<40 bpm)	Technical difficulties in monitoring ECG or SBP
Hypersensitivity to adenosine	Patient's request to stop

Modified with permission from Henzlova MJ, Cerqueira MD, Taillefer R, et al. ASNC Imaging Guidelines for nuclear cardiology procedures. *J Nucl Cardiol.* In press. Copyright © Elsevier.

mg/kg over 4 minutes), and the radiotracer is injected 4 minutes after the infusion is stopped. Side effects and contraindications are similar to adenosine. Aminophylline (50–250 mg IV) is more frequently administered for reversal of side effects given the longer half-life of dipyridamole.

Regadenoson

Regadenoson is an A2A adenosine receptor agonist. The recommended dose is 5 mL (0.4 mg regadenoson). It is given in a rapid (bolus) IV injection followed by saline flush. The radionuclide is administered 10 to 20 seconds after the saline flush. Side effects and contraindications are similar to adenosine. Aminophylline may be administered for reversal of side effects.

Dobutamine

Dobutamine stimulates beta-1 and beta-2 receptors resulting in an increase in heart rate, blood pressure, and myocardial contractility. It is infused at an initial rate of 5 to 10 μg/kg/min IV and increased in 10 μg/kg/min increments every 3 minutes to a maximum of 40 μg/kg/min. Its half-life is approximately 2 minutes. Similar to exercise testing, achieving more than or equal to 85% of the maximal age-predicted heart rate is a marker for adequate stress. If this is not achieved with maximum dose of dobutamine, atropine (0.5–2 mg IV) can be given in the absence of contraindications (prostatic hypertrophy, glaucoma). Side effects of dobutamine are palpitations, chest pain, headache, and dyspnea. Significant supraventricular or ventricular arrhythmias occur in 10% of patients, ischemic ST-segment depression is noted in roughly one-third of patients. Administration of a short-acting beta-blocker IV (e.g., Esmolol) may be necessary for severe side effects (Table 96-5).

TABLE 96-5 Contraindications and Indications for Early Termination of Dobutamine Pharmacologic Stress Testing

CONTRAINDICATIONS	EARLY TERMINATION CRITERIA
Recent (less than 1 wk) myocardial infarction	Similar to those for exercise testing
Unstable angina	
Hemodynamically significant left ventricular outflow tract obstruction	
Severe aortic stenosis	
Atrial tachyarrhythmias with uncontrolled ventricular response	
Prior history of ventricular tachycardia	
Uncontrolled hypertension (SBP >200 mm Hg and/or DBP >110 mm Hg)	
Aortic dissection or large aortic aneurysm	
Beta-blocker (heart rate and inotropic response to dobutamine will be attenuated)	

Modified with permission from Henzlova MJ, Cerqueira MD, Taillefer R, et al. ASNC imaging guidelines for nuclear cardiology procedures. *J Nucl Cardiol* 2009. Copyright © Elsevier.

Combination of Vasodilator and Low-Level Exercise Stress

The combination of vasodilator and low-level exercise stress (treadmill or handgrip) can be safely performed. Advantages are significant reduction in side effects of the vasodilator (i.e., hypotension) as well as improved image quality (i.e., less liver uptake of the radiotracer).

IMAGE ACQUISITION

Planar Imaging

With the advantages of SPECT imaging, planar imaging is infrequently performed, usually if SPECT imaging cannot be obtained (because of patient's body weight, claustrophobia).

Planar images usually including the left anterior oblique, anterior, and left lateral views can be acquired ungated and gated.

SPECT Imaging

Myocardial SPECT imaging is usually performed from an RAO to LPO angle covering 180 degrees (i.e., with a dual-headed camera, each camera head covers 90 degrees). Images are further processed, and the myocardium is reconstructed in the short axis (apex to base), vertical long axis (septum to lateral wall), and horizontal long axis (inferior to anterior wall). SPECT imaging has a superior spatial resolution compared to planar imaging and is more sensitive for detecting and localizing perfusion defects.

Gated Imaging

With gated SPECT acquisition, data collection is triggered by the QRS complex of the patient's ECG (i.e., R wave). The cardiac cycle is divided into a certain number (usually 8 or 16) of frames (of equal duration), each frame representing a specific phase of the cardiac cycle. Over time, data from several hundreds of cardiac cycles are obtained, and corresponding frames (1, 2... *n*) from all cardiac cycles are stored sequentially in their specific frame "bin" (1,2... *n*). After the acquisition is completed, each frame bin contains the summed data of the specific phase of the cardiac cycle. These summed frames (which contain the data of the entire study all added into one cardiac cycle) can then be displayed in a cinematic fashion. Consequently, left ventricular wall thickening and wall motion can be assessed, and LVEF (LV volumes at end diastole and end systole) can be calculated. Left ventricular function adds important information to perfusion imaging, and helps differentiating perfusion defects from artifacts. LVEF obtained by myocardial perfurion SPECT (MPS) is very reproducible and reasonably accurate. Especially in patients with relatively small ventricles, volumes (especially in end systole) maybe underestimated. The minimum number of frames for reliable LVEF assessment is 8. More frames (16, 24, or more) would improve temporal resolution, but the trade-off would be less favorable count statistics and/or a lengthier acquisition. A regular heartbeat is a prerequisite for gated imaging. Significant arrhythmias (atrial fibrillation, frequent ectopic beats) can lead to significant problems obtaining diagnostic quality images. Other difficulties may be artifact from skeletal muscle, pacemaker, or prominent T waves.

IMAGING RESULTS

NORMAL

With normal myocardial perfusion there is homogenous radiotracer uptake in the entire LV myocardium. The lateral wall may appear slightly brighter than the septum. Especially the basal septal wall has relatively decreased uptake (reflecting the membranous portion near the valve plane). The apex may have a small area of decreased uptake (so-called apical thinning). In addition, the areas of right ventricular (RV) insertion (7-o'clock and 11-o'clock positions on the short axis view) may also demonstrate slightly less uptake.

ABNORMAL

Stress myocardial perfusion imaging can differentiate between normal myocardium (normal perfusion at stress and rest), myocardial ischemia (so-called reversible defect: abnormal perfusion at stress which normalizes at rest) and myocardial scar (fixed defect: abnormal perfusion at stress that remains abnormal under resting conditions). Some stress perfusion defects are noted to be partially reversible at rest, meaning they show some but not complete normalization. Those defects may be a combination of scar and ischemia, or very severe ischemia, or a combination of ischemia and artifact. Besides evaluating for reversibility, characterization of a perfusion defect should include its location and extent (size and/or severity).

The location of a perfusion defect can be described according to vascular territory, myocardial wall, or segments involved (Table 96-6). The LAD typically contributes blood flow to the anterior, anteroseptal wall, and apex; the RCA supplies the inferior and inferoseptal wall; and the LCX the lateral wall. There is variability in blood supply of the posterior (inferolateral) wall depending on dominance (RCA vs. LCX), the apex (LAD vs. RCA), and anterolateral wall (LAD, LCX, or

TABLE 96-6 Commonly Used Segments in Myocardial Perfusion Imaging and Supply of Blood Flow from Coronary Arteries

	20-SEGMENT MODEL	17-SEGMENT MODEL	VASCULAR SUPPLY
Basal	Anterior	Anterior	LAD
	Anteroseptal	Anteroseptal	LAD
	Inferoseptal	Inferoseptal	RCA
	Inferior	Inferior	RCA
	Inferoletaral	Inferoletaral	LCX
	Anterolateral	Anterolateral	LCX
Mid	Anterior	Anterior	LAD
	Anteroseptal	Anteroseptal	LAD
	Inferoseptal	Inferoseptal	RCA
	Inferior	Inferior	RCA
	Inferoletaral	Inferoletaral	LCX
	Anterolateral	Anterolateral	LCX
Distal	Anterior	Anterior	LAD
	Anteroseptal	Septal	LAD
	Inferoseptal	Inferior	RCA
	Inferior	Lateral	LCX
	Inferoletaral		
	Anterolateral		
Apex	Anteroapical	Apical	LAD
	Inferoapical		

LAD, left anterior descending artery; RCA, right coronary artery; LCX, left circumflex artery.

TABLE 96-7 Summed Stress Score

Normal	0
Mildly reduced	1
Moderately reduced	2
Severely reduced	3
Absent	4

ramus intermedius). Evaluation of the extent/severity of a perfusion defect can be done based on visual assessment. In addition, there are several (semi)quantitative parameters (available from most software programs). The percentage of LV myocardium underperfused can be computed. The so-called summed stress score (SSS) applies scoring of the radiotracer uptake (Table 96-7). The lowest SSS is 0 (normal myocardium) and the most abnormal score is 68 (no radiotracer uptake in any segment). Using the SSS, a perfusion defect can be characterized as small (4–8), moderate (9–13), or large (greater than 13). Other parameters that have been used to describe the extent of myocardial perfusion abnormalities are the number of vascular territories involved (small: 0–1, moderate: 1–2, large: 2–3) as well as the percent of the left ventricular myocardium involved (small: less than 10%, moderate: 10%–20%, large: greater than 20%).

Low-Risk Parameters

Overall, patients with normal or near-normal myocardial perfusion images have a very low (less than 1%) annual cardiac event rate.

High-Risk Parameters

Several parameters observed during MPS are associated with a higher risk of cardiac events (greater than 5% per year). These include large stress-induced myocardial perfusion defects, perfusion defects in more than one vascular territory, substantial degree of reversibility of stress-induced perfusion defect, abnormal postexercise LVEF, transient left ventricular dilatation, abnormal rest LVEF (less than 40%), and increased lung uptake of thallium (lung/heart count ratio greater than 0.5). Thallium uptake in lungs is thought to reflect elevated LVED left ventricular dysfunction (importantly, lung uptake on a sestamibi scan does not have the same association). Other possible causes of thallium (or sestamibi) lung uptake could be inflammatory, infectious, or malignant conditions.

Accuracy

Depending on the exact imaging technique/protocol, patient population, and gold standard used, reported sensitivities, specificities, and normalcy rates of MPS are 80% to 85%, 65% to 81%, and 80% to 93% respectively.

Artifacts

Several artifacts can be observed in MPS. They can affect image quality and therefore diagnostic performance. The most frequent artifacts will be discussed as follows.

Attenuation

Attenuation describes the loss of photon signals when photons pass through tissue (lungs, soft tissue, bone) from the organ of interest (myocardium) to the detector. This can result in loss of count density (intensity) in the picture. Attenuation can be uniform or focal, depending on the patient's body habitus. Diaphragmatic attenuation may lead to inferior wall defects, whereas breast attenuation can affect the anterior (or apical, or lateral) wall. Attenuation artifacts are commonly present on both rest and stress images (fixed defects). To differentiate them from other forms of fixed defects (scar), one can either employ attenuation correction if available or review the gated images: a scar demonstrates abnormal wall motion, whereas attenuation artifacts will show normal motion and thickening. Imaging the patient in a different position (i.e., prone imaging) may also be helpful.

Motion

Patient motion (from respiratory variations, coughing, or inability to hold still) can be recognized by reviewing the raw projection images for unexpected steps or bouncing. Typical artifacts on the reconstructed tomographic slices are opposed defects on the contralateral walls (180 degrees apart), indistinct myocardial borders, or distortion of the heart shape with tails of radiotracer activity emanating from edges of a defect (this is sometimes called "hurricane sign"). If preventive measures (comfortable patient positioning, good immobilization, clear instructions, and sufficient delay of imaging after exercise) fail, one can apply motion correction or, if unsuccessful, repeat imaging.

Noncardiac Radiotracer Uptake

Noncardiac radiotracer uptake (namely, intense radiotracer uptake in the liver or GI tract adjacent to the myocardium) can lead to interfering hot spots. These hot spots can lead to hot spots in the adjacent myocardium itself by scattering radiotracer activity. Noncardiac radiotracer activity can also lead to cold spots in the myocardium when a ramp filter is used for reconstruction (a ramp filter applies negative values adjacent to [count dense] projection profiles to eliminate the star artifact). Therefore, intense noncardiac radiotracer uptake may lead to artificial perfusion defects or may mask actual perfusion defects or decrease reader confidence. Several measures to reduce or eliminate these artifacts are to delay imaging for better biliary and GI clearance, have the patient drink fluids, consider low-level exercise with pharmacologic stress testing, reimaging (possibly prone), or reprocessing.

PET MYOCARDIAL PERFUSION IMAGING

Radiopharmaceutical

Several PET radiotracers are used for myocardial perfusion imaging, including rubidium-82 chloride (Rb82), 13N ammonia, and O-15 water. Rubidium-82 is produced from an 82Sr/82Rb generator. It has a half-life of only 76 seconds. The usual dose is in the range of 30 to 60 mCi. Rb82 is a monovalent cation (potassium analog) that is taken up by the myocardial cells, similar to thallium, via active transport (Na+/K+ATPase). An onsite cyclotron is needed for the production of 13N ammonia (half-life 10 minutes) that is given at doses of 10 to 30 mCi. Another cyclotron-produced agent is O-15 water (half-life 2 minutes), which is only used in research settings.

Technique

Similar to SPECT imaging, there are various imaging protocols for myocardial perfusion with PET (rest/stress, stress/rest, etc). Cardiac PET perfusion studies can also be performed gated to assess for LV function and wall motion. Nevertheless, there are some general differences to SPECT imaging, mostly related to the short half-life of the currently available PET tracers and logistics involved. For example, pharmacologic stress is performed since exercise stress testing is typically not feasible; PET imaging can be performed with similar doses for the rest and stress studies (especially for Rb82); imaging can be completed in a shorter period of time overall; and a true peak stress LVEF can be calculated. Another advantage of PET is that attenuation correction is applied.

Interpretation

Like in SPECT imaging, PET perfusion studies are reviewed for the presence, reversibility, location, extent, and severity of perfusion defects.

Accuracy

Sensitivity of PET myocardial perfusion imaging is 90% (range, 83%–100%) with a specificity of 89% (range, 73%–100%). With PET, a true peak stress LVEF can be obtained (therefore, changes in LV function from rest to peak stress can be evaluated). Quantification of myocardial perfusion (in milliliter per minute per gram of tissue) and coronary flow reserve is feasible with PET, which may be particularly useful in patients with fairly balanced three-vessel disease or in the research arena.

MYOCARDIAL VIABILITY

CLINICAL BACKGROUND

In patients with coronary artery disease, left ventricular function/wall motion may be abnormal (ischemic cardiomyopathy). There can be various reasons for myocardium to be dysfunctional (Table 96-8). Hibernating myocardium is severely ischemic dysfunctional myocardium that is viable (meaning the abnormal contractility can be improved or even reversed when blood flow is restored). A myocardial scar on the other hand (which also demonstrates abnormal wall motion and perfusion) is nonviable (wall motion does not improve if blood flow is restored). If blood flow is not restored to an area of hibernating myocardium, it will eventually become a scar. Both hibernating and scarred myocardium (which have abnormal perfusion) should be distinguished from so-called stunned myocardium (which has normal perfusion). Stunned myocardium is myocardium with persistent wall motion abnormality following a period of ischemia despite restoration of perfusion. It is important to identify patients with hibernating (viable) myocardium. Patients with ischemic cardiomyopathy and viable myocardium have a better prognosis with revascularization (compared to medical therapy only). In most of these patients, revascularization improves wall motion (increased LVEF), and may also lead to increased survival, reduced cardiovascular events, arrhythmias, as well as relief of symptoms. Several imaging techniques are available to assess myocardial viability, including several nuclear medicine imaging procedures, echocardiography, and MRI.

TABLE 96-8 Myocardial Viability Pattern

	WALL MOTION	PERFUSION	FDG
Normal	Normal	Normal	Present*
Stunned	Abnormal	Normal	Present*
Hibernating	Abnormal	Abnormal	Present
Scar	Abnormal	Abnormal	Absent

*FDG uptake in normal or stunned myocardium may be variable. Both entities are not ischemic (perfusion is normal/preserved); therefore, FDG uptake does not add any information.

NUCLEAR IMAGING TECHNIQUES

THALLIUM

The underlying principle of viability imaging using thallium is the preservation of cell integrity needed for thallium uptake via active transport in viable myocardial cells. Although initial thallium uptake after injection is proportional to blood flow (normal myocardium has normal uptake, scar or hibernating myocardium has no/decreased uptake), thallium redistributes over time, meaning that myocardial Tl-201 is continuously exchanged with systemic Tl-201 as long as cells are viable. Thus, reversibility of a perfusion defect over time is a marker of viability. Several different protocols of assessing viability with thallium exist: initial imaging may be performed at rest or after stress; the redistribution image could be done at various time points after initial imaging (usually 3–4 hours after injection). Modifications are further delayed images (at 12, 24, or even 72 hours after injection). In addition, thallium reinjection to boost the available systemic thallium pool is an option. Although the PPV (if redistribution is observed, myocardium is indeed viable) is as high as 88%, the NPV is relatively poor, and a fixed defect does not necessarily rule out viability. Nevertheless, thallium SPECT imaging remains a commonly used technique because of its wide availability and overall good accuracy.

TC99M SESTAMIBI

The uptake of sestamibi is a marker of viability, because it requires certain degree of myocyte cell (membrane) and mitochondrial integrity for localization. For example, the degree of sestamibi uptake in dysfunctional myocardium compared to the maximum myocardial sestamibi uptake (using a cutoff of 50%–60% of maximum intensity) has been used to differentiate between viable myocardium and scar. This can be performed with or without nitroglycerin administration, but the latter may improve accuracy. Overall, sestamibi is less accurate than thallium (and FDG PET) imaging, and similar to thallium imaging, it underestimates the amount of viable myocardium.

F18 FLUORODEOXYGLUCOSE

In ischemic myocardium, metabolic substrate preference is shifted toward glucose (relative to fatty acid or lactate). Therefore F18-FDG, a marker of glucose metabolism, identifies preserved metabolic activity in regions of underperfused and dysfunctional myocardium.

TECHNIQUE

F18-FDG is a PET tracer with a half-life of 109 minutes. 18F-FDG is used to image metabolism of glucose (see Chap. 98 for details). The usual dose for cardiac imaging is 5 to 15 mCi. Normal myocardium preferentially utilizes free fatty acids in the fasting state, and the uptake of glucose (FDG) is usually low, although fairly variable. Therefore, when it comes to cardiac imaging with FDG, the goal is to stimulate the myocardium to utilize primarily glucose (take up FDG), which is usually accomplished by elevating glucose and insulin levels. For cardiac FDG imaging, patients fast for 6 to 12 hours. If the baseline blood glucose is less than 110 mg/dL, a standardized glucose load is administered (25–200 g, usually orally, although IV glucose is an alternative). In a normal individual, this stimulates the endogenous insulin response, and glucose is driven into the myocardial cells. Patient's blood glucose is monitored, and if it is less than 130 mg/dL approximately 1 hour after glucose load, FDG is administered IV. This protocol can be challenging in diabetic patients who may be unable to achieve a sufficiently low fasting blood glucose level, or have too high blood glucose levels after glucose administration. In these circumstances, exogenous insulin may be administered with further monitoring of blood glucose. FDG may be injected when blood glucose is trending down. Imaging is generally performed 45 to 60 minutes after FDG administration.

INTERPRETATION

Myocardial FDG uptake is assessed for its presence, distribution, and extent. Most importantly, comparison of FDG uptake (metabolism) and myocardial perfusion is performed to assess for areas of decreased or absent perfusion with concordant absence of FDG uptake (match) or discordant FDG uptake (mismatch). For such comparison, either a PET or SPECT myocardial perfusion study can be used.

ACCURACY

Reported sensitivities for FDG imaging to identify viable myocardium are 88% to 92%, with specificities of 73% to 89%, PPV of 68% to 100%, and NPV of 75% to 100%. Technical advantages of PET imaging (over SPECT) include reliable attenuation correction and very good spatial resolution. Disadvantages are relative limited availability of the technique and expertise, relative high cost, and challenges in diabetic patients. Viability imaging with FDG PET is rather extensively validated and currently the best (most sensitive) method in nuclear medicine and by many considered the gold standard.

OTHER IMAGING TECHNIQUES

ECHOCARDIOGRAPHY

Echocardiographic techniques assess myocardial wall thickness and motion. Viable myocardium demonstrates maintained contractile reserve (i.e., improvement in segmental wall motion with infusion of dobutamine). The hallmark of hibernating myocardium is a biphasic response during dobutamine infusion: after an initial improvement in segmental wall motion with infusion of low-dose dobutamine, worsening function during higher doses of dobutamine is observed (when the myocardium becomes more ischemic). Like SPECT imaging, it is frequently used because of the wide availability of the technique.

MRI

MRI allows evaluation of myocardial function, perfusion, and contrast enhancement. Scarred (nonviable) myocardium may demonstrate early hypoenhancement (perfusion defects on first-pass imaging), but the hallmark of scar tissue is late enhancement. Hibernating myocardium on the other hand is defined by the lack of late hyperenhancement.

RADIONUCLIDE VENTRICULOGRAPHY

Radionuclide ventriculography, also called gated blood pool study, radionuclide angiography, or multiple gated acquisition (MUGA) scan, is performed to evaluate global and regional ventricular function. Techniques include first-pass radionuclide angiography (FPRNA) and equilibrium radionuclide angiography (ERNA).

FIRST-PASS RADIONUCLIDE ANGIOGRAPHY

Overall, FPRNA is not frequently performed. It requires a fast compact bolus injection immediately followed by very rapid acquisition of data while the radiotracer passes through the central circulation. The main advantage of first-pass imaging is a more accurate assessment of RV function (compared to ERNA), since there is no overlapping radiotracer activity in other structures. Typically, images are obtained in the RAO view to assess the RV. Although FPRNA could be done with virtually any radiopharmaceutical (providing enough counts), it is usually performed in conjunction with ERNA (labeled red blood cells) or MPS (Tc99m sestamibi). For repeated acquisitions (i.e., baseline and peak stress), a tracer that is easily cleared, such as Tc-99m sulfur colloid or Tc-99m DTPA, may be preferable.

EQUILIBRIUM RADIONUCLIDE ANGIOGRAPHY

The radiopharmaceutical typically used for ERNA is Tc99m-labeled red blood cells (usual dose 10–20 mCi). Several methods for labeling of red blood cells exist (Chap. 93). In vivo labeling is sufficient for radionuclide ventriculography. Gated images are obtained in the left anterior oblique (this is usually not a fixed angle, but the view that allows for the best septal separation between RV and LV), anterior, and left lateral views (see gated imaging technique given earlier). Images are reviewed for visual assessment of chamber (LV, RV, atria) size, and function. At the state of equilibrium, radiotracer activity from a cardiac chamber is proportional to its volume. Therefore, ventricular function (LVEF) can be quantified. Regions of interest (ROI) are drawn either automatically or manually around the left ventricle at end systole (frame with fewest counts) and end diastole (frame with maximum counts). The left ventricular ejection fraction is calculated as follows:

$$\text{LVEF} = (\text{LVED} - \text{LVES}) / (\text{LVED} - \text{background})$$

The background ROT is usually a crescent shape adjacent to the LV. If a relatively hot structure (i.e., spleen) is included in the background ROI, the LVEF is falsely high (Table 96-9). A normal resting EF is usually $\geq$50% (50%–80%) The RVEF (normal 46%–70%) is usually slightly less than LVEF. Besides global ventricular function, regional wall motion is assessed. Wall motion is normally greatest in the apex and the free walls (and less in the septum). When wall motion is abnormal, the abnormality should be further described as akinesis (absence of motion), hypokinesis (diminished wall motion, which could be further classified as mild, moderate, or severe), or dyskinesis (paradoxical wall motion). Nowadays, exercise MUGA is rarely indicated. A normal response to exercise is an increase in LVEF by 5% or more. A failure to increase the LVEF by 5%, a decrease of LVEF from baseline, or the development of wall motion abnormalities (with or without chamber dilatation) indicates an abnormal response.

Quantitative (Fourier phase) analysis of a MUGA study reduces four-dimensional information for each

TABLE 96-9 Possible Sources of Error During Gated Blood Pool Imaging

	BACKGROUND ↑	BACKGROUND ↓	EDV ↑	EDV ↓	ESV ↑	ESV ↓
EF	↑	↓	↑	↓	↓	↑

↑, too high/overestimated; ↓, too low/underestimated

pixel into a two-dimensional image. These parametric images may be useful in evaluating regional variations of ventricular contractions. The so-called amplitude image shows cardiac contractility (how much each pixel moved during the cardiac cycle) color coded. In a normal patient, the LV should have a fairly uniform color. The phase image reflects the timing (sequence) of contraction (i.e., when each pixel moved in relationship to the R wave or other marker). The phase can be displayed as a color-coded image (the LV should have a fairly uniform color) or as a histogram (where a cardiac cycle is transformed into 360 degrees on the x-axis and number of pixels on the y-axis). This histogram should show the ventricles as a fairly narrow bell-shaped curve (widening would reflect abnormal wall motion); the ventricles and atria should be 180 degrees apart. The paradox image is the ED frame subtracted from the end-systolic frame (ES−ED). In a normal patient, the area of the LV should be a void. Any visible areas of the LV reflect dyskinetic areas. MUGA studies should be carefully reviewed for incidental findings such as splenomegaly, or a circular area of photopenia around the heart (which may be related to pericardial effusion).

CLINICAL APPLICATION

One of the main clinical applications nowadays is the assessment of patients who receive cardiotoxic therapy (specifically anthracyclines). Unfortunately, there are no universally excepted guidelines on how to follow these patients (i.e., how frequently to reassess LVEF, when/how to alter or discontinue therapy). Therefore there is some interinstitutional variation. Nevertheless, most people would agree that therapy should not be started if the baseline LVEF is less than 50% and that therapy should be discontinued if the LVEF falls to less than 50%. A decline in LVEF by more than 10% to 20% is also concerning. Other indications for gated blood pool studies are to follow patients with cardiomyopathy, especially if the LVEF is difficult to assess by other techniques or if the EF was borderline with another imaging technique prior to ICD implantation.

SUGGESTED READING

Gibbons RJ, Balady GJ, Bricker JT, et al. ACC/AHA 2002 guideline update for exercise testing: summary article: a report of the American College of Cardiology/American Heart Association Task Force on Practice Guidelines (Committee to Update the 1997 Exercise Testing Guidelines). *Circulation. 2002;106*(14):1883-1892. http://www.acc.org/qualityandscience/clinical/guidelines/exercise/exercise_clean.pdf. Accessed May 6, 2009.

Henzlova MJ, Cerqueira MD, Taillefer LH, Yao S-S. ASNC imaging guidelines for nuclear cardiology procedures: stress protocols and tracers. http://www.asnc.org/imageuploads/ImagingGuidelinesStressProtocols021109.pdf. Accessed May 6, 2009.

Iskandrian AE, Verani MS, eds. *Nuclear Cardiac Imaging. Principles and Applications*. 3rd ed. New York, NY: Oxford University Press; 2003.

Klocke FJ, Baird MG, Bateman TM, et al. ACC/AHA/ASNC 2003 guidelines for the clinical use of cardiac radionuclide imaging—executive summary: a report of the American College of Cardiology/American Heart Association Task Force on Practice Guidelines (ACC/AHA/ASNC Committee to Revise the 1995 Guidelines for the Clinical Use of Cardiac Radionuclide Imaging). *Circulation*. 2003;108(11):1404-1418. http://www.acc.org/qualityandscience/clinical/guidelines/radio/index.pdf. Accessed May 6, 2009.

Zaret BL, Beller GA, eds. *Clinical Nuclear Cardiology. State of the Art and Future Directions*. 3rd ed. Philadelphia, PA: Elsevier Mosby; 2005.

QUESTIONS AND ANSWERS

1. Which of the following radiopharmaceuticals for myocardial perfusion imaging has the highest extraction fraction?
   A. Thallium-201
   B. Tc-99m sestamibi
   C. Tc-99m tetrofosmin
   D. Tc-99m teboroxime

   ANSWER: D. Extraction fractions are as follows: Tc-99m teboroxime (>90%) > Tl-201(85%) > Tc-99m sestamibi(Tc-99m tetrofosmin) (55%–70%). (The most physiologic myocardial perfusion tracer with an extraction fraction of nearly 100% is O-15 water, a PET tracer.)

2. A 72-year-old male with chest pain and left bundle branch block presents for stress myocardial perfusion imaging (MIBI). He has a history of hypertension, diabetes, peripheral vascular disease (bilateral below the knee amputation). He received aspirin and metoprolol to manage his chest pain within the last 2 hours. Upon auscultation you notice wheezing. Concerning his stress test, which of the following is the best next step?
   A. Reschedule the test
   B. Perform the test using adenosine
   C. Perform the test using exercise
   D. Perform the test using dobutamine

   ANSWER: A. The test needs to be rescheduled. Certainly a patient with bilateral below the knee amputation would be unable to exercise. Vasodilator stress (adenosine) is contraindicated given active wheezing. Dobutamine is not an option because the patient recently received a beta-blocker dose and has a LBBB (this can lead to perfusion defects when the heart rate increases).

3. A 43-year-old diabetic female suffered an acute LAD myocardial infarction, which was treated with emergent stent. Besides occlusion of the proximal LAD, coronary angiogram at that time revealed mild to moderate disease in the LCX and RCA. Six months later, she presents with chest pain. Myocardial perfusion imaging reveals a stress-induced perfusion defect involving the lateral wall that is reversible at rest. LVEF is 50%. Which of the following is the best explanation for this finding?
   A. Acute LAD stent thrombosis
   B. Interval LCX infarct
   C. Interval progression of disease with ischemia in the LCX
   D. Interval progression of disease with ischemia in the LAD distal to the stent

   ANSWER: C. This is the only answer correctly describing the territory involved (the lateral wall receives blood supply from the left circumflex artery) and the nature of the perfusion defect (a stress-induced defect that is reversible at rest is ischemia). Especially in diabetic patients, coronary artery disease can progress relatively rapidly. An interval infarct may have been suspected if a fixed (nonreversible) defect was seen. LAD disease should involve the anterior, septal, or apical wall. Acute stent thrombosis usually occurs shortly after stent placement (not several months later).

4. A patient presents for exercise stress testing to evaluate for coronary artery disease. Baseline BP is 140/80 mmHg, HR 67 bpm, normal baseline ECG. At stage 2 of the BRUCE protocol, BP is 170/80 mmHg, HR 150 bpm. You proceed to stage 3. Which of the following is an absolute indication to terminate exercise tress testing?
   A. SBP decreases to 160 mm Hg, patient asymptomatic
   B. DBP decreased to 60 mmHg
   C. ECG shows 2 mm ST elevation in leads I, II, V1-V4.
   D. Greater than 10 PVCs per minute

   ANSWER: C. Absolute indications for early termination of exercise stress testing are decrease in SBP of greater than 10 mm Hg from baseline despite an increase in workload, when accompanied by other evidence of ischemia (not when asymptomatic, a false), ST elevation (≥1 mm) in leads without diagnostic Q waves, sustained ventricular tachycardia (not only several PVCs per minute). A decrease in DBP is a normal physiologic response to exercise.

5. Which of the patients described below does *not* have a high-risk myocardial perfusion scan pattern?
   A. A 35-year-old female with perfusion defects in the anterior and inferior wall and LVEF of 50%
   B. A 65-year-old male with lung/heart ratio of 0.3
   C. A 50-year-old male with moderate-sized anterior wall scar and LVEF of 30%
   D. A 42-year-old female with an SSS of 20

   ANSWER: B. Parameters that are associated with a high risk of cardiac events include stress-induced large myocardial perfusion defects (patient D), perfusion defect in more than one vascular territory (patient A), abnormal rest LVEF (<40%) (patient C), and increased lung uptake of thallium (lung/heart ratio >0.5). (option B is correct). Other high-risk parameters are large reversibility of stress-induced perfusion defect, abnormal postexercise LVEF, and transient left ventricular dilatation.

6. You review a radionuclide ventriculography on a patient with lymphoma and notice that the background ROI includes part of the spleen. The LVEF is likely
   A. underestimated
   B. overestimated
   C. not affected

   ANSWER: B. LVEF by ERNA is as follows: LVEF = (LVED − LVES) / (LVED − background).

   If a relatively hot structure (e.g., spleen) is included in the background ROI, the LVEF is overestimated. If a relatively photopenic area is included (i.e., stomach or large hiatal hernia), the LVEF is underestimated.

7. A patient with ischemic cardiomyopathy (LVEF 25%) undergoes sestamibi myocardial perfusion and FDG PET imaging. The MIBI scan shows severely decreased perfusion in the apex, anterior, septal, and inferior walls, and normal perfusion of the lateral wall. FDG uptake is noted in the anterior, anteroseptal, and lateral walls, and no FDG uptake is seen in the inferoseptal, inferior wall, and apex. Which of the following does this indicate?
   A. LAD scar, LCX hibernating, RCA scar
   B. LAD normal, LCX normal, RCA scar

C. LAD hibernating, LCX normal, RCA hibernating
D. LAD hibernating, LCX normal, RCA scar

ANSWER: D. The LAD territory (anterior wall and septum) has decreased perfusion, but preserved FDG uptake (viable); therefore it is hibernating. The LCX supplies the lateral wall, which has normal perfusion (normal). The RCA territory (inferior wall) has absent perfusion and no FDG uptake (match) indicating that this area is a scar. A matched defect involving the apex may indicate that it receives blood supply from the RCA (normal variant) or that there is a small distal LAD scar (nevertheless, most of the LAD territory is viable).

8. A patient with a baseline EF of 55% by MUGA received doxorubicin. A high-quality follow-up MUGA scan reveals an LVEF of 40%. Which of the following is the next best step?
   A. Confirm findings with transthoracic echocardiography
   B. Continue therapy with reduced dose and regular follow-up
   C. Continue therapy with same dose and short-term follow-up
   D. Discontinue doxorubicin

   ANSWER: D. Unfortunately there are no universally accepted guidelines on anthracycline cardiotoxicity; most people would agree that therapy should be discontinued if the LVEF falls below 50% (and no technical problems with the examination are identified). It is also important to use the same imaging technique (e.g., echocardiography or MUGA) for follow-up that was used for the baseline evaluation.

9. On a myocardial perfusion SPECT study, you notice decreased radiotracer uptake in the anterior wall at rest and stress (fixed defect) in a female patient. Gated images reveal preserved wall motion and thickening in the anterior wall. What does this represent?
   A. LAD ischemia
   B. LAD scar
   C. Attenuation artifact
   D. Gating artifact

   ANSWER: C. A fixed defect could represent a myocardial scar or an attenuation artifact. Breast tissue can lead to attenuation involving the anterior wall. To differentiate attenuation from scar, one can apply attenuation correction if available (attenuation artifacts should normalize, scar should not), or one can review gated images. A myocardial scar is associated with abnormal wall motion and thickening. Ischemia leads to reversible (not fixed) defects. There is no indication in the case that there is a gating problem.

97 THYROID AND PARATHYROID SCINTIGRAPHY

Sibyll Goetze

THYROID

INTRODUCTION

Patients with hyperthyroidism, thyroid nodules, or thyroid cancer are referred to the nuclear medicine department for the diagnosis and treatment of thyroid disease. Procedures performed in these patients may include thyroid (radioiodine) uptake, thyroid scintigraphy, and radioiodine therapy.

DIAGNOSTIC PROCEDURES

Thyroid Scintigraphy

Thyroid scintigraphy refers to a nuclear medicine procedure where images of the thyroid gland (or other thyroid tissue) are obtained after injection of a radiopharmaceutical that localizes to thyroid tissue, such as Tc-99m sodium pertechnetate (TcO_4^-) or radioiodine. Common indications for thyroid scintigraphy are to evaluate for typical patterns of radiotracer distribution in patients with hyperthyroidism (usually in combination with radioiodine uptake measurement), to investigate selected patients with a thyroid nodule, to locate ectopic thyroid tissue, assess neck or substernal masses, or to further investigate congenital hypothyroidism. Prior to the procedure, it is important to ensure that patients have not been exposed to interfering medications or agents (Table 97-1). Female patients must not be pregnant or nursing.

During thyroid scintigraphy, the patient is in the supine position with the neck extended. A gamma camera equipped with a pinhole collimator is typically used. A "distant" anterior image that includes the salivary glands and superior mediastinum is obtained first. Marker views to outline anatomical landmarks such as sternal notch, angle of the mandible, or other may be useful. Then with the camera centered over the thyroid

TABLE 97-1 Medications Potentially Interfering with Thyroid Imaging/Radioiodine Therapy and Recommended Time of Withdrawal

MEDICATION	TIME OF WITHDRAWAL
Antithyroid medications (PTU, methimazole)	>3–4 d
Thyroid hormone replacement	
Thyroxine	3–4 wk
Triiodinethyronine	2 wk
Multivitamins	1 wk (6 wk for thyroid cancer patients)
Topical iodine	2–3 wk (6 wk for thyroid cancer patients)
Amiodarone	>3–6 mo
Radiographic contrast media	
Intravenous water soluble (CT, angiography)	4 wk
Lipophilic agents	>1 mo
Lugol's solution, SSKI, Kelp, other	2–3 wk (6 wk for thyroid cancer patients)

bed, "close" images are obtained in the anterior and bilateral anterior oblique views. For the evaluation of thyroid nodules, marking of a palpable nodule should be performed. Interpretation of the examination should include an estimate of the overall intensity (compared to the salivary glands or background) and uniformity of radiotracer uptake within the thyroid gland. The presence, number, size, and location of any areas with significantly increased "hot" or decreased "cold" uptake are noted. Correlation with the patient's history, physical examination, laboratory values, and other imaging procedures is crucial. Sources of error are possible contamination (skin, hair, or clothing), interfering food, medications, technical errors, and esophageal activity (to clear radiotracer from the esophagus, patients may drink some water prior to imaging).

Tc-99m Sodium Pertechnetate (TcO_4)

Tc-99m pertechnetate (photopeak: 140 keV, half-life: 6 hours) is injected intravenously. Images are usually obtained 15 to 30 minutes after injection. Tc-99m pertechnetate is less expensive and more readily available than I-123. In addition, scintigraphy with pertechnetate can be completed in a shorter period of time (usually within 1 hour). Disadvantages of pertechnetate are that it is not organified by the thyroid cells (which may limit the evaluation of thyroid nodules) and activity in adjacent structures (esophagus, blood vessels) may be confusing. Images of the injection site to assess for dose infiltration should be obtained if the uptake in the thyroid gland is low.

Radioiodine

There are two forms of radioiodine used in nuclear medicine: I-123 (photopeak: 159 keV, half-life: 13 hours) and I-131 (photopeak: 364 keV, half-life: 8 days). Unlike pertechnetate, radioiodine is not only trapped by follicular thyroid cells, but also organified and incorporated into thyroid hormone, which reflects thyroid physiology somewhat more accurately. Radioiodine is administered orally. Since food may interfere with the procedure by slowing the absorption of radioiodine, it is recommended that patients fast for 2 hours before and after the radioiodine administration. After ingestion of I-123, imaging is typically performed at 4 to 6 hours. Since images are obtained several hours after radiotracer ingestion, the procedure using I-123 is longer compared to pertechnetate. Although I-123 is more expensive and less readily available than pertechnetate, it has several advantages including a more accurate characterization of thyroid nodules, better visualization of retrosternal thyroid tissue and more accurate/robust quantification of uptake (which is often requested in those patients). Beta-particle emission, high photon energy, and long half-life of I-131 all lead to a relatively high radiation dose to the thyroid (100 times more than I-123, Table 97-2). Therefore, I-131 should not be used for thyroid scintigraphy, unless radioiodine therapy is subsequently performed. It may also be useful in the evaluation of substernal masses (high-energy photons are even less attenuated by osseous structures).

Whole-Body Radioiodine Scans

Whole-body radioiodine scans are performed for the detection of residual thyroid and/or tumor tissue in patients with differentiated thyroid cancer. Patients are rendered hypothyroid (goal TSH greater than 30 mIU/L) to stimulate any potential thyroid or tumor tissue to trap radioiodine, which is nowadays often accomplished by administration of recombinant TSH (rTSH). Alternatively, thyroid hormone replacement therapy can be withdrawn (patient must discontinue T3 for 10–14 days and/or T4 for 3–4 weeks prior to imaging). Patients should also follow a low-iodine diet for 7 to 14 days. Diagnostic scans are performed with a relatively low dose of radioiodine. It has been suggested that higher doses of radioiodine (especially I-131) cause "stunning" of thyroid tissue (decreased uptake and efficacy of treatment doses of I-131 because of cell death or dysfunction). Planar anterior and posterior images from the top of the head to the lower extremities are usually obtained 24 hours (6–48 hours) after oral ingestion of 0.5 to 5.0 mCi of I-123 or 48 hours (24–72 hours) after 1 to 4 mCi of I-131. Spot images of the neck and as well as marker images to delineate anatomic structures (i.e., sternal notch, angle of the mandible) can be useful. SPECT or SPECT and CT may improve localization of iodine-avid tissue. Physiologic uptake includes the salivary glands, the oro- and nasopharynx, bowel, and bladder. There are

TABLE 97-2 Radiation Dosimetry for Thyroid and Parathyroid Imaging Agents in Adults

RADIOPHARMACE UTICAL	ADMINISTERED ACTIVITY (mCi)	RADIATION DOSE TO TARGET ORGAN (rad/mCi)	EFFECTIVE DOSE (remmCi)
Patients with thyroid gland (assuming 15% uptake)			
I-131 NaI	0.05–0.2 (scan) 0.004–0.01 (uptake)	780 (thyroid)	24.0
I-123 NaI	0.2–0.6 (scan) 0.1–0.3 (uptake)	7.0 (thyroid)	0.28
Tc-99m TCO4	2–10 (scan and uptake)	0.23 (large intestine)	0.048
Patients after thyroidectomy (0% thyroid uptake)			
I-131 NaI	1–5	3.0 (bladder wall)	0.41
I-123 NaI	0.5–5.0	0.33 (bladder wall)	0.048
Other			
18 F-FDG	10–20	0.59 (bladder wall)	0.07
Parathyroid imaging			
201 Tl chloride	2.0–3.5	2.0 (kidney)	0.85
99mTc sestamibi	5–25	0.14 (gallbladder)	0.031

Data modified from the Society of Nuclear Medicine procedure guidelines www.snm.org.

multiple pitfalls that should be kept in mind when interpreting radioiodine scans, the most common ones including contamination, breast, and thymic uptake. In addition, there are inflammatory conditions, other tumors, and even effusions or renal cysts that may also cause false-positive examinations and correlation with thyroglobulin (Tg) levels and other imaging procedures is often necessary. Diagnostic (low-dose) scans should be distinguished from posttherapy scans, which are obtained several days after radioiodine ablation/therapy. In addition to salivary glands, oro-/nasopharynx, bowel and bladder, the biodistribution of posttreatment scans includes mild diffuse uptake in the liver (secondary to metabolization of thyroid hormones). If a diagnostic whole-body scan is negative (no radioiodine-avid lesions identified), radioiodine-avid tissue/lesions may be detected on a posttreatment scan.

Radioactive Iodine Uptake Test

Radioactive iodine uptake (RAIU) is the measurement of the fraction of an administered radioiodine dose that accumulates in the thyroid gland. It is performed in patients with hyperthyroidism, especially to differentiate etiologies that may be treated with radioiodine (Graves disease, multinodular goiter (MNG), and hyperfunctioning adenoma) from those that can be followed clinically (thyroiditis, and iodine-induced hyperthyroidism). In patients who are deemed candidates for radioiodine therapy, the uptake measurement is frequently used to determine the individual patient treatment dose.

Similar to thyroid imaging, it is important to ensure that patients have not been exposed to interfering medications or agents (Table 97-1). Female patients must not be pregnant or lactating/nursing. Thyroid uptake measurements can be obtained with I-123 or I-131. To calculate a thyroid uptake, counts of the patient's neck at certain time point(s) after the dose administration in addition to counts of a calibrated standard (or patient dose) in a neck phantom, counts of the patient's thigh (patient background) and room background are necessary. Measurements can be taken early (2–6 hours) and/or late (18–24 hours). RAIU is calculated as follows (all in counts per minute).

$$\text{RAIU} = (\text{patient neck counts} - \text{patient background}) / (\text{administered or standard counts} - \text{room background}) \times 100\%$$

Reference normal values of RAIU are obtained from historical data and range from 5% to 15% at 4 hours and 10% to 35% at 24 hours. In most euthyroid patients, the uptake at 24 hours is greater than the 4-hour uptake. The historical reference values should not be strictly used since uptake may vary depending on laboratory (equipment used at different institutions) and specific population (varying levels of dietary iodine intake in different geographical regions). Radioiodine uptake values obtained should always be interpreted in the clinical context.

Although a thyroid uptake can also be determined with 99mTc pertechnetate using a gamma camera technique (drawing regions of interest over thyroid gland and background), this requires careful validation and is overall felt to be less accurate. Therefore it should be used with caution only in selected cases. Images of the injection site to assess for dose infiltration should be obtained if the uptake in the thyroid gland is low.

Radiation doses to target organs and effective doses are detailed (Table 97-2). It should be noted that the radiation dose increases with radioiodine avidity of the thyroid gland (i.e., the dose to the thyroid gland increases to 1300 rad/mCi of I-131 if the uptake is 25%). Effective doses are also higher in children compared to adults.

RADIOIODINE THERAPY

Therapy with I-131 in the form of sodium iodide given orally has been used for many years to treat benign (hyperthyroidism secondary to Graves disease, multinodular goiter, or autonomous adenoma) and malignant (thyroid cancer) conditions in adults and children. Regulations related to radioiodine therapy (licensure to administer I-131, release of patients after therapy, etc.) vary between jurisdictions.

Patient Preparation and Prerequisites

Prior to radioiodine therapy, patients must discontinue all potentially interfering medications (Table 97-1). For patients with hyperthyroidism, the avidity of the thyroid gland for radioiodine must be established, which is done by performing a radioiodine uptake test. Patients at increased risk for radioiodine-induced "thyroid storm" (patients with large thyroid glands, very high radioiodine uptake, patients receiving large amounts of radioiodine, and elderly patients with cardiovascular disease) will likely benefit from prophylactic beta-blocker therapy. Especially patients with thyroid cancer should follow a low-iodine diet 1 to 2 weeks prior to therapy. For female patients, a serum pregnancy test must be obtained. Breast-feeding must be discontinued at least 4 weeks prior to radioiodine therapy (to reduce radiation to the breast) and cannot be resumed after treatment for that child.

Side Effects and Associated Risks

Side effects and associated risks must be discussed with the patient by the performing physician, and informed consent must be obtained. Patients treated for hyperthyroidism will almost universally become hypothyroid (usually over a period of several months) and appropriate follow-up and lifelong thyroid hormone replacement therapy will be necessary. (Patients with thyroid cancer are usually already hypothyroid after thyroidectomy.) For patients with hyperthyroidism, other important possible side effects are related to radiation-induced thyroiditis and include transient hyperthyroidism (possible thyroid storm) and local tenderness (which may require steroid therapy in severe cases). In addition, patients with Graves orbitopathy may experience worsening of the eye disease, and prophylactic steroid administration should be considered.

It is possible that the initial radioiodine treatment is not completely efficient and a repeat treatment may be necessary. In patients with hyperthyroidism, the first treatment is usually effective in greater than 90% of patients. For thyroid cancer patients, the likelihood of subsequent radioiodine therapies depends on the stage and aggressiveness of the tumor. Thyroid remnant ablation in low-risk patients is successful with one treatment in more than 80% of patients.

For higher doses of radioiodine (thyroid cancer therapy), possible side effects also include mucositis, sialadenitis, and loss of taste. This is usually transient, but can be permanent in rare cases potentially leading to sicca syndrome (dry mouth and dry eyes) and increased risk of dental caries. Higher doses of radioiodine have also been associated with transient cytopenia, and high cumulative doses of I-131 (approaching 1 Ci) may lead to permanent bone marrow depression.

In male patients, temporary decrease in sperm counts has been observed following high doses of I-131. If cumulative doses exceed 400 mCi, sperm banking should be discussed with male patients. There has been no observed definite adverse effect of radioiodine treatment on female fertility and future pregnancies. All female patients are usually advised to avoid pregnancy for 6 months following radioiodine therapy to allow for time to achieve a stable euthyroid stage and to ensure that no repeat radioiodine therapy is necessary. Although there may be an increased risk of secondary malignancies (colon, bladder, breast cancer, and leukemia) after high doses of radioiodine, there is no definite threshold of I-131, and no recommendation of more intensive cancer screening other than usual age-appropriate screening is felt to be necessary.

Radiation Safety Precautions

Following radioiodine therapy, patients must follow precautions to protect any family members and the public from excess radiation. This includes increasing physical distance to other people (sleeping in separate beds), limiting time spent with others, and paying special attention to personal hygiene (prevent exposure of other people to body fluids that may contain I-131) following I-131 therapy.

I-131 Dose Determination

I-131 dose for Thyrotoxicosis: In general, multinodular goiter and autonomous adenomas are more resistant to radioiodine therapy than Graves disease. Therefore, multinodular goiter or single adenomas may require higher doses of I-131, and are more likely to require a second treatment. There are two different approaches to selecting I-131 dose for hyperthyroid patients. One is to empirically select a dose (5–10 mCi for patients with Graves disease and 15–29 mCi for patients with nodular goiters and adenomas). Another method is to determine a dose based on individual patient characteristics (size of the thyroid gland on physical examination and 24-hour radioiodine uptake) and desired activity to be delivered to the thyroid tissue as follows:

Treatment dose (mCi) = (thyroid gland size [g] × desired dose to be delivered to the thyroid [mCi/g])/(24-hour radioiodine uptake)

The desired dose to be delivered to the thyroid gland depends on the underlying condition and ranges from 80 to 200 μCi/g of thyroid tissue, with doses at the higher range selected for conditions that may be more resistant to I-131, such as nodular glands or very large goiters.

I-131 dose for Thyroid Cancer: Treatment doses are usually selected empirically based on clinical/histopathologic characteristics. While a dose of 75 to 100 mCi (or even as low as 30 mCi) should be administered for postsurgical remnant ablation in low-risk patients, patients at risk for residual/recurrent disease should be treated with higher doses (100–200 mCi). Metastatic disease is usually treated with I-131 doses of at least 150 mCi (locoregional metastasis) or 150 to 300 mCi (for distant metastasis). Alternatively, dosimetry may also be applied to determine a treatment dose. Although not frequently done, it may help to determine the highest possible dose that can be given without exceeding radiation to critical structures or to ensure that critical structures (lung or bone marrow) do not receive excess radiation with usual empiric doses (patients with extensive lung or bone metastasis). Radiation dose to the bone marrow should be less than 200 rads (whole-body retention at 48 hours less than 120 mCi). Whole-body retention at 48 hours should be less than 80 mCi in patients with diffuse lung metastases to prevent radiation pneumonitis and fibrosis.

CLINICAL SCENARIOS

THYROTOXICOSIS

There are many forms of thyrotoxicosis. Depending on the etiology, therapy and prognosis can vary. Sometimes, the etiology of thyrotoxicosis can be established based on clinical evaluation alone. If this is not the case, patients may be referred to the nuclear medicine department for further evaluation. For example, thyroid uptake helps to differentiate entities with increased radioiodine uptake (Graves disease, multinodular goiter, and autonomous adenoma) from thyrotoxicosis with decreased uptake (thyroiditis). This is important since thyroiditis is a benign self-limiting condition that usually does not require any specific treatment. Radioiodine uptake may be within the normal reference range, nevertheless it is inappropriately high in the setting of a recent low or suppressed TSH. This may be the case in patients with multinodular goiter and single adenoma, since there are areas of relatively hyperfunctioning and suppressed tissue, and the overall uptake can occasionally be normal. It may be difficult to distinguish these patients from patients with recovering thyroiditis (when radioactive iodine uptake returns to normal), and correlation with clinical data (duration of disease, TSH) and follow-up may be useful. In patients with Graves disease, uptake is typically well above the normal range. If further differentiation of the radioiodine-avid forms of thyrotoxicosis is necessary, a thyroid scan may help (diffuse uptake in Graves disease, heterogenous uptake in multinodular goiter, and a single hot focus in autonomous adenoma).

Graves disease, also called diffuse toxic goiter, is caused by IgG antibodies directed against TSH receptors on the cell surface of follicular thyroid cells. These antibodies stimulate the thyroid cells to increase the production of thyroid hormones (T4 and T3 are elevated, and TSH suppressed through feedback mechanism). Since iodine is needed for the thyroid hormone synthesis, radioiodine uptake is increased. In most patients, the 24-hour uptake is higher than the 4-hour uptake. On occasion, the 4-hour uptake may be higher than the 24-hour uptake. This is due to rapid turnover of radioiodine by the thyroid glands, usually in patients who are markedly hyperthyroid with very elevated radioiodine uptake (greater than 65%) at 4 hours. The autoimmune process is generally diffuse, leading to diffuse increased uptake on a thyroid scan. Treatment options for Graves disease are radioiodine therapy, antithyroid medications and, in selected patients (i.e., marked thyromegaly, or tracheal compression), surgery. Marine-Lenhart syndrome, a variant of Graves disease, basically represents Graves disease with coexistent multinodular goiter (also called nodular Graves disease). Radiotracer distribution on thyroid scintigraphy may be heterogenous.

Toxic autonomous nodule refers to thyrotoxicosis caused by one (or two) hyperfunctioning nodule that is no longer under the control of the pituitary-thyroid control mechanism and autonomously produces excessive amounts of thyroid hormone (T4/T3 increased/TSH low). Radioactive iodine uptake is usually mildly to moderately increased. Thyroid scan shows one (or two) distinct focus of increased radiotracer uptake, which may, or may not, suppress radiotracer uptake in the remainder of the normal thyroid tissue. I-131 therapy or surgery are treatment options.

Toxic multinodular goiter is a multinodular goiter associated with thyrotoxicosis. It is thought that several nodules of a multinodular goiter become hyperplastic and eventually function autonomously (T4/T3 normal to increased/TSH low). Radioactive iodine uptake is mildly to moderately increased, and the thyroid scan usually shows very heterogenous uptake with several areas of relatively increased and decreased uptake. Radioiodine therapy, surgery, or antithyroid therapy may be a treatment option.

Subacute thyroiditis (also called granulomatous thyroiditis, de Quervain thyroiditis, or giant cell thyroiditis) is presumed to be secondary to preceding viral infection. It may be associated with fever, systemic symptoms, thyroid tenderness/pain (erythrocyte sedimentation rate may be elevated). Inflammation of the thyroid gland leads to destruction of the follicular cell integrity with release of thyroid hormone (T4/T3 increased/TSH low) into the circulation. Radioactive iodine uptake is very low in the hyperthyroid phase because the follicular cells are damaged and unable to transport or organify iodine. The condition is self-limiting (resolving within several months), and symptomatic treatment with antiinflammatory medications may help. Silent thyroiditis (also known as painless thyroiditis, subacute lymphocytic thyroiditis, or atypical thyroiditis) may be a painless variant of subacute granulomatous thyroiditis or Hashimoto thyroiditis. If it occurs in the postpartum phase, it is called postpartum thyroiditis (5%–10% of pregnancies). An autoimmune process leads to destruction of the thyroid cells. The condition, although it can be recurrent, is self-limited, usually resolving within weeks to months. Radioactive iodine uptake is very low in the hyperthyroid phase secondary to cell damage. In the recovery phase of thyroiditis (after the acute thyrotoxic phase), radioactive iodine uptake (thyroid cell integrity) recovers and may be normal or even slightly elevated.

Iodine-induced hyperthyroidism is one end of the spectrum of iodine-induced thyroid disease (hypothyroidism is more common) and may be encountered following exposure to large amount of iodine, such as contrast agents or iodine-containing medication. The exact mechanism of iodine-induced thyrotoxicosis is not entirely understood, yet it may be related to underlying areas of autonomous nodular activity that are stimulated by the iodine to synthesize thyroid hormone. This is also called Jod-Basedow phenomenon. Radioactive iodine uptake is low, secondary to excess iodine saturating the thyroid gland.

Thyrotoxicosis secondary to extrathyroidal thyroid hormone can be seen in factitious thyrotoxicosis from (self) administration of excess thyroid hormone, metastatic thyroid cancer if the metastatic tissue produces sufficient amounts of thyroid hormone to cause thyrotoxicosis (very rare), or struma ovarii, a rare ovarian tumor that contains functioning thyroid tissue, which in rare cases produces excessive amounts of thyroid hormone.

Thyroid Nodules

It is important to understand that thyroid scintigraphy does not identify a nodule per se. It simply represents (differences) in radiotracer uptake (function) of thyroid tissue. Thyroid nodules can be diagnosed by physical examination or ultrasound (US), or other anatomical imaging. It is therefore wrong to interpret scintigraphic findings as nodules, unless proper correlation is made. In addition, thyroid scintigraphy has a very limited role in patients with thyroid nodules found on palpation or imaging tests. Thyroid scintigraphy may be useful if the TSH is low (to evaluate if the nodule is a hyperfunctioning adenoma) or if US-guided fine needle aspiration (FNA) was indeterminate and the clinical suspicion for cancer is not high (hot nodules could be followed). US is the imaging modality of choice to evaluate thyroid nodules.

If patients with a thyroid nodule are referred for scintigraphy, marking of a thyroid nodule is often necessary in addition to the routine thyroid scintigraphy procedure outlined earlier in the chapter. This helps to accurately correlate the scintigraphic findings/characteristics (decreased, normal, or increased uptake) with the palpable abnormality. For marking, palpation of the thyroid gland should be performed. If a palpable nodule remains palpable with the patient supine on the imaging table, a radioactive (hot) or radioopaque (cold) marker is placed exactly over the palpable nodule. Marker images should be obtained with the nodule/marker in the center of the field of view to avoid distortion from parallax effect. Duplicate views without the marker should also be obtained. Solitary nodules can be characterized depending on the intensity of radiotracer uptake compared to normal thyroid tissue as hot (increased), warm (isointense) or cold (decreased). Warm nodules are sometimes called equivocal. Hot nodules are almost certainly benign and most often represent a hyperfunctioning adenoma (malignancy rate less than 1%). Hyperfunctioning (hot) nodules may completely or partially suppress radiotracer uptake in normal thyroid tissue. Most solitary hypofunctioning (cold) nodules (90%) are benign and represent nonfunctioning adenomas, cysts, localized fibrosis, or thyroiditis. Nevertheless, up to 10% of solitary cold nodules are malignant and therefore require further evaluation. A dominant cold nodule in a multinodular gland could also be malignant (although less likely than a solitary cold nodule in an otherwise normal gland). Occasionally, a nodule will appear *not* cold (warm, or rarely hot) on a pertechnetate scan but in fact be cold on a radioiodine scan. This is when the lesion, although it can trap pertechnetate (or iodine), lacks the ability to organify iodine—it is called discordant nodule. Since very few nodules are discordant nodules, most experts feel that this does not warrant the routine use of I-123 in thyroid scintigraphy, given all the other advantages of Tc99m pertechnetate.

Thyroid Cancer

Introduction

Although an increasing incidence of thyroid carcinoma has been observed in recent years (at least partially secondary to early detection of disease), it remains a relatively infrequent entity. The typical presentation is a thyroid nodule incidentally found on examination or diagnostic imaging (US with FNA are generally used to establish the primary diagnosis), although patients may seek attention because of local symptoms or signs of metastatic disease. Thyroid carcinoma can be divided into several histologically different entities: differentiated tumors (including papillary and follicular carcinoma) are most common (70%–90%) with generally very good long-term prognosis. The remaining 10% to 30% are medullary carcinoma, anaplastic carcinoma, lymphoma involving the thyroid gland and metastases.

Differentiated Thyroid Cancer

Initial management for patients with differentiated thyroid cancer is typically total thyroidectomy. Usually postoperative radioiodine remnant ablation is performed several weeks after surgery. The treatment goals of radioiodine ablation/therapy (I-131 Rx) are to facilitate surveillance with iodine scans and stimulated Tg and decrease the risk of locoregional recurrence and cancer-related mortality.

TSH Stimulation

For radioiodine therapy (as well as for iodine scans), residual thyroid tissue needs to be maximally "stimulated" to take up iodine, which is usually achieved by making the patient hypothyroid (goal of TSH greater than 30 IU/mL). This can be reached either by thyroid hormone replacement withdrawal or by administration of rTSH in selected patients.

Whole-Body Iodine Scans

Pretherapy whole-body radioiodine scans are not generally recommended, but may be useful in patients in whom the extent of thyroid remnant tissue is unknown or when the results of the scan would alter the decision about I-131 Rx or the I-131 dose to be given. The use of I-123 or low-dose I-131 (3–5 mCi) is recommended for diagnostic whole-body radioiodine scans.

Posttherapy whole-body radioiodine scans (usually 7 days [3–14 days] after therapy) should be performed in all patients since it may detect new or additional metastases, alter staging or affect further management (in up to 15% of patients). In long-term management (6–12 months after I-131 therapy), diagnostic whole-body iodine scans may be of value in the follow-up of patients with high or intermediate risk of persistent disease. Low-risk patients clinically free of disease, negative stimulated Tg, and cervical US do not require routine iodine scans.

I-131 Dose for Ablation/Treatment

For initial (postsurgical) radioiodine ablation/treatment, a minimum effective dose (30–100 mCi) should be chosen, especially in low-risk patients, while a higher dose (100–200 mCi) may be appropriate for residual microscopic disease or a more aggressive tumor (e.g., tumor size greater than 1.5 cm, unfavorable histology [tall cell, sclerosing, and other variants], multifocal disease, lymphatic/vascular invasion, or positive margins). For lymph node and distant metastasis (lung bone), a dose of 150 to 200 mCi (or even 300 mCi) may be given. Radioiodine therapy doses can be selected empirically or calculated by dosimetry (this may be beneficial for pulmonary metastasis to limit radiation to the lung tissue). Since metastatic lesions may be stimulated after radioiodine is given, glucocorticoids should be administered prophylactically for patients with osseous or brain lesions that may predispose to increased risk for fractures or neurological compromise. In addition to I-131 therapy, other treatments such as surgery or external radiation should be considered in selected patients (local aerodigestive tract invasion, bone or brain metastasis). Persistent, recurrent, or metastatic disease can be treated with radioiodine (every 6–12 months) as long as disease continues to be radioiodine avid (visualized on posttreatment scans) and continues to respond to therapy (decrease in size of lesions, or declining Tg levels).

Long-Term Management

Following thyroidectomy and thyroid remnant ablation, disease-free status is defined by no clinical evidence of tumor, no imaging evidence of tumor, and undetectable serum Tg levels during TSH suppression and stimulation. Therefore, initial follow-up for low-risk patients should be based mainly on TSH-suppressed Tg and cervical US, followed by TSH-stimulated Tg (if the TSH-suppressed Tg is undetectable). Serum Tg levels (together with thyroglobulin antibodies [TgAb]) should be measure measured every 6 to 12 months. US of the thyroid bed and locoregional lymph nodes should be performed depending on patient's risk for disease and Tg status. Diagnostic whole-body iodine scans may be useful in a few selected patients.

Tg positive is defined by any detectable suppressed Tg level or a stimulated Tg more than 2 ng/mL (in the absence of interfering antibodies). Recommended evaluation for Tg-positive patients includes imaging of the neck (US) and chest (high-resolution noncontrast CT). If both are negative, empiric I-131 therapy should be considered; if either US or CT are positive, treatment options depend on results (surgery with or without I-131 therapy). Radioiodine can be repeated until the tumor is eradicated, no longer responds to treatment, or is no longer radioiodine avid. When disease is not radioiodine avid (negative posttreatment I-131 scan), patients may benefit from F18-FDG-PET (especially if suppressed Tg greater than 10 ng/mL).

Medullary Thyroid Cancer

Medullary thyroid cancer (MTC), a neuroendocrine malignancy originating from parafollicular C cells in the thyroid gland, is usually (75%) sporadic, although it can be seen as part of multiple endocrine neoplasia or isolated familial medullary thyroid cancer. It is usually managed surgically. After surgery, patients are followed with serum calcitonin and CEA levels. Imaging is obtained if these results are abnormal or if symptoms arise. Various imaging modalities have been used to evaluate medullary thyroid cancer including US, CT, MRI, as well as nuclear techniques, such as somatostatin receptor imaging with ^{111}In-pentetreotide and ^{131}I- or ^{123}I-MIBG. MIBG scintigraphy has a sensitivity of approximately 30%, while the sensitivity of somatostatin receptor imaging is in the range of 25% to 71%. Other radiopharmaceuticals (^{201}Tl, 99mTc-sestamibi, radiolabeled anti-CEA antibodies) are generally not used because of unsatisfactory results. The role of FDG-PET in patients with MTC is not established with reported wide ranges of accuracies and conflicting results. It may be useful in selected patients (serum calcitonin levels more than 1000 pg/mL, or if other imaging modalities are negative).

Anaplastic Thyroid Cancer

Anaplastic thyroid cancer is a very rare but very aggressive malignancy affecting mostly elderly patients. The use of nuclear (and other) imaging procedures for following patients with anaplastic thyroid cancer is very limited as the results do not change outcomes, which is typically quite poor.

Ectopic Thyroid Tissue

When the thyroid gland fails to completely descend to its location during embryologic development, thyroid tissue may remain along the course. Thyroid scintigraphy may be useful in confirming the presence of ectopic thyroid tissue, such as a lingual thyroid, thyroglossal duct remnant, or pyramidal lobe. For this indication, radioiodine is preferred over pertechnetate, given less salivary gland activity and higher tissue specificity.

In addition, thyroid scintigraphy may confirm that a mediastinal mass represents substernal goiter. For this indication, radioiodine is also preferred over pertechnetate because of less blood pool activity and higher-energy photons (less attenuation). Sometimes, the goitrous substernal tissue has impaired function (and is not very radioiodine avid) resulting in equivocal studies.

Neonatal Hypothyroidism

When the TSH screening test is abnormal in a neonate, thyroid scintigraphy may help differentiate between agenesis of the thyroid gland (nonvisualization of the thyroid gland), lingual thyroid or other ectopic tissue, and dyshormonogenesis (markedly increased radiotracer uptake by the thyroid gland).

PARATHYROID IMAGING

CLINICAL BACKGROUND

The most common cause of primary hyperparathyroidism is hyperfunctioning adenoma (80%–85%), followed by multiple gland hyperplasia (12%–15%), and parathyroid carcinoma (1%–3%). Parathyroid scintigraphy has been employed to localize parathyroid adenomas or other abnormal parathyroid tissue prior to surgery. Localizing imaging procedures are especially useful in patients who present with recurrent or persistent hyperparathyroidism after surgery, and patients at high surgical risk or presenting with life-threatening adenomas. Imaging is also helpful when minimally invasive surgery is considered.

IMAGING PROTOCOLS

Dual-Phase Sestamibi Imaging

Dual-phase imaging describes the acquisition of early and delayed images after injection of 99mTc sestamibi. Sestamibi localizes to tissue with relatively high blood flow (parathyroid adenomas are hypervascular) and localizes in mitochondria (oxyphil cells of parathyroid adenomas are rich in mitochondria). The principle of dual-phase Sestamibi imaging is that Sestamibi demonstrates faster washout from normal thyroid (and normal parathyroid) tissue, than from abnormal parathyroid glands. Therefore, abnormal parathyroid tissue becomes (more) prominent over time. Planar images of the neck and mediastinum are obtained early (approximately 10–15 minutes) and late (approximately 2–4 hours) after radiotracer injection. Additional images with a pinhole or converging collimator may be useful. SPECT (or SPECT/CT) imaging has become increasingly popular because of more precise anatomical localization. The accuracy of dual-phase Sestamibi parathyroid scintigraphy in the evaluation of parathyroid adenoma is greater than 90%. Relatively small size (500 mg or less) of a parathyroid gland may cause false-negative examinations. In addition, a number of parathyroid adenomas (as well as hyperplastic glands) have relatively fast washout characteristics. False-positive examinations may be caused by other lesions that have persistent Sestamibi uptake, such as thyroid nodules, other head and neck cancers, lymphadenopathy, or brown adipose tissue. Sestamibi can also be used for intraoperative lesion detection using a handheld gamma probe.

Dual-Isotope (Subtraction) Imaging

With dual-isotope or subtraction imaging, two different radiopharmaceuticals are used. One of the radiotracers utilized is taken up by both thyroid and parathyroid tissue (201-thallium chloride [half-life: 72 hours, photopeak: 69–83 keV], or 99mTc sestamibi) and the other radiotracer only accumulates in the thyroid gland (99mTc pertechnetate, or I-123). Similar to dual-phase Sestamibi imaging, images of the neck and mediastinum are obtained. The image of the thyroid specific tracer is subtracted from the thallium or sestamibi image—any remaining focus of radiotracer activity could represent a parathyroid adenoma. In addition to the sources of errors mentioned earlier in the chapter, patient motion/ misregistration is a particular problem with the subtraction imaging technique and may cause false-positive or negative examinations. Another potential problem may be agents interfering with thyroid scintigraphy (such as iodinated contrast). There is no clear consensus that dual-phase imaging is better than subtraction imaging technique.

Other Imaging Procedures

US has been used to localize parathyroid adenoma (hypervascular hypoechoic lesion). Advantage of US is that it is able to evaluate for coexisting thyroid abnormalities prior to neck surgery. Disadvantages are the inability to localize ectopic parathyroid glands (i.e., in the mediastinum) and difficulties in evaluating postsurgical neck.

CT and MRI may be useful in selected cases.

Suggested Reading

Carlisle MR, Lu C, McDougall IR. The interpretation of 131I scans in the evaluation of thyroid cancer, with emphasis on false positive findings. *Nucl Med Commun*. 2003;24:715-735.

Cooper DS, Doherty GM, Haugen BR, et al. The American Thyroid Association Guidelines Taskforce. Management guidelines for patients with thyroid nodules and differentiated thyroid cancer. *Thyroid*. Feb 2006;16(2):109-142.

Intenzo CM, dePapp AE, Jabbour S, et al. Scintigraphic manifestations of thyrotoxicosis. *Radiographics*. 2003;23:857-869.

Sandler MP, ed. *Diagnostic Nuclear Medicine*. 4th ed. Philadelphia, PA: Lippincott Williams & Wilkins; 2003.

Society of Nuclear Medicine. Procedure guideline for therapy of thyroid disease with iodine 131 (sodium iodide). Version 2.0 http://interactive.snm.org/docs. Accessed May 6, 2009.

Society of Nuclear Medicine. Procedure guideline for thyroid scintigraphy. Version 2.0, 1999. http://interactive.snm.org/docs. Accessed May 6, 2009.

Society of Nuclear Medicine. Procedure guidelines for thyroid uptake measurement. Version 3.0, 2006. http://interactive.snm.org/docs. Accessed May 6, 2009.

Society of Nuclear Medicine. Procedure guideline for scintigraphy for differentiated papillary and follicular thyroid cancer. http://interactive.snm.org/docs.

Society of Nuclear Medicine. Procedure guideline for parathyroid scintigraphy. Version 3.0, 2004. http://interactive.snm.org/docs. Accessed May 6, 2009.

Smith JR, Oates E. Radionuclide imaging of the thyroid gland: patterns, pearls, and pitfalls. *Clin Nucl Med*. Mar 2004;29(3): 181-192.

QUESTIONS AND ANSWERS

1. Which of the following is an appropriate I-131 dose for a 39-year-old female after total thyroidectomy with a 7-mm papillary (unifocal) thyroid carcinoma without clinical or imaging evidence of metastatic disease?
   A. 20 mCi
   B. 75 mCi
   C. 200 mCi
   D. Should be determined by dosimetry

   ANSWER: B. This patient (small unifocal papillary thyroid cancer) is at low risk for occult metastatic or recurrent disease. In these cases, a minimum dose that ensures effective thyroid remnant ablation should be chosen and is usually 75–100 mCi, although doses as low as 30 mCi have been utilized in selected patients. For this patient, 20 mCi would be inappropriately low and 200 mCi too high (200 mCi is usually used for patients with metastatic disease). Dosimetry is not necessary for this patient. It is usually applied in patients receiving doses of I-131 greater than 200–300 mCi or those who have extensive metastatic disease (lung, bones) to ensure that critical organs do not receive exceedingly high amounts of radiation.

2. Which of the following radiopharmaceuticals is *not* clinically used for thyroid scintigraphy or uptake measurements?
   A. Iodine-123
   B. Iodine-124

C. Iodine-131
D. 99mTc pertechnetate

ANSWER: B. Iodine-124 is a radioisotope of iodine. Although it could be used for PET imaging (half-life of 4.18 days), it is currently not clinically used for thyroid scintigraphy.

3. A clinically and biochemically euthyroid patient was found to have a 2-cm nodule when palpating the thyroid gland. Which of the following is the most appropriate imaging procedure for further evaluation?
A. Contrast-enhanced CT
B. F18 FDG-PET
C. US
D. I-123 scan

ANSWER: C. US is the imaging modality of choice for evaluating thyroid nodules. It can confirm the palpated abnormality is indeed a thyroid nodule, assess for the presence of other nodules (which may not be palpable), and assess the characteristics of the nodule (cystic component, calcifications, etc.). FNA may be performed with US guidance. Thyroid scintigraphy with I-123 may be useful if the patient is thyrotoxic, or if US-guided FNA was indeterminate and the clinical suspicion for cancer is not high. CT and PET have no role in the initial evaluation of a recently diagnosed thyroid nodule.

4. Which of the following is *not* a possible side effect of radioiodine therapy in a female patient with Graves disease?
A. Hypothyroidism
B. Infertility
C. Worsening of ophthalmopathy
D. Transient worsening of thyrotoxicosis

ANSWER: B. Treatment doses of I-131 for hyperthyroidism do not cause infertility in women. Radioiodine treatment can cause radiation-induced thyroiditis in the short term (transient worsening of thyrotoxicosis, neck pain) and hypothyroidism in the long term. Graves ophthalmopathy may develop or worsen in patients (especially smokers), and steroid prophylaxis or treatment may be necessary.

5. Which of the following statements about dual-phase Sestamibi parathyroid scintigraphy is *true*?
A. Early images are obtained at 4 hours, delayed images at 24 hours.
B. Should be considered in patients with recurrent hyperparathyroidism after parathyroidectomy.
C. Thyroid carcinoma may result in false-negative examinations.
D. An important step in the interpretation is the computer subtraction of the early from the delayed image.

ANSWER: B. Localization of an abnormal parathyroid gland is especially important prior to repeat surgery. Scintigraphic techniques (e.g., dual-phase Sestamibi imaging) are especially useful since an ectopic parathyroid adenoma may be found, and other imaging techniques may have limitations in the postsurgical neck. Early images are obtained at 10 to 15 minutes, delayed images at 2 to 4 hours. Thyroid carcinoma or adenomas may result in false-positive examinations. Using dual-phase Sestamibi imaging, no computer subtraction is necessary. Subtraction is performed when dual-isotope techniques are used.

6. Which of the following medications does *not* need to be discontinued prior to thyroid scintigraphy?
A. Levothyroxine
B. Methimazole
C. Propranolol
D. Propylthiouracil

ANSWER: C. Propranolol is a beta-blocker and does not need to be stopped prior to thyroid scintigraphy or radioiodine treatment.

7. Which of the following statements about Graves thyrotoxicosis is *true*?
A. Radioiodine uptake is typically uniformly increased.
B. Surgery is preferred over radioiodine therapy.
C. It is characterized by elevated levels of T4 and antinuclear antibodies.
D. It is a very rare cause of thyrotoxicosis.

ANSWER: A. Graves disease is a fairly common cause of thyrotoxicosis caused by stimulating TSH receptor antibodies (*not* antinuclear antibodies). Antithyroid medications and I-131 therapy are the main treatment modalities, and surgery is rarely indicated.

8. Which of the following combinations of clinical scenario and radioiodine uptake is correctly matched?
A. Factitious hyperthyroidism – normal
B. Graves disease – low
C. Silent thyroiditis – low
D. Struma ovarii – high

ANSWER: C. Radioiodine uptake is low in silent (lymphocytic) thyroiditis, subacute thyroiditis, factitious hyperthyroidism, iodine-induced hyperthyroidism, and ectopic hyperfunctioning tissue (struma ovarii). Radioiodine uptake is high in Graves disease. Radioiodine uptake is usually (inappropriately) high in toxic MNG and autonomous adenoma. *Caveat:* Radioiodine uptake could be normal in recovering thyroiditis.

9. A patient with locoregionally advanced papillary thyroid cancer (T3N2M0) presents 9 months after total thyroidectomy and radioiodine treatment (150 mCi). His stimulated Tg level is now 50 mg/dL. Cervical US shows nonspecific findings; noncontrast chest CT is negative. He receives 150 mCi I-131 for therapy. His posttreatment scan is negative. Which of the following would be the next most appropriate step?
   A. MRI of the neck
   B. Repeat CT of the chest with contrast
   C. FDG-PET
   D. Follow up in 6–12 months with Tg levels

   ANSWER: C. In a patient with elevated Tg levels and negative posttreatment iodine scan, FDG-PET is the most appropriate next step. The goal is to localize disease that could be managed by surgical resection or other local therapy (external vadiation therapy (XRT), radiofrequency ablation, chemo/alcohol embolization). FDG-PET has sensitivities of 45% to 100% and specificities of 90% to 100% for the diagnosis of recurrent thyroid cancer. PET/CT fusion imaging appears superior to PET alone. FDG-PET–positive patients who cannot be surgically treated, thyroid hormone suppression, chemotherapy, or monitoring without additional therapy may all be options. FDG-PET negative patients can be followed with serial FDG-PET and serial Tg measurements. Whether FDG-PET scanning (similar to radioiodine whole-body scans) should be performed under TSH stimulated conditions has not yet been definitively established. FDG-PET also has prognostic information: Patients with FDG-avid disease have a worse outcome compared to patients with negative FDG-PET scans.

10. Which of the following radiotracer combinations not appropriate for dual-isotope subtraction imaging in parathyroid scintigraphy is correctly matched?
   A. 99mTc pertechnetate – 99mTc sestamibi
   B. I-123 – 99mTc sestamibi
   C. Thallium – Pertechnetate
   D. 99mTc pertechnetate – I-123

   ANSWER: D. The principle of dual-isotope imaging is that a tracer that localizes in both thyroid and parathyroid glands (e.g., sestamibi, thallium) and a tracer that localizes to thyroid only are used. Images are obtained, while the patient remains in the same position, and are later computer subtracted. There are various combinations of radiopharmaceuticals, with doses varying depending on which one is used first and whether tracers with a different or similar photopeak are used. Pertechnetate and I-123 localize only to thyroid gland.

98 ONCOLOGY

Pradeep G. Bhambhvani and Sibyll Goetze

PET IMAGING

RADIOPHARMACEUTICAL: F18 FDG

18F fluorodeoxyglucose (FDG) is cyclotron produced. It has a (physical) half-life of 109 minutes. The radioactive component, 18F, decays via beta-positive emission to 18O. Like with any other positron emitter, upon annihilation of the positron with an electron, two gamma photons with energy of 511 keV are released. 18F-FDG is used to image the metabolism of glucose. It is a good imaging agent for applications in oncology because many tumor cells have increased glucose metabolism and therefore will demonstrate increased FDG uptake. FDG is injected intravenously and is taken up by the cells similar to glucose. Once intracellular, FDG undergoes phosphorylation by hexokinase to FDG-6-phosphatase. FDG-6-phosphatase cannot be metabolized further and is "trapped" in the cells (Fig. 98-1). Normal biodistribution of FDG includes the brain, the myocardium (which in the fasting state demonstrates variable FDG uptake), liver, spleen, GI tract, blood pool, lymphoid tissue, salivary glands, and testes. Since FDG is excreted through the urine, the urinary bladder (which is also the target organ) and renal collecting system accumulate FDG. Bowel uptake is thought to be secondary to uptake in smooth muscle, metabolically active mucosa, lymphoid tissue, swallowed secretions or FDG uptake by colonic bacteria or

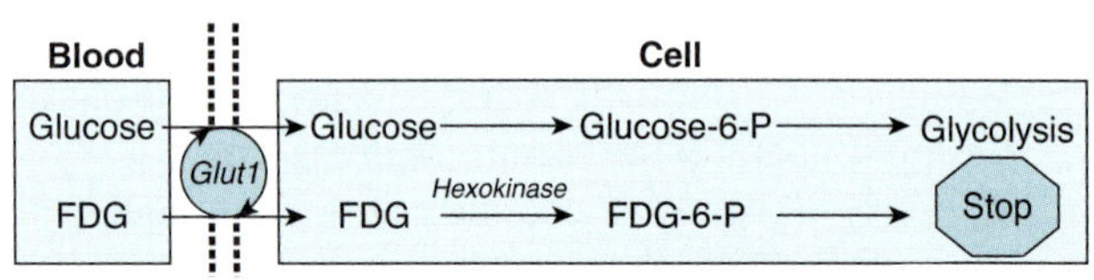

FIG. 98-1 Comparison between glucose and F18-FDG metabolism.

any combination—and therefore can be very variable in extent, intensity and overall pattern. Normal variants of FDG uptake are frequent and include uptake in muscles, bone marrow, breasts and ovaries (depending on patient's age, menstrual cycle), thymus and lymphoid tissue (especially in younger patients) among many others (Table 98-1). Uptake of FDG in the so-called brown adipose tissue (BAT), which can occasionally interfere with the assessment of the neck and thorax if intense, maybe reduced by keeping the patient in a warm room 30 to 60 minutes before injection, administration of a benzodiazepine like lorazepam or diazepam, or a beta blocker.

TABLE 98-1 Possible Sources of Error in FDG PET Interpretation

POTENTIAL FALSE POSITIVES	POTENTIAL FALSE NEGATIVES
Physiologic uptake and variants	**Tumor related**
Lymphoid tissue	Small size
Salivary glands	Necrotic (portion) of tumor
Brown adipose tissue (BAT)	Low-grade tumors
Thymus (thymic rebound/hyperplasia)	Serous/mucinous components
Breast tissue/gynecomastia	Some hepatocellular carcinomas
Muscle uptake	Some well-differentiated tumors (prostate, neuroendocrine, thyroid)
GI tract (GE junction, bowel)	Genitourinary carcinomas
GU uptake (extrarenal pelvis, bladder diverticulum)	Bronchioalveolar carcinomas
Female genital tract (endometrium, corpus luteum cyst)	Lobular carcinomas of the breast
Inflammatory processes	Peritoneal implant on bowel/liver
Atheromata, vascular grafts, venous thrombosis	**Patient related**
Surgical, biopsy, or ostomy site	Recent chemotherapy or radiotherapy
Hematoma	Hyperglycemia
Fracture	Hyperinsulinemia
Pneumonia	Artifact from patient motion
Postradiation (pneumonitis)	**Artifacts**
Postpleurodesis	Misalignment between PET and CT
Granulomatous processes (histoplasmosis, sarcoidosis, fungal, or mycobacterial disease)	
Subcutaneous injection sites	
Dose infiltration (and draining lymph node)	
Lymphadenitis	
Thyroiditis	
GI tract (diverticulitis or inflammatory bowel disease)	
Pancreatitis	
Cholecystitis	
Inflammatory arthropathy	
Osteomyelitis	
Benign tumor/disease	
Pituitary adenoma	
Adrenal adenoma/hyperplasia	
Thyroid adenoma	
Benign salivary gland tumors	
Colonic polyps and villous adenoma	
Benign ovarian lesions	
Benign bone lesions: aneurysmal bone cyst, Schmorl node, osteophyte, Paget disease	
Uterine leiomyoma	
Stimulated bone marrow (e.g., cytopenia or cytokine therapy)	
Fibrous dysplasia	
Artifacts	
Misalignment between PET and CT	
Attenuation correction artifacts	

Data modified from Delbeke D, Coleman RE, Guiberteau MJ, et al. Procedure guideline for tumor imaging with 18F-FDG PET/CT 1.0. *J Nucl Med.* 2006;47(5):885-895.

PATIENT PREPARATION AND IMAGING

To optimize uptake of FDG by the target (tumor), it is important that

- glucose which competes with uptake of FDG is kept within the normal range, and
- as much FDG as possible is available for uptake to the tumor (and not "shifted" to other organs).

Therefore, patients should be in a state of normal glucose and insulin levels since hyperinsulinemia would cause redistribution of glucose/FDG to muscle and myocardium. To achieve this goal, patients are asked to fast for at least 4 hours prior to the examination. Blood glucose (BG) is checked prior to injection of FDG and if BG >150 to 200 mg/dL, rescheduling of the patient should be considered. Patients should neither exercise nor perform strenuous activities for 24 hours prior to the examination to avoid uptake of FDG in musculature, reducing availability of FDG for tumor uptake. After injection of FDG (the usual dose for an adult ranging from 10–20 mCi for whole-body imaging), patients are resting quietly in a warm room for at least 45 minutes (usually 60–90 minutes) before imaging. For most applications in oncology, whole-body imaging from the skull base to the proximal thighs is performed. For cancer types with a high likelihood of lesions in the head or lower extremities, adjustments can be made. Increasingly, hybrid PET/CT machines (in contrast to standalone PET cameras) are used to ensure optimal fusion of physiologic (PET) and anatomic (CT) information. This leads to higher accuracy because it allows for better differentiation of FDG uptake by normal structures versus uptake by tumor. Besides aiding in the localization of FDG uptake, CT is also used for attenuation correction.

STANDARDIZED UPTAKE VALUE

For most clinical purposes, it is sufficient to assess the presence (and intensity) of FDG uptake visually and describe the intensity of uptake as mild, moderate, or intense in relation to background uptake (for example, in normal liver parenchyma). Nevertheless, for research purposes and certain clinical circumstances (for example, assessing solitary pulmonary nodule [SPN] or response to therapy), it maybe useful to include semiquantitative description of FDG uptake by tumor. Commonly used is the standardized uptake value (SUV). The SUV is defined as follows:

SUV = activity in region of interest in tumor (mCi/mL)/ (injected dose [mCi]/body weight [g]).

SUV can be expressed as maximum or mean SUV, and it can be adjusted for lean body mass (or BSA), which maybe preferably for circumstances where there are significant changes in body weight (e.g., follow-up of head and neck cancer patients under or after treatment). One should be careful in interpreting SUV since many factors influence its accuracy and reproducibility, such as the accuracy of the calibration of the PET scanner itself, strict adherence to clinical protocols, dose infiltration, time to imaging after radiotracer administration, type of reconstruction algorithm and attenuation map, the size of the selected region of interest, changes in uptake in other organs (e.g., bone marrow), and method of analysis (maximum vs. mean). The accuracy of the SUV also depends on the lesion size itself, and in lesions smaller than 1 cm FDG uptake maybe underestimated. There is no SUV value that definitely confirms or excludes malignancy. Fairly extensively evaluated is the value of SUV in the characterization of SPNs, where an SUV of less than 2.5 may best distinguish benign from malignant lesions. Nevertheless, this cannot be necessarily applied to other structures (liver, bone marrow, etc), and also depends on the prevalence of other (FDG-avid) disease processes.

CLINICAL APPLICATIONS

Solitary Pulmonary Nodule

SPN is defined as an approximately round lesion, less than 3 cm in diameter that is completely surrounded by lung parenchyma without other abnormalities. Overall 10% to 70% of these nodules maybe malignant. FDG imaging maybe helpful to characterize SPNs. For example, in low-risk patients (clinical likelihood of malignancy 20% or less), the negative predictive value (NPV) of a non–FDG-avid SPN is very high (decreasing the risk of malignancy to approximately 1%); nevertheless in high-risk patients, further evaluation of a SPN maybe necessary. An expert panel recently did not support the use of specific "quantitative thresholds." Several studies have used a cutoff of maximum SUV of 2.5 to differentiate benign from malignant nodules. Several studies have shown that FDG PET is useful for the evaluation of SPN with a sensitivity of 95% and specificity of 81%. There appears to be no major difference in accuracy whether visual assessment or SUV threshold was used. The positive predictive value (PPV) of FDG PET is higher than that of CT in characterizing a lesion as malignant. Specificity is affected by prevalence of other potentially FDG-avid disease such as histoplasmosis or fungal infections (Table 98-1).

Lung Cancer

In patient with non–small cell lung cancer (NSCLC), FDG PET is currently used for staging, restaging, evaluating recurrent disease, and assessing response to therapy. NSCLC is staged by the TNM system. Correct initial staging is important to determine treatment options (especially surgery) and prognosis. FDG PET is especially useful in evaluating nodal (N stage) and distant (M stage) metastasis. For example, normal-sized lymph nodes by CT maybe malignant and some enlarged lymph nodes maybe in fact benign. As far as correct staging of nodal status is concerned, PET has a sensitivity of 88% and specificity of 91% (compared to CT with a sensitivity of 63% and specificity of 76%). The fact that the specificity for PET is less than 100% is mostly related to FDG uptake in inflammatory nodes. One main impact of FDG PET is that surgery maybe avoided in patients who are "upstaged" when advanced disease is identified. Unsuspected metastatic disease has been found in 14% to 29% of patients with NSCLC undergoing FDG PET. Overall FDG PET seems to be reliable enough for the evaluation of bone metastasis that a bone scan (in addition to PET) is only recommended in special circumstances. One should keep in mind that FDG PET is not optimal for the evaluation of the T stage. In some cases, for example, FDG PET cannot clearly detect the level of invasion of adjacent structures, and CT (or MRI) is necessary in evaluating involvement of chest wall, mediastinum, pleura, and vascular structures. There are certain subtypes of NSCLC that may not be particularly FDG avid, such as bronchoalveolar cancer as well as carcinoid tumor. Although small cell lung cancer (like many aggressive cancer types) is FDG avid, PET imaging is not used in patients with small cell lung cancer because the disease tends to be advanced at the time of diagnosis. Therefore, therapy choices are usually limited, and curative treatment such as surgery is generally not an option.

Lymphoma

FDG PET imaging is used for both Hodgkin lymphoma and non-Hodgkin lymphoma (NHL). All grades and cell types may take up FDG with a substantial overlap of level of FDG uptake (therefore, PET imaging cannot replace histological grading). Especially low-grade lymphomas (MALT, marginal zone lymphomas, and small lymphocytic lymphomas) maybe less FDG avid. Nevertheless, PET maybe useful in individual patients with low-grade lymphoma suspected to have transformation to a more aggressive type to detect transformation and guide biopsy. For Hodgkin lymphoma and NHL, FDG PET is used for initial staging, monitoring response to therapy, detecting relapse and restaging. As far as initial staging is concerned, PET detects more lesions than CT (i.e., disease in lymph nodes that are not enlarged by CT). It changes staging and/or impacts patient management in 8% to 48% of patients in Hodgkin lymphoma and NHL. Overall hybrid PET/CT is more accurate than PET alone (accuracy of 84% and 94%, respectively). Splenic involvement may present as diffusely increased uptake or focal FDG-avid lesions. As far as the evaluation of bone marrow (BM) infiltration is concerned, FDG PET is complementary to bone marrow biopsy. Bone marrow biopsy and PET are concordant in 80% of cases. FDG-avid bone marrow lesions may need to be assessed by directed biopsy, while routine bone marrow biopsy is still necessary even if there are no FDG-avid lesions detected on PET imaging (since it maybe false negative). It has been shown that FDG detected BM disease that would have been missed by routine biopsy in 8% of patients, while 5% of patients had a positive bone marrow biopsy without abnormal FDG uptake (this may happen in lower-grade and non–FDG-avid lymphomas, or relatively less bone marrow involvement). Assessing response to therapy is more accurate with PET compared to CT mostly because of higher specificity (PET 86%, CT 31%) and better PPV (PET 100%, CT 42%). One of the strengths of PET is that it more correctly characterizes residual masses or enlarged lymph nodes as inactive disease if they are not FDG avid following treatment. FDG PET information has now been incorporated in *Revised Response Criteria For Malignant Lymphoma*, for example, defining a complete response as PET negative (of note, there are recommendations on how to standardize imaging techniques/interpretation and what exactly constitutes a "negative" PET). PET imaging also provides prognostic information: patients who have residual FDG-avid disease after therapy have a worse outcome in terms of overall survival than patients who have no detectable disease. Following therapy, an interval of 2 to 3 weeks (for chemotherapy) and 8 to 12 weeks (for radiation therapy) is recommended before obtaining a PET scan to avoid false-negative ("stunning" of viable cancer cells) and false-positive (from inflammatory response) results. The use of "midtherapy" (after several cycles of chemotherapy) PET scanning has been evaluated for Hodgkin lymphoma and NHL. It has been found that it is related to posttherapy scan results as well as event-free survival. In fact, presence (or absence) of FDG-avid disease was a stronger prognostic factor than any clinical parameter. With the information of midtherapy PET scans, therapy can be altered (intensified therapy for PET positive patients versus deescalation [avoiding toxicity] for PET-negative patients) with overall improved event-free survival.

Colorectal Cancer

Colorectal cancer is the third most common malignancy comprising 13% of all cancers. Similarly to lung cancer, the strength of FDG PET imaging is the evaluation of distant metastases, which may not be seen by conventional imaging. FDG PET is mostly used to stage patients with recurrent colorectal cancer. In this setting, it has a sensitivity of 97% and specificity of 76%. Patients with liver metastasis who are considered for curative resection should undergo PET to exclude other metastatic disease (to avoid futile surgery). FDG PET may detect unsuspected disease in 27% of patients (leading to changes in therapy in 37%), mostly avoiding surgery in patients who would not benefit from it. Another indication for PET is the evaluation of patients with elevated CEA levels and negative conventional imaging. In addition, FDG PET may also help differentiate between local recurrence (in the colon) and postsurgical scarring. False-negative studies maybe seen in patients with predominantly mucinous tumors. While FDG PET has no role in the screening/primary diagnosis of colorectal cancer, incidentally detected colorectal cancer during whole-body FDG imaging has been reported. Even though FDG uptake in the GI tract is very variable, focal intense uptake which can be seen in approximately 3% of patients requires further workup (e.g., colonoscopy) since there is a high likelihood of precancerous or cancerous lesions.

Breast Cancer

FDG PET should be added to conventional imaging to evaluate breast cancer patients with a clinical suspicion of metastatic disease or those with disease recurrence. FDG PET has currently no role for breast cancer screening and initial diagnosis of breast cancer or evaluation of breast masses; in fact there appears to be a high risk of false-negative results, for example missing early stage (small) lesions. Mammography and MRI (and US) are more accurate for these indications. In addition, FDG PET is usually not beneficial in assessing axillary lymph node involvement, and it cannot replace sentinel lymph node biopsy.

Head and Neck Cancer

Although overall a fairly rare malignancy, head and neck cancer is increasing in frequency, possibly related to its association with human papilloma virus. It is also linked to tobacco and alcohol use. FDG PET certainly has limitations in the evaluation of primary head and neck tumor (compared to contrast-enhanced CT or MRI), especially in defining the exact extent of the primary tumor and invasion of adjacent structures. Nevertheless, FDG PET is helpful in detecting nodal and distant metastasis and should be added to conventional imaging for staging head and neck cancer as well as for patients suspected to have recurrent disease. Even though the postsurgical neck is more difficult to evaluate given asymmetry of physiologic structures (muscles or salivary glands) and nonspecific inflammatory FDG uptake, PET appears more accurate than CT in this setting to assess for recurrent disease. FDG PET may also be useful in the detection of clinically suspected unknown head and neck primary tumors if conventional workup is negative. In this setting, if FDG-avid lesions are identified, directed biopsy should be performed, and if FDG PET is negative, further workup is required (e.g., biopsy of at risk sites or tonsillectomy).

Esophageal Cancer

FDG PET is very beneficial in staging of esophageal cancer because of its usefulness in detecting metastasis (M stage). Its accuracy for nodal disease (N stage) is only modest: the detection of local lymph node metastasis depends not only on the intensity of FDG uptake in the primary lesion and the involved lymph node but also the proximity of the lymph node to the primary lesion (intense FDG uptake in primary tumor may obscure the uptake in paraesophageal nodes). Overall accuracy for nodal staging with PET is 48% to 86%, while for CT/EUS it is 69% to 90%. FDG PET also lacks accuracy in evaluating the T stage with potential-false positive (secondary to FDG uptake in inflammatory lesions in the lower esophagus) as well as false-negative cases (small tumors, T1 stage). Endoscopy with EUS and/or contrast-enhanced CT is preferred for T and N staging. On the other hand, accuracy for detecting metastatic disease with FDG PET is 82% to 86%, while for CT it is 62% to 73%. PET is also used to assess response to therapy and to evaluate patients suspected (or known) to have recurrent disease.

Malignant Melanoma

Although FDG PET does not have a role in screening and diagnosis of melanoma and does not replace sentinel lymph node biopsy, it has a role in evaluating for metastatic disease. FDG PET has a sensitivity of approximately 96% and specificity of 87% for the detection of metastatic disease. Therefore, FDG PET should be considered in staging patients with "high-risk" melanoma (Breslow skin depth more than 1.5 mm, or metastatic disease at time of diagnosis), as well as for restaging at time of recurrence (especially with local recurrence if further surgery is considered an option). There are currently conflicting data on the routine use in patients with a positive sentinel lymph node biopsy. There are also emerging data on the usefulness of FDG PET in patients with elevation of S 100B markers. It should also be noted that MRI may perform better than PET in assessing metastatic lesions in the brain, liver, or bone marrow, and that small pulmonary lesions could possibly be more accurately detected by CT.

Thyroid Cancer

For the most part FDG PET is not useful for the diagnosis, follow-up, or surveillance of patients with differentiated thyroid carcinoma. FDG PET is currently recommended for patients with differentiated thyroid cancer (papillary or follicular cancer), after thyroidectomy and radioiodine ablation in the setting of detectable thyroglobulin levels (greater than 10 ng/mL), and a negative whole-body (posttreatment) radioiodine scan (with the goal of identifying patients who may benefit from specific treatment such as surgical excision or external beam radiation of FDG-avid disease). In this clinical setting, sensitivities of 45% to 100% and specificities of 90% to 100% for the diagnosis of recurrence were reported. FDG PET also reflects prognostic information: patients with FDG-avid disease have a worse prognosis compared to patients with negative FDG PET scans. Patients with Hürthle cell carcinomas (a rare, histologically distinct variant of follicular thyroid cancer) and patients with medullary thyroid cancer (a neuroendocrine malignancy that originates from parafollicular C cells of the thyroid gland) may benefit from FDG PET imaging in certain circumstances. Please see Chap. 97 for thyroid imaging.

Incidental Thyroid Uptake of FDG

Although FDG PET has no role in the detection/initial diagnosis of thyroid cancer or in the workup of thyroid nodules, focal FDG uptake in the thyroid gland is sometimes found incidentally (incidence of 1%–4%). If focal FDG uptake is detected in the thyroid gland, further evaluation (thyroid ultrasound with FNA or biopsy) is usually required, since there is a high likelihood of malignancy (up to 50% or more). Diffuse FDG uptake within the thyroid gland is seen in approximately 3% of patients undergoing FDG PET imaging. This phenomenon is most often benign and related to autoimmune (Hashimoto) thyroiditis or existing (or developing) hypothyroidism.

Brain Tumors

FDG PET has been helpful in differentiating between radiation necrosis (no FDG uptake) and persistent brain tumor (uptake), especially if other imaging is equivocal. FDG uptake has also been found to be related to the histological grade in certain tumors, providing noninvasive tumor grading and prognostic information. FDG PET may also facilitate guiding biopsy of brain tumors/ intracranial lesions. Because of the high physiologic FDG uptake in the brain, PET is relatively insensitive for the detection of intracranial metastasis, as metastasis maybe hyper- or hypo- or isometabolic. Amino acid PET tracers are more sensitive than 18F-FDG in imaging recurrent brain tumors, particularly low-grade tumors, in addition to differentiating between recurrent tumor and treatment-related changes.

Unknown Primary Tumor

If the anatomic origin of a biopsy-proven malignancy remains unidentified after diagnostic evaluation, it is called an unknown primary tumor. This may account for 2% to 7% of all malignancies. Approximately 25% of primary tumors are eventually localized by conventional imaging/workup. PET/CT maybe beneficial in the detection of occult primary lesions.

Other Tumors

Data about the use of FDG PET in many other cancers are evolving and various malignancies (pancreatic, cholangiocarcinoma, ovarian, endometrial cancer) maybe (and are) imaged using this technique. On some cancer types, data are insufficient at this point to make any specific recommendations about the use of FDG PET, such as sarcomas. Where PET is not universally advantageous are usually slow growing or well-differentiated tumors, such as differentiated thyroid cancer, neuroendocrine tumor, and prostate cancer. Other tumors are not FDG avid because of histologic characteristics (e.g., mucinous or clear cell tumors). Hepatocellular carcinoma (HCC) has varying degree of glucose-6-phosphatase and does not reliably retain FDG intracellularly (up to 59% of HCC are not FDG avid). Transitional cell cancer of the GU tract is potentially very FDG avid; nevertheless because of its location in the GU tract and the normal excretion of FDG in urine, imaging with PET is generally not useful (Table 98-1).

Bone Metastases

Since FDG PET is useful for the detection of distant metastatic disease in many cancer types, the question whether bone scintigraphy remains necessary for the evaluation of osseous metastatic disease arises. This question is not an easy one to answer. Certainly for malignancies where disease may be primarily located in the bone marrow space (lymphoma or multiple myeloma), FDG PET is more accurate than bone scintigraphy. For NSCLC, there appears to be enough evidence to support that bone scintigraphy is not necessary if a patient already undergoes PET imaging. For other cancers, for example breast cancer, FDG PET and bone scintigraphy are still complementary. Overall FDG PET/CT has a PPV for osseous metastatic disease of 61% to 98% (depending if lesions are concordant or discordant between the FDG and CT portion). Similar to bone scintigraphy, FDG PET has a lower PPV for solitary bone lesions, and further workup (MRI, biopsy) maybe necessary. Another PET tracer used to assess osseous metastatic disease is F-18 sodium fluoride. It has been found to have increased accuracy and efficiency (imaging 15–30 minutes after injection, duration 15–30 minutes) with a similar dosimetry compared to 99mTC-MDP. This tracer maybe more widely used in the future.

INDIUM-111 OCTREOSCAN

In-111 pentetreotide (Octreoscan) is the most commonly used agent for somatostatin receptor imaging. It can be useful in imaging patients with neuroendocrine tumors, such as carcinoids (80%–100% detection rate), gastrinomas, insulinomas, neuroblastomas, pheochromocytoma, paraganglioma, Merkel cell tumors, lymphomas, certain CNS neoplasms, small cell lung cancer, and medullary thyroid carcinoma. In-111 is chelated to octreotide, a somatostatin analogue using DTPA to form In-111 pentetreotide (Octreoscan). There are five somatostatin receptor subtypes (all of which bind somatostatin), but only subtypes 2 and 5 bind with pentetreotide. Pentetreotide has been shown to bind to somatostatin receptors on both tumor and nontumor sites throughout the body. Because 80% of enteropancreatic neuroendocrine tumors express subtype 2 receptors, a majority of these tumors are Octreoscan positive. The usual adult dose of In-111 pentetreotide is approximately 6 mCi. Normal uptake of In-111 pentetreotide occurs in the thyroid gland, liver, gallbladder, spleen, kidneys, urinary bladder, and the GI tract. SPECT is very useful in cases where the tumor is in the abdomen. Imaging is done usually at 4 and 24 hours. Early 4-hour images have the advantage of less or absent bowel activity; 48-hour images maybe done to clarify if abdominal activity is of GI origin. Uptake of octreotide is thought to be decreased with concurrent therapeutic somatostatin use, and may need to be discontinued prior to the scan.

METAIODOBENZYLGUANIDINE IMAGING

Metaiodobenzylguanidine (MIBG) is taken up by adrenergic tissue, as it is an analog of noradrenalin and guanethidine, and therefore the MIBG scan is considered as the first-choice imaging procedure in the evaluation of neuroendocrine tumors like pheochromocytoma, paraganglioma, and neuroblastoma. MIBG can be labeled with either I-131 or I-123. I-123 MIBG is preferable because it has a more favorable dosimetry and provides better image quality, while I-131 MIBG is cheaper, more easily available and has a longer half-life, therefore delayed images can be obtained, if needed. Certain medications interfere with the uptake and/or vesicular storage of I-MIBG, and include tricyclic antidepressants, sympathomimetic drugs (e.g., decongestants), antihypertensives including Labetalol, possibly calcium channel blockers and ACE inhibitors and certain antipsychotics. These drugs should be discontinued after consulting the referring physician for an adequate time prior to imaging. The thyroid gland needs to be blocked with Lugol iodine or perchlorate to prevent inadvertent radiation to the thyroid gland from bound and unbound I-131 or I-123. The usual dose given is 500 μCi of I-131 or 3 to 10 mCi I-123 labeled MIBG. Whole-body and spot images are obtained over 24 to 72 hours. SPECT images can be obtained if indicated. Normal biodistribution of MIBG includes the liver, spleen, urinary bladder, colon, salivary glands, heart, lung, and the thyroid gland. The adrenal glands maybe faintly visualized normally, more frequently with I-123 MIBG than with I-131 MIBG. Pheochromocytoma is seen as a focal area of MIBG accumulation in the adrenal gland or elsewhere. MIBG detects most of the adrenal and extraadrenal pheochromocytoma with an overall sensitivity of 80% to 90% and a specificity of 90% to 100%. Pheochromocytomas are known by the rule of "ten," 10% are malignant (tend to be larger lesions), bilateral, occur in pediatric patients, and are extraadrenal. The overall sensitivity and specificity of MIBG in the detection of neuroblastoma is approximately 90% and 94%, and MIBG is superior to MDP bone scan for detecting the presence of skeletal metastases in this condition, yet both studies maybe complementary.

GALLIUM-67 IMAGING

Gallium-67 had been used for many years in oncology imaging; however with improved technology in CT, MRI, and PET, uses of gallium in oncology have dramatically been curtailed. It has a half-life of 78.1 hours after intravenous injection gets bound to plasma proteins primarily transferrin. Its uptake in tumor tissue is thought to be related to presence of transferrin receptors on the tumor cells, which bind the Ga-67-transferrin complex. Normal biodistribution includes the nasopharynx, salivary glands, lacrimal glands, bone marrow, breast tissue, liver, spleen, bowel, and thymus. Kidneys and bladder may be seen in the initial 24 hours. Usual dose is 10 mCi for oncology imaging. Whole-body and spot images are usually obtained at 48 hours; additional images can be obtained in 24-hour intervals. SPECT imaging increases the sensitivity of lesion detection. Prior to the advent of PET, gallium-67 was widely used in the evaluation and follow-up of lymphoma.

RADIOIMMUNOTHERAPY

Radioimmunotherapy involves the use of monoclonal antibodies directed against specific tumor antigens labeled with a beta-particle emitting–radioisotope to deliver radiation directly to the tumor. The CD20 antigen on B lymphocytes is the target for the currently used radioimmunotherapies: yttrium-90, ibritumomab tiuxetan (Zevalin), and I-131 tositumomab (Bexxar) in refractory NHL.

Prerequisites to Therapy

The prerequisites to therapy include a platelet count more than 100 000, neutrophil count more than 1500 cells/cm^2, bone marrow involvement on biopsy less than 25%, no prior history of hypersensitivity reactions to murine antibodies, and satisfactory pretherapy biodistribution. Patients with prior myelotoxic therapies associated with autologous bone marrow transplantation or peripheral stem cell rescue and those with a history of prior external-beam radiation to more than 25% of the active marrow should be excluded at this time.

ZEVALIN (YTTRIUM-90 IBRITUMOMAB TIUXETAN)

Ibritumomab is an IgG1 kappa-monoclonal antibody directed against the CD20 antigen found on normal mature B lymphocytes and on more than 90% of malignant B lymphocytes in patients with B-cell NHL. The CD20 antigen is an ideal target for immunotherapy because it is absent from hematopoietic stem cells. Zevalin is a radiolabeled antibody therapy approved for treatment of relapsed or refractory, or CD20$^+$ transformed NHL. It has an overall response rate between 67% and 83%, with 15% to 37% of patients achieving complete remission. Zevalin consists of a murine monoclonal antibody attached to a metal chelator (Y-90). Y-90 is a pure beta-emitter that has a half-life of 64 hours. Unlike with I-131 Bexxar, no imaging can be performed as Y-90 has no gamma emission. The treatment is given on an outpatient basis, as the radiation exposure risk to family members is minimal. Unbound agent accumulates in bone so a stable antibody attachment is very important to limit bone marrow toxicity. Materials with a low atomic number, such as plastic or acrylics, are used for shielding so that the emitted beta particles will be completely absorbed in approximately 1 cm of these materials.

Protocol

A dose of unlabeled rituximab is used to block CD20-binding sites on B cells in the circulation and in the spleen thereby optimizing biodistribution of the radiolabeled agent. In-111 ibritumomab tiuxetan (5 mCi) is given IV to obtain a diagnostic scan for assessment of biodistribution. A whole-body scan is obtained between 48 and 72 hours following tracer administration, with subsequent optional scanning as needed. The normal biodistribution on the initial scan is good uptake in the blood pool, moderately high to high uptake in the normal liver and spleen, and moderately low to low uptake in the lungs, kidneys, and urinary bladder. Altered biodistribution is suggested when blood-pool activity is not visualized and when lung uptake exceeds liver activity, renal activity exceeds liver activity on posterior images, and greater uptake in the bowel than the liver. When altered biodistribution is suspected, whole-body images should be obtained at 90 to 120 hours to exclude delayed clearance or other abnormalities. Patients with altered biodistribution should not be treated with ^{90}Y-ibritumomab tiuxetan. If the biodistribution appears normal, then patients can be treated with ^{90}Y-ibritumomab tiuxetan. Dosing is calculated by patient body weight and baseline platelet count. The dose is 0.4 mCi/kg in patients with platelet counts greater than 150K, and 0.3 mCi/kg if the platelet count is between 100K and 150K. The maximum dose given is 32 mCi.

Toxicity

The primary adverse event is hematologic toxicity. The blood count nadir is usually between 7 to 9 weeks and counts normalize by 9 months posttreatment. Up to one-third of patients may later transform to an aggressive lymphoma. It is unclear if this represents therapy toxicity or the natural progression of the disease. Myelodysplasia or acute myelogenous leukemia has also been reported in a small minority (1.4%) of treated patients.

I-131 BEXXAR (I-131 TOSITUMOMAB)

Tositumomab is a murine monoclonal antibody that binds to the CD20 antigen expressed on the surface of malignant B lymphocytes. It is used in the treatment of rituximab refractory CD20$^+$ follicular NHL. Unlike Zevalin, the I-131 gamma emission is useful to evaluate the biodistribution of the agent and to calculate the treatment dose. Pretreatment with SSKI or Lugol's iodine is required to block thyroid uptake of I-131 that maybe released from the antibody. The patient is first treated with unlabeled tositumomab to block the excess CD20 sites and prevent unnecessary uptake in the reticuloendothelial system. Thereafter, a low dosimetry dose of I-131 tositumomab (5 mCi) is given; serial scans are obtained to calculate how fast the activity clears from the body. This along with platelet counts helps with calculating the therapy dose, which is given after repeat pretreatment of unlabeled tositumomab. The most common toxicity is hematologic; blood count nadir is reached between 3 to 7 weeks after therapy. Myelodysplasia can occur as can hypothyroidism from free I-131 effects on the thyroid gland. Approximately 63% of patients refractory to rituximab have some response to I-131 Bexxar and 29% have complete response.

Sentinel Node Detection

A sentinel node according to Morton's definition is a lymph node that receives afferent lymphatic drainage directly from a primary tumor. The purpose of lymphoscintigraphy in sentinel node detection is therefore to demonstrate the drainage pathway of the neoplasm. It is currently widely used in the evaluation of melanoma and breast cancer. Other indications of reported use include penile, vulvar, testicular, oral, urinary bladder, laryngeal cancers, and GI malignancies. Tc-99m sulfur colloid particles are most commonly used in North America for lymphoscintigraphy. The visualization of the sentinel node depends on the transport of the sulfur colloid particles from the injection site to the lymphatics, which drain into the sentinel node. In the node, these particles are trapped and phagocytosed by macrophages. The optimal particle size is between 10 and 50 nm. If the particles are too small, they enter the systemic circulation, and if they are too large, they are unable to enter the lymphatics.

Melanoma

The incidence of melanoma metastasis depends on the skin depth of tumor involvement. Node dissection is not usually required or does not make much sense for tumors less than 1 mm deep or more than 4 mm deep. Less than 1-mm deep tumors are seldom associated with lymphatic metastases, while 4 mm or deeper lesions are usually associated with distant metastases. In those with tumor depth between 1 and 4 mm, there is a high incidence of occult lymph nodal metastasis and a possible survival benefit associated with nodal dissection, therefore sentinel node detection is done. An intradermal injection of tracer is made at four or more sites surrounding the melanoma or the excisional biopsy scar; dynamic imaging and static images are acquired to identify the sentinel node followed by its localization and skin marking. The lymphatic drainage is usually predictable in the extremities, axillary, and inguinal in case of the upper and lower extremities. Popliteal nodes can be seen with melanoma on the calf, heel, or the lateral foot, while epitrochlear nodes are occasionally seen draining lesions on the forearm or hand. The drainage patterns are very unpredictable in case of the head and neck and trunk, where the drainage patterns may be bilateral, and in cases involving the trunk, drainage to the axilla, neck, or groin can be seen. An intraoperative gamma probe detector is frequently used to accurately localize the sentinel node at the time of surgery.

Breast Cancer

In addition to the size and grade of the primary breast tumor, the status of the axillary lymph node is an important factor for accurate staging and determines the need for adjuvant therapy. Clinical examination has a poor predictive value for the determination of axillary nodal involvement, and therefore histological examination of the lymph nodes is required for identification of metastatic disease. The axillary sentinel node can be accurately identified in 90% to 100% of patients with use of an intraoperative gamma probe and blue dye. Most of the breast lymphatic system drains to the axillary lymph nodes. Approximately 3% drains to the internal mammary chain nodes (usually from the medial portion of the breast), and a very small percentage drains to the posterior intercostal nodes. The standard surgical treatment in the past for breast cancer used to be radical mastectomy and axillary nodal dissection. The latter comes with a significant morbidity including pain, swelling, restricted range of motion, and paresthesias; also a majority of patients have no axillary metastasis and therefore have no benefit of this invasive surgical procedure. Sentinel node biopsy in the axilla involves removal of the sentinel node and other suspicious nodes. It is associated with less morbidity, shorter length of stay, and improved staging when compared with axillary nodal dissection. Tracer injection with Tc-99m sulfur colloid on the day of or even the day before could be superficial or deep. Superficial injections include intradermal, subcutaneous, periareolar, or subareolar. Deep injection techniques involve peritumoral (most common) and intratumoral approaches. Massaging the injection site facilitates migration of the sulfur colloid particles and aids in detection of the sentinel node. Prior to surgical biopsy, blue dye is also commonly injected around the margins of the tumor to aid in intra-operative detection of sentinel node.

Suggested Reading

Delbeke D, Coleman RE, Guiberteau MJ, et al. Procedure guideline for tumor imaging with 18F-FDG PET/CT 1.0. *J Nucl Med*. 2006;47(5):885-895.

Fletcher JW, Djulbegovic B, Soares HP, et al. Recommendations on the use of 18F-FDG PET in oncology. *J Nucl Med*. 2008;49(3):480-508.

Koopmans KP et al. ^{111}In-octreotide is superior to 123I-metaiodobenzylguanidine for scintigraphic detection of head and neck paragangliomas. *J Nucl Med*. 2008;49:1232-1237.

Lymphoscintigraphy in cutaneous melanoma: a total body atlas of sentinel node mapping. *Radiographics*. 2002;22:491-502.

Matthies A et al. Dual time point ^{18}F-FDG PET for the evaluation of pulmonary nodules. *J Nucl Med*. 2002;43:871-875.

Wahl RL, ed. *Principles and Practice of Positron Emission Tomography*. Philadelphia, PA: Lippincott Williams and Wilkins; 2002.

QUESTIONS AND ANSWERS

1. A 65-year-old male with history of refractory non-Hodkin lymphoma involving the mediastinal and

retroperitoneal nodal regions is referred for (Zevalin) Y-90 Ibritumomab therapy. Which of the following is a prerequisite to proceed with therapy?

A. Platelet count more than 100 000/μL
B. Renal activity greater than that of liver on the pretherapy indium scan
C. 10% bone marrow involvement with lymphoma
D. Uptake of Indium-111 ibritumomab in the mediastinal and retroperitoneal adenopathy

ANSWER: A. Zevalin is indicated in the treatment of refractory NHL. It is contraindicated if lymphoma involves greater than 25% of the bone marrow, if platelet count is less than 100 000, and if absolute neutrophil count is less than 1500 cells/cm^2. Prior to therapy with Y-90 Zevalin, a whole-body scan is obtained with In-111 ibritumomab to check for presence of altered biodistribution, which includes increasing activity in the lung, liver, heart, kidneys, and bowel. Although uptake of the tracer in involved lymph nodes can be seen occasionally, it is *not* a prerequisite.

2. Which of the following radiopharmaceuticals may be useful for localizing a pheochromocytoma?

A. I-131 meta-iodo-benzyl-guanidine
B. Gallium-67 citrate
C. I-131 tositumomab
D. Tc-99m mercaptoacetyl triglycine (MAG-3)

ANSWER: A. Neuroendocrine tumors including adrenal (pheochromocytomas) and extraadrenal paragangliomas arise from specific cells that originate from the embryonic neural crest. Most pheochromocytomas produce both epinephrine and norepinephrine, and clinically present with hypertension, headache, diaphoresis, tachycardia, and anxiety. Pheochromocytomas may occur as part of MEN-2A or 2B syndromes and are also seen with von Hippel-Lindau syndrome and neurofibromatosis. I-131 MIBG and In-111 pentetreotide are useful in imaging these tumors, though I-131 MIBG is the most common radiopharmaceutical used for adrenomedullary scintigraphy and detects most of the adrenal and extra adrenal pheochromocytomas. It is the preferred agent used for imaging adrenal pheochromocytomas, although there are some data to suggest that In-111 pentetreotide is more sensitive in detecting head and neck paragangliomas.

3. In cases of lymphoma, what is the implication of mild metabolic activity in the thymus gland on FDG PET-CT imaging?

A. Before treatment indicates a poor prognosis
B. Before and after treatment maybe a normal finding
C. After treatment indicates disease progression
D. Prior to treatment indicates involvement with lymphoma

ANSWER: B. Low-level thymic activity is commonly seen in young patients. Normal thymic activity is triangular or 'V' in configuration. Thymic hyperplasia or rebound represents an immunologic phenomenon seen following chemotherapy, especially in young patients. It is seen in up to 75% of children and in 5% to 16% of adults. Thymic activity is abnormal when the uptake is very focal, intense (some sources have suggested maximum SUV > 4) or when the typical triangular or V configuration is distorted.

4. A 45-year-old male has been recently diagnosed with a right lung mass, and bronchial carcinoid is suspected. Which of the following radiotracers should be employed for definitive diagnosis?

A. In-111 pentetreotide (Octreoscan)
B. F-18 FDG
C. Ga-67 citrate
D. Tc-99m sestamibi

ANSWER: A. Neuroendocrine tumors are derived from the cells of the embryonal neural crest. They have the ability to synthesize peptide hormones and neurotransmitters. Examples of these tumors include pituitary adenomas; medullary cancer of the thyroid gland; small cell lung cancer; pheochromocytomas (adrenal and extraadrenal); neuroblastomas; enteropancreatic tumors like gastrinomas, insulinomas, and carcinoid tumors. A variety of radiotracers are available to image these tumors. In-111 pentetreotide is widely used for somatostatin receptor imaging to evaluate several neuroendocrine tumors including carcinoid.

5. Which of the following statements regarding I-131 MIBG scanning in patients with suspected pheochromocytomas is *true*?

A. Usual dose of I-131 MIBG is 12 mCi.
B. Thyroid uptake of I-131 is blocked by Lugol iodine, which also reduces tumor uptake of I-131 MIBG.
C. Propranolol reduces tumor uptake of I-131 MIBG.
D. Over-the-counter decongestants (sympathomimetics) decrease tumor uptake of I-131 MIBG.

ANSWER: D. Sympathomimetics including over-the-counter decongestants like phenylpropanolamine, pseudoephedrine, and phenylephrine deplete the storage vesicles in the adrenergic tissues and therefore interfere with the uptake of MIBG and need to be discontinued prior to the MIBG scan. Additionally blood pressure medications like calcium channel blockers and labetalol also interfere with MIBG uptake and need to be discontinued prior to the examination. Lugol's iodine is given to saturate the thyroid gland with iodine and prevent uptake of I-131 by the thyroid gland. It however has no effect in the tumor uptake of MIBG. The usual dose of I-131 MIBG is 0.5 mCi.

6. A 56-year-old smoker is referred for a whole-body PET-CT scan for evaluation of a 1.5 cm left upper lobe SPN. Hypermetabolic activity (maximum SUV 3) is seen in the lung nodule at 60 minutes after 18-FDG injection, which increases to maximum SUV of 4.5 at repeat imaging performed 2 hours after tracer injection. Which of the following statements is accurate?
   A. Baseline SUV less than 1.0 is concerning for malignancy.
   B. Increasing SPN FDG activity is suggestive of an underlying malignancy.
   C. Increasing interval SUV is due to patient eating a snack in between the two images.
   D. Respiratory motion does not affect the standard uptake value.

   ANSWER: B. Improved detection of malignant lesions has been reported by performing "dual time point imaging." This technique is based on the observation that more commonly, tracer activity will washout of inflammatory or benign lesions, while malignant lesions retain or increase in FDG activity over time (although some inflammatory lesions occasionally also show increase over time). Lesions with a baseline SUV of less than 1 have a very high likelihood of being benign, and dual time point imaging is not required as it may result in false-positive examinations. Respiratory motion may produce lesion blurring and an apparent increase in lesion size. This results in a decrease in the activity concentration per pixel within the lesion and an underestimation of SUV.

7. All the following lung tumors may be falsely negative in an 18-FDG PET-CT scan with the exception of the following:
   A. Carcinoid
   B. Bronchoalveolar cell
   C. Adenocarcinoma
   D. Mucinous

   ANSWER: C. FDG PET scanning is not 100% sensitive in detection of tumors. Noteworthy exceptions include bronchoalveolar cell lung carcinoma (BAC), which may have a lower FDG uptake value and can result in a false-negative FDG PET-CT. Other pulmonary neoplasms that frequently have no significant uptake increased FDG include carcinoid and mucinous tumors. Carcinoid tumors are usually slow growing and well differentiated, therefore have low FDG retention while BAC and mucinous tumors have a low proportion of tumor cells within the matrix of fibrosis and mucin, resulting in decreased FDG retention. Lung cancer with the above exceptions is usually FDG avid.

8. A 60-year-old male with past history of colorectal cancer, postcurative resection 3 years ago, is noted to have gradually increasing CEA levels. 18-FDG PET-CT scan is done to evaluate for suspected recurrent disease. Which of the following is the most likely site for tumor recurrence?
   A. Within the abdomen/pelvis including the liver
   B. Lungs
   C. Skeletal system
   D. Brain

   ANSWER: A. Recurrent colorectal carcinoma occurs in 37% to 44% of patients within 2 years of curative resection. Local tumor extent and the presence or absence of adenopathy are important variables for determining prognosis and the risk for tumor recurrence. Serum levels of carcinoembryonic antigen (CEA) are frequently used as a tumor marker to monitor for the presence of recurrent tumor. However, the CEA test cannot localize the site of recurrent disease. Locoregional recurrence is more commonly encountered with rectal carcinoma, while colon carcinoma recurrence is more commonly seen in the liver or abdomen. FDG PET is also useful in distinguishing local tumor recurrence from postoperative scar.

9. Which of the following is the histological hallmark of Hodgkin lymphoma?
   A. Reed-Sternberg cell
   B. Schistocytes
   C. Smudge cells
   D. Plasmacytoma

   ANSWER: A. The characteristic histological finding in Hodgkin lymphoma, a B-cell neoplasm, is the Reed-Sternberg cell. These are large cells with a characteristic clear area surrounding the nucleoli, giving an "owl-eye" appearance to the nuclei, seen in the lymph node surrounded by a dense inflammatory infiltrate. Patients usually present in their third or seventh decades with palpable adenopathy and constitutional symptoms (B symptoms) of fever, night sweats, pruritus, and weight loss. There are four subtypes of Hodgkin disease: nodular sclerosis (most common form), mixed cellularity, lymphocyte predominant (favorable prognosis), and lymphocyte depleted (worst prognosis). PET-CT is useful in staging, restaging, and monitoring of response to therapy in lymphoma and also in directing site of diagnostic biopsy. It has replaced gallium-67 in the evaluation and follow-up of patients with lymphoma, because of its higher sensitivity and specificity, resolution, and favorable scan times (takes several days for completion of the gallium scan). Plasmacytomas are tumors containing plasma cells such as multiple myeloma. Smudge cells are histologically seen in chronic lymphocytic leukemia, while schistocytes are noted in hemolytic conditions like DIC and TTP.

10. Which of the following is a contraindication to the surgical treatment of NSCLC?
    A. Ipsilateral hilar adenopathy
    B. Tumor which is larger than 2 cm from the carina, without carinal invasion
    C. Ipsilateral peribronchial adenopathy
    D. Ipsilateral supraclavicular adenopathy

    ANSWER: D. Surgical resection is the treatment of choice of early stages of NSCLC and therefore accurate staging is crucial. The decision about resectability of NSCLC is based among other variables on which lymph nodes are involved with the tumor. In general, ipsilateral adenopathy (N2 disease) is an acceptable indication for surgical resection of tumor, while contralateral involvement (N3 disease) or metastatic cervical and supraclavicular adenopathy are contraindications to surgical treatment.

99 LABORATORY NUCLEAR MEDICINE AND MOLECULAR IMAGING

Jon A. Baldwin

INTRODUCTION

This chapter first reviews two nonimaging studies performed in nuclear medicine laboratories—measurement of thyroid uptake and the Schilling's test. (Laboratory measurements of ERPF and GFR are discussed in Chap. 85.) A brief outline and review of the concepts of molecular imaging follow. The end of the chapter contains summary charts and tables that residents will find to be useful for preparing for written and oral board examinations.

NUCLEAR MEDICINE LABORATORY STUDIES

THYROID UPTAKE

Measurement of radioactive iodine uptake is a useful test to help differentiate nonmalignant thyroid diseases, and to determine the amount of ^{131}I that will be used to treat a condition such as Graves disease. In this test, a small amount of either ^{123}I (50–100 μCi) or ^{131}I (5–10 μCi) is administered orally to the patient. If 200 to 400 μCi of ^{123}I is used, imaging of the thyroid gland can also be performed. Recall that because of the dose to the patient and poor imaging characteristics, ^{131}I is not used in routine diagnostic imaging of the thyroid gland. Sodium pertechnetate is generally not used to determine thyroid uptake because of technical challenges and near-universal preference for the radioiodine method. Regardless of which radiotracer is used, the device which most commonly measures the thyroid uptake is the same—a thyroid probe, which operates on the same principle as an NaI well counter. A gamma camera can be used to determine thyroid uptake, as well as perform whole-body dosimetry (i.e., to estimate doses to particular organs), but is not terribly practical in most clinical applications.

Before radioiodine is administered to the patient, several patient preparation factors should be considered. The patient should be NPO for at least 4 hours to promote GI absorption of the radiotracer. More importantly, it should be verified that the patient has been off any medications that can interfere with thyroid uptake for the proper amount of time. The length of time these medications must be discontinued varies with the physiologic duration of their effect on the thyroid gland. In general, these medications will decrease radioiodine uptake. A list of some common medications, and the length of time they should be discontinued before a thyroid uptake study is attempted, is listed in Table 99-1. Once it is established that these patient preparations have been followed, the probe is used to count the background radiation in the room. The radioiodine sample is usually contained within a capsule, but can be in liquid form. Capsule is preferred to avoid aerosolization or loss of the dose, and it can also easily be placed in the neck phantom. The radiotracer is placed in a Lucite neck phantom, and that phantom is counted for 1 to 2 minutes. The probe is placed at a distance of 25 to 30 cm from the surface of the phantom. The dose is administered to the patient, and the patient will have their neck counted at a specified time after administration. The "gold standard"

TABLE 99-1 Drugs Affecting Radioiodine Uptake, and the Amount of Time They Should Be Discontinued Before Radioactive Uptake Study Is Performed

MEDICATION	TIME MEDICATION SHOULD BE DISCONTINUED
Propylthiouracil (PTU)	3–5 d
Methimazole (Tapazole)	5–7 d
Triiodothyronine (Cytomel—T_3)	2–3 wk
Iodinated contrast	2–4 wk
Amiodarone	2–4 wk
Lugol's solution or SSKI	2–4 wk
Thyroxine (Synthroid—T_4)	4–6 wk
Iodine supplements	4–6 wk

is to have the neck counted at 24 hours, but many centers will count their patients at anywhere from 2 to 6 hours. Whenever the patient is counted, room background will be again counted (before the patient is in the room). Counts of the patient will be performed for 1 to 2 minutes with the probe 25 to 30 cm anterior to their neck. Counts of the patient's thigh will also be performed, to correct for the background within the patient (i.e., to "subtract" counts in the neck that are coming from structures other than the thyroid). The formula used to compute radioiodine uptake is counts per minute, or cpm.

$$\frac{\text{Neck counts (cpm)} - \text{thigh counts (cpm)}}{\text{Administered counts (cpm)} - \text{room background counts (cpm)}} \times 100\%$$

The administered counts in the denominator are decay corrected for the amount of time that has elapsed since the neck phantom was counted. In the past, this was accomplished by counting a "standard" of similar activity in the phantom at the time the patient was counted. In most facilities, the radioiodine probe systems have computer software that will make this calculation automatically.

Normal radioiodine uptake values will vary based on the time that is chosen to count the patient. The normal values at 4 hours as reported by the Society of Nuclear Medicine's *Procedure Guideline for Thyroid Uptake Measurement* are 6% to 18%; at 24 hours, the normal values are 10% to 35%. These values will vary from institution to institution. Causes for abnormally high or low radioiodine uptake values are summarized in Table 99-2.

SCHILLING TEST

This nuclear medicine study does not require imaging. The patient is given a radioactive substrate, and a sample is taken from the patient at a set time after its administration and measured. The Schilling test is an effective physiological method of assessing cobalamin (vitamin B_{12}) absorption, although it is not performed very often anymore (Table 99-3). The cobalamins have a cobalt-containing corrin ring, a nucleoside base projecting off one face of the ring, and a beta-group of variable composition attached to the cobalt on the opposite side of the ring. The four varieties of vitamin B_{12} in tissue are the metabolically active forms methylcobalamin and deoxyadenosylcobalamin, and hydroxocobalamin and cyanocobalamin. The last two are converted in vivo into active metabolites. All mammals require vitamin B_{12} in their diet; none can synthesize it in vivo. There are only two reactions in humans known to require vitamin B_{12}. It is required in specific metabolic pathways responsible for deoxyribonucleic acid (DNA) synthesis and for the integrity of myelin. Methylcobalamin is an essential cofactor for the enzyme that produces tetrahydrofolic acid, which is required for the conversion of deoxyuridine monophosphate to deoxythymidine monophosphate. Vitamin B_{12} is involved in the isomerization of methylmalonyl coenzyme A to succinyl coenzyme A. Vitamin

TABLE 99-2 Causes of Increased or Decreased Radioiodine Uptake

INCREASED RADIOIODINE UPTAKE	DECREASED RADIOIODINE UPTAKEE
Hyperthyroidism	Subacute thyroiditis
Graves disease	Drug induced
Multinodular goiter	Increased iodine pool
Solitary hyperfunctioning adenoma (RAIU often normal)	Iodinated contrast
Hashitoxicosis	Lugol's/SSKI
Iodine deficiency	Iodine/mineral supplements
Recovery phase of subacute thyroiditis	Amiodarone
Tumors secreting TSH-like substances (rare)	Interference with thyroid function
Pituitary adenoma	PTU/Tapazole
Hydatidiform mole	Cytomel/Synthroid
Trophoblastic tumors	Hypothyroidism (primary or secondary)
Choriocarcinoma	Ectopic secretion of thyroid hormone (rare)
Metastatic thyroid carcinoma	Struma ovarii

TABLE 99-3 Interpretation of Findings in Schilling Test

FINDING	CAUSE
Part I Shilling test: Urinary excretion ≥6%–9%	Dietary insufficiency
Part I Shilling test: Urinary Excretion <6%–9%	Pernicious anemia Intestinal malabsorption Generalized (e.g., sprue) Specific to terminal ileum (e.g., Crohn disease) Pancreatic insufficiency
Part II Shilling test: Urinary excretion ≥6%–9%	Pernicious anemia
Part II Shilling test: Urinary excretion <6%–9%	Intestinal malabsorption Pancreatic insufficiency

B_{12} deficiency leads to increased levels of methylmalonate, which can lead to formation of abnormal fatty acids; these may be incorporated into neuronal lipids, leading to a predisposition to myelin breakdown. Vitamin B_{12} is plentiful in meat and dairy products, and only minute quantities are sufficient for biological processes (only a few micrograms per day are needed). Body stores are typically 3 to 4 mg. One is unlikely to have a deficiency based on inadequate intake (sometimes seen in strict vegans). Deficiency therefore is usually due to absorption problems, and is typically insidious in onset. Patients with vitamin B_{12} deficiency typically have moderate to severe megaloblastic anemia, leukopenia with hypersegmented granulocytes, mild-to-moderate thrombocytopenia, and neurologic changes related to involvement of the posterolateral spinal tracts. These can present as spastic paraparesis, sensory ataxia, and severe paresthesias in the lower limbs. Initially the vitamin B_{12} is released from its protein-bound form in animal foods by the action of pepsin in the acidic environment of the stomach. The liberated vitamin B_{12} is bound to salivary vitamin B_{12}-binding proteins ("R binders"). These R binders protect the vitamin B_{12} from degradation by stomach acid. The R binder is dissolved by pancreatic proteases in the duodenum. Vitamin B_{12} next binds to intrinsic factor (IF), which is produced by parietal cells in the stomach, forming an IF-vitamin B_{12} complex. This complex is transported to the ileum, where it adheres to IF receptors on the ileal cell membranes. It is then transported in the plasma bound to transcobalamin II. There are several steps along this process in which vitamin B_{12} absorption can be interfered with. The Schilling's test is used to differentiate if vitamin B_{12} deficiency is due to lack of IF (pernicious anemia) or malabsorption. It can be performed as either a two-step procedure (with ^{57}Co-vitamin B_{12}) or a one-step procedure (with ^{57}Co-vitamin B_{12} and ^{58}Co-vitamin B_{12}). In preparation for the Schilling test, the patient should be NPO after midnight, and remain fasting for 2 hours after oral administration of the test dose. This is because the amount of vitamin B_{12} in a meal can significantly affect the fractional absorption of the test dose. The patient should not receive parenteral vitamin B_{12} for at least 3 days before the study. Biliary excretion of that parenteral vitamin B_{12} into the GI tract may also significantly affect the fractional absorption of the test dose. It is also important to be aware if the patient has had other recent radionuclide studies, particularly if these radiotracers are excreted through the kidneys. The patient is administered a 0.5 mCi dose of ^{57}Co-vitamin B_{12} orally. The radiolabeled vitamin B_{12} dose ranges from 0.5 to 2.0 μg—you do not want to saturate the limited IF-mediated mechanism for cobalamin absorption. The patient is given 1 mg intramuscular nonradioactive vitamin B_{12} between 0 and 2 hours. This promotes blocking of vitamin B_{12}-binding sites (i.e., transcobalamin), which will lead to excretion of a large portion of the radioactive vitamin B_{12} into the urine. The patient will collect their urine for 24 hours following administration of the ^{57}Co-vitamin B_{12}. Ideally the urine collection should be at least 1 L. Patients with poor function (Cr ≥2.5) will require longer collection times of 48 or 72 hours. The patient's urine sample, a standard, and a background sample will be counted. If radioactive cobalamin excretion is normal (≥ 6%–9% of administered dose is recovered in urine), there is no evidence of malabsorption, and dietary deficiency is suspected. If excretion is diminished, then the patient should proceed with phase II Schilling test. The procedure for the phase II study is essentially the same, except now IF is given orally with the radioactive vitamin B_{12}. This serves to differentiate IF deficiency from IF-independent causes of malabsorption. If the excretion is still more than 6% to 9%, then IF deficiency is not the cause. If a cause such as pancreatic insufficiency, bacterial overgrowth, tapeworm infection, or if interfering medications are suspected, phase III and phase IV Schilling tests can be performed after oral pancreatic enzymes are added and antibiotic therapy is completed, respectively. Needless to say, this is rarely performed. There are several pitfalls in this test, the most important of which is urine collection. Improper urine collection (e.g., insufficient volume) can falsely lower results. Several sources of error can stem from patient preparation. Another drawback is if the excretion percent is low, then more testing has to be done determine the cause. To help avoid doing a phase II study, a dual isotope Schilling test can be performed. This can be done because the two radioactive cobalts used have different photopeaks (^{57}Co, 122 keV; ^{58}Co, 811 and 511 keV—one must correct for the downscatter from the ^{58}Co into the ^{57}Co window). In this procedure, the patient is given a capsule containing 0.25 μg of 0.8 mCi radiolabeled ^{58}Co-vitamin B_{12} and 0.25 μg of 0.5 mCi ^{57}Co-vitamin B_{12} bound to IF. The patient preparation and collection procedure is the same. If the B_{12}-IF to B_{12} ratio is greater than 1.4, the cause is IF-dependant vitamin B_{12} deficiency. In this study, one is more interested in the IF-bound vitamin B_{12} to free vitamin B_{12} ratio, so urine collection errors are not as important as in phase I Schilling's test. Another benefit of the dual isotope test is it is a shorter test, and generally additional testing is not needed. The drawbacks include greater dose to patient, increased cost, and potentially performing a test with IF that was not needed. Falsely low B_{12} without true B_{12} deficiency can be caused by folate deficiency, myeloma, aplastic anemia, pregnancy, oral contraceptives, and transcobalamin I deficiency. Falsely normal B_{12} with true B_{12} deficiency can be seen with liver disease, chronic myelogenous leukemia, transcobalamin II deficiency, and recent B_{12} injection.

MOLECULAR IMAGING

Molecular imaging is the ability to characterize and quantify biological processes in living organisms at the cellular or even subcellular level. Based on how much molecular imaging is being touted at national meetings and in the literature, one might think that molecular imaging has only been around for a short time. This is not the case, as in the strictest sense molecular imaging has been around as long as nuclear medicine has been in existence. Following the distribution of radioactive $Na^{131}I$, ^{99m}Tc MDP, ^{18}F-FDG, or numerous other radiotracers in physiologic and pathophysiologic processes is molecular imaging that has been around for decades. What has changed in recent times are the scale and the targets of the processes being imaged. As technology has improved, the ability to deliver, image, and resolve smaller molecules has become reality. In addition, the understanding of genetics and molecular biology has aided us in where to target our probes to best image a disease process. This section will review the basic genetic structure and function, as well as the basic design of molecular probes that can target the different processes in the expression of genetic expression.

GENETIC STRUCTURE AND THE CENTRAL DOGMA

It has been more than 50 years since Watson and Crick first determined the molecular structure of DNA, which was known as early as the 1940s to be the primary repository of our genetic information. Four nucleotide bases—adenine, cytosine, guanine, and thymine—are the building blocks of DNA structure. It is these four bases that are arranged in long sequences to form our genetic code. These bases are made up of a phosphate group, a cyclic deoxyribose sugar, and either a purine base (adenine and guanine) or pyrimidine base (cytosine and thymine). The purine and pyrimidine bases are able to form hydrogen bonds with a specific partner: adenine with thymine and cytosine with guanine. Two strands of nucleotides with complementary base pairs are twisted into shape of double helix. This double helical configuration is achieved through base pair interaction and stacking. It is the sequence of these base pairs in particular locations on the DNA strand, called genes, that are expressed to educe the information contained within the DNA into a functional structure to interact with its environment. Genes make up a genotype, or the hereditary constitution of an organism. These genes, when expressed, lead to the phenotypical appearance of an organism, as a result of the interaction of its genotype and its environment. In the eukaryotic cell, the genetic information is contained within the nucleus. The enormous amount of genetic material (more than three billion base pairs) in the human genome is organized into nucleosomes, the basic unit structure chromosomes. DNA strands are wrapped around positively charged proteins called histones (which are attracted to the negatively charged phosphate groups on the DNA molecule) to ultimately form the nucleosomes. These structures are unwound and compacted as needed for the processes of replication and transcription.

DNA replication typically occurs during the S phase of the cell cycle. The DNA strand itself is unwound and separated by the enzyme DNA helicase. DNA replication is said to be semiconservative, which is to say that each of the two strands of DNA is used as a template for the formation of a new complimentary DNA strand. During replication, deoxyribonuclide triphosphates (dATP, dCTP, dGTP, and dTTP) complimentary to the template are added sequentially. The growth occurs only in the 5′ to 3′ direction. DNA polymerases facilitate these reactions. The DNA strand that is read in the 3′ to 5′ direction is called the leading strand, because replication can grow in the complimentary 5′ to 3′ direction without interruption. The original complimentary DNA (in the 5′ to 3′ direction), however, must be read as a short sequence at a time because of its direction. This is the lagging strand, and its replication results in so-called Okazaki fragments, that are later spliced together by DNA polymerase ε. Despite the enormity of the task, there is excellent fidelity in the replication process, with only about 1 error per 10 to 100 billion bases.

The "central dogma" of molecular biology is that DNA is transcribed to RNA, which is then translated to protein. The information contained in the genetic code of DNA will ultimately be expressed as proteins, which contributes to the structure or function of the organism. As one can imagine, control of this process is intricate and complex.

DNA is sequestered in the nucleus of the cell (there is some extranuclear DNA in the cell, located in the mitochondria—its control and function is beyond the scope of this review). Protein synthesis occurs outside the nucleus, in the ribosome. To deliver the genetic message to this protein factory, the cell will make a copy of a portion of its DNA, but make that copy with RNA. In transcription—the message is the same, it is written in a slightly different "language." RNA is similar to structure to DNA, the differences being that ribose is the cyclical sugar (as opposed to deoxyribose in DNA), and that pyrimidine base uracil is used instead of thymine. The process of transcription itself is accomplished by RNA polymerases. RNA polymerase II is the polymerase that will produce the RNA template—messenger RNA, or mRNA—that will ultimately lead to protein production. RNA polymerase II will also produce snRNA, which will aid in the processing of mRNA. RNA polymerase I will transcribe DNA to produce particular subunits of ribosomal RNA (rRNA), while RNA polymerase III will transcribe DNA to produce other rRNA subunits and transfer RNA (tRNA). Transcription begins when the RNA polymerase binds to the promoter site, a specific sequence of DNA bases located upstream of the DNA to be transcribed. After this, the DNA is unwound, and transcription can begin. Only one strand of the DNA is used in the transcription process; it is called the template or antisense strand. The other complimentary DNA strand is called the coding or sense strand. This strand will have the same code as the transcribed mRNA (with the appropriate thymine—uracil substitutions, of course). The RNA polymerase moves in the 3' to 5' direction. In eukaryotic cells, there are a host of other DNA-binding sites, as well as proteins called transcription factors that interact with RNA polymerase and adjacent areas within the chromatin, that contribute to the process of transcription. There are sequences on the DNA upstream of the main promoter that will bind proteins to further promote and enhance transcription. These enhancers will increase the level of transcription. There are also sequences that will reduce the amount of transcription called repressor sequences.

The mRNA that results from the process of transcription is not the mRNA that will leave the nucleus to be translated into protein. Instead, this "pre-mRNA" must first be processed to its final form. First, a cap (in the form of 7-methylguanosine) is placed on the 5' end of the pre-mRNA to make it resistant to degradation. Next, a polyA tail (numerous adenine residues) is added to the end of the transcript. This pre-mRNA as originally transcribed consists of areas that will ultimately used (exons) and ultimately discarded (introns). This splicing will be accomplished by the spliceosome—a complex of numerous proteins and snRNA. Specific nucleotide sequences in the intron key the spliceosome as to where to cut. Splicing must be precise, as the leaving behind or deletion of even one nucleotide can change the protein that would be ultimately produced. Where the splice does occur can change in a tightly regulated process depending on the needs of the cell, enabling many different proteins to be produced from a particular sequence of DNA.

Once transcribed and modified, this mRNA is free to leave the nucleus and travel to the ribosome. It will be translated there into the language of amino acids and proteins. It is interesting to contemplate that the incredible complexity of an organism is in essence the result of precise combinations of just 20 amino acids (and that these are directed by sequential combinations of four bases). The proteins produced either provide cell and organ structure, or will catalyze reactions as enzymes to further the function and form of the organism.

The "interpreters" that translate the mRNA message are the ribosomes. Ribosomes are a combination of proteins and rRNA. There are different subunits that come together to form a complete ribosome: in the eukaryotic cell they are the 60 S and 40 S subunits (where S represents the Svedberg unit, a measure of sedimentation coefficient). The complete ribosome has binding sites for mRNA and for tRNA. There are two binding sites for tRNA in the ribosome, the so-called P (for *p*eptidyl) site and A (for *a*minoacyl) site. These sites are adjacent to each other, allowing the reading of two adjacent codons. The tRNAs are the molecules that carry individual amino acids. There is a specific tRNA for each possible codon (triplets of bases read from the mRNA), except for the three stop codons. There is only one start codon, and this codon codes for the amino acid methionine. Beyond the 4 just mentioned, there are 60 other possible triplet combinations. Recall that there are only 20 amino acids—more than 1 codon can code for a particular amino acid. In this way, the genetic code is said to be "degenerate." The degeneracy is located at the third position in the codon—for example, UGU and UGC both code for the amino acid cysteine. Amino acids are added to their specific tRNA by the enzyme aminoacyl-tRNA synthetase to form aminoacyl-tRNA.

In order for the process of translation to begin, recognition of the start codon by the ribosome, as well as an additional specific sequence near the start codon, must be achieved. Once the mRNA-ribosome-methionine-tRNA complex is formed, additional factors are needed to begin and continue the process of translation. These factors are initiation factors, elongation factors, and termination (or release) factors. Once the initiation complex is formed, and the methionine-tRNA occupies the P site of the ribosome, the tRNA with the complimentary anticodon to the next mRNA codon finds its way to the A site on the ribosome. A combination of elongation factors and enzymes present in the ribosome will form a peptide bond between the two amino acids. Once this occurs, additional enzyme/factors will eject the tRNA at the P site, while passing its amino acid to the aminoacyl-tRNA at the A site. This complex is then moved to the P site, and the mRNA is moved one codon. This process repeats itself until a stop codon is reached. At that time, release factors will recognize the stop codon, and the polypeptide chain is transferred to a water molecule. The mRNA is released, to be either translated again or degraded.

As purine and pyrimidine bases were the unit structures of DNA and RNA, amino acids are the unit structures of proteins. They all have a central carbon atom, to which is attached a hydrogen, a carboxyl group, and an amino group. Where they differ is at the fourth position, the side chain. These are grouped into nonpolar, polar, acidic, and basic side chains based on their chemical properties. The chain of amino acids, called a polypeptide, will eventually form a particular three-dimensional structure. There are four levels of structure in a protein. The first is the amino acid sequence itself. This will ultimately determine the form the polypeptide will have in the aqueous environment of the cell. The secondary level of protein structure is determined by hydrogen bonding between the amino and carboxyl groups of nearby amino acids. The most common forms of secondary structure in proteins are the alpha-helix and the beta-pleated sheet. The R side chain interactions, along with folding and interacting of the alpha-helices and the beta-pleated sheets, will contribute to the three-dimensional shape, or tertiary structure, of the polypeptide. Quaternary structure of a protein is the result of interactions of multiple polypeptides.

Once a protein is formed, it can be further modified by the apparatus of the cell. Disulfide bonds can be formed to strengthen tertiary or quaternary structure; sugars and/or lipids can also be added to specific amino acid residues in posttranslational modification of the protein. These proteins can then be used in the cell as enzymes or structural proteins, incorporated into the cell membrane for a variety of functions, or secreted from the cell.

MOLECULAR IMAGING PROBES

In general, current imaging for disease processes requires that the pathologic process be of a sufficient macroscopic size (usually on the order a few millimeters), or sufficiently disruptive of function (e.g., altered blood flow leading to contrast enhancement), that it can be detected by conventional imaging modalities. It would be considerably better for the patient if the disease process could be found before it led to these macroscopic changes. If a way could be found to target mutations in genetic material for a particular disease, one could potentially catch a disease at an earlier stage, where treatment could be more effective. Of course, the next logical step would be to tailor a treatment to fix or eradicate that same aberrant gene or genes. First things first, though, although there have been many advancements in a relatively short time, there is still progress that needs to be made in the development of probes for a particular target, delivery systems to the target, and systems capable of imaging these probes. Molecular imaging can be defined as is the in vivo visualization of normal and abnormal cellular processes at a molecular or genetic level of function. It is used to provide characterization and measurement of biological processes in both spatial and time relations. Targets that can be imaged range from genes to mRNA to proteins. While it might seem to make the most sense to target a particular gene directly, there are many more copies of the transcripts or translations of that gene available for the probe to attach to. The molecular target that has the most copies available is the protein. The protein target may be a membrane receptor, an intracellular receptor, an enzyme, or a transporter. Some examples of this are already widely used in nuclear medicine. ^{111}In pentetreotide (Octreoscan) is a chelated peptide that targets somatostatin receptors, ^{111}In capromab pendetide (ProstaScint) is a monoclonal antibody that targets the prostate-specific membrane antigen, and ^{111}In ibritumomab tiuxetan (Zevalin) is a monoclonal antibody that targets the B-lymphocyte CD20 receptor (and is used as part of a regimen to treat non-Hodgkin lymphoma). ^{18}F FDG is transported across a cell's membrane by GLUT-1 transporter. Once inside the cell, it is phosphorylated to ^{18}F-FDG-6-phosphate by hexokinase. Further metabolism of this substrate is not possible by the cell; it is trapped inside the cell. ^{18}F-FDG therefore is used to measure glucose metabolism, "targeting" the increased expression and activity of the GLUT-1 transporter and hexokinase. Targeting is in quotations, as unlike the first two examples, it is not directed at a particular object, but rather is the nonspecific process of glucose metabolism, which can be seen in physiologic, inflammatory, or malignant processes. Targeted probes are specific in that they bind with high affinity with the substrate of interest. Ideally, they are cleared from background tissues quickly (giving good target-to-background ratio) and have minimal nonspecific or random binding.

Radiopharmaceuticals listed in the chapter demonstrate the common configuration that all molecular probes share, whether in nuclear medicine, or using other imaging modalities. First, there has to be a substrate that will bind to or otherwise interact with the target to properly localize the event that one wishes to image. The second part of the probe is the "beacon," a substrate that can send a signal to allow for localization within an organism. In nuclear medicine, this is a radionuclide, but chelated Gd^{+3} (for T1 contrast) or superparamagnetic iron oxide nanoparticles have been used in molecular beacons in MRI. It is also possible to make molecular probes for optical imaging. Optical imaging uses fluorescent and bioluminescent probes that emit radiation in the visible or near-infrared wavelengths, which can be scanned by optical cameras. Unfortunately, light can travel only a few millimeters through tissue so it is limited to imaging skin, breast, and small animals (for research applications), as well as in surgical and endoscopic procedures. Near-infrared fluorescence is preferred, as there is the least absorption from tissues at this wavelength. Fluorescence from the tissues themselves is minimal at this wavelength as well. This wavelength can penetrate a depth of a few centimeters.

As of now, targeted molecular probes in ultrasound remain in the realm of research. However, nontargeted microbubbles made of lipids or proteins, and filled with a nonreactive gas that has low solubility in tissues, can be used in clinical practice to determine parameters such as blood flow and volume (e.g., tumor angiogenesis) in particular structures. By placing, for example, antibodies on the surface of the microbubbles, one can gain the specificity for a particular process or substrate to make it a targeted molecular probe.

So-called smart probes have been developed that will only function when particular parameters are met, such as the presence of a particular enzyme to catalyze a reaction. These smart probes are frequently used in optical imaging, although some MRI smart probes have been developed. The beacon does not "light" until acted on by a particular physiologic condition (e.g., change in pH) or more often, until a particular enzyme is present. Because of this, there is excellent target-to-background ratio. The most common example is the use of a smart probe to detect a particular protease. When this protease has not been expressed by the cell or organism, there is no detectable signal. If, however, the protease is present, it will cleave a specific site on the probe, removing a "quencher" and allowing the fluorescent molecule to become visible.

REVIEW MATERIALS

The last four tables in this chapter are charts that have been put together for both radiology and nuclear medicine residents to help summarize the myriad radionuclides and studies they struggle to master over the course of their residency. Table 99-4 is a list of acronyms used in nuclear medicine. Table 99-5 summarizes common radionuclides used in nuclear medicine, listed in alphabetical order. It includes half-lives, photopeaks, and chemical forms of the radionuclides. Table 99-6 is sorted by nuclear medicine study, and includes radiopharmaceutical used, route of administration, and other information specific to the study. Table 99-7 lists ^{99m}Tc radiopharmaceuticals and their applications.

TABLE 99-4 Acronyms Used in Nuclear Medicine

Instrumentation/Terms	
ADC	Analog-to-digital converter
AOR	Axis of rotation
COR	Center of rotation
CPU	Central processing unit
CRT	Cathode ray tube
DICOM	Digital communication standard
EDTA	Ethylenediaminetetra-acetic acid
ERPF	Effective renal plasma flow
FWHM	Full width at half maximum
LEAP	Low-energy all-purpose (collimator)
MUGA	Multigated acquisition
PET	Positron emission tomography
PHA	Pulse height analyzer
PMT	Photomultiplier tubes
RAM	Random-access memory
ROM	Read-only memory
ROR	Radius of rotation
SDAT	Senile dementia, Alzheimer's type
SPECT	Single-photon computed tomography
Radiotracers	
18-FDG	18-F fluorodeoxyglucose
DMSA	Dimercaptosuccinic acid
DTPA	Diethylenetriaminepentaacetic acid
EDC	Ethylene L-cysteinate dimer (Neurolite)
HMPAO	Hexamethylpropyleneamine oxime (Ceretec)
IDA	Iminodiacetic acid
MAA	Macroaggregated albumin
MAG3	Mercaptoacetyltriglycine
MDP	Methylene diphosphonate
MIBG	Metaiodobenzylguanidine
MIBI	Sestamibi (Cardiolite)
OIH	Orthoiodohippurate
SC	Sulfur colloid

TABLE 99-5 Common Radionuclides Used in Nuclear Medicine

NUCLIDE	Z	P*	T1/2	DECAY‡	MAJOR EMISSIONS§	CHEMICAL FORM(S)	USES
Carbon-11	6	A	20 m	β+	γ 511 keV, β+.96MeV	^{11}C acetate; ^{11}C palmitate; ^{11}C carfentanil	PET metabolic agents; receptor binding
Chromium-51	24		27.8 d	EC	γ 320 keV	51Cr EDTA	Red cell mass
Cobalt-57	27	A	272 d	EC	γ 122 keV	^{57}Co vitamin B_{12}	Schilling test
Fluorine-18	9	A†	109 m	EC, β+	γ 511 keV: β+.64 MeV	^{18}F- fluorodeoxyglucose;	Metabolic/tumor agent
						^{18}F sodium fluoride	Metabolic agent
Gallium-67	31	A	78 h	EC	γ 93, 184, 296, 388 keV	Gallium citrate	Inflammatory disease detection; tumor localization
Gallium-68	31	G†	68 m	EC, β+	γ511 keV	Gallium citrate	
Indium-111	49	A	67 h	EC	γ172, 247 keV	Labeled WBC; labeled antibodies, proteins and peptides	Inflammatory disease detection; tumor localization
						^{111}In pentetreotide (OctreoScan)	Somatostatin receptor analog
						^{111}In DTPA	Cisternogram; liquid phase gastric emptying
Iodine-123	53	A	13 h	EC	γ159 keV	Sodium iodide	Thyroid scintigraphy; thyroid uptake/function
						Iodoamphetamine	Cerebral perfusion scintigraphy
Iodine-131	53	R	8 d	β−	γ 284, 364, 637; β− 0.19 MeV	Sodium iodide	Thyroid CA scintigraphy; thyroid uptake/function
						Tositumomab (Bexxar)	Treatment of relapsed/refractory NHL
						NP-59, MIBG	Adrenal imaging
Molybdenum-99	42	R	66.7 h	β−	γ 181, 740, 778 keV	Ionically bound to alumina (Al_2O_3) column	Technetium 99 m generator
Nitrogen-13	7	A	10 m	β+	γ 511 keV	^{13}N ammonia; ^{13}N glutamate	PET perfusion agent; metabolic agent
Oxygen-15	8	A	124 s	β+	γ511 keV	^{15}O- CO_2, ^{15}O- water; ^{15}O- oxygen	PET perfusion agents; metabolic agent
Phosphorus-32	15	R	14 d	β−	β− 695 keV, 1.7 MeV	Sodium phosphate	Palliation of bone metastases; PCV therapy
Rubidum-82	37	G†	1.3 m	EC, β+	γ511 keV, 777 keV	^{82}Ru chloride	PET cardiac perfusion agent
Samarium-153	62	A	1.9 d	β−	β− 233 keV; γ 103 keV	^{153}Sm- lexidronan/ ^{153}Sm- EDTMP	Palliation of bone metastases
Strontium-89	38	R	50.5 d	β−	β− 1.46 MeV	^{89}Sr- chloride	Palliation of bone metastases
Technetium-99 m	43	G	6 h	IT	γ 140 keV	Multiple	Variable
Thalium-201	81	A	73 h	EC	69–81 keV¶	Thallous chloride	Myocardial perfusion scintigraphy; tumor imaging
Xenon-133	54	R	5.3 d	β−	γ 81 keV	Inert gas	Pulmonary ventilation scintigraphy
Yttrium-90	39	R	64.2 h	β−	β− 937 keV	^{90}Y- ibritumomab tiuxetan (Zevalin)	Treatment of relapsed/refractory NHL

*Produced: A = accelerator; G = generator; R = reactor.

†Given the fact that this isotope is generator produced and/or has a (relatively) long half-life, a cyclotron need not be on premises for use of this nuclide.

‡β+ = positron; β− = negatron or beta decay; EC = electron capture; IT = isomeric transformation.

§Underlined value is the commonly imaged photopeak(s).

¶Major emissions are characteristic x-rays of daughter product, mercury-201 (^{201}Hg).

TABLE 99-6 Brief Summary of Nuclear Medicine Study Parameters

STUDY	RADIOPHARMACEUTICAL	ADMINISTERED	DOSE TO IMAGE TIME	SPECIAL
Adrenal medullary	^{131}I MIBG/^{123}I MIBG	IV	24–72 h	Lugol solution for patient
Bone marrow	^{99m}Tc sulfur colloid	IV	Immediate	
Bone scan	^{99m}Tc MDP	IV	Immediate (3 phases), 2–3 h	
Brain death	^{99m}Tc HMPAO or ECD	IV	Flow and immediate static	
Brain SPECT	^{99m}Tc HMPAO or ECD	IV	15 min or later	
Cardiac PET	^{18}F-FDG	IV	45–60 min	Cardiac viability; glucose loading + insulin needed
Cardiac PET	^{82}Rb	IV	Immediate	Cardiac perfusion
Cardiac SPECT	^{99m}Tc sestamibi	IV	1–4 h	Planar–increase dose
Cardiac SPECT	^{99m}Tc tetrofosmin	IV	30 min–1 h	Planar–increase dose
Cardiac SPECT	^{201}Tl chloride	IV	Immediate (poststress), 3–4 h	Cardiac viability, 4- to 24-h delays
Cisternogram	^{111}In- DTPA	Subarachnoid	2, 6, 24, 48, 72 h as needed	Pledgets for CSF leak
Gallium	^{67}Ga citrate	IV	48–72 h	Use 5 mCi for infection, image at 24 h
Gastric emptying	^{99m}Tc sulfur colloid	PO(with egg)	Immediate, image 1 h	Use ^{111}In DTPA for liquid phase
GI bleed	^{99m}Tc tagged RBCs	IV	Immediate (3-h delay if needed)	Can also use ^{99m}Tc SC
Hemangioma	^{99m}Tc tagged RBCs	IV	Immediate	SPECT improves sensitivity
HIDA	^{99m}Tc DISDA or mebrofenin	IV	Immediate (3-h delay if needed)	Vary dose with bilirubin
LeVeen shunt	^{99m}Tc MAA	Intraperitoneal	Immediate, 1-h delay (lungs)	
Liver/spleen	^{99m}Tc sulfur colloid	IV	20 min	Rib margin marker on AP images
Lung perfusion	^{99m}Tc MAA	IV	Immediate	Lower dose if done before vent.
Lung ventilation	^{133}Xe	Inhaled	Immediate	Posterior views
Lung ventilation	^{99m}Tc DTPA aerosol	Inhaled	Immediate	
Lymph Node scintigraphy	^{99m}Tc filtered sulfur Colloid	Intradermal	Immediate up to 1 h	Identify sentinel LN
Meckel's	^{99m}Tc Na pertechnetate	IV	Immediate	
MUGA	^{99m}Tc tagged RBCs	IV	Immediate	Gated images
Octreotide	^{111}In pentetreotide	IV	4 h and 24 h	SPECT improves sensitivity
Parathyroid	^{99m}Tc sestamibi	IV	15 min, 2 h (and 4 h if needed)	Pinhole or SPECT improve detection
PET oncology	^{18}F-FDG	IV	1 h	
ProstaScint	^{111}In capromab pendetide	IV	96 h	Will need ^{99m}Tc tagged RBC too
Renal-cortical	^{99m}Tc DMSA	IV	1–3 h	Also ^{99m}Tc glucoheptonate
Renal-GFR	^{99m}Tc DTPA	IV	Immediate	
Renal-tubular	^{99m}Tc MAG-3	IV	Immediate	Used to approximate ERPF
Testicular	^{99m}Tc Na pertechnetate	IV	Immediate and 15 min delayed	
Thyroid scan	^{99m}Tc Na pertechnetate	IV	15–30 min	Trapped but not organified
Thyroid scan	Na^{123}I	PO	4–24 h	Trapped and organified
Thyroid uptake	Na^{131}I	PO	4 h and 24 h if needed	If probe used, no pictures obtained
Thyroid uptake	Na^{123}I	PO	4 h and 24 h if needed	If probe used, no pictures obtained
Thyroid WB	Na^{131}I	PO	24–72 h	Withdraw Sythroid or give rTSH
Thyroid WB	Na^{123}I	PO	24–48 h	Withdraw Sythroid or give rTSH
Thyroid WB	Na^{131}I	PO	7 d	Post high-dose therapy
WBC scan	^{99m}Tc HMPAO	IV	1 and 4 h (24 h if needed)	Also ^{111}In WBC

TABLE 99-7 Nuclear Medicine Studies Sorted by Technetium Agent

^{99m}Tc AGENT	APPLICATION*
^{99m}Tc arcitumomab (CEA scan)	[Monoclonal antibody for colorectal cancer evaluation]
^{99m}Tc bicisate (Ethylene L-cysteinate dimer or ECD)†	SPECT cerebral perfusion imaging
^{99m}Tc bromotriethyl IDA (Mebrofenin)	Hepatobiliary scintigraphy
^{99m}Tc diethylenetriamine-pentaacetic acid (DTPA)	Lung ventilation (aerosol), renal scintigraphy, GFR, cisternography, shunt patency [brain scintigraphy; blood volume]
^{99m}Tc dimercaptosuccinic acid (DMSA)	Renal cortical scintigraphy
^{99m}Tc diphosphonate (MDP)	Skeletal scintigraphy
^{99m}Tc disopropyl IDA (DISIDA)	Hepatobiliary scintigraphy
^{99m}Tc exametazine (HMPAO)‡	SPECT cerebral perfusion imaging, tagging agent for WBC studies
^{99m}Tc glucoheptonate	Renal scintigraphy [brain/CSF]
^{99m}Tc macroaggregated albumin (200–600 k particles)	Pulmonary perfusion scintigraphy
^{99m}Tc mercaptoacetyltriglycine (MAG3)	Renal scintigraphy, ERPF
^{99m}Tc red blood cells	GI bleeding detection, ventriculography (MUGA), hepatic hemangioma detection
^{99m}Tc sestamibi (Cardiolite)	Myocardial perfusion imaging {15–30 mCi (2-d protocol); 8–10 mCi rest/20–30 mCi stress (1-d protocol)}; parathyroid scintigraphy [breast cancer imaging]
^{99m}Tc sodium pertechnetate	Thyroid gland scintigraphy, Meckel diverticulum detection, testicular imaging [salivary gland scintigraphy]
^{99m}Tc sulfur colloid (filtered particle size.3 to 1.0 μm)	Liver/spleen (RES) scintigraphy, GI bleeding detection (tagged RBC is preferred method), gastric emptying, bone marrow scintigraphy
^{99m}Tc sulfur colloid (filtered particle size.03 to.1 μm)	Lymphoscintigraphy
^{99m}Tc tetrofosmin (Myoview)	Myocardial perfusion imaging (see sestamibi protocols)

*Applications in square brackets, "[ ]", indicate rarely used or historical uses of the agent. Numbers in set brackets, "{ }", are ranges of activity for adult patients; pediatric doses are often weight based.
†Neurolite (trade name)
‡Hexamethylpropylenamine oxime or Ceretec (trade name)

Suggested Reading

Li KCP et al. A primer on molecular biology for imagers. *Acad Radiol.* 2004;11:S7.

QUESTIONS AND ANSWERS

1. A patient has laboratory findings consistent with hyperthyroidism, with an elevated T_4 and suppressed TSH. When a radioactive iodine uptake test is performed, the uptake is 4%. Which of the following conditions does the patient likely have?
   A. Graves disease
   B. Toxic multinodular goiter
   C. Toxic hyperfunctioning adenoma
   D. Subacute thyroiditis

   ANSWER: D. Subacute thyroiditis. It is not unusual that by the time the patient has the radioactive iodine uptake study, the T_4 released as a result of the thyroiditis has caused a feedback decrease in TSH secretion. This would lead to decreased radioiodine uptake. All of the other choices would most likely result in an elevated radioiodine uptake.

2. Of the following agents, which will interfere with radioactive iodine uptake for the *longest*?
   A. Propylthiouracil
   B. Thyroxine
   C. Intravenous iodine contrast
   D. Triiodothyronine

   ANSWER: B. Thyroxine (Synthroid), which is T_4, will interfere the longest.

3. What is the purpose of administering 1-mg intramuscular nonradioactive vitamin B_{12} immediately after administering the radiolabeled vitamin B_{12}?
   A. This promotes radiolabeled vitamin B_{12} uptake in the gut.
   B. This interferes with radiolabeled vitamin B_{12} uptake in the gut.
   C. This promotes urinary excretion of radiolabeled vitamin B_{12}.
   D. This will stimulate IF production in the patient.

   ANSWER: C. This promotes urinary excretion of radiolabeled vitamin B_{12}. If the patient was given vitamin B_{12} within 3 days before the test, this may decrease the fractional absorption of the test dose. This is due to biliary excretion of that parenteral vitamin B_{12} into the GI tract.

4. When handing you the results of a patient's radioactive iodine thyroid uptake, the technologist tells you that he just realized that he forgot to include the counts from the patient's thigh in his calculations. How would this affect the computed radioiodine uptake value?
   A. Result will be underestimated compared to the true value.
   B. Result will be overestimated compared to the true value.
   C. Will not affect the result
   D. Cannot know what effect it will have on the result

   ANSWER: D. Cannot know what effect it will have on the result. In this situation, the only body part counted in the patient is the neck. The thigh counts are used to account for activity in the neck that is not coming from the thyroid gland, but rather from background activity in the other structures of the neck. If the thyroid uptake was high, then you in essence have thyroid counts/(standard in phantom − room background) and there would be a slight underestimation. If the thyroid uptake is low, then patient background would be high, meaning there would be counts coming from the neck that were not really coming from the thyroid, overestimating the uptake.

5. Which of the following will *not* result in an abnormal part I Schilling test?
   A. Dietary deficiency
   B. Pernicious anemia
   C. Crohn's disease
   D. Sprue

   ANSWER: A. Dietary deficiency. Pernicious anemia would cause the uptake of ^{57}Co vitamin B_{12} to be low in the part I test; it would be normal in part II, when IF is provided. Malabsorption from either Crohn's disease or sprue would interfere with ^{57}Co vitamin B_{12} uptake in the ileum.

6. A referring physician calls you to ask how long their patient should discontinue their methimazole. What would your response be?
   A. No need to discontinue
   B. 1 day
   C. 1 week
   D. 1 month

   ANSWER: C. 1 week.

7. The genetic code is said to be degenerate because
   A. Error rate of DNA is 1 in each 10–100 million bases.
   B. More than one triplet can specify the same amino acid.
   C. Only 1% to 2% of the three billion base pairs in the human genome encodes for proteins.
   D. It probably will never amount to much.

   ANSWER: B. More than one triplet can specify the same amino acid. Fidelity in DNA replication is excellent, with 1 error per 10 to 100 billion bases. While it is true that only 1% to 2% of the base pairs in the human genome encode for proteins, this is not why the code is called degenerate.

8. The central dogma of molecular biology is that:
   A. DNA is transcribed to mRNA, which is translated to protein.
   B. DNA is translated to mRNA, which is transcribed to protein.
   C. DNA is translated to rRNA, which is transcribed to protein.
   D. The genetic code is degenerate.

   ANSWER: A. DNA is transcribed to mRNA, which is translated to protein.

9. ProstaScint is a type of molecular probe used to detect prostate cancer. It is a monoclonal antibody that targets __________, and uses __________ as its beacon.
   A. Prostate-specific antigen (PSA); ^{111}In
   B. Prostate-specific membrane antigen (PSMA); ^{111}In
   C. Prostate-specific antigen (PSA); ^{99m}Tc
   D. Prostate-specific membrane antigen (PSMA); ^{99m}Tc

   ANSWER: B. ProstaScint is a monoclonal antibody directed against a glycoprotein expressed by prostate epithelium known as prostate-specific membrane antigen (PSMA). It uses ^{111}In as its radionuclide.

10. Which of the following wavelengths is the best choice for optical imaging molecular probes?
    A. All wavelengths are equally useful
    B. Ultraviolet
    C. Visible light
    D. Near-infrared

    ANSWER: D. Near-infrared has the least absorption by organs and tissues, and has better penetration in tissues.

Section 11
PEDIATRIC RADIOLOGY

100 PEDIATRIC MUSCULOSKELETAL SYSTEM

Brenton D. Reading and
Robert P. Nuttall

DEVELOPMENTAL/IDIOPATHIC ABNORMALITIES

BLOUNT DISEASE

Blount disease is a developmental deformity of the tibia, also known as tibia vara. Its etiology uncertain but it is likely caused by sequelae of developmental bowing, which does not correct. Normal bowing is seen up to 3 years of age, which then progresses to genu valgum in 3 to 5 years of age. Subsequently, normal posture should be achieved. If not, surgical correction with epiphysiodesis is often required to correct the persistent bowing.

DEVELOPMENTAL DYSPLASIA OF THE HIP

Developmental dysplasia of the hip (DDH) can range from mild acetabular dysplasia to irreducible dislocation of the femoral head. The incidence is approximately 1:1000 and is more common in girls than boys (8:1). The left hip is much more commonly affected than the right hip (70%–75%). There is bilateral involvement in 5% of patients. Ultrasound is the study of choice in children younger than 6 months of age as radiographs are not very useful. However, after 6 months of age, ossification of the femoral head makes ultrasound less useful. High-risk patients include those with a family history of DDH, breech delivery, oligohydramnios, as well as neuromuscular and foot abnormalities. Physical findings include positive hip click with dislocation and relocation (Barlow and Ortolani maneuvers respectively), shortened leg with decreased abduction, and asymmetric gluteal folds.

Radiographic features of DDH include late or asymmetric femoral head ossification (normal femoral head ossification typically occurs between 3 and 7 months, earlier in girls; 90% are ossified by 7 months); positioning of the femoral head lateral to the Perkins line and superior to the Hilgenreiner line; and abnormal curve of Shenton line. The Hilgenreiner line is a horizontal line drawn through the triradiate cartilage; the Perkins line is drawn perpendicular to the Hilgenreiner line at the outer acetabular edge; the Shenton line is a sinuous arch extending along obturator foramen to the medial femoral neck. US indicators of DDH are an alpha angle less than 60 degrees and a shallow acetabulum.

JUVENILE RHEUMATOID ARTHRITIS (JUVENILE IDIOPATHIC ARTHRITIS)

Juvenile rheumatoid arthritis (juvenile idiopathic arthritis) is a chronic polyarthritis, most commonly involving large joints such as the knees and wrists. This most commonly presents within the first 5 years of life and is more common in females than males. Erosion of the dens and atlantoaxial subluxation can occur. The systemic form is called Still disease, with symptoms including polyarthritis, splenomegaly, myocarditis or pericarditis, lymphadenopathy, and fever.

LEGG-PERTHES

Legg-Perthes is an idiopathic avascular necrosis of the femoral head. It usually presents with knee pain and limp. It is more frequent in boys than girls (5:1), and it is bilateral approximately 15% of the time. Onset before 6 years of age usually results in better outcome. Early radiographic findings include a patchy trabecular pattern, widening of the joint space, crescent sign, marrow edema on MRI, and contrast enhancement. Chronic findings include coxa plana and coxa magna, fragmentation/collapse of the capital femoral epiphysis, physeal growth arrest, and short femoral neck.

NEWBORN PERIOSTEAL REACTION

Newborn periosteal reaction may be normal or pathologic. Physiologic periosteal reaction is usually symmetric and commonly occurs in the first few months of life, typically involving the long bone diaphyses. Prostaglandin use and TORCH infections (Table 100-1) can cause periosteal reaction. Caffey disease is an idiopathic, self-limiting condition usually occurring in the first few months of life with periosteal new bone and adjacent soft-tissue swelling. The areas involved include the mandible, ribs, scapula, clavicles, femurs, humerus, radius, and ulna. In addition, metastatic disease, especially from neuroblastoma must also be considered as a cause for diffuse periosteal reaction.

OSGOOD-SCHLATTER DISEASE

The etiology of Osgood-Schlatter disease is controversial. The most likely cause is related to traction on the tibial tuberosity during growth resulting in microfractures with avulsion and tearing at the insertion of the patellar tendon. The tibial tubercle region is commonly irregular with multiple bony fragments.

PROXIMAL FOCAL FEMORAL DEFICIENCY

Proximal focal femoral deficiency is a congenital abnormality involving variable degrees of deficiency of the proximal portions of the femur. This can also involve the acetabulum and the femoral head in severe cases. The patient presents with leg-length discrepancy. The fibula may be absent and the foot is often deformed.

TABLE 100-1 TORCH Infections

Toxoplasmosis
Hepatitis B
Syphilis
Varicella-Zoster
HIV
Parovirus
Rubella
Cytomegalovirus
Herpes virus

SCOLIOSIS

Congenital scoliosis is secondary to congenital spinal anomalies such as hemivertebra and butterfly vertebra. Neuromuscular scoliosis is common in cerebral palsy. It is typically a C-shaped scoliosis without a compensatory curve because of the lack of weightbearing. Idiopathic scoliosis has a typical S-shaped curve, consisting of a thoracic dextroscoliosis and a lumbar levoscoliosis. Multiple forms of idiopathic scoliosis exist including infantile, juvenile, and adolescent types. Adolescent is the most common type and frequently occurs in females. Surgical treatment is generally reserved for greater than 40-degree curvature. Nonidiopathic scoliosis has numerous causes including spinal pathology such as tethered cord, syrinx, and tumor; spinal bony lesions such as osteoid osteoma and osteoblastoma; metastatic disease; osteomyelitis; Langerhans cell histiocytosis; neurofibromatosis; postirradiation changes; and leg-length discrepancy.

SLIPPED CAPITAL FEMORAL EPIPHYSIS

Slipped capital femoral epiphysis (SCFE) is similar to a Salter-Harris I fracture involving the proximal femoral physis which presents in adolescents with hip or knee pain. It is twice as common in males and is usually idiopathic or occasionally posttraumatic. Bilateral involvement is not rare but often presents in an asynchronous pattern. There is increased incidence in renal osteodystrophy, hypothyroidism, and hypopituitarism, as well as obesity. Femoral head displacement is posterior and medial. A frogleg view is crucial for diagnosis; the neutral view can appear normal. A line drawn tangential to the lateral cortex of the femoral neck should intersect a portion of the femoral head; if not, SCFE is likely. Surgical intervention involves pin fixation. Avascular necrosis, premature osteoarthritis, and chondrolysis are potential complications.

TALIPES EQUINOVARUS (CLUBFOOT)

The frequency of clubfoot is approximately 1 to 4:1000, with occurrence in males approximately twice that in females. The feet are affected bilaterally approximately 30% to 50% of the time. Clubfoot presents with hindfoot equinus with a decreased lateral talocalcaneal angle less than 35 degrees, hindfoot varus with a decreased talocalcaneal angle less than 20-degrees AP, and forefoot varus with medial displacement of first metatarsal relative to the long axis of the talus. Clubfeet may be corrected with manipulation, casting, and splinting alone. Cases that respond poorly to splinting and manipulative treatment require operative management.

TOXIC SYNOVITIS

Toxic synovitis is a diagnosis of exclusion. It is most common in children younger than 10 years. Joint effusion is present but no evidence of bacteria, virus, or inflammatory change is identified. The etiology is likely viral. The associated pain usually subsides with rest.

INFECTION

DISCITIS

Discitis is often secondary to hematogenous seeding and commonly involves adjacent vertebral endplates. It is most common in children from 6 to 10 years of age and is most common in the lumbar region. Vertebral body osteomyelitis is more common in adults since adult disks are avascular.

OSTEOMYELITIS

The typical locations of osseous infection are age-related. In infants, the primary site is metaphyseal with potential extension to the epiphyses. Epiphyseal involvement can occur up to approximately 18 months of age, at which time the appearance of epiphyseal ossification centers prevents access to these regions. In children up to the age of skeletal maturity, a metaphyseal location is most common because of slow blood flow in this region. The femur is the most frequently affected bone, followed by the tibia and humerus. Multifocal involvement can be seen in neonates and infants.

Bony changes may not be seen for 10 to 14 days or routine radiographic analysis. A nuclear medicine bone scan is more sensitive in this time period. Modes of transmission include hematogenous; direct extension secondary to cellulitis and sinusitis; and direct implantation secondary to open injury, foreign body penetration, and postoperative complications. Common pathogens include *Staphylococcus aureus*, group B *streptococcus*, especially in neonates, as well as *Salmonella* or *Strep pneumoniae* in sickle cell patients. Fungal or mycobacterial involvement can also be seen in immunocompromised patients. Joint space involvement can occur with intra-articular metaphyses, such as the hip, elbow, and shoulder. Brodie abscesses are chronic, circumscribed areas of osteomyelitis which most commonly occur in the femur or tibia and are more commonly metaphyseal than diaphyseal.

SEPTIC ARTHRITIS

Septic arthritis is bimodal in distribution typically occuring in infants or teenagers and most cases occur in children younger than 3 years of age. The most commonly affected joints are the hip and knee. Septic arthritis presents with pain on joint movement and refusal to walk. *S. aureus* and group A *streptococcus* are the most common agents. There is significant potential for joint destruction. Spread is typically from the adjacent metaphysic with hematogenous seeding of the synovial vasculature. Radiographic findings are related to effusions and synovial inflammation. Findings at the hip include an increased teardrop distance measured from medial cortex of femoral metaphysis to "teardrop" of acetabulum. A distance of greater than 2 mm compared with the uninvolved hip is worrisome.

METABOLIC BONE DISEASE

RICKETS

Rickets in children is the result of a disruption in the pathway of either vitamin D or phosphate metabolism. Defective mineralization in developing bone causes osteomalacia. The most common cause is a vitamin D deficiency. A diet lacking in calcium or phosphorus may also produce rickets. Widening and cupping of the metaphyses is noted, most prominent at the knee because growth is most rapid in this location. Noncalcified osteoid along the shaft leads to the appearance of periosteal lifting. Coarsening of trabeculae is noted in contrast to the ground glass osteopenia of scurvy. Bones may become bowed because of softening and weight-bearing as well as green stick type fractures. Similar findings are seen in pediatric renal osteodystrophy and secondary osteopenia.

NEOPLASMS

BENIGN OSSEOUS LESIONS

For benign osseous lesions, see Tables 72-1 to 72-3.

ENCHONDROMAS

These are benign cartilaginous growths, most frequently seen between 10 and 40 years of age. The radiographic findings of an enchondroma consist of a pathognomonic pattern of a lucent lesion with calcifications in rings and arcs. However, radiographs may not depict the calcified matrix, particularly in the hands and feet. Enchondromas are the most common cystic lesion involving the phalanges, but are most commonly seen in the humerus and femur.

Fibrous Cortical Defect

This is a nonaggressive fibrous lesion of bone, which is referred to as nonossifying fibroma (NOF) if larger than 3 cm. The lesions are most commonly seen in the distal femur and proximal tibia and are estimated to be present in 30% to 40% of all children. These lesions are typically well-defined, eccentric, lucent lesions with a sclerotic margin that may not extend around the entire lesion. The lesions should not be painful and there should be no periosteal reaction unless a pathologic fracture is present. The natural course is gradual regression, often associated with increasing sclerosis without treatment. These are considered "do not touch" lesions, as no further imaging or intervention is indicated.

Fibrous Dysplasia (Lichtenstein-Jaffe Disease)

This is a fibro-osseous lesion in which medullary bone is replaced by fibrous tissue. It is usually seen in the lower extremities although skull involvement is not uncommon. Fibrous dysplasia is most frequently seen in pediatric patients between 5 and 20 years of age and may be associated with hyperparathyroidism and hyperthyroidism. Radiographic findings include lucent osseous lesions (often in the diaphysis or metaphysis) with a smooth and homogeneous matrix "ground glass" appearance, endosteal scalloping, lack of periosteal reaction, and expansion of outer cortex with cortical thinning in skull lesions. There is a low risk of malignant transformation. Monostotic fibrous dysplasia is the most common type (85%), most frequently involving the skull, ribs, and femurs.

Langerhans Cell Histiocytosis (histiocytosis-x)

There are multiple forms of this disease process ranging from systemic disease to focal lesions. Eosinophilic granuloma (EG) is the most common presentation and has the best prognosis. Findings include lytic lesions most commonly involving the skull (punched-out lesions), mandible (floating teeth), and vertebral bodies (vertebra plana). EG should always be included in the differential diagnosis for a pediatric lytic lesion of bone as these lesions may at times be aggressive in appearance with periosteal reaction, pain, and associated soft-tissue involvement. Letterer-Sewe generally presents prior to age 2 years with multisystem involvement and is often fatal. Associated findings include, cutaneous rash, hepatosplenomegaly, lymphadenopathy, and pulmonary disease. Hand-Schuller-Christian usually presents by age 5 with high morbidity and approximately 15% mortality. There is chronic diffuse involvement of the skull and orbits with associated findings of diabetes insipidus, hepatosplenomegaly, and marrow involvement.

Osteochondroma

This is a cartilage-capped exostosis, which grows away from the joint. There is cortical and medullary continuity with the parent bone. Growth continues until the growth plate closes. These are typically metaphyseal and tend to occur in long bones such as the femur and tibia. However, many other locations are possible especially when multiple lesions are present. These are more common in males than females and are not intrinsically painful but associated mass effect on adjacent structures can be symptomatic. These lesions are most commonly seen in the first three decades of life.

Osteoid Osteoma

Most common in teenagers, and more frequent in males than females, these are cortically based lesions which present with night pain relieved by aspirin. The femur and tibia are common locations. Plain films may show a sclerotic focus with or without the more lucent cortical nidus, which is clearly demonstrated on CT. Nuclear medicine may also be helpful. Surgical excision or thermal ablation is curative if the nidus is completely treated.

Osteoblastoma

Osteoblastoma (giant osteoid osteoma) lesions are also more common in males than females and most frequently occur in the second and third decades. A common location is the posterior elements of the spine. The main symptom is pain and the treatment is surgical curettage.

MALIGNANT OSSEOUS LESIONS

Ewing Sarcoma

This is the second most common primary bone malignancy in children, often presenting in the second decade with a 2:1 male-to-female ratio. Metastatic disease to the lung, lymph nodes, and bones is common at presentation. Flat bones and long bones such as the femur, pelvis, and ribs are commonly involved with a permeative pattern of bone destruction. Aggressive (onion skin) periosteal reaction is commonly seen and there is usually a prominent soft-tissue component.

Osteosarcoma

This is the most common primary pediatric bone malignancy. The age range is 10 to 25 years with typical symptoms of pain and swelling. Fifty to seventy-five percent are found in the region of the knee with the proximal humerus also being a common site. These are pearly metaphyseal lesions with aggressive periosteal reactions. Approximately 15% of affected individuals present with bony metastasis at the time of diagnosis. Multiple types exist, including the classic medullary type, as well as parosteal, periosteal, telangiectatic, multifocal, and radiation- or chemotherapy-induced osteosarcoma.

TRAUMA

ELBOW TRAUMA

Supracondylar fractures are the most common elbow fractures in skeletally immature patients: while radial head fractures are more common in skeletally mature young adults. Lateral condyle fractures are the second most common type of pediatric elbow fracture.

There are six ossification centers at the elbow joint. It is important to understand that these centers ossify in a specific sequence. A mnemonic to remember the order is CRITOE: Capitellum, Radial head, Internal (medial) epicondyle, Trochlea, Olecranon, External (lateral) epicondyle. Knowing this order is particularly helpful in recognizing a medial epicondyle avulsion fracture, the third most common pediatric elbow fracture. The fracture fragment may become trapped in the joint and could be misinterpreted as the trochlear ossification center if the order of I (medial epicondyle) before T (trochlea) was not remembered.

Elbow fractures may be difficult to see. Elevation of the posterior fat pads is consistent with a joint effusion and should cause high suspicion for a fracture. If a fracture is not seen, repeat films in 7 to 10 days may be helpful. If the anterior humeral line does not pass through the middle one-third of the capitellum, supracondylar fracture is suspected.

Nursemaid elbow is a very common injury in infants and small children in which the radial head slips from the annular ligament and no longer aligns with the capitellum. This typically presents as refusal to move the arm with no associated history of trauma.

GROWTH PLATE INJURIES

The growth plate is the weakest part of the bone and is therefore susceptible to injury. Accounting for approximately 15% to 20% of all pediatric fractures, physeal injuries are more common in males than females. Five types are commonly discussed as described by Salter and Harris (Table 100-2). Types I, II, and III have an excellent prognosis; types IV, and V can disrupt the growth plate or cause asymmetric growth, possibly leading to limb shortening or angulation. Osteochondritis dissecans is an osteochondral injury that can be considered a type VII fracture, involving only the epiphysis.

TABLE 100-2 Salter-Harris Fracture Classification

Type I	Growth plate (slipped capital femoral epiphysis)
Type II	Growth plate and adjacent metaphysis; most common growth plate injury (50%–75%)
Type III	Growth plate and the epiphysis; most commonly in the distal tibia (juvenile Tillaux fracture)
Type IV	Growth plate, metaphysis, and epiphysis; common sites are the distal humerus and tibia
Type V	Crush-type injury

NONACCIDENTAL TRAUMA

Skeletal findings are only present in about one-third of child abuse cases. However, skeletal findings are the most commonly discovered radiologic manifestation of child abuse. Once suspicion of abuse has been raised, a skeletal survey is the primary method of evaluation. Nuclear medicine bone scan can also be useful, especially when a skeletal survey is negative but clinical suspicion remains high. The fractures most suspicious for abuse involve the posterior ribs; long bones in nonambulatory children, especially the femur; metaphyseal corners; scapula; and sternum. Fractures with moderate specificity include complex skull fractures, fractures of different ages, and multiple bilateral fractures. Fractures with low specificity involve the skull (linear), clavicle, and long bones in ambulatory children. Periosteal reaction usually appears within 10 days of the original insult and is nonspecific; however, in possible nonaccidental trauma, it should be viewed with suspicion. Conditions, which can mimic child abuse include osteogenesis imperfecta (OI), rickets, scurvy, and infantile cortical hyperostosis (Caffey syndrome).

OTHER DISTINCT PEDIATRIC FRACTURES

Because of relatively compliant bones, pediatric fractures may not completely traverse the bony shaft. Bowing fractures have no visible fracture line and are most common in the forearm. Greenstick fractures disrupt only one cortex and are fairly uncommon. Buckle or torus fractures are common cortical fractures frequently occuring in the distal forearm cortical deformity. These fractures demonstrate angulation of the bone and are often only evident on one view, most commonly the lateral view. Toddler fracture is a nondisplaced tibial fracture, usually in the distal third, and typically presenting between 9 months and 3 years. These fractures are often spiral or oblique and may be seen well on only one projection. Toddlers with this fracture often present with a refusal to walk and therefore an evaluation of the entire extremity is often required to exclude other pathology. Pediatric stress fractures of the calcaneus and cuboid may also occur.

SKELETAL DYSPLASIAS

ACQUIRED SKELETAL DYSPLASIAS

Acquired disorders are more common than congenital dysplasias. For normal osseous development, growing bones require physiologic muscle tension and gravitational loading. Any process that interferes with this normal stress may lead to osseous dysplasia. Examples of disease processes causing acquired skeletal dysplasia include paraplegia or quadriplegia, chronic bedrest (leukemia, juvenile chronic arthritis, etc.), and neuromuscular diseases (cerebral palsy, Duchenne muscular dystrophy, poliomyelitis, etc.). Affected individuals may demonstrate extremely gracile (long and thin) bones, coxa valga, pelvic malformation, and diminished muscle mass. While the clinical distinction between the etiologies for acquired skeletal dysplasias is generally straightforward, in the absence of specific findings such as articular erosions to suggest juvenile rheumatoid arthritis, the radiographic appearance may be very similar and clinical history is key. Poorly healed fractures or postoperative deformities can also appear severely dysmorphic and should be on the differential for acquired bone dysplasias.

CONGENITAL SKELETAL DYSPLASIAS

The congenital skeletal dysplasias are a group of more than 200 disorders consisting of abnormalities in cartilage and bone growth. The overall incidence of skeletal dysplasias is approximately one case per 4000 to 5000 births. The most common congenital skeletal dysplasias are achondroplasia, osteogenesis imperfecta (OI), and thanatophoric dysplasia (TD). In general, no racial predilections are described. Other than the X-linked recessive disorders, males and females are equally affected by most skeletal dysplasias.

ACHONDROGENESIS

Achondrogenesis is an autosomal, recessive, lethal chondrodystrophy characterized by the following triad: severe micromelic dwarfism, craniomegaly with normal-to-decreased calvarial ossification, and poor vertebral body ossification. Achondrogenesis is divided into two main categories: type I (Houston-Harris syndrome and Parenti-Fraccaro disease) with abnormal enchondral and membranous ossification and type II (Langer-Saldino syndrome) with abnormal enchondral ossification.

The prognosis of all types of achondrogenesis is very poor with death occurring either in utero or shortly after birth because of respiratory failure. The differential considerations include homozygous achondroplasia, short rib-polydactyly syndromes, and TD.

ACHONDROPLASIA

The most common nonlethal form of chondrodysplasia is achondroplasia. This rhizomelic form of dwarfism is autosomal dominant in inheritance and de novo mutations account for 75% to 80% of cases. Affected individuals generally have normal intelligence and motor function. However, because of the narrowing of osseous foramina, neurologic deficits may occur.

The diagnosis is based on typical clinical and radiologic features. The radiologic features are best evaluated with a skeletal survey. Radiographic findings include a contracted skull base with small foramen magnum, normal trunk length, rhizomelic shortening of the limbs with trident hands and brachydactyly, thoracolumbar gibbus in infancy, large calvarial bones in contrast to the small cranial base and facial bones, limited elbow extension, progressive interpedicular narrowing at the lumbar spine, short pedicles (which can cause spinal stenosis), genu varum, short femoral necks, metaphyseal flaring, dysplastic ilium, narrow sacroiliac groove, and flat-roofed acetabula. The prognosis of achondroplasia is generally good with a long life expectancy. The potential differential diagnosis list includes achondrogenesis, thanatophoric dwarfism, and chondroectodermal dysplasia (Ellis-van Creveld syndrome).

ASPHYXIATING THORACIC DYSTROPHY (FAMILIAL ASPHYXIATING THORACIC DYSTROPHY, JEUNE SYNDROME)

Jeune syndrome, a potentially lethal congenital form of dwarfism, is a rare genetically heterogeneous disorder with autosomal recessive inheritance. The classic findings of Jeune syndrome include a narrow thorax and micromelia, respiratory and renal manifestations (associated with bilateral microcystic kidney disease), and retinal degeneration.

The most common cause of death in Jeune syndrome is respiratory failure with 60% to 70% fatality among affected individuals in infancy and early childhood. However, respiratory symptoms vary widely ranging from respiratory failure and infantile death to latent phenotype with respiratory symptoms. In affected individuals with respiratory failure, alveolar hypoventilation is caused by impaired chest expansion as a result of short ribs. The few patients who survive into early adolescence face an increased risk for development of chronic renal failure. The differential considerations include TD, short-limb polydactyly syndrome, and achondroplasia.

CAMPOMELIC DYSPLASIA (CAMPTOMELIC DYSPLASIA)

Campomelic dysplasia is an autosomal, recessive disorder with occasional sporadic autosomal dominant mutations, which results in bowing of the long bones. The most characteristic radiographic sign is marked anterior bowing of the femur and tibia. At times, bowing may be so severe that the angulation can mimic fracture. Additional findings include bell-shaped narrow chest, hypoplasia of the midthoracic vertebral bodies, scoliosis, and talipes equinovarus.

Polyhydramnios and anomalies of the central nervous, cardiac, and renal systems are also associated with campomelic dysplasia. The prognosis is poor with death generally occurring before 5 months of age related to respiratory insufficiency.

CHONDRODYSPLASIA PUNCTATA

Chondrodysplasia punctata is a group of syndromes with characteristic osseous sclerotic calcifications near the articulations from birth. Associated findings include short limb segments, dysmorphism with hypoplastic nose, skin lesions, and cataracts. Other associated anomalies vary depending on the subtype. The types can be divided into five groups: autosomal dominant (including dysplasia epiphysealis congenital, stippled epiphyses, chondrodysplasia punctata dominant type, chondrodysplasia epiphysealis punctata, and chondrodystrophia calcificans congenital); autosomal recessive; X-linked dominant (Conradi-Hunermann syndrome); X-linked recessive, and Sheffield type.

The autosomal dominant form is the most common type and most cases are the result of a de novo mutation. The major criteria for diagnosis include craniofacial dysmorphism, symmetric frontal bossing, flat nasal bridge, dysplastic auricles, mongoloid palpebral fissures, hypertelorism, and high arched palate. Other associated abnormalities include ocular abnormalities, cutaneus abnormalities, skeletal abnormalities (e.g., asymmetric mild shortening and bowing of long bones, vertebral anomalies, and clubfoot deformity), and miscellaneous abnormalities (e.g., pulmonary artery stenosis, ascites, and polyhydramnios). Although occasionally associated with mild mental retardation, the prognosis is excellent and affected individuals usually have a normal lifespan and intelligence.

The autosomal recessive or rhizomelic type results in radiologic findings of symmetric shortening of the proximal bones, punctate calcific deposits in infantile cartilaginous skeleton, and coronal clefts in the vertebra. This type is associated with mental retardation. The prognosis is poor as most fetuses die in utero or shortly after birth, and the few that survive longer suffer severe debility and profound mental retardation. Death then ensues in the first decade of life.

The X-linked dominant type (Conradi-Hunermann type subgroup B) is a very uncommon syndrome with possible lethality in the hemizygous male. The prognosis is extremely variable ranging from neonatal death to near undetectability of the disorder in the adult. The X-linked recessive type is a very rare disorder with radiologic findings resembling the nonrhizomelic type. The Sheffield type or chondroplasia punctata mild form is also very rare. The clinical manifestations include failure to thrive, mental retardation, and typical facies with flattened tip of the nose and depressed nasal bridge.

CHONDROECTODERMAL DYSPLASIA (ELLIS-VAN CREVELD SYNDROME)

Ellis-van Creveld syndrome is an autosomal, recessive form of acromesomelic dwarfism with an increased incidence among individuals of Old Order Amish descent. The clinical tetrad of Ellis-van Creveld syndrome consists of chondrodystrophy, polydactyly, ectodermal dysplasia, and cardiac anomalies. Chondrodystrophy affects the tubular bones leading to a disproportionate dwarfism with progressive distal limb shortening of the forearms and lower legs. In addition, congenital cardiac anomalies occur in 50% to 60% of patients.

The radiographic findings include acromesomelia, which is most prominent in the hands, ulnar postaxial polydactyl, syndactyly, short ribs with thoracic narrowing, delayed bone maturation, valgus deformity of the knee, and clinodactyly of the fifth finger. The prognosis is poor with death occurring in the first month of life in up to 50% of cases because of respiratory/cardiac complications. The differential includes asphyxiating thoracic dysplasia and short rib polydactyly syndromes.

CLEIDOCRANIAL DYSOSTOSIS (CLEIDOCRANIAL DYSPLASIA)

Cleidocranial dysostosis (cleidocranial dysplasia) is an autosomal dominant disorder, which results from an abnormality in membranous and enchondral bone formation with a tendency to affect midline structures. Common findings include macrocephaly with delayed suture closure, wormian bones, hypertelorism, a small face, dental dysplasia, hypoplasia/aplasia of the clavicles, narrow pelvis, and spinal anomalies. Despite the tendency to affect midline structures, other bones are often involved including the ossicles of the ear and the extremities. The prognosis is good with a normal life expectancy. Possible complications associated with this syndrome include dental anomalies, hearing loss, scoliosis, and dislocations of the shoulder, radial head, or hip.

CRANIOSYNOSTOSIS

Sagittal stenosis is the most common type resulting in a boat-shaped calvarium referred to as dolichocephaly/scaphocephaly. Coronal synostosis is often associated with a so-called Harlequin eye, with elongation of the superior/lateral orbit. A brachiocephalic contour of the calvarium is present if bilateral synostosis occurs. This condition can be seen with associated abnormalities, such as Apert syndrome (coronal synostosis with syndactyly) and Crouzon disease (coronal synostosis with craniofacial dysostosis). Metopic synostosis results in a pointed forehead (trigonencephaly). Lambdoid synostosis results in brachycephaly if bilateral and plagiocephaly if unilateral. Kleeblattschädel (cloverleaf skull) results from pansutural synostosis.

ENCHONDROMATOSIS

Enchondromas are ectopic hyaline cartilage rests within intramedullary bone. Multiple enchondromas may occur in three distinct disorders: Ollier disease, Maffucci syndrome, and metachondromatosis. Ollier disease is a nonhereditary disorder with multiple enchondromas, which can grow large, become disfiguring, and generally occur in a unilateral distribution. There is an increased risk for degeneration to chondrosarcoma in affected individuals. Maffucci syndrome is also nonhereditary and is less common than Ollier disease, presenting with both multiple hemangiomas and enchondromas. The soft-tissue hemangiomas typically have numerous phleboliths, visible on radiographs. There is an increased risk for degeneration to chondrosarcoma as well as increased risk for other malignancies of the CNS and abdomen. Metachondromatosis is autosomal dominant in transmission and presents with multiple enchondromas and osteochondromas. However, these osteochondromas differ from conventional osteochondromas in that they point toward rather than away from the joint. Although in most cases, chondrosarcoma has aggressive features, low-grade chondrosarcoma may be indistinguishable from an enchondroma and if symptomatic then concern for chondrosarcoma is increased.

POLYOSTOTIC FIBROUS DYSPLASIA (MCCUNE-ALBRIGHT SYNDROME)

Polyostotic fibrous dysplasia may involve any bone but most commonly affects the long bones, ribs, and skull. Females are much more commonly affected than males. Lesions range from asymptomatic areas detectable only by bone scan to markedly disfiguring lesions. The larger lesions can result in frequent pathologic fractures and impingement on vital nerves. McCune-Albright syndrome is described with café au lait skin pigmentation and autonomous endocrine hyperfunction. In this syndrome, adrenocorticotropic hormone (ACTH)–independent Cushing syndrome results in growth failure and hypertension in infancy, hyperthyroidism typically occurs because of one or more autonomous hyperfunctioning nodules, and growth hormone excess from somatotroph adenomas in the pituitary can occur resulting in gigantism and/or acromegaly. Precocious puberty is a result of gonadotropin-independent autonomous ovarian or testicular function and girls as young as 4 months with McCune-Albright syndrome can have breast development or vaginal bleeding. Excess estrogen can result in a marked advancement in skeletal maturity.

The craniofacial form of fibrous dysplasia (Leontiasis Ossea) occurs in 10% to 25% of patients with the monostotic form and in 50% with the polyostotic form. The frontal, sphenoid, maxillary, and ethmoidal bones are the most commonly affected and involvement of the occipital and temporal bones is less common. Lesions in the maxillofacial bones and skull base may result in neurologic deficits related to narrowed cranial foramina. Cherubism (familial fibrous dysplasia) is an autosomal dominant variant with variable penetrance, which occurs in children and is more severe in males. The findings consist of a broad and protruding jaw with symmetric fibrous dysplasia involving the maxilla. Regression of this form may occur after adolescence.

When assessing for polyostotic fibrous dysplasia with a skeletal survey, total radiation exposure can be decreased if a focused skeletal survey is preceded by a bone scan. The differential considerations are broad and include Paget's disease, fibrous cortical defect/nonossifying fibroma, hyperparathyroidism, giant cell tumor, EG, and hemangioma.

GAUCHER SYNDROME

Often occurring in Ashkenazi Jews, this autosomal, recessive disorder has no gender predilection and results in accumulation of sphingolipids in the reticuloendothelial cells. The result is hepatosplenomegaly and osseous infarcts because of increased intramedullary pressure causing occlusion of the intramedullary veins. In approximately 50% of patients, osteonecrosis may also develop in a subchondral location such as the femoral head, leading to subchondral collapse and early arthrosis. Other osseous findings include flaring in the metaphyses (Erlenmeyer flask deformity), possibly related to packing of Gaucher cells. Affected individuals may also be at increased risk for osteomyelitis. The usual form of the disorder is associated with a normal life span, although infantile and juvenile forms may result in mental retardation and early mortality.

HYPOPHOSPHATEMIC RICKETS (X-LINKED HYPOPHASPHATEMIA)

This X-linked dominant syndrome is caused by a hereditary defect of the renal tubules, which causes decreased reabsorption of phosphate and reduced serum phosphate levels. This decreased reabsorption does not respond to usual amounts of vitamin D. The disorder exhibits rachitic epiphyseal and metaphyseal abnormalities predominantly in the lower limbs. Affected individuals may also demonstrate a generalized bone remodeling abnormality causing short, squat bones.

MARFAN SYNDROME

Marfan syndrome is an inherited connective tissue disorder transmitted as an autosomal dominant trait, which primarily involves the eye, skeleton, and cardiovascular system. Although sporadic cases occur, most cases are owing to autosomal dominant gene with a high degree of penetrance. Affected individuals are characteristically tall and thin with disproportionately long limbs in respect to the trunk, greatest peripherally with the appearance of "arachnodactyly." Ocular abnormalities are common and associated cardiac and vascular abnormalities lead to a shortened life expectancy.

METAPHYSEAL CHONDRODYSPLASIAS

This heterogeneous group of intrinsic dysplasias is characterized by flaring in the metaphyses of the short and long tubular bones (Erlenmeyer flask deformity), while the epiphyses remain normal. The osseous deformity is caused by abnormal, physeal, proliferative,and hypertrophic zones. Hypercalcemia is commonly seen and these disorders are also associated with neutropenia, lymphopenia, immunodeficiency, pancreatic exocrine insufficiency, Hirschsprung's disease, and intestinal malabsorption. The metaphyseal chondrodysplasias are often recognized in early childhood with waddling gait, lumbar lordosis, genu varum, short stature, retardation, joint contractures, and exophthalmic eyes. Radiographic findings include enlarged metaphyses and widened cupped physes (similar to rickets), and coxa vara without associated bowed femur.

Multiple epiphyseal dysplasia is predominantly autosomal dominant in transmission and is related to imperfect articular cartilage that is unable to withstand normal loading. Involvement of the hips must be differentiated from Perthes' disease and unlike Perthes', there is generally symmetric involvement and the acetabulum is often irregular. However, there may be superimposed osteonecrosis (AVN) of the hip. In Schmid type, affected individuals demonstrate mild short stature; greater involvement of the lower extremities with leg pains, varus deformities of the knees and ankles, and genu varum, which may be severe. Jansen type is an extremely rare, progressive disorder with variable range and severity of symptoms, most commonly occurring because of random spontaneous de novo mutations. Pyle disease is a mild form of metaphyseal dysplasia and affected individuals are often tall and asymptomatic. The McKusick type is autosomal recessive and presents with sparse brittle hair, light pigmentation, shortening of long bones, cupped widened metaphyses, and widened costochondral junctions.

Differential consideration primarily includes rickets. Many affected individuals will initially be thought to have a hypophosphatemic vitamin D-resistant rickets, which can lead to the inappropriate administration of vitamin D.

MULTIPLE HEREDITARY EXOSTOSIS (FAMILIAL OSTEOCHONDROMATOSIS)

Multiple hereditary exostosis (familial osteochondromatosis) is an autosomal dominant disorder. The average age at diagnosis is 3 years. Numerous sites are affected simultaneously. Malignant transformation is a significant risk. Chondrosarcoma has been reported in up to 20% of cases in some series. The lesions at greatest risk for sarcomatous degeneration are those occurring near the pelvis, scapula, proximal humerus, proximal femur, and spine. A change in size of the exostosis or onset of pain in an affected skeletally mature individual is cause for concern and investigation. Growth abnormalities caused by joint involvement as well as mass effect on adjacent vessels and nerves can be significant. Multiple cartilaginous exostoses are seen arising from the metaphyses, pointing away from epiphysis, and extending down the diaphysis during growth. The osteochondromas may increase in size and number with growth, but generally become latent at maturity. In over 90% of cases, the distal tibia, proximal tibia, proximal femur, and proximal humerus are involved. Other common sites of involvement include the iliac crests, scapulae, and ribs. Clinical problems include pathologic fracture, pressure of exostosis on surrounding soft tissues, and neurovascular compromise.

NEUROFIBROMATOSIS

This autosomal dominant disorder affects the bones, the nervous system, soft tissue, and the skin. There are two genetic disorders with at least eight different clinical phenotypes. Neurofibromatosis 1 (NF1) is the most common subtype and is referred to as peripheral NF. The characteristics of NF1 include six or more café au lait macules larger than 5 mm in diameter prepubertal and larger than 15 mm postpubertal, two or more neurofibromas or one plexiform neurofibroma, axillary/inguinal freckling, optic glioma, two or more Lisch nodules, a distinctive osseous lesion (sphenoid dysplasia or thinning of the long bone cortex) with or without pseudoarthrosis, and a first-degree relative with NF1. Neurofibromatosis 2 (NF2) or central NF characteristics include bilateral masses of the eighth cranial nerve seen with appropriate imaging techniques (e.g., CT, MRI), a first-degree relative with NF2, and either a unilateral mass of the eighth cranial nerve or two of the following: neurofibroma, meningioma, glioma, schwannoma, or juvenile posterior subcapsular opacity.

The skeletal findings of NF include pseudoarthrosis of the tibia; bowing of the long bones, orbital defects; dysplasia of the sphenoid wings with resulting herniation of the temporal lobe through the enlarged superior orbital fissure and pulsating exophthalmos; thoracic cage asymmetry with flaring or prominence of the inferior ribs; and abnormalities of cortical diaphyseal structure, density, and metaphyseal modeling. The mortality rate is higher than that of healthy population because of increased potential for malignant transformation of diseased tissues and the development of neurofibrosarcoma.

OSTEOGENESIS IMPERFECTA

OI is an autosomal dominant congenital syndrome with increased bone fragility. The sclera ranges from white to blue. Type I OI is the mildest form. Affected individuals generally have no long-bone deformity. Over a lifetime, the numbers of fractures can range from 1 to 60. Affected individuals have a high tolerance for pain. Other possible findings include kyphoscoliosis, hearing loss, premature arcus senilis, and easy bruising. Type II OI is the most severe form and is often lethal. All patients have in utero fractures, which may involve the skull, long bones, and/or vertebrae. The cause of death is usually related to the extreme fragility of the ribs resulting in pulmonary hypoplasia or occasionally cranial injury with CNS hemorrhage. Individuals with type III OI may have joint hyperlaxity, muscle weakness, chronic unremitting bone pain, and skull deformities (e.g., posterior flattening) caused by bone fragility during infancy. In utero fractures are common. Limb shortening and progressive deformities can occur. Type IV OI is not clearly defined. Dentinogenesis imperfecta may be present. Fractures usually begin in infancy, but in utero fractures may occur. The long bones are usually bowed.

OSTEOPETROSIS

This clinical syndrome is characterized by failure of osteoclasts to resorb bone, resulting in skeletal fragility despite increased bone mass. Osseous overgrowth may also cause hematopoietic insufficiency, disturbed tooth eruption, nerve entrapment syndromes, and growth impairment. This is a heterogeneous disorder with different molecular lesions and a range of clinical features. However, all forms share a single pathogenic etiology in the osteoclast. If untreated, infantile osteopetrosis usually results in death by the first decade of life owing to severe anemia, bleeding, or infection. Adults with osteopetrosis are usually asymptomatic and have good long-term survival rates. Radiologic features are usually diagnostic and include generalized osteosclerosis, uniformly sclerotic bones, alternating sclerotic and lucent bands in the iliac wings and near ends of long bones, bone within bone appearance (endobone), thickened and dense skull especially at the base, small and underpneumatized sinuses, and extremely dense vertebrae with alternating bands (Rugger-Jersey sign). Pycnodysostosis is a rare, autosomal, recessive syndrome with similar presentation because of failure of osteoclasts to resorb bone.

SHORT-RIB POLYDACTYLY SYNDROME

This is a group of autosomal recessive lethal skeletal dysplasias with micromelic dwarfism, short-ribbed narrow thorax, and ulnar/fibular polydactyly. The prognosis is poor with death occurring in utero or shortly following birth because of respiratory failure. Four types are described: type I (Saldino-Noonan syndrome), type II (Majewski syndrome), type III (Verma-Naumoff syndrome), and Beemer-Langer syndrome. Other associated findings include poorly ossified vertebral bodies with notchlike ossification defects, cleft lip/palate, widened metaphases (type III), syndactyly, as well as cardiac, GI, and GU malformations. Differential considerations include TD, camptomelic dysplasia, and OI.

THANATOPHORIC DYSPLASIA

This is the most common form of lethal skeletal dysplasia in the neonatal period. This severe rhizomelic (micromelic) dwarfism is most commonly caused by de novo dominant mutations. TD is nearly always lethal in the neonatal period because of respiratory insufficiency secondary to reduced thoracic capacity or related to compression of the brainstem. There are two clinically defined subtypes. TD type 1 is the most common subtype with a normally shaped skull and curved long bones shaped like a telephone receiver. The femurs are most affected. TD type 2 presents with a cloverleaf-shaped skull (kleeblattschadel) and straight femurs. Radiographic findings include narrow chest, small scapula, normal clavicles, short ribs with flared ends, rhizomelic shortening of the long bones, telephone receiver-shaped femurs, flattened vertebral bodies with wide intervertebral spacing, and enlarged skull. The prognosis is poor with death often occurring in utero or shortly after birth because of respiratory failure. Differential considerations include homozygous achondroplasia, short-rib polydactyly syndrome, and achondrogenesis

THROMBOCYTOPENTA-ABSENT RADIUS SYNDROME

This is a rare condition with bilateral radial aplasta and episodes of thrombocytopenta, which begin in the neoratal pertad. There are associated abnormalities in some affected individuals involving the lower extremities, heart, and face. Differential considerations include VACTERL, Holt-Oram syndrome, and Fanconi syndrome.

SUGGESTED READING

Dighe et al. Fetal skeletal dysplasia: an approach to diagnosis with illustrative cases. *Radiographics*. 2008;28:1061-1077.

Fayad LM, Johnson P, Fishman EK. Multidetector CT of musculoskeletal disease in the pediatric patient: principles, techniques, and clinical applications. *Radiographics*. 2005;25(3):603-618.

Schlesinger AE, Hernandez RJ. Diseases of the musculoskeletal system in children: imaging with CT, sonography, and MR. *AJR Am J Roentgenol*. 1992;158:729-741.

Slovis TL. *Caffey's Pediatric Diagnostic Imaging*. 11th ed. Philadelphia, PA, Mosby; 2008.

Taybi H, Lachman RS. *Radiology of Syndromes, Metabolic Disorders, and Skeletal Dysplasias*. 4th ed. Chicago, IL: Year Book; 1996.

QUESTIONS AND ANSWERS

1. What is the most common form of skeletal dysplasia?
   A. Achondroplasia
   B. Thanatophoric dysplasia
   C. Acquired skeletal dysplasia
   D. Osteogenesis imperfecta

   ANSWER: C. Acquired skeletal dysplasias are the most common cause for skeletal dysplasias, more common than all of the congenital skeletal dysplasias combined. Achondroplasia is the most common congenital skeletal dysplasia. Thanatophoric dysplasia is the most common skeletal dysplasia, which is lethal in the neonatal period.

2. An 8 month-old male infant is greater than three standard deviations below normal size with the following radiographic findings: contracted skull base with small foramen magnum, rhizomelic shortening of the limbs with trident hands and brachydactyly, progressive interpedicular narrowing at the lumbar spine, short pedicles, and flat-roofed acetabula. What is the most likely diagnosis?
   A. Achondrogenesis
   B. Chondroectodermal dysplasia
   C. Thanatophoric dysplasia
   D. Achondroplasia

   ANSWER: D. The described findings are classic for achondroplasia. The other congenital skeletal dysplasias listed are generally fatal in the neonatal period. The clinical tetrad of chondroectodermal dysplasia (Ellis-van Creveld syndrome) consisting of chondrodystrophy, polydactyly, ectodermal dysplasia, and cardiac anomalies was not described.

3. What is the most common cause of death in Jeune syndrome?
   A. Craniocervical junction impingement
   B. Intracranial hemorrhage
   C. Respiratory failure
   D. Electrolyte imbalance

   ANSWER: C. The skeletal dysplasias with a narrow thorax (Jeune syndrome, thanatophoric dysplasia, short-limb polydactyly syndrome, etc.) often are often fatal in the neonatal period because of respiratory failure from alveolar hypoventilation caused by impaired chest expansion.

4. What is the most common etiology of rickets?
   A. Vitamin D deficiency
   B. Low dietary intake of calcium
   C. Low dietary intake of phosphorus
   D. Decreased renal tubular reuptake of phosphorus

   ANSWER: A. Vitamin D deficiency is the most common cause of rickets. Low dietary intake of calcium and phosphorus may also cause rickets. Decreased renal tubular uptake of phosphorus is the cause of hypophosphatemic rickets (X-linked hypophosphatemia).

5. Which of these fractures is most likely to result in asymmetric growth?
   A. Displacement of the distal radius epiphysis through the growth plate
   B. Fracture through the distal femoral physis extending through the metaphysis
   C. Fracture through the lateral distal tibial physis extending through the epiphysis

D. Lateral condylar physeal fracture extending through the capitulotrochlear groove

ANSWER: D. A lateral condylar physeal fracture extending lateral to the trochlea through the capitulotrochlear groove is a SH type IV fracture. SH type IV and V fractures have the highest risk of growth disturbance. The remaining fractures are types I to III.

6. What region of the bone is usually initially involved in pediatric osteomyelitis?
   A. Epiphysis
   B. Metaphysis
   C. Physeal plate
   D. Diaphysis

   ANSWER: B. Pediatric osteomyelitis most commonly begins in the metaphysis because of rich vascular supply and slow blood flow in this region. The epiphysis may be involved up until ossification occurs at approximately 18 months of age.

7. A patient with sickle cell disease presents with osteomyelitis. What is the most likely organism?
   A. *Staphylococcus aureus*
   B. *Streptococcus pyogenes*
   C. *Pseudomonas aeruginosa*
   D. *Salmonella*

   ANSWER: A. Although Salmonella osteomyelitis is frequently associated with sickle cell disease, the most common etiology for osteomyelitis remains *Staphylococcus aureus.*

8. Which of these fractures is most characteristic of nonaccidental trauma?
   A. Linear skull fracture
   B. Clavicular fracture
   C. Posterior rib fractures
   D. Complex skull fracture

   ANSWER: C. Highly suspicious fractures for abuse include posterior rib fractures, long bone fractures in nonambulatory children, metaphyseal corner fractures, scapular fractures, and sternal fractures. Fractures with moderate specificity include complex skull fractures. Fractures with low specificity include linear skull fractures and clavicle fractures.

9. Which of the following lesions should be biopsied?
   A. Painful lucent lesion with calcifications in rings and arcs
   B. Sclerotic cortical lesion with a central nidus and pain at night relieved by aspirin
   C. Well-defined proximal tibial, eccentric, lucent lesion with a sclerotic margin
   D. Cartilage-capped exostosis that grows away from the joint with open physes

   ANSWER: A. An enchondroma cannot be differentiated radiographically from a low-grade cartilaginous neoplasm and pain suggests the possibility of low-grade chondrosarcoma. A sclerotic lesion with a central nidus suggests an osteoid osteoma. A well-defined lucent lesion in the proximal tibia likely represents a nonossifying fibroma. A cartilage-capped exostosis growing away from the joint is consistent with an osteochondroma and the possibility of sarcomatous degeneration is raised with continued growth after skeletal maturity.

10. Which of the following does *not* increase the risk for developmental dysplasia of the hip?
    A. Breech delivery
    B. Male infant
    C. Oligohydramnios
    D. Family history of DDH

    ANSWER: B. High-risk patients include those with a family history of developmental dysplasia of the hip, breech delivery, oligohydramnios, as well as neuromuscular and foot abnormalities. Females are affected more commonly than males.

101 PEDIATRIC CHEST

Richard S. Martin and Christopher J. Guion

NEONATAL CHEST

TUBES AND LINES

Evaluating the placement of all the various support devices is an important function of the pediatric radiologist. Some line placement is unique to the neonatal period.

Both the umbilical arterial and venous catheters enter through the umbilicus. The course of the umbilical artery catheter is from the umbilical artery to the internal iliac artery (hypogastric artery) to the aorta. The tip of the catheter can be left high (T6–T9) or low (L3–L4). These positions are chosen so as to avoid the origins of the celiac axis, superior mesenteric artery, and the renal arteries. The course of the umbilical venous catheter is from the umbilical vein to the left portal vein, then through the ductus venosus to the inferior vena cava to the right atrium. The correct position of the tip is above the right diaphragm projected over the right atrium. Beware of common malpositions of the umbilical venous catheter. The catheter tip overlying the right upper quadrant and directed toward the patient's right indicates right portal vein placement. An abrupt caudad reversal of the catheter below the level of the diaphragm indicates middle hepatic vein placement. Advancement beyond the right atrium frequently crosses through a patent foramen ovale into the left atrium. From the left atrium, the tip can actually enter a pulmonary vein.

Extracorporeal membrane oxygenation (ECMO) is used as pulmonary bypass. ECMO is a therapy of last resort for patients with a reversible disease and a chance of survival. There are two forms: venovenous and arteriovenous. With venovenous ECMO, a single, large cannula is seen with its tip overlying the right atrium. Blood is removed from the right atrium, travels through a membrane oxygenator, and is returned to the venous system. With the arteriovenous form, two cannulas are seen. The arterial catheter is placed into the right carotid artery with its tip overlying the aortic arch. The venous catheter is placed via the right internal jugular vein to the right atrium. The right common carotid artery and right internal jugular vein are sacrificed during arteriovenous ECMO.

In general, the endotracheal tube tip should be placed in the center of the trachea halfway between the inferior margins of the clavicles and the carina. In the term, newborn ideal endotracheal tube placement equates to 2 cm above the carina. Keep in mind that in this early stage of life, the trachea is quite short. Helpful phone calls to the intensive care unit regarding tube malposition should be reserved for a tube tip terminating above the thoracic inlet, within the main bronchi, or an esophageal intubation.

AIR LEAK IN THE NEONATE

Air leak is used as a general term to describe rupture of the alveolus or pulmonary interstitium, generally resulting from an increase in alveolar pressure with some type of air block. The term includes pneumothorax, pneumomediastinum, pneumopericardium, and pulmonary interstitial emphysema. Infants are imaged supine; therefore, pleural air in a pneumothorax collects anteriorly and medially. A pleural line is often very difficult to see. The majority of neonatal pneumothoraces are noted medially. They may appear as a lucency along the cardiac margin. One should suspect a pneumothorax when there is a hyperlucent lung or a "deep sulcus sign." Pneumomediastinum can be recognized when there is uplifting of the thymus causing a "sail sign." Cross-table lateral or decubitus imaging may help to differentiate an anterior pneumothorax from a pneumomediastinum. On cross-table lateral imaging, air will often surround the thymus, while on decubitus imaging, air will rise and outline the pleural surface. With pneumomediastinum, air can appear to surround the heart, creating the "continuous diaphragm sign." In pneumopericardium, air outlines the heart. The air is limited superiorly by the pericardial reflection of the great vessels.

Pulmonary interstitial emphysema results from barotrauma, which causes alveolar tears. Air then tracks into the perivascular spaces and lymphatics. Pulmonary interstitial emphysema is seen as well-defined, linear, and bubblelike lucencies, which can be either focal or diffuse. These lucencies may coalesce into cystic air collections. Findings are typically transient but serve as a warning for possible impending pneumothorax or pneumomediastinum.

PULMONARY PATHOLOGY ASSOCIATED WITH THE NEONATE

Respiratory distress syndrome (RDS) (also referred to as hyaline membrane disease or surfactant deficiency) is a disease of the premature infant caused by the inability of the premature type II pneumocytes to produce enough surfactant. Surfactant coats the alveoli and lowers the surface tension. A deficiency or lack of surfactant leads to alveolar collapse and decreased pulmonary compliance. Classically, the chest radiograph demonstrates low lung volumes and diffuse, bilateral granular opacities. Since the larger bronchi do not collapse, air bronchograms are visualized. Severity is inversely proportional to gestational age. RDS is rarely seen after 36 weeks gestation. Treatment is with intratracheal administration of exogenous surfactant. Possible complications of surfactant therapy include pulmonary hemorrhage and increased risk of developing a patent ductus arteriosus.

Bronchopulmonary dysplasia (BPD) (also referred to as chronic lung disease of infancy) is a common complication of prematurity and was initially described by Northway et al. as having four stages. Because of changes in therapy, the four stages are not typically seen today. Mechanical ventilation and oxygen toxicity are felt to be the cumulative agents in the development of BPD. Premature infants requiring prolonged ventilatory support are most at risk for developing BPD. By the beginning of the third week of life, hazy densities are seen throughout the lungs. Over weeks to months, coarse lung markings, bubbly lucencies, and areas of asymmetric aeration develop.

Transient tachypnea of the newborn (TTN) (also referred to as retained fetal fluid and wet lung disease) is a condition seen in near-term, term, and postterm infants. The condition results from delayed clearance of the fetal pulmonary fluid. Conventional wisdom holds that the thoracic squeeze during passage through the birth canal helps expel this fluid from the lungs. Therefore, infants delivered by cesarean section are at increased risk. This condition is also seen following maternal sedation and also in infants of diabetic mothers. The typical clinical course is the onset of respiratory distress by 6 hours after birth, peaking of symptoms at around 24 hours after birth, and resolution of symptoms by 48 to 72 hours after birth. Radiographically, a proximal humeral head ossification center is seen in these term or postterm infants. There are prominent interstitial markings, indistinct pulmonary vasculature, fluid in the fissures, and pleural effusions. The heart size is usually normal.

Meconium aspiration syndrome is seen in the term or postterm infant. Meconium is usually passed during the first 24 hours after birth. Intrapartum or intrauterine aspiration of meconium can result from advanced gestational age, fetal distress, preeclampsia, maternal drug abuse, and placental insufficiency, among others causes. The thick meconium causes airway obstruction, surfactant insufficiency, and chemical pneumonitis. The radiograph demonstrates areas of asymmetric hyperinflation, as well as, atelectasis. "Ropey" perihilar densities can be seen. As these are term or postterm infants, the proximal humeral head ossification center will be present. Air leak phenomena including pneumothorax or pneumomediastinum can be seen. Severe cases may require ECMO. Fatalities still occur from this condition.

Persistent pulmonary hypertension of the neonate (also referred to as persistent fetal circulation of the neonate) is a physiologic condition in which there is continuation of high pulmonary vascular resistance and failure of the normal transition to low pulmonary vascular resistance. Persistent pulmonary hypertension of the neonate occurs as an idiopathic primary form and a secondary form related to hypoxemia (seen with meconium aspiration syndrome, congenital diaphragmatic hernia, and neonatal pneumonia). Right-to-left shunting may occur through the foramen ovale or ductus arteriosus. The chest radiograph may be normal or show pulmonary oligemia. There can be mild cardiomegaly and hepatomegaly.

Patent ductus arteriosus results from delayed closure of the ductus arteriosus. The normal ductus arteriosus typically closes by day 2 after birth, but it may remain patent in hypoxic infants. Initially, there is right-to-left shunting, but as the pulmonary vascular resistance begins dropping at the end of the first week, a left-to-right shunt develops. The radiograph shows an increase in heart size and prominent pulmonary vascularity. The vessels start to become ill-defined as the interstitial edema increases. The prostaglandin inhibitor, indomethacin, is used to close the ductus. Transcatheter occlusion or surgery may be required.

Chylothorax is the most common cause of a large pleural fluid collection in the newborn period. Initially, lymph accumulates in the pleural space, becoming chylous after the ingestion of lipids in milk or formula. Most affected infants will have developed symptoms by the end of the first week of life. The majority of cases occur on the right; however, bilateral cases are encountered. There is a male gender predilection. While the etiology is usually unknown, thoracic duct rupture is the presumed causative agent. Chest radiograph demonstrates a pleural fluid collection. In extreme cases, there is complete opacification of the hemithorax with contralateral shift of the mediastinal contents. Widening of the ipsilateral ribs may be seen. Treatment is by thoracentesis.

Congenital Tracheobronchial Abnormalities

Tracheal atresia is a rare condition in which there is usually absence of the entire trachea. The bronchi or, if present, the distal trachea connects to the esophagus. Chest radiograph may show absence of the tracheal air column.

Tracheal stenosis can be congenital or acquired. The rare congenital form is because of complete cartilaginous rings. Congenital tracheal stenosis may be either focal or diffuse. The VACTERL association (Vertebral anomalies, Anal atresia, Cardiac anomalies, Tracheo-esophageal fistula, Renal anomalies, and Limb anomalies) may be seen in these patients. The acquired form may result from intubation or traumatic suctioning.

Bronchial atresia is most often seen in lobar or segmental bronchi. There is an upper lobe predilection. In the neonatal period, a fluid density "mass" is seen in one of the upper lobes. There is an association with other bronchopulmonary foregut malformations.

A tracheal bronchus (also referred to as a pig bronchus) is present in a small percentage of the population. In this condition, the entire right upper lobe segment or the apical segment of the right upper lobe is supplied by a bronchus arising directly from the trachea. Complications include recurrent pneumonia, atelectasis, and/or air trapping within the portion of the right upper lobe supplied by the ectopic bronchus.

Congenital Pulmonary Anomalies

In pulmonary agenesis, there is complete absence of the lung. An equal frequency of occurrence is seen between the left and right lung. Right lung agenesis has a higher association with cardiac anomalies than does left-sided agenesis. In cases of true agenesis, no bronchus is present on the affected side. In cases of aplasia, a small atretic bronchus is present. Chest radiograph reveals a small, opaque hemithorax with mediastinal shift toward the affected side. In addition to cardiac anomalies, there are multiple other associated anomalies, including renal agenesis and imperforate anus.

There is a specific form of right lobar agenesis/aplasia called scimitar syndrome or venolobar syndrome. An abnormal pulmonary vein drains into the superior vena cava, creating the so-called scimitar shadow seen in the right chest. The right pulmonary artery is either small or absent. There is systemic arterial supply to the abnormal lung from the aorta. There may be absence of the inferior vena cava.

Pulmonary hypoplasia classically involves the right lung. There is typically a small or absent pulmonary artery. The chest film reveals a small hemithorax with mediastinal shift toward the affected side. In classic right-sided pulmonary hypoplasia, the lateral view demonstrates a soft-tissue stripe anterior and/or posterior to the lung. This stripe is created by extrapleural areolar soft tissue. This areolar tissue also leads to a loss of the right heart border on the frontal view.

Congenital lobar emphysema is a condition in which there is progressive hyperexpansion of a lobe. The left upper lobe is most commonly affected, followed by the right middle lobe, followed by the right upper lobe. The lower lobes are much less commonly involved. The etiology remains elusive. While there is over distension of a lobe, no true alveolar wall destruction occurs. Initially, a soft-tissue density is seen in the affected lobe secondary to fetal fluid. As the fetal fluid begins to clear, progressive hyperexpansion of the lobe is seen. Treatment is by lobectomy.

Congenital cystic adenomatoid malformation (also referred to as congenital pulmonary airway malformation) is an intrapulmonary mass consisting of a proliferation of hamartomatous tissue. These masses have both solid and cystic components. The cysts usually communicate with the tracheobronchial tree. There would appear to be no lobar predilection, as upper and lower lobe preference have been reported by different authors. The commonly used classification system is based on cyst size at imaging. In common parlance, there are three types (Table 18-1). Type I lesions have at least one dominant cyst greater than 2 cm in diameter. Type II lesions contain numerous small cysts of more uniform size measuring up to 2 cm in diameter. Type III lesions are the least common and are solid in appearance, being composed of microcysts. Type I lesions are rarely associated with other congenital malformations. Type II lesions are associated with other congenital malformation in approximately 50% of the cases. The prognosis in type III congenital cystic adenomatoid malformation is poor. Depending on the age at imaging (presence or absence of retained fetal fluid) and the type, there is a varied appearance. The lesion can be cystic, mixed cystic and solid, or solid. These lesions have the potential for malignancy in the form of rhabdomyosarcoma and are therefore resected.

Pulmonary sequestration is a congenital mass of abnormal pulmonary tissue, which receives its blood supply from the systemic circulation and has no normal communication with the bronchial tree. The systemic arterial supply is from the aorta. There are two forms of sequestration: intralobar and extralobar. Differentiation of the two forms cannot be reliably made by imaging. In general, the characteristics of intralobar sequestration include no separate pleural covering, venous drainage by way of pulmonary veins, the vast majority being in the lower lobe (left greater than right), and an uncommon association with other anomalies. Extralobar sequestration has its own pleural covering, the majority are left-sided, and venous drainage is to the azygous. Diagnosis is earlier than the intralobar form. Extralobar sequestration has a greater than 50% association with other anomalies. Radiographically, the lesion first appears as a radiopaque mass. Once infection has occurred gas may be present, giving a multiloculated cystic appearance. In both types, the lesion is most commonly seen in the left lower lobe.

Bronchogenic cysts occur with equal frequency within the lung parenchyma and the mediastinum. They initially appear as smoothly marginated, thin-walled, homogeneous masses of soft-tissue density. Once infected, gas may be seen within the lesion.

PEDIATRIC CHEST INFECTION

Growth of the airway occurs throughout fetal development and for years after birth. The development of the terminal bronchi has occurred by the 16th week of gestation. The aveoli developes between the 16th and 24th weeks of gestation and continues through 8 years of age, although the majority have developed by 3 years. Although the tracheal cartilage is developed at birth the posterior noncartilaginous aspect of the trachea, the pars membranacea, may allow for compression of the posterior tracheal air column. This allows for the appearance of near AP collapse of the trachea in a crying infant with expiration. On inspiration the tracheal air column should be easily recognized on chest radiographs. The course of the trachea may change with inspiration and expiration in infants, buckling away from the aortic arch with expiration.

LARYNGEAL AND SUBGLOTTIC INFLAMMATORY DISEASE

Croup occurs often with parainfluenza virus and causes subglottic edema and narrowing. The term encompasses laryngotracheobronchitis. It is common in young children from 6 months to 3 years of age. Tracheal bacteria infections may cause crouplike symptoms and are frequently staphylococcal in origin. Epiglottitis is associated with *Haemophilus influenzae* type B. This often occurs during winter months and predominately affects the 3- to 6-year-old age group. Swelling of the epiglottis and aryepiglottic folds may cause life-threatening airway obstruction, whereas croup is less likely life threatening. Retropharyngeal hemorrhage caused by trauma may have a similar appearance. Foreign bodies most commonly produce more distal bronchial occlusion rather than upper airway obstruction. These entities may be exacerbated in smaller children because of the small caliber of the upper airway.

Masses within the subglottic airway of young children may be secondary to manipulation such as intubation or tracheostomy causing granulation tissue. Entities such as airway papillomatosis are secondary to infection with papilloma virus, which can be acquired at birth. Soft-tissue mass such as subglottic hemangioma may involute similarly to cutaneous hemangiomas over several years.

AGE-RELATED RESPIRATORY INFECTION

Respiratory infections affect about one-quarter of children younger than 2 years of age. Several respiratory infections are age related. Tracheobronchitis and bronchiolitis peak at 6 to 12 months of age. Entities such as cytomegalovirus may be acquired in utero. Infectious agents such as group B streptococcus and chlamydia may be acquired at birth. Respiratory synsytial virus may cause bronchiolitis in neonates and young infants. Parainfluenza and croup are more commonly seen in 2- to 3-year-old. *Mycoplasma pneumoniae* is more common in schools-age children. Many radiologists note it is difficult to differentiate bacterial and viral pneumonia, as there is considerable overlap in appearance. Some patterns may be helpful. Central parabronchial edema and atelectasis is more suggestive of a viral etiology or entities such as mycoplasma or chlamydia infection. Diffuse fluffy infiltrates, which extend to the lung periphery or lobar consolidations, are more commonly seen with bacterial infection.

Recurring pneumonia should suggest evaluation for chronic conditions. Cystic fibrosis, immunodeficiency congenital or acquired, and conditions such as chronic granulomatous disease, asthma, asplenia, or sickle cell disease with functional asplenia may be considered. Congenital anomalies such as pulmonary sequestration, congenital cystic adenomatoid malformation, or anomalous bronchi are also in the differential diagnosis. Extrinsic compression by mass or intrinsic obstruction such as foreign body needs to be excluded (Table 101-1).

VIRAL DISEASE

Viral bronchiolitis continues to be one of the most common indications for imaging in children with airways disease. Hyperinflation with peribronchial edema and areas of subsegmental atelectasis are common. Hilar lymphadenopathy may be present and does not have the

TABLE 101-1 Respiratory Infection

Pneumonia in newborns	Group B *Streptococci*
	Escherichia coli and *Klebsiella pneumoniae*
	Chlamydia
Viral	RSV, influenza, parainfluenza, adenoviruses, myxo- and paramyxoviruses
	Epstein Barr virus, HIV, Varicella-Zoster, measles
	Cytomegalovirus (CMV) and Varicella-Zoster, consider immunocompromised patients
Bacterial	*Streptococcus pneumonia* (most common), *Haemophilus influenzae, Hemolytic streptococcus, Staphylococcus aureus*, gram-negative bacilli, *Mycobacterium tuberculosis*, atypical mycobacteria, *Legionella*, Actinomyces, Nocardia
	Pseudomonas, *Haemophilus influenzae*, and Aspergillus, consider in children with respiratory compromise such as cystic fibrosis
Nonviral, nonbacterial	*Mycoplasma pneumoniae*
	Chlamydia pneumoniae
Fungal	*Blastomycosis dermatitidis*
	Histoplasma capsulatum
	Coccidioidomycosis
	Aspergillus, candida, consider immunocomprised patient

ominous significance when seen in the adult setting. The etiology of upper respiratory infection is viral in 95% of preschool children younger than 5 years of age. Although viruses are still most common in school-age children older than 5 years, *M. pneumoniae* may be seen in up to 30% of cases and streptococcal pneumoniae has been seen more frequently. Pleural effusions are relatively uncommon in viral lower airways disease. Respiratory syncytial virus is highly contagious and more severe in children younger than 2 years of age. It accounts for 60% of respiratory infections below the age of 5 years and is known to peak in the late fall and winter months. Respiratory infection associated with measles is less common in developed countries with immunization. Children with measles pneumoniae may be prone to superimposed infection with *H. influenzae*, *Staphylococcus aureus*, and *Streptococcus pyogenes*.

M. pneumoniae has a variable appearance and may be reticular nodular, interstitial, or involve a single lobe, making it difficult to distinguish from viral or bacterial infections. Hilar lymphadenopathy may be common and pleural effusion is uncommon. Pneumonia associated with cytomegalovirus and Varicella Zoster commonly affects immunosuppressed patients.

BACTERIAL PNEUMONIA

Round pneumonia may appear as a well-defined, round opacification and may simulate a mass but should not cause mass effect on adjacent structures. This is often seen in up to 8 years of age and is commonly *S. pneumoniae*. *S. aureus* and *H. influenza* are also commonly seen. *Pneumocystis carinii* and *pertussis* would be atypical. In this age group, the collateral pathways of air circulation (channels of Lambert and Pores of Kohn) are not well developed. This decreases the spread of infection giving the "round" appearance. Although the differential diagnosis may include entities such as foregut duplication cyst, or even neuroblastoma in the posterior mediastinum, these may cause mass effect. Pneumonic complications may result, depending upon the severity and distribution. Abscess, pneumatocele, cavitary necrosis, or bronchopleural fistulas may occur. Cavitary necrosis is currently most commonly seen with *S. pneumoniae*. A retrocardiac opacity needs to be differentiated from a hiatal hernia or entities such as foregut malformation, or neurogenic tumors.

In bacterial infection, pleural effusions are seen in approximately 20% of *S. pneumoniae* and are more common in younger children. Pleural effusions may be seen in up to 80% of *S. aureus* pneumonia. Suppurative complications of pneumonia may require CT to help differentiate complex fluid collections, cavitary necrosis, lung abscess, or pericarditis. Lung infection associated with a chest wall mass may occur with both infection and neoplasm. Differential may include such as actinomycosis, blastomycosis and tuberculosis, or neoplastic lesions such as Ewing sarcoma, rhabdomyosarcoma, or PNET. Rib osteomyelitis may be seen with both bacterial infection and tuberculosis. In cases of multiple lung abscesses, septic emboli must be considered as well as children with aspiration and/or periodontal disease.

TUBERCULOSIS

Tuberculosis is seeing a comeback in children with decreased immunizations and resistant strains. It is still a major cause of morbidity and mortality in developing countries and may complicate HIV infection. Primary tuberculosis in children is acquired through droplet infection usually from adults with cavitary disease. Children younger than age 5 are more susceptible and a more disseminated form is seen in children younger than 2 years of age. Primary tuberculosis may heal with calcified hilar lymphadenopathy (Ranke complex). Bronchial compression from adjacent lymphadenopathy may be seen. Both pleura effusion and thin walled cavitation is common. Rib and chest wall involvement is usually from hematogenous spread rather than direct extension. Hematogenous dissemination is most common in the 3 to 6 months age group. Tuberculous meningitis is common. Pneumonia associated with lymphadenopathy should raise the concern for TB testing. CT is more sensitive than plain radiographs for demonstrating findings of primary tuberculosis.

Histoplasmosis may cause granulomatous disease simulating pulmonary tuberculosis. It is a fungus found in the soil most commonly in the Mississippi river Delta and South Western United States. Long-standing infection, which crosses lung and pleura to involve chest wall should raise the specter of other fungal entities such as blastomycosis, actinomycosis, and aspergillosis.

SUGGESTED READING

Berrocal T, Madrid C, Novo S, et al. Congenital anomalies of the tracheobronchial tree, lung, and mediastinum: embryology, radiology, and pathology. *Radiographics.* 2004;24(1):17.

Chernick V. *Disorders of the Respiratory Tract in Children.* Philadelphia, PA: W.B Saunders Company; 1990;(1):3-18.

Ferguson EC, Krishnamurthy R, Oldham SA. Classic imaging signs of congenital cardiovascular abnormalities. *Radiographics.* 2007;27(5):1323-1334.

John SD, Ramanathan J, Swischuk LE. Spectrum of clinical and radiographic findings in pediatric mycoplasma pneumonia. *Radiographics.* 2001;21(1):121-131.

Lobo L. The neonatal chest. *Eur J Radiol.* 2006;60(2):152-158.

Northway WH Jr., Rosan RC. Radiographic features of oxygen toxicity in the newborn: bronchopulmonary dysplasia. *Radiology.* 1968;91:49-58.

Rand T, Kirchner L, Puig S, et al. Lines and tubes in neonatal intensive care patients. *Radiologe.* 2000;40(1):52-57.

Rosado-de-Christenson ML, Frazier AA, Stocker JT, et al. From the archives of the AFIP. Extralobar sequestration: radiologic-pathologic correlation. *Radiographics.* 1993;13(2):425-441.

Shady K, Siegel MJ, Glazer HS. CT of focal pulmonary masses in childhood. *Radiographics.* 1992;12(3):505-514.

QUESTIONS AND ANSWERS

1. Which of the following is most likely to communicate with the tracheobronchial tree?
   A. Sequestration
   B. Congenital lobar emphysema
   C. Bronchogenic cyst
   D. Abscess

   ANSWER: B. Congenital lobar emphysema communicates with the bronchial tree at birth. Bronchogenic cysts may develop a communication with the airway caused by infection. Sequestration and abscess do not have a normal connection to the bronchial tree.

2. Concerning umbilical arterial catheter placement, which of the following is *incorrect*?
   A. Line placement between T6 and T9
   B. Line placement between T9 and L2
   C. Line placement between L3 and L4

   ANSWER: B. The UAC is placed either high (T6–9) or low (L3–4) in order to avoid the origin of the celiac axis, superior mesenteric artery, and the renal arteries.

3. Pulmonary interstitial emphysema serves as a warning for what possible impending condition?
   A. Necrotizing enterocolitis
   B. Heart failure
   C. Pneumothorax
   D. Pneumonia

   ANSWER: C. PIE serves as a warning for possible impending pneumothorax or pneumomediastinum.

4. What is the typical clinical course of transient tachypnea of the newborn?
   A. Onset of respiratory distress by 6 hours after birth, peaking of symptoms around 24 hours after birth, and resolution by 48 to 72 hours
   B. Onset of respiratory distress by 24 hours after birth, peaking of symptoms around 48 hours after birth, and resolution by 4 days
   C. Onset of respiratory distress by 48 hours after birth, peaking of symptoms around 3 days after birth, and resolution by 1 week

   ANSWER: A. Transient tachypnea of the newborn is also reformed to as retained fetal fluid or wet lung disease and is seen in postterm infants. It is because of a delayed clearance of fluid with onset of respiratory distress within 8 hours of birth, peaking around 1 day, and resolution by 48 to 72 hours.

5. What is the most common cause of a large pleural fluid collection in the newborn period?
   A. CHF
   B. Congenital lobar emphysema
   C. Pneumonia
   D. Chylothorax

   ANSWER: D. Chylothorax is the most common cause of a large pleural effusion in the newborn period, usually within the first week of life. It is usually right-sided but can be bilateral.

6. A 6-week-old infant presents with fever, hyperinflation of the lungs, and peribronchial cuffing. What is the most likely diagnosis?
   A. Chlamydia
   B. *Parainfluenza*
   C. *Staphylococcus pneumoniae*
   D. *Streptococcus pneumoniae*
   E. *Mycoplasma pneumoniae*

   ANSWER: B. Viral pneumonia and parainfluenza commonly present with the above symptoms in this age group. Effusion may occur. Consolidation is rare. Bacterial pneumonia in the neonate is often caused by *Streptococcal pneumoniae*.

7. What causes membernous croup?
   A. *Staphylococcus aureus*
   B. Hematolysis influenza
   C. Parainfluenza
   D. Streptococcus
   E. Pseudomonas

   ANSWER: A. Membranous croup or exudative tracheitis is a bacterial infection, most commonly *staphylococcal* in etiology. Membranous croup is an uncommon bacterial inflammation involving the larynx, trachea, and bronchi. Patients are generally older and sicker than children with viral croup. Viral croup or laryngotracheobronchitis is commonly parainfluenza.

8. What is the most common cause of round pneumonia in children?
   A. *S. aureus*
   B. *Streptococcus*

C. Pseudomonas
D. Klebsiella

ANSWER: B. *Streptococcus* and *staphylococcus* are both causes of round pneumonia. *Streptococcus* is more common in the young age ranging from 1 to 3 years. Round pneumonia appears round because of poorly developed collateral pathways (pores of Kohn and channels of Lambert). With time, initial round pneumonia may develop in more typical consolidation.

102 PEDIATRIC CARDIOVASCULAR DISEASE

Eric J. Howell

CHEST RADIOGRAPHY

HEART SIZE

The heart size is often difficult to assess on the frontal image because of the relatively large thymus in infants and small children and poor inspiration, as a result, the cardiothoracic ratio is of little use. In older children, this ratio is usually less than 50%. The lateral view is more useful in evaluation of cardiac size; posterior cardiac margin approaching the spine suggests cardiac enlargement. Gross cardiomegaly is seen in volume overloading of the heart, as in severe valve regurgitation (Ebstein anomaly), cardiomyopathy, pericardial disease, and mediastinal masses.

PULMONARY VASCULATURE

Pulmonary vasculature is also often difficult to assess considering the frequent supine positioning and expiratory phase. Normally, the pulmonary artery branches are the same size as the accompanying bronchi. The right descending pulmonary artery should be the same or less than the width of the trachea, and no pulmonary vessels should be seen in the peripheral one-third of the lung. Normal vasculature can be present in valvular defects without shunting, in small-to-moderate shunts, and in balanced complex congenital heart disease.

Increased vasculature is seen in pulmonary to systemic shunts greater than 2:1. Decreased pulmonary vasculature is seen in cyanotic lesions with right-to-left shunt. Pulmonary venous hypertension is another pattern recognized by hyperinflation of the lungs, perihilar vessels that are poorly defined, septal lines, and frank alveolar edema. Asymmetrical pulmonary flow can be seen with pulmonary arterial stenosis or hypoplasia and disturbances in ventilation with secondary vasoconstriction.

AORTA

Identifying the side and size of the aorta is often difficult secondary to overlap from the thymus. The trachea usually deviates away from the side of the aortic arch, which may help. A prominent ascending aorta is usually abnormal in children.

SITUS

The position of the stomach and liver should be assessed on chest radiographs when there is concern for congenital heart disease.

BONE ABNORMALITIES

Abnormalities such as scoliosis, segmentation anomalies, and rib anomalies are often associated with congenital heart disease. Rib notching is present in older children having coarctation of the aorta and intercostal collateral vessels. A bifid manubrial ossification center may be present in Down syndrome (80% trisomy 21, 20% normal children).

CT ANGIOGRAPHY

ADVANTAGES

CT offers the best global assessment of intrathoracic structures including the lungs and airways. Sedation is less often needed relative to MR vascular imaging; CT can be performed with support devices such as pacemakers. Images can be reconstructed in multiple planes.

DISADVANTAGES

CT results in relatively high radiation doses to the pediatric patient. CTA has a similar dose to routine chest CT; however, functional evaluations using gated CT have a greater dose than limited diagnostic catheter angiography or nongated CTA. CT also requires use of intravenous contrast, which carries a small risk of significant adverse reactions.

CONTRAST

Low osmolar, nonionic iodine, 300 mgI/mL is typically used. The dosage is 1.5 mL/kg with maximum total volume 125 to 150 mL. If additional scanning is needed, the study can be repeated with an additional 1 to 1.5 mL/kg.

The suggested rates of administration are 1.5 mL/s with a 24-gauge angiocath, 2.0 to 2.5 mL/s with a 22-gauge angiocath, and 3.0 to 4.0 mL/s with a 20-gauge angiocath. The use of a power injector is preferable for optimal bolus formation. The timing of the delay in scanning relative to contrast administration is empiric in small children, usually 6 to 7 seconds after the onset of contrast administration. For large children, the delay is 50 seconds or alternatively, bolus tracking may be used.

SCAN TECHNIQUE

The highest possible number of detector rows and the thinnest reconstructed slice thickness should be employed. The pitch is 1.3 to 1.75. The tube current varies depending on patient size and as many units automatically modulated base on patient thickness. The peak kilovoltage is 80 kVp for infants, 100 kVp for young children, and 120 kVp for older children.

MAGNETIC RESONANCE IMAGING

FUNCTIONAL ASSESSMENT

MR is used to assess the ventricles, specifically end-diastolic and end-systolic volumes, ejection fraction, stroke volumes, cardiac output, cardiac index, and shunt sizes.

TECHNIQUES

A combination of spin echo and gradient echo imaging is used to assess morphology. Recently, double inversion recovery morphologic imaging with flowing blood having signal void has been used. Another common technique used is gadolinium-enhanced magnetic resonance angiography with time of flight SPGR sequence. The steady-state free procession sequence (SSFP) is used for evaluating cardiac motion and function.

INDICATIONS

Most lesions are not evaluated with MR initially. Postop MR can be useful to assess the repair of transposition and evaluate various shunts (Glenn and Fontan) for patency or stenosis. MR has been used to evaluate right ventricular arrhythmogenic dysplasia. It can help demonstrate myocardial fat deposition, focal myocardial thinning, and microaneurysm formation. Wall motion abnormalities are also well shown by MR. The evaluation of the peripheral pulmonary arteries, which is difficult by echocardiography, is well shown by MR. MR is also a useful tool in diagnosing aortic abnormalities, such as coarctation, aneurysm, and vascular rings.

PATHOLOGY

ACYANOTIC CONGENITAL HEART DISEASE

All left-to-right shunts have increased pulmonary blood flow (Table 102-1).

TABLE 102-1 Acyanotic Congenital Heart Disease

Atrial septal defect (ASD)	Right-sided enlargement; secundum defect most common
Ventricular septal defect (VSD)	Right-sided and left atrial enlargement; membranous most common
Patent ductus arteriosus (PDA)	Right-sided, left atrium and aortic enlargement
Endocardial cushion defect (ECD)	Right-sided enlargement; trisomy 21
Aortic stenosis	Valvular most common
Aortic coarctation	"3" sign; associated with Turner syndrome
Pseudocoarctation	High aortic arch
Cor triatriatum	Ventricular enlargement with edema
Pulmonic stenosis	Dilatation of main and left pulmonary artery with right ventricular hypotrophy
Absence of the pulmonic valve	Dilatation of main and right pulmonary; Tetralogy

Atrial Septal Defect

With atrial septal defect, there is right-sided enlargement, but no left atrial enlargement. The secundum defect at the foramen ovale is the most common type, accounting for approximately 80% of ASD. The primum defect, which is below the foramen ovale, is less common, accounting for approximately 10% of cases. The sinus venosus type, posterior to the foramen ovale, accounts for the remaining 10%. Sinus venous type ASD is associated with partial anomalous pulmonary venous return of the right lung.

Ventricular Septal Defect

In ventricular septal defects, there is right-sided enlargement and left atrial enlargement. The membranous type is the most common (75%–80%), followed by muscular (10%–15%), and supracristal or conal (5%–10%). VSD may be isolated or associated with other complex congenital heart malformations.

Patent Ductus Arteriosus

There is an increased incidence of PDA in premature infants, infants with asphyxia, and congenital rubella. Radiographic findings include enlargement of the aorta and left atrium, in addition to right-sided enlargement. Indomethacin can be used to treat this defect. Transcatheter closure can be used for small-to-moderate lesions in term infants. Surgery is usually reserved for large defects in term infants and defects in preterm infants.

Endocardial Cushion Defect

This type of defect results from abnormal development of the endocardial cushions. The defect can be partial (ostium primum ASD and cleft mitral valve) to complete atrioventricular (AV) canal (primum ASD, large VSD beneath AV valves, common AV valve with five leaflets). There is right-sided enlargement secondary to interatrial or interventricular shunting. Left atrial enlargement may be present if there is mitral insufficiency. The defect is associated with trisomy 21, and 40% of these patients have congenital heart diseases and of these 40% have ECD. This subset of patients more commonly develops pulmonary hypertension with this defect.

Outflow Obstruction Lesions

Aortic Stenosis

Valvular aortic stenosis is the most common type of outflow obstruction. Seventy-five percent of these patients have a normal chest radiograph. A dilated ascending aorta may be identified, and there may be an abnormal number of leaflets or stenosis of a normal valve. Supravalvular stenosis is uncommon (1%–2%). This form is associated with Williams syndrome. Muscular subvalvular stenosis accounts for 8% to 20% of cases.

Aortic Coarctation

Aortic coarctation has narrowing of the descending thoracic aorta adjacent to the site of the ductus ateriosus and just distal to the left subclavian artery origin. There is always a juxtaductal discrete narrowing, but there may also be varying degrees of tubular hypoplasia of the transverse arch and isthmus. Associated anomalies are frequent, and there is an inverse relationship between age at presentation and presence of other lesions, such as bicuspid aortic valve, VSD, PDA, and other left-sided obstructive lesions. There is an increased frequency of coarctation associated with Turner syndrome.

There are two theories for the development of aortic coarctation. The ductal sling theory postulates that there is an abnormal extension of contractile ductal tissue that forms a shelf. The blood flow theory describes decreased blood flow through the aortic isthmus in fetal life, secondary to left-sided obstructive lesions and as a result, there is abnormal aortic development and coarctation. Radiographic findings include the "3" sign upper convexity of the dilated aorta, narrowing at the coarctation and the lower convexity representing poststenotic dilatation. A "reverse 3 sign" is seen with a barium-filled esophagus. Occasionally, rib notching can be seen in children older than 5 years, as a result of dilated intercostal arteries. Both CT and MRI can assess coarctation and collateral blood flow. There is controversy regarding treatment of native coarctation with balloon angioplasty with stent or surgery. The former is the preferred procedure for recurrent coarctation.

Pseudocoarctation

There is a high aortic arch in pseudocoarctation. Though the thoracic aorta is kinked, it is not obstructed.

Cor Triatriatum

Cor triatriatum is a rare lesion and is associated with other lesions in 12% to 50% of cases. It results from an anomaly of pulmonary vein development in which the pulmonary veins connect to an accessory chamber of the left atrium. The accessory chamber is separated from the true left atrium by a fibromuscular septum that has a small, obstructed opening. An ASD may be present. There is pulmonary venous obstruction. On radiographs, there is right ventricular enlargement, pulmonary edema, and a large left atrial shadow representing both chambers. MR can be used to show the left atrial anatomy and the size and course of pulmonary veins.

Pulmonic Stenosis

Radiographs may be normal in pulmonic stenosis if there is only mild narrowing. More severe narrowing creates poststenotic dilatation of the main and left pulmonary artery, right ventricular hypertrophy with elevation, uplifting of the cardiac apex on the frontal film, and filling in of the upper retrosternal clear space on the lateral view. The main pulmonary artery may be prominent in adolescence and there needs to be a correlation between imaging findings and clinical examinations.

Absence of the Pulmonic Valve

Absence of the pulmonic valve may be isolated or occur with other lesions, most commonly tetralogy of Fallot (TOF). Regurgitant blood flow results in aneursymal dilatation of the main, right and left pulmonary arteries with compression/narrowing of the central and peripheral tracheobronchial tree. CTA and MRA studies can assess both the vascular abnormality and associated caliber and compression of the tracheobronchial tree.

CYANOTIC CONGENITAL HEART DISEASE

Tetralogy of Fallot

TOF is the most common cyanotic congenital heart disease and is associated with trisomy 21, DiGeorge syndrome, and Alagille syndromes (Table 102-2). There is a right aortic arch in 25% of cases. Tetralogy has four components: right ventricular outflow tract obstruction, right ventricular hypertrophy, VSD, and overriding aorta. There is a normal to slightly enlarged heart size with a boot shape on radiographs as the right-sided changes elevate the cardiac apex. The main pulmonary artery segment is concave, creating a left heart margin concavity. Pulmonary vascularity is diminished to a varying degree depending on morphology and can be disorganized if multiple systemic to pulmonary collaterals are present. Preoperative CT and MR can be helpful in delineating the pulmonary artery anatomy and caliber and systemic to pulmonary collaterals. Cardiac MR assesses right ventricular size and function.

TABLE 102-2 Cyanotic Congenital Heart Disease

Tetralogy of Fallot	Most common cyanotic defect; trisomy 21, DiGeorge and Alagille syndromes 1. Right ventricular outflow tract obstruction 2. Right ventricular hypertrophy 3. VSD 4. Overriding aorta
Tricuspid atresia	
Pulmonary atresia with intact ventricular septum	
Pulmonary atresia with VSD	Severe tetralogy of Fallot
Ebstein anomaly	Abnormal tricuspid valve
Transposition of the great vessels	D- and L-types; "egg-on-a-sting"
Truncus arteriosus	CATCH 22 syndrome
Total anomalous pulmonary venous return	
Double outlet right ventricle	
Hypoplastic left heart	Males; under development of left ventricle w/ obstruction of inflow and outflow.

Tricuspid Atresia

In tricuspid atresia, there is an absence of the tricuspid valve with no blood flow from the right atrium to the right ventricle. Associated lesions include transposition, pulmonary hypoplasia/stenosis, coarctation of the aorta, ASD, patent foramen ovale, and VSD. Seventy percent of cases have ventriculoarterial connections that are concordant with severe pulmonary or subpulmonary stenosis. Thirty percent of cases have ventriculoarterial connections that are discordant with transposition and associated mild pulmonary stenosis and aortic obstruction. There is variable radiographic appearance depending on the type and associated lesions. The heart is usually normal to mildly large with normal-to-decreased pulmonary vascularity. CT and MR are useful postoperatively to evaluate patients after Fontan repair.

Pulmonary Atresia with Intact Ventricular Septum

In this entity, there is right ventricular outflow obstruction with variable development of the right ventricle. The central pulmonary arteries and branching pattern are normal. There are variable tricuspid valve abnormalities with severe stenosis and insufficiency. These patients may have massive cardiomegaly if insufficiency is present.

Pulmonary Atresia with VSD

Pulmonary Atresia with VSD is felt to represent the most severe form of TOF.

Ebstein Anomaly

The development and positioning of the tricuspid valve leaflets are abnormal in this anomaly. There is apical displacement of the septal and posterior valve leaflets into the right ventricle, resulting in partitioning of the right ventricle into an atrialized upper segment and apical outflow chamber. The anterior leaflet is normal in position, but redundant. Almost all patients have ASD or a patent foramen ovale. Tricuspid insufficiency leads to elevated right atrial pressure and right-to-left shunting at the atrial level with cyanosis. The classic radiographic appearance shows a globular-shaped heart with normal-to-diminished pulmonary vascularity. MR reveals valve position, evaluates right ventricular function, and assess degree of shunting and regurgitation.

Transposition of the Great Vessels

In transposition, there is an abnormal relationship between the great vessels and the ventricles.

There are two main types of transposition: d-transposition and l-transposition. In d-transposition, the ascending aorta is anterior and to right of the main pulmonary artery. The aorta is connected to the right ventricle and the main pulmonary artery to the left ventricle. The coronary arteries arise from the ascending aorta. There are resulting parallel circuits, which require mixing of blood to maintain life. The cardiac apex is usually left-sided, and there is atrial situs solitus. Fifty percent of patients have simple transposition of the great vessels with a patent foramen ovale and/or PDA and no other anomalies. Twenty-five percent of patients have VSD. Twenty-five percent of patients have VSD and pulmonary stenosis or subpulmonary left ventricular outflow tract obstruction. Right aortic arch is present in 4% of simple lesions and in 16% of patients with VSD. There are variable radiographic findings. The classic appearance is described as an "egg on a string" heart with narrowed superior mediastinum from thymic atrophy and altered great vessel arrangement. Pulmonary vasculature is normal in neonates, then increases, as pulmonary vascular resistance decreases unless pulmonary stenosis is present. MR can be useful in evaluating older switch procedures. CTA is also useful in evaluating postoperative stenosis.

In l-transposition (congenitally corrected type), there is ventriculoarterial discordance and ventricular inversion. There is leftward and anterior positioning of the aorta relative to the pulmonary artery. The anatomic left ventricle is to the right of the anatomic right ventricle. In 20% to 50% of patients, mesocardia or dextrocardia is present. Most patients have additional abnormalities, including VSD (80%), pulmonary stenosis (30%–50%), abnormal tricuspid valve, conduction abnormalities, coarctation, and ventricular hypoplasia. On radiographs, there may be an abnormal straightening of the mid and upper left heart border because of the position of the aorta.

Truncus Arteriosus

This is a conotruncal defect with a single vessel arising from the ventricles, which overrides a VSD that supplies the systemic, pulmonary, and coronary circulations. There is one semilunar valve with two to four leaflets that are often abnormal. One-third of cases are associated with deletions in the genes of chromosome 22q11. This has been linked with the CATCH 22 syndrome, which has cardiac anomalies, abnormal facies, thymic hypoplasia, cleft palate, and hypocalcemia. There is an increased incidence of truncus arteriosus in infants of diabetic mothers and retinoic acid exposure.

The truncal valve insufficiency and/or regurgitation lead to heart failure. Radiographs reveal a large heart with increased vascularity, pulmonary edema, right aortic arch, and thymic atrophy. Most patients are adequately assessed with echocardiography without the need for CT or MR. The Collett and Edward classification is used to describe the specific truncal abnormality (Table 102-3).

Total Anomalous Pulmonary Venous Return

In this anomaly, all pulmonary veins connect to the systemic venous circulation or directly to the right atrium rather than the left atrium. The four pulmonary veins may form a common pulmonary vein or connect separately. The male-to-female ratio is 3 to 4:1. One-third of cases have been associated with other cardiovascular malformations, especially heterotaxia syndromes.

Darling classification is an anatomic-based description of location of the pulmonary venous drainage (Table 102-4). All type III lesions are obstructed, while only 50% of type I lesions are obstructed. Without venous obstruction, the physiology is similar to a large ASD. In type I lesions, there is a widened mediastinum with increased blood flow through the vertical vein, left brachiocephalic vein, and SVC. This gives the classic "snowman" heart in older children. There is cardiomegaly and increased pulmonary vasculature. With

TABLE 102-3 Collett and Edwards Classification of Truncus Arteriosus

Separate origins from lateral aspects of the truncus	6%–10%
Separate origins of pulmonary arteries directly from the posterior surface of the truncus	29%–48%
Short main pulmonary trunk arising from the left side of the truncus	48%–68%
Pseudotruncus: pulmonary atresia with bronchial collateral vessels off the descending aorta (complete sixth arch development failure)	

TABLE 102-4 Darling Classification

I, Supracardiac	50% of patients with TAPVR
	Four pulmonary veins form a common pulmonary vein behind the left atrium. This empties into a left vertical vein, which goes to the left innominate vein, which leads to the right-sided SVC
II, Cardiac	20%
	Pulmonary veins drain to the right atrium or as a common pulmonary vein to the coronary sinus
III, Infracardiac	20%
	Veins form a common pulmonary vein, which courses below the diaphragm to empty into the portal vein, ductus venosus, hepatic vein, or IVC
IV, Mixed type	10%
	All patients have a patent foramen ovale or ASD which maybe small and contribute to obstruction. Thes obstruction may be intrinsic or extrinsic

obstructive lesions, pulmonary venous hypertension and congestion are seen. There is an edema pattern with normal-sized heart, pleural effusions, thymic atrophy, and lung hyperinflation. CT and MR are useful in depicting the pulmonary veins and connections.

Double Outlet Right Ventricle

Double outlet right ventricle results from a conotruncal defect. The aorta and pulmonary artery arise from the right ventricle. A VSD is present and is the outlet from the left ventricle. A classification system has been developed based on VSD position. In the subaortic, type accounting for 50% of lesions, the blood from the left ventricle preferentially enters into the aorta. One-half of these patients also have pulmonary stenosis. Subpulmonary (Taussig-Bing) type accounts for 30% of cases. In this type, the blood from the left ventricle preferentially enters into the pulmonary artery. Thirty-five percent of these cases have associated aortic obstruction. Doubly committed accounts for 5% of lesions. In this type, the VSD is beneath the aortic and pulmonary valves with blood flow from the left ventricle to both the aorta and pulmonary artery. Noncommitted accounts for the remaining 10% of cases. The VSD is remote from the outflow and not committed to either great artery. There is no classic pattern on radiograph for all forms of double outlet right ventricle. The clinical presentation, physiology, radiographic appearance is dependant on the VSD position and associated stenosis. It may resemble VSD, TOF, or transposition.

Hypoplastic Left Heart

There is a spectrum of anomalies associated with hypoplastic left heart syndrome. These include underdevelopment of the left ventricle with obstruction or atresia of the inflow and outflow of the left ventricle. Two-thirds of cases occur in males. Findings include a hypertrophied left ventricular myocardium with a small chamber, hypoplastic ascending aorta, aortic valve atresia or stenosis, mitral atresia or stenosis, and a PDA. There often is a patent foramen ovale or ASD. Coarctation is present in 80% of cases. Both pulmonary and systemic circulations depend on the right ventricle. When the ductus constricts, there is decreased systemic perfusion, myocardial ischemia, and shock. Radiographic findings are variable ranging from normal to marked cardiomegaly. There may be an edema pattern in the lungs. MR may be useful to assess the anatomy if a two-ventricle repair is being considered. Treatment involves a staged reconstruction procedure, usually a Norwood procedure, followed by a bidirectional Glenn shunt, and then a Fontan shunt. Alternatively, cardiac transplantation has been used.

OPERATIVE PROCEDURES FOR CONGENITAL HEART DISEASE

Blalock-Taussig Shunt

The original Blalock-Taussig shunt operation created an end-to-side subclavian artery to pulmonary artery anastomosis. The modified procedure is a graft between the subclavian artery and PA.

Glenn Shunt

The Glenn shunt is a unidirectional connection from the superior vena cava to the right pulmonary artery. The right pulmonary artery is divided from the main and left pulmonary artery. The bidirectional Glenn shunt is an end-to-side anastomosis of the superior vena cava to the right pulmonary artery, which remains in continuity and therefore provides blood flow to both sides.

Fontan Procedure

The classic Fontan procedure is a connection of the right atrium to the main pulmonary artery with a direct anastomosis or conduit. The new modified procedure has an anastomosis between the inferior vena cava and pulmonary arteries with a conduit or lateral atrial tunnel patch. The Fontan procedure is used for treatment of single ventricles and tricuspid atresia. Complications with this procedure include elevated systemic venous pressures, right heart chamber thrombosis, pulmonary arterial-venous malformation, arrhythmias, and protein losing enteropathy.

Jatene Arterial Switch

The arterial switch procedure is used to repair d-transposition. The pulmonary artery and aorta are returned to normal position after transection above the valves and switching. The coronary arteries are transplanted to the systemic vessel.

Mustard/Senning Procedure

Prior to the use of the switch procedure, the Mustard/Senning procedure was used to repair d-transposition, but is rarely used today. In this procedure, the systemic blood flow is redirected from the superior and inferior vena cava through a baffle or tunnel into the left (pulmonary) ventricle. The Mustard procedure uses a pericardial baffle and the Senning uses a right atrial flap. Pulmonary venous blood flow is redirected into the right (systemic) ventricle. Complications include baffle obstruction and leak, right ventricular failure, arrhythmia, and tricuspid insufficiency.

Rastelli Procedure

The Rastelli procedure is used in patients with d-TGV and a large VSD. An external conduit connects the right ventricle to the pulmonary artery. Blood flows from the LV to the ascending aorta through a VSD.

Norwood Procedure

The Norwood procedure is used in hypoplastic left heart syndrome. The Norwood procedure has several components, which include atrial septectomy, transection of the pulmonary trunk proximal to the pulmonary bifurcation, and anastomosis of the pulmonary trunk to the aorta. A patch homograft is used to augment the ascending aorta and aortic arch. The patent ductus is ligated and a modified Blalock-Taussig shunt is placed to provide pulmonary blood flow.

Ross Procedure

The Ross procedure is used in aortic stenosis for severe dysplasia or insufficiency. There is translocation of the pulmonary valve to the aortic position as an aortic root replacement and then use of a pulmonary homograft.

CARDIAC AND VISCERAL MALPOSITION

Abnormalities of Visceral Situs

Situs solitus is the normal arrangement in the body. In situs inversus, there is a mirror image of normal. This arrangement has a slightly increased incidence of congenital heart disease (3%–5%), such as right aortic arch, atrioventricular discordance, and transposition of the great vessels. Situs ambiguous or heterotaxy encompasses all other arrangements. It is typically divided into right (asplenia) and left (polysplenia) isomerism. Radiographs, CT, MR, and US are used for evaluation.

Asplenia

Asplenia is more common in males. There are bilateral trilobed lungs with bilateral minor fissures and eparterial bronchi. There are bilateral systemic atria. The liver is horizontal and centrally placed. Bowel malrotation is common with the stomach in an indeterminate position. The spleen is absent. The abdominal aorta and inferior vena cava are located on the same side of the spine. There is complex congenital heart disease in all patients, typically single ventricle, transposition, common atrioventricular canal, and pulmonary outflow obstruction.

Polysplenia

Polysplenia is more common in females and has a better prognosis than asplenia. There are bilateral bilobed lungs with hyparterial bronchi, with bilateral pulmonary atria. The liver is central in the abdomen. Bowel malrotation is common with the stomach in an indeterminate position. There are multiple spleens present in the upper right or left abdomen. There is interruption of the inferior vena cava with azygous continuation. Cardiac anomalies are present in 50%, typically anomalous systemic venous return, ASD, VSD, atrioventricular canal, double outlet right ventricle, and total or partial anomalous venous return.

VASCULAR RINGS AND SLINGS (GREAT VESSEL ANOMALIES)

Left Aortic Arch with Aberrant Right Subclavian Artery

This is the most common aortic arch anomaly with a 0.5% incidence. It is typically asymptomatic. There is a posterior impression on the esophagus as evidenced on esophagography.

Innominate Artery Compression

In this condition, the innominate artery originates to the left of midline and passes in front of the trachea. There is an anterior tracheal impression 1 to 2 cm above the carina. No esophageal impression is seen on esophagography. It rarely causes symptoms of respiratory obstruction.

Right Aortic Arch, Mirror Image Branching

Congenital heart disease is present in almost all patients; typically the lesions are cyanotic. The arch anomaly itself is not symptomatic.

Right Aortic Arch with Aberrant Left Subclavian Artery

This type of right aortic arch is rarely associated with congenital heart disease. A ring exists that is completed by the ligamentum arteriosum. There may be a diverticulum of Kommerell giving origin to the aberrant left subclavian artery. The vascular ring is typically loose and many patients have only mild or no symptoms.

Double Aortic Arch

In this anomaly, there are bilateral patent arches or atresia of one arch. Two vessels arise from the ascending aorta, joining posteriorly and having a left descending aorta in 80% of cases. The right arch is usually more superior in location, posterior, and larger, and there usually are no associated cardiac anomalies.

Pulmonary Artery Sling

In pulmonary artery sling, an anomalous vessel originates from the right pulmonary artery, passes between the trachea and esophagus, and supplies the left lung. It is accompanied by hypoplasia or dysplasia of the tracheobronchial tree in 65% of cases. It creates an indentation on the anterior wall of the esophagus at the level of the carina on esophagography. Initially, the right lung is opaque, but in older neonates and children, it becomes hyperlucent.

Suggested Reading

Hubbard AM, Fellows KE, Miller WT, et al. MRI of the heart. *Semin Roentgenol.* 1998;33(3).

Link KM, Lesko NM, et al. Cardiac imaging. *Radiol Clin North Am.* 1994;32(3).

Gaca AM, Jaggers JJ, Dudley LT, Bisset GS. Repair of congenital heart disease: a primer—part 1. *Radiology.* 2008;247: 617-631.

Gaca AM, Jaggers JJ, Dudley LT, Bisset GS. Repair of congenital heart disease: a primer—part 2. *Radiology.* 2008;248: 44-60.

QUESTIONS AND ANSWERS

1. Which type(s) of atrial septal defect is *not* commonly associated with anomalous pulmonary venous return?
   A. Primum
   B. Secundum
   C. Sinus venosus
   D. All types of atrial septal defect can be associated with anomalous pulmonary venous return

   ANSWER: B. The sinus venosus type is associated with anomalous connection of the right pulmonary veins especially the upper lobe veins to either the right atrium or superior vena cava. The ostium primum defect is associated with multiple other anomalies including total anomalous venous return.

2. What is the most common type of ventricular septal defect?
   A. Conal
   B. Membranous
   C. Supracristal
   D. Muscular

   ANSWER: B. Approximately 80% of VSD occur in the membranous septum.

3. Which type of aortic stenosis is associated with Williams syndrome?
   A. Valvular
   B. Subvalvular
   C. Supravalvular
   D. None of the above

   ANSWER: C. Williams syndrome is a sporadic genetic condition associated with distinctive facies and behavior, hypercalcemia, hyperacusis, and cardiovascular anomalies especially supravalvular aortic stenosis.

4. What is the proposed mechanism for development of coarctation?
   A. Reduced blood flow
   B. Abnormal cardiac looping
   C. Ductal sling
   D. Both A and C

   ANSWER: D. Although neither theory has been proven to be definitive, both the reduced blood flow and ductal sling have been proposed as mechanisms in formation of coarctation.

5. What percentage of patients with hypoplastic left heart have coarctation?
   A. 25%
   B. 50%
   C. 80%
   D. 100%

   ANSWER: C. Aortic coarctation is present in 80% of patients with hypoplastic left heart syndrome.

6. Which of the following is *not* a component of tetralogy of Fallot?
   A. ASD
   B. VSD
   C. Right ventricular hypertrophy
   D. Pulmonary outflow obstruction

ANSWER: A. Tetralogy of Fallot consists of a defect in the anterior ventricular septum, obstruction of the right ventricular outflow tract, overriding aortic root above the VSD, and right ventricular hypertrophy.

7. Which of the following is the most common type of cyanotic congenital heart disease?
   A. Truncus arteriosus
   B. Tetralogy of Fallot
   C. Transposition of the great vessels
   D. Tricuspid atresia

   ANSWER: B. Tetralogy of Fallot is the most common accounting for nearly 10% of all congenital heart lesions.

8. Massive cardiomegaly can be seen in all of the following *except*:
   A. Pericardial effusion
   B. Ebstein anomaly
   C. Pulmonary atresia with an intact septum
   D. Total anomalous pulmonary venous return with obstruction

   ANSWER: D. Total anomalous venous return with obstruction. With this lesion there is normal cardiac configuration and size. The other lesions listed can have massive enlargement of the heart shadow.

9. Which of the following is associated with right aortic arch?
   A. Truncus arteriosus
   B. Tetralogy of Fallot
   C. Ebstein anomaly
   D. Both B and C
   E. Both A and B

   ANSWER: E. Truncus arteriosus and tetralogy of Fallot have right-sided aortic arch usually the mirror image branching type as an associated anomaly.

10. Which of the following is *not* a procedure used for treating transposition?
    A. Jatene switch
    B. Mustard
    C. Senning
    D. Ross
    E. Rastelli

    ANSWER: D. The Ross procedure is used in treating aortic stenosis.

103 PEDIATRIC GASTROINTESTINAL TRACT

Martha M. Munden and Daniel W. Young

CONGENITAL DIAPHRAGMATIC HERNIAS

A Bockdalek hernia is a large, posterolateral defect in the diaphragm, with an estimated frequency of 1 per 2 to 5000 births. These occur more often on the left than the right side. Bowel can occupy the chest, shifting the heart and mediastinal structures to the opposite side, and ipsilateral and contralateral pulmonary hypoplasia is associated because of this space-occupying process. The pulmonary hypoplasia is more severe on the ipsilateral side. However, there are new developing theories that congenital diaphragmatic hernia is secondary to disruption of normal mesenchymal differentiation, with abnormal formation of the diaphragm affecting bronchial development, thus the pulmonary hypoplasia. Pulmonary hypertension commonly complicates congenital diaphragmatic hernias. Extracorporeal membrane oxygenation (ECMO) may be implemented in the newborn period (The other frequent reasons for ECMO are meconium aspiration and persistent pulmonary hypertension in the newborn).

A Morgagni hernia is a congenital anterior diaphragmatic hernia. This form of congenital hernia is much rarer than the Bockdalek hernia. The Pentology of Cantrell is a rare, associated condition (Table 103-1).

A hiatal hernia is an upward extension of cardia and fundus of the stomach into the chest through the diaphragmatic hiatus.

ESOPHAGUS

Gastroesophageal reflux (GER) can lead to symptoms and/or pathologic changes, which are referred to as

TABLE 103-1 Pentology of Cantrell

Omphalocele
Anterior diaphragmatic hernia
Sternal cleft
Ectopia cordis
Intracardiac defect: either a ventricular septal defect or a diverticulum of the left ventricle

TABLE 103-2 GERD Symptoms

GERD Symptoms
Poor growth (decreased nutritional intake from vomiting)
Irritability or refusing to feed because of pain
Blood loss from esophagitis
Breathing problems and recurrent respiratory illness
Globus sensation
Acidic or sour taste in the mouth (water brash)
Dysphagia

gastroesophageal reflux disease (GERD). GER is a normal part of life in the newborn to some extent. There are many, varied symptoms of GERD (Table 103-2).

Most healthy infants have GER within the first 6 months of life, with prevalence decreasing with age, and spontaneous resolution is typical. The incidence is higher in premature infants. Those with neurologic disorders also have an increased incidence, partly because of reduced lower esophageal pressures with elevated intracranial pressure and abnormal esophageal peristalsis because of CNS dysfunction. In normal infants, transient relaxation of the distal esophagus occurs with the passage of food content and is initiated by peristalsis. The high-pressure zone of the intra-abdominal esophagus is important to prevent reflux. The integrity of the high-pressure zone depends on an adequate length of intra-abdominal esophagus, normal diaphragm, an intact phrenoesophageal ligament, and adequate gastric emptying. Anatomic predisposition to GER includes hiatal hernia, tracheosophageal fistula, and esophageal atresia.

The Nissen fundoplication is the most commonly performed procedure out of the antireflux procedures and creates a 360-degree wrap of the gastric fundus around the distal esophagus creating an antireflux "valve." This is now being performed laparoscopically on a more routine basis. Complications can arise when the esophageal wrap slips above the diaphragmatic hiatus, or there may be partial slippage above the diaphragm with a paraesophageal hernia. These conditions are associated with a reoccurrence of GER and dysphagia. The wrap is intended to be below the level of the hemidiaphragm. Additional problems include gastric bloat related to the inability to belch after the fundoplication, dysphagia, recurrent reflux, and others.

Esophageal atresia is highly associated with tracheoesophageal fistula (TEF). Esophageal atresia commonly presents with proximal esophageal atresia with distal TEF. The dilated proximal pouch is classically associated with tracheomalacia. The surgical repair usually occurs on the side opposite from the aortic arch. Therefore, since most patients have a left-sided aortic arch, a right thoracotomy is most often performed. This entity is associated with VATER/VACTERL (Vertebral defects, Anorectal malformations, Cardiovascular defects, Tracheoesophageal defects, Renal anomalies, Limb deformities [radial ray abnormalities]). The distal esophageal segment in primary esophageal repair is known to have diminished peristaltic properties. There is usually stenosis at the site of primary anastomosis, which can cause obstruction of large foreign bodies or food. Balloon dilatation therapy is frequently performed to treat the narrowing at the anastomotic site. Proximal esophageal atresia with a distal TEF occurs in 82%, with proximal and distal esophageal atresia present in 9%, "H" type fistula with no esophageal atresia in 6% of patients, esophageal atresia with proximal and distal TEF in 2% and esophageal atresia with proximal fistula in 1%.

Swallowed foreign bodies can lodge at the level of the aortic arch or the thoracic inlet in the normal esophagus. Most small foreign bodies that reach the stomach pass out of the GI tract without harm in the fecal stream. Foreign bodies that need special mention include batteries and multiple magnets. Any time, more than one swallowed magnet passes beyond the stomach, they can attract each other through walls of adjacent loops of intestine, leading to obstruction with reported cases of necrosis and perforation. These foreign bodies may need endoscopic or surgical removal. Another concern is the penny minted after 1982 with a high zinc content. If it becomes lodged in the stomach, it may corrode because of a reaction of zinc with hydrochloric acid. Therefore, swallowed foreign objects should be monitored to ensure passage within about 2 days. Also of concern are the small disk batteries, which can cause mucosal injury if lodged in the esophagus in as short a time as 1 hour.

It is possible to perforate the back of the pharynx at the site of Killian dehiscence with a nasogastric tube. One should realize that patients with esophageal atresia have a proximal pouch that terminates near the T3 level or above. If the nasogastric tube cannot pass and is below the T3 level, consider traumatic perforation of the esophagus. Instillation of air through the tube with radiography can be helpful in diagnosing this condition.

STOMACH, SMALL BOWEL, AND COLON

A bezoar consists of an accumulation of undigested foreign material within the stomach. It is classified by the type of accumulated foreign material within the stomach (Table 103-3). It occasionally leads to obstruction.

TABLE 103-3 Bezoar

Lactobezoar	Congealed milk or formula. This is the most common bezoar of infants
Trichobezoar	Swallowed hair
Phytobezoar	Plant fibers, persimmon fibers

Bezoars can be seen occasionally on conuentional radiographs UGI examination, US, and CT.

Duodenal atresia can result in obstruction of the proximal duodenum and is associated with the "double-bubble" sign on radiographs. Duodenal atresia has a high association with Down syndrome but is not associated with a microcolon.

Jejunal and ileal atresia results in complete obliteration of the lumen. Proximal atresias may have a normally formed colon because of the passage of the succus entericus. Ileal atresia and distal jejunal atresia are frequently associated with microcolon. Ileal atresia may be seen in cases of complicated meconium ileus.

Meconium ileus presents with inspissated thick black enteric material in the distal small bowel and has a high association with cystic fibrosis. It can be treated with careful water-soluble contrast enemas. The hyperosmolar properties of water-soluble contrast allow water to be drawn into the GI tract to facilitate passage of meconium. Complications with meconium ileus occur in 30% to 50% of cases and include volvulus, perforation, atresia, peritonitis, and pseudocyst.

Meconium peritonitis is secondary in utero GI tract perforation in which meconium is expelled into the peritoneum. The meconium calcifies and can be a tell-tale sign. Meconium peritonitis is highly associated with meconium ileus. It is important to remember that calcifications may be seen in the scrotum in this condition because of the concomitant presence of a patent processus vaginalis.

Meckel diverticulum (omphalomesenteric duct remnant) is an antimesenteric outpouching of distal ileum, which has a fibrous connection with the umbilicus. These fibrous bands may be associated with internal hernia and volvulus. The Meckel diverticulum can bleed if it contains a sufficient amount of gastric tissue, which is diagnosed with the technetium-99m pertechnatate scan. The bleeding occurs on the wall opposite from the Meckel diverticulum due to ulceration resulting from acid production.

Small intramural nodules of lymphoid tissue are seen in the small bowel in patients with lymphoid hyperplasia. There is an association with IgA immunodeficiency.

Necrotizing enterocolitis (NEC) is an inflammatory condition of premature neonates and infants characterized by intramural air (pneumatosis intestinalis). There can be portal venous gas and free intraperitoneal air associated with GI tract perforation. NEC has no definitive known cause but is strongly associated with prematurity. A combination of factors including prematurity with the immaturity of the immune system, alteration in mesenteric blood flow, and feeding may be associated, as NEC is usually seen after, not before, the beginning of feeding. It often presents with increased residuals, distention of the abdomen, and bloody stools.

Hirshsprung disease implies aganglionosis of the colon, resulting in a transition zone. The distal bowel is frequently of normal to slightly small caliber with a transition to dilated proximal bowel. There may be irregular contractions in the distal segment; the most common transition zone is near the recto sigmoid junction, which is deficient in submucosal and intramural ganglion cells of neural crest origin. There is an association of Hirshsprung disease with other neurocristopathies such as neuroblastoma, Ondine curse (central hypoventilation syndrome), and Waardenburg syndrome (white forelock, deafness). With total colonic aganglionosis, the entire colon and parts of the distal small bowel may be void of ganglion cells. If a newborn has a perforated appendicitis, one should suspect total colonic aganglionosis.

Meconium plug syndrome is a form of colonic dysmaturity in which meconium plugs obstruct the colon. Hirshsprung disease needs to be excluded in order to make this diagnosis. A suction rectal biopsy is usually sufficient. This disorder may also be seen in patients whose mothers have received magnesium sulfate for eclampsia.

Neonatal small left colon syndrome is a form of colonic dysmaturity and has an association with infants of diabetic mothers. No surgery is needed, as this condition is typically outgrown. Colon atresia is a rare cause of microcolon.

Cystic fibrosis is the most common autosomal, recessive disorder of whites. (Sickle cell disease is the most common autosomal, recessive disorder of African Americans.) Cystic fibrosis occurs secondary to a sodium chloride transport gene regulation abnormality and is associated with cirrhosis of the liver, pancreatic insufficiency; sinusitis, increased sweat chloride, sinusitis, infertility, and increased incidence of pneumonia, bronchiectasis, and tracheobronchiomegaly. Embolotherapy may be necessary in patients who have uncontrolled hemoptysis. Fifteen percent of patients have a history of meconium ileus. Fibrosing colonopathy can be seen in patients with cystic fibrosis that receive pancreatic enzyme replacement therapy. Distal intestinal obstruction syndrome, formerly called meconium ileus equivalent, is a condition in which stool fecal material becomes so viscous that it causes

TABLE 103-4 VACTERL/VATER Syndrome

Vertebral defects
Anorectal malformations
Cardiovascular defects
Tracheoesophageal defects
Renal anomalies
Limb deformities

bowel obstruction. A water-soluble contrast enema may be used therapeutically to treat this.

Imperforate anus is classified: as high, intermediate, or low. High imperforate anus is anal atresia with the point of atresia above the levator sling muscles. High imperforate anus is associated with rectourethral fistula in the male and rectovaginal fistula in the female. Patients with rectourethral fistula may have intraluminal meconium calcification. This is thought to be because of an alteration of pH secondary to the mixture of urine and meconium. High imperforate anus is treated by colostomy and a subsequent rectal pull through procedure. A fistula closure may also be required. Low imperforate anus may be treated with anoplasty. Intermediate imperforate anus occurs when the patient has external signs of a low lesion with a fistula to the urethra. Imperforate anus is associated with VACTERL/VATER (Table 103-4) and Currarino triad (Table 103-5).

HETEROTAXY

The term "situs solitus" refers to the normal arrangement of the systemic atria on the right, a right-trilobed lung, right-sided liver, and IVC. Situs inversus refers to the mirror image of situs solitus with the systemic atria on the left, a left-sided trilobed lung, left liver, left IVC, right-sided cardiac apex, stomach, spleen, and aorta. Heterotaxy, or "situs ambiguous," refers to malpositioning of the viscera with indeterminate atrial arrangement. A variety of terms are used to describe the "ambiguous" visceral arrangement such as asplenia, right isomerism, bilateral right-sidedness and polysplenia, bilateral left-sidedness, or left isomerism. There is a high association of congenital heart disease with heterotaxy (50%–100%).

TABLE 103-5 Currarino Triad

Imperforate anus
Presacral mass, such as anterior meningocele
Teratoma
Rectal duplication
Sacral anomaly

Classic heterotaxy with asplenia has been used to describe bilateral trilobed lungs with bilateral minor fissures and eparterial bronchi, bilateral systemic atria, and central/midline liver. The stomach may be midline and small. The IVC and aorta are on the same side of the spine. These patients commonly have complex, severe cardiac anomalies and carry a worse prognosis.

Heterotaxy with polysplenia typically indicates bilateral bilobed lungs, bilateral pulmonary atria, a midline liver, stomach in variable position (though always on the same side as the spleen), and multiple spleens. The IVC may be interrupted with azygous or hemiazygous continuation. Heterotaxy with polysplenia tends to have less common and less severe cardiac anomalies. There is some association with biliary atresia. Both asplenia and polysplenia can be associated with midgut malrotation. Cardiac ECHO, abdominal US, MRI, and even CT may be indicated to define the full extent of the visceral and cardiac anomalies in these patients as the features of situs ambiguous are inconsistent.

EMERGENT PEDIATRIC ULTRASOUND

HYPERTROPHIC PYLORIC STENOSIS

Idiopathic hypertrophic pyloric stenosis (IHPS) was first described in 1627, though the etiology remains unknown. Infants with IHPS are clinically normal at birth and develop projectile, nonbilious emesis over a short time internal. IHPS typically occurs within the first 2 to 12 weeks of life. The incidence is two to five per 1000 births per year in the white populations and is less common among African Americans and Asian populations. It occurs more frequently in males, with ratios varying from 2.5:1 to 5.5:1. While there is a known hereditary link, it is likely polygenic with male and female children of affected mothers carrying an increased risk of developing IHPS. The risk is less for those children of an affected father.

The muscle in IHPS has been found to be deficient in the number of nerve terminals and markers for nerve-supporting cells, nitric oxide synthase activity, messenger RNA production for nitric oxide synthase, interstitial cells of Cajal, with increased insulin-like and platelet-derived growth factors. The abnormal muscle innervations may lead to failed relaxation of the muscle with secondary hypertrophy and obstruction. Interestingly, these levels return to normal months after surgical treatment.

The symptoms develop over a short period of time, progressively worsening until projectile emesis occurs after all feedings. The gastric contents are nonbilious, but may be blood-tinged with protracted vomiting caused by gastritis. Eventual hypochloremic alkalosis develops with sodium and potassium deficits. With delayed diagnosis, extensive weight loss can occur. In severe cases, an emaciated infant may present with visible vigorous peristalsis noted in the epigastric region.

When IHPS occurs, the normal pyloric ring is no longer present, replaced by an elongated channel lined by thickened muscle that abruptly changes caliber from the normal 1 mm thickness of the gastric wall. The muscle wall thickness ranges from 3 to greater than 6 mm. Normal muscle wall thickness is less than 2 mm. There is also a redundant gastric mucosa associated with IHPS, which obstructs the elongated, thickened pyloric channel. The channel length is variable and can measure from 1.5 to well over 2 cm.

An experienced pediatric surgeon can palpate the "olive," which represents the thickened, elongated pyloric channel. However, this is an art that is slowly being lost with increasing reliance on radiologic diagnosis. While the UGI examination was the mainstay in years past, it is now more of an accidental finding when the symptoms suggesting IHPS were not elicited prior to its performance. Typically, if suspicion is high, or a preliminary abdominal radiograph shows a distended stomach, US is performed, as it is a rapid diagnosis when positive.

Pylorospasm is a transient spasm of the pylorus. Similar to IHPS, patients present with emesis. However, upper GI examination and US show antral narrowing with delayed, intermittent, gastric emptying, not obstruction. On US, the single muscle wall thickness is normal as is the channel length.

Prostaglandin E therapy is used to maintain the patency of the ductus arteriosus in ductal dependent cardiac lesions and can lead to hyperplasia of the gastric mucosa. This can result in gastric outlet obstruction and an elongated pyloric channel on upper GI. However, on US, the muscle thickness will be normal and the obstruction is caused by mucosal hyperplasia. This disappears when the prostaglandin E therapy is discontinued.

Midgut malrotation occurs with a variety of abnormal rotations of the gut, which result in a foreshortened mesentery. The abnormal short mesenteric base allows excessive mobility of the small bowel and can result in midgut volvulus, where the small bowel rotates around the superior mesenteric artery (SMA) axis. Volvulus of the midgut or Ladd bands (which cross the third portion of the duodenum) can lead to obstruction. While upper GI is the primary mode for diagnosis, findings can be seen on US. With malrotation, the third portion of the duodenum is malpositioned anterior to the SMA, not in its normal retroperitoneal location. The normal anatomic position of the third portion of the duodenum is between the SMA and aorta. In malrotation with midgut volvulus, the sonographic whirlpool sign is seen, representing a branch of the jejunal vein wrapping clockwise around the SMA. Demonstration of the normal retromesenteric position of the third portion of the duodenum between the SMA and aorta sonographically has been shown to be a reliable finding that the bowel is in its normal anatomic position.

DUPLICATION CYSTS

Congenital duplication cysts are a relatively uncommon but well-known congenital abnormality. They can occur anywhere along the digestive tract along the mesenteric side with the small intestine the most frequent site: ileum, then jejunum, and then duodenum. (Small intestine: approximately 45%, colon,15%; gastric, 7%; duodenum, 5%; thoracic, 4%). Duplication cysts are firmly attached to the intestine, sharing a common wall and mesenteric blood supply with the gut. They can present with obstructive type symptoms or a palpable abdominal mass. A duplication cyst can be complicated by intussusception, volvulus, perforation, and rarely malignancy (frequency highest with those occurring within the colon in adults). US is probably the most common imaging modality and a duplication cyst has the characteristic sonographic appearance of the echogenic inner mucosal layer with hypoechoic outer muscular layer (the "gut signature"). The wall gut signature may not be circumferential as the layers are not uniform in thickness. If seen during a barium study, the cyst will show mass effect extending into the lumen of the portion of bowel. Gastric mucosa occurs in a reported 17% to 36% of duplication cysts and can lead to ulceration and GI bleeding. Those containing gastric mucosa can be demonstrated using Tc-99m sodium pertechnetate, similar to the uptake within a Meckel diverticulum. Sensitivity of Tc-99m imaging is reported to be 75%. At CT, a duplication cyst will be seen as a nonenhancing cystic mass. Fluid within the lumen typically has low Hounsfield units unless complicated by hemorrhage or proteinaceous material. Treatment is surgical excision.

GALLBLADDER

The incidence of gallstones in pediatrics is approximately 1.5%. Some of the more common etiologies of cholelithiasis in pediatrics include Lasix therapy, malabsorption, TPN, sickle cell disease, spherocytosis, thalassemia, and cystic fibrosis. Imaging findings are the same as those for adults. The normal gallbladder length in the neonate and young infant is less than 3 cm and the width is less than 1 cm. From 2 to 16 years of age, the length is less than 8 cm and width is less than 3.5 cm. Wall thickness is 3 mm or less. The common bile duct is significantly smaller in children than adults. The common bile duct is less than 1.2 mm in children 3 months of age and younger, less than 2 mm in infants up to 1 year of age, and less than 4 mm in older children.

Kawasaki disease (mucocutaneous lymph node syndrome) is associated with a hydropic gallbladder and focal artery dilatation, most worrisome being the coronary arteries.

Ascending cholangitis is a common finding in patients who have had the Kasai procedure, caused by the lack of a sphincter preventing the upward migration of bowel organisms into the biliary system.

Alagille syndrome (also known as arteriohepatic dysplasia) is an autosomal dominant (variable expression) disorder with characteristic facial features including a pointed chin, elongated nose, and broad forehead. Patients typically present with cholestatic jaundice in early infancy. Elevated serum bile acids often result in severe pruritis and xanthomas. Additional associated abnormalities include pulmonary stenosis, butterfly vertebrae, growth and mental retardation, eye and kidney involvement, as well as hypogonadism.

The histologic finding in liver biopsy in Alagille syndrome an increased portal tract to bile duct ratio reflecting the bile duct paucity. The bile paucity may not be present in the newborn and the clinical picture may suggest neonatal hepatitis. Other features of the syndrome help in making the diagnosis. Treatment of the cholestasis includes choleretic agents, partial external biliary diversion when indicated for severe pruritus and xanthomas, and liver transplant when indicated for end-stage liver disease.

BILIARY ATRESIA AND NEONATAL HEPATITIS

Biliary atresia and neonatal hepatitis are common causes of conjugated hyperbilirubinemia. Neonatal hepatitis is a nonspecific hepatic inflammation with different etiologies including infection (CMV, toxoplasmosis, spirochetes, rubella, herpes, syphilis, protozoa), metabolic defects (such as alpha-1 antitrypsin deficiency, galactosemia, and glycogen storage disease), familial recurrent cholestasis, and errors of metabolism such as nesidioblastosis (idiopathic hyperinsulin hypoglycemia of infancy). Both biliary atresia and neonatal hepatitis present around 3 to 4 weeks of age with jaundice. Biliary atresia is characterized by obliteration or disruption of the extrahepatic biliary system with obstruction to bile flow. The perinatal subtype form of biliary atresia is seen in 65% of cases and has isolated biliary atresia, while approximately 35% have the fetal subtype with multiple congenital abnormalities including polysplenia, malrotation, azygous continuation of IVC, situs inversus, preduodenal portal vein, bilobed right lung, complex congenital heart disease, choledochal cyst. Additional subtypes based on location of involvement include type I biliary atresia, which is rare with focal involvement. In type II, uncommon as well, there is atresia of the intrahepatic bile ducts and in type III (by far the most prevalent seen in greater than 90%), there is atresia of the right and left hepatic ducts to the level of the portal hepatis.

Distinguishing between biliary atresia and neonatal hepatitis is important, as biliary atresia requires early biliary diversion and neonatal hepatitis is managed medically. If the distal common bile duct is obstructed, an anastomosis between the extrahepatic biliary tree and intestine is performed. However, the majority require the Kasai procedure in which a portion of small bowel is attached to the portal region to allow bile drainage. The success of the Kasai procedure is 90% when performed in infants younger than 2 months and 50% when performed between 2 and 3 months of age, dropping even further after 3 months; thus the importance of a rapid diagnosis. Both entities may have some coarsening and increased echogenicity of liver parenchyma at US. With biliary atresia, the "triangular cord" sign, representing the fibrous remnant of the bile duct at the portal hepatis in extrahepatic biliary atresia, is fairly specific if present. Also, in biliary atresia the gallbladder is typically small or absent, though can be normal in about 10% of patients. Often with biliary atresia, the gallbladder is shrunken and irregular with poorly developed gallbladder wall, measuring less than 15 mm in length. Change in gallbladder size after a milk-feeding, indicating patency of the common bile duct is seen only with neonatal hepatitis. Scintigraphic examination will show tracer uptake by hepatic parenchyma, but no excretion in biliary atresia, while parenchymal uptake is decreased in neonatal hepatitis, but there will be excretion.

CHOLEDOCHAL CYST

Choledochal cyst is an uncommon cause of obstructive jaundice, more frequently seen in females and Asian infants, thought to be related to an abnormal insertion of the common bile duct into the pancreatic duct with reflux of pancreatic enzymes into the pancreatic duct causing chemical cholangitis and subsequent dilatation of the common bile duct. Some may present with the classic triad of pain, jaundice, and a right upper quadrant mass while some are asymptomatic. Choledocal cyst is typed according to the Todani classification (Table 51-1).

INSPISSATED BILE SYNDROME

Inspissated bile syndrome is an uncommon cause of jaundice in neonates. Inspissated bile is echogenic but does not cause shadowing. In can obstruct extrahepatic bile ducts. Inspissated bile may be associated with TPN, cystic fibrosis, massive hemolysis, and increased enterohepatic circulation with Hirshsprung disease intestinal atresias, and intestinal stenoses.

Spontaneous perforation of the extrahepatic bile ducts is a rare entity, affecting infants younger than 3 months of age presenting with jaundice and ascites. The perforation is usually at the junction of the cystic and common hepatic ducts. At US, ascites and a loculated fluid collection at the portal hepatis are typical. Scintigraphy confirms the bile leakage.

PORTAL HYPERTENSION

Portal hypertension results from an increase in pressure gradient between the portal venous sytem and the hepatic veins or IVC. Most often, it is caused by intrinsic liver disease, but can be because of posthepatic etiology such as right-sided heart failure, constrictive pericarditis, and Budd-Chiari syndrome. Prehepatic causes include portal vein thrombosis (such as those resulting from umbilical venous catheter induced thrombus), portal mass effect by adjacent tumors. An uncommon etiology in portal hypertension is an underlying arteriovenous malformation. Imaging findings in portal hypertension include an enlarged portal vein (normal for children younger than 10 years is 8.5 +/−2.7 mm and 10 +/− 2 mm from 10 to 20 years of age), decreased or reversal of portal venous flow (normal velocity is between 20 and 30 cm/s with respiratory variation), increased flow within hepatic artery, varices, splenomegaly, a thick lesser omentum, and ascites. Hemorrhage from varices is an important complication of portal hypertension. The left gastric vein drains the distal esophagus and proximal stomach and courses through the lesser omentum, entering the portal venous system near the splenoportal junction. The normal lesser omentum lies behind the left lobe of the liver and contains the left gastric artery and vein. The diameter of the lesser omentum in children is nearly constant. The lesser omental AP diameter can be related to the diameter of the aorta and does not exceed 1.7 times the adjacent aortic caliber. In the absence of fatty infiltration or adenopathy (other contents within the lesser omentum), if the lesser omental/aorta ratio exceeds 1.7:1, portal hypertension should be considered.

Portal vein thrombosis can result from thrombosis induced by umbilical vein catheters, sepsis, dehydration, or tumor invasion (usually hepatoblastoma). Acutely, the portal vein is enlarged and can be easily demonstrated by US, CT, or MRI. Chronic portal vein thrombosis results in periportal collateral vein formation (cavernous transformation). Cavernous transformation has been shown to develop within 6 to 20 days after an acute thrombosis. A mass of collateral vessels around the main portal vein forms with intrahepatic extension of collaterals in some patients. Portosystemic collaterals form mainly through the left gastric and perisplenic veins and portoportal from the periportal or pericholecystic venous channels to the intrahepatic portal veins. Despite the recruitment of collaterals, portal hypertension usually occurs.

BUDD-CHIARI SYNDROME

Budd-Chiari syndrome is an uncommon, yet potentially fatal if untreated, condition resulting from acute hepatic vein obstruction and is characterized clinically by ascites, abdominal pain, jaundice, tender hepatomegaly, and liver failure. Etiologies include tumor thrombus extension from Wilms tumor radiation, chemotherapy, coagulation disorders, congenital webs. Obstruction of large or small caliber veins leads to hepatic congestion, causing hepatocellular injury. Type I Budd-Chiari syndrome is obstruction at the IVC level, type II is obstruction at the level of the major hepatic veins, and type III is obstruction at the level of the small centrilobular venules (veno-occlusive disease). Imaging by CT or US shows occlusion of hepatic veins, increased caudate enhancement, and patchy enhancement of the remaining hepatic segments. Ascites and gallbladder wall edema are present.

VENO-OCCLUSIVE DISEASE

Veno-occlusive disease consists of occlusive fibrosis of small, intrahepatic, centrilobular, and sublobular venules. Hepatic veins and IVC are patent. It is one of the most frequent serious complications after stem cell transplantation, occurring in 5% to 60% in children who have had stem cell transplant. The primary site of injury is the sinusoidal endothelial cells of hepatic venules with eventual complete venular obliteration, hepatocellular necrosis, and widespread fibrous change. Veno-occlusive disease has a high-associated morbidity and mortality in post-transplant patients. Those at increased risk include those with preexisting liver disease, second myeloablative stem cell transplant, prior certain chemotherapy agents, prior conditioning with busulfan, melphalan, or both, and osteopetrosis. The principle cause in most cases is the toxicity of the preparative regiment for bone marrow transplant. Early symptoms include weight gain, tender hepatomegaly, ascites, and edema. The diagnosis can be challenging, as there are a lack of sensitive laboratory and imaging diagnostic studies. The imaging study of choice is abdominal Doppler with findings including slow or reversed portal venous flow (hepatofugal flow), decreased or reversal of diastolic flow in the hepatic arteries (increased resistance), ascites, hepatomegaly, and a thick gallbladder wall.

HENOCH-SCHONLEIN PURPURA

Henoch-Schonlein purpura is an IgA-mediated vasculitis of small vessels that affects the bowel, skin, joints, and kidneys. Patients often present with abdominal pain with a rash. Hemorrhage into the bowel wall resulting in thickening can act as a lead point for intussusceptions. Seventy-five percent of cases occur between the ages of 2 and 11 years. Bowel wall thickening, ascites, and secondary intussusceptions can be seen sonographically.

APPENDICITIS

The role of the appendix, thought for years to be a troublesome vestigial remnant, is now being studied in the etiology of ulcerative colitis and for its role in the development of gut associated lymphoid tissue. Some hypothesize that appendicular lymphoid tissue may contribute to the development of colitis. Inflammation of the appendix is the most common cause for emergent abdominal surgery in childhood. The use of ultrasound in the evaluation of underlying appendicitis is well documented throughout the literature.

Inflammation of the appendix results from luminal obstruction caused by lymphoid hyperplasia of submucosal follicles, obstruction caused by an appendicolith or hard concretions, and rarely foreign bodies, parasites, and so on. Mucus production increases intraluminal pressure, bacteria proliferate, and the appendix distends. Venous congestion, edema ensues and by about 12 hours, inflammatory process may become transmural. If untreated, arterial flow is reduced causing ischemia and eventual necrosis with perforation. Perforation typically will occur within 48 to 72 hours with complications that include abscess formation, peritonitis, sepsis, infertility, adhesions, and even death.

The lifetime risk for appendicitis is approximately 7% in females and 9% in males and appendicitis is much more common in developed countries. The peak incidence of appendicitis is highest in males from 10 to 14 years of age and 15 to 19 years in females. The classic symptoms of periumbilical pain that migrates to the right lower quadrant accompanied by anorexia, mild nausea, and several episodes of emesis, only occurs in around one-third of patients. In the very young, those younger than 3 years of age, when idiopathic intussusception is a common etiology for abdominal pain, the diagnosis of appendicitis is more difficult than in the child who can provide a history of pain in the right lower quadrant. Most children present with perforation younger than 3 years of age.

In clinically equivocal cases, imaging can improve the accuracy of diagnosis. Prompt diagnosis is necessary to prevent delay in treatment, perforation, and its complications. Plain films are nonspecific and insensitive in the diagnosis of appendicitis and can be normal or show decreased gas in the right lower quadrant, scattered air-fluid levels, an indistinct psoas margin, or mildly dilated small bowel loops. The presence of a calcified appendicolith has a high-positive predictive value for appendicitis in the presence of abdominal pain, but can be detected on plain films in only around 5% to 10% of cases. Most consider plain films to be of little value for routine evaluation.

US and CT have served to reduce the false-negative rate of appendectomies, with rates of 20% to 30% now around 4% to 8%. While CT does have an overall increased sensitivity and specificity compared to US, CT does not come without the cost of ionizing radiation and can be difficult to interpret in the very young child with little or no intra-abdominal fat. Limited and low-dose CT is being utilized to expedite the diagnosis of appendicitis in clinically equivalent cases. However, with the lack of fat in the young pediatric patient, most would agree that US, in experienced hands, is the best route for initial examination for suspected appendicitis in the infant and nonobese pediatric patient.

The use of graded-compression US in the diagnosis of appendicitis was first described by Puyleart in 1986. A high-resolution linear transducer is placed at the site of maximal tenderness indicated by the patient to compress and displace bowel loops to identify the appendix. The location of the appendix is highly variable and the anatomic position determines the symptoms and site of tenderness when the appendix is inflamed, thus the importance in examining the region indicated by the patient. Graded compression is utilized to locate either a normal or inflamed appendix to exclude or confirm the diagnosis of appendicitis. The normal appendix, which is a blind-ending tubular structure that compresses, is usually found anterior to the psoas muscle. The normal appendix has a thin, echogenic inner layer of mucosa and submucosa surrounded by a peripheral hypoechoic layer of muscularis propria. It is important to follow the suspected appendix back to the cecum, where the appendix arises about 1 to 2 cm below the terminal ileum and follow it along its length to the tip to ensure that an inflamed terminal ileum is not mistaken for an inflamed appendix. This is also necessary to include those with inflammation limited to the tip of the appendix. The abnormal appendix is identified as a blind ending, noncompressible, tubular structure measuring greater than 6 mm in maximum transverse diameter. In early appendicitis, the echogenic line, which corresponds to the mucosa and submucosa, is maintained. Loss of this echogenic line may be one of the earliest signs of perforation. With increasing inflammation, the appendix becomes hyperemic and increased flow can be seen by color Doppler. Signs of perforation include increasing echogenicity of the surrounding inflamed fat, adjacent fluid with varying degrees of increased echogenicity, as well as widespread echogenic fluid, abscess formation, and secondary small bowel obstruction.

Absolute exclusion of appendicitis by US is more difficult and the drawback for performing ultrasound to diagnose appendicitis is the operator dependency and the increasing incidence of obesity in childhood. In experienced hands, ultrasound has reported negative predictive value of 96%, but the overall reported sensitivity varies widely. In a recent publication of a study of sonographic techniques by Lee et al. in diagnosing acute appendicitis in a group, which included pediatric and adult patients, they were able to visualize the appendix in 98% of their control group and 99% in their patient group. In addition to the upward-graded compression, using a linear transducer to push the cecum and appendix out of the pelvis, they utilized several additional maneuvers to increase the visibility of the appendix. A forced extrinsic compression by the examiners left hand on the posterior aspect of the cecum, while graded compression with the linear transducer anteriorly was used. They also increased their sensitivity by turning the patient into the left lateral oblique decubitus position to displace the cecum and appendix medially.

The patient with a short history of signs and symptoms suggesting appendicitis, but an inconclusive US examination, can undergo a repeat limited US examination within a short period of time. This is in accordance to the ALARA principle.

Obesity in childhood has become an increasing problem in the US and can severely limit the ability to evaluate for appendicitis sonographically. Hormann et al showed that the higher the body mass index-for-age percentile (BMI-FAP), the more difficult it was to detect the appendix, not an unexpected finding. Age is not adequate to use for a cut-off in the decision as to whether to use US or CT in the clinically inconclusive patient as even the very young can be extremely obese; while, an older, thin patient may be an ideal candidate for an US examination. A significant decrease in US sensitivity occurs beyond a BMI threshold of 25. The decision of whether to proceed with CT or to attempt a limited US in a larger patient is dependent on the resources of the individual institution.

Pitfalls in the diagnosis of appendicitis by ultrasound include the inability to identify inflammation localized to the tip of the appendix, thus the importance of searching for the tip. With a recent perforation, the appendix may reseal at the tip or rupture such that no appendix can be identified, another cause for a false-negative examination. Presentation too early in the course of inflammation, such as in the patient with only 6 to 8 hours of pain, may lead to a false-negative US examination. In this case, if there is continued clinical suspicion and an inconclusive examination, the patient can be held for observation with repeat limited scan of the right lower quadrant within about 8 to 12 hours because appendicitis usually "declares" itself in 24 to 36 hours.

Omental infarction, an entity becoming more prevalent with the increasing incidence of childhood obesity, can lead to a confusing examination with echogenic, inflamed omentum at the site of tenderness, which may decrease the ability to find a normal appendix. Adnexal pathology including pelvic inflammatory disease, ovarian torsion, and hemorrhagic ovarian cysts can mimic appendicitis clinically and the inflammation related to pelvic inflammatory disease can extend to the appendiceal region. Mesenteric adenitis (a cluster of three or more ileocolic nodes measuring greater than 5 mm short axis diameter with a normal appendix) and even an inflamed Meckel diverticulum can mimic appendicitis. A dilated ureter obstructed by a distal stone may be mistaken as the appendix by the inexperienced sonographer.

False-positive studies can result from bowel inflammation adjacent to the normal appendix. It is important to follow the complete course of the appendix to prevent terminal ileum thickening from Crohn disease from mimicking appendicitis. The bowel wall thickening associated with Henoch-Schonlein purpura can be confused with appendicitis. The vasculitis of Henoch-Schonlein purpura can cause intramural thickening, which can be difficult at times to differentiate from both appendicitis and intussusception. Bowel wall thickness usually ranges from 5 to 8 mm with Henoch-Schonlein purpura. In addition, the appendix in cystic fibrosis can be of much greater diameter and incompressible because of mucoid material in its lumen without being related to appendicitis.

INTUSSUSCEPTION

Intussusception occurs when a loop of bowel (intussusceptum) invaginates into a more distal loop of bowel (intussuscipiens). Idiopathic intussusceptions generally occur from about 3 months of age to 2 years, with males affected about three times more frequently than females. Classic symptoms occur in only about 50% and include intermittent severe abdominal pain with interval periods of lethargy, palpable abdominal mass, and "currant jelly" stools. While only about half have the classic triad of symptoms, most (75%) have stools that test positive for occult blood.

The large majority of idiopathic intussusceptions are ileocolic or ileoileocolic and occur secondary to lymphoid hyperplasia within Peyer patches in the terminal ileum, leading to the intussusceptum invaginating into the intussuscipiens. The mesentery is drawn with the intussusceptum, which becomes compressed causing compromise of venous drainage with subsequent bowel edema, possible ischemia, obstruction, and infarction. Ischemia of the mucosa causes bleeding and mucus outpouring, resulting in the "currant jelly." If treated, mortality is only 1% to 3%. Delayed treatment leads to bowel necrosis and even death. Recurrence rates range from 5% to 20%.

Predisposing illness leading to lymphoid follicular hyperplasia include recent URI or diarrheal illness, particularly adenovirus, and enterovirus, thus the more seasonal variation in presentation with idiopathic intussusception. Intussusception with underlying lead points (less than 5%) is uncommon in infants and more common in neonates and children older than 5 years, as well as those with small bowel intussusceptions. Intussusceptions within small bowel can be associated with Henoch-Schonlein purpura, indwelling gastric or gastrojejunostomy tubes, polyps in Peutz-Jeghers syndrome, and recent intraperitoneal or retroperitoneal resection. Lead points also include duplication cysts, Meckel diverticula, lymphoma, and even trauma.

The consequence of missing the diagnosis of intussusception can be disastrous for the patient. Plain film findings include small bowel obstruction, decreased gas in the right lower quadrant, a gasless abdomen, findings, which are generally nonspecific. The "target sign" is more specific, representing a soft-tissue mass containing a circular area of lucency representing the mesenteric fat of the intussusception. This is often seen in the right upper quadrant. The meniscus sign consists of a crescent of gas within the colon lumen outlining the intussusception. Plain films are often not useful in the diagnosis of intussusceptions. However, plain films can be useful to evaluate for complications of intussusception such as small bowel obstruction or intestinal perforation.

Ultrasound is readily available and has become the imaging modality of choice to evaluate for intussusception, along with other suspected etiologies of acute abdominal pain in the emergency department setting. Sensitivity in detection of intussusception is reported to be 98% to 100%· In a prospective study, Verschelden et al. reported ultrasound to have a negative predictive value of 100%, meaning no patient having a negative US examination was found to have an intussusception by enema. This applies in the case of ileo and ileoileocolic intussusception where the peripheral location of the colon is easily evaluated sonographically. In the case of intussusceptions limited to the small bowel, these numbers do not necessarily apply given the limitation of central detail by bowel gas, especially in the postoperative patient.

On US examination, the typical findings of an intussusception are a mass from 3 to 5 cm or greater in size located in the distribution of the colon, usually on the right side. In the study of Verschelden et al., most of their examinations were performed by third and fourth year residents who had completed several months of training. Use of high frequency linear transducers is recommended for optimal bowel detail. An excellent description of the appearance of an intussusception on transverse and longitudinal imaging is provided by del-Pozo et al. Transversely, an intussusception produces a target sign with multiple hypoechoic concentric rings of alternating layers of collapsed intussusceptum lumen and the bowel wall signature of the intussusceptions surrounding an echogenic center of the mesenteric fat often containing lymph nodes, or the "doughnut" sign with echolucent outer ring surrounding an echogenic center. In longitudinal views, the intussusception has been characterized as having a "pseudokidney" sign, where the intussuscipiens has a hypoechoic rim and the more central intussuscepting mesenteric fat is more echogenic, similar to the kidney.

Clearly defined echogenic/echolucent alternating rings correspond to less edematous bowel and typically better success of reduction. Enlarged mesenteric lymph nodes are commonly seen in children with gastroenteritis and following various viral syndromes. These mesenteric nodes are commonly pulled with the mesentery into the intussusception and are commonly seen sonographically within the central echogenic mesentery at US. The mesentery is dragged between the loops and is maximum at the base of the intussusception and absent at the apex. Sonographic signs associated with irreducibility include interloop fluid with a thickened outer hypoechoic ring with "doughnut "pattern and absence of blood flow in an intussusception. This pattern holds true, both with ileocolic and small bowel intussusceptions. The lymph nodes, along with edematous mesentery, are thought to impede the exit of the intussusceptum. Identification of a lead point is valuable information provided sonographically for decisions in further management of the patient.

Not only should the right lower quadrant and distribution of colon be studied with abdominal pain, but small bowel should be briefly studied as well. Often transient small bowel intussusceptions are found incidentally and complete resolution should be documented. CT and US studies have shown that benign, transient small bowel intussusceptions tend to be less than 3.5 cm in length; nontransient ones are often associated with lead points. Their appearance is similar, though more midline in location, and they can be multiple in patients with polyps associated with Peutz-Jeghers syndrome. Symptoms are often more chronic than acute, not the classic signs of idiopathic intussusception.

INTUSSUSCEPTION PITFALLS

Causes of the occasional false-positive US examination include any condition leading to bowel wall thickening, such as vasculitis leading to intramural hematoma in Henoch-Schonlein purpura. The characteristic appearance on transverse imaging of eccentric, hyperechoic mesenteric fat, and lymph nodes should not be present in these conditions, which can serve to differentiate bowel wall thickening from an intussusception.

In conclusion, if a child has all three classic signs and symptoms of an intussusception, the most cost-effective approach for the next evaluation would be to perform a contrast enema examination, as this has the potential both to confirm the diagnosis and to treat the problem. However, if the diagnosis is less straightforward, ultrasound is the ideal modality to identify which children would be appropriately treated by enema reduction for an intussusception. Ultrasound also has the advantage of identifying an underlying lead point when present and can serve to help one judge the reducibility of an intussusception by its appearance.

SUGGESTED READING

Addis DG, Shaffer N, Fowler BS, et al. The epidemiology of appendicitis and appendectomy in the United States. *Am J Epidemiol.* 1990;132:910-925.

Alloo J, Gerstle T, Shilyansky J, Ein SH. Appendicitis in children less than 3 years of age: a 28 year review. *Pediatr Surg Int.* 2004;19(12):777-779.

Applegate K, Goske M, Pierce G, Murphy D. Situs revisited: imaging of the Herotaxy syndrome. *Radiographics.* 1999;19: 837-852.

Bernard H, Azadeh S, Coppens E, et al. Intrathoracic migration of the wrap after laparoscopic nissen fundoplication—radiologic evaluation. *AJR Am J Roentgenol.* 2002;178: 859-862.

Blickman H. *The Requisites: Pediatric Radiology.* 2nd ed. St. Louis: Mosby; 1998.

Buonomo C, Taylor GA, Share JC, Kirks DR. Gastrointestinal tract. In: Kirks DR, ed. *Practical Pediatric Imaging: Diagnostic Radiology of Infants and Children.* 3rd ed. Philadelphia, PA: Lipponcott-Raven; 1998:946.

Canon C, Morgan D, Einstein D, et al. Reflux disease: what the radiologist needs to know. *Radiographics.* 2005;25:1485-1499.

Carrico CW, Fenton LZ, Taylor GA, et al. Impact of sonography on the diagnosis and treatment of acute lower abdominal pain in children and young adults. *AJR Am J Roentgenol.* 1999;172: 513-516.

Daneman A, Navarro O. Intussusception part 1: a review of diagnostic approaches. *Pediatr Radio.* 2003;33:79-85.

Daneman A, Navarro O. Intussusception part 2: an update on the evolution of management. *Pediatr Radio.* 2004;34:97-108.

del-Pozo G, Albillos JC, Tejedor D, et al. Intussusception in children: current concepts in diagnosis and enema reduction. *Radiographics.* 1999;19:299-319.

del-Pozo G, Gonzalez-Spinola J, Gomez-Anson B, et al. Intussusception: trapped peritoneal fluid detected with US—relationship to reducibility and ischemia. *Radiology.* 1996;201(2): 379-383.

Diley A, Wesson D, Munden M, et al. The impact of ultrasound examinations on the management of children with suspected appendicitis: a 3 year analysis. *J Pediatr Surg.* 2001;36:303-308.

Eklof OA, Johanson L, Lohr G. Childhood intussusception: hydrostatic reducibility and incidence of leading points in different age groups. *Pediatr Radiol.* 1980;10:83-86.

Farkas SA, Hornung M, Sattler C, et al. Preferential migration of CD62L cells into the appendix in mice with experimental chronic colitis. *Eur Surg Res.* 2005;37(2):115-122.

Fefferman NR, Bomsztyk E, Yim AM, et al. Appendicitis in children: low-dose CT with a phantom-based simulation technique—initial obserations. *Radiology.* 2005;237:641–646.

Gebbers JO, Laissue JA. Bacterial translocation in the normal human appendix parallels the development of the local immune system. *Ann N Y Acad Sci.* ;2004;1029:337-343.

Gubernick JA, Rosenberg HK, Ilaslan H, Kessler A. US Approach to jaundice in infants and children. *Radiographics.* 2000;20: 173-195.

Hernandez JA, Swischuk LE, Angel CA. Validity of plain films in intussusception. *Emerg Radio*. 2004;10(6):323-326.

Hernanz-Schulman M. Infantile hypertrophic pyloric stenosis. *Radiology*. 2003;227(2):319-331.

Hormann M, Scharitzer M, Stadler A, et al. Ultrasound of the appendix in children: is the child too obese? *Eur Radiol*. 2003;13:1425-1431.

Kaneko K, Tsuda M. Ultrasound-based decision making in the treatment of acute appendicitis in children. *J Pediatr Surg*. 2004;39(9):1316-1320.

Koumanidou C, Vakaki M, Pitsoulakis G, Kakavakis K, and Mirilas P. Sonographic detection of lymph nodes in the intussusception of infants and young children. *AJR Am J Roentgenol*. 2002;178:445-450.

Lee JH, Jeong YK, Park KB, et al. Operator-dependent techniques for graded compression sonography to detect the appendix and diagnose acute appendicitis. *AJR Am J Roentgenol*. 2005;184:91-97.

Lim HK, Bae SH, Lee KH, et al. Assessment of reducibility of ileocolic intussusception in children: usefulness of color Doppler sonography. *Radiology*. 1994;191(3):781-784.

Lvoff N, Breiman RS, Coakley FV, Lu Y, Warren RS. Distinguishing features of self-limiting adult small-bowel intussusception identified at CT. *Radiology*. 2003;227:68-82.

Menten R, Lebecque P, Saint-Martin C, Clapuyt P. Outer diameter of the vermiform appendix: not a valid sonographic criterion for acute appendicitis in patients with cystic fibrosis. *AJR Am J Roentgenol*. 2005;184:1901-1903.

Mercado-Deane MG, Burton EM, Brawley AV, Hatley R. Prostaglandin-induced foveolar hyperplasia simulating pyloric stenosis in an infant with cyanotic heart disease. *Pediatr Radiol*. 1994;24:45-46.

Munden MM, Bruzzi J, Coley BD, Munden RF. Sonography of pediatric small-bowel intussusception: differentiating surgical from nonsurgical cases. *AJR Am J Roentgenol*. 2007;188:275-279.

Navarro OM, Daneman A, Chae A. Intussusception: the use of delayed, repeated reduction attempts and the management of intussusceptions due to pathologic lead points in pediatric patients. *AJR Am J Roentgenol*. 2004;182:1169-1176.

Pracros JP, Tran-Minh VA, Morin DE, et al. Acute intestinal intussusception in children: contribution of ultrasonography (145 cases). *Ann Radiol (Paris)*. 1987;30:525-530.

Puylaert JBCM. Acute appendicitis: US evaluation using graded compression. *Radiology*. 1986;158:355-360.

Ripolles T, Garcia-Aguayo J, Martinez M, Gil P. Gastrointestinal bezoars—sonographic and CT characteristics. *AJR Am J Roentgenol*. 2001;177:65-69.

Schlesinger AE, Dorfman SR, Braverman RM. Sonographic appearance of omental infarction in children. *Pediatr Radiol*. 1999;29:598-601.

Siegel MJ, Friedland JA, Hildeboldt CF. Bowel wall thickening in children: differentiation with US. *Radiology*. 1997;203:631-613.

Sivit CJ, Siegel MJ. Gastrointestinal tract. In: Siegel MJ, ed. *Pediatric Sonography*. 3rd ed. Philadelphia, PA: Lippincott Williams & Wilkins; 2002:278.

Sivit CJ, Siegel MJ. Gastrointestinal tract. In: Siegel MJ, ed. *Pediatric Sonography*. 3rd ed. Philadelphia, PA: Lippincott Williams & Wilkinds; 2002:337-383.

Sivit CJ. Imaging the child with right lower quadrant pain and suspected appendicitis: current concepts. *Pediatr Radiol*. 2004;34:447-453.

Taylor GA. Suspected appendicitis in children: in search of the single best diagnostic test. *Radiology*. 2004;231(2):293-295.

Theriot JA, Sayat J, Franco S, Buchino JJ. Childhood obesity: a risk factor for omental torsion. *Pediatrics*. 2003;112(6):460.

Vershelden P, Filiatraut D, Garel L, et al. Intussusception I children: reliability of US in diagnosis-aprospective study. *Radiology*. 1992;184:741-744.

Wiersma F, Sramek A, Holscher HC. US features of the normal appendix and surrounding area in children. *Radiology*. 2005;235(3):1018-1022.

Yousefzadea DK. The position of the duodenojejunal junction: the wrong horse to bet on in diagnosing or excluding malrotation. *Pediatr Radiol*. 2009;39:S172–S177.

QUESTIONS AND ANSWERS

1. What is the most important anatomic landmark in the pediatric upper GI examination?
   A. Gastric fundus
   B. Duodenojejunal junction
   C. Pyloric channel
   D. Gastric antrum

   ANSWER: B. The location of the duodenojejunal junction, which determines if there is midgut malrotation and therefore risk for midgut volvulus.

2. Which of the following diagnoses is suggested with bilious vomiting?
   A. Hypertrophic pyloric stenosis
   B. Biliary atresia
   C. Midgut volvulus
   D. Gastric volvulus

   ANSWER: C. This can be an important clue of the possible diagnosis of malrotation–and midgut volvulus. Bilious vomiting suggests the diagnosis is located distal to the ampulla, as in midgut volvulus. Gastric outlet obstruction, such as from pyloric stenosis or gastric volvulus would have nonbilious vomiting.

3. What is the best test for the diagnosis of malrotation?
   A. UGI examination
   B. Ultrasound
   C. CT
   D. MRI

   ANSWER: A. Upper GI, because it specifically locates the duodenojejunal junction.

4. What is a sonographic finding of malrotation?
   A. Preduodenal portal vein
   B. Short pancreas

C. Microgastria
D. Inversion of the SMA/SMV relationship

ANSWER: D. Inversion of the SMA/SMV relationship. A "whirlpool" sign can be seen with midgut twisting around the vessels, midgut volvulus.

5. What would be the safest contrast material to use to evaluate the proximal pouch in a patient with esophageal atresia and distal tracheoesophageal fistula?
A. Gastrografin
B. Barium agent
C. Air
D. Non–ionic water-soluble contrast

ANSWER: C. Air. Instill a few cubic centimeters of air into the Replogal catheter used to drain or decompress the proximal pouch.

6. Which one is associated with microcolon?
A. Meconium ileus
B. Scarring
C. Infants of diabetic mothers
D. Midgut volvulus

ANSWER: A. A microcolon is a small unused colon and is seen in the setting of meconium ileus, ileal atresia, colonic atresia, and megacystis-microcolon-hypoperistalsis syndrome. Jejunal atresia may not be consistently included on this list since the succus entericus produced by the small intestine may be associated with a normal caliber colon.

7. Intraperitoneal calcifications are identified in the abdominal cavity and scrotum. What is the most likely diagnosis?
A. High imperforate anus
B. Meconium peritonitis
C. Hypercalcemic state
D. Hyperparathyroidism

ANSWER: B. Meconium peritonitis. This implies that there has been a GI tract perforation in utero and scrotal calcifications prove patent processes vaginulus.

8. If a contrast enema is being used to treat meconium ileus, what contrast should be used?
A. Barium
B. Air
C. Water-soluble contrast
D. Lipiodol

ANSWER: C. Water-soluble contrast media, such as contrast media used for VCUG. Its hypertonicity draws fluid into the bowel lumen, helping cleanse the inspissated thick, black material.

9. What are contraindications to the performance of an air or contrast enema to reduce ileocolic intussusceptions?
A. Pain
B. Small bowel obstruction
C. Perforation and peritonitis
D. Hypothermia

ANSWER: C. Perforation and peritonitis.

10. If a patient is felt to have meconium plug syndrome, what underlying disorder should still be considered?
A. Cystic fibrosis
B. Meconium ileus
C. Meconium peritonitis
D. Hirshprung disease

ANSWER: D. Meconium plug syndrome is a form of colonic dysmotility and is transient. Clinically, it can be indistinguishable from Hirshsprung disease, which is a permanent motility disruption due to segmental absence of colonic ganglion nerve cells.

104 PEDIATRIC GENITOURINARY TRACT

Jeremy T. Royal and Stuart A. Royal

ADRENAL GLAND

Neonatal adrenal hemorrhage is associated with coagulopathy, birth trauma, sepsis, and asphyxia and can typically be seen in infants of diabetic mothers who are large for gestational age. It is bilateral in 10% and more common on the right (85% in one study). Typical sonographic features include nonvascular hematoma that involutes over months to years and may develop calcification. Adrenal insufficiency is extremely rare.

Neuroblastoma is the most common solid, extracranial childhood malignancy with a peak age of 2 years. Three-fourths occur in the abdomen, with two-thirds of these occurring in the adrenal medulla. One-third of these occur in the extra-adrenal retroperitoneum, with 20% in the posterior mediastinum, 3% in the presacral pelvis (Table 104-1), and 5% in the neck. Neuroblastoma encases adjacent upper abdominal arteries and extra-adrenal neuroblastoma invades the epidural space via the neural foramina. Metastases (50% at diagnosis) are common to the liver and bone, though extremely rare

TABLE 104-1 Pediatric Presacral Mass

CYSTIC	SOLID
Cystic sacrococcygeal teratoma	Solid sacrococcygeal teratoma
Duplication cyst	Neuroblastoma
Anterior meningeal cyst	Rhabdomyosarcoma
	Primary sacrococcygeal bony tumors

to lung. Calcification in abdominal neuroblastoma is seen in 85% via CT scanning and 30% via radiography. Radionuclide bone scan demonstrates uptake in the primary mass in 75% and is performed at diagnosis in addition to radiographic bone survey. MIBG has uptake in 70%. Ultrasound and CT of the primary area with supplemental MR is typically utilized for complete staging. Stage IV-S neuroblastoma is seen in infants younger than 1 year of age with skin, liver, and bone marrow but no osseous cortical abnormality. Multiple syndromes are classified based upon metastasis (Table 104-2).

The overwhelming majority of patients have elevated catecholamines at diagnosis. Better prognosis includes lower stage, stage IV-S, thoracic primary, Shimada histologic grade, high-DNA index, low N-MYC amplification, and age younger than 1 year.

KIDNEYS

CONGENITAL ABNORMALITIES

Ureteropelvic junction (UPJ) obstruction is the most common form of urinary tract obstruction in pediatrics. It is four times more common in newborn boys than girls and bilateral in 10% to 20%. It is seen in association with horseshoe kidney, inferior renal ectopia, and the lower pole of a complete duplex collecting system. Patients may be diagnosed prenatally with sonography. Postnatally, UPJ obstruction is the most common cause of a palpable abdominal mass. Patients may present with urinary tract infection (UTI), intermittent abdominal pain, vomiting, or hematuria. On nuclear scans with a diuretic challenge, a T1/2 washout from peak activity greater than 20 minutes is diagnostic of obstruction. A T1/2 washout of 10 to 20 minutes is indeterminate.

TABLE 104-2 Metastatic Neuroblastoma Syndromes

Hutchinson syndrome	Primary adrenal neuroblastoma
	Skeletal metastases (skull)
	Proptosis
	Bone pain
Pepper syndrome	Primary adrenal neuroblastoma
	Hepatomegaly secondary to metastases
Blueberry-Muffin syndrome	Primary adrenal neuroblastoma
	Multiple metastatic skin lesions

Multicystic dysplastic kidney (MCDK) is a nonfunctioning kidney, which is replaced by multiple, noncommunicating cysts with intervening dysplastic parenchyma. It is the most common cause of a unilateral, cystic kidney in a neonate, and it is the second most common abdominal mass in a neonate. The classic form results from pelvoinfundibular atresia. Up to 40% of these patients have a contralateral abnormality, commonly contralateral UPJ obstruction, and 25% have contralateral reflux. In 85%, the affected kidney tends to involute over time. MCDK is typically diagnosed with ultrasound, but nuclear scintigraphy can be helpful to confirm the diagnosis by demonstrating absence of renal function.

Renal ectopia represents normal renal tissue in an abnormal location. Kidneys that fail to ascend, generally maintain some degree of anterior orientation. Variations of renal ectopia include horseshoe kidney, crossed fused ectopia, pelvic kidney, iliac (ptotic) kidney, and thoracic kidney. Pelvic kidney is the most common form of ectopia, accounting for about 60% of cases. Malpositioned kidneys are at a higher risk for vesicoureteral reflux (20%–30%), trauma, obstruction (usually UPJ), infection, stones, and a slight increase in the incidence of Wilms tumor. Aberrant and multiple renal arteries and veins are also common. Horseshoe kidney may be associated with genital anomalies, VACTERL anomalad (vertebral, anorectal, cardiac, tracheoesophageal, renal, limb abnormalities), and Turner syndrome, among others.

Renal agenesis may occur bilaterally or unilaterally. Bilateral renal agenesis is lethal. Males are affected three times more often than females. This condition produces profound oligohydramnios, and the kidneys, which can usually be seen by the 15th week of gestation by ultrasound, are not present. If the diagnosis is not made until birth, the child will manifest with Potter syndrome: pulmonary hypoplasia (usually with spontaneous pneumothoraces), abnormal facial features, and deformity of the limbs. Unilateral renal agenesis may be detected prenatally, postnatally, or may be silent until puberty, when associated genital tract anomalies become apparent. The association of unilateral renal agenesis with genital tract anomalies in females, especially the absence or hypoplasia of the vagina, is called Mayer-Rokitansky-Kuster-Hauser syndrome. Seminal vesical cyst can be seen in males with unilateral renal agenesis. Unilateral renal agenesis is frequently seen in association with anomalies of the cervical and lumbosacral spine, and/or anorectal anomalies. The contralateral kidney should be measured to evaluate for compensatory hypertrophy.

Autosomal recessive polycystic kidney disease (ARPKD) is a genetic disorder characterized by bilateral, symmetric cystic renal disease involving the distal convoluted tubules and collecting ducts. The kidneys are typically bilaterally enlarged and hyperechoic with poor corticomedullary differentiation and may fill the flanks and displace adjacent organs. Small, discreet cysts (less than 1 cm) may or may not be visible. There is usually a history of oligohydramnios. Small biliary ductal ectasia and liver fibrosis are always present, with Caroli disease seen in a small number of patients. Twenty to forty-five percent of patients with ARPKD present in the second decade of life with renal failure and require dialysis or renal transplantation. Late complications include portal hypertension secondary to hepatic fibrosis.

Autosomal dominant polycystic kidney disease (ADPKD) is a genetic disorder characterized by bilaterally macrocystic kidneys and is associated with other systemic abnormalities. The kidneys are typically within two standard deviations of normal in size at diagnosis in childhood. The cysts tend to be larger than 1 cm in size. Occasionally, pediatric patients with ADPKD may have diffusely hyperechoic kidneys similar to ARPKD. Cysts may also involve the liver (50%) and the pancreas (9%). Noncystic manifestations include cardiac valvular disorders, hernias, colonic diverticula, and congenital "Berry" aneurysms (15%). Tuberous sclerosis can rarely have renal cystic disease, which is similar in appearance to ADPKD. Patients with ADPKD most commonly present in the fourth or fifth decade of life with renal failure or hypertension.

RENAL TUMORS

Wilms tumor is the most common abdominal tumor of childhood with a peak age of 3 years. Typical triphasic pathology occurs with epithelial, blastemal, and stromal elements, though anaplasia is a high-risk histologic feature. Staging includes CT imaging of the chest. Bone metastases are uncommon so that bone imaging is not usually performed. Stage V includes bilateral synchronous tumors, which are associated with nephroblastomatosis. Calcification is present in 9% of radiographs and 15% of CT examinations. Pulmonary metastases are present in 20% of children at time of diagnosis. Nephroblastomatosis, secondary to persistent metanephric blastema in the kidneys, is a risk for developing Wilms tumor. Perilobar nephroblastomatosis is located in the subcortical region and is associated with Beckwith-Wiedemann syndrome (also at risk for hepatoblastomas and adrenal carcinoma), hemihypertrophy, Perlman syndrome, and trisomy 18 (Table 104-3). Intralobar nephroblastomatosis is located deep within the kidney and is associated with Drash syndrome, sporadic aniridia, WAGR syndrome, and has a high risk for degeneration into Wilms tumor. Imaging includes evaluation of the inferior vena cava, as extension into the renal vein is common and alters surgical approach. Follow-up imaging for metachronous tumor in the contralateral kidney (10%) and pulmonary metastases is key. Screening recommendation for the follow-up of Wilms tumor in high-risk patients is renal ultrasound at 3-month intervals up to 8 years of age.

Congenital mesoblastic nephroma is the most common solid renal tumor less than 3 months of age. This benign lesion should not metastasize and is unilateral. A cellular variant can have a more aggressive clinical course. The gross appearance is similar to a uterine fibroid. Entrapped normal renal tissue can mimic function in these lesions.

TABLE 104-3 Wilms Tumor Versus Neuroblastoma

	WILMS TUMOR	NEUROBLASTOMA
Frequency	Most common abdominal solid tumor	Most common overall extracranial solid tumor
Metastasis	Pulmonary	Bone cortex
Prognostic indicators	Anaplasia-worse	Shimada class, better with age <1 y Increased DNA index, Low N-MYC, thoracic primary
Unique staging parameters	Stage V-bilateral kidneys	Stage 4S-bone marrow but no bony cortex metastasis. Ninety percent resolve spontaneously
Associated syndromes	Beckwith-Wiedemann, DRASH, Sporadic Aniridia, WAGR	None
Calcification	15% on CT	50%–85% on CT
Vascular invasion	40% Renal Vein/IVC	Rare

Clear-cell sarcoma is the bone-metastasizing renal tumor of childhood, so that bone imaging is required at diagnosis and in follow-up. Features are similar to Wilms tumor otherwise.

Rhabdoid tumor is a highly aggressive, usually fatal primary renal tumor that occurs in children typically younger than 1 year of age. It is associated with hypercalcemia and is associated with CNS tumors most common in the posterior fossa, usually PNET.

Renal cell carcinoma is typically seen in adolescents, where 50% of primary renal tumors are Wilms tumor and 50% are renal cell carcinoma. Appearance and workup is otherwise typical for Wilms tumor.

Multilocular cystic nephroma is a multicystic focal mass in the kidney, which can encompass benign lesions such as multilocular cyst to cystic Wilms tumor (cystic partially differentiated nephroblastoma). Imaging cannot distinguish a benign multicystic primary renal mass from a malignant one, so that removal of the lesion is required. They can occasionally herniate into the renal pelvis.

Renal medullary carcinoma occurs in adolescents with sickle cell trait and is highly aggressive and usually fatal.

ACQUIRED ABNORMALITIES

Renal vein thrombosis, more common in the left kidney, is most common in dehydrated or septic infants and infants of diabetic mothers. The thrombosis starts in the intrarenal venules and propagates centrally. Ultrasound demonstrates heterogeneous echogenicity of the enlarged kidney, poor corticomedullary differentiation, and may show focal hemorrhages. Renal artery Doppler demonstrates reversed diastolic flow.

Urolithiasis in childhood is most commonly caused by idiopathic hypercalciuria. Important other causes include type I renal tubular acidosis (RTA), furosemide treatment for bronchopulmonary dysplasia (BPD), stasis with hydronephrosis, Lesch-Nyhan syndrome with uric acid stones, metabolic diseases such as cystinuria, xanthinuria, oxalate stones, cystic fibrosis, Crohn disease, and infection stones (struvite–calcium magnesium ammonium phosphate). Medullary nephrocalcinosis (Table 104-4) can give an increased echogenic pyramid appearance with a differential diagnosis including medullary cystic disease, ARPKD, Beckwith syndrome, Sickle cell disease, Bartter syndrome, acute renal failure, and protein deposition such as Tam-Horsfall proteinuria and hemoglobinuria/myoglobinuria.

TABLE 104-4 Hyperechoic Renal Medulla

Medullary nephrocalcinosis
ARPKD
Beckwith syndrome
Medullary sponge kidney
Tamm-Horsfall protein
Bartter syndrome
Acute renal failure
Sickle cell disease

URETERS, BLADDER, AND URETHRA

Vesicoureteral reflux (VUR) is common, with lower incidence in African Americans. It is thought to occur secondary to a shortened submucosal tunnel within the bladder with a lateralized ureteral orifice. Children with VUR have twice the incidence of pyelonephritis. Since VUR is seen in approximately 25% of asymptomatic siblings of affected children, screening of siblings is recommended. There is a correlation of renal scarring and lack of spontaneous resolution of reflux with increasing grade of reflux. VUR is graded as follows:

Grade I-reflux into a ureter that does not reach the renal pelvis.
Grade II-reflux reaching the pelvis but not blunting the calyces.
Grade III-reflux reaching the calyces causing mild blunting.
Grade IV-reflux reaching the calyces causing moderate blunting.
Grade V-dilated and tortuous ureter with complete calyceal blunting.

Radiographic voiding cystourethrography (VCU) is recommended in boys with their first UTI and with complex anatomy (suspected duplex collecting system). Radionuclide cystogram is recommended in first time UTI in girls, follow-up male and female for known reflux, postoperative reflux assessment, and sibling reflux screening. Ultrasound is the most common method of upper tract assessment in UTI evaluation. Radionuclide cystogram has a 1/100 radiation dose compared to fluoroscopic VCU. Eighty percent of children with grade I to II reflux spontaneously resolve with age. Reflux and infection are felt to be independent phenomena though may affect one another. Similar statements for bladder outlet obstruction related to reflux can be made. Postnatally, sterile VUR typically does not cause scarring. Complications of renal scarring include hypertension, renal insufficiency, and proteinuria. If the patient is noncompliant, develops resistant infection, has high-grade reflux, or develops progressive scarring, treatments consist of ureteral reimplantation or advancement procedures, or STING procedure (subureteric transurethral injection).

With acute pyelonephritis, 30% to 50% are associated with vesicoureteral reflux. Scarring occurs most commonly in children younger than 1 year of age and is rare after onset greater than 3 years of age. DMSA scanning, CT, and MRI are more sensitive than sonography or IVP for this diagnosis. Acute pyelonephritis most commonly appears as a wedge-shaped, segmental defect, less commonly rounded, and is frequently polar where compound calyces occur. Ultrasound is used initially in hospitalized UTI patients to exclude an obstructed infected system (pyonephrosis).

Ureteral duplication is the most common anomaly of the urinary tract and may be partial or complete. In complete duplication, the ureter draining the upper pole of the kidney inserts into the bladder inferior and medial to the ureter draining the lower pole (Weigert-Meyer rule). The upper pole ureter tends to obstruct (75% from a ureterocele). The lower pole ureter has a short submucosal tunnel and tends to reflux. Complete duplication is bilateral in approximately 25% of cases. Ultrasound and VCU are the first-line imaging modalities for diagnosis. MR urography with heavily T2-weighted sequences can occasionally be a supplemental tool for imaging the ureters. In symptomatic patients, the type of surgery depends on the function of the upper pole.

Posterior urethral valves (PUV) is a form of chronic urethral obstruction secondary to fusion and prominence of the plicae colliculi, normal concentric folds of the urethra. It occurs exclusively in males and is the most common cause of congenital bladder outlet obstruction. The diagnosis is typically made on VCUG and demonstrates an abrupt transition from a dilated posterior urethra to a small, bulbous urethra at the level of the valves. Bladder wall trabeculation/muscular hypertrophy is commonly seen. PUV is associated with vesicoureteral reflux (50%), urinary ascites, and urinomas in newborns. Despite increased prenatal detection and improved surgical interventions, approximately one-third of patients will eventually develop renal insufficiency.

Ureterocele is congenital cystic dilation of the distal submucosal portion of the ureter. An intravesical ureterocele occurs when the ureterocele is completely contained within the bladder. An extravesicle ureterocele occurs when part of the cyst extends to the urethra, bladder neck, or perineum. An orthotopic (simple) ureterocele has its orifice located in a normal anatomic position at the trigone of the bladder and is usually seen in single systems. An ectopic ureterocele has its orifice located anywhere else, though the ureterocele presents as an intravesicle mass. Ectopic ureterocele is five times more common in girls than boys, is bilateral in 10% of cases, and is the most common cause of bladder outlet obstruction in girls. Cecoureteroceles are a subtype of ureterocele, which is elongated by tunneling under the trigone and the urethra. Treatment of ureteroceles includes cystoscopic fenestration of the ureterocele and/or resection and reimplantation of the ureterocele or heminephroureterectomy depending on upper pole function. Ureteroceles are best seen with ultrasound, which also evaluates the ureters and kidneys. With VCUG, early filling images are essential for demonstrating ureteroceles.

An ectopic ureter is one that drains outside the posterolateral angle of the trigone, either within the bladder or extravesically. It is associated with ureteral duplication anomalies in 80% of cases. In cases of an ectopic ureteral insertion, the ureter may insert infrasphincteric in girls and lead to chronic wetting. In boys, the ectopic ureter is suprasphincteric and does not lead to wetting, but may insert into the epididymis, vas deferens, or spermatic cord and cause epididymitis.

Primary megaureter is a dilated ureter, which is secondary to functional obstruction of the distal, adynamic, normal caliber ureteral segment. The functionally obstructed ureter may be associated in 20% of cases with coexisting vesicoureteral reflux. This entity can lead to decreased renal function, but renal function is usually more preserved than in other cases of congenital obstructive uropathy. Primary megaureter is associated with ipsilateral and contralateral UPJ obstruction.

Urachal anomalies are secondary to persistence of the midline connection between the bladder dome and the umbilicus, which is a remnant of the fetal allantoic stalk. A urachal fistula (patent urachus) is an open channel from the bladder to the umbilicus through which urine can leak. A urachal sinus is persistence of a superficial segment of the channel opening onto the skin surface. A urachal diverticulum is persistence of the deep segment creating a diverticulum of the anterosuperior bladder. A urachal cyst is persistence of the intermediary segment with a fibrous attachment to the bladder wall and umbilicus. The urachal remnant is treated with resection secondary to a small risk of malignant conversion to adenocarcinoma, not transitional cell carcinoma. Associated abnormalities include prune-belly syndrome, PUV, urethral atresia, and cloacal anomalies.

Bladder diverticulum is a protrusion of the mucosa of the bladder through a defect in the muscular wall (pseudodiverticula). A "Hutch" diverticulum occurs in a periureteral location, typically laterally and cephalad to the ureteral orifice. It may be associated with single system VUR, infection, hematuria, or stone formation. Primary diverticula are idiopathic and may be seen with several syndromes including cutis laxa, Menkes, and Ehlers-Danlos syndrome. Secondary bladder diverticula are the result of chronically increased intravesical pressure with hypertrophy of the bladder musculature and may be seen in patients with severe lower urinary tract obstruction, such as PUV, and in patients with neurogenic bladders. VCUG is the best imaging modality for diagnosis.

Prune-belly (Eagle-Barrett) syndrome occurs in boys with laxity of the abdominal wall musculature, urinary tract dilation, and cryptorchidism. It is thought to be because of mesodermal arrest. The posterior urethra is dilated secondary to prostatic hypoplasia. Varying degrees of hydronephrosis and renal dysplasia may be seen. Pulmonary hypoplasia secondary to oligohydramnios can be an important component in severe cases. VCUG may show posterior urethral dilation or urethral diverticulum (persistent prostatic utricle) without PUV.

Neurogenic bladder (most commonly related to myelodysplasia in children) can be classified into two types:

1. Hyperreflexic contractile bladders—Trabeculated, thick wall with normal to small volumes and bladder sphincter dyssynergia.
2. Overflow neurogenic bladder—Smooth wall large capacity bladder, frequently with incontinence because of sphincteric weakness.

The key treatment protocol is to establish bladder emptying, either with intermittent catheterization or spontaneous voiding. Without success, 50% have upper tract deterioration with hydronephrosis, infection, and eventual chronic renal failure. Differential diagnosis of the hyperreflexic neurogenic bladder includes William syndrome, Menkes syndrome, and cutis laxa or Ehlers-Danlos. There is an increased incidence of urolithiasis and autonomic dysreflexia. Other treatment options include medications, bladder augmentation surgery, and operations for continence. Patients with dysfunctional voiding (severe form with nonneurogenic, neurogenic bladder-Hinman syndrome) have a form of bladder sphincter dyssynergia, which can mimic neurogenic bladders of defined etiologies. The "spinning top" urethra is a typical morphology for dysfunctional voiders, especially in females.

Urethral duplication is a rare, congenital anomaly that occurs more often in males than females. In the epispadiac type, an incomplete accessory channel has a dorsal opening in the phallus and ends blindly. The complete or partial form originates from the bladder or proximal urethra and courses through the dorsal aspect of the penis to end in an epispadiac position anywhere between the glans and the root of the penis. The ventral urethra, which is always associated with the urinary sphincter, is normally positioned and ends in the glandular meatus. In the hypospadiac type, an incomplete accessory channel has a ventral opening in the phallus and ends blindly in the periurethral tissue similar in appearance to a urethral diverticulum or Cowper duct. Hypospadias is associated with cryptorchidism.

The prostatic utricle is in the midline verumontanum and is associated with hypospadias, prune-belly syndrome, imperforate anus, and Down syndrome. The prostatic utricle fills with contrast during VCUG. A Mullerian duct cyst is rare and is a large mass originating from the verumontanum and does not communicate with the urethra on VCUG.

TUMORS

Rhabdomyosarcoma originates most commonly in children in the head and neck. Genitourinary tract (GU) is the second most common location and extremities the third. The GU tumors most commonly involve the bladder (sarcoma botryoides), the prostate in periadolescent males, and rarely the vagina and the uterus. Another rare location includes the retroperitoneal pelvis. Spread is local, lymphatic, and hematogenous to lungs, liver, and bone. The bladder tumors have a typical intraluminal polypoid extension. Rare associations include neurofibromatosis, Li-Fraumeni syndrome, Beckwith Wiedemann syndromes, and postradiation. The majority of patients are younger than 5 years of age.

Sacrococcygeal teratoma can present as a presacral mass with typical imaging features of teratoma, and the classification is type I primarily external (47%), type II dumbbell (34%), type III (9%) primarily within the abdomen and pelvis, and type IV (10%) entirely internal. The more cystic varieties are typically benign, while solid components indicate malignancy. Alpha-feta protein produced in endodermal sinus components should be measured to gauge malignancy. Surgical resection requires coccygeal removal to prevent recurrences. These can be associated with the Currarino triad (presacral mass, anorectal stenosis, sacral anomalies), which has an autosomal dominant inheritance pattern and can present with polyhydramnious or high output cardiac failure from arterovenous shunting.

MALE GENITAL TRACT

Testicular torsion is twisting of the testis and spermatic cord within the scrotum, resulting in vascular occlusion or infarction. It is most commonly seen between 11 and 18 years of age. The testicle twists medially in two-thirds of cases, and the axis of the testes may change from a vertical to horizontal orientation. Diagnosis is made on ultrasound by demonstrating decreased or absent blood flow within the testicle. Extratesticular flow may be increased. In recent torsion, the testicle parenchyma may be completely normal. Otherwise, the testicle may be enlarged and demonstrate a heterogeneous or hypoechoic echotexture. Hydrocele may be seen. Testicular torsion is associated with an abnormally high attachment of the tunica vaginalis, resulting in a "bell-clapper" deformity. Prenatal testicular torsion almost invariably presents with testicular infarction. Viable torsed testes undergo orchiopexy, while nonviable testes are removed. Preventative orchiopexy is typically performed on the contralateral, nontorsed testis. Surgical salvage rates are 80% to 100% if the patient is found within 6 hours of pain and quickly decline after 12 hours.

Torsion of the testicular appendage is spontaneous twisting of one of the pedunculated vestigial remnants of tissue extending from the testicle or epididymis, causing ischemia and pain and is typically treated nonsurgically. It occurs most commonly between 6 and 12 years of age. Ultrasound shows an enlarged appendage (greater than 5 mm), spherical in shape, with periappendiceal hyperemia but no flow in the appendix. A reactive hydrocele is common. The "blue dot" sign of an ischemic appendage is seen through the scrotal wall in a minority of patients.

Epididymo-orchitis is infectious inflammation of the epididymis, testicle, or both. On ultrasound, there is enlargement of the affected tissue with accompanying hyperemia and a small reactive hydrocele. It is most often caused by *Staphylococcus aureus*, *E. coli*, or viruses, especially mumps. It is the most common cause of acute, painful scrotum in the postpubescent male. Elevation of the affected hemiscrotum relieves the pain of epididymitis (Prehn sign) and exacerbates torsion.

If the newborn has an enlarged scrotum and multiple calcifications around the testes, meconium peritonitis with a patent processus vaginalis should be a strong consideration.

MALE GENITAL TUMORS

Testicular neoplasms are unusual in infants and children, representing around 1% of all childhood malignancies. Of those that occur in children, 60% occur at age 2 or younger. These tumors typically present as painless, nontender, firm scrotal masses of weeks to months duration. Scrotal ultrasound typically demonstrates a mass, which can be confused for infarct, granuloma, and focal orchitis. Reactive hydroceles may be seen in 15% to 20% of cases. Color Doppler typically demonstrates increased vascularity.

Germ cell tumors represent around 70% of all testicular tumors in children. Yolk sac tumors are by far the most common germ cell tumor in children, representing 80% to 90% of cases. Of those, 75% are diagnosed by 2 years of age. These tumors are frequently complicated by hemorrhage. Serum alpha-fetoprotein levels are elevated in 90% of affected patients. Testicular teratoma is the second most common germ cell tumor in children, usually developing between 3 months and 5 years of age. This appears as complex solid and cystic mass on ultrasound and is derived from elements of all three germ cell layers. Bony elements/dental structures are hyperechoic with posterior shadowing and are often visible on conventional radiographs. Prepubertal teratomas are typically benign (85%), while postpubertal teratomas are more frequently malignant, with elevated serum hCG levels.

Gonadal stromal tumors are almost always benign and represent around 25% of pediatric testicular masses. Leydig cell tumors and Sertoli cell tumors are the most common gonadal stromal tumors of childhood. Leydig cell tumors represent 45% of these and are the most common testicular neoplasm in African American children. These are typically diagnosed in 2- to 9-year-old, but may be associated with hormone production and premature virilization if androgens are produced and gynecomastia if estrogen is produced. Sertoli cell tumors represent 20% of nongerm cell tumors, half are diagnosed by the first year of life, and gynecomastia caused by estrogen production may occur.

FEMALE GENITAL TRACT

CONGENITAL ABNORMALITIES

In hydrometrocolpos, there is dilatation of the vagina and/or uterus either secondary to imperforate hymen (no associated anomalies) or vaginal atresia (high incidence of renal anomalies and other anomalies). This presents as a mass prolapsing through the introitus (imperforate hymen) or abdominal/pelvic mass between the bladder and rectum. Secondary hydronephrosis is an important complication. Echogenic debris within the dilated vagina can be related to mucus secretion or infection. Rare peritoneal calcification is related to reflux of secretions out the fallopian tubes. A key imaging feature is to identify the small uterus attached to the top of the vagina in hydrometrocolpos to distinguish from other pelvic masses. Hydrometrocolpos has a bimodal age presentation, either in infancy or in periadolescent age group. In adolescents, it presents with monthly pain associated with lack of menstrual periods. It can have associated vertebral and cardiac anomalies in addition to mullerian duct fusion anomalies.

Patients with intersex disorders and ambiguous genitalia benefit from a complete evaluation including chromosomes, gonadal assessment, external and internal genital anatomy, hormonal assessment, rearing, and psychosocial orientation. Ultrasound is helpful to demonstrate the infantile uterus, and ovaries can frequently be identified. VCUG and vaginogram are important to demonstrate the anatomy of the bladder, the urethra, vagina, and urogenital sinus. MRI occasionally is utilized to identify the internal genital anatomy. The most common etiology for female intersex is congenital adrenal hyperplasia. Other causes include maternal androgen ingestion or masculinizing ovarian tumor in the mother. Male intersex or pseudohermaphroditism is frequently from testicular feminization or lack of Mullerian regression factor secretion. Deficiency of enzymes such as 5-alpha-reductase deficiency can produce this syndrome. Gonadal dysgenesis such as XY gonadal dysgenesis is a variant of Turner syndrome producing ambiguous genitalia. In the Drash syndrome (gonadal dysgenesis, nephropathy, and Wilms tumor), ambiguous genitalia are present. True hermaphroditism is rare, where both testicular and ovarian tissue occur in the same patient.

Precocious puberty occurs in females developing signs of puberty before 8 years of age and in males before 9 years of age. Isosexual precocious puberty can be related to hamartoma of the tuber cinereum. These patients can also present with gelastic seizures. Rare other CNS tumors can provoke precocious puberty. Females with precocious puberty can have autonomous ovarian cysts stimulating estrogen secretion, rare estrogen secreting adrenal tumors, and McCune-Albright syndrome associated with polyostotic fibrous dysplasia, cafe-au-lait spots, and precocious puberty.

Males with isosexual precocious puberty are evaluated for hypothalamic hamartoma (a mass at the base of the hypothalamus, which is isointense to gray matter on T1 and T2 images and does not enhance). Rare androgen-secreting adrenal carcinomas or testicular tumors in males occur. Males can have congenital adrenal hyperplasia that mimics sexual precocity. Leydig tumors of the testes and rare HCG secreting tumors can occasionally cause precocious puberty in boys. HCG secreting tumors occur in hepatoblastomas, some teratomas of the mediastinum and the retroperitoneum, intracranial germinomas, and pineablastomas.

Ovarian torsion is also termed adnexal torsion including torsion of the ovary, fallopian tube, or both. It produces unilateral enlarged ovary with peripheral cysts, typically best seen on ultrasound though also seen on CT or MR, which can also show additional fallopian tube twisting or thickening. This entity in pediatrics is most common without underlying mass or tumor and is in the differential diagnosis of right lower quadrant pain including appendicitis. Salvage of the ovary is more common than in testicular torsion.

FEMALE GENITAL TUMORS

Ovarian dermoid tumor (two germ cell lines) and teratoma (three germ cell lines) are the most common ovarian tumors. They can be bilateral in up to 25% and malignant degeneration in approximately 10%. CT, MR, and ultrasound can demonstrate calcifications, fat, hair, teeth, and cysts. Teratomas are most commonly sacrococcygeal (7%) and gonadal (29%) with ovarian more common than testicular. Complications include torsion and spontaneous rupture and malignant degeneration.

Rhabdomyosarcoma of the vagina is typically botryoides and extend out the introitus (interlabial mass) (Table 104-5), producing a differential diagnosis with hydrometrocolpos, prolapsing ureterocele, urethral prolapse, and urethral cyst. Vaginal primaries are more common than the rare uterine primary tumors. It is included as one of the small blue round cell tumors including neuroblastoma, Ewing sarcoma/PNET, and leukemia/lymphoma. Endodermal sinus tumor is a rare vaginal tumor of infancy. Clear cell adenocarcinoma of the vagina (also termed mesonephroma) can present in a patient with or without exposure to DES and mimic rhabdomyosarcoma.

Sixty percent of pediatric ovarian neoplasms are germ cell tumors (70% teratomas, 25% dysgerminomas—most common pediatric ovarian malignancy, and 5% endodermal sinus tumors). Twenty percent are epithelial neoplasms including cystadenoma (80%) and cystadenocarcinoma (10%) and 10% are sex cord tumors. Granulosa cell tumors are the most common ovarian cause of isosexual precocious puberty in females. One-third of pediatric ovarian neoplasms are malignant. Most do not have specific imaging features and are best initially evaluated with ultrasound. CT and MRI scanning are helpful for evaluation of peritoneal involvement, lymphatic spread, or hematogenous pulmonary metastases.

Ovarian cystadenoma is the second most common ovarian neoplasm in children after mature teratoma. It may arise in dysgenetic gonads but less commonly than gonadoblastoma. Leydig cell tumors rarely produce androgens causing virilization in females.

The most common intra-abdominal neonatal mass in a female is an ovarian cyst caused by placental hormonal stimulation of the in utero ovary. These may torse or infarct and are followed clinically with occasional surgical intervention. Ovarian cysts greater than or

TABLE 104-5 Bulging Mass at the Introitus

Ectopic ureterocele
Hydrometrocolpos
Rhabdomyosarcoma
Urethral cyst/Skene gland cyst
Urethral prolapse

equal to 3 cm in size in older children and adolescents can be symptomatic alone or with torsion occasionally. Hemorrhage into ovarian cysts will produce echogenic material with fluid–fluid level or debris on ultrasound and can mimic appendicitis in presentation.

Suggested Reading

Beckwith JB. Questions and answers: Wilms' tumor screening. *AJR Am J Roentgenol.* 1995;164:1294.

Berrocal T, Lopez-Pereira P, Arjonilla A, et al. Anomalies of the distal ureter, bladder, and urethra in children: embryologic, radiologic, and pathologic features. *Radiographics.* 2002;22:1139-1164.

Donnely L et al. *Diagnostic Imaging: Pediatrics.* Philadelphia, PA: Amirsys Publishing; 2005.

Gordon I, Riccabona M. Investigating the newborn kidney- update on imaging techniques. *Semin Neonatol.* 2003;8:269-278.

Karmazyn B, Steinberg R, Kornreich L, et al. Clinical and sonographic criteria of acute scrotum in children: a retrospective study of 172 boys. *Pediatr Radiol.* 2005;35:302-310.

Kawashima A, Sandler CM, Wasserman NF, et al. Imaging of urethral disease: a pictorial review. *Radiographics.* 2004;24(suppl 1): S195-S216.

Kocaoglu M, Frush DP. Pediatric sacral masses. *Radiographics.* 2006;26:833.

Kraus SJ, Lebowitz RL, Royal SA. Renal calculi in children: imaging features that led to diagnoses: a pictorial essay: *Pediatr Radiol.* 1999;29:624.

Kushner BH. Neuroblastoma: a disease requiring a multitude of imaging studies. *J Nucl Med.* 2004;45:1172.

Lonergan GJ et al. "From the Archives of the AFIP: neuroblastoma, ganglioneuroblastoma, and ganglioneuroma: radiologic-pathologic correlation." *Radiographics.* 2002;22:911-934.

Lowe LH, Isuani BH, Heller RM, et al. Pediatric renal masses: Wilms' tumor and beyond. *Radiographics.* 2000;20:1585.

McHugh K, Pritchard J. Problems in imaging of three common pediatric solid tumors. *Eur J Radiol.* 2001;37:72.

Retani R, Cohen HL, Firoe E. Pediatric gynecologic ultrasound. *Ultrasound Q.* 2004;20:127-139.

Slovis T et al. *Caffey's Pediatric Diagnostic Imaging.* 11th ed. Philadelphia, PA: Mosby Elsevier Publishing; 2008.

Troiano RN, McCarthy Sm. Mullerian duct anomalies: imaging and clinical issues. *Radiology.* 2004;233:19-34.

Wu HY, Snyder HM III. Pediatric urologic oncology: bladder, prostate, testis. *Urol Clin North Am.* 2004;31:619-627.

QUESTIONS AND ANSWERS

1. A newborn presents with an enlarged scrotum. On ultrasound, multiple irregular calcifications are noted within the scrotum. Which of the following is the most likely diagnosis?
   A. Neuroblastoma
   B. Tuberculous peritonitis
   C. Teratoma
   D. Meconium peritonitis
   E. Hemangiomatosis

   ANSWER: D. Meconium peritonitis (typically secondary to in utero bowel perforation) can lead to scrotal calcifications in the case of a patent processus vaginalis. Noting that this surrounds the testicle and is not within the testicle would exclude testicular teratoma, and this is not a location for neuroblastoma. Tuberculous peritonitis is rare and would be unlikely to have this appearance. Hemangiomatosis could be considered if there were phleboliths present.

2. What is the most likely testicular tumor in a 1-year-old?
   A. Seminoma
   B. Mixed germ cell tumor
   C. Yolk sac tumor
   D. Embryonal tumor
   E. Teratoma

   ANSWER: C. Yolk sac tumor is the most common testicular tumor in a young boy. Teratoma is the second most common testicular tumor. Other germ cell line tumors are less common. Stromal tumors are less common overall than germ cell tumors.

3. A newborn infant has bilaterally enlarged, hyperechoic kidneys on ultrasound and a history of oligohydramnios. What is the most likely diagnosis?
   A. Autosomal dominant polycystic kidney disease
   B. Autosomal recessive polycystic kidney disease
   C. Multicystic dysplastic kidney
   D. Wilms tumor
   E. Lymphoma

   ANSWER: B. Autosomal recessive polycystic kidney disease is the most common etiology of bilaterally enlarged, hyperechoic kidneys. ADPKD kidney would rarely present in the newborn period and would most commonly have multiple, enlarged cysts. Bilateral MCDK is a fatal disease. Wilms tumor and lymphoma do not present in the newborn period.

4. What is the most common location of GU obstruction in a neonatal male?
   A. Bulbous urethra
   B. Prostatic urethra
   C. Ureterovesicle junction

D. Distal ureter
E. Ureteropelvic junction

ANSWER: E. Ureteropelvic junction obstruction is the most common cause of hydronephrosis in the newborn male. PUV and UVJ obstructions are less common.

5. A 2-year-old girl presents for the first time with burning micturition, fever, pyuria, and flank pain. What is the most appropriate study?
   A. Renal ultrasound and radionuclide cystogram
   B. MR Urography and fluoroscopic voiding cystourethrogram
   C. DMSA scan and radionuclide cystogram
   D. Contrast-enhanced CT and voiding cystourethrogram
   E. Intravenous pyelogram and radionuclide cystogram

   ANSWER: A. Renal ultrasound and radionuclide cystogram is the most appropriate combination of studies in a young girl with a first-time UTI or suspected acute pyelonephritis. Radionuclide cystograms are preferred to fluoroscopic VCUs because of radiation concerns. MR urography, DMSA, and contrast-enhanced CT are occasionally used as supplemental tests in this scenario. IVP is not used in this setting.

6. In a 3-month-old, what is the most likely etiology of an echogenic renal mass?
   A. Multicystic dysplasia
   B. Wilms tumor
   C. Neuroblastoma
   D. Mesoblastic nephroma
   E. Rhabdoid tumor

   ANSWER: D. Mesoblastic nephroma is the most common solid renal mass in early infancy. Multicystic dysplasia should be detected either in utero or perinatally. Wilms tumor occurs at an older age. Neuroblastoma, though the most common solid extracranial tumor of childhood, is not a renal mass. Rhabdoid tumor is rare compared to mesoblastic nephroma.

7. What is the most likely etiology of a mass between the rectum and bladder in a 1-day-old female?
   A. Rectal duplication
   B. Sacrococcygeal teratoma
   C. Hydrometrocolpos
   D. Neuroblastoma
   E. Rhabdomyosarcoma

   ANSWER: C. Hydrometrocolpos with an enlarged vagina presenting as a mass between the rectum and bladder would be the best diagnosis. Rectal duplications are rare and usually occur retrorectal. Sacrococcygeal teratoma and neuroblastoma occur in the presacral space. Congenital rhabdomyosarcoma would be extremely rare.

8. In a 3-year-old female with isosexual precocious puberty and an echogenic ovarian mass, what is the most likely etiology?
   A. Brennan tumor
   B. Granulosa cell tumor
   C. Krukenberg tumor
   D. Benign ovarian cyst
   E. Dysgerminoma

   ANSWER: B. Granulosa cell tumor. This is the most common pediatric tumor causing isosexual precocious puberty in a female. Brennan tumor, Krukenberg tumor, and dysgerminoma do not produce precocious puberty. Autonomous ovarian cysts can produce isosexual precocious puberty though would not be an echogenic mass.

9. What condition has surveillance imaging because of high risk for Wilms tumor?
   A. Hereditary aniridia
   B. Beckwith-Wiedemann syndrome
   C. Neurofibromatosis type I
   D. Horseshoe kidney
   E. Infants of diabetic mother

   ANSWER: B. Beckwith-Wiedemann syndrome. Sporadic aniridia, not hereditary aniridia, requires surveillance imaging for high-risk Wilms tumor. Although neurofibromatosis type I and horseshoe kidney statistically have a slight increased incidence of Wilms tumor, we do not use surveillance imaging for them. Infants of diabetic mothers are not at risk for Wilms tumor.

10. What disorder has increased medullary echogenicity in a newborn?
    A. Fanconi syndrome
    B. Tam-Horsfall proteinuria
    C. Multicystic dysplastic kidney
    D. Caroli disease
    E. Autosomal dominant PCKD

    ANSWER: B. Tamm-Horsfall proteinuria. This causes transient oliguria in the newborn because of Tamm-Horsfall protein deposition in the tubules causing a medullary hyperechoic appearance. This does not occur in Fanconi syndrome, multicystic dysplastic kidney, Caroli disease, or ADPKD (could be seen in ARPKD).

105 PEDIATRIC NEUROIMAGING

Shyamsunder B. Sabat and Yoginder N. Vaid

PEDIATRIC BRAIN

NORMAL MYELINATION

At term birth, the white matter is largely unmyelinated. Myelination of the brain proceeds from posterior to anterior, central to peripheral, and inferior to superior directions. Also, sensory pathways myelinate earlier than motor, projection pathways earlier than association, and proximal pathways earlier than distal. Until 6 months of age, T1-weighted images and after 6 months, T2-weighted images are best for assessment of myelination. On T1 images, myelination is complete by 8 months and by 18 months on T2-weighted images.

CONGENITAL ANOMALIES

Schizencephaly

Schizencephaly refers to gray matter-lined clefts extending from the cortical surface to the ventricles. It can be unilateral (60%) or bilateral (40%). The clefts can be open lip (65%–85%) or closed lip (15%–35%) depending on their position (focally or throughout). Most clefts occur around the pre- and postcentral gyrus. Patients present with seizures, hemiparesis, and variable developmental delay. Bilateral cases have more severe symptoms. Unilateral closed type has the best developmental outcome. Optic nerve hypoplasia and consequent blindness are present in one-third of patients with schizencephaly. The septum pellucidum is often absent in cases of bilateral schizencephaly. Thus, many patients with schizencephaly (especially bilateral) have septo-optic dysplasia. While open lip schizencephaly is easy to diagnose, closed lip may mimic transmantle heterotopia and deep infoldings of polymicrogyria. A dimple on the lateral ventricular wall, where the cleft opens into the ventricle may help identify such subtle cases.

Polymicrogyria

Polymicrogyria is a disorder of neuronal organization, resulting in formation of multiple small gyri. It can be focal, multifocal, or diffuse, and unilateral or bilateral. The posterior portion of the Sylvian fissure is the most common location, followed by parietal and temporal locations. The commonest syndrome associated with polymicrogyria is congenital bilateral perisylvian syndrome consisting of bilateral opercular polymicrogyria presenting with pseudobulbar palsy, seizures, and developmental delay.

Lissencephaly ("smooth brain")

Lissencephaly ("smooth brain") refers to paucity of gyral and sulcal development on the brain surface. Agyria (classic lissencephaly) is complete lack of sulcation and pachygyria (incomplete lissencephaly) is decreased sulcation with few broad, flat gyri. The latter is more common than the former. The sulci in pachygyria are normal with corresponding anatomic names, while the ones seen in polymicrogyria do not correspond to established anatomic sulci. Also in pachygyria, the cortex-white matter junction is smooth, while in polymicrogyria it is irregular. Lissencephaly is associated with various gene mutations such as L1S1, DCX, and syndromes such as Miller-Dicker, Walker-Warburg. Lissencephaly can also be caused by in utero CMV infection. There is a "figure-of-eight" appearance on cross-sectional images because of shallow, vertical sylvian fissures. Cobblestone lissencephaly has a characteristic pattern with irregular cortical projections into the white matter and is seen in various congenital muscular dystrophies (Walker-Warburg syndrome, Fukuyama muscular dystrophy).

Heterotopia

Heterotopia is ectopic gray matter in locations other than the cortex or other normal anatomic locations. Patients almost always present with seizures, variable delay, and motor weakness. Heterotopic gray matter is isointense to gray matter on all MRI pulse sequences.

Heterotopia falls into one of three types. Subependymal heterotopia occurs along the inner ventricular lining and must be differentiated from subependymal nodules of tuberous sclerosis. Focal subcortical heterotopia is subcortical and results in overlying cortex being thin with shallow sulci. It can have mass effect mimicking tumor but does not enhance or have edema. It is often associated with abnormalities such as callosal dysgenesis and dysplastic basal ganglia. Mantle heterotopias is a subtype, which has linear gray matter deposit extending from cortex to ventricular margin but lacks the characteristic dimple on the outer ventricular margin seen in schizencephaly. Band heterotopia (double cortex) is more common in females (90%). It can be complete around the cortex or partial, commonly in the frontal region. Overlying cortex shows normal thickness with shallow sulcation. This heterotopia is hypermetabolic on FDG-PET and shows increased blood flow on BOLD imaging.

Focal cortical dysplasia presents with seizures. Focal cortical dysplasia with balloon cells (Taylor-type dysplasia) shows focal cortical thickening with blurring of gray-white matter junction. Focal cortical dysplasia without balloon cells most commonly appears as a region of thin cortex with volume loss and T2 hyperintensity of underlying white matter. Focal retraction of the cortex with prominent overlying vein (cortical vein sign) if present, aids in the diagnosis of focal cortical dysplasia.

Hemimegalencephaly

Hemimegalencephaly describes hamartomatous overgrowth of part or whole cerebral hemisphere. Imaging features include dysplastic cortex with broad gyri, shallow sulci, ipsilateral enlarged ventricle, white matter signal abnormalities, and heterotopias. It is seen in many disorders like epidermal nevus syndrome, Proteus syndrome, NF1, Klippel-Treunaunay-Weber syndrome, and tuberous sclerosis.

Holoprosencephaly

Holoprosencephaly describes a group of heterogeneous disorders characterized by failure of cleavage of the cerebrum by varying degrees. It is mostly caused by maternal diabetes or by genetic syndromes like trisomy 13 (Patau syndrome) and trisomy 18 (Edward syndrome). Depending on increasing levels of cleavage, it can be divided into alobar, semilobar, and lobar types. In globar holoprosencephaly, the cerebrum is pancake-like with no Sylvian or interhemispheric fissure, and no falx cerebri, septum pellucidum, or corpus callosum. Also absent are the optic tracts, olfactory bulbs (arrhinencephaly), internal cerebral veins, vein of Galen, superior and inferior saggital sinuses. The thalami and basal ganglia are fused and the third ventricle is absent. There is a single monoventricle with wide communication with a large dorsal cyst filling most of the posterior cranium. The cerebellum and brainstem are relatively normal. Discrete middle and anterior cerebral arteries are usually absent, and when present, the latter are fused to form a single azygous anterior cerebral artery. Facial abnormalities can include a cyclopia (single midline orbit, arhinia, and proboscis: a fleshy appendage in forehead), cebocephaly (hypotelorism, single-nostril nose), and ethmocephaly (hypotelorism, proboscis, absent nose). In semilobar holoprosencephaly, there is partial separation of cerebral hemispheres with rudimentary temporal and occipital lobes. The frontal lobes are fused. There is a monoventricle with a partial falx present posteriorly. Septum pellucidum is absent and thalami are partially fused. The corpus callosum consists of only the splenium (only brain anomaly with presence of splenium in absence of anterior corpus callosum). Facial anomalies are mild, like cleft lip and palate. In the lobar form of holoprosencephaly, brain appears normal but frontal horns are fused with absent septum pellucidum. Bodies of lateral ventricles are apposed closely. The falx is present although it is hypoplastic anteriorly; thalami are separate. Face often has only hypotelorism. Lobar holoprosencephaly may be a spectrum of septo-optic dysplasia.

Septo-optic Dysplasia

Septo-optic dysplasia is believed to be a mild form of lobar holoprosencephaly; it consists of absent septum pellucidum with hypoplasia of optic nerve/optic chiasm and of the hypothalamus. It may be associated with Chiari II malformation, aqueductal stenosis, schizencephaly, and corpus callosum agenesis. Hypothalamic pituitary dysfunction is present in two-thirds of patients with septo-optic dysplasia (Demorsier syndrome).

Hydranencephaly

Hydranencephaly is an encephaloclastic porencephaly presumably because of in utero occlusion of bilateral internal carotid arteries. It is thought secondary to infection such as CMV or caused by a genetic cause. A midline falx is present. Differential diagnosis includes severe hydrocephalus in which a thin rim of cortical mantle is present and alobar holoprosencephaly in which falx is absent and thalami are fused.

Agenesis/Dysgenesis of Corpus Callosum

Corpus callosum has rostrum, genu, body, and splenium, which develop from anterior to posterior direction beginning with the genu. Rostrum develops last. Partial agenesis may result in variable formation of anterior structures (except rostrum). Imaging features of complete agenesis include absent cingulate sulcus with gyri appearing to radiate from a high-riding third ventricle. The lateral ventricles are parallel, nonconverging with dilated occipital horns (colpocephaly). There is medial concavity of the frontal horns because of indentation by the bundle of Probst (longitudinal tracts which would have crossed over) and enlargement of the temporal horns. Pericallosal lipomas and interhemispheric cysts, which may or may not communicate with the high-riding third ventricle may be found. Associated malformations include Dandy-Walker syndrome, cephalocele, heterotopia, and coloboma. Callosal agenesis can be seen in Aicardi, Klinefelter, and fetal alcohol syndromes.

Dandy-Walker Syndrome

The Dandy-Walker complex consists of posterior fossa cystic malformations, which includes Dandy-Walker malformation, Dandy-Walker variant, megacistern

TABLE 105-1 Dandy-Walker Complex

Megacistern magna
Dandy-Walker variant
Dandy-Walker malformation
Blake pouch cyst

magna, and Blake pouch cyst (Table 105-1). The Dandy-Walker malformation consists of an enlarged posterior fossa with high position of the tentorium, hypo- or agenesis of the cerebellar vermis and cystic dilatation of the fourth ventricle. The foramina of Magendie and Luschka are absent. Male-to-female ratio is 1:3 and hydrocephalus is often present. Associated malformations may include with dysgenesis or lipoma of the corpus callosum, heterotopias, polymicrogyria, holoprosencephaly, and occipital encephalocele. The Dandy-Walker variant is more common and has variable inferior vermian hypoplasia and varying enlargement of the fourth ventricle but posterior fossa volume remains normal. Megacistern magna consists of a normal vermis but an enlarged cisterna magna. Blake pouch cyst represents posterior ballooning of the inferior medullary velum (posteroinferior wall of the fourth ventricle) into the cisterna magna and is secondary to failure of perforation of the foramen of Magendie. There is no vermian hypoplasia and the posterior fossa is enlarged. The above malformations may be difficult to differentiate from each other but the outcome is related not to the nature of the malformation but the degree of cerebral abnormalities and hydrocephalus.

A large posterior fossa arachnoid cyst, although developmentally unrelated, can mimic the above entities. Posterior fossa is usually enlarged and the vermis is not hypoplastic. It can also be differentiated from Dandy-Walker complex by the fact that it does not communicate with the fourth ventricle (as seen on thin heavy T2-weighted images and CSF flow studies).

Chiari Malformations

Chiari I malformation consists of downward herniation of peg-like cerebellar tonsils through the foramen magnum into the upper cervical spine. It is secondary to short, flat clivus with small posterior fossa. Patients have occipital headache on straining and sometimes have downbeat nystagmus. It can be associated with craniovertebral junction anomalies like basilar invagination, occipitalization of C1, and Klippel-Feil syndrome. Patients can develop hydrocephalus and syringohydromyelia. Tonsillar ectopia because of chronic intracranial hypotension can be differentiated by a sagging third ventricle, enlarged dural sinuses and marked dural enhancement.

Chiari II (Arnold-Chiari malformation) also shows a very small posterior fossa, downward tonsillar and vermian herniation, caudal displacement of the fourth ventricle, and medulla, forming a characteristic cervicomedullary kink. MRI also reveals upward cerebellar herniation with wrapping of cerebellar tissue around the brainstem, midbrain collicular fusion into a beak-like projection (tectal beaking), and fenestrations of falx. Skull films show Luckenschadel or lacunar skull, (which disappears by 6 months of age), scalloped clivus, and absent/hypoplastic posterior arch of C1. Associated abnormalities include lumbar myelomeningocele (90%–100%), dysgenesis of corpus callosum (80%–85%), absence of septum pellucidum (40%), aqueductal stenosis, obstructive hydrocephalus (60%–90%), and syringohydromyelia. It is the single most common cause of hydrocephalus in children constituting approximately 40% of all hydrocephalus.

Chiari III malformation consists of a midline occipital bone defect/posterior spina bifida at C1, C2 with a high cervical/low occipital encephalocele with many of the other intracranial features of Chiari II.

Cephaloceles

Cephalocele is a term given to herniation of intracranial contents through defects in the skull. They are named for the location of bone defects through which they pass. Occipital (70%), parietal (10%), frontoethmoidal (9%), and nasopharyngeal (1%) are the commonest types. Frontoethmoidal is the commonest in Southeast Asia. They are identified as meningoceles if they contain CSF-filled meninges and encephaloceles if they contain brain tissue. MRI shows the contents of the sac and CT depicts the exact osseous defects. Atretic cephaloceles are involuted true cephaloceles and present as subscalp palpable masses in the midline in parietal or occipital regions with focal bone defect. Persistent falcine sinus, a normal accessory sinus, usually obliterated by birth is usually present. Occipital cephaloceles are associated with Chiari malformations, Dandy-Walker malformation, callosal anomalies, heterotopias, and imaging is indicated to pick up these, as well as the relation of the cephalocele to the dural sinuses. Frontoethmoidal cephaloceles show contiguous brain tissue/CSF within it with an absent crista galli. These should be differentiated from other midline masses like nasal dermoid and nasal glioma. Nasal dermoid is bright on T1, suppresses on fat suppression, and shows a split crista galli. Nasal glioma (a misnomer; actually nasal cerebral heterotopia) is dysplastic brain tissue in the nasal cavity or subcutaneous tissue with no intracranial connection. There is no split in the crista galli. Sphenoidal cephaloceles are rare and present as a nasopharyngeal mass. Coronal CT shows midline split in the sphenoid body.

Neurocutaneous Syndromes

A heterogeneous group of disorders affecting nervous system and other ectodermally developed structures. Common ones are neurofibromatosis, tuberous sclerosis, Sturge-Weber syndrome, and von Hippel-Lindau disease. All are autosomal dominant except Sturge-Weber syndrome, which is developmental and not hereditary. Neurofibromatosis is associated with mutation in chromosome 17. Neurofibromatosis type 1 has multiple peripheral nerve neurofibromas (hypointense on T1, hyperintense on T2/FLAIR, and show homogenous enhancement), cranial nerve schwannomas (mostly fifth), craniofacial plexiform neurofibromas (pathognomonic for neurofibromatosis), optic nerve gliomas, cerebral gliomas (tectum, brainstem), CNS hamartomas (unidentified bright objects on T2-weighted images), occlusion/stenosis of distal ICA/proximal MCA with Moya-Moya phenomenon, dumb-bell neurofibromas of spinal nerves with widening of neural foramen, lateral/anterior thoracic meningoceles, dural ectasia with posterior vertebral body scalloping. Skeletal manifestations include orbital dysplasia with bare orbit sign (because of lateral displacement of the innominate line on frontal skull radiograph), perilambdoid skull defects, kyphoscoliosis, pseudoarthrosis of tibia, multiple nonossifying fibromas, and hemihypertrophy. Other systemic manifestations include lower lung interstitial fibrosis, pheochromocytoma, parathyroid adenomas, renal artery stenosis/aneurysms, neurofibromas in wall of intestine, Lisch nodules (hamartomas) in iris, café-au-lait spots, and axillary freckling in skin. Neurofibromatosis type 2 is associated with deletion in chromosome 22. It has multiple meningiomas, bilateral vestibular schwannomas, schwannomas of other cranial nerves, and spinal ependymomas.

Tuberous sclerosis presents as seizures and mental retardation. CNS imaging shows multiple subcortical and subependymal hamartomas (hypodense, nonenhancing on CT and hypointense on T1, hyperintense on T2/FLAIR, calcify after first year of life). Subependymal giant cell astrocytoma is a growing hamartoma at the foramen of Monroe with astrocytic neoplastic transformation and resultant hydrocephalus. It shows uniform enhancement. Interval growth (not enhancement) is the definitive sign of neoplastic transformation. Other manifestations include skin angiofibromas, ash-leaf patch, shagreen patch, gingival fibromas, renal angiomyolipomas (fat-containing tumors), multiple renal cysts, cardiac rhabdomyomas, bone islands, thick periosteal reaction in distal phalanges, lymphangioleiomyomatosis, and repeated pneumothorax/chylothorax.

Sturge-Weber syndrome presents as seizures, bupthalmos and unilateral facial angioma in distribution of V1 and V2 segments of trigeminal nerve (port wine stain). Imaging shows ipsilateral leptomeningeal venous angioma with or without gyral calcification, overlying calvarial thickening, atrophy of underlying brain parenchyma because of vascular steal and enlargement of adjacent choroid plexus.

Von Hippel-Lindau disease consists of single or multiple cerebellar and/or spinal hemangioblastomas (can be cystic with solid enhancing mural nodule/only cyst/only enhancing nodule; tubular flow voids in the nodule are common). Multiple hemangioblastomas are pathognomonic. Other imaging manifestations are retinal angiomas, endolymphatic sac carcinomas, renal cell carcinomas, renal cysts, pheochromocytomas, pancreatic islet cell tumors/cysts/cyst adenomas, epididymal cystadenomas, and cysts in liver, spleen, adrenal, lung, and bones.

Aqueductal Stenosis

It is the most frequent cause of congenital hydrocephalus. Occlusion occurs at the level of superior colliculus or intercollicular sulcus. Most common cause is postinflammatory (50%), secondary to perinatal infections such as TORCH, mumps, influenza, syphilis, or intracranial hemorrhage. It can also be developmental because of aqueductal forking (a condition in which it branches into dorsal and ventral channels and the dorsal in turn divides into several ductules) or aqueductal web. Neoplastic occlusion of the aqueduct can result from tectal/quadrigeminal or pineal masses. MRI shows loss of CSF flow void in the aqueduct. MRI with or without CSF flow studies can be used for diagnosis.

Craniosynostosis

Craniosynostosis refers to premature fusion of the cranial sutures and can be primary as a developmental anomaly or secondary to lack of brain growth. More than three-fourths involve a single suture and are nonsyndromic. The skull shape depends on the suture that prematurely fuses as follows (Table 105-2). CT reveals sutural sclerosis and bony bridging of the sutures.

TABLE 105-2 Craniosynostosis

INVOLVED SUTURE	CEPHALIC SHAPE
Sagittal	Dolichocephaly
Metopic	Trigonocephaly
Unilateral coronal	Anterior plagiocephaly
Unilateral lambdoid	Posterior plagiocephaly
Bilateral coronal with lambdoid	Brachycyphaly/turricephaly
Bilateral coronal with lambdoid	Oxycephaly
All sutures	*Kleeblattschadel* (cloverleaf skull)

Three-dimensional shaded-surface reconstruction is superior to conventional radiographs and CT for diagnosis. Raised ICT, hydrocephalus, proptosis, and optic atrophy are important complications.

INFECTIOUS/INFLAMMATORY DISORDERS

TORCH Infections

Table 100-1.

Congenital CMV is the most common serious viral infection among newborns and results from transplacental infection. Early second trimester infection results in microcephaly, lissencephaly, cerebellar hypoplasia, delayed myelination, hydrocephalus, extensive periventricular calcifications, and lenticulostriate vasculopathy. The latter is seen on US as perivascular calcification along lenticulostriate arteries. In mid second trimester infections, the cortical abnormality is polymicrogyria and all the other above findings, but slightly milder. In late gestation infection, there are no neuronal migrational abnormalities and other findings are milder.

Toxoplasmosis is also acquired transplacentally and imaging shows microcephaly, periventricular and intraparenchymal calcifications, hydrocephalus (often severe), porencephaly, and hydranencephaly (if severe). Unlike CMV infection, cortical malformations are rare.

Rubella is extremely rare in the developed world and can have similar imaging features as toxoplasmosis.

Herpes simplex infection in newborns is acquired while passage through the birth canal and is caused by HSV type 2. There is a diffuse necrotic meningo-encephalitis without predilection for the frontal and temporal lobes unlike in adults. Imaging shows mild meningeal enhancement and signal abnormalities beginning in the white matter which spread to the gray matter over 2 days. Diffusion-weighted MRI shows the earliest changes. Fifty percent have deep gray matter involvement, hemorrhage or cerebellar involvement. Eventually, there is multicystic encephalomalacia and diffuse cerebral atrophy.

Bacterial Meningitis

It is the most common CNS infection in children. Group B *streptococci* and *Escherichia coli* are the most common organisms in neonates, while *Haemophilus influenzae* type 2, *Streptococcus pneumoniae*, *E.coli* and *Neisseria meningitidis* are the culprits in the postneonatal period. Imaging is useful when the diagnosis is in doubt or to identify complications like hydrocephalus (communicating), venous thrombosis (empty delta sign), venous infarcts (do not show restricted diffusion like arterial infarcts), arterial infarcts (seen in basal ganglia, brainstem and is because of arteritis), subdural effusions, and empyemas (empyemas show restricted diffusion while effusions do not), cerebritis, abscess, postmeningitic deafness (for evaluation for cochlear implant; calcification in the cochlea/cochlea stenosis is a poor indicator for success).

Cerebritis and Brain Abscess

Both cerebritis and brain abscess have similar imaging characteristics as in adults, including restricted diffusion. The frontal lobe is the most common location for brain abscess in children. The temporal lobe and cerebellum are preferred sites for otogenic abscesses. Brain abscess in infants has poor capsule formation resulting in rapid enlargement and relatively large size. Also, they are commonly periventricular with high incidence of intraventricular rupture.

Tuberculous Meningitis

Tuberculous meningitis is uncommon in United States and is commonly secondary to miliary tuberculosis. Imaging demonstrates hydrocephalus with marked enhancement of the basal cisterns because of extensive basal exudates. Intraparenchymal tuberculomas (tubercular abscesses) may be seen and the cerebellum is a common location.

Acute Postinfectious Encephalitis

Acute demyelinating encephalomyelitis/ADEM is autoimmune in nature and can occur after common trivial bacterial/viral upper respiratory or gastrointestinal infection or even vaccination. Mortality rate is 10% to 20%. Imaging shows restricted diffusion and scattered T2/FLAIR hyperintensities in bilateral cerebral white matter and also in the thalami and basal ganglia. Sparing of the corpus callosum and deep gray matter involvement distinguish it from multiple sclerosis. Brainstem, cerebellum, and spinal cord are involved in one-third to one half of the cases.

HIV Infection

Approximately 90% of HIV infection is acquired by vertical transmission. Median age of disease onset is approximately 8 months. Imaging shows global atrophy, basal ganglia calcifications, and subcortical white matter calcifications (most common in frontal lobes). As opposed to adults, intracranial neoplasms and infections are relatively rare. Lymphoma is the most common neoplasm, typically involving the basal ganglia/thalamic region and often associated with systemic disease. CMV disease and progressive multifocal leukoencephalopathy are the most common infections. HIV vasculopathy can manifest as vascular ectasia, (seen at base of the brain), vasculitis, and thrombosis. Acquired HIV disease has similar manifestations as in adults.

Rasmussen Encephalitis

Rasmussen encephalitis is chronic localized encephalitis of unknown origin and one of the most important causes of intractable partial seizures. There is T2/FLAIR hyperintensity in the cortex and subcortical white matter involving a part (frontal/temporal) or the whole hemisphere with no contrast enhancement. Eventually, there is atrophy/encephalomalacia of the affected region with progressive dilatation of the adjacent ventricle. MR spectroscopy shows reduced NAA in the affected white matter. FDG-PET imaging reveals diffusely decreased activity in the region. It is treated by antiepileptics and subtotal/total hemispherectomy.

NEOPLASMS

Medulloblastoma

Medulloblastoma arises from the cerebellar vermis and is the most common posterior fossa tumor in children, accounting for 15% to 20% of all intracranial tumors and 30% to 40% of all posterior fossa tumors. They are the most common brain tumor in 6 to 11 year age group with male to female ratio of 3:1. CSF dissemination is very frequent; most common intracranial locations include the vermian and basilar cisterns. Spinal "drop metastasis" are seen in 40% of patients, most commonly in the thoracic and lumbosacral levels. Systemic metastasis can rarely occur to the bones, lymph nodes, and lung. On noncontrast CT, the tumor is slightly hyperdense (best diagnostic sign); on T2-weighted images, the solid portion is isointense to gray matter. Calcifications are seen in 20%; solid portion enhances, and cystic/necrotic areas are seen in up to 50% of cases. Hemorrhage is rare.

Astrocytoma

It the most common brain tumor in children, comprising of 40% to 50% of all brain tumors. Forty percent occur in the cerebellum, 20% in the brainstem and the remaining 40% are supratentorial. Most of the cerebellar astrocytomas are juvenile pilocytic astrocytomas, WHO grade 1. Cerebellar astrocytomas occur in the cerebellar hemisphere and approximately two-thirds of these tumors are cystic with a solid well-enhancing mural nodule. The remaining one-third are solid, enhancing with central nonenhancing cystic region. Supratentorial astrocytomas have varying WHO grades with variable solid/cystic components; they often involve the deep nuclei and have a worse prognosis than cerebellar pilocytic astrocytoma.

Ependymoma

Ependymoma comprises 8% to 15% of posterior fossa tumors. It arises from the floor/roof of the fourth ventricle and has a tendency to grow through the midline foramen of Magendie into the cisterna magna (a specific sign seen in 60%) or through the lateral foramina of Lushka into the CPA cisterns. It is a predominantly solid mass with calcifications in approximately 50% and small cysts in 20%. Hemorrhage and CSF dissemination occur in approximately 10%. On CT it is iso to mildly hyperdense and isointense to gray matter on T2-weighted images. They show moderate heterogeneous enhancement.

Brainstem Gliomas

Brainstem gliomas comprise approximately 15% to 20% of brain tumors and 20% to 30% of posterior fossa tumors. They are most commonly located in the pons, cause expansion of the brainstem and thus present with multiple cranial nerve palsies. Two-thirds have indistinct margins; correspond to WHO grade III/IV and show minimal or no enhancement. One-third are focal and are either grade I/II.

Craniopharyngioma

Craniopharyngiomas account for 50% of suprasellar tumors in children. Ninety percent have cysts, 90% with calcification, and 90% have contrast enhancement (peripheral rim enhancing). They may erode into the dorsum sellae or may grow into the sella with widening of the sella.

Primitive Neuroectodermal Tumors

Primitive neuroectodermal tumors are large tumors that occur in deep cerebral white matter and have distinct margins. The solid portion is hypodense on CT and isointense to gray matter on T2/FLAIR images; cystic areas and punctate calcification are common. When a large, solid, and sharply delineated mass is seen in a young child, the diagnosis of PNET is most likely, particularly when the mass is markedly heterogeneous.

Dysembryoblastic Neuroepithelial Tumor (DNET)

Dysembryoblastic neuroepithelial tumor (DNET) is seen in children or young adults. It presents with longstanding, refractory epilepsy. Sixty percent occur in the temporal lobe and 30% in the frontal. Imaging demonstrates a well-demarcated, lobulated cortical mass, hypodense on CT, hypointense on T1-weighted, and hyperintense on T2-weighted images with cystic or microcystic components in 30% to 40% of the cases. Calcification is present in 30% of cases. Scalloping of the inner table of the calvarium may be seen. Enhancement, usually patchy, can be seen 30% of tumors. They are metabolically inactive with no significant activity on FDG-PET.

Choroid Plexus Papilloma

Choroid plexus papilloma soccur mainly in infants, cause severe secretory hydrocephalus, and have marked male predominance. It is a lobulated intraventricular mass, most commonly in the atrium of the lateral ventricle. The surface of the mass has papillary appearance on MRI that differentiates it from other intraventricular tumors like meningioma and ependymoma, which have a smooth surface. It is iso-/mildly hyperdense on CT with punctate foci of calcification and homogeneous contrast enhancement. The central portion is hypointense on T2-weighted images. Choroid plexus carcinoma has a tendency to invade the ventricle walls with adjacent vasogenic edema.

Pineal Tumors

Germinomas account for more than 50% of all pineal tumors. Male to female ratio is 10:1. Peak occurrence is in later part of second decade. It presents as a round/lobulated mass with iso-to hyperdensity on CT, T2-weighted/FLAIR hypointensity on MRI, and shows homogeneous contrast enhancement. CSF dissemination to the brain and spine is common.

Pineocytomas are uncommon in children. Pinealoblastoma is the second most common tumor of the pineal gland in the pediatric age group. They are highly malignant and can invade the cerebellar vermis, the walls of the third ventricle, and often have CSF dissemination. There usually iso-to-hyperintense on T2-weighted/FLAIR images. Necrotic or cystic areas may be present in larger pineoblastomas. Typically, there is intense but heterogeneous contrast enhancement. They are larger, more irregular and show more heterogeneous enhancement than pineocytomas or germinomas.

METABOLIC DISORDERS

Demyelinating/Dysmyelinating Disorders

Metachromatic leukodystrophy, typically presents between infancy and 5 to 7 years of age. There is diffuse demyelination with subcortical white matter sparing. Krabbe disease (mean age 3–6 months) shows bilateral hyperdense thalami, caudate nuclei, corona radiata, and cerebellar dentate nuclei with T1 hyperintensity in these structures. Enhancement of cranial nerves and the cauda equina may be seen. Adrenoleukodystrophy is an X-linked disorder, affecting males 5 to 7 years of age and shows predominately bilateral occipital white matter and splenium of corpus callosum involvement. Canavan disease (neonatal period) is commonly seen in Ashkenazi Jews and presents with macrocephaly with diffuse white matter disease and early involvement of subcortical U fibers. MRS shows a very high NAA peak, which is highly specific for this disorder. Alexander disease (infancy) also shows macrocephaly with predominately frontal white matter involvement associated with involvement of bilateral caudate nuclei and parietal white matter. MELAS (Mitochondrial myopathy Encephalopathy with Lactic Acidosis and Stroke) shows fluctuating T2 hyperintensities involving both gray and white matter predominantly in the occipital and parietal lobes, evolving into well-defined strokes, or resolving completely. MRS shows elevated lactate peak. Leigh disease is a mitochondrial disorder with characteristic, bilateral, nonenhancing, putaminal CT hypodensities and T2 hyperintensities with elevated lactate levels in basal ganglia.

MISCELLANEOUS DISORDERS

Mucopolysaccharidosis shows patchy white matter T2 hyperintensities in bilateral cerebral hemispheres and corpus callosum with prominent perivascular spaces. Hallervorden-Spatz disease shows markedly T2 hypointense globus pallidus with central hyperintensity (eye of the tiger sign). Wilson disease reveals CT hypodensity and T1 hyperintensity in bilateral basal ganglia, while phenylketonuria shows nonspecific periventricular white matter hyperintensity on T2.

Trauma

CT scan is the modality of choice in imaging acute head trauma. Epidural hematoma in children is the result of tear of dural veins rather than arterial injury. Epidural and subdural hemorrhages have imaging characteristics similar to adults.

Nonaccidental Head Injury

Nonaccidental head injury (NAHI) is the most common cause of severe head injury in infants. Children younger than 3 years are most vulnerable and shaking is the most common mechanism. Characteristic imaging findings include bilateral subdural hemorrhages, subarachnoid hemorrhage, interhemispheric subdural hemorrhage, subdural hemorrhage of various ages, and severe head injury in absence of fracture, diffuse axonal injury, and cerebral atrophy in later stages. Bilateral retinal hemorrhages are frequent; macrocephaly, bilateral posterior rib fractures, and metaphyseal fractures can also be seen. Skull fractures are common and are frequently located at the vertex, communicated, depressed, and often cross sutures. Husbands, boyfriends, and caretakers are the most common perpetrators, and greater than three-fourths of the perpetrators are unemployed. History frequently is insufficient to explain the severity of injury. Coagulopathies need to be ruled out. Glutaric aciduria type 1 can mimic NAH1 and also has macrocephaly, bilateral subdural, effusions, and retinal hemorrhages, but neuromotor abnormalities are almost always present.

VASCULAR DISORDERS

Vein of Galen Aneurysm/Malformation

Aneurysm is a misnomer. Vein of Galen aneurysm/malformation is a central AVM occurring between intracranial arteries, usually choroidal, thalamoperforate, and anterior cerebral arteries and the vein of Galen and is probably secondary to intrauterine straight sinus thrombosis with recanalization. Male to female ratio is 2:1. It is detectable in utero after 30 weeks gestation as a hypoechoic aneurysmally dilated vein of Galen. Rim calcification with variable thrombus can be seen on CT and MRI. It usually presents as intractable neonatal heart failure, macrocrania with obstructive hydrocephalus or headaches and intracranial hemorrhage beyond infancy. There can be areas of encephalomalacia secondary to steal and ischemia. Neonatal heart failure, if present has a high mortality despite treatment.

Moya-Moya Syndrome

Is characterized by progressive occlusion of terminal internal cerebral and proximal middle cerebral arteries with development of multiple collaterals consisting of thalamoperforate and lenticulostriate arteries giving rise to the classic "puff of smoke" appearance on angiography. Various diseases can give rise to moyamoya type of circulation: NF1, tuberous sclerosis, mucopolysaccaridoses, recurrent thromboembolism, Down syndrome, radiation therapy, sickle cell disease, glycogen storage disease type Ia, and HIV. MRI shows multiple flow voids in the basal ganglia, thalami, and base of brain with subarachnoid hemorrhage and cerebral infarcts.

Sickle Cell Disease

CT contrast agents may precipitate sickling and are to be avoided. MR contrast agents are however safe. Imaging in sickle cell disease reveals thickened calvaria, infarctions, encephalomalacia from previous ischemic episodes, and moya-moya type of circulation.

Juvenile Angiofibroma

Juvenile angiofibroma occurs in the adolescent males and presents as recurrent, often refractory epistaxis. Imaging shows a nasopharyngeal mass with multiple flow voids and intense enhancement. The mass often causes bowing of the lateral wall of the maxillary sinus (antral sign). Epistaxis is controlled by endovascular embolization.

Hereditary Hemorrhagic Telangiectasia (Osler Weber Rendu Disease)

Multiple tiny telangiectasias in the nasal mucosa cause recurrent and refractory epistaxis and are often the initial presentation in patients with Osler-Weber-Rendu disease, usually manifesting in the second decade. Control of epistaxis is best done by endovascular means.

Hypoxic Ischemic Injury in the Newborn

Hypoxic ischemic injury in the newborn in premature manifests as either germinal matrix hemorrhage or perivertricula leucomalacia. Germinal matrix hemorrhage occurs in newborns younger than 34 weeks in the region of the caudothalamic groove. There may or may not be intraventricular extension, hydrocephalus, or less commonly, intraparenchymal extension. This type of hemorrhage is hyperechoic on US. Periventricular leukomalacia is ischemia occurring in frontal white matter near foramen of Monroe or in peritrigonal location. Subsequent cavitation occurs in approximately 3 weeks. Before cavitations, periventricular leukomalacia appears as indistinct, globular hyperechoic areas. Subsequent cavities are typically tiny and clustered. CT and MRI later reveal T2/FLAIR hyperintensity with paucity of periventricular white matter and ventriculomegaly.

In full-term newborns, mild-to-moderate hypotension causes ischemia in the watershed territories of ACA-MCA and MCA-PCA (called parasaggital injury). Profound hypotension irrespective of age infarcts the basal ganglia, thalami, and perirolandic cortex, which are the most metabolically active areas of the brain.

PEDIATRIC SPINE

CONGENITAL ANOMALIES

Aplasia or Hypoplasia of Odontoid

Complete failure of formation of dens results in aplasia while partial formation is referred to as dens hypoplasia. Aplasia of os terminale results in a notch at the tip of the odonto is old process. Os terminale appears at 6 years of age and fused with rest of dens by 10 to 12 years. During this age group, it should not be confused for a fracture.

Os Odontoideum

Os odontoideium is felt to be a variant resulting from enlargement of the os terminale part of odontoid, associated with enlarged anterior arch of C1. It also mimics a fracture of odontoid. Instability at cranio-cervical junction and C1-2 should be checked by flexion extension views. There is an association with Down, Morquio, and Klippel-Feil syndromes.

SEGMENTATION ANOMALIES

Block Vertebra or failure of sclerotome segmentation results in fused vertebrae at one or multiple levels, lumbar more common than cervical spine, which is more common than thoracic spine. Narrowing (waist) at the level of rudimentary disc and fused posterior elements are typical findings. Differential diagnosis includes postsurgical changes, juvenile chronic arthritis, postdiscitis and ankylosing spondylitis. There may be associated other anomalies: hemivertebra, butterfly vertebra, rib fusion anomalies, and posterior arch anomalies. This can be an isolated finding or associated with syndromes like Klippel-Feil syndrome.

KLIPPEL-FEIL SYNDROME

Klippel-Feil syndrome includes failure of segmentation of cervical somites creating block vertebra at one or multiple levels in cervical spine. Clinically, patients present short neck with limited neck motion and low posterior hairline (40%–50%). There is an association with Sprengel shoulder (20%–30%), congenital scoliosis (60%), and neurologic problems such as synkinesia (20%).

VATER ASSOCIATION (VACTERL ASSOCIATION)

Nonrandom association of anomalies of multiple organ systems (except brain) is referred to VATER syndrome: Vertebral, Anorectal/auricular, Tracheoesophageal fistula, Esophageal atresia, Renal/radial/rib, limbanomalies. It is diagnosed when three or more of these coexist.

Vertebral anomalies including block vertebra, hemivertebra, and butterfly vertebra are associated with sickle sacrum, caudal regression, and cardiac anomalies (VSD (30%), PDA (26%), ASD (20%).

SPINAL DYSRAPHISM

Congenital anomalies of spine are usually associated with tethering of spinal cord. Nonoccult includes meningocele (only meninges) and myelomeningocele (meninges and spinal elements). Occult anomalies are skin covered or nearly skin covered with dimple, dermal sinus tract, lipoma, skin tag (tail), tuft of hair, or hemangioma.

Underlying cord abnormalities include tethered cord, split cord (diastematomyelia), and terminal myelocystocele. Rarely cord may terminate high (stump ending). Intrathecal lesions can include dermoid, epidermoid, hemangioma, and anterior meningocele. Spinal ultrasound is best for initial screening, and MRI is further definitive evaluation.

DIASTEMATOMYELIA

Diastematomyelia (split cord malformation) is a type of occult dysraphism. It occurs as a sagittal split of the cord by a fibrous, cartilaginous, or osseous (less than 50%) bar. There may be associated segmentation anomalies, widened interpediculate distance. Most are located in the lumbar or lower thoracic spine. Split cord may reunite or stay split, and a syrinx is identified in up to 50% of cases. The cord abnormalities will need to be untethered, and there is good prognosis following spur resection with untethering.

CAUDAL REGRESSION SYNDROME

Caudal regression syndrome describes a series of anomalies, including partial or complete agenesis of sacrum, thoracic, and lumbar spine. It is secondary to defective induction of caudal cell mass before seventh week of gestation and occurs in 1% of all diabetic pregnancies. There is an association with VACTRL.

CURRARINO TRIAD

Currarino triad includes partial sacral agenesis (scimitar sacrum), imperforate anus, and anterior meningocele. It may be associated with teratoma, or cyst in presacral region.

INFLAMMATORY DISORDERS

Discitis is an inflammatory process of disc space. *Staphylococcus aureus* is the most common agent. Initially, patient presents with low back pain and typically have negative radiographs. Bone scan is usually positive at presentation revealing increased uptake in bodies on either side of the disc. Radiographic findings will eventually include a narrow disc with endplate irregularity of the vertebral bodies.

MRI reveals low T1 signal in marrow on adjacent bodies, decreased disc space, and loss of cortical low signal. T2-weighted images demonstrate high signal in marrow, loss of high signal of disc, and edema of paravertebral tissues. Gadolinium confirms the diagnosis with enhancement of the vertebral bodies and disc margins as well as the paravertebral soft tissues.

TUBERCULOUS SPONDYLITIS

Although, rare in the United States, incidence is on rise with increasing immigration from Southeast Asia and Latin America. Caudal thoracic or lumbar spine is the most common site of involvement. Anterior vertebral body initially affected with spread to the disc and adjacent vertebra. Posterior elements are relatively spared (gibus deformity).

Radiographs reveal lytic lesion in anterior body with disc narrowing. Multiple vertebral bodies may be affected, and the disc space and posterior elements may be spared. Paraspinal soft tissue with cold psoas abscess is the classic finding. Contrast-enhanced MRI depicts the extent of disease more accurately, specially the soft-tissue abscesses.

NEOPLASMS

Ewing Sarcoma

Ewing sarcoma is a malignant lesion of primitive neuroectodermal (small blue cell tumor) origin, arising from vertebral body with almost purely destructive nature. There is usually associated soft-tissue mass. Patients may present with localized pain, fever and leukocytosis.

Radiography shows permeative destruction, vertebra plana, and multiple vertebral bodies may be involved. MRI is the best modality for staging. Differential considerations include Langerhans cell histiocytosis, osteomyelitis, other small blue cell tumors and sarcoma.

METASTASES

Metastatic disease to the spine is usually from leukemia, lymphoma, rhabdomyosarcoma, neuroblastoma, Wilms tumor, and PNET. Langerhans cell histiocytosis will have similar appearance. Radiography reveals lytic or sclerotic lesions, compression of vertebral bodies, and paraspinal masses. On MRI, there is variable signal on T1-weighted and increased signal on T2-weighted images. Fat suppressed, postcontrast images demonstrate the tumor infiltration.

Leukemia is the most common malignancy of childhood. Acute lymphoblastic leukemia is much more common than acute myeloblastic leukemia. Imaging findings are nonspecific, characterized by osteopenia, compression deformities, and pathologic fractures. Soft-tissue masses (chloromas) in the paraspinal region are more commonly seen in acute myelogenous leukemia.

Imaging findings in Hodgkin and non-Hodgkin lymphoma are also nonspecific in nature with multiple focal lesions, usually lytic and rarely sclerotic nature. Soft-tissue masses in the paraspinal region and adenopathy may be helpful additional findings.

ANEURYSMAL BONE CYST

Aneurysmal bone cyst (ABC) is a benign cystic expansile mass with loculated appearance on conventional radiography. Up to one-third occur in the spine, usually arising in the posterior elements and may extend into the body. Absent spinous process or pedicle on frontal radiograph and expansile mass in the lamina on lateral view are classic findings. CT demonstrates multiple fluid/fluid levels because of hemorrhage. There is natural zone of transition. Septal enhancement may be seen on postcontrast CT. MRI demonstrates the products of hemorrhage more clearly.

OSTEOBLASTOMA

Osteoblastoma (giant osteoid osteoma) is an expansile lesion arising in the posterior elements of spine. It is greater than 2 cm in size, characterized by single lytic with and variable sclerosis of its margins. It may be difficult to identify on conventional radiographs. CT demonstrates narrow zone of transition. The appearance is similar to a large osteoid osteoma. MR demonstrates variable signal on T1- and T2-weighted sequences. Rarely fluid/fluid levels similar to aneurysmal bone cyst may be seen. Enhancement on postcontrast scan is variable. The patient may present with painful scoliosis.

LANGERHANS CELL HISTIOCYTOSIS

Langerhans cell histiocytosis is a nonneoplastic condition characterized by monoclonal proliferation of Langerhans cells. There is vertebral body involvement sparing the adjacent discs (thoracic greater than lumbar greater than cervical spine). On electron microscopy, cytoplasmic inclusion bodies (Birbeck granules) are identified.

Imaging features include severe compression deformity of the vertebral bodies, resulting in vertebra plana. The posterior elements, usually spared, are more commonly affected in cervical region. Small paraspinal soft-tissue mass can be seen. Commonly affected regions include the skull, spine, pelvis, and extremity bones. Lytic lesions with variable sclerosis are seen.

Conventional skeletal survey is more sensitive than bone scan. MRI demonstrates that spinal soft-tissue masses and mass effect on the spinal cord more accurately. The disc shows no involvement in this condition, even in the presence of extensive compression deformity of adjoining vertebral bodies.

TRAUMA

Fractures and dislocations of the spine are less common than in adults but are important to diagnose, as they are associated with significant morbidity and mortality. Developmental structures can mimic trauma. Primary centers of ossification begin to appear after

8 weeks of gestation. Secondary centers appear around puberty and fuse by 25 years of age. The atlas has one ossification center for its anterior arch and two for the posterior arch. Anterior arch is seen only in 20% of patients in first year. The axis has five primary centers, one for body, one for each neural arch, and two for the dens. The subdental synchondrosis should not be confused for a fracture. It begins close after 3 years of age in girls and by 5 years of age in boys. The terminal center for dens appears by 6 years of age and fuses by 10 to 12 years. C3 through C7 have three primary ossifications centers (one for body and one for each arches). The synchondroses fuse by 3 to 6 years of age.

Each vertebra has five secondary centers, one for transverse process, one for spinous process, and one for superior and inferior epiphyseal ring. They appear by puberty and close by 25 years of age. Horizontal orientation of the facet joints makes the spine in younger children susceptible to subluxation and dislocations. After 8 to 11 years, the nature of injuries becomes similar to adults. Pseudosubluxation of C2 over C3 and C3 over C4 can be seen up to age 11. Normal alignment of the posterior spinolaminar line helps to differentiate from the true subluxation. Injuries in the upper cervical spine are more common, because of higher fulcrum in younger children (C2–3) than adults (C5–6). Heavier head and poorer support by weaker ligaments make upper cervical spine more susceptible to distraction, subluxation, and dislocation. Spinal cord injuries without radiographic abnormalities (SCIWORA) is more common in children than in adults.

Atlanto-occipital dislocation is seen in young children involved in high-speed motor vehicle collisions. Typically, there is anterior displacement of the skull relative to the spine. On lateral view of the cervical spine, the dens to basion distance (DB) should be between 5 and 12 mm. Powers ratio (BC/OA) should be less than one.

SPONDYLOLYSIS/SPONDYLOLISTHESIS

Spondylolysis is a break in pars interarticularis, felt to be a stress- or trauma-related. L5 and L4 are the commonest sites. Most are bilateral (less than 15% unilateral). This is best demonstrated on an oblique view of the spine as a break in the "Scotty dog's neck." Bone scan with SPECT is the most sensitive modality for initial diagnosis. Axial and sagittal CT is used for anatomic localization. MRI shows low signal on T1-weighted and high signal on T2-weighted images through the region of pars interarticularis.

MISCELLANEOUS

Scheurmann Disease

Scheurmann disease (juvenile kyphosis) is a disease of children characterized by kyphosis with pain in the thoracolumbar region. Children between the age of 13 and 16 years are most commonly affected. Etiology is uncertain, but pathologically, there is osteochondrosis of the secondary centers of ossification of the vertebral bodies. Metabolic, mechanical, and endocrine causes have been proposed. Males are affected more than females, and it may be hereditary, autosomal dominant.

Radiographs demonstrate thoracic kyphosis, wedging of the vertebrae, irregular end plates of the vertebral bodies because of herniation of the nucleus pulposus (Schmorls nodes). Limbus vertebra may also be seen. Diagnostic criteria: (Sorenson) include hyperkyphosis greater than 40 degrees, with irregular upper and lower vertebral endplates, loss of disc space height, wedging of 5 degrees or more in three consecutive vertebrae. Differential considerations include congenital kyphosis, trauma, Langerhans cell histiocytosis, osteoporosis because of chronic glucocorticoid steroid therapy, ankylosing spondylitis, and generalized skeletal displasia.

Scoliosis

Scoliosis is defined as lateral curvature of spine greater than 10 degrees. It is idiopathic, characterized by dextrocurvature of the thoracic spine with levocurvature of the lumbar spine. Females are affected seven times more commonly than males. Atypical idiopathic scoliosis has levothoracic and dextrolumbar curvature. Congenital scoliosis is caused by segmentation or formation anomalies or a combination of the two. It is typically characterized by short segment acute scoliosis. Neuromuscular scoliosis is typically C-shaped. Infections of tuberculous or pyogenic origin, benign and malignant tumors, trauma, and radiation therapy are other common etiologies for scoliosis.

Conventional radiography best demonstrates the nature of scoliosis. Method of Cobb is utilized for measurement: the angle between two lines drawn perpendicular to the endplates of the terminal vertebrae is measured. MRI may be used to rule out underlying spinal cord anomalies including tethering, tumor, syrinx or infection among etiologies. CT and three-dimensional reconstruction are useful for surgical planning.

Intervertebral Disc Calcification

Intervertebral disc calcification is of unknown etiology. Infection and trauma have been implicated. Typically patients present with fever, neck pain, elevated sedimentation rate, and leukocytosis. Biochemical abnormalities of the nucleus pulposus and abnormal vascular supply of the disc are also proposed mechanisms of disease. Cervical and thoracic spine are most common sites of disc calcification, and C6-7 is the most common site for symptomatic disc calcification. Overall, it is a self limiting condition, rarely requiring surgical intervention.

Radiographs readily demonstrate disc calcification. CT or MR is used to demonstrate mass effect on the cord. Of the symptomatic patients, a little more than one-third of the patients may demonstrate posterior disc protrusion.

Sacrococcygeal Teratoma

Sacrococcygeal teratoma is a germ cell tumor containing elements of all three germ cell layers located in the coccyx. It usually presents as a large mass in distal end of body in a newborn or diagnosed on prenatal sonography. Males are affected four times more than females. Eighty percent are benign. Tumors are staged based upon the tumors' relative location (inside, outside) the body (Table 105-3).

Radiography reveals a soft-tissue mass, many with calcifications. Ultrasound reveals a complex cystic/solid mass. CT and MRI show complex mass with cystic, solid, hemorrhagic and calcified components and heterogeneous enhancement. Differential considerations include anterior meningocele, neuroblastoma, rhabdomyosarcoma, and rarely chordoma.

Astrocytoma of Cord

Astrocytoma of cord is the most common intramedullary primary tumor of cord of childhood; most are low-grade gliomas, although subarachnoid spread has been seen. It is associated with NF 1 and 2. It is an asymmetric infiltrating mass with homogeneous enhancement and no tendency for hemorrhage. Differential considerations include other tumors of cord, syringohydromyelia, acute inflammatory myelitis, cord ischemia, vascular malformations.

Ependymoma of Cord

Ependymoma of the cord most commonly occurs in cervical region as an expansile intramedullary mass with hemorrhagic features. It is slow growing with widening of osseous canal, increased interpediculate distance, and posterior vertebral scalloping. Symmetrical expansion of cord is typical. Myxopappilary ependymoma is a separate entity that arises from filum terminale. It is an enhancing mass that is also slow growing with expansion of bony canal similar to intramedullary type. It has a much better prognosis than intramedullary type.

TABLE 105-3 Staging of Sacro/Coccygeal Teratoma

STAGING	TUMOR RELATIVE TO BODY
I	Primarily external (47%)
II	Dumb-bell shaped, equally external and internal (34%)
III	Primarily internal (9%)
IV	Totally internal (10%), mostly malignant

Neuroblastoma

Neuroblastoma arises from primitive neural crest cells and has variable differentiation and malignant tendency. Ganglioneuroma is the most differentiated and most benign; ganglioneuroblastoma, a mixture of neuroblasts and ganglion cells; neuroblastoma, most poorly differentiated and most malignant therefore, it presents as paraspinal abdominal mass with weight loss, fatigue, irritability (paraneoplastic syndrome). Neuroblastoma accounts for 65% to 70% intra-abdominal paraspinal masses. Radiography shows paraspinal soft-tissue widening with calcifications and osseous bony destruction. MRI shows paraspinal enhancing mass with or without intraspinal extradural extension and cord compression. MRI is best for diagnosis; presurgical planning incorporates PET with FDG. Bone scan is also good for staging while MIBG is good for staging as well as postsurgical surveillance.

Neurofibroma

Type 1 neurofibromatosis (NF1), an autosomal dominant (chromosome 17) mesodermal dysplasia associated with nerve root neurofibroma, plexiform neurofibroma or malignant peripheral nerve tumors is more common in children (1/5000). Spinal manifestations include, kyphoscoliosis, multiple nerve root tumors and lateral meningocele (dural ectasias).

Type 2 neurofibromatosis (NF 2) is more common in adults, (1/50 000), and is an autosomal dominant (chromosome 22) dysplasia characterized by multiple inherited schwanomas (nerve VIII most common), intraspinal meingiomas and intramedullary ependymomas. More than 80% have intraspinal tumors at diagnosis.

Hydrosyringomyelia

A general radiographic term used to describe a cavitory lesion of cord in (hydromyelia) or around (syringomyelia) the spinal central canal. Patients present with loss of pain and sensation with preservation of propisception, position, and light touch. Etiologies include Chiari malformation I or II, trauma, infection, and spinal cord tumor. Imaging reveals a linear, cystic, sometime septated lesion. Contrast enhancement is useful in differentiation and demonstration of associated tumor.

Suggested Reading

Chao CP, Zaleski CG, Patton AC. Neonatal hypoxic-ischemic encephalopathy: multimodality imaging findings. *Radiographics*. 2006;26(suppl 1):S159-S172.

Donnelly LF. *Diagnostic Imaging Pediatrics*. Vol 7. 1st ed. Salt Lake City: Amirsys (Philadelphia : Elsevier);2005:38-45.

Gerber P, Coffman K. Nonaccidental head trauma in infants. *Childs Nerv Syst*. 2007;23(5):499-507.

Hedlund GL. Neuroradiology of the central nervous system in childhood. *Neurol Clin*. 2002;20(4):965-981.

Herron J. Intra-cranial manifestations of the neurocutaneous syndromes: pictorial review. *Clin Radiol*. 2000;55:82-98.

Holland BA, Haas DK, Norman D, Brant-Zawadzki M, Newton TH. MRI of normal brain maturation. *AJNR Am J Neuroradiol*. 1986;7:201-208.

Hunter JV, Wang ZJ. MR spectroscopy in pediatric neuroradiology. *Magn Reson Imaging Clin N Am*. 2001;9(1):165-189.

Osborn RE, Byrd SE, Naidich TP, Bohan TP, Friedman H. MR imaging of neuronal migrational disorders. *AJNR Am J Neuroradiol*. 1988;9(6):1101-1106.

Vézina LG. Imaging of central nervous system tumors in children: advances and limitations. *J Child Neurol*. 2008;23(10):1128-1135.

QUESTIONS AND ANSWERS

1. What is the normal progression of myelination in a newborn?
   A. Cranial to caudal
   B. Posterior to anterior
   C. Motor to sensory
   D. Peripheral to central

   ANSWER: B. Myelination characteristically occurs from posterior to anterior, caudal to cranial, and central to peripheral. Also, sensory and projection pathways myelinate before association pathways.

2. Which of the following can mimic child abuse?
   A. Canavan disease
   B. Phenylketonuria
   C. Homogentisic aciduria
   D. Glutaric aciduria

   ANSWER: D. Glutaric aciduria type I shows characteristic signs of child abuse head injury like bilateral subdural effusions, large head, and bilateral retinal hemorrhages. The most striking finding on brain imaging is the presence of very wide CSF spaces anterior to the temporal lobes and within the sylvian fissures. Widening of the sylvian fissures is a very characteristic finding in this disorder. Abnormal neuromotor development is almost always present and is a clue to the diagnosis.

3. Which of the following is closely related to septo-optic dysplasia?
   A. Hydranencephaly
   B. Lobar holoprosencephaly
   C. Lissencephaly
   D. Colpocephaly

   ANSWER: B. Septo-optic dysplasia is closely related lobar holoprosencephaly and shares many of its features. In fact many consider many cases of lobar holoprosencephaly to be a subtype of septo-optic dysplasia.

4. What is most commonly associated with corpus callosal agenesis?
   A. Dandy-Walker malformation
   B. Holoprosencephaly
   C. Lissencephaly
   D. Schizencephaly

   ANSWER: A. The most common malformation associated with callosal agenesis is Dandy-Walker malformation. Syndromes in which callosal agenesis is seen are Aicardi syndrome, fetal alcohol syndrome. Lissencephaly is commonly seen in congenital muscular dystrophies. Holoprosencephaly is seen in Edward and Patau syndromes.

5. In which of the following is CSF dissemination *not* seen?
   A. Ependymoma
   B. Medulloblastoma
   C. Choroid plexus papilloma
   D. Pinealoblastoma

   ANSWER: C. CSF dissemination is seen in all except in choroid plexus papilloma. Germinomas that occur typically in suprasellar/pineal region can also have CSF dissemination. CSF dissemination is most commonly present at the time of presentation in medulloblastoma.

6. In which of the following diseases are Hyperdense thalami seen on CT?
   A. Metachromatic leukodystrophy
   B. Alexander disease
   C. Wilson disease
   D. Krabbe disease

   ANSWER: D. Krabbe is an autosomal recessive sphingolipidosis. The thalami, central white matter, and cerebellum, which show hyperdensities on CT are seen on MR as decreased signal intensity on T2-weighted images and increased on T1-weighted images. These findings are attributed to alterations in the ratio of lipids, water, and proteins in response to breakdown of myelin and the associated astrogliosis with fine microcalcifications.

7. In which of the following diseases can Moya-moya disease be seen?
   A. Sickle cell disease
   B. Amyloidosis
   C. Myelofibrosis
   D. Multiple myeloma

   ANSWER: A. Moyamoya is seen in sickle cell disease. It is associated with nonatherosclerotic intimal thickening and occlusion of terminal ICA, proximal MCA, and ACA. It can also be seen in NF1, protein C/S deficiency, radiation injury, Down syndrome, systemic lupus erythematosis, and polyarteritis nodosa.

8. Which of the following diseases are spinal ependymomas associated with?
   A. Chiari II malformation
   B. NF2
   C. Von Hippel-Lindau disease
   D. Tuberous sclerosis

   ANSWER: B. NF2 has associated multiple meningiomas, bilateral eighth nerve and multiple cranial nerve schwannomas, spinal cord ependymomas, multiple paraspinal schwannomas/neurofibromas. The ependymomas usually occur in the cauda.

9. In what percentage of patients with Chiari II malformation Myelomeningocele is seen ?
   A. 0%–10%
   B. 10%–20%
   C. 50%–60%
   D. 90%–100%

   ANSWER: D. Myelomeningocele is seen in almost all cases of Chiari II syndrome and is located in the lumbar region. The cord is low lying and tethered. Lipomyelomeningocele can also be found. Other spinal dysraphisms can also be associated.

10. Children born to diabetic mothers are at risk for which of the following diseases?
    A. Sacrococcygeal teratoma
    B. Diastematomyelia
    C. Caudal regression syndrome
    D. Hydromyelia

    ANSWER: C. Caudal regression syndrome is a congenital defect, characterized by the absence of the sacrum and defects of variable portions of lumbar spine. Majority of cases are sporadic, and it occurs in up to 1% of pregnancies of women with diabetes and up to 22% of cases of CRS are associated with either type 2 or type 2 diabetes. Femoral hypoplasia, clubbed feet, and flexion contractures of the lower extremities are also commonly seen. Additionally, caudal regression syndrome is often associated with anomalies of the gastrointestinal tract, genitourinary tract, and heart, as well as with neural tube defects. Sirenomelia, which was thought to be the most severe form of caudal regression syndrome (today it is considered a different entity), is the main differential diagnosis. Fusion of the lower extremities is a typical finding of sirenomelia and is absent in caudal regression syndrome.

INDEX

C

D

G

H

N

O

S

U

V